Introduction for Educators:

Start your students off right!

Your students need to begin thinking like nurses from the moment they walk into your program. Authors Judith Wilkinson and Karen Van Leuven help them with a fresh new approach to teaching *Fundamentals of Nursing* with their innovative 2-volume presentation.

Volume 1: Theory, Concepts and Applications contains the material you'll cover in your classroom. It stresses knowledge mastery, critical thinking, evidence-based practice, and is case based. The content of this volume, as well as the *Electronic Study Guide* on CD-ROM packaged with it, is meticulously cross referenced to

Volume 2: Thinking and Doing in which the critical thinking introduced in *Volume 1* is applied to clinical procedures, and which uses a multi-generational, multi-cultural family as the basis for a case study threaded through *Volume 2*. This approach best suits the way you teach—and no other textbook has it!

The Wilkinson and Van Leuven "think like a nurse" learning suite also includes:

⇒ *Electronic Study Guide* bound into the back of *Volume 1* with
- Learning Outcomes
- Answers and suggested responses to the exercises in *Volume 1* and *Volume 2*
- Additional exercises and suggested supplemental readings
- Knowledge Maps, Care Plans, and Care Maps
- Practice test bank for students
and much more!

⇒ *Instructor's Resource Disk* (for adopters) that includes: a test bank, an instructor's guide, an image bank, and a PowerPoint Presentation.

⇒ *Online Resources at DavisPlus* for instructors and students—see page iv for more information.

⇒ *Procedure Checklists for Fundamentals of Nursing* – a separate print version as a convenience for you and your students. Its content is also available and customizable on the *Electronic Study Guide* and on the *Instructor's Resource Disk*.

⇒ *Fundamentals Packages* – When thinking of resources for your students' coursework, think about saving them money too. You have a choice of packages of essential F.A. Davis texts and references that include:
- *Taber's Cyclopedic Medical Dictionary*,
- *Davis's Drug Guide for Nurses*,
- *Davis's Comprehensive Handbook of Laboratory and Diagnostic Tests with Nursing Implications*,
and other titles fundamental to your students' success!

The next few pages present an overview to illustrate the key features of this unique text.
A more in-depth description is presented in the authors' *Preface*.

Toward Thinking Like a Nurse

Theories on learning have shown that students learn better if they can see how the content will be useful to them. They understand better when presented with something concrete in addition to tackling the abstract definitions and theory. *Volume 1* emphasizes the relationship between theoretical knowledge and practical knowledge to encourage each of your students to think like a nurse. This approach allows you to emphasize either theory or practice as it suits you and your students.

Follow the layout of the chapters to see the real difference inherent in this book:

27 CHAPTER

Urinary Elimination

Learning Outcomes

After completing this chapter, you should be able to:

* Describe the normal structure and function of the organs in the urinary system.

* Describe the processes of urine formation and elimination.

* Discuss factors that affect urinary elimination.

* Describe the contents of a nursing assessment and physical examination focused on urinary elimination.

Each chapter starts with **Learning Outcomes**—a checklist of what your students should know once they've completed the chapter.

Meet Your Patient, also at the opening of each chapter, introduces your students to the patient they will follow and whose experiences illustrate the principles presented throughout the chapter, thus capturing their interest with real-life scenarios.

MEET Your Patient

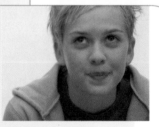

During your assigned clinical experience at University Hospital, the RN asks you to complete the admission process for Jessica, a 22-year-old university student who is complaining of frequent, painful urination. As you interview her, Jessica becomes embarrassed. "It's really hard to talk about this. Do you really need all these details?" she inquires. Then, she asks to use the bathroom. You ask her to give you a midstream clean-catch urine sample while she is in the restroom. When she returns, she gives you a small specimen of pink-colored, strong-smelling urine. "I feel like I have to go so bad and then I hardly have any urine. It's a little bloody, and I'm not having my period," she states.

You close the door and interview Jessica in private about her usual urination pattern and current symptoms. Your calm approach and straightforward manner put her at ease. She confides that she has recently become sexually active and that her symptoms began after spending the weekend with her new partner. You take her vital signs: oral temperature 99.4°F (37.4°C), radial pulse 88 bpm, respiratory rate 20, and blood pressure 108/72 mm Hg.

After you report your assessment data to the RN, the emergency department (ED) physician asks you to perform a dipstick urinalysis on the urine sample and to send the urine sample to the lab for culture and sensitivity. He asks you: "Well, what do you think we need to do next?" How would you answer his question?

As you gain theoretical and practical knowledge in this chapter, we will return to this case study to discuss how you might answer the physician's question and support Jessica's recovery. You will also have the opportunity to evaluate your feelings about giving care that patients may regard as highly personal or even embarrassing.

Care Plans and Care Maps throughout!

☞ **See examples in Chapter 27, pages 627-631.**

Theoretical Knowledge
knowing why

A variety of factors, including personal hygiene, age, nutrition, stress, sexual activity, and medications, play a role in urinary health. That's why it is vitally important that you take a holistic approach to patients who have altered urinary elimination patterns. Such an approach requires theoretical knowledge of normal urinary physiology, factors that influence urinary elimination, and common alterations in urinary function.

HOW DOES THE URINARY SYSTEM WORK?

To understand problems affecting the urinary system, you'll need to first understand how the urinary system functions in a healthy individual. The organs of the urinary system include the kidneys, ureters, bladder, and urethra (Figure 27–1).

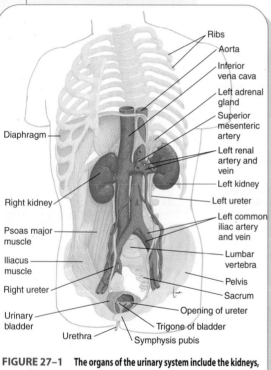

FIGURE 27–1   The organs of the urinary system include the kidneys, ureters, bladder, and urethra.

Chapters are divided into two sections. **Theoretical Knowledge—Knowing Why** and **Practical Knowledge—Knowing How** reflect how information is communicated in real life and enable your students to focus on just the **why** or the **how**. This is where the text's conversational tone is truly evident—the authors sound as if they are talking to your students rather than lecturing them. Headings (often phrased as questions that highlight students' concerns about the information), bulleted lists, boxes, and figures break up the text and make it more visually engaging.

The Kidneys Filter and Regulate

The kidneys filter metabolic wastes, toxins, excess ions, and water from the bloodstream and excrete them as urine. If kidney function is impaired, these substances reach toxic levels and begin to poison the body's cells. The kidneys also help to regulate blood volume, blood pressure, electrolyte levels, and acid-base balance by selectively reabsorbing water and other substances. Secondary functions of the kidneys are to produce erythropoietin, secrete the enzyme renin, and activate vitamin D_3 (calcitrol). The kidneys are located against the posterior abdominal wall behind the peritoneum (they are **retroperitoneal**). The average kidney weighs about 5 ounces and is the shape of a kidney bean (see Figure 27–1).

The outer layer, or **cortex,** of the kidney is composed of millions of microscopic functional units called *nephrons* (Figure 27–2). The inner layer, or **medulla,** consists of 8 to 10 wedge-shaped cones called the *renal pyramids*. The renal pyramids are made up of bundles of collecting tubules. The innermost area is the **renal pelvis.** Funnel-shaped extensions known as **calyces** (singular: **calyx**) enclose the central portion of each renal pyramid and direct urine into the renal pelvis.

Practical Knowledge
knowing how

As a nurse, you will monitor and assist clients with urinary elimination, teach them about body function, and work collaboratively with the healthcare team to facilitate normal urinary function. In the remainder of the chapter we will discuss these activities. Also see the Nursing Care Plan and the Care Map.

| Assessment |

To assess urinary elimination, you will use data from the nursing history, physical examination, and diagnostic and laboratory reports.

Nursing History

Because urination patterns vary among individuals, you will need a nursing history to determine what is normal for a particular client. As you interview the client, pay attention to her reaction to your questions. Many people are embarrassed about discussing urination. Tailor your assessment to the client's needs, and use language that makes the client comfortable.

For a set of interview questions,

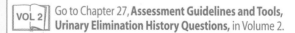

VOL 2   Go to Chapter 27, **Assessment Guidelines and Tools, Urinary Elimination History Questions,** in Volume 2.

For clients with a urinary diversion, you should also gather data on the client's usual care of the stoma, use of appliances, and adjustment to the ostomy.

Physical Assessment

Physical assessment for urinary elimination includes examination of the kidneys, bladder, urethra, and

Links That Help Your Students Think Like Nurses

The didactic material that you'll cover in your classroom is contained in *Volume 1: Theory, Concepts and Applications*. The content of this volume is systematically linked to *Volume 2: Thinking and Doing* in which the critical thinking introduced in *Volume 1* continues to be applied, this time to a single unifying case study, to chapter content, and to the clinical procedures that are the core of *Volume 2*.

- *Sutures* ("stitches") are the traditional wound closures. Several types of suture materials are available. *Absorbent* sutures are used deep in the tissues, for example, to close an organ or **anastomose** (connect) tissue. Because they are made of material that will gradually dissolve, there is no need to remove absorbent sutures. *Nonabsorbent* sutures are placed in superficial tissues and require removal, often by a nurse. Suturing leads to small puncture wounds along the track of the laceration or incision. For instructions on removing sutures and staples,

 Go to Chapter 34, **Technique 34–2: Removing Sutures and Staples,** in Volume 2.

Icons meticulously incorporated throughout the text indicate cross references between the "theory, concepts, and applications" in *Volume 1* and the "thinking and doing" in *Volume 2*.

- *Surgical staples* are made of lightweight titanium. They provide a fast, easy way to close a
- *Surgical glue* is a relatively new meth closure. It is safe for use in clean, wounds. It is an ideal wound closure me tears.
- *In vacuum-assisted wound closure,* a in the wound is attached by a tube t pressure pump to remove wound drai subatmospheric pressure to improve h a clean and moist environment, and fo to bacterial infection. The vacuum devi erized and can be programmed for con termittent negative pressure.
- *Compression stockings* are used with ulcers of the lower extremities. They a ous pressure to the veins, which facili return and allows the ulcers to heal.

Critical Thinking questions ask your students to apply what they've just learned to the patient introduced earlier in the chapter, to a new patient, or to their own lives.

TECHNIQUE 34–2 Removing Sutures and Staples

Removing Sutures

1. Obtain a suture removal kit.
2. Use the forceps to pick up one end of the suture.
3. Slide the small scissors around the suture, and cut near the skin. This helps you avoid pulling the exposed portion of the suture through the underlying tissue.
4. With the forceps, gently pull the suture in the direction of the knotted side to remove it.

Removing Staples

1. Obtain a staple remover.
2. Place the staple remover under the center of each staple, and slowly close it. This spreads the ends of the staples apart, freeing them from the skin.
3. Remove every other staple, and check the tension on the wound.
4. If there is no significant pull on the wound, remove the remaining staples. Consider placing a piece of gauze nearby so that you have a place to deposit the staples as you remove them.

Suture types

Plain interrupted

Mattress interrupted

Plain continuous

Mattress continuous

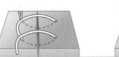

Removing interrupted sutures

Removal techniques

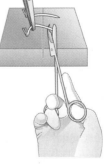

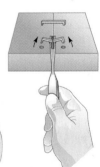

Removing staples

CriticalThinking 34–4

Review the Braden and Norton scales. Apply these risk assessment scales to Mr. Harmon ("Meet Your Patient").

- What additional information, if any, do you need to complete these assessments?
- Which scale do you find most useful?

Chapters include **Knowledge Checks**, questions designed to allow your students to check their recall of the material they've just read and that are cross referenced to the corresponding answers on the *Electronic Study Guide* on CD-ROM.

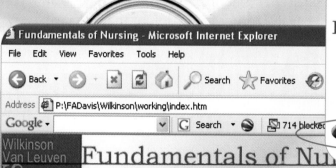

- *Depth of the wound.* **Superficial wounds** involve only the epidermal layer of the skin. The injury is usually the result of friction, shearing, or burning. **Partial-thickness wounds** extend through the epidermis into the dermis. **Full-thickness wounds** extend into the subcutaneous tissue and beyond (Sussmen & Bates-Jensen, 2001). The descriptor **penetrating** is sometimes added to indicate that the wound involves internal organs. Wound depth is a major determinant of healing time: The deeper the wound, the longer the healing time.

KnowledgeCheck 34–3

- Explain the difference between an acute and a chronic wound.
- Describe the wound categorization system based on contamination.
- How does wound depth affect healing?

Go to Chapter 34, **Knowledge Check Response Sheet and Answers,** on the Electronic Study Guide.

Fundamentals of Nursing - Microsoft Internet Explorer

File   Edit   View   Favorites   Tools   Help

Back   ✕   🔁   🏠   Search   ⭐ Favorites

Address P:\FADavis\Wilkinson\working\index.htm

Google ▾   G Search ▾   714 blocked

Wilkinson
Van Leuven   Fundamentals of Nu

Electronic Study Guide

■ Chapter & Resources   ■ Additional Resources

Knowledge Check 34-3

- Explain the difference between an acute and a chronic wound.

  Answer:
  Acute and chronic wounds have different durations and causes.
  - **Acute** wounds are expected to be of short duration. Acute wounds may be intentional (surgical incisions) or unintentional (trauma).
  - Wounds are classified as *chronic* when they exceed the anticipated length of recovery. Chronic wounds include pressure, arterial, venous, and diabetic ulcers. These wounds are frequently colonized with bacteria, and healing is very slow because of the underlying disease process. A chronic wound may linger for months or years.

- Describe the wound categorization system based on contamination.

  Answer:
  Wounds are categorized based on four levels of contamination:
  - **Clean** wounds are uninfected wounds with minimal inflammation. They may be open or closed and do not involve the gastrointestinal, respiratory, or genitourinary tracts (these systems frequently harbor bacteria). There is very little risk of infection for these wounds.
  - **Clean-contaminated** wounds are surgical incisions that enter the gastrointestinal, respiratory, or genitourinary tracts. There is an increased risk of infection for these wounds, but there is no obvious infection.
  - **Contaminated** wounds include open, traumatic wounds or surgical incisions in which a major break in asepsis occurred. The risk of infection is high for these wounds.
  - **Infected** wounds are wounds with evidence of infection, such as purulent drainage or necrotic tissue. Wounds

---

| toward evidence-based practice |

Gibson, M.C., Keast, D., Woodbury, M.G., Black, J., Goettl, L., Campbell, K., et al. (2004). Educational intervention in the management of acute procedure-related wound pain: A pilot study. *Journal of Wound Care, 13*(5), 187–190.

This pilot study investigated the use of an educational intervention to manage acute pain associated with wound care in an outpatient clinic. Five patients aged 65 years or older with a history of pain during wound treatments were included in this pilot study. Each had a chronic wound that required dressing changes or debridement. Before the wound treatment, the nurse gave the patients information about the procedure, discussed strategies

they could use to make it as comfortable as possible, and explained how to use a rating scale to indicate their pain or emotional discomfort. Three out of five patients reported reduced pain and/or distress following the wound treatment.

---

1. How would you apply the findings of this pilot study to your clinical practice?

2. How might these findings be further investigated?

Go to Chapter 34, **Toward Evidence-Based Practice Suggested Responses,** on the Electronic Study Guide.

Toward Evidence-Based Practice boxes describe important research that applies to the topic at hand and ask your students to consider higher cognitive level questions about the study or studies. Suggested responses appear on the *Electronic Study Guide.*

Online Resources at *DavisPlus*

DavisPlus makes it quick and simple to locate all of F.A. Davis's online resources by serving as an easy-to-navigate centralized hub. Wilkinson and Van Leuven's *Fundamentals of Nursing* offers robust online teaching tools for you and learning tools for your students at http://davisplus.fadavis.com. In addition to the clinically relevant resources presently available, updated content that will keep your students thinking like nurses will be developed and posted as well.

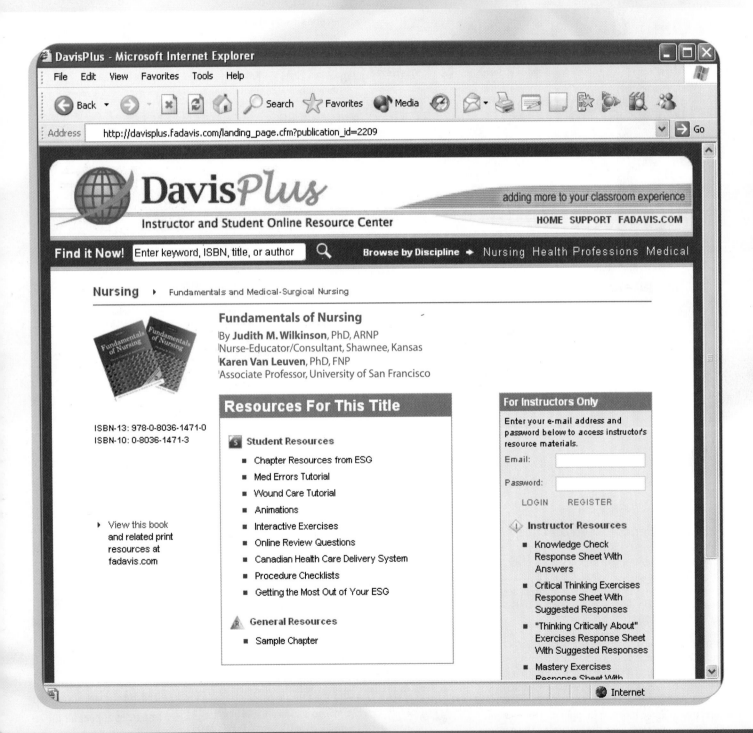

Fundamentals of Nursing

Theory, Concepts & Applications

VOLUME 1

JUDITH M. WILKINSON, PHD, ARNP
Nurse Educator/Consultant
Shawnee, Kansas

KAREN VAN LEUVEN, PHD, FNP
Associate Professor
University of San Francisco
San Francisco, California

Family Nurse Practitioner
Oakland, California

 F. A. Davis Company/Publishers   Philadelphia

F. A. Davis Company
1915 Arch Street
Philadelphia, PA 19103
www.fadavis.com

Printed in the United States of America

Last digit indicates print number: 10 9 8 7 6 5 4

Acquisitions Editor: Lisa B. Deitch
Content Development Manager: Darlene D. Pedersen
Special Projects Editor: Shirley A. Kuhn
Senior Project Editor: Danielle Barsky

As new scientific information becomes available through basic and clinical research, recommended treatments and drug therapies undergo changes. The author(s) and publisher have done everything possible to make this book accurate, up to date, and in accord with accepted standards at the time of publication. The author(s), editors, and publisher are not responsible for errors or omissions or for consequences from application of the book, and make no warranty, expressed or implied, in regard to the contents of the book. Any practice described in this book should be applied by the reader in accordance with professional standards of care used in regard to the unique circumstances that may apply in each situation. The reader is advised always to check product information (package inserts) for changes and new information regarding dose and contraindications before administering any drug. Caution is especially urged when using new or infrequently ordered drugs.

Library of Congress Cataloging-in-Publication Data

Wilkinson, Judith M., 1939–
    Fundamentals of nursing: theory, concepts & applications/Judith M.
Wilkinson, Karen Van Leuven.
        p. cm.
    Includes index.
    ISBN 0-8036-1197-8—ISBN 0-8036-1198-6
    1. Nursing.   I. Van Leuven, Karen.   II. Title.
    RT41.W56 2007
    610.73—dc22

                                        2006016419

Vol. 1: ISBN 10: 0-8036-1197-8
Vol. 1: ISBN 13: 978-0-8036-1197-9

Set: ISBN 10: 0-8036-1471-3
Set: ISBN 13: 978-0-8036-1471-0

Dedications

We dedicate this book to:

The many nursing students we have had the privilege of assisting along their professional path.

My husband, Franklin Hiam, who carried computers, books, and files to the four corners of the earth so I could have working "vacations" with him. Also to Mason, Emily, Aubrey, and Jeffrey Wilkinson, who have not had as much quality time with Grandmom as they and I would have liked.

Judith Wilkinson

My parents, Eileen and Edsel Van Leuven, who always encouraged me to follow my dream; and my family, Robert, Sarah, and Scott Bradsby, who supported me at every step in this process.

Preface

We chose our book title carefully. We have used the words *theory, concepts, application, thinking,* and *doing* because we believe that excellent nursing requires an equal mix of knowledge, thought, and action. It is knowledge and its application—not just the tasks nurses do—that delineate the various levels of nursing. Even so, skillful performance of tasks is essential to full attainment of the nursing role.

We chose the word *fundamentals* because this text, and its concomitant course, is truly that: the foundation for all that follows. In that sense, and because this basic content will be used throughout the nurse's career, we believe it is—or should be—the most important course students will take. We want them to say, "Everything I need to know, I learned in Fundamentals—all I needed to know about how to think, what to do, and how to be (at least at a basic level)." You will see those themes integrated throughout each chapter.

ORGANIZATION

We have organized the learning package into two volumes to make it easier for on-the-go students to have at hand the material they need in either the classroom or the clinical setting. The content of Volumes 1 and 2 is comprehensive. However, to minimize weight and bulk, and to keep the content manageable for students, we have put some enrichment material on the Electronic Study Guide packaged in Volume 1 for students who need it or who wish to pursue a subject in more depth. Our chapters are self-contained and rich in cross-references so that teachers and students can use them in any order that fits their needs.

Content within each chapter is generally organized into two major sections: "Theoretical Knowledge (Knowing Why)" and "Practical Knowledge (Knowing How)." There is some overlap in these concepts because the two types of knowledge are interdependent. We have made the general distinction because many nursing programs begin with content learned in supporting prerequisite classes and then layer on additional theoretical knowledge to explain the rationale for nursing actions and activities (practical knowledge). This distinction also affords more flexibility in teaching fundamentals. For example, it should be as useful to teachers who believe students are more motivated when they present first the concrete (practical knowledge), and then the abstract

(theoretical knowledge) as to those who teach from the theoretical to the practical.

We have endeavored to write a text that can be used as a reference throughout the student's career—one that is comprehensive but not overwhelming. To that end, for example, in Chapter 9 we present a brief overview of growth and development in Volume 1. Many students take a separate growth and development course, and we believe they do not need a fundamentals course to teach the same subject matter. But for teachers who wish to teach it, or students who need to review it, we include a comprehensive version of Chapter 9 on the Electronic Study Guide.

FEATURES

The chapters have numerous pedagogical features to facilitate student learning:

- *"Learning Outcomes," "Chapter Overview," and a summary feature titled "What Are the Main Points in This Chapter?"*—These focus the student's study and provide repetition to facilitate review retention of material.

- *Interactive approach*—The text is written in an engaging style that speaks directly to the student. Recall and critical-thinking questions occur frequently to break chapters up into small, manageable segments and maintain interest. Volume 2 provides white space for students to answer questions or take notes.

- *"Meet Your Patient"*—This chapter-opening feature in Volume 1 introduces one or more patients. The scenario is used throughout the chapter to illustrate theoretical points and make the content "come alive." These patients are often followed in the critical-thinking activities in Volume 2.

- *"Knowledge Check"*—These questions allow students to test their recall of the material presented in the text. Answer sheets and answers are provided on the Electronic Study Guide (ESG).

- *"Critical Thinking" exercises*—Thought-provoking questions in both volumes allow the student to synthesize content and explore personal beliefs. Response sheets are provided on the ESG; suggested responses are found on the Instructor's Resource Disk.

- *"Evidenced-Based Practice" boxes*—In every chapter, we describe research related to the chapter topic and pose critical-thinking exercises for students to examine these findings. The concept of evidence-based practice is introduced in Chapter 8 (Theory and Research) and mentioned frequently in other chapters as well.

- *"Care Plans"*—Sixteen care plans integrating NANDA, NIC, and NOC are found in Volume 1 and the ESG. They are based on case studies that allow students to see the nursing process in action. Evidence-based rationales are provided for interventions.

- *"Care Maps"*—Care maps associated with each care plan allow visual learners to grasp the connection between the phases of the nursing process. They also provide an alternative method of care planning.

- *"Critical Aspects" boxes*—The critical aspects of all chapter procedures are presented in bullet format in Volume 1 and at the beginning of each procedure in Volume 2. These boxes serve as a reference for the "Practical Knowledge" content in Volume 1; in Volume 2 they provide a quick review just before the student performs a procedure in the clinical area.

- *"Teaching: Self-Care" boxes*—Self-care boxes appear throughout Volume 1. They are similar to the traditional "teaching boxes" and focus on equipping patients to perform self-care.

- *"Home Care" boxes*—These provide guidelines for safely modifying care for delivery in the home.

- *"Complementary and Alternative Modalities (CAM)" boxes*—Included in several Volume 1 chapters, these describe a complementary therapy related to the chapter topic or present research concerning a therapy (e.g., prayer, in Chapter 14).

- *"Caring for the Garcias"*—This feature begins the critical-thinking exercises in every chapter of Volume 2. It allows students to become familiar with a single family and to experience vicariously the continuity of care they may encounter in outpatient settings. Space has been provided so that students can jot notes.

- *"Thinking Critically About" [Sections.]*—These clinically based exercises guide students to safely practice their critical thinking skills in preparation for doing so in the clinical area. Frequently, these clinical exercises further analyze material related to the "Meet Your Patient" scenario in Volume 1.

- *"Knowledge Maps"*—In Volume 2, every chapter that does not have a clinical procedure *does* have a knowledge map of Volume 1 theoretical content. This helps students learn the skill of mapping chapter content as a study aid.

- *"Diagnostic Testing" boxes*—These are found in Volume 2, in applicable chapters. We believe it is more meaningful to place the diagnostic test information near the related content rather than in an isolated chapter. If students need a reference source, we recommend a comprehensive diagnostic testing book.

THEMES

The following are themes that are integrated and stressed throughout both volumes of this text, some of them in every chapter:

- *Critical thinking and the full spectrum model of nursing.* In addition to the critical-thinking questions and exercises in Volumes 1 and 2, concepts in Volume 1 are often presented in an inductive manner, or pose a question to the student (e.g., "What would happen if. . .?"). The full spectrum model of nursing is a comprehensive approach to care that uses critical thinking in all aspects of care. It is not rigidly overlaid on each chapter. Because students cannot focus on everything at once, different parts are stressed at different times. Sometimes they are asked, "What theoretical knowledge do you need to. . .?" In other instances they might be asked, "What biases do you have that might interfere with. . .?"

- *Nursing process.* Nursing process is related to critical thinking in Chapter 2; Chapters 3 through 7 are a comprehensive presentation of the nursing process, which is presented as reflexive rather than linear. The "Practical Knowledge" sections of Volume 1 are organized according to the nursing process phases; the procedures in Volume 2 have assessment and evaluation components. In addition, many of the questions and exercises provide opportunity for using the nursing process.

- *NANDA, NIC, and NOC standardized languages.* Thorough discussion of these taxonomies occurs in the nursing process and other chapters. NOC outcomes and NIC interventions are included in every chapter of Volume 1, as appropriate to chapter content; many are presented in tables in Volume 2. The Omaha System and the Clinical Care Classification are also used in the community and home health chapters, respectively.

- *Caring.* Caring is thoroughly integrated in many chapters. Chapter 1 provides historical examples of nursing as a caring profession. Chapter 8 describes the important caring theories. The case study in Chapter 8 introduces Watson's theory, and that theory is used throughout the chapter to illustrate how theory is applied in nursing.

- *Wellness.* Many examples used in this text refer to people who are not ill. Chapter 10 emphasizes health, and Chapter 41 talks about the nurse's role in health promotion.

- *Culture.* Cultural diversity is highlighted throughout the text in clinical scenarios, illustrations, and theoretical discussion. Chapter 13 focuses on culturally sensitive nursing care. The "Caring for the Garcias" feature in Volume 2 features a multicultural extended family, and ethnic variations are described, as applicable, in procedures.

- *Developmental stage.* The "Theoretical Knowledge" section in most chapters devotes a section to discussing the effects of developmental stages on the chapter topic. In Volume 2, procedures include variations for children and older adults.

- *Spirituality.* Chapter 14 is probably the most extensive presentation of spiritual care available in a fundamentals text. Spirituality is integrated within various chapters in scenarios and examples.

- *Documentation.* All chapters include reference to documentation, where relevant. The procedures in Volume 2 all have guidelines for documentation and examples of how to document the procedure.

- *Delegation.* Delegation is introduced early, in the nursing process chapters, and is reinforced in most Volume 1 chapters. Chapter 38, Leading and Managing, also discusses delegation. In Volume 2, all procedures have guidelines for delegating.

- *ANA standards.* Nursing and other healthcare standards (e.g., JCAHO, Medicare) are frequently referenced. Links to pertinent web sites are given.

- *Ethics.* In addition to the comprehensive treatment in Chapter 44, ethical knowledge is an aspect of our full-spectrum model. As such, many of the critical-thinking exercises ask students to grapple with ethical issues. A good example is found in Chapter 6, Volume 2.

- *Legal issues.* Chapter 45 is devoted to legal issues in nursing. Legal issues (e.g., licensing) are integrated in many other chapters, as well.

- *Community and home health care.* Chapters 42 and 43 are devoted exclusively to these topics. Clinical scenarios and examples involve nurses in these settings; Volume 1 has special feature boxes regarding these topics; procedures in Volume 2 have sections for adapting skills to home care.

- *Complementary therapies.* Nursing is presented as holistic throughout. Chapter 40 is devoted exclusively to complementary and alternative therapies; and several chapters in Volume 1 (e.g.,

Chapter 13, Culture) contain material related to this topic.

- *Contemporary issues.* We have included information about bioterrorism (Chapter 20, focused on infection and asepsis; Chapter 42, focused on community health; and in the "Meet Your Nurse Role Model" scenario in Chapter 39, focused on informatics). The chapter on safety (Chapter 21) includes ways to cope with gang violence in the healthcare setting.

- *Technology and computers.* Chapter 39 is an excellent introduction to nursing informatics. Standardized languages and computerized care planning and documentation are interspersed throughout the book (for example, in Chapter 23, Administering Medications).

THE TEXT AS A RESPONSE TO CHANGE

This book was developed to address the needs of today's beginning nursing students and in response to several changes in nursing education and practice.

Changes in Students

- **Nontraditional students.** Students range from traditional, younger students to older, second-career students. Many students are older and have work or family responsibilities that compete with school.

  To address this change, we have followed two principles of adult learning: that learning must be relevant and efficient. For example, we have divided the content into two volumes devoted to the classroom and clinical setting, respectively. We have made great use of the Electronic Study Guide as well as the web site to deliver enhancements to the printed text, knowing that highly motivated and computer-literate students will welcome the chance to use these technologies to maximize their learning.

- **Wide variety in learning styles.** Students learn in different ways.

  We have used over 1200 photos and as many diagrams to assist visual learners. Sound files of heart sounds and many other clinical assessment findings are included on the Electronic Study Guide for auditory learners. To teach psychomotor skills, we have, in addition to step-by-step procedures, checklists students can print out for practicing procedures or teachers to use in evaluations.

  Because learning improves when content is meaningful to the learner, each chapter opens with a patient scenario or story of a practicing nurse. This story is woven throughout the chapter to show how concepts are applied and how nurses

think. We stress practical application throughout the text because adults want to apply knowledge to circumstances. The case study of the Garcia family, which is introduced in and continues throughout all chapters of Volume 2, is a prime example of this approach.

- **Reading comprehension.** For many reasons—changes in admission requirements, for example, or the increasing numbers of students for whom English is a second language—some schools are finding the reading abilities of today's students to be lower than those of the past.

  We addressed this change by writing in an informal style, addressing the student directly ("you will . . ."). We have not made the content more elementary, but we have made reading about it more inviting and user-friendly. We define new terms at their first use in each chapter and include a glossary on the Electronic Study Guide for additional terms the student may not know.

  To aid in retention, we have interspersed "Knowledge Checks" and "Critical Thinking" questions frequently throughout Volume 1 to allow students to check their recall and understanding of the material presented as they progress through the chapters. Recognizing that repetition aids retention, We list "Learning Outcomes" at the beginning of each chapter in Volume 1. In addition, each chapter in Volume 2 includes an "Overview" of chapter content and a list titled "What Are the Main Points in This Chapter?" In more than half of the chapters, there is also a full-page "Knowledge Map" of the chapter content.

- **The technology generation.** The newer generation of students is accustomed to using technology and to multi-tasking.

  To hold their attention, we have presented information in an easy-to-read style, in an interactive manner, and in relatively short segments interspersed with review questions and critical-thinking questions. For this same reason, the text frequently directs students to find related information on the Electronic Study Guide and on the Internet.

Changes in Curriculum

- **Teachers say they do not have enough time to "cover the content."** One way to address this problem is to not reteach material students have had in other classes. We provide, for example, enough anatomy and physiology in each chapter to aid students who need to review A&P or who are taking A&P concurrently with nursing courses. You should not need to "cover" it in class. Most students do take a separate course in growth and develop-

ment, so we have included most of that material (Chapter 9) on the Electronic Study Guide.

- **Some curricula have deemphasized mental health; mental health may be taught in other (e.g., medical-surgical) clinical areas, with no separate mental health course.** In response to pleas from educators, we have expanded the mental health content in Chapter 11 and included tools for psychosocial assessment. In addition to the usual concepts of self-concept and self-esteem, we have included basic assessments and interventions for anxiety and depression, which students will encounter regularly in all areas, not just on mental health units. In Chapter 18, Communication & Therapeutic Relationships, we have expanded the content on the nurse-patient relationship and communication techniques that mental health teachers find so essential. Chapter 25, Stress & Adaptation, includes information about defense mechanisms.

- **The curriculum does not include separate pharmacology, nutrition, ethics, or nursing process courses.** Because all nurses need grounding in these topics, we have provided extensive coverage both in Volume 1 and the ESG. Chapter 23, Administering Medications, provides in-depth pharmacology information. Chapter 26, Nutrition, provides a good basic foundation for understanding patients' nutritional needs. Chapter 44 is a comprehensive look at nursing ethics. We have, arguably, the most useful and thorough presentation of nursing process available in a fundamentals text. These chapters, as well as most others, will be a valuable reference for students when they take other clinical nursing courses.

Changes in Nursing and Health Care

- **Nursing role is increasingly complex, requiring management, delegation, and supervision skills early in the career.** To address this change, we have included a comprehensive discussion of leadership and management in Chapter 38. Delegation is presented early, in the nursing process chapters, and stressed in the rest of the chapters in Volume 1, as applicable. Each clinical procedure in Volume 2 contains a "Delegation" section.

- **Health care has moved increasingly from the hospital to the home and community.** To address this change, we have included a provocative discussion about the evolving healthcare system in the supplementary material for Chapter 1 on the Electronic Study Guide. In addition, Chapters 42 and 43 focus on home care and community care, respectively. Home and community care are

integrated throughout Volume 1 (e.g., Chapter 34 cites *Healthy People 2010* public goals for reducing pressure ulcers); and each procedure in Volume 2 includes home care adaptations, as well as patient teaching points that will enable patients and caregivers to assume more responsibility for care.

- **Nurses need to be critical thinkers and lifelong learners.** To address this change, we have organized the text around a model of full-spectrum nursing, a comprehensive approach to care that uses critical thinking in all aspects of care. Critical thinking is integrated throughout both volumes of the text, both in discussion and in critical thinking exercises. Discussion of this model follows.

The Full-Spectrum Model of Nursing

We believe that nursing knowledge is a fusion of theoretical knowledge, practical knowledge, self-knowledge, and ethical knowledge. To function at the highest level, nurses use critical thinking and the nursing process to blend thoughts and actions to put caring into action. We refer to this blend as *full-spectrum nursing*. We have organized our learning package to reflect this philosophy. This model is presented in Chapter 2 and referred to and used throughout the text.

The Learning Package

This is a well-integrated and cross-referenced package containing a two-volume text, an Electronic Study Guide, an Instructor's Resource Disk, and an associated web site. Although any item can be used either in classroom or clinical settings, Volume 1 will usually be used in the classroom setting and in preparing for clinical, whereas Volume 2 will usually be used in the clinical setting or learning lab. Icons in Volumes 1 and 2 guide students to material on the Electronic Study Guide, the Internet, or the companion volume (1 or 2).

Volume 1

Volume 1 contains all the theoretical and conceptual material typically present in a fundamentals text; however, it is presented in a clinically focused, user-friendly manner, incorporating many examples. This presentation allows students to see how the content will be useful to them in practice. In Chapters 8 through 45, the nursing process is used as the model to organize the "Practical Knowledge" section.

Unit 1—focuses on how nurses think. It begins by showing the evolution of nursing: how our history relates to our present. Chapter 2 focuses on critical thinking, and Chapters 3 through 7 provide an exten-

sive treatment of the nursing process. This unit prepares students to follow the organization of subsequent chapters and provides the thinking tools and processes they need to apply the content of the other chapters. Chapter 8 contains an overview of the processes of theory building and nursing research.

Unit 2—focuses on the internal and external factors that affect an individual's health (e.g., family, culture, spirituality, and life stage). Internal factors are personal beliefs or attributes that influence how the client views health, health care, and nursing. A groundbreaking feature is Chapter 10, which describes the health-illness-wellness continuum in an experiential way, promoting self-knowledge, personal growth, and affective learning of that content.

Unit 3—examines essential nursing interventions. We consider these skills "essential" because nurses use some or all of these skills in *all* areas of nursing, regardless of setting or patient diagnosis. The unit begins with documentation and includes communication, teaching, taking vital signs, physical assessment, asepsis, safety, hygiene, and medication administration.

Unit 4—concentrates on nursing care that supports physiological function. We examine broad categories of physiological function (e.g., nutrition, elimination, oxygenation) and discuss related nursing care.

Unit 5—explores diverse nursing functions. For example, we look at leadership and management, the use of technology and informatics, and health promotion activities. Chapter 39 is a more thorough introduction to informatics than typically found in a fundamentals text. We are especially proud of Chapter 40, which provides a deeper treatment of holistic healing than you will typically find. We believe that a fundamentals book, overall, provides all concepts needed for a holistic view of the patient—just scan our chapter titles to see what we mean by that. We just went one step farther with Chapter 40.

Unit 6—looks at the context for nurses' work. This includes chapters on community and home care, as well as the ethical and legal contexts for nursing work. In addition, we include, on the Electronic Study Guide, an excellent chapter (Chapter 46) on Canadian Healthcare Delivery Systems, written by respected Canadian nurse authors.

Volume 2

Volume 2 is designed primarily, but not exclusively, for use in the skills lab and clinical setting. As does Volume 1, it includes both thinking and doing. The critical-thinking exercises require students to use their thinking skills and the nursing process to apply theoretical knowledge to specific patient situations.

The clinical procedures, assessment tools, clinical forms, diagnostic testing information, and standardized language tables comprise the practical knowledge sections. Throughout Volume 2, students have access to a simulated experience known as "Caring for the Garcias," through which they learn about the nursing role, the healthcare system, and the real-world application of the content in Volume 1.

Electronic Study Guide

The Electronic Study Guide, on the CD included in Volume 1, contains expanded discussions of some of the Volume 1 material, mastery questions, answers to the Volume 1 "Knowledge Checks," a panel of 300 NCLEX-style test questions, a glossary, additional care plans and care maps, and procedure checklists. The ESG contains forms that students can print out to write their answers to "Knowledge Checks," "Critical Thinking" questions, mastery questions, and the Volume 2 critical-thinking exercises. On the CD, the questions themselves have expandable space so that answers can be typed in on the CD and then printed out.

The large glossary provides definitions of all bolded terms used in the text as well as supplementary terms that may be helpful to students.

Procedure checklists can be used to study for skills lab or clinical, or as a means to assess skill mastery. Checklists are provided in two formats: one is a detailed list of steps for each procedure; another is a generic, principles-based list that instructors can use to evaluate all procedures.

Instructor's Resource Disk

The Instructor's Resource Disk contains everything that is on the Electronic Study Guide plus a number of features to assist faculty. These include an image bank of illustrations from the book, lesson plans, PowerPoint lecture outlines, teaching strategies to accompany each chapter, suggested responses for the critical-thinking exercises in Volumes 1 and 2, instructions for using concept mapping, and a test bank of over 1000 NCLEX-style questions, many of which are in the new NCLEX formats.

Web Site

The text web site, for both students and teachers, is housed on the F. A. Davis server available at www.fadavis.com. The site contains many of the materials you will find on the Electronic Study Guide, as well as additional content mastery activities and clinical animations.

You are fortunate to be able to work with students at perhaps the most formative point in their nursing education. We are certain that each of you will bring your own special style to the teaching of this most important nursing course and that you will find new and creative ways to use the many teaching and learning features we have provided. We hope your enjoyment of this learning package is equal to our pride in it.

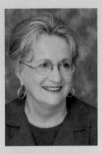

Judith Wilkinson

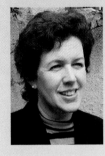

How to Use This Learning Package (for Teachers)

For suggestions about how to use this integrated learning package,

 Go to **How to Use This Learning Package,** on the Instructors Resource Disk.

Getting the Most Out of This Learning Package (for Students)

For ideas about how to use your textbooks and the Electronic Study Guide to get the best results from your studying,

 Go to **Getting the Most Out of This Learning Package,** on the Electronic Study Guide.

Acknowledgments

We wish to extend sincere thanks to the exceptional team that helped us create this package:

- Lisa Biello Deitch, Acquisitions Editor and friend, for her vision in imagining the broad concept for this work, and for her support in allowing us the freedom to flesh out that idea in ways that are true to our own vision.

- Patti Cleary, Editor in Chief of Nursing, whose wise counsel was often sought.

- Shirley Kuhn, Special Projects Editor; Danielle Barsky, Senior Project Editor; and Darlene Pedersen, Content Development Manager, who always went the extra mile in the development phase of this textbook. We appreciate their long hours and their willingness to take on an enormous amount of work, and we are grateful for their ability to keep quality always in mind, even when working at maximum speed.

- Wendy Earl of Wendy Earl Productions, and Sandie Sigrist of Techbooks for their gentle nudging and support that allowed this project to become a reality.

- Ted Clow and Mark Lozier, photographers, who worked with us tirelessly to get the job done, as well as Barbara Proud, photographer, for her multigenerational family and other photos.

- Sally Peyrefitte, copyeditor extraordinaire.

- Bettina Borer, Art Editor, for her artist's eye and meticulous attention to detail.

- Betty Paulanka, EdD, RN, Dean and Professor of the College of Health Sciences at the University of Delaware; Elaine Burkett, BSN, RN, Clinical Simulation Laboratory Coordinator at the University of Delaware; and Meredith Bishop, Pediatric Clinical Simulation Laboratory Coordinator at the University of Delaware, for the use of their state-of-the-art nursing lab, coordination of student models, and time spent organizing supplies and providing consultation on procedures.

- Patricia M. Dillon, RN, MSN, DNSc; and Temple University, Philadelphia, Pennsylvania, for the use of the nursing lab and her help in providing models for photos and her generous assistance with procedures and illustrations.

- Professor DaNell C. Moore, M.Ed., M.S.N., Lab Coordinator, Department of Nursing, Armstrong Atlantic State University, Savannah, Georgia, for use of nursing lab supplies and equipment.

- Joanne DaCunha, RN and Acquisitions Editor, for her expertise and the generous use of her time in obtaining photos demonstrating procedures.

Contributors

The following people contributed material that has been used in developing this learning package. We are grateful for their assistance.

We wish to express special thanks to **Diane Bligh** and **Kathy Shepard,** whose "can do" attitude allowed them to take on a variety of writing tasks and complete them well and on time, and to **Collette Hendler** for her assistance with the test bank and procedures.

Recognizing that all work echoes and builds on that which came before it, we are grateful to **Ann Haffer** and **Bonnie Raingruber** for their creative use of Stephen Brookfield's work in their writings. It helped us to build on our own work in that area, significantly enriching the model of critical thinking we used in this text.

Nancy R. Ahern, RN, MSN
Instructor
Brevard Campus
School of Nursing
University of Central Florida
Cocoa, Florida
Chapters 13 and 14

Rachel E. Albert, PHD, RN
Director and Associate Professor of Nursing
University of Maine at Fort Kent
Fort Kent, Maine
Chapter 18

Mary Ann Anderson, PHD, APRN, BC
Associate Professor, Retired
College of Health Professions
Weber State University
Ogden, Utah
Chapter 8

Diane M. Bligh, RN, MS, CNS
Associate Professor, Nursing
Front Range Community College
Westminster, Colorado
Concept Maps, Care Maps, Test Questions, Procedures

Mary Beth Bohli, BSN, MSN
Assistant Professor
Onondaga Community College
Syracuse, New York
Chapter 4

Christine Dimartile Bolla, RN, DNSC
Nursing Faculty
Dominican University of California
San Rafael, California
Chapter 37

Carol Boswell, RN, EDD
Associate Professor, School of Nursing
Texas Tech University HSC
Odessa, Texas
Chapter 4

Clara Boyle, RN, EDD
Associate Professor of Nursing
Salem State College
Salem, Massachusetts
Chapter 25

Mary Anne Bright, EDD, APRN, BC
Associate Professor Emerita
University of Massachusetts Amherst
Amherst, Massachusetts
Chapter 40

Patricia Carroll, RN, CEN, RRT, MS
Educational Medical Consultant
Meriden, Connecticut
Care Plans

Traudel B. Cline, AD, BS, MS, PHD
Nurse Educator/Staff Nurse
Milwaukee Area Technical College
Milwaukee, Wisconsin
Chapter 22

Pamela Sue Combs, RN, MSN
Clinical Faculty
University of Louisville
Louisville, Kentucky
Chapter 16

Leanne Cowin, BN, MNS, PHD
University of Western Sydney
Sydney, Australia
Chapter 11

Kathleen Crawford, BS, LVN
Adult Nurse Practitioner Candidate
Yale School of Nursing
New Haven, Connecticut
Chapter 45

Patricia Marie Dillon, DNSc, RN
Assistant Professor
Temple University
Philadelphia, Pennsylvania
Procedures

Maggie Thurmond Dorsey, RN, MSN, EDD
Assistant Professor
University of South Carolina, Aiken
Aiken, South Carolina
Chapter 28

June S. Goyne, RN, MSN, EDD
Chair, Department of Nursing and BSN Program Director
Columbus State University
Columbus, Georgia
Chapter 35

Janice Harris, RN, MSN
Associate Professor; Coordinator, RN-BSN Program
Columbus State University
Columbus, Georgia
Chapter 21

Annette Hayes, MSN, RNC, CS
Assistant Director, School of Nursing
Ohio Valley General Hospital
McKees Rocks, Pennsylvania
Chapter 9

Collette Bishop Hendler, RN, BS, CCRN
Clinical Leader, Med Care
Abington Memorial Hospital Intensive Care Unit
Abington, Pennsylvania
Test Questions, Procedures

Patricia Holden-Huchton, RN, DSN, ACRN
Associate Professor
University of Nevada
Reno, Nevada
Supplemental Materials for Chapter 1

Anita Huse, RN, MSN, EDD
Department of Nursing Education
Tufts-New England Medical Center
Boston, Massachusetts
Chapter 30

Melba Ingram, RN, MSN
Faculty
Texarkana College
Texarkana, Texas
Chapter 41

Kathleen Jones, MSN, APRN, BC
Associate Professor of Nursing
Walters State Community College
Johnson City, Tennessee
Procedures

Lori Klingman, MSN, RN
Faculty
Ohio Valley General Hospital School of Nursing
McKees Rocks, Pennsylvania
Chapter 9

Susan Jeanne Lamanna, RN, MA, MSN, ANP
Associate Professor, Nursing
Onondaga Community College
Syracuse, New York
Chapter 15

Sandra Dahl McHenry, DNSc, RN
Associate Professor; Chair, Special Education
Services/Instruction
Rowan University
Glassboro, New Jersey
Chapter 32

Gary J. Measom, APRN, PHD, CCRN
Assistant Professor
Utah Valley State College
Orem, Utah
Chapter 31

Kristen S. Montgomery, PHD, RN
Assistant Professor of Nursing
University of South Carolina
Columbia, South Carolina
Chapter 12

Kathleen Ahern Nieubuurt, RN, MS
Nursing Faculty
Chemeketa Community College
Salem, Oregon
Test Questions

Barbara Nubile, RN, MSN
Assistant Dean, Division of Nursing
Yavapai College
Prescott, Arizona
Procedures

Mary O'Keefe, RN, PHD, JD
Assistant Professor of Nursing
Texas Tech University
Houston, Texas
Chapter 45

James C. Pace, DSN, MDiv, APRN-BC, FAANP
Professor of Nursing; Coordinator, ANP/Palliative Care
Program
Vanderbilt University School of Nursing
Nashville, Tennessee
Chapter 14

Cindy Parsons, DNP, ARNP, BC
Assistant Professor of Nursing
University of Tampa
Tampa, Florida
Test Questions

Linda Pasto, MS, RN
Professor of Nursing and Health
Tompkins Cortland Community College
Dryden, New York
Chapter 24

Joyce W. Pompey, RN, MSN
Instructor
University of South Carolina, Aiken
Aiken, South Carolina
Chapter 28

Debbie J. Rahn, RN, MSN, CNE
Curriculum Coordinator
The Reading Hospital School of Nursing
West Reading, Pennsylvania
Chapter 18

Bonnie Raingruber, PHD, MS, BS, CNS
Director, Center for Health and Human Services
Research and Professor of Nursing
California State University, Sacramento
Nurse Researcher
University of California, Davis
Sacramento, California
Concept Maps, Mapping Tutorial

Judith P. Ruland, PHD, RN
School of Nursing
College of Health and Public Affairs
University of Central Florida
Orlando, Florida
Chapter 44

Debra Anne Schilleman, RN, BSN, LSAC
CNA Program Coordinator
Davis Applied Technology College
Kaysville, Utah
Chapter 33

Michelle Seale
Kettering College of Medical Arts
Kettering, Ohio

Kathy Shepard, RN, CWS
Infection Control Nurse, Employee Heath Nurse,
Education Coordinator, Certified Wound Specialist
HealthSouth Hospital of Terre Haute
Terre Haute, Indiana
Procedures

Joellen H. Shumway, RN, ADN
CNA Program Coordinator/Instructor
Davis Applied Technology College
Kaysville, Utah
Chapter 27

Marlene Smadu, RN, BSCN, MADED, EDD
Associate Dean, Regina Site, College of Nursing
University of Saskatchewan
Regina, Saskatchewan
Chapter 46

Pamela Smith, PHD, RN
Chair and Professor, Division of Nursing
MidAmerica Nazarene University
Olathe, Kansas
Chapter 10

Susan Smith, BSN, RNC
Brandywine Hospital
Coatesville, Pennsylvania
S. K. Smith Consulting
Warriors Mark, Pennsylvania
Chapter 23

Joanne Thanavaro, DNP, MSN (R), APRN-BC
Associate Professor of Nursing
Barnes-Jewish College of Nursing
ANP-Independent Practice
Patterson Medical Clinic
St. Louis, Missouri
Chapter 19

Lisa Theriault, RN, MSN, APRN
Assistant Professor of Nursing
University of Maine at Fort Kent
Fort Kent, Maine
Chapter 26

Deborah Weaver, RN, PHD
Associate Professor
Valdosta State University
Valdosta, Georgia
Chapter 3

Diane Whitehead, EDD, RN
Department Chair, Nursing
Nova Southeastern University
Fort Lauderdale, Florida
Chapter 38

Bruce K. Wilson, PHD, LVN, RN, CNS
Associate Professor of Nursing
University of Texas-Pan American
Edinburg, Texas
Chapter 20

Paige Wimberley, MSN, RN-CS
Faculty, Department of Nursing
Arkansas State University
Jonesboro, Arkansas
Chapter 34

Kathleen M. Young, MA, RN
Instructor of Nursing
Western Michigan University
Kalamazoo, Michigan
Chapter 39

Reviewers

Rachel E. Albert, PHD, RN
Director and Associate Professor of Nursing
University of Maine at Fort Kent
Fort Kent, Maine

Ivy Alexander, PHD, C-ANP
Associate Professor
Yale University School of Nursing
New Haven, Connecticut

Janet G. Alexander, RN, MSN, EDD
Associate Professor of Nursing
Samford University
Birmingham, Alabama

Anita D. Althans, RNC, MSN
Assistant Professor of Nursing
Our Lady of Holy Cross College
New Orleans, Louisiana

Gina M. Ankner, RN, ANP, BC
College of Nursing
University of Massachusetts–Dartmouth
North Dartmouth, Massachusetts

Allen M. Backman, MSc, PHD
Chair, Health Services Management Specialization
University of Saskatchewan College of Commerce
Saskatoon, Saskatchewan

Michele A. Baqi-Aziz, MS, CNS, FNP, RN
Clinical Instructor/Lecturer
University of Pennsylvania School of Nursing
Philadelphia, Pennsylvania

Nina Beaman, RNC, CMA, MS
Program Director
Bryant and Stratton College
Richmond, Virginia

Mary Beth Bohli, BSN, MSN
Assistant Professor
Onondaga Community College
Syracuse, New York

Carol Boswell, RN, EDD
Associate Professor of Nursing
Texas Tech University Health Sciences Center
Odessa, Texas

Meg Brown, MSN, APRN, BC, CNAA
Assistant Professor of Nursing
Alcorn State University
Natchez, Mississippi

Carmen Bruni, MSN, RN, CNA, BC
Assistant Professor of Nursing
Texas A&M International University
Laredo, Texas

Jan A. Buker, RN, MSN, CNOR
Faculty
Norfolk General Hospital
Norfolk, Virginia

Beverly Bye, MS, MED, RN, CRNP, FNE-A, CES
Clinical Assistant Professor
Towson University
Towson, Maryland

Faye Carlson, RN, MS, CCRN, CNRN
Nursing Faculty
Boise State University
Boise, Idaho

Joan Carnosso, RN, BSN, MSN
Assistant Professor of Nursing
Boise State University
Boise, Idaho

Barbara A. Caton, RN, MSN
Assistant Professor of Nursing
Missouri State University
West Plains, Missouri

Regina Cavin, RN, MSN
Assistant Professor of Nursing
Alcorn State University
Natchez, Mississippi

Jennifer Kay Cipolla, RN
Staff Nurse/House Supervisor
St. Joseph Medical Center
Kansas City, Missouri

Lissa Shelby Clark, BS, MSN, RN
Instructor in Nursing
University of Nebraska Medical Center
Omaha, Nebraska

Traudel B. Cline, AD, BS, MS, PHD
Nurse Educator/Staff Nurse
Milwaukee Area Technical College
Milwaukee, Wisconsin

Karen Cummins, RN, MSN, CRNP
Nursing Faculty
Community College of Allegheny County
Pittsburgh, Pennsylvania

Lynn M. Czaplewski, RN, BC, CRNI, BSN, OCN
Clinical Instructor
Columbia College of Nursing
Milwaukee, Wisconsin

Diana Davidson Dick, RN, MED
Dean of Nursing
Saskatchewan Institute of Applied Science & Technology
Saskatoon, Saskatchewan

Marcie L. Davis, RN, BC, BSN
Nursing Instructor
Ulster County BOCES Career & Technical Center
Port Ewen, New York

Mardell Davis, RN, MSN, PHD
Assistant Professor of Nursing
University of Alabama
Birmingham, Alabama

Sheila A. Dunn, RN, MSN, C-ANP
Nurse Practitioner
Veterans Affairs Outpatient Clinic
Belleville, Illinois

Marlys Eggum, RN, FNP, ANCC
Nursing Instructor
Miles Community College
Miles City, Montana

Susan Eldred, RN, BSCN, MBA, PHN
Professor of Nursing
University of Ottawa
Ottawa, Ontario

Sally E. Erdel, RN, MS
Assistant Professor of Nursing
Bethel College
Mishawaka, Indiana

Carolyn D. Foster, RN, MA, MN
Associate Dean
Presbyterian Hospital School of Nursing
Charlotte, North Carolina

Pauline Freedberg, MSN, RN
Professor of Nursing
Westmoreland County Community College
Youngwood, Pennsylvania

Beth Furlong, PHD, JD, RN
Associate Professor, School of Nursing
Creighton University
Omaha, Nebraska

Lynn M. Gaddis, BSN, MSN, PHD
Associate Professor/Fundamentals Coordinator
Cuyahoga Community College Nursing Program
Cleveland, Ohio

Lucille Gambardella, PHD, RN, CS, APN-BC
Chair, Department of Nursing
Wesley College
Dover, Delaware

Deborah R. Garrison, RN, BS, MS, PHD
Chair, Nursing Programs
Wilson School of Nursing
Wichita Falls, Texas

Lynette Graesing, RN, BSN
Nursing Faculty
Iowa Lakes Community College
Emmetsburg, Iowa

Anita M. Hakala, RN, MSN
Nursing Faculty
Central Maine Community College
Auburn, Maine

Connie Ann Hall, RN, MSN, EDD
Instructor of Nursing
Penn State University
Uniontown, Pennsylvania

Karen Hamilton, RNC, MSN
Assistant Professor of Nursing
University of South Alabama
Mobile, Alabama

Brenda Hamilton-Anderson, RN, MSN, APRN, BC, NP-C
Family Nurse Practioner
Tifton, Georgia

Nicole Harder, RN, BN, MPA
Coordinator, Learning Laboratories
University of Manitoba
Winnipeg, Manitoba

Robin Harwood, RN, MN, CNS-MH
Professor of Nursing
Johnson County Community College
Overland Park, Kansas

Carol Haus, RN, BSN, MSN, PHD
Assistant Director
Western Pennsylvania Hospital School of Nursing
Pittsburgh, Pennsylvania

Annette Hayes, MSN, RN, CS
Nursing Faculty
Pueblo Community College
Durango, Colorado

Carole Heath, EDD, MSN, CHN, PHN
Professor of Nursing
Sonoma State University
Rohnert Park, California

Caroline Helton, BSN, MSN
Instructor in Nursing
Missouri State University
Springfield, Missouri

Rosanna M. Henry, MSN, RN
Lab Supervisor, Instructor in Nursing
Duquesne University
Pittsburgh, Pennsylvania

Marie J. Hunter, BSN, MSN
Assistant Professor of Nursing
Utah Valley State College
Orem, Utah

Connie A. Ilkiw, RN, MSN
Associate Professor
Cox College of Nursing & Health Sciences
Springfield, Missouri

Marie C. Infante, RN, MS, MBA, JD
Member, Health Section
Mintz, Levin, Cohn, Ferris, Glovsky & Popeo
Washington, DC

Beverly K. Johnson, PHD, RN
Associate Professor
Seattle University College of Nursing
Seattle, Washington

Kathleen C. Jones, MSN, APRN, BC
Associate Professor of Nursing
Walters State Community College, Health Programs
Division
Morristown, Tennessee

Jill B. Keller, RN, MSN
Associate Professor
Henderson Community College
Henderson, Kentucky

Gretchen A. Kelley, RN, PHD
Educator, Perinatal Services
Memorial Hermann Healthcare
Houston, Texas

Anita G. Kinser, RNC, EDD
Assistant Professor of Nursing
California State University–San Bernadino
San Bernadino, California

Mary Lee Kirkland, MSN, EDD, RN
Associate Professor of Nursing
Medical University of South Carolina
Charleston, South Carolina

Diane K. Kjervik, RN, JD, FAAN
Professor/Associate Dean
University of North Carolina School of Nursing
Chapel Hill, North Carolina

Lori Klingman, MSN, RN
Faculty
Ohio Valley General Hospital School of Nursing
McKees Rocks, Pennsylvania

Linda Ann Kucher, MSN, RN, CMSRN
Assistant Professor of Nursing
Gordon College
Barnesville, Georgia

Carla Lee, RN, EDS, MN, PHD, FAAN
Assistant Professor of Nursing
Holy Names University
Oakland, California

Karol B. Lindow, RN, CNS, MSN
Associate Professor of Nursing
Kent State University–Tuscarawas
New Philadelphia, Ohio

Juliene G. Lipson, PHD, RN, FAAN
Professor Emerita, Community Health Systems
University of California–San Francisco
San Francisco, California

Brenda S. Lohri-Posey, EDD, RN
Assistant Professor of Nursing
Belmont Technical College
St. Clairsville, Ohio

Luana Martindale, BSN, MSN
Associate Professor of Nursing
University of Arkansas at Little Rock
Little Rock, Arkansas

Maureen McDonald, MS, RN
Professor of Nursing
Massasoit Community College
Brockton, Massachusetts

Tom McIntosh, PHD
Assistant Professor
University of Regina
Regina, Saskatchewan

Diana E. McMillan, RN, PHD
Assistant Professor, Faculty of Nursing
University of Manitoba
Winnipeg, Manitoba

Gary J. Measom, APRN, PHD, CCRN
Assistant Professor
Utah Valley State College
Orem, Utah

DeAnne Messias, PHD, RN
Associate Professor
College of Nursing and Women's Studies
University of South Carolina
Columbia, South Carolina

Karima F. Miller, BSN, MSN, FNP-C
Family Nurse Practitioner
Long Beach City College
Long Beach, California

Diana Mixon, BSN, MSN
Associate Professor of Nursing
Boise State University
Boise, Idaho

Susan A. Moore, PHD, RN
Associate Professor of Nursing
New Hampshire Community Technical College
Manchester, New Hampshire

Sandra G. Nadelson, RN, MSN, MED
Nursing Faculty
Community College of Southern Nevada
Las Vegas, Nevada

Mary Elizabeth S. Nelson, MSN, APRN-BC
Nurse Practitioner, Physical Medicine and Rehabilitation
Medical College of Wisconsin
Milwaukee, Wisconsin

Troy Nelson, ADN, BSN, APRN
Instructor in Nursing
Utah Valley State College
Orem, Utah

Deborah L. Newquist, RN, MED, MS
Instructor of Nursing
Western Wisconsin Technical College
La Crosse, Wisconsin

Patricia Nutz, MSN
Instructor in Nursing
St. Francis Hospital
New Castle, Pennsylvania

Francine Opfar, NP, APRN
Assistant Professor of Nursing
Utah Valley State College
Orem, Utah

Jan G. Overman, RN, MSN
Dean of Health Technologies
Forsyth Technical Community College
Winston-Salem, North Carolina

Cindy Parsons, DNP, ARNP, BC
Assistant Professor of Nursing
University of Tampa
Tampa, Florida

Roxanne Perucca, MSN, CRNI
Nurse Manager
University of Kansas Hospital
Kansas City, Kansas

Thomas Petricini, RN, MSN
Nursing Instructor
Sharon Regional Health System
Sharon, Pennsylvania

Suzanne Porfyris, APN, NP, MSN, PNP
Pediatric Nurse Practitioner
Children's Memorial Hospital
Chicago, Illinois

Karen Przytulski, MS, RD
Director of Dietary
Doctors Hospital of Jackson
Jackson, Mississippi

Larry D. Purnell, PHD, RN
Professor of Nursing
University of Delaware
Newark, Delaware

Ruth Remington, PHD, RN
Assistant Professor of Nursing
University of Massachusetts–Lowell
Lowell, Massachusetts

Carina Rew-Markham, RN, BSN, MS
Legal Nurse Consultant
Robins, Kaplan, Miller & Ciresi
Minneapolis, Minnesota

Judith A. Robertson, RN, MN
Instructor in Nursing
Seminole Community College
Sanford, Florida

Jane S. Roman, RN, MED
Chair, Surgical Technology Certificate Program
Bunker Hill Community College
Chelsea, Massachusetts

Nancy L. Rowley, RN, MSN, CCRN
Visiting Assistant Professor of Nursing
Miami University of Ohio
Hamilton, Ohio

Patricia F. St. Hill, PHD, RN, MPH
Professor, Bellevue School of Nursing
Hunter College of the City University of New York
New York, New York

Jo Ann L. St. Romain, MSN, RN
Professor
Delgado Community College
New Orleans, Louisiana

Shelia Savell, MSN, RN
Clinical Instructor
College of Nursing
University of Arkansas for Medical Sciences
Little Rock, Arkansas

Patricia Schafer, PHD, RN
Associate Professor, Kirkhof College of Nursing
Grand Valley State University
Grand Rapids, Michigan

Vivian C. Schrader, RN, MS
Assistant Professor of Nursing
Boise State University
Boise, Idaho

Jalee Scott, RN, MSN, OCN
Nursing Faculty
Methodist Medical Center College of Nursing
Peoria, Illinois

Gale P. Sewell, RN, MSN
Assistant Professor
Kent State University
Ashtabula, Ohio

Judith Shamian, RN, MPH, PHD
President & CEO, VON Canada
University of Toronto
Ottawa, Ontario

Kathy Shepard, RN, CWS
Infection Control Nurse, Employee Heath Nurse,
Education Coordinator, Certified Wound Specialist
HealthSouth Hospital of Terre Haute
Terre Haute, Indiana

Margaret Sherer, MS, RN, CEN
Nursing Faculty
Portland Community College
Portland, Oregon

Deborah Witt Sherman, RN, FAAN, BSN, MSN, PHD
Associate Professor
New York University College of Nursing
New York, New York

Frances Snodgrass, JD, MA, MS, RN
Associate Professor/Chair, School of Nursing
West Virginia Institute of Technology
Montgomery, West Virginia

Lillian Sonnenschein, MSN, APRN, BC
Assistant Professor of Nursing
Bristol Community College
Fall River, Massachusetts

Karen A. Stemler, MS, RN, APRN, FNP
Program Instructor in Nursing/Adult Nurse Practitioner
Yale University
New Haven, Connecticut

Genine Schwinge, MS, APRN
Adjunct Instructor, Nursing Department
Suffolk County Community College, Ammerman Campus
Selden, New York

Catherine B. Talley, MSN, RN, PAHM
Associate Professor of Nursing
University of South Carolina–Spartanburg
Spartanburg, South Carolina

Rebecca A. Terranova, MA, RN, C.
Nursing Arts Laboratory Manager
New York University College of Nursing
New York, New York

Roselena Thorpe, RN, PHD
Professor & Nursing Department Chair
Community College of Allegheny County
Pittsburgh, Pennsylvania

Jeannette Tomanka, BSN, MS, NP-C
Medical Writer
ICOS Corporation
Bothell, Washington

Gladdi Tomlinson, RN, MSN
Nursing Professor
Harrisburg Area Community College
Harrisburg, Pennsylvania

Janice V. Tramel, PA-C, NP
Testing & CME Coordinator, Physician Assistant
Program
University of Southern California Keck School
of Medicine
Alhambra, California

Kuei-Shen Tu, RN, MSN
Assistant Professor of Nursing
University of Alabama-Birmingham
Birmingham, Alabama

Barbara Ullman, MSN, RN, FNP-C
Director, Nurse Practitioner Program
University of Phoenix
Phoenix, Arizona

Linda Vanni, RN, MSN, CS
Clinical Nurse Specialist
Karmanos Cancer Center, Karmanos Pain Service
Detroit, Michigan

Mary Walden, RN, BSN, CWOCN, MSN
Wound Center Nurse Director
Gilmore Memorial Hospital
Amory, Mississippi

Linda S. Wallace, EDD, MSN, RN
Associate Professor and Director of International Studies
Indiana University Kokomo School of Nursing
Kokomo, Indiana

Virginia S. Wangerin, MSN, RN
Director of Nursing Education
Des Moines Area Community College
Ankeny, Iowa

Mina Wayman, MSN, RN, GNP
Assistant Professor of Nursing
Utah Valley State College
Orem, Utah

Deborah L. Weaver, RN, PHD
Associate Professor of Nursing
Valdosta State University
Valdosta, Georgia

Bonnie K. Webster, RN, MS, BC
Instructor, Nursing School
University of Texas Medical Branch
Galveston, Texas

Jacqueline C. Williams, RN-C, MSN
Instructor in Nursing
Shelton State Community College
Tuscaloosa, Alabama

Patricia Moran Woodbery, BSN, MSN, ARNP, CS
Professor of Nursing
Valencia Community College
Orlando, Florida

Kathleen M. Young, MA, BSN, BCRN
Master Faculty Specialist
Western Michigan University
Kalamazoo, Michigan

Detailed Contents

CHAPTER 7
Nursing Process: Implementation & Evaluation 119

CHAPTER 8
Nursing Theory & Research 138

CHAPTER 15
Loss, Grief, & Dying 263

UNIT 3

Essential Nursing Interventions 287

CHAPTER 16
Documenting & Reporting 288

CHAPTER 17
Measuring Vital Signs 304

CHAPTER 18
Communicating & the Therapeutic Relationship 337

CHAPTER 23
Administering Medications 472

CHAPTER 24
Teaching Clients 527

UNIT 4
How Nurses Support Physiological Functioning 549

CHAPTER 25
Stress & Adaptation 550

CHAPTER 26
Nutrition 574

CHAPTER 27
Urinary Elimination 618

CHAPTER 28
Bowel Elimination 650

CHAPTER 29
Sensory Perception 679

CHAPTER 30
Pain Management 698

CHAPTER 35
Oxygenation 844

CHAPTER 36
Fluids, Electrolytes, & Acid-Base Balance 886

CHAPTER 37
Perioperative Nursing 922

UNIT 5

Nursing Functions 951

CHAPTER 38
Leading & Managing 952

Special Features

Complementary and Alternative Modalities Boxes

Toward Evidence-Based Practice Boxes

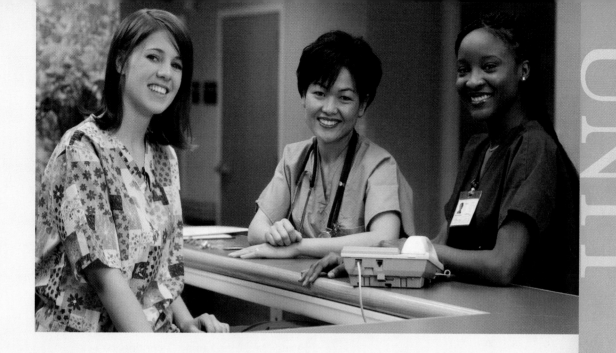

How Nurses
Think

CHAPTER 1

Evolution of Nursing
Thought & Action

Learning Outcomes

After completing this chapter, you should be able to:

* Describe the role of religion in the development of nursing.

* Identify the factors that led to the change of nursing from a vocation of men and women to a predominantly female profession.

* Explain the role of the military in the development of the nursing profession.

* Define *nursing* in your own words.

* Discuss the transitions nursing education has undergone in the last century.

* Differentiate between the various forms of nursing education for licensed practical/vocational nurses and registered nurses.

* Discuss the regulation of nursing practice.

* Give four examples of influential nursing organizations.

* Identify the recipients of nursing care.

* Name the four focuses of nursing care.

* Identify nine expanded roles for nursing. See the Electronic Study Guide.

* Compare and contrast the places where nurses work.

* Delineate the forces and trends that are affecting contemporary nursing practice.

Then & Now

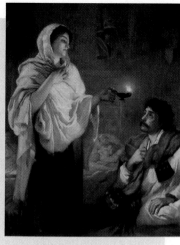

Time: 1854, Üsküdar (now part of Istanbul, Turkey) in the Crimea

The hospital tent is set up away from the battlefield. The injured and dying soldiers are lying caked in dried blood and filth upon the bare earth. Outside, the air is cool, yet the tent is stifling and the air rank with the smell of disease and death. Scanning the scene, Florence Nightingale gathers her staff of 38 nurses. They review the conditions of the hospital tent, the health problems of the soldiers, and the supplies and equipment they have to work with. First, they open the tent to allow in fresh air. Then they clean the tent, prepare clean bedding, and bathe the wounded. They assess and dress the wounds, feed the soldiers a nutritious meal, and comfort those dying or in pain. They offer encouragement to the healthier soldiers and help them to write letters home. Within a brief period of time the mortality rate drops from 47% to 2% and morale improves immeasurably.

Time: 2006, Your local hospital

While standing at the bedside mixing an antibiotic solution, Susan listens to the ventilator cycle. She notes that her patient has begun to trigger breaths on his own. In the background she hears the cardiac monitor. It has become increasingly irregular over the last hour. She mentally runs through her assessment of the patient. "Why is his heart so irritable?" she thinks. She calls the lab and asks if the morning blood work results are available. When the lab technician faxes the results to the unit, she notes that the potassium level is low at 2.9 mEq/L. She calls the attending physician and informs him of the lab results and the cardiac irritability. Susan tells the physician, "His potassium is low from the diarrhea he's had since we began the antibiotics." Susan and the physician develop a plan to administer IV KCl (potassium chloride, a medicine frequently used to raise the serum potassium level) and check the potassium level every 8 hours. She starts the KCl replacement. Several hours later she charts that the *ectopy* (irregular heartbeat) has decreased.

Time: 2025, A local home

Yesterday, Mr. Samuels underwent cardiac surgery. He was discharged home this morning and is now under your care. As a home care nurse, your role is to assess his condition, provide skilled care, teach Mr. Samuels how to care for himself, instruct his family about his care, and coordinate any required additional services. Mrs. Samuels greets you at the front door. She tells you that her husband is in a lot of pain and that the chest drainage system appears full. She looks frightened and says, "When my father had cardiac surgery 15 years ago, he spent 5 days in the hospital. The nurses took care of him in the hospital. I don't understand why my husband got sent home so quickly." You explain that changes in technology and the healthcare system allow you to take care of clients in the home who would previously have been in the hospital. As you begin your assessments, you tell Mrs. Samuels, "After I've gathered more information, we'll make a plan for his care that will make all of us more comfortable."

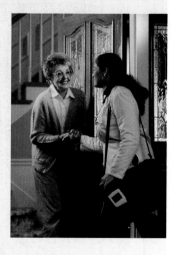

In each of these scenarios, the nurses engaged in *full-spectrum nursing;* that is, they used their minds and their hands to improve the client's comfort and condition. As the scenarios illustrate, nursing roles have undergone many changes over time. Yet nursing remains a profession dedicated to care of the client.

NURSING IMAGES THROUGHOUT HISTORY

An understanding of the past can lend insight into the present. In the next few pages we will review the portrayal of nursing in art and popular culture at different periods in history, and relate the images to the reality of contemporary nursing. This will help you appreciate the rich traditions of nursing and give you insight into the major forces that have shaped nursing as it is today. Pay close attention to the rate of change in recent years, and keep in mind that nursing and health care are poised for even more rapid change in the future.

When you think of nursing, what picture comes to mind? As you think of each of the three scenarios at the opening of this chapter, what do you see when you try to picture the story? Is this the same image you get when you imagine yourself as a nurse?

Artwork, television, popular stories, advertisements, and greeting cards have all portrayed nurses in many ways. Some of these images are flattering, and others are demeaning. Whether accurate or not, they influence how people view nursing. Some of these images may have figured in your decision to become a nurse, in either a positive or negative way. In the next section we will discuss these images and explore the truth and fiction behind each of them.

Angel of Mercy

One common image is the nurse as an angelic creature. The angel-nurse is serene and content and shown with a halo or other religious symbols. This image is so pervasive that even uniform shops and medical supply houses sell cups, T-shirts, and pins that feature the angelic nurse. There is some truth to this stereotype.

History demonstrates a strong link between nursing and religious orders. In ancient Egypt, Greece, and Rome, the temples were health centers as well as places of worship. In the temples, priests and priestesses treated the ill with a mixture of physical care, prayer, and magic spells.

The Vedas, the most ancient sacred books of the Hindu faith (circa 1200 B.C.E.), provide a detailed description of Indian healthcare practices and are some of the earliest writings to describe a distinct nursing occupation. In these texts, Charaka and Samhita, a physician and surgeon team, detail the roles of the physician, drugs, nurse, and the patient. Their writings indicate that nurses of that period were always male and were part of a priestly order. Nursing responsibilities included knowledge of the preparation, compounding, and administration of drugs; wisdom; purity; and devotion to the patient.

From the first to the tenth centuries, lay deacons and deaconesses in the Christian church began to visit the sick in their homes and to function as nurses. Initially the sick were brought to the local bishop's house for care, but this led to overcrowding as care of the sick outside the home became popular. Eventually early Christian hospitals developed. The earliest known Christian hospital appeared in the first century. The oldest continuously existing hospital, Hôtel Dieu in Lyons, France, was founded in 542 C.E. (Figure 1–1). In the United States, all training programs for nurses

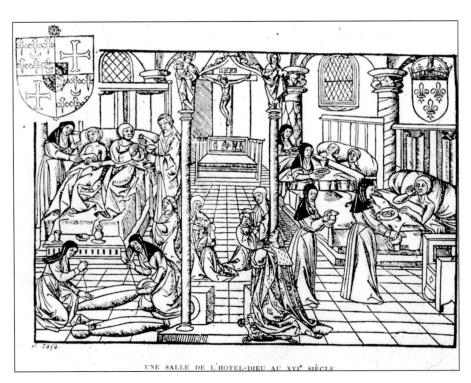

UNE SALLE DE L'HOTEL-DIEU AU XVIe SIÈCLE

FIGURE 1–1 Hôtel Dieu in Lyons, France, the oldest continuously existing hospital.

were affiliated with religious orders until well after the Civil War, and to this day, many healthcare institutions are owned and operated by religious groups.

Another reason for the association between nursing and spirituality is the fact that, *until about 100 years ago, nurses cared for patients at great risk to their own lives.* Today we have an advanced understanding of germ theory, infectious diseases, and sanitation. But this information is relatively new. Prior to the development of sophisticated microscopes and techniques for culturing microorganisms in the 19th century, people who entered nursing placed themselves at risk for exposure to diseases that were poorly understood and often could not be cured. Providing care in spite of these risks was considered self-sacrificing, much like the call to serve in religious life. Even as recently as the 1950s, antibiotics were not readily available, and the chief cause of **mortality** (death) was infectious disease.

The association of nursing with religion has not always been positive. Early Christianity did benefit nursing by creating nursing orders, establishing hospitals, and honoring the service provided by nurses. However, from the 15th to the 19th century, the influence of Christianity in general society began to wane. This period marked a transition from medieval to modern civilization. In medicine this time was associated with major advances in anatomy and physiology and a growing understanding of communicable disease. Art, music, literature, and science flourished, but as the influence of the church began to be challenged, nursing orders were often persecuted. Many nurses within religious orders fled them to avoid imprisonment or death.

From the 19th century onward, religious groups gradually re-emerged as influential in society and in nursing. Today many nursing programs, universities and colleges, and healthcare institutions are affiliated with religious groups. Examples include the University of Notre Dame, the Seventh Day Adventist hospital system, and the American Baptist nursing home system. Although most of these organizations have mission statements or guidelines that incorporate charitable values such as compassion and caring, they no longer require religious dedication from their nursing students.

CriticalThinking 1–1

Which aspects of the nurse-as-angel appeal to you most when you think about the way you will practice nursing? Why?

Handmaiden

Another widely recognized stereotype is that of the nurse as handmaiden to the physician. This stereotype depicts the nurse as a woman assisting a male physician at the bedside of a patient. The physician is shown in the dominant role, with the nurse waiting in

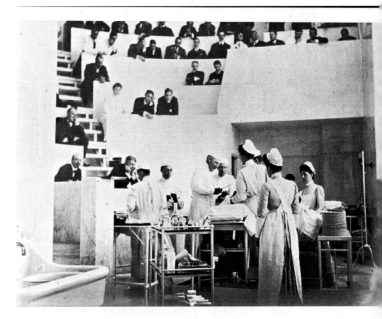

FIGURE 1–2 Handmaiden image of nursing.

anticipation for the physician's orders or supporting the patient while the physician provides care (Figure 1–2).

The validity of this image has changed over time. Initially the role of the nurse was limited to bathing, feeding, and supporting the patient; keeping the patient environment clean and orderly; and providing support for the physician. Today nurses collaborate with all members of the healthcare team, providing care not only at the direction of physicians but along with them (Table 1–1). Many current nursing activities were once performed only by physicians. For example, there was a time when only physicians used a stethoscope and took blood pressure readings. Nurses now routinely perform these assessments. Nurses also give medications by intravenous and injectable routes, but this was not the case 50 years ago. Although injectable penicillin began to be used during World War II, allowing many soldiers to survive injuries that would have been fatal in the past, only physicians and medics in the battlefield hospitals were allowed to administer it. The aunt of one of the authors is a retired RN who vividly recounts how proud she was to administer her first penicillin injection without direct physician supervision—several years after the war. Today this story may seem comical because nurses perform so many complex and critical tasks.

Although nursing has become more complex and somewhat more autonomous, the physician remains the final decision maker about most patient care. Much of this power is derived from legal and financial authority.

Put simply, the legal definition of medicine has carved out a broad role for physicians, including the supervision of nurses and other health professionals. In contrast, nursing practice acts are not as broad and inclusive. Barbara Safriet, a legal expert on healthcare issues, has extensively studied the boundaries between

TABLE 1-1   Examples of Nursing Activities

Dependent Activities	Independent Activities
Administering medicines ordered by the physician	Evaluating the patient's response to the medicine and withholding the next dose if the patient has a negative reaction
Performing an ordered test	Teaching the patient what to expect from the test; preparing the patient for the test (e.g., shaving a site); supporting the patient during the test
Administering intravenous fluids	Evaluating the patient's response to treatment; monitoring the flow rate; evaluating the site for redness or leakage
Ensuring that the patient receives the ordered diet	Teaching a pregnant woman about the additional nutrients needed in her diet

healthcare providers as well as the pros and cons of these boundaries when attempting to reform health care. She states that physicians, who traditionally came from the wealthy and learned class, wrote and lobbied for legislation early in the history of their discipline that gave them sweeping powers and assured their control of health care. Now it is very difficult to challenge these laws. Safriet's 1994 landmark paper on the impediments to expanding nursing's role is cited on the Electronic Study Guide.

 Go to Chapter 1, **Reading More About Evolution of Nursing Thought & Action,** on the Electronic Study Guide.

Physicians also retain significant power because they generate income for healthcare institutions. People enter a hospital, nursing home, or home service as patients of physicians. The patients—or their insurers—then pay the facility to deliver care that is ordered by the physician. Without physicians, the institution does not make money. In contrast, nurses are usually employees of healthcare institutions and therefore may be considered a healthcare expense. Many advanced practice nurses are authorized to order care and bill for services and therefore have some power in healthcare decision making; however, this is not true for most nurses.

Although the handmaiden image may have been more widespread in the past, *many nurses never considered themselves to be handmaidens of physicians.* For example, the publications, letters, and diaries of Florence Nightingale, who is revered as the founder of modern nursing, indicate that she considered nurses the colleagues of physicians rather than their servants. In a letter to Elizabeth Blackwell, who later went on to become the first female physician, Nightingale wrote:

No man, not even a doctor, ever gives any other definition of what a nurse should be than this—

'devoted and obedient'. This definition would do well for a porter. It might even do for a horse. . . . (Chambers, 1958, p. 130)

At the age of 24, Florence Nightingale became convinced that her mission in life was to be with the sick (Figure 1–3). Nightingale met resistance from her wealthy, upper-class family, who stated that nursing was beneath her social station. Hospitals at that time were filthy and provided care only for the poor; the affluent cared for their sick in the home. In spite of her family's protests, Nightingale went on to study nursing in Germany.

When Nightingale returned to England to begin her work as a nurse, she immediately set out to lobby politicians and physicians on the importance of nursing and the need for public health reform. She was able to illustrate the importance of nursing and public health through her work in the Crimean War. In Scutari, now Turkey, Nightingale and her staff completely revamped the services offered to the wounded. It was at Crimea that Nightingale became known as the "Lady of the Lamp" because she walked through the camp at night providing care to the sick and wounded. Nightingale's major contributions include:

• The establishment of nursing as a distinct profession
• Introduction of a broad-based liberal education for nurses
• Major reform in the delivery of care in hospitals
• The introduction of standards to control the spread of disease in hospitals
• Major reforms in health care for the military

The employment status of most nurses is another factor that must be considered when looking at the validity of the handmaiden image. As we discussed earlier, most nurses work for healthcare institutions

rather than directly for physicians. If nurses have indeed been handmaidens, perhaps it has been to the institutions that employ them. Nurses are actively working to combat the handmaiden stereotype; for instance, they are forming unions to improve their working conditions and benefits. It is interesting that, with recent changes in the healthcare system, more physicians are becoming employees of healthcare institutions as well—and some, like nurses, are forming unions. The increasing costs of health care, coupled with decreasing reimbursement for health services, appears to be driving these changes.

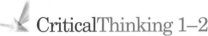

CriticalThinking 1–2

What similarities or differences do you see between the angelic and handmaiden images of nursing?

Battle-Ax

In the 1975 film *One Flew Over the Cuckoo's Nest,* Nurse Ratched personifies the contemporary image of the nurse as the battle-ax or torturer, treating her patients with cruelty and disdain. Charles Dickens gave an earlier version of the abusive nurse in his 1844 novel *Martin Chuzzlewit,* in the character of Sairy Gamp. Mrs. Gamp personified the view of nurses that many people held at that time: she was corrupt, harsh, and frequently intoxicated. How did these negative images come about? And why does this image persist? Again, history may provide insight.

The values of service and devotion to the patient were lost when, from the 14th to the 16th century, (a period known as the Renaissance), the influence of Christianity faded. Prior to this time, religious-affiliated nursing orders provided most care for the sick. However, as religion was abandoned and replaced by science and philosophy, nursing orders dissolved, and the knowledge of caring for the sick was lost. Municipal authorities took over hospitals, and criminals, sentenced to care for the sick in the hospitals in lieu of going to jail, assumed the nursing role. Forced to care for large numbers of patients without the benefit of training, supplies, assistance, or time off, these criminals often managed their workload by treating patients harshly and drinking while on duty. Most patients who entered such hospitals did not leave alive. Such practices persisted until the 1860s in Europe and until after the Civil War in the United States. It is no wonder, then, that the battle-ax image of nurses endured so long.

Caregiving activities may also contribute to the persistence of the battle-ax image. Giving injections, cleaning and dressing wounds, drawing blood, and starting intravenous lines are examples of nursing activities that, although performed to preserve the patient's health, may cause significant pain. Unfortunately,

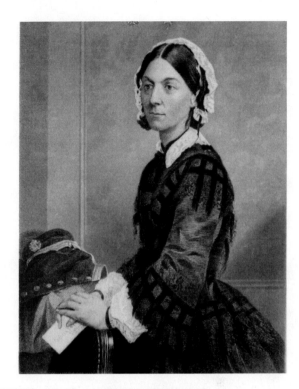

FIGURE 1–3   Florence Nightingale (1820–1910).

this association with pain helps to perpetuate the image of nurses as unfeeling. Aware of the power of this image, nurses on pediatric units typically wear colorful uniforms with child-friendly patterns such as balloons or circus clowns to avoid frightening children who may associate "nurse" with "pain."

Ironically, the image of the nurse as a battle-ax is in direct opposition to the image of the angel of mercy. These opposite images have co-existed for centuries.

Naughty Nurse

The sexy, risqué nurse was an image that arose in the early part of the 20th century with burlesque shows and persists in popular culture today. For example, in the 1980s, a prime-time television show called *The Nightingales* portrayed nurses as sexy, mindless women. The long-running (1972–1983) hit series *M*A*S*H* prominently featured Hot Lips Houlihan and other nurses, who were potential dates for the bright and talented surgeons. Get-well cards often portray nurses in short skirts, fishnet stockings, high heels, and cap, as do dime-store novels, comic books, and even CDs.

To see how pervasive this image is, go online and search under the term *nurse.* This search will yield many links to nursing organizations, nursing education programs, and nursing journals. However, it will also yield a large number of pornographic web sites featuring women who are supposedly nurses. Their role is implied through props—a nursing cap, a stethoscope, or a uniform—in the background.

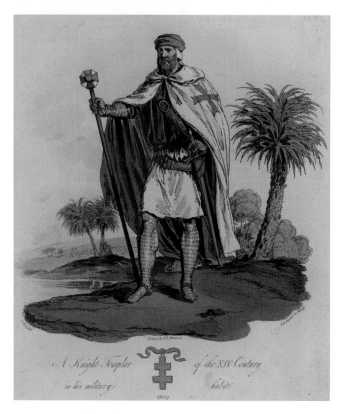

FIGURE 1–4   A hospitaler at the time of the Crusades.

Why is this so? What gives this image its power? As trusted health professionals, nurses frequently provide care that involves exposure of the patient's body, contact with bare skin, and discussion of intimate aspects of the client's life. In addition, hospitalized patients are in a weakened, vulnerable state, and the nurse may seem quite powerful by contrast. Thus, despite the fact that nurse-patient contact is professional and does not involve sexual intimacy, the "naughty nurse" stereotype may express a forbidden desire for intimate contact with a stranger in a position of power.

In addition, the traditionally female nurse's collaboration with traditionally male physicians may reinforce the stereotype of the nurse in a sexual role. In television shows and romance novels, compliant nurses are "rewarded" with marriage to the handsome surgeon, whereupon they "escape" nursing and retire to life as "the doctor's wife." Of course, it is true that nurses work closely with physicians and other healthcare providers. This close association may lead to socialization, friendships, and sometimes even marriages among healthcare professionals, but this is the exception rather than the rule. The "naughty nurse" stereotype may be popular, but it is not founded on truth.

CriticalThinking 1–3

- How do the images of the nurse as a battle-ax or sex object affect your view of nursing?
- As a nurse, what can you do to counteract these images?

Military Image

Nursing imagery is often military. Throughout the last century, nurses were frequently portrayed in uniform providing support at the battlefield, and nurses are still often depicted as warriors fighting disease. What is the history of these two military images?

Nurses on the Battlefield

Nurses' involvement in the military dates from 27 B.C.E., as the Roman Empire began to consolidate its dominion. Prior to this time, wounded soldiers depended on the charity of private citizens or religious persons. However, because the Roman Empire relied on the success of military excursions to extend its domain, the survival and well-being of its soldiers were critical. One of the great contributions of the Roman Empire was thus the development of the military hospital and the practice of providing first aid on the battlefield.

During the Middle Ages the two largest influences on nursing were the military and religion. These two threads fused in the Crusaders, soldiers who went to battle to conquer Islamic lands and spread Christianity throughout the world. Among the Crusaders were **hospitalers,** specialized soldiers who at the end of battle returned to the outposts to care for the sick and injured (Figure 1–4). Among the hospitalers, three orders predominated: (1) the Knights of St John, which established men's and women's branches throughout Europe—one of which still exists in England; (2) the Teutonic Knights, a strictly male order; and (3) the Knights of St Lazarus, which was established to care for lepers.

Throughout time nursing has had a presence on the battlefield. This trend has continued in modern history. In 1861, at the outbreak of the Civil War, the U.S. government established the Army Nursing Service. Its role was to organize nurses and hospitals and coordinate supplies for the soldiers. Many trained nurses joined the Army Nursing Service from religious orders that provided nursing education through a mentorship approach. Thousands of laypersons also volunteered. Among the lay nurses was Clara Barton, who organized her own nursing efforts. Rather than providing care in base hospitals, far removed from the battlefield, Barton and her volunteers provided care in tents set up close to the fighting. Barton was indiscriminate in provision of care, nursing soldiers from the North and South, black and white. When the war was over, Barton continued this universal care through the establishment of the American Red Cross. Other notable figures who served as nurses include Harriet Tubman, who helped slaves escape to freedom on the Underground Railroad; the poet Walt Whitman; the author Louisa May Alcott; and Dorothea Dix, the Union's Superintendent of Female Nurses during the Civil War.

Nurses also served in World War I, World War II, Korea, Vietnam (Figure 1–5), and the Gulf War. In these wars the nurses were all formally trained. Formal training for nurses became widespread in Europe in the 1860s after the widely publicized success of Nightingale in the Crimea. In the United States the first formal training program was established in 1873.

Nurses Fighting Disease

A second military image portrays nurses as warriors in the fight against disease. This image is commonplace in public awareness campaigns against infectious diseases. Florence Nightingale's contributions in public health and **epidemiology** (the study of the distribution and origins of disease) were among the first such efforts. In her *Notes on Hospitals* (1863), Nightingale stated that air, lighting, nutrition, and adequate ventilation and space assist the patient to recuperate. The hospitals she designed to incorporate these ideas were associated with decreased mortality, decreased rate of **nosocomial infection** (an infection associated with a healthcare facility), and decreased length of hospital stay.

Another notable event in the fight against disease occurred in 1893 when Lillian Wald and Mary Brewster founded the Henry Street Settlement in New York to improve the health and social conditions of poor immigrants. This is considered the start of public health nursing in the United States. Since then, nurses have played an important role in improving health and preventing illness by promoting safe drinking water, adequate sewage facilities, and proper sanitation measures in communities.

Figure 1–6 shows the nurse as a warrior in the fight against disease. In this figure, a nurse is slaying a beast that represents tuberculosis. The nurse is dressed in white and stands out clearly, whereas the monster is a dark and shadowy beast crawling over the globe.

In spite of the historical association of nursing with the military, currently only a small percentage of licensed U.S. nurses work in the armed services. Similarly, despite the powerful image of the nurse slaying tuberculosis, only approximately 10% of nurses work in community and public health agencies (HRSA, 2000).

Caucasian Women

As you looked at the preceding images of nurses, did you notice that all of them are white women? Women of color and men of any race are rarely shown as nurses.

Only about 6% of nurses in the United States and 5% in Canada are men (Rasmussen, 2001), and men are a minority of the total nursing population worldwide (Figure 1–7). This is ironic considering that many ancient nursing orders were exclusively male. In early Christianity, deacons provided nursing care to parish men while deaconesses provided care to

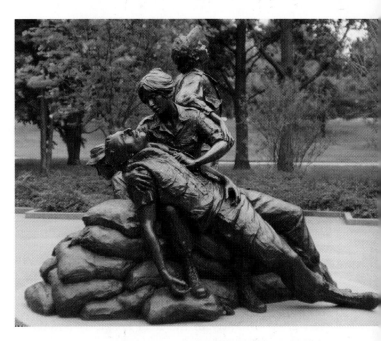

FIGURE 1–5 Women's Memorial for the Vietnam War. Copyright 1993, Vietnam Women's Memorial Foundation, Inc. Glenna Goodacre, sculptor.

women. During the Crusades, male hospitalers provided nursing care to their fellow soldiers who were injured in battle, and even today the majority of medics and hospital corpsmen who provide battlefront first aid are men. Female nurses in the military are

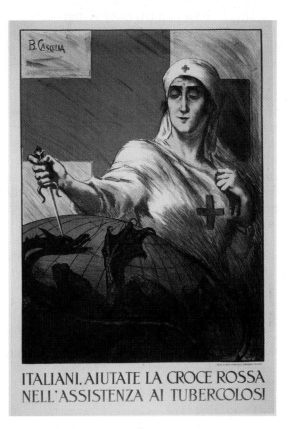

ITALIANI, AIUTATE LA CROCE ROSSA NELL'ASSISTENZA AI TUBERCOLOSI

FIGURE 1–6 Fighting disease. In this poster, the nurse is portrayed as a dragon slayer, fighting the monster of tuberculosis.

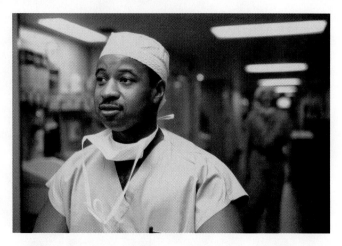

FIGURE 1–7 The roles of men in nursing are now as varied as those for women, and the opportunities for personal and professional fulfillment are as great.

TABLE 1-2 Race and Ethnicity Among Registered Nurses in the United States

Race/Ethnicity	1996	2000
Caucasian	90	86.6
African American	4.0	4.9
Asian/Pacific Islander	3.4	3.7
Hispanic/Latino	1.4	2.0
Native American	0.4	0.5
2 or more races	Not assessed in 1996	1.2

Source: March 2000 National Sample Survey of Registered Nurses, Division of Nursing, BHPR, Health Resources and Service Administration (HRSA).

seen predominantly in the field hospitals and away from the battlefront.

Popular media often reflect cultural beliefs. In the 2000 film *Meet the Parents,* Ben Stiller plays the role of a nurse. His future in-laws, who cannot understand why he would choose nursing as a profession, continually challenge him to defend his position and intelligence. This stereotype has not aided in the recruitment of men into the profession. Ironically, since the women's movement, women have received support as they moved into traditional male occupations such as physician, engineer, and scientist. However, many men perceive that they have not been welcomed into female-dominated fields (Meadus, 2000).

People of all colors and races work as nurses around the world. In the United States, Canada, and many European countries, most nurses are Caucasian; however, the recent trend is toward a slightly more diverse nurse workforce (Table 1–2). Major nursing and healthcare organizations agree on the need to increase diversity in nursing. One proposed solution is to increase the representation of minorities in advanced practice nursing and faculty positions so that they will serve as role models and mentors for incoming nurses. This solution may also be effective with the recruitment of men into nursing; however, it is also essential that practicing nurses embrace these changes and welcome others into the field.

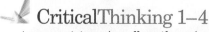

CriticalThinking 1–4

In your opinion, what efforts, if any, should nursing organizations take to recruit a more diverse workforce?

Full-Spectrum Nurse

Nurses are often shown actively caring for the patient—dressing wounds, bathing, giving medications—but the intellectual or thinking side of nursing is rarely portrayed. To be safe providers, nurses must carefully consider their actions. The angel of mercy and military stereotypes reinforce the idea that nursing is a duty and that nurses are carrying out orders. The naughty nurse, the battle-ax, and the handmaiden images suggest a woman who is prone to action but may not be carefully considering her actions.

In reality, a substantial portion of the nursing role involves thinking. Nursing requires careful thought about the patient, the treatment plan, the healthcare environment, the patient's support system, the nurse's support system and resources, and safety. Nurses use clinical judgment, critical thinking, and problem solving as they care for patients.

Clinical judgment involves observing, comparing, contrasting, and evaluating the client's condition to determine whether change has occurred. It also involves careful consideration of the client's health status in light of what is expected based on the client's condition, medications, and treatment. These actions, collectively known as assessment, are discussed in Chapters 3 and 19, and in each of the clinically focused chapters.

Critical thinking is a reflective thinking process that involves collecting information, analyzing the adequacy and accuracy of the information, and carefully considering options for action. Nurses use critical thinking in every aspect of nursing care. Critical thinking is discussed at length in Chapter 2 and applied in every chapter in this text.

Problem solving is a process by which nurses consider an issue and attempt to find a satisfactory solution. This process is used constantly in professional and personal life. The nursing process (see Chapters 2 through 7) is one type of problem-solving process.

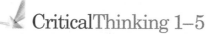

CriticalThinking 1–5

In the three scenarios of "Nurses Make a Difference: Then & Now," what image of nursing predominates?

CONTEMPORARY NURSING PRACTICE: EDUCATION, REGULATION, AND ORGANIZATION

As students about to enter a new field, you need to understand the reality of your chosen career. The remainder of this chapter discusses the current state of nursing, nursing education, and the trends affecting nursing.

How Is Nursing Defined?

As the preceding section shows, there are many images of nursing. These images are only loosely based on fact and sometimes conflict. They make it difficult to convey to the public the reality of nursing—and they are confusing to nurses and other members of the healthcare team as well. In addition, the constantly changing nature of nursing, health care, and society further complicate the definition of nursing. Therefore, it is important for nurses to articulate clearly, for themselves and for the public, what nursing is and what nurses do. The following are the views of three important nursing organizations on the question, "What is nursing?"

International Council of Nurses Definition

In 1973 the International Council of Nurses (ICN), an organization representing nurses throughout the world, defined nursing according to the beliefs of respected theorist Virginia Henderson:

> The unique function of the nurse is to assist the individual, sick or well, in the performance of those activities contributing to health or its recovery (or to peaceful death) that he would perform unaided if he had the necessary strength, will or knowledge. (Henderson, 1966, p. 15)

In the decades since the adoption of this definition, nursing throughout the world has changed. Advances in health care have altered the type of care required by clients. Nurses have taken on expanded roles, and once again there is renewed interest in providing care outside the hospital. To reflect these changes, the ICN has revised their definition of nursing. Currently, the ICN defines nursing as follows:

> Nursing encompasses autonomous and collaborative care of individuals of all ages, families, groups and communities, sick or well and in all settings. Nursing includes the promotion of health,

prevention of illness, and the care of ill, disabled and dying people. Advocacy, promotion of a safe environment, research, participation in shaping health policy and in patient and health systems management, and education are also key nursing roles. (ICN, 2003)

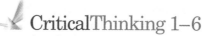

CriticalThinking 1–6

Look at the three scenarios of "Nurses Make a Difference: Then & Now." What nursing actions did the nurses perform that are represented in the ICN definition of nursing?

Nursing Association Definitions

Similar changes can be seen in the approach of the American Nurses Association (ANA) and the Canadian Nurses Association (CNA). In 1980, the ANA defined nursing as "the diagnosis and treatment of human responses to actual and potential health problems" (p. 2). Attempts to refine this definition have been fraught with difficulty. Nurses are a heterogeneous group of people with varying skills who perform activities designed to provide care ranging from basic to complex in a growing number of settings. It is very difficult to describe the boundaries of the profession. In 2003, the ANA acknowledged six essential features of professional nursing:

1. Provision of a caring relationship that facilitates health and healing;
2. Attention to the range of human experiences and responses to health and illness within the physical and social environments;
3. Integration of objective data with knowledge gained from an appreciation of the patient or group's subjective experience;
4. Application of scientific knowledge to the processes of diagnosis and treatment through the use of judgment and critical thinking;
5. Advancement of professional nursing knowledge through scholarly inquiry; and
6. Influence of social and public policy to promote social justice (p. 5).

As a result, the ANA redefined professional nursing as:

> The protection, promotion, and optimization of health and abilities, prevention of illness and injury, alleviation of suffering through the diagnosis and treatment of human response, and advocacy in the care of individuals, families, communities, and populations (ANA, 2004, p. 6).

In Canada a task force on the scope of practice stated:

> . . . [I]t will never be possible to define, precisely and in great detail, which activities are inside and which are outside the boundaries of nursing. This is partly because the 'state of the art' of healthcare and

BOX 1-1　What Is Nursing?

- I use the word nursing, for want of a better. It has been limited to signify little more than the administration of medicines and the application of poultices. It ought to signify the proper use of fresh air, light, warmth, cleanliness, quiet, and the proper choosing and giving of diet—all at the least expense of vital power to the patient (Nightingale, 1876, p. 5).

- Events that give rise to higher degrees of consideration for those who are helpless or oppressed, kindliness and sympathy for the unfortunate and for those who suffer, tolerance for those of differing religion, race, color, etc.—all tend to promote activities like nursing which are primarily humanitarian (Dock & Stewart, 1938, p. 3).

- Nursing has been called the oldest of the arts and the youngest of the professions. As such, it has gone through many stages and has been an integral part of societal movements. Nursing has been involved in the existing culture—shaped by it and yet helping to develop it. (Donahue, 1985, p. 3)

- Nurses provide care for people in the midst of health, pain, loss, fear, disfigurement, death, grieving, challenge, growth, birth, and transition on an intimate front-line basis. Expert nurses call this the privileged place of nursing (Benner & Wrubel, 1989, p. xi).

- Nursing　The care and nurturing of healthy and ill people, individually or in groups and communities (Venes & Thomas, *Taber's cyclopedic medical dictionary*, 2001).

nursing are changing so rapidly that such lists become outdated almost before they are completed, and partly because the field has become far too complex to be reduced to lists of tasks and procedures. As the nursing profession matures and the body of nursing knowledge expands, it will become easier to clearly describe the principles, models and functions that are the basis of nursing. (CNA, 1993, pp. 17–18)

You may wonder why there has been so much emphasis on creating a definition. Many organizations and leaders have pushed for accurate definitions to help the public understand the value of nursing, to describe what activities and roles belong to nursing versus other health professions, and to help students and practicing nurses understand what is expected of them. From our brief review of nursing history, you can see that nursing has undergone tremendous change, from the provision of mere kindness and support to full-spectrum work that is based in science but still focuses on care and nurturing. Undoubtedly nursing will continue to change as nursing knowledge increases and society changes. Box 1–1 lists several additional definitions of nursing for you to consider.

As a student entering nursing, you can use definitions and descriptions to understand what is expected of you. To aid you in this task, Table 1–3 reviews the essential components of the nursing role. While in the clinical setting, you will observe nurses functioning in each of these capacities. Nursing is a flexible career that requires you to move effortlessly between these areas to meet the needs of the patient.

KnowledgeCheck 1–1

- What factors make it difficult to define nursing?
- Based on the ICN definition of nursing, what does a nurse do?

 Go to Chapter 1, **Knowledge Check Response Sheet and Answers,** on the Electronic Study Guide.

Is Nursing a Profession, Discipline, or Occupation?

One strategy used to describe a field is to categorize it as a profession, discipline, or occupation. Although the term *profession* is freely used, a group must meet the following criteria to be considered a **profession** (Starr, 1982):

- The knowledge of the group must be based on technical and scientific knowledge.
- The knowledge and competence of members of the group must be evaluated by a community of peers.
- The group must have a service orientation and a code of ethics.

Nursing appears to meet all criteria of a profession as defined by Starr. Entry-level nursing education requires coursework in basic and social sciences as well as humanities, arts, and general education. Nursing education and practice are increasingly based on research from nursing and related fields. State or provincial regulatory bodies have defined the criteria that nurses must meet to practice, and they monitor members for adherence to standards. Nursing is clearly focused on providing service to others, and the major professional organizations have developed ethical guidelines to guide the practice of nursing.

Donaldson and Crowley (1978) define a **discipline** as "a unique perspective, a distinct way of viewing all phenomena, which ultimately defines the limits and nature of its inquiry" (p. 113). To be considered a discipline, a profession must have a domain of knowledge that has both theoretical and practical boundaries. The theoretical boundaries of a profession are the questions that arise from clinical practice and are then investigated through research. The practical boundaries are the current state of knowledge and research in the field (Meleis, 1991). This is the known, or the facts that dictate safe practice.

A case can be made that nursing is both a profession and a discipline. It is a scientifically based, self-governed

TABLE 1-3 Roles and Functions of the Nurse

Role	Function	Examples
Direct care provider	Addressing the physical, emotional, social, and spiritual needs of the client.	Assessing the client Giving medications Patient teaching
Communicator	Using interpersonal and therapeutic communication skills to address the needs of the client, to facilitate communication in the healthcare team, and to advise the community about health promotion and disease prevention.	Counseling a client Discussing unit staffing needs at a meeting Providing HIV education at a local school
Client/family educator	Assessing and diagnosing the teaching needs of the client, group, family, or community. Once the diagnosis is made, nurses plan how to meet these needs, implement the teaching plan, and evaluate its effectiveness.	Preoperative teaching Prenatal education for siblings Community classes on nutrition
Client advocate	Supporting clients' right to make healthcare decisions when they are able to voice their opinions and protecting clients from harm when they are unable to make decisions.	Helping a client explain to his family that he does not want to have further chemotherapy
Counselor	Counseling clients on health-related issues through the use of therapeutic communication skills.	Counseling a client on weight-loss strategies
Change agent	Advocating for change that enhances health. The nurse may use counseling, communication, and educator skills to accomplish this change. Change may be advocated on an individual, family, group, community, or societal level.	Working to improve the nutritional quality of the lunch program at a preschool
Leader	Inspiring others by setting an example of positive health, assertive communication, and willingness to improve	Florence Nightingale Walt Whitman Harriet Tubman
Manager	Coordinating and managing the activities of all members of the team.	Charge nurse on a hospital unit (e.g., assigns patients and work to staff nurses)
Case manager	Coordinating all care delivered to a client.	Coordinator of services for clients with tuberculosis
Research consumer	Incorporating research into practice to provide the most appropriate care, to identify clinical problems that warrant research, and to protect the rights of research subjects.	Reading journal articles Attending continuing education; seeking additional education

profession that focuses on the ethical care of others. It is also a discipline that is driven by theoretical and practical aspects, demanding thorough knowledge of its scientific basis and clinical skills. Put simply, nursing requires theoretical knowledge and practical skills.

In spite of meeting criteria for both designations (profession and discipline), nursing is often described as an occupation or job. Unlike physicians, most of whom are in control of their practice environment, working conditions, and schedule, most nurses are

hourly wage earners. The employer, not the nurse, decides the conditions of practice and the nature of the work. Nurse practice acts do not preclude nurses from functioning more autonomously, however. The following may improve the status of nursing:

- Standardizing the educational requirements for entry into practice
- Enacting uniform continuing education requirements
- Encouraging the participation of more nurses in professional organizations
- Educating the public about the true nature of nursing practice

 CriticalThinking 1–7

How do you evaluate the status of nursing? Is nursing a respected profession? Give examples to support your opinion.

How Do Nurses' Educational Paths Differ?

The transition into the nursing profession involves formal and informal processes. The formal process consists of completing the initial and continuing education required for licensure. The informal process involves a gradual progression in skill and clinical judgment that allows the nurse to advance in the profession.

Formal Education

When the patient calls out "Nurse!", who can respond? To legally use the title *nurse,* one must be a graduate of an accredited nursing education program and have successfully passed a licensure exam. Students may enter nursing through two portals: as a practical nurse or a registered nurse. Other personnel may respond to the patient's call, but they cannot legally be considered nurses.

Practical and Vocational Nursing Education

Practical nursing education prepares nurses to provide bedside care to clients. Practical nurses are known as licensed practical nurses (LPNs) or licensed vocational nurses (LVNs). In the United States a student who wishes to become an LPN/LVN may attend one of approximately 1100 approved programs given at technical schools and community colleges. Educational programs for LPN/LVNs offer both classroom and clinical teaching and usually last 1 year. After completing the practical nursing education program, the student must pass the NCLEX-PN exam. Practical nurses work under the direction of the registered nurse (RN) or the physician.

Registered Nursing Education

Currently, five educational pathways lead to licensure as a registered nurse (RN). Graduates of all these programs must successfully complete the NCLEX-RN exam to practice as an RN.

- *Diploma programs.* Until the 1960s, diploma programs were the mainstay of nursing education. These programs are usually given under the auspices of a hospital. The typical program lasts 3 years and focuses on clinical experience in direct patient care. Since the 1960s the number of diploma programs has steadily decreased. In the year 2000, a total of 1666 RN programs existed in the United States. Of those, only 86 were diploma programs.
- *Associate degree programs.* Most associate degree (AD) programs are centered in community colleges. Although the nursing component typically lasts 2 years, students are required to take numerous other courses in liberal arts and the sciences. Associate degree programs account for 53% of all RN programs in the United States. The student is prepared to provide direct patient care. Many AD graduates enter RN-to-BSN (or RN "completion") programs to obtain a baccalaureate degree in nursing. The length of time required to complete the BSN varies according to the program and to the number of credits each student can transfer.
- *Baccalaureate degree programs.* Students in baccalaureate programs pursue a course of study like that of other undergraduate students. The course of study lasts at least 8 semesters. Students are prepared to provide direct patient care, to work in community care, to use research, and to enter graduate education. Of the 1666 accredited RN programs, 695 programs prepare students at the baccalaureate level.
- *Master's entry programs.* These programs provide a specialized pathway into nursing. The typical student has a baccalaureate degree in another field and has entered nursing as a second career. Programs usually last 3 years. At the completion, the student is eligible to sit for the licensing exam and is awarded a master's degree in nursing.
- *Doctoral entry.* This is the most unusual entry pathway into nursing. The nursing doctorate (ND) path parallels the pathway through which physicians enter the healthcare field. This entry path has very limited enrollment.

For several decades, nursing leaders have debated about the most appropriate educational pathway for entry into the profession. For an overview of this debate,

 Go to Chapter 1, **Supplemental Materials: Entry into Practice Debate,** on the Electronic Study Guide.

Graduate Nursing Education

Graduate nursing education prepares the RN for advanced practice, expanded roles, or research. In master's

and doctoral education programs, coursework is concentrated in the nursing major.

Master's degree programs prepare RNs to function as advanced practice nurses (APNs), to teach, or to function in a more independent role. Programs typically last 2 or more years and are at the university level. For additional discussion on expanded nurse roles,

 Go to Chapter 1, **Expanded Career Roles,** on the Electronic Study Guide.

Doctoral programs in nursing offer professional degrees. Typically the student has completed a baccalaureate and master's degree prior to entry into a doctoral program. Degrees awarded are usually the DNS (doctor of nursing science) or PhD (doctor of philosophy). The DNS program prepares the nurse for advanced clinical practice. The PhD is a research degree.

Other Forms of Education

Advances in health care have a strong influence on nursing practice. To stay current after graduating, you must participate in ongoing education. **Continuing education** is a professional strategy to keep up with current clinical knowledge. Continuing education programs are available at the work site, at local colleges and universities, through privately run educational groups, on the Internet, and in professional journals. In 22 states, renewal of the nursing license requires successful completion of a specified number of continuing education courses. Some states allow nurses to take any approved coursework, while others have specific requirements in special areas such as HIV/AIDS and domestic violence. The rules regarding continuing education are rapidly changing. When you receive your initial license, you will be notified by your state board of registered nursing (BRN) about the current continuing education requirements, if any. Thereafter the BRN will notify you by mail of any changes in the requirements. For an overview of the continuing education requirements for license renewal in the United States,

 Go to Chapter 1, **Supplemental Materials: Expanded Career Roles,** on the Electronic Study Guide.

Another form of ongoing education is **in-service education.** These programs are offered at the work site. In-service education may focus on the use of new equipment or the introduction of new policies, or it may resemble traditional continuing education programs.

Informal Education

As you have learned, entry into the profession is accomplished by successful completion of an accredited nursing education program. Entry into practice also requires socialization into the profession. **Socialization** is the informal education that occurs as you move into your new profession. It is the knowledge gained from direct experience, observation in the real world, and informal discussion with peers and colleagues. This socialization begins when you enter the educational program and continues as you gather expertise. In essence, informal education complements formal education and creates clinical competence.

Patricia Benner (1984) described the process by which a nurse acquires clinical skill and judgment. As this process shows, expertise is not merely evidence of skilled application of knowledge, but rather a personal integration of knowledge that requires technical skill, thoughtful application, and insight. This is what we mean in this text when we use the term *full-spectrum nursing*. Expertise requires both thinking and doing skills.

Stage 1: Novice. This phase begins with the onset of education. The novice is receptive to education and is learning the rules.

Stage 2: Advanced beginner. After considerable exposure to clinical situations, nurses improve in performance and begin to recognize the elements of a situation. The result is progression to the advanced beginner stage. The nurse functioning at this level begins to use more facts and is more sophisticated with use of the rules. A new graduate usually functions at this level.

Stage 3: Competence. Nurses achieve competence after several years of practice. Competent performers have gained additional experience and wrestle with more complex concerns. They are able to handle their patient load and prioritize situations. They are also more involved in their caregiving role and may be emotionally involved in the clinical choices made.

Stage 4: Proficient. Proficient nurses are a resource for newer nurses. They are able to see the "big picture" and can coordinate services and forecast needs. They are much more flexible and fluent with their role. Proficient nurses plan intuitively as much as consciously.

Stage 5: Expert. Expert nurses are able to see what needs to be achieved and how to do it. They trust in and use their intuition. They have expert skills and are often consulted when others need advice or assistance.

Benner's model deals with the development of clinical wisdom. It is important to keep in mind that this progression is not automatic. Nurses do not simply move through the stages as they gain experience. Instead, this model assumes that, to improve in skill, nurses must not only gain experience but must also be attuned to the clinical situation. This requires an ability to take in information from a variety of sources

1-2 Nursing Values and Behaviors

- The nurse's primary concern is the good of the patient.
- Nurses need to be competent.
- Nurses demonstrate a strong commitment to service.
- Nurses illustrate a belief in the dignity and worth of each person.
- Nurses constantly strive to improve their profession.
- Nurses work collaboratively within the profession.

and to notice subtle variations. Although expertise is a goal, not everyone can achieve this level of skill.

The ANA and other organizations are also involved in helping nurses to continue to improve their practice (e.g., by setting standards and articulating nursing values). For example, in the Code for Nurses, the ANA provides guidelines for nurses to conduct themselves in their day-to-day practice. These guidelines describe behaviors and values that help improve practice and participation in the profession. See Chapter 44 for further discussion of the ANA Code for Nurses. Box 1–2 also presents values and behaviors associated with nursing.

How Is Nursing Practice Regulated?

Nurse practice acts are laws that regulate nursing practice. In the United States, each state enacts its own nurse practice act. In Canada, this is done on a provincial level. The state or provincial board of nursing is the agency responsible for regulating nursing practice. Although there are minor variations, each board of nursing is responsible for:

- Defining the practice of nursing
- Establishing criteria that allow a person to be considered a registered nurse (RN) or licensed practical or vocational nurse (LPN/LVN)
- Determining activities that are in the scope of practice of nursing and that nurses may perform (and by implication, those they may not); and those that may be performed only by licensed nurses
- Enforcing the rules that govern nursing

To practice nursing, an individual must be licensed as a nurse. Licenses are issued by the state. All states require attendance at an approved nursing program and successful completion of the National Council Licensure Exam (NCLEX). To receive licensure in another state, the nurse simply applies for reciprocity. For further details about licensing and the regulation of nursing practice, see Chapter 45.

Nursing is also governed by standards of practice. **Standards** "provide a means by which a profession clearly describes the focus of its activities, the recipients of service, and the responsibilities for which its practitioners are accountable" (ANA, 2004, p. vii). Standards are used by individual nurses, employers of nurses, professional organizations, and other professions.

As a student of nursing, you may use the ANA or CNA standards of nursing practice to get a better understanding of nursing. Practicing nurses use the standards to judge their own performance, develop an improvement plan, and understand what employers expect of them. Employers incorporate the standards into annual evaluation tools at hospitals and health facilities. Professional organizations use the standards to educate the public about nursing, to plan for continuing education programs for nurses, and to guide their efforts at lobbying and other activities that advocate for nurses. Finally, other professions read the standards of practice to examine the boundaries between nursing and other health professions. Table 1–4 presents the ANA standards, and Box 1–3 presents examples of provincial standards in Canada.

 CriticalThinking 1–8

What additional information have you learned about nursing from your review of the ANA and CNA standards of practice?

What Are Some Important Nursing Organizations?

Numerous organizations are involved in the profession of nursing. Some of the most influential are discussed here.

American and Canadian Nurses Associations

The American Nurses Association (ANA) and the Canadian Nurses Association (CNA) are the official professional organizations for registered nurses in their respective countries. Both of these organizations were formed in 1911 from an organization previously known as the Nurses' Associated Alumnae of the United States and Canada.

Originally these organizations focused on establishing standards of nursing to promote high-quality care and work toward licensure as a means of ensuring adherence to the standards. The ANA and CNA continue to update their standards. In addition, they are important representatives of nurses and nursing concerns in the political arena. As such, they track healthcare legislation, serve as a liaison with national government representatives to inform them of how current and proposed legislation will affect nursing, and develop and sponsor legislation that will have a positive effect on nursing and on patient care.

TABLE 1-4   American Nurses Association: Standards of Clinical Nursing Practice

Standards of Care

Standard 1	Assessment	The registered nurse collects comprehensive data pertinent to the patient's health or the situation.
Standard 2	Diagnosis	The registered nurse analyzes the assessment data to determine the diagnoses or issues.
Standard 3	Outcome Identification	The registered nurse identifies expected outcomes for a plan individualized to the patient or situation.
Standard 4	Planning	The registered nurse develops a plan that prescribes strategies and alternatives to attain expected outcomes.
Standard 5	Implementation	The registered nurse implements the identified plan.
Standard 5A	Coordination of Care	The registered nurse coordinates care delivery.
Standard 5B	Health Teaching and Health Promotion	The registered nurse employs strategies to promote health and a safe environment.
Standard 5C	Consultation	The advanced practice registered nurse and the nursing role specialist provide consultation to influence the identified plan, enhance the abilities of others, and effect change.
Standard 5D	Prescriptive Authority and Treatment	The advanced practice registered nurse uses prescriptive authority, procedures, referrals, treatments, and therapies in accordance with state and federal laws and regulations.
Standard 6	Evaluation	The registered nurse evaluates progress toward attainment of outcomes.

Standards of Professional Performance

Standard 7	Quality of Practice	The registered nurse systematically enhances the quality and effectiveness of nursing practice.
Standard 8	Education	The registered nurse attains knowledge and competency that reflects current nursing practice.
Standard 9	Professional Practice Evaluation	The registered nurse evaluates one's own nursing practice in relation to professional practice standards and guidelines, relevant statutes, rules, and regulations.
Standard 10	Collegiality	The registered nurse interacts with and contributes to the professional development of peers and colleagues.
Standard 11	Collaboration	The registered nurse collaborates with patient, family, and others in the conduct of nursing practice.
Standard 12	Ethics	The registered nurse integrates ethical provisions in all areas of practice.
Standard 13	Research	The registered nurse integrates research findings into practice.
Standard 14	Resource Utilization	The registered nurse considers factors related to safety, effectiveness, cost, and impact on practice in the planning and delivery of nursing services.
Standard 15	Leadership	The registered nurse provides leadership in the professional practice setting and the profession.

Source: American Nurses Association. (2004). *Standards of nursing practice.* Silver Spring, MD: Author.

BOX 1-3   Canadian Nurses Association Standards of Nursing Practice

CNA standards are set by the individual provinces and serve as the benchmark to evaluate professional practice.

- Professional service to the public. Nursing has a commitment to provide quality care to the public.
- Knowledge-based practice. Each nurse bases his/her practice on nursing science and the related humanities and sciences.
- Continuing competence. Each nurse is personally responsible for maintaining professional competence.
- Ethical practice. The nurse complies with the CNA Code of Ethics.
- Professional responsibilities and accountability. The nurse is personally responsible for ensuring his/her practice meets the standards of the profession and legislative requirements.

Sources: Summarized and adapted from Alberta Association of Registered Nurses. (1998). *Bylaws.* Edmonton, Alberta, Canada: Author; Canadian Nurses Association. (1987). *A definition of nursing practice. Standards for nursing practice.* Ottawa, Ontario, Canada: Author; Association for Registered Nurses in Newfoundland and Labrador. (2002). *Standards for nursing practice.* St. John's, Newfoundland, Canada: Author; College of Nurses of Ontario. (1996). *Professional standards for registered nurses and registered practical nurses in Ontario.* Toronto, Ontario, Canada: Author; Northwest Territories Registered Nurses Association. (1995). *Standards of practice for registered nurses.* Yellowknife, Northwest Territories, Canada: Author; Nurses Association of New Brunswick. (1998). *Standards for nursing practice.* Fredericton, New Brunswick, Canada: Author; Registered Nurses Association of British Columbia. (1998). *Standards for nursing practice in British Columbia.* Vancouver: Author; and Registered Nurses Association of Nova Scotia. (1996). *Standards for nursing practice.* Halifax, Nova Scotia, Canada: Author.

The ANA is composed of 54 state and territorial organizations. Individuals belong to state- or territory-level nursing organizations, and these belong to the ANA. The ANA has a national convention every 2 years. Representatives are elected from the local branches of the state organizations to bring their concerns to the national level. At the national office, an elected board of directors conducts the work of the organization with the assistance of paid staff. The ANA publishes many materials on nursing issues and standards and is also responsible for publication of the *American Journal of Nursing.*

The CNA is organized similarly. It is composed of a federation of provincial organizations with individual members participating at the provincial level. CNA activities are similar to those of the ANA; however, the CNA is also responsible for administering the nursing licensure exam in Canada (the state Boards of Nursing are responsible for this in the United States) and for publishing *Canadian Nurse.*

National League for Nursing

Originally founded as the American Society of Superintendents of Training Schools for Nurses in 1893, the National League for Nursing (NLN) was the first nursing organization with a goal to establish and maintain a universal standard of education. The NLN sets standards for all types of nursing education programs, evaluates nursing education programs, studies the nursing workforce, lobbies and participates with other major healthcare organizations to set policy for the nursing workforce, aids faculty development, and funds research on nursing education.

International Council of Nursing

The International Council of Nursing (ICN) is composed of a federation of national nursing organizations from over 120 nations. The ICN represents nursing on a global level. The organization aims to ensure quality nursing care for all, supports global health policies that advance nursing and improve worldwide health, and strives to improve working conditions for nurses throughout the world.

National Student Nurses Association

The National Student Nurses Association (NSNA) represents nursing students in the United States. It is the student counterpart of the ANA. The organizational structure and function parallel those of the ANA. The NSNA sponsors yearly conventions to address the concerns of nursing students and publishes *Image,* a journal dedicated to nursing student issues. Local chapters are usually organized at individual schools. In Canada, the Canadian University Student Nurses Association serves in the same capacity as the NSNA.

Sigma Theta Tau International

Sigma Theta Tau International (STTI) is the national honor society for nursing. Members are sought from the nursing community as well as from senior level baccalaureate and graduate programs. The goal of this organization is to foster nursing leadership and research.

Specialty Organizations

Numerous specialty organizations have developed around clinical specialties, group identification, or similarly held values. Here are some examples:

- *Clinical specialty.* Association of Operating Room Nurses (AORN); Association of Nurses in AIDS Care (ANAC); Hospice and Palliative Nurses Association (HPNA); Emergency Nurses Association (ENA); American Association of Women's Health, Obstetric and Neonatal Nurses (AWHONN)
- *Group identification.* National Association of Hispanic Nurses (NAHN), American Assembly for Men in Nursing (AAMN), National Black Nurses Association (NBNA)
- *Similar values.* Nurses Christian Fellowship (NCF), Nursing Ethics Network (NEN)

Web sites of a variety of nursing organizations are identified on your Electronic Study Guide.

 Go to Chapter 1, **List of Nursing Organizations,** on the Electronic Study Guide.

CONTEMPORARY NURSING PRACTICE: CARING FOR CLIENTS

Although a comprehensive definition of nursing is difficult to formulate, all definitions agree that nursing is about caring.

Who Are the Recipients of Nursing Care?

The ANA defines the recipients of nursing care as "individuals, groups, families, or communities. . . . The recipient(s) of nursing care can be referred to as patient(s), client(s), or person(s)" (ANA, 1995, p. 2). Nurses may work independently or with other healthcare providers to care for patients. **Direct care** involves personal interaction between the nurse and clients (e.g., giving medications, dressing a wound, or teaching a client about medicines or care). Nurses deliver **indirect care** when they work on behalf of an individual, group, family, or community to improve their health status (e.g., restocking the code blue cart [an emergency cart], ordering unit supplies, or arranging unit staffing). A nurse may use independent judgment to determine the care needed or may work under the direct order of a primary care provider.

What Are the Purposes of Nursing Care?

Nurses provide care to achieve the goals of health promotion, illness prevention, health restoration, and end-of-life care. Together these aspects of care represent a range of services that cover the spectrum from complete well-being to death.

Health Promotion

The World Health Organization defines **health** as "a state of complete physical, mental, and social well-being, and not merely the absence of disease or infirmity" (WHO, 1984). This inclusive definition can be applied to individuals, groups, families, or communities. **Health promotion** activities are any activities that foster the highest state of well-being of the recipient of the activities. For example, you might counsel a pregnant client about the importance of adequate prenatal nutrition to promote health at the individual level. Group and family-level health promotion activities might include teaching about nutrition during pregnancy in prenatal classes and in family education programs. On a community level your nursing activities would be focused on reaching a larger number of people. For example, you could advocate for prominent billboards highlighting the importance of prenatal care and nutrition, post signs in grocery stores recommending food sources for pregnant women, and lobby for labeling of substances that should be avoided in pregnancy.

Illness Prevention

Illness prevention focuses on avoidance of disease. Activities are targeted to decrease the risk of developing an illness or to minimize the risk of exposure to disease. To avoid disease, people must know the causes of disease and the route of disease transmission. For example, pneumonia causes many deaths every year. Those affected are society's most vulnerable: the very young, the very old, and the very ill. Some nursing activities to decrease the risk of pneumonia include:

- Teaching the importance of hand washing to decrease the transmission of infection
- Advocating for and administering pneumonia immunizations to those at high risk

Health Restoration

Health restoration encompasses activities that foster a return to health for those already ill. To restore health, the nurse provides direct care to ill individuals, groups, families, or communities. This aspect of care is what most people think of when they envision the nursing role. Recall that health has physical, mental, and social dimensions. When you engage in health-restoration activities, your care should address each of these dimensions. Health-restoration activities include the following:

- Providing hygiene and nutrition for someone unable to do so independently
- Assessing an ill client's health status
- Performing diagnostic tests on a client
- Administering medications or treatments

- Counseling individuals or groups
- Tracking clients with a communicable disease to ensure that they receive appropriate therapy
- Lobbying for community changes to decrease the prevalence of disease within a community

End-of-Life Care

Not all nursing activities can be directed toward promoting or restoring health, or preventing disease. Death is an inevitable consequence of life. Nurses have been active in promoting the respectful care of those who are terminally ill or dying. Nursing activities for the dying are designed to promote comfort, maintain quality of life, provide culturally relevant spiritual care, and ease the emotional burden of death. Nurses work with dying individuals, their family members and support persons, and with organizations that focus on the needs of the terminally ill.

KnowledgeCheck 1–2

Recall the last time that you had a cold. Identify health-promotion, illness-prevention, and health-restoration activities for individuals, families, groups, and communities in relation to the common cold.

 Go to Chapter 1, **Knowledge Check Response Sheet and Answers,** on the Electronic Study Guide.

Where Do Nurses Work?

As a nurse you will have the opportunity to work in a variety of settings. During your education you will be placed in many settings and clinical units that will allow you to see some of the possible options available to you upon graduation. Approximately 60% of nurses work in hospitals. The remaining 40% work in extended care facilities, ambulatory care, and community or home health settings.

Hospitals provide services to clients who require round-the-clock nursing care. This type of care is frequently referred to as *acute care*. Length of stay is limited to the amount of time that the client requires 24-hour observation.

Extended care facilities provide care for clients for an extended period of time—usually longer than 1 month. These facilities include skilled nursing facilities (SNF, also known as convalescent hospitals) and rehabilitation facilities. Clients may begin receiving care at these sites directly or may be transferred there for ongoing care after hospitalization.

Ambulatory care is synonymous with outpatient care. Clients reside at home or in non-hospital settings and come to the site for care. Ambulatory care sites include private health and medical offices, clinics, and outpatient therapy centers.

Home care is provided to clients who are homebound or unable to get themselves to ambulatory care centers for services. Services are usually coordinated by a home health or visiting nurse service and include nursing care as well as various therapies and home assistance programs. Home care services may also be employed when the client or family decides that home is the preferred site of care—particularly when the client is terminally ill. Home care is also appropriate when clients still requiring skilled care are discharged from the hospital because their reimbursable length-of-stay has expired.

| toward evidence-based practice |

Brush, B. L, & Capezuti, E. (2001). Historical analysis of siderail use in American hospitals. *Journal of Nursing Scholarship 33*(4), 381–385.

This study used social historical research methods to examine the pattern of siderail use, the value attached to siderails, and attitudes about raising siderails over time. Siderails on an adult bed were a rarity until the 1930s; continual watchfulness was employed to ensure safety. Siderails now have become a permanent fixture of the hospital bed. Initially their use was for temporary protection of confused patients; the siderails were appendages that had to be attached to the bed when it was judged that they would benefit the patient. However, litigation against hospitals and nurses for fall-related injuries began to appear in the 1930s. In addition, recurrent nurse shortages, and the move away from ward structure toward semi-private and private rooms promoted the use of siderails instead of nursing observation. Recent research has demonstrated that siderail-induced injuries may occur, especially entrapment, and that sustained bedrest has negative physical and emotional consequences. In spite of these recent research-based findings, ongoing siderail use remains the norm in promoting patient safety.

1. What trends and factors currently affecting nursing might influence whether siderail use changes in the near future?

2. What additional information would you like to know before advocating for a change in siderail use?

 Go to Chapter 1, **Toward Evidence-Based Practice Suggested Responses,** on the Electronic Study Guide.

Community health deals with provision of care for the community at large. Community health nurses provide services to at-risk populations and devise strategies to improve the health status of the surrounding community. Examples of community health programs include health care for the homeless and school-based programs designed to decrease the incidence of teen pregnancies. Community and home care are discussed separately in Chapters 42 and 43, respectively.

For an expanded discussion of these workplaces and services, as well as the organization and regulation of the healthcare delivery system in the United States (including quality assurance and quality improvement),

 Go to Chapter 1, **Supplemental Materials: The Healthcare Delivery System,** on the Electronic Study Guide.

 Go to Chapter 46, **Canadian Healthcare Delivery System,** on the Electronic Study Guide.

WHAT FACTORS INFLUENCE CONTEMPORARY NURSING PRACTICE?

Two types of factors influence contemporary nursing practice: those in society at large and outside the profession, and those within nursing and health care.

Trends in Society

As you have seen, our historical roots strongly influence current nursing practice and will inevitably continue to influence its future development. In addition, nursing is currently influenced by trends in the economy, increased consumer knowledge, legislation, the women's movement, and collective bargaining:

- *The national economy* has a tremendous impact on nursing. In every country except the United States, health care is provided as a right of citizenship. In the United States, health insurance coverage is linked to full-time employment in large companies with health insurance benefits. Thus, as unemployment figures rise, the number of people without insurance escalates. Fearing the high costs of medicines and health care, many uninsured people delay seeking needed care. The effect is that clients are often sicker when they enter the healthcare system. This taxes the system's resources and raises the level of nursing care required. Another consideration is that the healthcare industry—even in a strong economy—is very expensive to operate. Downturns in the economy affect institutional investments and profits, and may limit medications and services available. Similarly, the salaries of healthcare providers are influenced by national economic trends.

- *The role of the healthcare consumer* also affects nursing. Historically, patients relied on the knowledge and decision making of the healthcare team. Now, however, consumers are demanding greater choice in the decisions that affect their health.

  Patients have access to vast amounts of health and medical information, particularly through the Internet. Web sites such as WebMD and PubMed, and online medical and health journals give consumers accurate and up-to-date health information. This access has allowed consumers to be active participants in discussions about their health problems and therapy options.

  Direct-to-consumer marketing is another form of health information, in which companies advertise medicines and therapies directed at the potential user. Advertisements appear in magazines, on television, on billboards, and in the newspaper. Pharmaceutical companies rely heavily on this advertising to generate interest in new therapies. Clients may make direct requests for therapies they have heard about in the media. Nurses need to be prepared to address the truthfulness of the advertisements and to present balanced information to clients.

- *Consumer interest has also generated legislation* that affects nursing care. Legislation directed at patients' rights (Patients' Bill of Rights), the patient's right to know (informed consent), and the patient's right to a dignified death (living will/advanced directives) all govern the care that nurses render to patients. These acts are further discussed in Chapters 44 and 45.

- *The women's movement* has also influenced the nursing profession and those considering a career in nursing. Historically, women were allowed to practice nursing only while they remained single. As the women's movement gained momentum, women began to enjoy more equitable treatment and were no longer forced out of nursing if they chose to have a family. However, the women's movement also opened up more career choices for women, and nursing has become just one of many options as opposed to a preferred career pathway. Also, as you have seen, societal views of nursing as a women's profession affect men's entry into nursing.

- *Collective bargaining* is a form of negotiating that allows nurses to seek better wages and working conditions as a group rather than individually. A union or organization that represents the nurses usually conducts collective bargaining. Collective bargaining has resulted in major improvements in wages, benefits, and working conditions for nurses. These improvements have made nursing more attractive as a career choice. Not all states have collective bargaining groups for nurses.

Trends in Nursing and Health Care

Many trends in nursing and health care also affect contemporary practice. We discuss the most significant of these trends here.

Increased Use of Complementary and Alternative Medicine

The National Institutes of Health define healthcare treatments or services outside the traditional healthcare system as **complementary and alternative medicine (CAM).** They include medical systems, such as homeopathy, naturopathy, chiropractic, and traditional Chinese medicine, as well as specific treatments, such as herbal medications, dietary changes, massage therapy, yoga, aromatherapy, prayer, and hypnotism. See Chapter 40. Many of these therapies have evolved alongside traditional health care. For example, many powerful drugs are derived from herbs, and conventional physicians have always prescribed dietary remedies for certain ailments. The following factors have contributed to this interest in CAM:

- Rising costs of traditional care, including prohibitive insurance costs.
- Widespread reporting of treatment errors in the media. Some people are now uncertain about the validity of traditional health care.
- Growing distrust of the role of insurance and managed care organizations in determining treatment options.
- Ever-changing health recommendations over the last 20 years. For example, there have been numerous studies to examine the pros and cons of hormone replacement therapy for post-menopausal women.
- Increasing cultural diversity of the population, and the accompanying exchange of information about therapies from different cultural traditions.
- Creation of the National Center for Complementary and Alternative Medicine at the National Institutes of Health. This recognition has given CAM a legitimacy it formerly lacked.

Expanded Variety of Settings for Care

Over 40% of nurses now work outside the hospital setting, as compared to 20% in 1980 (Jonas & Kovner, 2002). This trend toward increased diversification in practice sites is expected to continue. As the site of employment shifts away from the hospital, nurses must be prepared to function in these alternative settings. This change requires entry-level education programs to prepare nurses for this type of work (Wilkinson, 1996). For those already in the field, it may require retooling to deal with this change. In the hospital, nurses have access to support personnel, consultation with other nurses and healthcare providers, ready access to equipment and diagnostic testing services, and increased access to the patient. As more care is delivered in outpatient, community, or home settings, nurses must be prepared to function more autonomously and creatively. Nurses must adapt care to the equipment available at the site, and they must rely heavily on the skills of patients and family members to detect change and report the need for additional services.

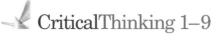

CriticalThinking 1–9

What is your nursing program doing to prepare you to work outside the hospital setting?

Increased Autonomy and Advanced Practice Roles

The growing role of nursing outside the hospital, the increasing complexity of care, the limited supply of nurses, and the increased use of technology have changed nursing from a largely supportive role to one of increasing responsibility. In addition, the increased use of advanced practice nurses (APNs) has resulted in greater public exposure for nurses. Professional and public reports demonstrate high patient satisfaction with APNs. Studies have also shown comparable, and at times superior, patient outcomes over physician-provided care (e.g., better understanding of and compliance with treatment regimen, and fewer hospitalizations). This positive exposure has resulted in increased acceptance and support for all nurses.

Increased Use of Unlicensed Assistive Personnel

Unlicensed assistive personnel (UAP) are healthcare providers who help nurses and physicians provide patient care. Common UAP roles include nurse aide, assistant, orderly, and technician. UAPs may perform simple nursing tasks (e.g., bathing, taking temperatures, or making beds) under the direction of the licensed nurse. This redistribution of workload has prompted much controversy.

Although it may seem appropriate to allow the UAP to assume the simple tasks, this change distances the licensed nurse from many aspects of direct patient care. The nurse retains ultimate responsibility for the patient yet may have to base important patient care decisions on information obtained by someone else. Unfortunately many nurses now in practice were never taught in their formal nursing programs about delegation and supervision. This can create problems on nursing units, because some nurses are uncertain about what can safely and legally be delegated and how much responsibility they retain. To remedy this problem, many schools are now adding coursework on delegation to their curricula, and textbooks such as this one are including information about delegation.

As you progress through your program, you will notice that nurses often gather different information from a client encounter than someone without nursing experience. For example, a nursing aide may provide a bedbath to an elderly client. The aide will be able to tell the RN that there are no open areas on the skin. However, a nurse performing the same task would be able to do an extensive client assessment while giving the bath. The nurse would be able to comment on the client's level of cognition (orientation to surroundings and self), the client's tolerance for activity, breath sounds, heart sounds, bowel sounds, and the condition of the skin. The nurse might use the time during the bath to educate the client about his condition or to gather information about the client's home and support system that can be used for discharge planning.

Influence of Nurses on Healthcare Policy

Professional nursing organizations have been actively involved in politics at the local, state, and national levels. Each of the major professional organizations actively lobbies and educates elected and appointed officials about the role nursing plays in health care. Nursing organizations sponsor legislation that promotes the interest of the profession and supports changes that positively influence health outcomes. Nurse-sponsored legislation has addressed safe staffing in hospitals, needle-exchange programs to decrease the transmission of HIV, and funding to increase nursing enrollment during times of nursing shortages.

As individuals, nurses should vote, lobby their elected representatives, and run for political office. Together, nurses represent the largest health professional group; as a voting block, they have strong political power. Many nurses have also promoted nursing by organizing local nursing groups to support candidates or legislation, or by speaking out in the community on health and nursing issues. Nurses are typically trusted and respected political candidates, running successful campaigns at the local, state, and national level. You should consider all of these political activities as you move into the profession.

Divergence Between High-Tech and High-Touch

Recent advances in healthcare technology have prolonged the lives of patients who are critically ill, such as premature newborns and elderly patients with advanced cardiovascular, pulmonary, or renal disease. The increasing use of this technology has led to numerous legal and ethical dilemmas, particularly about end-of-life care. This trend is in sharp contrast to the concurrent trend toward holism and high-touch therapies, which often avoid technology. One of the biggest challenges in health care is integrating these two divergent trends. For an excellent discussion on these colliding values, read *Holistic Health and Healing* by Mary Anne Bright (2002).

 Go to Chapter 1, **Resources for Caregivers and Health Professionals,** on the Electronic Study Guide.

 Suggested Readings: Go to Chapter 1, **Reading More About the Evolution of Nursing Thought & Action,** on the Electronic Study Guide.

 Bibliography: Go to Volume 2, Bibliography.

CHAPTER 2

Critical Thinking
& the Nursing Process

Learning Outcomes

After completing this chapter, you should be able to:

✺ Give one definition and one example of critical thinking.

✺ List at least six critical-thinking skills and attitudes.

✺ Explain ways in which nurses use critical thinking.

✺ List the six overlapping and interdependent phases of the nursing process.

✺ Describe what the nurse is doing in each phase of the nursing process.

✺ Explain how critical thinking is used in the nursing process.

✺ Discuss, and give examples of, the difference between practical/procedural knowledge and theoretical knowledge.

✺ Name the main concepts of the full-spectrum nursing model.

✺ Explain how nursing knowledge, nursing process, and critical thinking work together in full-spectrum nursing.

Your Nursing Role

It's a pleasant Saturday afternoon, and you're meeting with an old friend that you haven't seen in 2 years. She asks, "I hear you've decided to be a nurse. What made you choose that?"

CriticalThinking 2–1

How would you reply to her question?

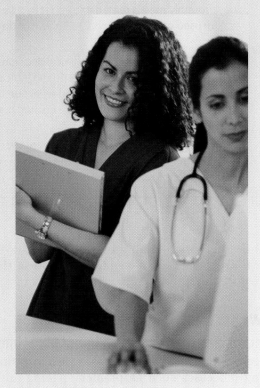

She listens to your answer with interest. "I don't think I could do that. I couldn't be around people who are sick and in pain. Hospitals are such sad places.'" To respond to this statement, you will need to consider your motivation for entering nursing and your beliefs about the profession.

CriticalThinking 2–2

- What factors or persons influenced your decision to be a nurse?
- Have others asked you why you chose to become a nurse? How have the reactions you received before colored your explanation of your career choice?
- What makes this situation similar to or different from your prior experiences?
- What's important in this situation?
- Of the possible answers you are considering, which answer best reflects your true feelings about your career choice? Why are the other answers not appropriate?
- What beliefs and assumptions are coloring your response?

If you are able to answer these questions, then you have used critical thinking to guide your decision making. Critical thinking involves careful consideration of a situation to arrive at a solution, based on analysis of the data. Critical thinking is vital when considering important decisions. This is the kind of thinking you will use as a nurse.

WHAT IS YOUR VIEW OF NURSING?

Chapter 1 introduced you to the roles and responsibilities of nurses, activities that nurses engage in, and the career of nursing. Throughout this text, you will learn much more. Thus, your view of nursing may change as you progress in your studies. To track your progress, establish a baseline by examining your current view of nursing.

CriticalThinking 2–3

What is your image of nursing? List at least five attributes a nurse should have, and at least five responsibilities that you consider to be a part of nursing.

In this exercise, when you listed some nursing responsibilities, you may have mentioned activities such as, "gives medications," or "performs tests and treatments." And you were correct—partially. A big

part of nursing is about *doing*. Nursing is activity oriented. However, now more than ever, the emphasis is on *thinking*. So, another way to describe nursing is to say that *nursing involves both thinking and doing*.

The scientific basis for providing health care changes daily. Research is constantly uncovering new information that changes the practice of all healthcare providers. Therefore, you should know up front that you cannot possibly learn everything about health care and nursing in nursing school. In fact, to be a safe and competent nurse you will need to constantly update your knowledge and skills. To aid your lifelong learning, you will need to develop and refine your critical-thinking skills. Critical thinking helps you to know what is important about each patient's situation, when you need more information, and when you need help to make the best decision.

Theoretical Knowledge
knowing why

WHAT IS CRITICAL THINKING?

If critical thinking is so important, then you might be wondering, what exactly is it? One humorous definition is that critical thinking is "the art of thinking about your thinking while you are thinking in order to make your thinking better: more clear, more accurate, or more defensible" (Paul, 1988). Upon closer study, this definition makes an important point. It tells us that we should reflect on the thinking process we are using to figure something out: "Why did I ask those particular questions? Do I have enough information to decide, or have I jumped to a conclusion? Have I considered all the possibilities?"

Box 2–1 provides several definitions of critical thinking, or you may want to use the following definition:

> **Critical thinking** is a combination of reasoned thinking, openness to alternatives, an ability to reflect, and a desire to seek truth.

There are many definitions of critical thinking because it is a complex concept and people think about it in different ways—none of them "wrong." In fact, any situation that requires critical thinking is likely to have more than one "right" answer. You do not need critical thinking to add 2 + 2 and come up with the answer. However, you do need critical thinking to "problem-solve" important decisions.

Critical thinkers are flexible, nonjudgmental, inquisitive, honest, and interested in seeking the truth. They possess intellectual skills that allow them to use

---

BOX 2–1 Some Definitions of Critical Thinking

- Critical thinking is the disciplined, intellectual process of applying skillful reasoning as a guide to belief or action (Paul, Ennis & Norris, 1996).
- Critical thinking is careful and deliberate determination of whether to accept, reject, or suspend judgment (Moore & Parker, 2001).
- Critical thinking is a dynamic, purposeful, analytic process that results in reasoned decisions and judgments (Assessment Technologies Incorporated, 1998).
- Critical thinking, as the term is generally used these days, roughly means reasonable and reflective thinking focused on deciding what to believe or do (Ennis, 2000).
- In nursing, critical thinking for clinical decision-making is the ability to think in a systematic and logical manner with openness to question and reflect on the reasoning process used to ensure safe nursing practice and quality care (Heaslip, 1992).
- Critical thinking is disciplined, self-directed, rational thinking that supports what we know and makes clear what we don't know (Wilkinson, 2001, p. 36).

---

their curiosity to their advantage, and they have critical attitudes that motivate them to use those skills responsibly.

What Are Critical-Thinking Skills?

Skills in critical thinking refer to the cognitive (intellectual) activities and processes used in complex thinking processes such as problem solving and decision making. In this example, the skills are italicized, and the complex thinking process is in bold type:

> When planning nursing care, nurses *gather information* about the client and then **draw tentative conclusions about the meaning of the information** *to identify the client's problems*. Then they *think of several different actions* they might take to help **solve or relieve the problem.**

The following are a few examples of critical-thinking skills:

- Objectively gathering information on a problem or issue
- Recognizing the need for more information
- Recognizing gaps in one's own knowledge
- Listening carefully, reading thoughtfully

- Separating relevant from irrelevant data; important from unimportant data
- Organizing or grouping information in meaningful ways
- Making inferences (tentative conclusions) about the meaning of the information
- Integrating new information with prior knowledge
- Visualizing potential solutions to a problem
- Objectively evaluating the likelihood that each potential solution will work
- Exploring the advantages, disadvantages, and consequences of each potential action
- Evaluating the credibility and usefulness of sources of information

What Are Critical-Thinking Attitudes?

Attitudes are not the same as intellectual skills. They are more like feelings and traits of mind. Your attitudes and character determine whether you will use your thinking skills fairly and with an open mind. Without a critical attitude, people tend to use thinking skills to justify narrow-mindedness and prejudice, and to benefit themselves rather than others. The following are some critical-thinking attitudes (Paul, 1990):

- **Independent thinking.** Critical thinkers do not believe everything they are told; they do not just go along with the crowd. They listen to what others think and they learn from new ideas. They do not accept or reject an idea before they understand it. Nurses should challenge actions and policies that have no logical support.
- **Intellectual curiosity.** Critical thinkers love to learn new things. They are always curious and frequently think or ask, "What if . . . ," "How could we do this differently," and "How does this work?"
- **Intellectual humility.** Critical thinkers are aware that they do not know everything, and they are not embarrassed to ask for help when they don't know. They re-evaluate their conclusions or chosen course of action in light of new information and are willing to admit when they are wrong.
- **Intellectual empathy.** Critical thinkers try to understand the feelings and perceptions of others. They try to see a situation as the other person sees it.
- **Intellectual courage.** Critical thinkers consider and examine fairly their own values and beliefs, as well as beliefs of others, even when this is uncomfortable. They are willing to rethink, and even reject, previously held beliefs that are not well justified. Without intellectual courage, people become resistant to change.
- **Intellectual perseverance.** Critical thinkers don't settle for the quick, obvious answer. They do not jump to conclusions. Important questions are usually complex, and critical thinkers are willing to give them serious thought and research, even when this takes a great deal of effort and time.
- **Fair-mindedness.** Critical thinkers try to make impartial judgments. They treat all viewpoints fairly, realizing that personal biases, customs, and social pressures can influence their thinking. They examine their own biases each time they make a decision.

Critical thinking can be used in all aspects of your life. Any time you are trying to reach an important decision, reasoned action (critical thinking) is called for. Everyday uses of critical thinking might include deciding where you should live, choosing which nursing programs you should apply to, and deciding between several job offers. The rest of this chapter shows you why critical thinking is important to you in your chosen career, nursing.

Knowledge Check 2–1
- Define *critical thinking* in your own words.
- List five skills or attitudes that reflect critical thinking.

 Go to Chapter 2, **Knowledge Check Response Sheet and Answers,** on the Electronic Study Guide.

WHY IS CRITICAL THINKING IMPORTANT FOR NURSES?

Nurses use complex critical-thinking processes (e.g., problem solving, decision making, and clinical reasoning) in every aspect of their work (Table 2–1). Nurses constantly assess their patients and determine how they are responding to nursing interventions and medical treatments. Because nurses care for a variety of patients with a multitude of concerns, the patients' response to therapy may not always be apparent. Reasoning and reflection are required for the nurse to decide what interventions to use, determine whether they worked, and, if not, figure out why.

Nurses Deal with Complex Situations

Critical thinking is important for nurses because they deal with complex situations daily. One such situation is that of caring for clients with **comorbidities** (concurrently occurring health problems). These greatly influence client responses. For example, if a healthy 9-year-old fell and broke his right arm, he would experience pain and discomfort. However, with proper casting and time to heal, the child would recover. While recovering, he may have to eat using

TABLE 2-1   Complex Thinking Processes

Problem solving	Identifying a problem and finding reasonable solutions to it. Requires critical-thinking skills such as organizing data, identifying relevant and important data, making inferences, making decisions, projecting consequences of actions, and applying theoretical knowledge to a specific patient context. The nursing process is a problem-solving process.
Decision making	Choosing the best action to take. In nursing, this is usually the action likely to produce the desired patient outcome. Requires thinking skills such as making judgments (e.g., about what is important) and making choices. Important in problem solving; however, many decisions are made that are not related to problem solving.
Clinical reasoning	Reflective, concurrent, creative thinking about patients and patient care. Clinical reasoning is used in the nursing process. Reasoning is logical thinking that links thoughts together to create meaning.

his left hand or limit the use of his injured arm. However, the adjustments would be quite different for an older adult who has had a stroke (a comorbidity) that limits the use of his left arm. With decreased function in the left arm, a right-arm fracture would severely affect an older person's ability to care for himself. The 9-year-old child would likely be discharged home from the emergency department or clinic in the care of his parents or guardians. The nurse's primary interventions would be to teach parents the home care needed by the child. However, the nurse caring for the older adult would need to evaluate whether the client requires care in the hospital or in a skilled-care facility and what support services the client will need as he convalesces. In the inpatient setting, nursing interventions might initially include assisting the client with eating, bathing, and toileting.

Clients Are Unique

Critical thinking is important also because each client is unique. Their *individual differences* (e.g., type of illness, culture, and age) make it impossible to provide strict rules for all client care. Research-based care plans and protocols identify guidelines for providing care; however, nurses must evaluate and modify these guidelines to be sure they are appropriate for each client.

Consider the following example: You have undoubtedly been told to drink plenty of fluid when you have a cough. Staying well hydrated keeps the secretions moist so that you can cough them up. Now imagine yourself at work as a nurse. You are caring for a client in renal failure. Your client no longer urinates and is being considered for dialysis. You notice that this client has a persistent cough. Should you encourage this client to drink as much fluid as possible? Do you see how you could cause harm to a client by unthinkingly doing as you have been told? Nurses must always think, "How will that work in *this* instance?" "How is this like or different from similar situations?"

Culture is another thing that makes a client unique. Nurses must think critically to give culturally sensitive care. Ethnic and cultural differences affect the client's and family's view of health and the healthcare system, as well as their responses to health problems. Cultural beliefs strongly influence how people define sickness, at what point they seek healthcare services, what type of healthcare provider they see, and the type of treatment they consider acceptable. The excellent nurse is adept at assessing the client's and family's cultural beliefs and adapting care so that it is responsive to their needs.

A client's *role* also influences when, how, and why a person seeks health care. A single mother with young children may ask to be discharged from the hospital early to meet the needs of her family. Clients with extensive support from family or friends may be willing to take more time to convalesce when they are ill. Nurses take these things into consideration, for example, when determining why a nursing intervention was (or was not) successful.

Other factors may influence how a person responds to illness or to healthcare intervention:

- *Age.* Each of us was raised with a set of beliefs and knowledge that were strongly influenced by the prevailing views of our times.
- *Personal bias.* Clients may have set beliefs about health and illness.
- *Previous experience* with healthcare problems. For example, a boy who has experienced a painful injection in the past may be terrified when he sees the nurse approach with a syringe.

Nurses Apply Knowledge to Provide Holistic Care

In addition to the need to individualize care for each patient, there are some things about nursing itself that require the nurse to be a critical thinker.

- *Nursing is an applied discipline.* This means that nurses must *apply* their knowledge, not just memorize

and regurgitate facts. Nurses deal with complex, ill-defined, and sometimes confusing problems—not well-defined ones such as you find in a math book.

- *Nursing uses knowledge from other fields.* Nurses use information from chemistry, physiology, psychology, social sciences, and other disciplines to identify and plan interventions for patient problems.

- *Nursing is fast-paced.* Nurses deal with situations that may be hectic. A patient's condition may change hour to hour or even minute to minute, so "knowing the routine" may not be adequate. Critical thinking is essential to respond appropriately under stress.

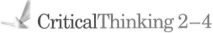 CriticalThinking 2–4

Write a short scenario (story) about a nurse that illustrates one of the reasons why nurses need to be critical thinkers.

WHAT ARE THE DIFFERENT KINDS OF NURSING KNOWLEDGE?

Critical thinking does not occur in a vacuum—one must have something to think about and with: one's knowledge base. Nurses use various kinds of knowledge: theoretical, practical, personal, and ethical. Every chapter of this text is designed to help you gain practical knowledge and theoretical knowledge. Put very simply, that is "knowing what" (to do) and "knowing why" (to do it). In fact, the chapters are organized according to those two types of knowledge.

Each chapter begins by presenting theoretical knowledge. **Theoretical knowledge** consists of information, facts, principles, and theories in nursing and related disciplines (e.g., anatomy and psychology). This kind of knowledge consists of research findings and rationally constructed explanations of phenomena. You will use it to describe your patients, explain their health status, provide your reasoning for choosing interventions, and predict patient responses to interventions and treatments.

Each chapter then provides the practical knowledge that enables you to apply your theoretical knowledge to caring for patients. **Practical knowledge**—knowing what to do and how to do it—consists of processes (e.g., the decision process and the nursing process) and procedures (e.g., how to give an injection).

In addition to theoretical and practical knowledge, nurses use **personal knowledge;** that is, self-understanding. To think critically, you must be aware of your beliefs, your values, your cultural and religious biases, and so on. This kind of knowledge helps you to find errors in your thinking and enables you to

"tune in" to your patients. You can gain this knowledge by developing self-awareness—by reflecting (asking yourself), "Why did I do that?" or "How did I come to think that?"

Finally, nurses use **ethical knowledge;** that is, knowledge of obligation, or right and wrong. Ethical knowledge consists of information about moral principles and processes for making moral decisions. It helps you to fulfill your ethical obligations to patients and colleagues. Chapter 44 will add to your ethical knowledge.

A MODEL FOR CRITICAL THINKING

A **model** is a set of interrelated concepts that represent a particular way of thinking about something—much in the same way that the shape of a lens affects what you see. For example, you would look through a telescope to view a distant star. Looking at the star through reading glasses or a magnifying glass would give a different view. The critical thinking model used throughout this book provides one way of looking at critical thinking. This model organizes critical thinking into five major categories. Table 2–2 defines each category and provides questions to help you focus your thinking in patient care situations. You can use some of the questions when deciding what to think and do; you can use others when analyzing a situation after it happens (reflecting). Figure 2–1 is a simpler representation of the model, relating it to the nursing process, which is introduced on page 31.

This model is not meant to be all-inclusive; there is much more to critical thinking than just the questions listed in Table 2–2. It is intended to be a guide when you are faced with clinical decisions or unfamiliar situations. The questions can help you to "think about your thinking" as you apply principles and knowledge from myriad sources to a current problem. This should help you to achieve good outcomes for your patients. You do not need to ask yourself every question in every situation—just those that are relevant. And you do not proceed from top to bottom in the table. The processes do not occur "sequentially," so you may jump back and forth between them.

Let's apply the model to a situation faced by all nursing students. In a short while you will begin your clinical rotations, if you have not already done so. Many students find clinical rotations exciting, yet somewhat frightening. How could you use the five points of the critical-thinking star to approach your first clinical day so that you will be well prepared and able to function safely?

One of the first things you need to consider is your usual response to new experiences. How do you react

TABLE 2–2 Critical-Thinking Model

Process	Definition	Questions for Focusing
Contextual awareness (deciding what to observe and consider)	This includes an awareness of what's happening in the context of the situation, including values, cultural issues, and environmental influences.	• What is going on in the situation that may influence the outcome? • What factors may influence my behavior and others' behavior in this situation? • What about this situation have I seen before? What is different? • Who should be involved in order to improve the outcome? • What else was happening at the same time that affected me in this situation? • What happened just before this incident that made a difference? • What emotional responses influenced how I reacted in this situation? • What changes in behavior alerted me that something was wrong?
Inquiry (based on credible sources)	This involves applying standards of good reasoning to your thinking when analyzing a situation and evaluating your actions.	• How do I go about getting the information I need? • What framework should I use to organize my information? • Do I have enough knowledge to decide? If not, what do I need to know? • Have I used a valid, reliable source of information (e.g., patient, other professionals, references)? • Did I (do I need to) validate the data (e.g., with the client)? • What else do I need to know? What information is missing? • Are the data accurate? Precise? • What's important and what's not important in this situation? • Did I consider professional, ethical, and legal standards? • Have I jumped to conclusions?
Considering alternatives	This involves exploring and imagining as many alternatives as you can think of for the given situation.	• What is one possible explanation for [insert what is happening or what happened]? • What are other explanations for what is happening? • What is one thing I could do in this situation? • What are two more possibilities/alternatives? • Are there others who might help me develop more alternatives? • Of the possible actions I am considering, which one is most reasonable? Why are the others not as reasonable? • Of the possible actions I am considering, which one is most likely to achieve the desired outcomes?
Analyzing assumptions	This involves recognizing and analyzing assumptions you are making about the situation, and examining the beliefs that underlie your choices.	• What have I (or others) taken for granted in this situation? • Which beliefs/values are shaping my assumptions? • What assumptions contributed to the problem in this situation? • What rationale supports my assumptions? • How will I know my assumption is correct? • What biases do I have that may affect my thinking and my decisions in this situation?
Reflecting skeptically and deciding what to do	This involves questioning, analyzing, and reflecting on the rationale for your decisions.	• What aspects of this situation require the most careful attention? • What else might work in this situation? • Am I sure of my interpretation in this situation? • Why is (was) it important to intervene? • What rationale do I have for my decisions? • In priority order, what should I do in this situation and why? • Having decided what was wrong/happening, what is the best response? • What might I delegate in this situation? • What got me started taking some action? • What priorities were missed? • What was done? Why was it done? • What would I do differently after reflecting on this situation?

Sources: Model based on Brookfield, S. D. (1991). *Developing critical thinkers.* San Francisco: Jossey-Bass; McDonald, M. E. (2002). *Systematic assessment of learning outcomes: Developing multiple-choice exams.* Boston: Jones and Bartlett Publishers; Paul, R. W. (1993). *Critical thinking: What every person needs to survive in a rapidly changing world* (3rd ed.). Santa Rosa, CA: Foundation for Critical Thinking; Raingruber, B. & Haffer, A. (2001). *Using your head to land on your feet.* Philadelphia: F. A. Davis Company; and Wilkinson, J. M. (2001). *Nursing process and critical thinking* (3rd ed.). Upper Saddle River, NJ: Prentice Hall.

to change? What other tasks or assignments do you have that will dictate the timing of your preparation? Have you had any previous experiences that will aid or hamper you in your preparation? As you consider these questions, you are addressing **contextual awareness.**

You need to gather information about the clinical experience. It is important to use **inquiry based on credible sources** as you gather data. For example, you may want to ask your instructor for guidance on how to prepare. You may also wish to consult a student who has successfully completed the same course. If you have been assigned to provide care for a client, you need to gather accurate information about the client. You could use the client's chart and your textbooks to prepare. You should use only knowledgeable, reliable sources of information—for example, you should get your information from nursing texts and nursing journals, not lay (nonprofessional) magazines such as *Readers Digest* or *Ladies Home Journal*. After you have more information, you should go back and analyze your response to the situation. You may find that you are feeling less anxious already! All of this is a part of inquiry.

Now that you know something about the clinical experience, you can plan your day. You need to **consider alternatives** and **analyze your assumptions** about the experience. What is expected of you? What do you expect from the experience? How should you approach your client? How will you introduce yourself? What skills do you have? How will you apply them to caring for your client?

After you feel that you have addressed these concerns, you need to quickly review your preparation **(reflective skepticism).** Have you gathered enough information to feel comfortable in the situation? Have you left anything out? Do you need more information?

This was a demonstration of how you might apply the critical thinking model to a real experience. In this example you also used theoretical, practical, personal, and ethical knowledge.

KnowledgeCheck 2–2

In the preceding example, identify the actions that demonstrate use of each of the four types of knowledge.

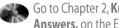 Go to Chapter 2, **Knowledge Check Response Sheet and Answers,** on the Electronic Study Guide.

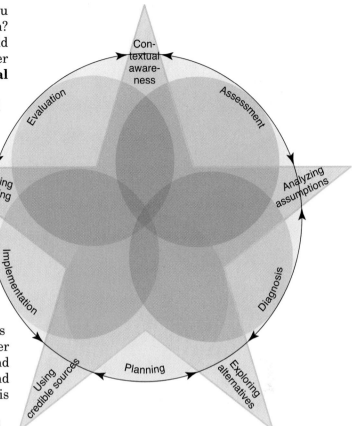

FIGURE 2–1   Model of critical thinking and the nursing process.

Practical Knowledge
knowing how

WHAT IS THE NURSING PROCESS?

The **nursing process** is a systematic problem-solving process that guides all nursing actions. It is the type of thinking and doing nurses use in their practice. In fact, the American Nurses Association (ANA) organizes its standards of care around the nursing process (ANA, 2004). The Canadian Nurses Association in 1987 published standards for practice that were also organized around the nursing process. More recently standards in Canada have been developed by provincial and territorial associations. They, too, usually include the nursing process and critical thinking in their standards for practice (Alberta Association of Registered Nurses, 1999; Registered Nurses Association of British Colombia, 2000).

CriticalThinking 2–5

Practice your critical thinking. What questions should you ask about the last paragraph you have just read?

Look at Figure 2–1 and Table 2–2. When evaluating the last paragraph, you should ask about the credibility of the sources cited, and you should ask yourself

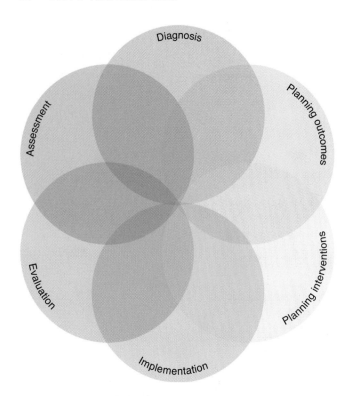

FIGURE 2–2   The phases of the nursing process.

whether you have enough information about them to judge their credibility. Do you know what the ANA and the CNA are? What do they do? Who belongs to them? What are standards of practice, and who decides what will be in them? What effect do they have on what you will be doing as a nurse? Those are the kinds of questions you should ask when you see such statements. If you have read Chapter 1, you can probably answer most of these questions. You will see standards of care and practice quoted in chapters throughout this book, beginning in Chapter 3.

All nurses apply the nursing process, to well clients and ill clients alike, in any setting (e.g., homes, clinics, hospitals). The purpose of the nursing process is to help the nurse provide goal-directed, client-centered care. The nursing process, like nursing itself, involves both thinking and doing. Nurses must have good psychomotor and interpersonal skills, and they must use a sound knowledge base and good judgment to determine when and how to use their skills.

What Are the Phases of the Nursing Process?

The nursing process consists of six phases (or steps): assessment, diagnosis, planning outcomes, planning interventions, implementation, and evaluation (Wilkinson, 2001). A model illustrating these phases is shown in Figure 2–2. Note, though, that experts organize the phases in different ways. Many have a five-step

process, combining outcomes and interventions into one planning phase. Some even have a four-step process; they combine assessment and diagnosis into one phase that they call "assessment." There is no "right" way to do it because you do not use the steps separately anyway. Your text presents them separately to make it easier for you to learn how the process works.

Assessment is the first phase of the nursing process. This is the data-gathering stage. Information may come from many sources: the client via history or physical exam, the client record, lab or test data, other health professionals, the client's family or support system, as well as the professional literature. In this phase your purpose is to gather information that you will use to draw conclusions about the client's health status.

Diagnosis is the second phase of the nursing process. In this step you will identify the client's health needs (usually stated in the form of a problem) based on careful review of your assessment data. You need to analyze all your data, synthesize and cluster information, and hypothesize about your client's health status. The term *diagnosis* has been thought of as medical, such as a diagnosis of cancer, diabetes, or tonsillitis. However, nurses also formulate diagnoses. Nursing diagnoses reflect the client's responses to actual or potential health problems and are different from medical diagnoses, as you will discover in Chapter 4.

Planning is involved in the third and fourth steps of the nursing process. Planning can be divided into two phases: planning (predicting) outcomes and planning interventions. The finished product of the planning phases is a holistic nursing care plan, individualized to reflect the client's problems and strengths. A care plan is a written or computerized document containing detailed instructions for a client's nursing care (see Figure 5–3).

Planning outcomes is the step in which you work with the client to decide goals for your care—that is, the client outcomes you want to achieve through your nursing activities. These outcomes will drive your choice of interventions. Here is an example of an outcome statement you might find in a care plan:

> Nutritional status will improve as evidenced by a weight gain of 3 lb by July 1.

See Chapter 5 for other ways to write goal/outcome statements.

Planning interventions is the phase in which you develop a list of possible interventions based on your nursing knowledge and then choose those most likely to help the client to achieve the stated goals. The best interventions are those that are supported by sound research.

Implementation is the action phase. In this phase you carry out or delegate the actions that you previously planned. You may delegate an action to

another member of the healthcare team only if it is an action that may safely and legally be carried out by that team member. Delegation is further discussed in Chapter 7, "Implementing and Evaluating," and Chapter 38, "Leading and Managing." In this phase you also document your actions and the client's responses to them.

Evaluation is the final phase of the nursing process. In this phase you judge whether your actions have successfully treated or prevented the client's health problems. You need to determine whether the desired outcomes have been achieved. You then modify the care plan as needed. For example, if a problem has been resolved, you delete it from the care plan; if outcomes have not been achieved, you determine why. It may be that a new intervention is needed. If so, you add it.

Notice that the nursing process is not intended to be linear. Instead it is a cyclical process that follows a logical progression. You will find that you go back and forth between the steps, especially as you gain nursing experience. In addition to being cyclical, the steps may be concurrent. That means that some of the steps may occur at the same time. For example, while inserting a urinary catheter (implementation step), the nurse also observes the urine that returns through the tube (assessment step). You will learn about each nursing process phase in depth in Chapters 3 through 7.

KnowledgeCheck 2–3

- List the six phases of the nursing process.
- In which stage does the nurse collect data?
- Which stage involves problem identification?
- What does the nurse do in the evaluation step?

 Go to Chapter 2, **Knowledge Check Response Sheet and Answers,** on the Electronic Study Guide.

How Is the Nursing Process Related to Critical Thinking?

Critical thinking and the nursing process are interrelated, but not identical:

- Nurses use critical thinking for decisions unrelated to the nursing process (e.g., to decide how many nurses are needed to staff the unit).
- Some nursing activities (e.g., applying a cardiac monitor, inserting a urinary catheter), although they must be done skillfully, do not require reflective critical thinking.

The nursing process is essentially a problem-solving process. As such, it is one of the *complex* critical-thinking skills (see Table 2–1). Inherent to complex skills such as the nursing process are many individual critical-thinking skills (see Table 2–2 and Figure 2–1). The following section illustrates how nurses use critical thinking, as well as nursing knowledge, in each phase of the nursing process.

WHAT IS FULL-SPECTRUM NURSING?

Caring is an important nursing value. **Full-spectrum nursing** is a unique blend of thinking and doing that translates caring into action. It is performed by nurses who fully develop and apply nursing knowledge, critical thinking, and the nursing process to benefit patients.

What Concepts Are Used in the Model?

Remember that, in critical thinking, one must have something to think about. When nurses think, they use the nursing knowledge that they have stored in their memory. In addition, they think about patient information (or the *patient situation*), which they acquire through use of the nursing process. In summary, in full-spectrum nursing you bring critical thinking and the nursing process to bear on nursing knowledge and patient information (Figure 2–3). Thus, the four primary concepts of full-spectrum nursing are:

Critical thinking
Nursing process
Nursing knowledge
Patient situation

The full model involves everything you have learned about these four concepts, summarized as follows:

Critical thinking
Contextual awareness
Reflecting critically
Considering alternatives
Examining assumptions
Inquiry based on credible sources

Nursing knowledge
Theoretical knowledge
Practical knowledge
Personal knowledge
Ethical knowledge

Nursing process
Assessment
Diagnosis
Planning outcomes
Planning interventions
Implementation
Evaluation

Patient situation
Patient information/data
Patient "story"
Everything you know about the patient
Holistic data about medical diagnosis, life situation, and physical, emotional, psychosocial, and spiritual needs

You can see that a full-spectrum nurse needs excellent thinking skills because there is so much to think *about* and so much to *do*.

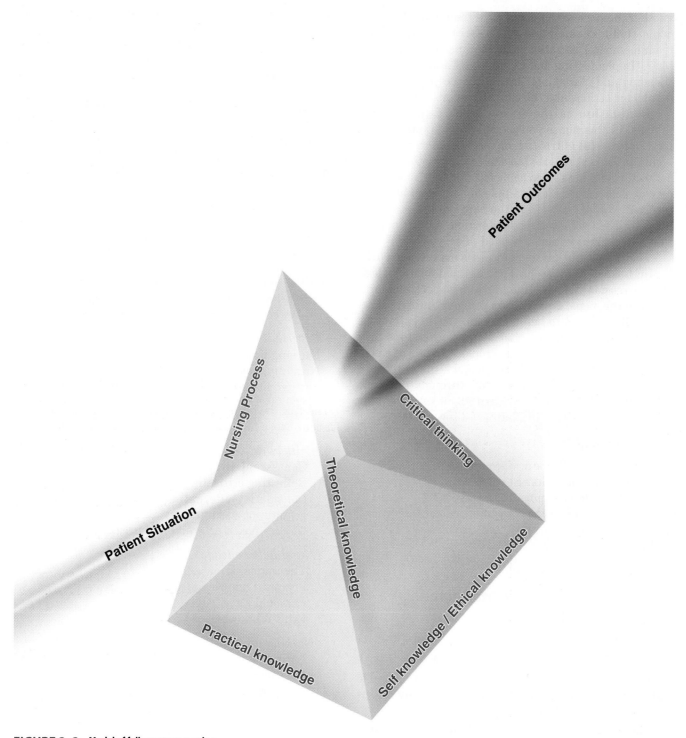

FIGURE 2–3   Model of full-spectrum nursing.

How Does the Model Work?

The full-spectrum nursing model is used throughout this text, so it is important that you understand how it works. The following examples illustrate how the four main concepts of full-spectrum nursing work together. The examples are organized according to nursing process steps. As you read, remember that nursing process and problem solving are themselves complex critical-thinking skills.

> **Assessment.** When taking a patient's temperature, a nurse sees a glass of ice water on the overbed table.

> *Nursing knowledge.* The nurse realizes that a cold drink can change the temperature reading (theoretical knowledge). The nurse uses her interviewing

skills to get more information from the patient; she uses a psychomotor skill when she finally measures the patient's temperature (practical knowledge).

Nursing process. The nurse observed the glass of ice water on the table. The nurse asks, "How long since you've taken a drink of water?"

Critical thinking. This nurse has recognized relevant information and identified the need for more information. The nurse uses the patient's answer to decide what to do.

Patient situation. The nurse knows that the water was within the patient's reach and that the patient was physically capable of reaching it. The patient's answer to her question provides more information for the nurse to process.

Diagnosis. A nurse sees that a patient is crying and twisting a tissue in her hand. The patient is going to surgery soon, and she has no family or friends with her.

Nursing knowledge. The nurse knows that crying and physical agitation are symptoms of anxiety; but he also realizes that he needs more information to be certain (theoretical knowledge). The nurse uses his interviewing skills to get more information from the patient (practical knowledge).

Nursing process. The nurse has recognized a pattern of cues that may indicate a diagnosis of Anxiety. He says, "You seem upset. Can you tell me what's going on?" When the patient says she is worried about surgery, the nurse confirms his nursing diagnosis of Anxiety.

Critical thinking. This nurse recognized a pattern of cues, made a tentative inference that the patient is fearful or anxious, and identified the need for more information.

Patient situation. The nurse has the information that the patient is going to surgery and has no family or friends with her.

Planning outcomes. A nurse is developing expected outcomes (goals) for an elderly man with a fractured leg and a nursing diagnosis of Impaired Walking. Realizing that the man also has a medical diagnosis of emphysema and is usually short of breath, the nurse phrases the outcome to take that into consideration and writes, "Will walk across room, using walker, by 7/11, with no change in oxygen saturation." For a client with no comorbidity, the nurse would probably have written this outcome as: "Will walk across room unassisted, using walker, by 7/11."

Nursing knowledge. The nurse has theoretical knowledge: (1) the usual interval before a patient with a fracture begins to walk, (2) the effects of aging on

mobility and strength, (3) the effects of emphysema on oxygenation, (4) the fact that walking requires strength and uses oxygen. When the nurse helps the patient to walk, he draws on his procedural knowledge of assisting with ambulation.

Nursing process. The nurse developed an achievable, measurable outcome criterion by which to evaluate the patient's progress.

Critical thinking. Generating evaluation criteria is a critical-thinking skill. The nurse also used the skill of considering context (the patient situation) when developing the outcome and the skill of making interdisciplinary connections (e.g., from knowledge of pathophysiology, developmental stages, and mobility concepts).

Patient situation. The nurse knows that the man has emphysema, is often short of breath, has a newly fractured leg, and will be using a walker.

Planning interventions. When planning nursing activities for a man with clinical depression, the nurse recalls from a psychology class that low self-worth is a source of depression. In addition, she has heard the man make several negative comments about himself, such as "I'm no good." The nurse plans activities that will allow the client to have some successes so that his self-esteem will increase.

Nursing knowledge. The nurse has theoretical knowledge of depression and self-worth, or self-esteem. The nurse probably used practical knowledge (interviewing skills) when assessing the patient's self-esteem.

Nursing process. Undoubtedly, the nurse has already assessed the patient, made a nursing diagnosis of Low Self-Esteem, and written a goal such as "Will improve his self-esteem, as evidenced by making fewer than two negative comments about self per day." The nurse then chooses interventions to achieve the goal.

Critical thinking. The nurse made interdisciplinary connections by applying theory to a specific patient situation. Also, the nurse undoubtedly considered alternatives (e.g., which interventions to use, what the results of each intervention are likely to be) when choosing the activities.

Patient situation. The nurse obtained data about the patient situation through the nursing process: the patient is depressed and exhibits low self-esteem.

Implementation. A nurse realizes that heat is lost through evaporation. Therefore, when a client has a fever, she wipes his face with a cool, damp cloth.

| toward evidence-based practice |

Demarco, R., Hayward, L., & Lynch, M. (2002). Nursing students' experiences with and strategic approaches to case-based instruction: A replication and comparison study between two disciplines. *Journal of Nursing Education, 41*(4), 165–174.

This is phase II of a three-part study looking at case-based instruction among health disciplines. Case-based instruction is often used to foster critical thinking. In this phase, senior-level nursing students enrolled in a leadership and management course were instructed using case scenarios rather than traditional lectures. The researchers examined the students' experiences with this style of learning. Learning through case study was viewed as a real-world experience and was valued as a way to learn. Students found this style of learning very motivating. They experienced learning as "emerging from within" the class and small groups. Students also noted that group dynamic issues affected the learning experience. Overall, students found case-based study a positive experience.

1. Based on the results of this study, if you were an instructor would you use case-based learning to teach a course in fundamentals of nursing? Why or why not?

2. How is a fundamentals course similar to and different from the course described in this study? How does that affect your decision to use case-based learning in your fundamentals course?

 Go to Chapter 2, **Toward Evidence-Based Practice Suggested Responses,** on the Electronic Study Guide.

Nursing knowledge. The nurse used theoretical knowledge of the principles and mechanisms of heat loss. She also used practical knowledge to take the patient's temperature and to apply the cool, damp cloth.

Nursing process. The nurse has assessed that the patient has a fever. The unstated goal is to bring the temperature down to normal. The intervention is to wipe the patient's face with a cool, damp cloth; the nurse implements that activity.

Critical thinking. The nurse has applied a principle (evaporation creates heat loss) to a specific patient situation (fever).

Patient situation. The patient has a fever. Apparently the patient is not well enough to apply his own moist compresses, since the nurse is doing it.

Evaluation. Thirty minutes after giving a pain medication, a nurse checks with the patient to see whether the pain has been relieved. The nurse is using the desired outcome ("States pain relief is adequate . . .") as a criterion for evaluating the effectiveness of the nursing activity.

Nursing knowledge. The nurse has theoretical knowledge of the interval before the medication takes effect. The nurse undoubtedly used practical knowledge when administering the medication.

Nursing process. The nurse has apparently assessed the patient, identified a nursing diagnosis of Acute Pain, set a desired outcome, implemented an intervention, and is planning to evaluate its effect—all the steps of the nursing process.

Critical thinking. Criterion-based evaluation is a critical-thinking skill.

Patient situation. All we know from this scenario is that the patient is in pain and has received medication for it. From the way the goal is stated, we can assume that the patient can talk. The patient may be in an inpatient setting because he is not administering his own medication, and the nurse expects to be able to check on him in 30 minutes. Certainly the nurse has all that information. After evaluating the effects of the medication, she will also know how well this medication works for this individual.

So, as you can see, you need to learn about critical thinking and the nursing process because they are essential to your practice. Nursing process, critical thinking, and nursing knowledge will enable you to translate your caring into action.

 Suggested Readings: Go to Chapter 2, **Reading More About Critical Thinking & the Nursing Process,** on the Electronic Study Guide.

 Bibliography: Go to Volume 2, Bibliography.

Nursing Process:
Assessment

Learning Outcomes

After completing this chapter, you should be able to:

✳ Define nursing assessment including the four features common to all definitions.

✳ Compare medical and nursing assessments (similarities and differences).

✳ Explain how assessment is related to each of the other steps of the nursing process.

✳ State the ANA position on delegating assessment.

✳ Name three JCAHO requirements regarding patient assessment.

✳ Use assessment skills to gather data during a nursing assessment.

✳ Define initial assessment, ongoing assessment, comprehensive assessment, and focused assessment.

✳ Explain the importance of discharge planning assessment.

✳ List five special needs assessments and state when or why you would use them.

✳ Identify the following types of data: subjective, objective, primary source, secondary source.

✳ Explain the importance of observation in a nursing assessment.

✳ Explain the purpose of a nursing interview.

✳ Identify at least four components of a nursing health history and state the purpose of each.

✳ State the difference between directive and nondirective interviewing.

✳ Compare and contrast open-ended and closed questions, including definitions, uses, advantages, and disadvantages.

✳ Describe how to prepare for an interview.

✳ List and give examples of six guidelines for conducting interviews.

✳ Describe three circumstances in which you should validate data.

✳ Describe two frameworks for organizing data.

✳ State four guidelines for documenting data.

✳ Explain the difference between a cue and an inference.

✳ Compose three questions to ask yourself when you are evaluating the quality of your assessments.

MEET Your Patient

As the intake nurse in a community-based clinic in Miami, Florida, your role is to complete a comprehensive nursing assessment and initiate a plan of care for the clients. Your first client is a 24-year-old single woman, Sami, who is requesting clinic services for her general healthcare needs. Sami is Hispanic and lives alone in a one-bedroom apartment in this neighborhood. She works as a fitness trainer at the local YMCA. Her family lives in Tampa, Florida. Sami's earnings place her at the poverty level, but she realizes that she must have health care to prevent illness and to detect and receive treatment of illnesses should they arise. You will be asked to apply full-spectrum thinking to Sami's case throughout the chapter as you learn the concepts of assessment.

ASSESSMENT: THE FIRST STEP OF THE NURSING PROCESS

Assessment is the systematic gathering of information related to the physical, mental, spiritual, socioeconomic, and cultural status of an individual, group, or community. Although various definitions exist, all definitions of assessment include the following features:

• Collecting data
• Using a systematic and ongoing process
• Categorizing the data
• Recording the data

The purpose of assessment is to obtain enough data to allow you to be of help to the patient. The nursing interview and the physical assessment findings become a part of the **patient database** (all the pertinent patient data obtained by nurses and other health professionals). You will use the facts, impressions, and contextual information obtained in your assessment to develop a plan of care.

How Is Assessment Related to Other Steps of the Nursing Process?

Assessment is the first phase of the nursing process. Data must be accurate and complete, because the remainder of the nursing process rests on this foundation of data. Assessment is related to other nursing process steps as follows (Figure 3–1):

• Assessment provides the data necessary for identifying the client's actual or potential health problems and strengths (*diagnosis phase*).

• When *planning outcomes,* data about the person's motivation, family, and available resources helps you formulate realistic goals.

• Assessment data also helps you to choose the *interventions* most likely to be acceptable to and effective for the client.

• *Implementation* offers another opportunity for you to gather data by observing the client's responses as you perform the intervention. For example: While helping a client ambulate, you might observe that she becomes short of breath. If this is new data, you might then identify a new diagnosis of Activity Intolerance.

• In the *evaluation* stage, you assess client responses to interventions that were performed for existing problems. This *reassessment* provides the basis for changes in the care plan.

How Does Nursing Assessment Fit into Collaborative Care?

As a nurse, you will focus on your clients' *responses* to illness: their physical responses, their understanding of the illness, the effects of the illness on their lives and their ability to care for themselves, and their emotional responses and concerns. This is different from medical assessments, which focus on disease. You will also use assessment with healthy clients, to help identify ways they can maintain their current level of wellness and prevent disease. Again, this is different from the traditional medical model, in which assessment typically focuses on detection of disease.

The database created from the nursing assessment findings can be accessed and used by other healthcare professionals. In some settings, the nurse looks at the database and delegates or makes referrals to other professionals with expertise in a particular area of health care. This helps ensure that clients receive the proper care by qualified individuals at the time it is needed.

To illustrate further, we will use Sami's case: Sami has not had a gynecological (female) examination for 5 years. In the interview Sami tells you that her mother has had breast cancer and that her sister is being treated for endometriosis. After asking whether, because of any religious or other beliefs, she would be offended by a frank discussion, you also ask about her sexual activity, assuring her that you will keep all information confidential. As a result of this interview, you encourage Sami to get a women's health examination as soon as possible. She agrees, and you refer her to a women's clinic, where she will be charged according to her ability to pay.

What Do Professional Standards Say About Assessment?

Complete, skillful, and timely assessment of all clients is an important skill for nurses in all healthcare settings. Standards of governmental agencies, professional organizations, and accrediting bodies, such as the following, all address assessment.

The American Nurses Association (ANA) standards for clinical practice, which apply to all nurses, identify assessment as a professional responsibility (Box 3–1).

Canadian provincial nursing organizations mention assessment as one dimension of professional practice (Box 3–1).

Nurse practice acts regulate the practice of nurses in individual states. The National Council of State Boards of Nursing (2002) *Model Nursing Practice Act* also asserts that the scope of nursing includes surveillance and comprehensive assessment of the health status of individuals and groups.

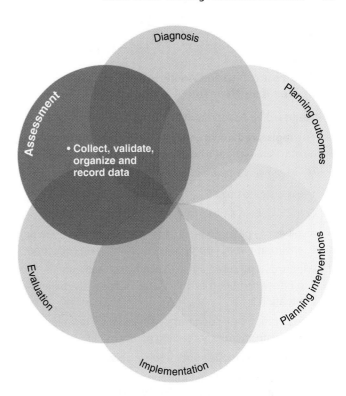

FIGURE 3–1 Nursing process: Assessment phase.

The Joint Commission on Accreditation of Healthcare Organizations (JCAHO, Section 1: Assessment of Patients [PE], 2000) identifies assessment as an essential element of patient care. In agencies where there is an RN on staff, the JCAHO requires that an RN assess patients' needs for nursing care. The JCAHO provides detailed standards regarding what and when to assess, including standards that require agencies to provide evidence that:

- Assessments are written, comprehensive (physical, psychological, and social status), and used to identify and assign priorities for care
- Agency policy designates (1) when each patient is to be reassessed and (2) which disciplines can make which assessments
- All patients are assessed for pain

KnowledgeCheck 3–1

- What are the four features common to all definitions of assessment?
- How is a nursing assessment similar to a medical assessment?
- How is it different?

 Go to Chapter 3, **Knowledge Check Response Sheet and Answers,** on the Electronic Study Guide.

Can I Delegate Assessments?

For data to be reliable, someone with education and experience must perform the assessment. Nurse aides or other unlicensed assistive personnel (UAP) may

BOX 3-1 Professional Standards for Assessment

American Nurses Association Standards of Nursing Practice

Standard 1. Assessment

The registered nurse collects comprehensive data pertinent to the patient's health or the situation.

Measurement Criteria

The registered nurse:

Collects data in a systematic and ongoing process.

Involves the patient, family, other healthcare providers, and environment, as appropriate, in holistic data collection.

Prioritizes data collection activities by the patient's immediate condition, or anticipated needs of the patient or situation.

Uses appropriate evidence-based assessment techniques and instruments in collecting pertinent data.

Uses analytical models and problem-solving tools.

Synthesizes available data, information, and knowledge relevant to the situation to identify patterns and variances.

Documents relevant data in a retrievable format.

Source: Reprinted with permission from American Nurses Association, *Nursing: scope and standards of practice* (3rd ed.). © 2004 American Nurses Publishing, American Nurses Foundation/American Nurses Association, 600 Maryland Are., SW, Suite 100 W, Washington, DC 20024–2571.

Canadian Provincial Standards of Practice (Examples)

In Canada, practice standards are set by each province. The following are examples that apply to assessment.

Province of Alberta

The registered nurse continually strives to acquire knowledge and skills to provide competent, evidence-based nursing practice. The registered nurse:

Accesses appropriate information and resources that enhance patient care and achievement of desired patient outcomes.

Demonstrates critical thinking in collecting and interpreting data, planning, implementing, and evaluating all aspects of nursing care.

Documents timely, accurate reports of data collection, interpretation, planning, implementing, and evaluating care.

Source: Alberta Association of Registered Nurses. (1999). *Nursing practice: Professional conduct: Nursing practice standards.* Retrieved January 17, 2003, from http://nurses.ab.ca/profconduct/npa.html

Province of Nova Scotia

The registered nurse demonstrates competencies relevant to own area of nursing practice. Each registered nurse applies appropriate knowledge and skills to assess, plan, intervene and evaluate services, and revises plan as needed.

Source: Registered Nurses' Association of Nova Scotia. (1997). *Standards for nursing practice.* Retrieved January 17, 2003, from http://www.rnans.ns.ca

collect information such as temperature, height, and weight. However, as a nurse, it is your responsibility to assign those tasks, validate the data collected, conduct the interview, and complete the physical assessment. The ANA's *Code of Ethics for Nurses*, Provision 4 (2001) states: "The nurse . . . determines the appropriate delegation of tasks consistent with the nurse's obligation to provide optimum patient care." See Chapters 7 and 38 for a thorough discussion of delegation of tasks to UAPs. The following resources can guide you in deciding which caregivers are qualified to perform parts or all of an assessment.

- *State nurse practice acts.* Each state has a nurse practice act that specifies which portions of the assessment can legally be completed by individuals with different credentials. Look for statements related to

delegation. For example, the definitions in the NCSBN *Model Nursing Practice Act* (2002) differentiate between assessments by RNs and LPNs/LVNs (Box 3–2).

- *Agency policies/procedures.* Each facility has policies and procedures that state which caregivers can collect and document specified data.
- *Accrediting agencies.* These agencies also provide guidelines for who can perform assessments and document the findings (e.g., JCAHO, 2000, Section 1: PE).
- *The American Nurses Association (ANA).* The ANA provides definitions of nursing and *Scope and Standards of Practice* (2004) to further guide who is ultimately responsible and qualified to collect assessment data.

CriticalThinking 3–1

Think about the following situations, then answer the questions. More than one answer may be acceptable. Compare your ideas with those of other students or nurses, or consult your instructor.

- Suppose you are an RN in a healthcare setting where the policy states that UAPs can take vital signs (blood pressure, pulse, temperature, and respirations). You have a patient who is critically ill and whose condition is changing rapidly. Would you take the vital signs or delegate the task to the UAP? Why?
- Imagine that you are an RN in the same hospital on a different day. All but one UAP has called in sick today because of an influenza outbreak. This UAP is inexperienced and overwhelmed by her tasks. Would you bathe the patients in your caseload (even though that is usually done by a UAP) or would you ask the UAP to do it? Why?

It is obvious from these examples that you must use good judgment when applying standards and policies and deciding when to delegate assessments.

Sources of Data

Subjective data (*covert data, symptoms*) is information told to the nurse by the client, family, or community. Subjective data reveals the perspective of the person giving the data, and includes thoughts, feelings, beliefs, and sensations. Thus, subjective data from two different people can vary. For example, people with insomnia often report getting much less sleep than their sleep partner says they do. Subjective data can also be used to clarify objective data (e.g., "How did you get this scar?"). Some people (e.g., infants) are unable to provide subjective data. Others can give subjective data, but you might question its accuracy. For example, what would you do if an obviously obese person told you his weight is 135 lb? What could you do to be sure?

Objective data (*overt data, signs*) is gathered through a physical assessment or from laboratory or diagnostic tests. It can be measured or observed by the nurse or other healthcare providers. Examples are vital signs, x-ray test results, skin color, and urine output. One use of objective data is to validate (check) subjective data. In the preceding example, if you thought 135 lb was inaccurate, you might weigh the person. You may also gather objective data when the subjective data seems accurate but indicates that more information is needed. For example, when Sami told you her family and sexual history, you learned that she has significant risk factors for breast and cervical cancer and referred her for a gynecological exam. The results of the breast exam and Pap smear (Papanicolaou test, a smear of cervical cells) provide objective data related to these risk factors.

Primary data is the subjective and objective data obtained from the client: what the client says or what you observe. **Secondary data** is obtained "second-hand," for

---

BOX 3–2 Delegation Model Nursing Practice Act (Revised 2002), Selected Definitions Related to Nursing Assessment

Comprehensive assessment by the RN   An extensive data collection (initial and ongoing) for clients, families, groups and communities addressing anticipated changes in client conditions as well as emergent changes in a client's health status; recognizing alterations to previous client conditions; synthesizing the biological, psychological and social aspects of the client's condition; evaluating the impact of nursing care; and using this broad and complete analysis to make independent decisions and nursing diagnoses; plan nursing interventions; evaluate need for different interventions; and the need to communicate and consult with other health team members.

Focused assessment by the LPN/VN   An appraisal of the client's status and situation at hand, contributing to ongoing data collection, and deciding who needs to be informed of the information and when to inform.

Source: Reproduced from the NCSBN web site (*www.ncsbn.org*) and used by permission from the National Council of State Boards of Nursing (NCSBN), Chicago, IL © 2002.

---

example, from the medical record or from another caregiver. For example, a client's husband may say, "She seems more confused than usual." Or the UAP may report, "Mr. Atlas's heart rate was 100 beats per minute this morning." If you count the heart rate yourself, though, it is primary data. Table 3–1 provides further examples of types and sources of data.

KnowledgeCheck 3–2

During Sami's appointment at the women's clinic, she has a Pap smear, breast exam, and blood work. She also informs the nurse practitioner that her menstrual flow is very heavy and that she experiences severe abdominal cramping. All of this data is added to the database as reference for future visits. Sami's Pap smear results and breast exam are normal, but she is moderately anemic (she has a low hemoglobin level). When the nurse practitioner sees the lab results, she suspects that the heavy flow may be causing Sami's anemia. According to clinic protocol, she prescribes birth control pills for Sami to control her heavy, painful periods and provide contraception. Ongoing assessment will include visits every 6 months to manage her birth control pills and monitor the anemia. State whether the following data are primary or secondary, subjective or objective:

- You see in the chart that Sami's breast exam was normal.
- Sami tells the nurse practitioner that she experiences cramping with her menstrual cycle. *For the nurse practitioner,* is this primary or secondary, subjective or objective data?

TABLE 3-1   Examples of Data Types

Data Types	
Subjective Data	**Objective Data**
"I have been having a lot of pain in my abdomen."	Suprapubic area firm to light palpation. Lower abdomen semi-soft.
"My throat hurts to swallow."	White patches noted at the back of the throat and tonsillar area is reddened and swollen.
"Our children have no place to go after football games. That is why they get into so much trouble."	In a windshield survey, no public facility was open after football games to allow young people to socialize under supervision.

Data Sources	
Primary Source (Client)	**Secondary Sources (Everything Else)**
Pulse rate 100 bpm.	From chart: WBC count 14,000.
States feeling short of breath.	In transfer report, nurse states that the surgical dressing is dry.
Abdomen tender on palpation.	Client's wife states that he has been tired a lot lately.

- The nurse practitioner tells you that Sami is anemic.
- You check the results of the Pap smear on the computer and see that it is normal.

 Go to Chapter 3, **Knowledge Check Response Sheet and Answers,** on the Electronic Study Guide.

Types of Assessment

Assessment can be broad and general or very specific. The type of assessment you do depends on the client's status. In acute care settings such as the emergency department, the assessments are rapid and focused on the presenting problem. In inpatient settings, you may perform an initial comprehensive assessment at admission and other, more focused assessments over time, according to the client's needs.

Initial and Ongoing Assessments

An **initial (admission) assessment** is completed when the client first presents to the healthcare agency. First obtain data related to the person's reason for seeking nursing or medical assistance. Then complete a comprehensive assessment if the client's condition permits. Data gathered from the initial assessment provides guidance for care and determines the need for

further assessment. Initial assessment data tends to be static; for example, demographic data (marital status, occupation) is not likely to change often.

Ongoing assessment is performed as needed, at any time after the initial database is completed. Ideally, you will make at least some observations at every contact with a client. You use data from ongoing assessments to identify new problems or to follow up on previously identified problems. In comparison to the initial assessment, ongoing assessment data reflects the dynamic state of the client. For example, vital signs may change rapidly and serve as important indicators of developing or resolving problems.

Comprehensive and Focused Assessments

A **comprehensive assessment** (also called a *global assessment, patient database,* or *nursing database*) provides holistic information about the client's overall health status. It includes data about the client's body systems and functional abilities, emotional status, and psychosocial situation, including information about the family and community. It also requires assessment of client strengths related to the mind, body, and spirit. The assessment tools (forms) used in most healthcare settings require comprehensive data. Gathering comprehensive data helps you to be sensitive to a patient's culture, values, beliefs, and economic situation.

A **focused assessment** is performed to obtain data about an actual, potential, or possible problem that has been identified. It focuses on a particular topic, body part, or functional ability rather than on overall health status. For example, focused assessments can center on pain, nutrition, spiritual health, social support, lifestyle, and family assessment. These specialized assessments add to the database created by the comprehensive initial assessment.

An *initial focused assessment* is used to follow up on client symptoms or unusual findings during the first exam (e.g., on admission to a hospital). *Ongoing focused assessment* is used to evaluate the status of existing problems and goals. Consider the following examples:

Initial focused assessment. When the nurse asks Mr. Jacobs why he has come to the clinic today, he replies, "I can't get rid of this pain in my foot." The nurse asks questions to get in-depth information about this symptom. For example: When did it begin? On a scale of 1 to 10, how severe is it? What makes it worse? What do you do to make it feel better? She also examines the foot for joint mobility, redness, edema, and tenderness to touch.

Ongoing focused assessment. After surgery, Ms King has a nursing diagnosis of Acute Pain secondary to abdominal incision. The nurse assesses her pain level at least every 2 hours and before and after administering pain medication.

CriticalThinking 3–2

- Give examples of each type of assessment (initial, ongoing, comprehensive, focused) using patients you have observed or cared for or your own personal experiences as a patient.
- How might age and developmental stage make a difference in your assessment of a patient?
- Suppose you are the triage nurse at the community clinic in the Meet Your Patient scenario. What kind of assessment do you perform at Sami's first visit (initial, ongoing, comprehensive, focused)? What type will the care provider at the women's clinic perform?

Special Needs Assessments

A **special needs assessment** is a type of focused assessment. It provides in-depth information about a particular area of client functioning and often involves using a specially designed form. Some special needs assessments (e.g., of nutrition status and pain) are required by JCAHO for all clients. In some settings, such as hospice, home health, and rehabilitation settings, other special needs assessments (e.g., of functional abilities) are also required. You should perform a special needs assessment any time assessment cues suggest risk factors or problems in an area of client functioning.

Special needs assessments can be quite lengthy; therefore, you need to carefully consider when and how to use them. You need enough data to provide holistic care, but you must balance this need against the need not to intrude on the client's privacy. The data you obtain should enhance the care provided to the client and add to the comprehensive assessment. The following are some special needs assessments:

Nutritional assessment. You should perform a nutritional assessment when data suggests that the client is undernourished, is at risk for Imbalanced Nutrition, or requires nutritional therapy as an intervention (as in a person newly diagnosed with diabetes). In addition to information about food intake, it includes information related to personal, psychosocial, and economic problems that may affect nutrition. See Chapter 26 for more information about nutritional assessment.

Pain assessment. In addition, good nursing care and accrediting agency standards require you to perform a thorough pain assessment on all patients during the initial assessment and in ongoing assessments (JCAHO Standard PE:1.4, 2000). For more information on pain assessments, see Chapter 30.

Functional ability assessment. Functional ability is especially important in discharge planning and home care. Future rehabilitation needs are derived from initial and ongoing functional ability assessments. These three functional assessment tools are commonly used:

BOX 3–3 Questions for Assessing Independence in Activities of Daily Living

Mobility

Does the client require objects (e.g., cane, crutches, walker, wheelchair) for support?

Transfer

Can the client get in and out of bed and in and out of a chair without assistance?

If not, how much help does the client need?

Is the client completely confined to bed?

Bathing

Can the client perform a sponge bath, tub bath, or shower bath with no help?

If not, specifically what assistance does the client need?

Dressing

Can the client get all necessary clothing from drawers and closets and get completely dressed without help?

If not, specifically what assistance does the client need?

Feeding

Can the client feed self without assistance?

If not, specifically what assistance does the client need (e.g., help with cutting meat, tube feeding)?

Toileting

Can the client go to the bathroom, use the toilet, clean self, and rearrange clothing without help?

If a night bedpan or commode is used, can the client empty and clean it independently?

If the client needs help with these activities, specifically what does it include?

Continence

Does the client independently control urination and bowel movements?

If not, how often is the client incontinent of bladder or bowel?

Does the client require an indwelling urinary catheter?

- The Katz Index of ADL scale (1963). This instrument assesses the client's independent performance in these very basic areas: bathing, dressing, toileting, transfer, continence, and feeding. Nurses often use the data to plan staffing and appropriate placement of clients. See Box 3–3 for questions to use when assessing activities of daily living (ADLs).
- Lawton Instrumental Activities of Daily Living scale (IADL) (1969). This easy-to-use tool is

particularly helpful in assessing a person's ability to independently perform the more sophisticated tasks of everyday life, such as shopping.

You will find the Lawton scale in

 Go to Chapter 3, **Assessment Forms: Lawton IADL,** in Volume 2.

- The Karnofsky Performance Scale (Karnofsky & Burchenal, 1949). This tool is used primarily in palliative care settings to assess functional abilities at the end of life.

 Go to Chapter 3, **Supplemental Materials: Karnofsky Performance Scale,** on the Electronic Study Guide.

Cultural assessment. A heightened awareness of cultural influences should guide your assessment and nursing care, but be careful not to stereotype clients based on culture. To be culturally competent, you must be able to assess and honor each person's diversity. For content included in a cultural assessment, see Chapter 13.

Spiritual health assessment. Spiritual health contributes to overall well-being. For ill persons, spirituality can be a problem or a source of support. To gather useful information, you must do more than ask the client's religious preference. Spiritual health assessment provides insight into how a client interprets life events and health. See Chapter 14 for further information.

Psychosocial assessment. In a psychosocial assessment, you gather information about lifestyle, normal coping patterns, understanding of the current illness, personality style, previous psychiatric disorders, recent stressors, major issues related to the illness, and mental status (Gorman, Raines, & Sultan, 2002). You should perform a focused psychosocial assessment if initial assessment data indicates that social and emotional needs are not being met (e.g., if the client is very anxious or exhibiting symptoms of stress), or if sociocultural factors (e.g., unemployment, environmental pollution) present a risk to health. See Chapter 11.

Wellness assessment. Health promotion focuses on activities of a healthy person to achieve a higher level of health. When supporting wellness behaviors, you assume that people can identify their own health needs, so most assessment tools are self-administered by the client. In addition to assessing spiritual health, social support, and nutrition, a wellness assessment includes data about physical fitness, a life-stress review, health beliefs, and lifestyle. See Chapter 41 for a more detailed discussion of assessing wellness.

Family assessment. Health behaviors and beliefs generally have their beginnings in family interactions. Therefore, a family assessment provides a better understanding of the client's health-related values, beliefs, and behaviors. Family assessment is discussed in Chapter 12.

Community assessment. Community assessment provides information about community demographics, resources, health concerns, points of referral, environmental risks, and community norms and values. See Chapter 42 for more information about community assessment.

 CriticalThinking 3–3

Based on the data you have so far about Sami, consider the need to perform any of the special purpose assessments. What is your rationale for using or not using a special needs assessment?

WHAT IS INCLUDED IN A COMPREHENSIVE ASSESSMENT?

A **comprehensive assessment** consists of a nursing history and physical examination. It contains both subjective and objective data. Figure 3–2 shows what information is gathered in an initial comprehensive assessment (database) and how it fits into the broad concept of assessment in the nursing process. You will find an example of a form for recording a comprehensive assessment in Volume 2. Nurses collect data through the use of all their senses. Whether assessment is initial or ongoing, comprehensive, or focused, you will use the skills of observation, physical examination, and interviewing.

 Go to Chapter 3, **Assessment Forms: Nursing Admission Data Form,** in Volume 2.

Observation

Observation refers to the deliberate use of all five of your senses to gather and interpret patient and environmental data. All that you see, hear, feel, smell, or sense becomes data in the context of assessment. You should make systematic observations each time you are with a patient. In other words, you should try to use the same sequence of observation at each patient contact. The mnemonic (memory aid) in Box 3–4 may help you.

Physical Assessment

Physical assessment (or *physical examination*) produces primarily objective data and makes use of the following techniques, which are described in detail in Chapter 19.

- **Inspection.** Observation and visual examination of the client, as well as use of equipment such as an otoscope or ophthalmoscope.

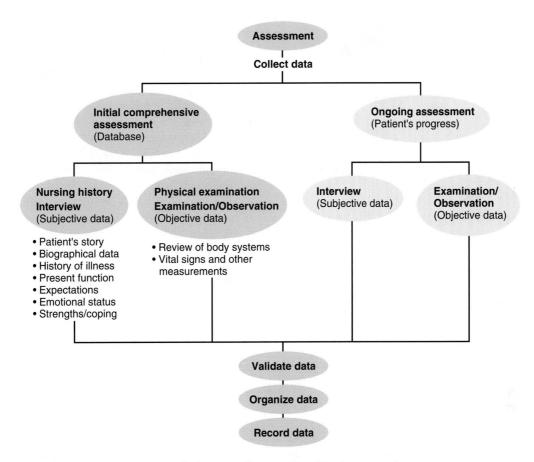

FIGURE 3–2 **Overview of assessment content and methods.** *Source:* Wilkinson, J. M. (2001). *Nursing process and critical thinking* (3rd ed.), p. 88. Reprinted by permission of Pearson Education, Inc., Upper Saddle River, NJ.

- **Palpation.** Light touch, progressing to deeper touch, using the pads of the fingers.
- **Percussion.** The striking of a body surface with the tip of a finger, which produces different vibrations and sounds depending on what is under the area that is tapped (air, fluid, or solid).
- **Auscultation.** Listening with the unaided ear for sounds made by the client (*direct auscultation*) and then listening with the use of a stethoscope (*indirect auscultation*) for normal and abnormal sounds within the body.

KnowledgeCheck 3–3

Give at least two more examples of data you might obtain with each of the following senses. One example is provided for each.

- Touch (example: bladder distention)
- Vision (example: facial expression of pain)
- Smell (example: fecal odor)
- Hearing (example: bowel sounds)

 Go to Chapter 3, **Knowledge Check Response Sheet and Answers,** on the Electronic Study Guide.

BOX 3-4 **Mnemonic for Observing**

Use the first letter of each word to help you observe systematically as you enter a patient's room.

Do Help Every Patient Deliberately (DHEPD)

Distress. Observe first for signs of distress (e.g., pain, pallor, labored breathing)

Hazards. Next look for safety hazards (spills, equipment cords, sharps)

Equipment. Is all equipment working: IV running? Catheter draining? Oxygen working?

People. Who are the people in the room? Family? Other caregivers? What are they doing?

Details. Look more closely. Examine the patient thoroughly for appearance, breathing, condition of dressings, correct positioning, skin color and condition, odors, condition of linens, and any other clues that might indicate a need for care.

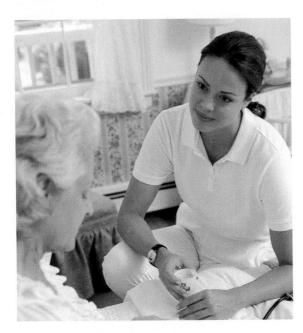

FIGURE 3–3 The nurse conducts an informal interview.

The Nursing Interview

A **nursing interview** is purposeful, structured communication in which you question the patient to gather subjective data for the nursing database (Figure 3–3). The admission interview is planned, but during ongoing assessment, the interview may be informal, brief, and narrowly focused.

What Are the Components of a Nursing Health History?

The nursing health history covers some of the same topics as the medical history, but the rationale for the questions is different. For example, if an elderly man has a fractured hip, the physician would be interested in the cause of the fracture, the extent of the injury, and any preexisting medical problems that might make the client a poor surgical risk. As the nurse, you would also ask about the cause of the injury, but you would also want to know what effect the injury has on the man's ability to perform his everyday activities. You would also identify supports and strengths to begin planning for his eventual discharge and self-care.

Health history forms vary among agencies and according to purpose (e.g., inpatient, clinic, surgery, medical, emergency room, or newborn care), but most include the following information:

Biographical data. This is relatively unchanging information such as name, address, age, gender, race, religion, marital status, and occupation. The person's responses to these questions reflect his mental status and ability to communicate.

Chief complaint / reason for seeking health care. This is the client's perception or reason for seeking medical or nursing advice. From this, you will be able to target your assessment to gather the most relevant and important data. Ask the client specifically what caused him to seek help (e.g., checkup, chest pain), and document the answer in the client's words.

History of present illness. Find out when this illness or problem began, how the client's health has changed from his usual status, and what effect the illness has had on his daily life.

Client's perception of health status and expectations for care. This includes the client's knowledge about his illness and its potential effects on his life. For example, does a client with arterial insufficiency think his foot will be "normal" again? Also, what does the client think will be done for him (e.g., does he know that his foot will be amputated)? And what does he want the nurses to do to help (e.g., leave a light on at night, bring my medicines)?

Past medical history. This includes childhood diseases and immunizations, previous hospitalizations, and previous surgeries. The past medical history helps guide your assessment and helps you to understand some of the data you obtain. For example, if Sami tells you she had her appendix out when she was 5 years old, you would expect to find a scar on her abdomen.

Family and social history. In addition to family medical history, this includes information about family and other relationships, economic status, occupations, exposure to toxic materials, home conditions, and ethnicity. Family medical history includes data on first-degree blood relatives such as mother, father, siblings, and maternal and paternal grandparents. Risk factors for various illnesses and disorders are often tied to multigenerational problems. Social history includes information on tobacco, alcohol, and drug use as well as exercise habits.

Medication (nutritional supplements, herbs) history and current use. Past medication usage may uncover some medical history the client has forgotten to disclose. As you continue with the assessment, you can direct questions toward previous episodes of medical treatment. Current medications are of utmost importance because (1) they may interact with newly prescribed medications and (2) some may affect certain body symptoms, causing abnormalities in your assessment findings (e.g., skin color, laboratory values). Also inquire about vitamin and nutritional supplements and the use of alternative-therapy medications such as homeopathic preparations and herbal remedies. Many herbs interact with prescription medications.

Complementary/alternative modalities (CAM). These are therapies used instead of or in addition to the allopathic therapies recommended by physicians—for example, chiropractic care, homeopathy, aromatherapy, music therapy, massage therapy, energy work (therapeutic touch, Reiki), and acupressure or acupuncture. Such therapies can support or interfere with conventional therapies, so this is important information.

Review of body systems and associated functional abilities. This is subjective data regarding body systems (e.g., Do you have a productive cough?). It includes functional abilities (e.g., difficulties with dressing, bathing, eating, and elimination). You can obtain this data during the physical assessment as well as in the interview.

Types of Interviews

Interviews may be directive or nondirective. Use **directive interviewing** to obtain factual, easily categorized information (e.g., age, sex), or in an emergency situation. In this type of interview, you control the topics and ask mostly closed questions to obtain specific information. **Closed questions** are those that can be answered with a "yes," "no," or other short, factual answer. They usually begin with *who, when, where, what, do (did, does),* and *is (are, were).* Closed questions are useful for patients who are very anxious or who have communication difficulties.

When you want to promote communication, build rapport, or help the patient to express feelings, use **nondirective interviewing.** This means that you allow the patient to control the subject matter. Your role is to clarify, summarize, and ask mostly open-ended questions that facilitate thought and communication. **Open-ended questions** specify a topic to be explored, but phrase them broadly to encourage the patient to elaborate. Subjective data is best obtained by asking open-ended questions.

Both types of interview have advantages and disadvantages. Directive interviewing is efficient but may cause you to miss topics of importance to the patient. Nondirective interviewing allows you to find out what is important to the patient, but it is time-consuming and can produce much irrelevant data.

A successful interview includes closed and open-ended questions. Use broad, open-ended questions to guide the patient to talk about certain topics. From the answers to the broad questions, you can decide which topics to clarify or follow up with specific, closed questions. Part of the interview with Sami might have gone like this:

Nurse	When was your last physical examination? *(closed question)*
Sami	I had a female exam about 5 years ago.

TABLE 3-2 Examples of Closed and Open-Ended Questions

Closed Questions	Open-Ended Questions
Are you having any pain?	Tell me about your pain.
Do you ever drink excessively?	Tell me about your use of alcohol.
Why did you come to this clinic?	I am glad to see you here today. Could you tell me a little bit about why you decided to come see us?
Do you have any family history of heart disease?	Tell me about your family members and what kind of experiences they may have had with heart disease or problems with circulation.
Are there any parks where you can walk safely?	Tell me about safe places here in your community where you might go to take a walk.

Nurse	What problems have you had in that area? *(open-ended question)*
Sami	None, really.
Nurse	What about other women in your family? *(open-ended question)*
Sami	Well, my mother had breast cancer about the same time that I went for my checkup. She's OK now though.
Nurse	Go on . . . *(open-ended question)*
Sami	And my sister has been taking some pills for endometriosis. She hasn't been able to get pregnant because of that.
Nurse	Are you sexually active? *(closed question)*
Sami	Yes.
Nurse	Tell me about that. *(open-ended question)*

See Table 3–2 for other examples of closed and open-ended questions.

Preparing for the Interview

While they are learning, some students feel uncomfortable interviewing patients. You may have one of the following concerns:

• You may feel that you are imposing on the patient, who clearly needs rest more than you need information. This may be because you believe a "real nurse" has already obtained the information, or because you don't have a clear idea of how the information will be used. This problem can be relieved by good preparation.

- You may worry that the patient won't be receptive to answering personal questions from a stranger (you). To help set the tone for the interview, be sure to tell your patients that the information given will be kept confidential and that they can refuse to answer any question. Remember that the patient can choose what to tell and what to withhold from you. Also, be aware that the patient may have been feeling the need to talk about something, has not known how to bring it up, and is relieved that you have introduced the topic.

- You may be afraid that some of your questions will upset the patient—that the person will cry or become angry. Remember that patients usually feel better after expressing their emotions. Expressions of strong emotion are hard to accept, but you must learn to do it. You will have large gaps in your data if you avoid all difficult topics, and your patients will not get the help they need.

Your interviews will go more smoothly if you take time to prepare yourself and your patient before you begin asking questions.

Preparing Yourself

The following will help you to prepare yourself:

- *Be sure you know why you are conducting the interview and how the data will be used.* As a student, this may simply mean preparing thoroughly for your clinical assignment.

- *Read the patient's chart.* This will give you an idea of where to start with the interview and keep you from covering topics already assessed by other caregivers. Be careful to keep an open mind though. If you approach an interview with preconceived ideas, you may overlook important data.

- *Form some goals and think of some opening questions* for the interview.

- *Schedule some uninterrupted time* for the interview.

- *Gather the necessary assessment forms and equipment,* such as your stethoscope, pen, pencil, blood pressure cuff, and thermometer.

- *Take a deep breath and compose yourself* before entering the room.

Preparing the Space

The following will help you to prepare a comfortable environment for the interview:

- *Provide privacy* (e.g., ask visitors to wait outside, shut the door). In some interviews, the client's significant others will offer information that may or may not be pertinent. Keep the focus on the client, but do not ignore the information provided by others. Also, realize that the presence of even a close family member may inhibit the client in some situations. For example, suppose that you are taking an obstetrical history. A wife may not want her husband to know that she had a miscarriage before they were married. Unless you need information from the visitor (e.g., when the client cannot communicate clearly) you may wish to postpone the interview until it can be done in private.

- *Remove distractions* (e.g., turn off the television, arrange for someone to watch the children for a while if they are present).

- *Position yourself at the same level as your client,* even if the client is in bed. Sit down. Do not hover over the bed.

Preparing the Patient

The following actions will help to ensure that the patient is ready for the interview:

- *Introduce yourself* to the patient and others in the room.

- *Call the patient by name; ask what name the patient prefers.* Don't use endearing terms like "grandma," "dear," and "sweetie." You may think you are being friendly or expressing your caring, but many people feel belittled by these terms.

- *Tell the patient what you will be doing and why.* Explain that you will be taking notes and that you will keep all information confidential. If you wish to record or videotape the interview, be sure to obtain permission from the patient.

- *Assess readiness to discuss health issues.* If the patient indicates that now is not a good time, reschedule. For example, if the patient has just received some bad news about his condition, or in his personal life, he may need some time to process that information before he can concentrate on interview questions.

- *Assess and provide for comfort* (e.g., assess and medicate for pain, offer the bedpan, offer a drink of water).

- *Assess for anxiety.* Be sure the patient is comfortable emotionally as well as physically. A very anxious person cannot provide good information, so you may need to intervene to relieve anxiety before proceeding.

Conducting the Interview

The following guidelines will help you to obtain complete and reliable information:

- *Individualize your approach* based on the client's age, developmental level, and cultural background. Ask yourself, "What approach is best considering my client's age?" Respect the generational differences of a person older or younger than you, and be sensitive to cultural differences (e.g., comfort with eye contact, the need for space).

- *Begin with neutral topics,* such as the biographical data (e.g., address, contact person, occupation). Ask more personal or sensitive questions after you and the client are more comfortable with each other.

- *Use active listening.* This is the most important interviewing technique. Focus intently on trying to understand what the client is saying, rather than thinking ahead to what your response to the statement will be. Use the mnemonic FOLK to remember other active listening behaviors:

  Face the patient (either sitting or standing).
  Open, relaxed posture (arms and legs uncrossed).
  Lean toward the patient.
  Keep eye contact.

- *Don't get caught up in note taking.* Excessive writing interferes with eye contact and may inhibit the client's responses, especially when you are discussing personal issues such as sexuality or drug and alcohol use.

- *Pay attention to nonverbal communication.* For example, body language may signal that the person is tired or in pain but is too polite to say so. If the person is fatigued, you may need to end the interview and finish it at another time.

- *Use open-ended questions* as much as possible, to encourage the client to talk.

- *Don't ask too many questions.* If you do, you may seem merely curious instead of interested in the client. Use neutral statements instead (e.g., instead of "How many children do you have?" say "Tell me about your family.")

- *Avoid asking "why"* (e.g., "Why have you stopped taking your pills?"). "Why" causes some people to become defensive. Parents frequently ask their children, "Why did you do that?" For some people, "why" suggests disapproval.

- *Don't use healthcare jargon* (e.g., "I want to take your vital signs"), but don't "talk down" to the client (e.g., "How often do you go potty?" asked of an adult).

- *Confirm that clients understand terminology* they use. If a client says, "It's the inflammation that causes me the trouble, you know," you might say, "Tell me where the inflammation is and what happens when you have it." People may repeat words they hear from care providers without really knowing what the words mean.

- *Refocus the client* when her story becomes scattered or does not produce useful information. Allow the client to talk about the topics of importance to her, but direct her to topics that need to be covered (e.g., "We haven't talked about your surgery. What do you expect to happen?").

- *Curb your curiosity.* Don't get caught up in the details of the client's story. Focus on the information you need to plan care.

- *Don't give advice or voice approval or disapproval* (e.g., "It's good that you were firm with your daughter" or "You should take your pills on time"). Even if the advice is good, it may cause the client to be less open with you and interfere with your ability to gather data.

Closing the Interview

The following guidelines will help ensure that the interview has accomplished both your goals and the patient's goals:

- *Prepare the patient for closure.* Inform the patient that the interview is nearly finished.

- *Summarize* the key points of the interview.

- *Be sure you have recorded all the important data.* Ask the patient, "Is there anything else you would like to tell me?" or "Is there anything else we should talk about?"

- *Thank the patient for answering the questions.*

- *Encourage the patient to keep you informed.* For example, you might say, "Please let us know if you think of anything else we should know."

- *Tell the patient what to expect next.* Tell the patient when you will be leaving, when you will see him again, and what he can expect for the rest of the day (e.g., tests, treatments).

- *Ask, "Is there anything I can do for you before I leave?"*

KnowledgeCheck 3–4

- What are the nine components of a nursing history and why are they important?
- What are two things you should do to prepare yourself before an interview?
- List several things you could do to be sure that the client is comfortable before the interview.
- State four guidelines that will help you to obtain complete and accurate data when conducting an interview.

 Go to Chapter 3, **Knowledge Check Response Sheet and Answers,** on the Electronic Study Guide.

HOW AND WHEN SHOULD I VALIDATE DATA?

Suppose a patient has told you that he has never had high blood pressure (BP), but you obtain a BP reading of 180/98 mm Hg. What would you do? Would you record the 180/98 mm Hg reading, or would you:

- Ask the patient some more questions, such as, "What do you mean when you say you have never had high blood pressure?" or "What have you been doing in the last 15 minutes?"

- Ask another nurse to double-check your findings?

- Check when the sphygmomanometer was last calibrated?
- Retake the BP using a different sphygmomanometer?
- Compare the reading to previous entries in the chart?
- Check the BP in the patient's other arm?
- Wait a few minutes and take the reading again in the same arm?

All of those are ways to **validate** your data—to verify it or double-check it. Validating data helps to ensure that it is accurate, complete, and factual and that you have not jumped to conclusions. If the patient tells you that he was running late and had just jogged the two blocks from the parking lot, you would know that 180/98 does not reflect his usual BP and that you need to check it again.

Not all data must be validated. You can usually assume, for example, that laboratory results are correct and that the patient has given you correct information about data such as height, weight, and birth date. You should validate data under the following circumstances (Wilkinson, 2001):

1. Subjective and objective data do not agree, or do not make sense together.
   Example: In the preceding situation, the subjective data was "never had high BP," but the objective data, BP 180/98 mm Hg, indicates that the BP is elevated.
2. The patient's statements differ at different times in the interview.
   Example: A patient tells you that he follows a low-cholesterol diet. However, later when describing his usual daily food pattern, he includes eggs for breakfast, a cheese sandwich for lunch, and a hamburger for dinner.
3. The data falls far outside normal range.
   Example: A patient has no symptoms of infection or high fever, but you obtain an oral temperature reading of 106°F (41.1°C). (Hint: Ask him if he has just had something warm to drink.)
4. Factors are present that interfere with accurate measurement.
   Example: The patient has extremely small arms, and there are no pediatric BP cuffs available. The BP will probably not be accurate; you should take it again when appropriate equipment is available.

HOW CAN I ORGANIZE DATA?

Professional standards require systematic data collection (see Box 3–1). This means that you collect and record data in predetermined categories, not just at random. Data in most initial (e.g., admission) assessments is automatically categorized by the agency's data-collection form. For ongoing assessments, you may need to provide your own organizing structure, or

framework. Because a **framework** represents a particular way of thinking about clients and health, it indicates which information is significant and guides you in deciding which patient data to observe. The major concepts of a model/framework help you to cluster data and find patterns.

Nonnursing Models

ANA professional standards state that nursing data collection should be holistic. Many agencies use a **body systems (medical) framework** for at least a section of the assessment form. This model is useful for identifying medical problems, but it needs to be combined with other models (e.g., a nursing model or Maslow's Hierarchy) to provide the holistic data you need to identify both nursing and medical problems. **Maslow's Hierarchy of Needs** (1970) groups data according to human needs and states that the basic needs must be met before higher needs can be addressed. Maslow's categories of needs, from most basic to highest, are:

Physiological. Basic survival needs (e.g., oxygen, water, food, and shelter)
Safety and security. The need to be safe and comfortable (e.g., safe from falls and treatment side effects as well as the need for psychological security)
Love and belonging. The need for love and affection (e.g., family, social supports)
Esteem and self-esteem. The need to feel good about oneself (e.g., body image, pride in achievements, admiration from others)
Self-actualization. The need to achieve one's potential; the need for growth and change (e.g., extent to which goals are achieved, role performance)

See Chapter 8 for a more complete discussion of Maslow's model.

Nursing Models

Nurse theorists have developed many different theories and models for thinking about nursing, clients, health, and the environment. Nursing models produce a holistic database that is useful in identifying nursing rather than medical diagnoses. Several nursing theories are described in Chapter 8. The accompanying box (3–5) identifies the major concepts of five models frequently used to structure nursing assessments. The concepts are the categories that you would use to gather and cluster data.

HOW SHOULD I DOCUMENT DATA?

The ANA *Scope and Standards of Practice* (2004) and JCAHO standards (2000) stress the importance of documenting assessment findings in a retrievable format.

BOX 3-5 Assessment Models: Major Concepts

Gordon's Functional Health Patterns   Describes common patterns of behavior and describes them as functional or dysfunctional. This is intended as a model for nursing assessment and diagnosis, not a complete nursing theory. The functional health patterns are major model concepts:

Health perception/health management

Nutritional/metabolic

Elimination

Activity/exercise

Cognitive/perceptual

Self-perception/self-concept

Sleep/rest

Role/relationship

Sexual/reproductive

Coping/stress tolerance

Value-belief

Source: Adapted from Gordon, M. (1994). *Nursing diagnosis: Process and application* (3rd ed.). St. Louis, Mosby, p. 70.

The NANDA Nursing Diagnosis Taxonomy II   Consists of functional patterns and is a modified version of the Gordon model. It is intended as a model for categorizing nursing diagnoses, not as a fully developed theory of nursing. The NANDA domains (categories) are:

Health Promotion

Nutrition

Elimination

Activity/Rest

Perception/Cognition

Self-Perception

Role/Relationships

Sexuality

Coping/Stress Tolerance

Life Principles

Safety/Protection

Comfort

Growth/Development

Source: Adapted from NANDA International. (2004). *NANDA nursing diagnoses: Definitions & classification 2005–2006*. Philadelphia: Author.

The Taxonomy of Nursing Practice (NANDA/NOC/NIC)
Intended as a model for categorizing nursing diagnoses, client outcomes, and nursing interventions. It consists of four domains and 28 classes.

Functional domain. Activity exercise, comfort, growth and development, nutrition, self-care, sexuality, sleep/rest, values/beliefs

Physiological domain. Cardiac function, elimination, fluid and electrolytes, neurocognition, pharmacological function, physical regulation, reproduction, respiratory function, sensation/perception, tissue integrity

Psychosocial domain. Behavior, communication, coping, emotional, knowledge, roles/relationships, self-perception

Environmental domain. Health care system, populations, risk management

Source: Dochterman, J., & Jones, D. (Eds.). (2004). *Unifying nursing languages: The harmonization of NANDA, NIC, and NOC*. Washington, DC: American Nurses Association, NursesBooks.org.

The Roy Adaptation Model   Conceptualizes patients as adapting constantly to internal and external demands within a biological and psychosocial context. Using this model, you would look at the person's ability to achieve balance in the following "adaptive modes":

Activity and rest

Nutrition

Elimination

Fluid and electrolytes

Oxygenation

Protection

Temperature regulation

Regulation of the senses

Physical self-concept

Personal self-concept

Role function

Interdependence

Source: Adapted from Roy, C., & Andrews, H. (1991). *The Roy adaptation model: The definitive statement*. Norwalk, CT: Appleton & Lange, pp. 15–17.

Orem's Self-Care Model   Conceptualizes health as the ability to perform self-care. Using this model, you would gather data to identify the following universal self-care deficits that require nursing assistance.

Maintenance of a sufficient intake of air, water, and food.

Maintenance of a balance between activity and rest

Maintenance of a balance between time alone and time with others

Provision of care associated with elimination processes and excrements

Prevention of hazards to human life, functioning, and well-being

Promotion of human functioning and development within social groups in accord with human potential, limitations, and desire to be normal (as determined by science, culture, and social values)

Source: Adapted from Orem, D. (1991). *Nursing: Concepts of practice* (4th ed.). St. Louis: Mosby-Year Book, p. 126.

Accurate, timely, and clear documentation of all assessment findings benefits patients by providing the basis for planning effective nursing care. Furthermore, since the nursing database is a permanent part of the client's record, documentation protects you, the nurse, by establishing that you actually performed the needed assessments. Malpractice lawsuits are not unusual in our society, and court cases may be presented years after you care for a patient. Your documentation is the only evidence supporting the care you gave. The assumption in malpractice cases is, "If it isn't documented, it wasn't done."

Guidelines for Recording Assessment Data

Follow these guidelines when recording assessment data:

- Document as soon as possible after you perform the assessment.
- Write neatly, legibly, and in ink.
- Use only agency-approved abbreviations.
- Write the patient's own words, when possible, in quotation marks. If the comments are too long, summarize what the patient says (e.g., Patient states that he is sleepy).
- Record only the most important patient words. If you record everything the patient says, the narrative will probably be too long and contain too much irrelevant data. For example, write "Patient states, 'I hardly slept at all last night'" even though what the patient actually said was, "I hardly slept at all last night. I tossed and turned and people kept waking me up. Then the thunder and lightning came, and then I had to get up to go to the bathroom, and my wife called early this morning."
- Use concrete, specific information rather than vague generalities such as *normal, adequate, good,* and *tolerated well.* For example, what does it mean to say, "Patient slept well"? Did she fall asleep easily and sleep for 6 hours? Did she fall asleep with difficulty, but sleep for 8 hours? Did she sleep only 4 hours, but state that she feels well rested? It is much better to write, "Patient fell asleep before 9:00 P.M. and slept until 6:00 A.M. She states that she woke up only once during the night and feels rested now. Observed sleeping three times during the night."
- Record *cues,* not *inferences.* **Cues** are what the client says and what you observe. **Inferences** are judgments and interpretations about what the cues mean. In other words, just the facts, Jack (or Jill). For example:

Cues	Inferences
"My head hurts."	Patient has a headache.
Incision red, draining pus, edges separated.	Incision is infected.
Tearful. States that father died of a heart attack. Trembling.	Anxious about scheduled cardiac catheterization.
States, "I hate my mother. I wish I was dead."	Patient is angry and suicidal.

Tools for Recording Assessment Data

Each agency or facility has its own forms and formats for documentation of initial and ongoing assessments. You will record data on a variety of documents, including nurses' notes and the following:

Graphic flow sheet. Includes vital signs such as blood pressure, pulse, respirations, and temperature so that trends over time can be seen clearly. See Figure 3–4.

Intake and output sheet. May be on the graphic sheet, as in Figure 3–5, or separate. This form has spaces for all intake: oral, intravenous, and tube feedings. There is also space to record all output: urine, fluid from drainage tubes, wound drainage, and bowel movements.

Nursing admission assessment. Although agency forms differ in appearance and framework, all collect similar data as specified by JCAHO standards for initial assessment. You can see an example of an admission assessment form in Volume 2.

 Go to Chapter 3, **Assessment Forms: Nursing Admission Data Form,** in Volume 2.

Nursing discharge summary. May be a part of the initial assessment form because data obtained at admission is used for discharge planning.

Special purpose forms. Examples are diabetic flow sheets and medication administration forms.

Computer documentation. In some facilities, initial data and ongoing assessment data are entered into a computer program for organization and easy retrieval. See Figure 3–5 for an example of data documented on a computer.

REFLECTING CRITICALLY ABOUT ASSESSMENT

After gathering and recording patient data, use critical thinking to help you evaluate the quality of your assessment. See Chapter 2 for a review of critical thinking, as needed. The following are questions to guide your final judgments about your data.

1. Are my data complete?
   - Have I completed all areas of the assessment form?
   - Is there anything else I need to know to identify or rule out a nursing diagnosis?

Teaching Self Assessment

As you learned in Chapters 1 and 2, it is essential for nurses to provide information that will help clients to care for themselves. One important aspect of self care is performing regular self assessments to detect symptoms of disease.

Important assessments every person needs to know:

- Breast self exam or testicular self exam—monthly
- Skin assessment—daily but at least weekly
- Feet assessment—daily if diabetic, otherwise weekly

Before you begin teaching:

- Assess the readiness of your client to be taught some type of assessment and willingness to learn.
- Assess current knowledge or understanding of the topic to be discussed.

See Chapter 19 for details of these assessments.

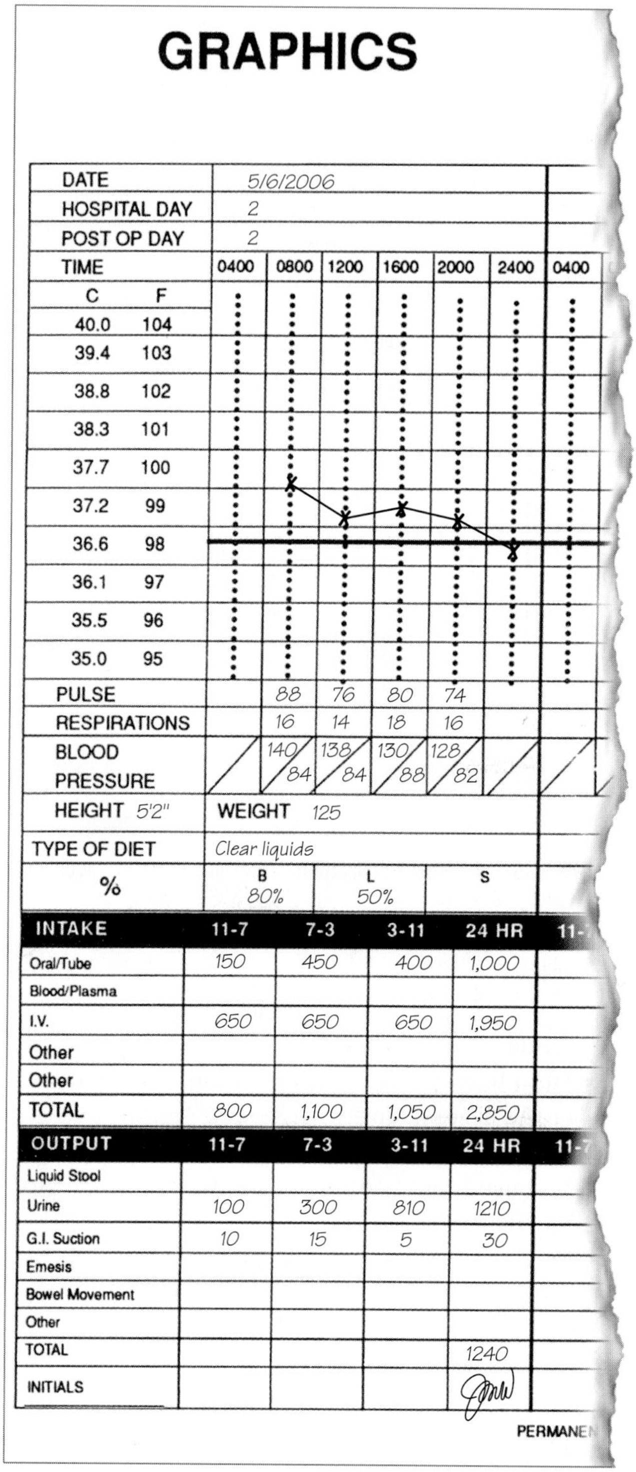

GRAPHICS

DATE	5/6/2006						
HOSPITAL DAY	2						
POST OP DAY	2						
TIME	0400	0800	1200	1600	2000	2400	0400

C	F
40.0	104
39.4	103
38.8	102
38.3	101
37.7	100
37.2	99
36.6	98
36.1	97
35.5	96
35.0	95

	0400	0800	1200	1600	2000	2400	0400
PULSE		88	76	80	74		
RESPIRATIONS		16	14	18	16		
BLOOD PRESSURE		140/84	138/84	130/88	128/82		

HEIGHT 5'2" WEIGHT 125

TYPE OF DIET Clear liquids

%	B 80%	L 50%	S

INTAKE	11-7	7-3	3-11	24 HR	11-
Oral/Tube	150	450	400	1,000	
Blood/Plasma					
I.V.	650	650	650	1,950	
Other					
Other					
TOTAL	800	1,100	1,050	2,850	

OUTPUT	11-7	7-3	3-11	24 HR	11-7
Liquid Stool					
Urine	100	300	810	1210	
G.I. Suction	10	15	5	30	
Emesis					
Bowel Movement					
Other					
TOTAL				1240	
INITIALS				Jmw	

PERMANEN

FIGURE 3–4 Graphic flow sheet. *Source:* Courtesy of Smith Northview Hospital, Valdosta, GA.

- Have I collected holistic data: physical, emotional, interpersonal, spiritual, and cultural?
2. How do I know the data is accurate?
3. Have I recorded data rather than conclusions (cues, not inferences)?
4. Did I validate any data that does not make sense? Does any of the data conflict with other data?
5. Did I record the data in clear, specific terms, using the patient's words, when possible, for subjective data? Did I avoid vague terms such as "normal," "good," and "slept well"?
6. Have I followed up with in-depth special needs assessments when appropriate?
7. Have I included only relevant data, taking care to protect the client's privacy?
8. The assessment interview:
   - Did I use therapeutic communication during the assessment?
   - Did I avoid asking too many questions and using too many closed questions?
   - How comfortable was I during the interview?
   - What signals did I get from the client in response to my questions? Did I follow up?
9. Physical assessment, observation, and examination
   - Did I miss something in the environment?
   - How did the client and significant others respond to me verbally and nonverbally?
   - Did I pay attention to detail?
   - How were my techniques (palpation, percussion, auscultation, inspection)?

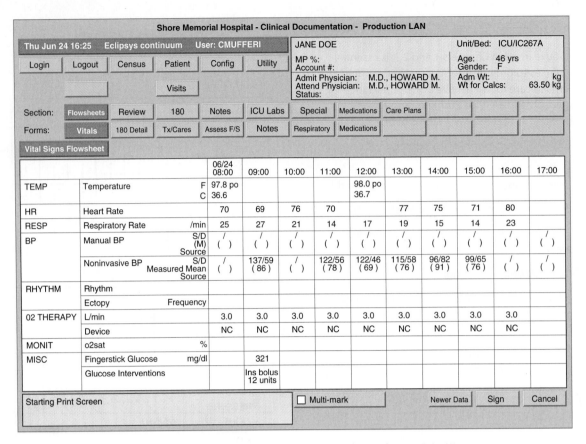

Shore Memorial Hospital - Clinical Documentation - Production LAN

Thu Jun 24 16:25	Eclipsys continuum	User: CMUFFERI				JANE DOE		Unit/Bed: ICU/IC267A

Login	Logout	Census	Patient	Config	Utility

MP %:
Account #:

Age: 46 yrs
Gender: F

		Visits			

Admit Physician: M.D., HOWARD M.
Attend Physician: M.D., HOWARD M.
Status:

Adm Wt: kg
Wt for Calcs: 63.50 kg

Section:	Flowsheets	Review	180	Notes	ICU Labs	Special	Medications	Care Plans			
Forms:	Vitals	180 Detail	Tx/Cares	Assess F/S	Notes	Respiratory	Medications				

Vital Signs Flowsheet

			06/24 08:00	09:00	10:00	11:00	12:00	13:00	14:00	15:00	16:00	17:00
TEMP	Temperature	F	97.8 po				98.0 po					
		C	36.6				36.7					
HR	Heart Rate		70	69	76	70		77	75	71	80	
RESP	Respiratory Rate	/min	25	27	21	14	17	19	15	14	23	
BP	Manual BP	S/D (M) Source	/ ( )	/ ( )	/ ( )	/ ( )	/ ( )	/ ( )	/ ( )	/ ( )	/ ( )	/ ( )
	Noninvasive BP	S/D Measured Mean Source	/ ( )	137/59 (86)	/ ( )	122/56 (78)	122/46 (69)	115/58 (76)	96/82 (91)	99/65 (76)	/ ( )	/ ( )
RHYTHM	Rhythm											
	Ectopy	Frequency										
02 THERAPY	L/min		3.0	3.0	3.0	3.0	3.0	3.0	3.0	3.0	3.0	
	Device		NC	NC	NC	NC	NC	NC	NC	NC	NC	
MONIT	o2sat	%										
MISC	Fingerstick Glucose	mg/dl		321								
	Glucose Interventions			Ins bolus 12 units								

Starting Print Screen		☐ Multi-mark	Newer Data	Sign	Cancel

FIGURE 3–5   Computer screen capture: Assessment data. *Source:* Courtesy of Shore Memorial Hospital, Somers Point, NJ.

10. Memory

- Did I have to ask questions in the sequence found on the forms?
- Did I have to depend on the forms for all aspects of the assessment?
- Did I have to repeat any area of assessment because I could not remember what I saw, heard, smelled, or felt?

If you have followed the recommended processes and reflected critically on your assessment, you should have the data necessary to create a holistic plan of care individualized to meet the client's needs.

 Go to Chapter 3, **Resources for Caregivers and Health Professionals,** on the Electronic Study Guide.

 Suggested Readings: Go to Chapter 3, **Reading More About Nursing Process: Assessment,** on the Electronic Study Guide.

 Bibliography: Go to Volume 2, Bibliography.

Nursing Process:
Diagnosis

Learning Outcomes

After completing this chapter, you should be able to:

* Define the following terms: *diagnosis, nursing diagnosis, diagnostic reasoning, diagnostic label, defining characteristics, related factors, risk factors, health problem.*

* Explain how nursing diagnosis is related to the rest of the nursing process.

* Relate the history of nursing diagnosis since the 1950s, including the role of the American Nurses Association and NANDA.

* Differentiate between nursing diagnoses, medical diagnoses, and collaborative problems.

* Explain the differences between actual, risk, possible, syndrome, and wellness nursing diagnoses.

* Describe a process for determining a nursing diagnosis.

* Differentiate between a cue and an inference.

* Explain why an etiology is always an inference.

* Describe at least two frameworks for prioritizing nursing diagnoses.

* Describe errors of theoretical and self-knowledge that may occur in diagnostic reasoning.

* Define the terms: *standardized language* and *taxonomy.*

* Explain how you can know which of the NANDA labels to use to describe a patient's problem.

* Write nursing diagnosis statements and collaborative problem statements in correct format, using format variations when appropriate.

* Clarify the relationship between nursing diagnoses and goals/interventions.

* State at least five criteria for judging the quality of a diagnostic statement.

* Recognize issues associated with the NANDA diagnostic labels and with standardized language in general.

Your Patient

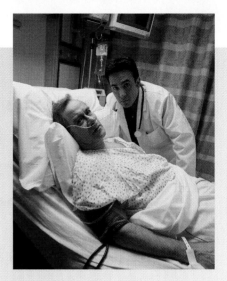

On your evening shift at an acute care facility, you will be admitting a client, Todd, from the emergency department (ED). Todd's ED nurse telephones you to give report about him. The ED nurse tells you that Todd's admitting medical diagnosis is chronic renal failure. He is married, 58 years old, currently employed, and has a medical history of type II diabetes mellitus. In the past 3 days, he has developed decreased sensation in his bilateral lower extremities with slight mobility impairment.

You still have many questions concerning Todd's immediate and long-term needs. You will need to ask Todd about his medication regimen, his compliance with his diabetes treatment plan, and the extent to which his family is involved. You will also need to find out what laboratory tests have been completed and how severe his renal dysfunction has become. After you obtain the necessary data, you will organize and analyze it to form some initial impressions about what it means. Some initial impressions might be:

- His admitting diagnosis is chronic renal failure; so you can anticipate a problem with fluid balance.

- He has been admitted to the hospital and is acutely ill, so he may be anxious and fearful.
- He has decreased sensation in his lower extremities, so he may have a mobility or a safety problem.
- He has diabetes, so he is at risk for impaired skin and tissue integrity.
- Because diabetes and renal failure require complex regimens and patient self-care, it is possible that Todd may not be managing his therapy effectively, either because he is not motivated to do so or because he lacks the knowledge to do so.

When Todd and his family arrive on your unit, you begin gathering additional data. Armed with comprehensive data, you then make a list of Todd's health problems, in priority order. These actions illustrate the diagnosis phase of the nursing process phase. The purpose of diagnosing is to identify the client's health status, from which you will create your plan of care.

Theoretical Knowledge
knowing why

Professional standards of practice identify diagnosing as the unique obligation of the professional nurse (Box 4–1). Although many nursing activities may be delegated, diagnosis cannot. To meet practice expectations and professional obligations, you must assume the role of diagnostician and make clinical judgments.

DIAGNOSIS: THE SECOND STEP OF THE NURSING PROCESS

Diagnosis is the second step of the nursing process. It is the phase in which you determine the meaning of your assessment data. Using your critical-thinking skills, you identify patterns in the data and draw conclusions about the client's health status, including strengths, problems, and factors contributing to the problems. As in all phases of the nursing process, you should involve the patient and family as much as possible in the diagnostic process.

As you can see in Figure 4–1, diagnosis overlaps with the other nursing process steps. Most nurses actually begin diagnostic reasoning during the assessment phase. For example, you probably formed your initial impressions about Todd while you were still gathering data. Upon hearing the medical diagnosis, chronic renal failure, you would have immediately considered the diagnosis Risk for Imbalanced Fluid Volume, but you would have obtained more data before actually recording that as a nursing diagnosis. So your tentative diagnostic conclusion would actually lead you to collect more data: Is he still producing urine? What is his oral intake? Does he have edema? Do you see how you would move back and forth between assessment and diagnosis? The two stages are not

BOX 4-1 Professional Standards for Diagnosing

American Nurses Association Standards of Nursing Practice

Standard 2. Diagnosis

The registered nurse analyzes the assessment data to determine the diagnoses or issues.

Measurement Criteria:

The registered nurse:

Derives the diagnoses or issues based on assessment data.

Validates the diagnoses or issues with the patient, family, and other healthcare providers when possible and appropriate.

Documents diagnoses or issues in a manner that facilitates the determination of the expected outcomes and plan.

Note: There are additional measurement criteria for advanced practice registered nurses.

Source: Reprinted with permission from American Nurses Association, *Nursing: Scope and standards of practice* (3rd ed.). 2004. American Nurses Publishing, American Nurses Foundation/American Nurses Association, 600 Maryland Ave., SW, Suite 100 W, Washington, DC 20024-2571.

Canadian Provincial Standards of Practice (Example)

In Canada, practice standards are set by each province. The following is one example that applies to diagnosis. Note that the standards mention interpretation of data but do not specifically use the term *diagnosis.*

Province of Alberta

The registered nurse continually strives to acquire knowledge and skills to provide competent, evidence-based nursing practice. The registered nurse:

Demonstrates critical thinking in collecting and interpreting data, planning, implementing, and evaluating all aspects of nursing care.

Documents timely, accurate reports of data collection, interpretation, planning, implementing, and evaluating care.

Source: Alberta Association of Registered Nurses. (1999). *Nursing practice: Professional conduct: Nursing practice standards.* Retrieved January 17, 2003, from http://nurses.ab .ca/profconduct/npa.html

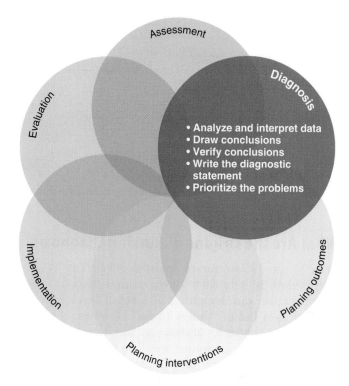

FIGURE 4–1 Nursing diagnosis: Second phase of the nursing process.

separate at all, but we present them that way to make it easier for you to learn.

Diagnosis is critical because it links the assessment step, which precedes it, to all the steps that follow it (Figure 4–2). Assessment data must be complete and accurate for you to make an accurate nursing diagnosis. Accuracy is essential because the nursing diagnosis is the basis for planning client-centered goals and interventions.

You will find the term **diagnosis** used in the nursing literature to refer to:

• The second phase of the nursing process

• The reasoning process used in interpreting assessment data

You will also see the term **nursing diagnosis** used to refer to:

• A formal diagnostic statement of the client's health status, containing both the problem and etiology (factors contributing to the problem).

• The list of standardized terms (labels) used to write diagnostic statements. Those terms are actually problem labels; you must add a second part (etiology) in order to create a complete diagnostic statement.

 Go to Chapter 4, **NANDA Taxonomy II: Domains, Classes, and Diagnoses (Labels),** in Volume 2.

Table 4–1 summarizes and provides examples of how nursing diagnosis terminology is used in this text.

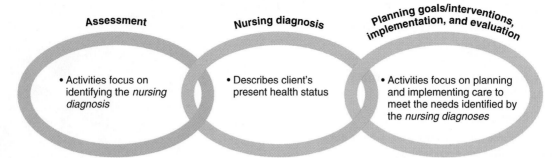

FIGURE 4–2 Diagnosis links the assessment phase to the rest of the nursing process.

What Are the Origins of Nursing Diagnosis?

Prior to the 1950s, nurses assisted physicians by collecting data to help them diagnose and treat disease. Nursing care was thought of as a set of tasks and organized as a list of "things to do." However, nursing leaders saw the need to describe the knowledge and work that are unique to nursing. The term *nursing diagnosis* was first used to differentiate nursing from medicine in 1953, when Fry stated that a nursing diagnosis identifies the client's needs for nursing rather than for medical care. During the 1960s, nursing schools began to teach diagnosis as a part of the nursing process but were still careful to explain that nurses were not usurping medical authority by using diagnostic thinking. Until the early 1970s, nursing diagnosis was not widely used in nursing practice, but two major events in 1973 spurred change:

1. The First Conference on Nursing Diagnosis was held (Gebbie, 1976). A national task force was formed to begin developing a language to describe the health problems treated by nurses.
2. The American Nurses Association (ANA) *Standards of Nursing Practice* included nursing diagnosis as an expectation of professional nurses.

In 1980, the ANA published *Nursing: Social Policy Statement*, which characterized nursing as "the diagnosis and treatment of human response to actual or potential health problems" (ANA, 1980, p. 2). As a result of this definition and the work of the nursing diagnosis task force, most state nurse practice acts began to designate nursing diagnosis as an exclusive responsibility of registered professional nurses. Nursing diagnosis is now widely used in nursing education and practice. The formal list of nursing diagnostic labels

TABLE 4–1 Nursing Diagnosis Terminology

Term and Existing Meanings	Terminology Used in This Book	Example
Diagnosis		
1. The second phase of the nursing process.	1. *Diagnosis*	With Todd ("Meet Your Patient"), you used *diagnostic reasoning* in order to *diagnose* and list his problems. This was the *diagnosis phase* of the nursing process.
2. The reasoning process used in identifying patient problems and strengths.	2. *Diagnostic process, diagnostic reasoning* or *diagnosing*	
Nursing Diagnosis		
1. The end product of the diagnostic reasoning process: a full diagnostic statement describing client health status. It contains both problem and etiology.	1. *Nursing diagnosis, diagnostic statement*	For Todd, you might have made a *nursing diagnosis* of Excess Fluid Volume secondary to renal failure. To write that statement, you would have used the *NANDA label* Fluid Excess Volume.
2. A standardized problem label from the NANDA taxonomy (e.g., Anxiety).	2. *Label, NANDA label, problem label, diagnostic label*	

describes health problems that can be addressed by independent nursing actions and, in that sense, forms the body of knowledge that is unique to nursing.

Since the first conference, the nursing diagnosis group has continued to meet every 2 years. In 1982 it adopted the name North American Nursing Diagnosis Association (NANDA). In 2002 the organization changed its name to NANDA International, to reflect its large number of members from countries outside the United States and Canada. NANDA continues to review and refine the diagnostic labels and to discuss new and revised labels at each biannual conference. They encourage individual nurses and nursing organizations to submit new and revised diagnoses. The diagnoses on the official list are approved for clinical use and further study; they are not intended to represent finished products, because most have very little basis in research.

KnowledgeCheck 4–1

- Why is the diagnosis step so critical to the other phases of the nursing process?
- What two nursing organizations have been responsible for making diagnosis a part of the professional nursing role?

 Go to Chapter 4, **Knowledge Check Response Sheet and Answers,** on the Electronic Study Guide.

What Are Health Problems?

A **health problem** is any condition that requires intervention to promote wellness or to prevent or resolve disease or illness. When you identify a health problem, you must then decide how to treat it: independently or in collaboration with other health professionals. The answer determines whether it is a nursing diagnosis, a medical diagnosis, or a collaborative problem. See Table 4–2 for a comparison of these problem types.

Recognizing Nursing Diagnoses

A **nursing diagnosis** is a statement of client health status that nurses can identify, prevent, or treat independently. It is stated in terms of **human responses** (reactions) to disease, injury, or other stressors, and it can be either a problem or a strength. Human responses can be biological, emotional, interpersonal, social, or spiritual. For example, Todd's medical diagnosis is chronic renal failure. A *physical response* to renal failure might be Excess Fluid Volume. Admission to the ED is also a stressor, to which his *emotional response* might be Anxiety or Fear. What other actual or possible responses were identified for Todd in the situation? Take a moment to write them down.

Recall that Todd has a stressor, decreased sensation in his lower extremities, to which he has responded with slight impairment of mobility. Perhaps you identified

that possible responses for Todd might include falling (safety), impaired skin integrity and impaired tissue integrity, and ineffective management of his therapy. All of those are responses to disease, illness, or stressors. Also note that besides being a stressor, the decreased sensation in Todd's lower extremities can be considered a physical response to type II diabetes mellitus. Was this response on the list you just made?

 ## CriticalThinking 4–1

Imagine that you have been in an automobile accident. You have internal injuries and broken bones and will be hospitalized for at least 2 weeks, right before your final exams. What human responses (physical, emotional, interpersonal, social, spiritual) would you have?

In 1990, NANDA officially defined *nursing diagnosis* as "a clinical judgment about individual, family, or community responses to actual or potential health problems/life processes. Nursing diagnosis provides the basis for selection of nursing interventions to achieve outcomes for which the nurse is accountable" (NANDA, 2003, p. 263). This definition emphasizes the clinical judgment aspect of diagnosing.

Recognizing Medical Diagnoses

A **medical diagnosis** describes a disease, illness, or injury. The purpose of a medical diagnosis is to identify a disease process or pathology so that appropriate treatment can be given. It is more narrowly focused than a nursing diagnosis. Todd has two medical diagnoses: chronic renal failure and type II diabetes.

Except for advanced practice nurses, nurses cannot legally diagnose or treat medical problems. Your assessment data will help the medical team to identify disease states and evaluate the effects of medical therapies. For example, if your assessment indicates that a medication does not adequately relieve a patient's pain, you would inform the primary care provider, who would prescribe a different medication or dosage. You need to know the pathophysiology of the patient's illness to understand and evaluate the effects of medical treatments and to know how to focus your assessments. The following are differences between medical and nursing diagnoses:

- *You cannot predict a patient's nursing diagnoses just by knowing his medical diagnosis or pathology.* Nursing diagnoses are human responses; and human responses are complex and unique to each person. A medical diagnosis, in contrast, remains the same as long as a particular injury or pathology is present. Todd's medical diagnosis of type II DM will not change because his body cannot use glucose normally. This is not true for his nursing diagnoses. Suppose Todd has a nursing diagnosis of Noncompliance

TABLE 4-2

Comparison of Nursing Diagnoses, Medical Diagnoses, and Collaborative Problems

	Nursing Diagnosis	Medical Diagnosis	Collaborative Problem
Definition	A clinical judgment about individual, family, or community responses to a health problem	Disease, illness, injury, or condition validated by signs and symptoms and medical diagnostic studies	Certain potential physiological complications that are always associated with a disease, test, or treatment
Focus	The individual/person	Disease, pathology, and medical treatments/ procedures	Pathophysiology (complications caused by the disease process)
Characteristics	Holistic; describes physiological, psychological, social, interpersonal, and spiritual responses	Describes disease or pathology; does not consider the broader range of human responses	Describes potential physiological complications only; not holistic
Who Diagnoses?	Professional nurse	Physicians, advanced practice nurses, physician's assistants	Nurses
Who Orders Treatment?	Professional nurse, primarily	Physician, advanced practice nurse, physician's assistants	Physician orders primary interventions; however, nurse can order some as well
Problem Status	Can be actual, potential, or possible	Actual or possible ("rule out")	Always potential; if the problem actually develops, it is then a medical diagnosis
Purpose of Nursing Interventions	Treat or prevent the problem; relieve the symptoms	Carry out medical orders for treatment; monitor for improvement or worsening of the condition.	Monitor for development of the complication; institute some, but not all, preventive interventions
Example of Diagnostic Statement	Ineffective Denial related to difficulty coping with new diagnosis of "heart attack"	Myocardial infarction	Potential complication of myocardial infarction: congestive heart failure
Example of Data to Support the Diagnosis	Waited more than 6 hours before coming to hospital. Minimizes symptoms, refuses pain medications. States, "I've got to get back to work. I can't stay in the hospital." Laughing, joking, saying, "It's nothing."	Cardiac enzymes elevated; has had severe chest pain; elevated white blood cell count; ECG and echocardiogram diagnostic of cardiac muscle ischemia	58-year-old man with diagnosis of myocardial infarction (MI); acknowledges chest pain; ECG and lab work diagnostic of MI

with diabetic diet related to lack of knowledge about food groups. If he learns about the foods and begins following his diet, he would no longer have this nursing diagnosis. But he would still have the medical diagnosis of type II DM.

- *A medical diagnosis, disease, or pathological condition can have any number of nursing diagnoses associated with it.* For example, in response to his type II DM, Todd might have nursing diagnoses of Noncompliance and Risk for Impaired Skin Integrity.

- *Clients with the same medical diagnosis may have different nursing diagnoses.* Another client with type II DM may not have a diagnosis of Noncompliance, but instead may have a diagnosis of Ineffective Denial because he simply cannot accept that that he truly has diabetes. Other patients with type II DM might have diagnoses of Anxiety, Deficient Knowledge, Disturbed Body Image, and perhaps others, depending on their unique responses to the stressor, type II DM.

Recognizing Collaborative Problems

Collaborative problems are "certain physiologic complications [of diseases, medical treatments, or diagnostic studies] that nurses monitor to detect onset or changes in status" (Carpenito, 2002, p. 21). They have the following characteristics:

- *All patients who have a certain disease or treatment are at risk for developing the same complications.* That is, the collaborative problems (complications) are determined by the medical diagnosis or pathology. Consider these examples:

    Todd, because he has type II DM, has the collaborative problem Potential Complication of type II DM: hyperglycemia and/or hypoglycemia. All other patients with type II DM also have those potential complications.

    All patients having surgery have the collaborative problem Potential Complication of surgery: infection

    Use your theoretical knowledge of anatomy, physiology, microbiology, pathophysiology, and so on, as the basis for identifying the complications associated with a particular disease or treatment.

- *A collaborative problem is always a potential problem.* If it becomes *actual*, then it is no longer a collaborative problem, but a medical diagnosis requiring physician interventions. Consider what would be needed if the preceding potential complications became actual problems:

    Actual hyperglycemia (high blood glucose) or actual hypoglycemia (low blood glucose)

    Actual infection of a surgical incision

    Either condition would require medical intervention to prevent serious harm to the patient.

- *If you can prevent the complication with independent nursing interventions alone, it is not a collaborative problem.* Collaborative problems require both physician-prescribed and independent nursing interventions to prevent them or minimize the complications. Independent nursing interventions are primarily to monitor for onset of the complication, although nurses can provide some independent preventive measures.

See Figure 4–3 for an algorithm to help you differentiate nursing diagnoses from medical diagnoses and collaborative problems.

KnowledgeCheck 4–2

State whether each of the following represents a nursing diagnosis, medical diagnosis, or collaborative problem:

- All women after giving birth to a baby are at risk for developing postpartum hemorrhage.
- A patient has signs and symptoms of appendicitis, which must be treated with surgery and antibiotics.

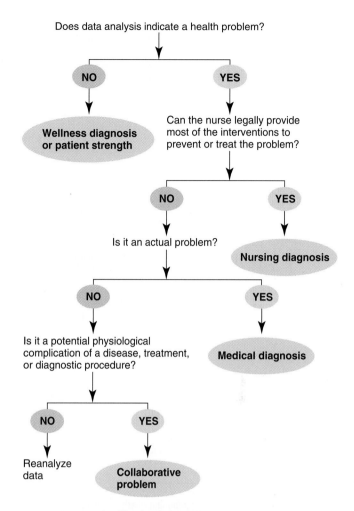

FIGURE 4–3 Algorithm for distinguishing among nursing, medical, and collaborative problems.

- A client is at risk for constipation because he postpones defecation and also does not get enough dietary fiber and fluids. The problem can be prevented by patient teaching, which the nurse is licensed to do.

 Go to Chapter 4, **Knowledge Check Response Sheet and Answers,** on the Electronic Study Guide.

Types of Nursing Diagnoses

You must determine the "status" of each nursing diagnosis—that is, is it an actual, potential, or possible problem; a wellness diagnosis; or a syndrome? This is important because each status requires (a) different wording in the diagnostic statement and (b) different nursing interventions. See Figure 4–4.

Actual Nursing Diagnosis: Problem Is Present

An **actual nursing diagnosis** is a problem response that exists at the time of the assessment. You identify it by the signs and symptoms (cues) that are present. Todd ("Meet Your Patient") may have at least one actual nursing diagnosis (Impaired Walking or perhaps

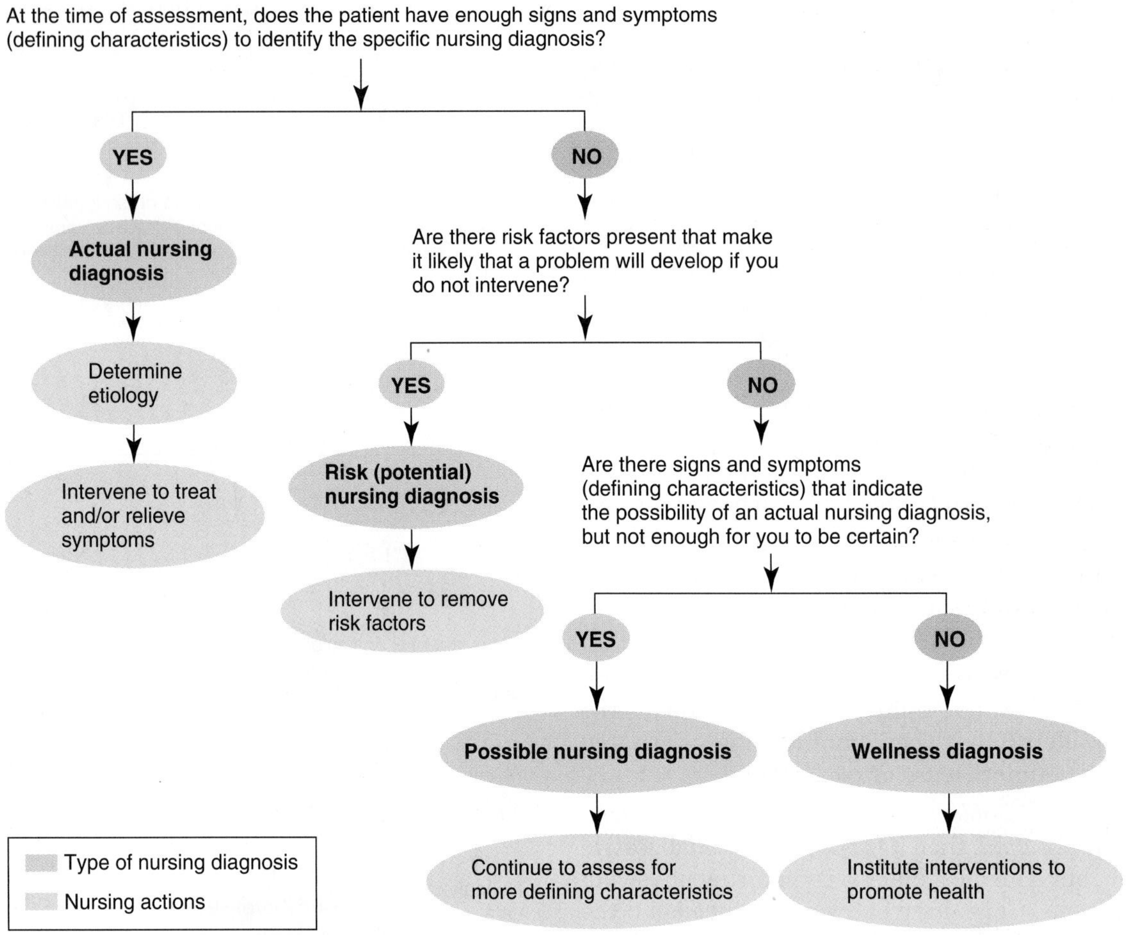

At the time of assessment, does the patient have enough signs and symptoms (defining characteristics) to identify the specific nursing diagnosis?

YES

NO

Actual nursing diagnosis

Are there risk factors present that make it likely that a problem will develop if you do not intervene?

Determine etiology

YES

NO

Intervene to treat and/or relieve symptoms

Risk (potential) nursing diagnosis

Are there signs and symptoms (defining characteristics) that indicate the possibility of an actual nursing diagnosis, but not enough for you to be certain?

Intervene to remove risk factors

YES

NO

Possible nursing diagnosis

Wellness diagnosis

Type of nursing diagnosis

Nursing actions

Continue to assess for more defining characteristics

Institute interventions to promote health

FIGURE 4–4   Algorithm for determining whether a nursing diagnosis is an actual diagnosis, a risk (potential) diagnosis, a possible diagnosis, or a wellness diagnosis.

Impaired Physical Mobility), related to his lack of peripheral sensation; however, no signs and symptoms were given in the scenario to support that diagnosis.

Risk Nursing Diagnosis: Problem May Occur

A **risk nursing diagnosis** describes a problem response that is likely to develop in a vulnerable patient if the nurse does not intervene to prevent it. You will identify a risk diagnosis when the patient does not have signs/symptoms of a problem, but does have risk factors present that increase his vulnerability. For example, Todd's loss of lower limb sensation is a risk factor for a diagnosis of Risk for Falls; however, Todd has no symptoms or history of falling.

Use risk nursing diagnoses only for patients who have more susceptibility to the problem than others in the same or comparable setting. For example, all surgical patients have at least some risk for developing infection, so you should not routinely write Risk for Infection on every surgical care plan. You would, instead, write Potential Complication of surgery: infection (incision and systemic). Use the nursing diagnosis Risk for Infection for patients who are *unusually* susceptible

to infection (e.g., one who is undernourished or one with a compromised immune system).

Possible Nursing Diagnosis: Problem May Be Present

A **possible nursing diagnosis** exists when your intuition and experience direct you to suspect that a diagnosis is present, but you do not have enough data to support the diagnosis. The main reason for including this type of diagnosis on a care plan is to alert other nurses to continue to collect data to confirm or rule out the problem. Todd ("Meet Your Patient") has a symptom of slightly impaired mobility. This could indicate the diagnoses Impaired Physical Mobility, Impaired Walking, or Risk for Falls. You need more data in order to decide which nursing diagnosis is appropriate, so you might write a nursing diagnosis of Possible Risk for Falls related to decreased sensation in both legs.

Syndrome Nursing Diagnosis: Several Related Problems Are Present

A **syndrome nursing diagnosis** represents a collection of nursing diagnoses that usually occur together. For example, the NANDA label Risk for Disuse Syndrome is

used to represent all the complications that can occur as a result of immobility (e.g., pressure ulcer, constipation, stasis of pulmonary secretions, thrombosis, body image disturbance).

Wellness Nursing Diagnosis: No Problem Is Present

You will use a **wellness diagnosis** when an individual, group, or community is in transition from one level of wellness to a higher level of wellness. A wellness diagnosis describes health status, but it is not a health problem. For you to make a wellness diagnosis, two conditions must be present: (1) The client's present level of wellness is effective, and (2) the client wants to move to a higher level of wellness.

KnowledgeCheck 4–3

- What are the five types of nursing diagnoses?
- What kind of nursing diagnosis is each of the following?
  - a. Jane Thomas regularly engages in exercise but tells you she would like to increase her endurance.
  - b. Mrs. King has several of the signs and symptoms (defining characteristics) of the nursing diagnosis Ineffective Coping.
  - c. Alicia Hernandez seems anxious, but you are not sure. You would like to have more data in order to diagnose or rule out a diagnosis of Anxiety.
  - d. Charles Oberfeldt has no symptoms of constipation. However, he reports that he does not include many fiber-rich foods in his diet and drinks few liquids. In addition, he is now fairly inactive because of a back injury. These are all risk factors for a diagnosis of Constipation.

 Go to Chapter 4, **Knowledge Check Response Sheet and Answers,** on the Electronic Study Guide.

WHAT IS DIAGNOSTIC REASONING?

A comprehensive patient assessment produces a great deal of data. **Diagnostic reasoning** is the thinking process that enables you to make sense of it. In diagnostic reasoning, you will use your critical thinking to analyze and interpret data, draw conclusions about the patient's health status, verify problems with the patient, prioritize the problems, and record the diagnostic statements.

This text presents diagnostic reasoning in separate steps so that it is easier to learn, but that is not the way it really occurs (Figure 4–5). When you first begin to use diagnostic reasoning, use the steps "in order" so that you will not miss anything. But just as you move back and forth between assessing and diagnosing, you will soon find yourself moving back and forth between the steps of diagnostic reasoning, skipping steps, returning to previous steps, and doing some steps simultaneously.

Analyzing and Interpreting Data

As you analyze and interpret the data, you will gradually narrow the quantity of data you must deal with.

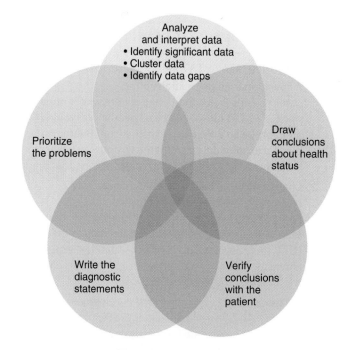

FIGURE 4–5   The diagnostic reasoning process.

But even as you narrow the field of data to the significant points and patterns, you will note the need for new information and further assessments. To analyze and interpret data, follow three steps: (1) identify significant data, (2) cluster cues, and (3) identify data gaps and inconsistencies.

1. Identify Significant Data

Significant data (also called **cues**) are data that influence your conclusions about the client's health status. A cue should alert you to look for other cues that might be related to it (form a pattern). You may be thinking, "How will I recognize a cue?"

A cue is usually an unhealthy response. One way to recognize cues is to draw on your theoretical knowledge (e.g., of anatomy, physiology, psychology, and so on) and compare each piece of data to standards and norms. For example, suppose you have noted that a woman's pulse rate is 110 beats per minute (bpm). Is this an unhealthy response—a cue? You would of course use as one standard the average rate (80 bpm) and normal range (60–100) for an adult pulse. But this woman is a long-time cigarette smoker who also drinks coffee and colas (both caffeinated beverages). These habits increase pulse rate, so 110 bpm may be a normal finding for this client. See Box 4–2 for other indications of cues.

KnowledgeCheck 4–4

- What is a cue?
- What are five ways you can recognize a cue?

 Go to Chapter 4, **Knowledge Check Response Sheet and Answers,** on the Electronic Study Guide.

BOX 4-2　Recognizing Cues

The following may indicate cues.

1. A deviation from population norms.
   Example: For a well-conditioned athlete who is not a smoker, a heart rate of 120 beats per minute would probably be an unhealthy response (cue). But remember that in addition, you must always consider whether the response is normal for the patient or the situation.

2. Changes in usual health patterns that are not explained by developmental or situational changes.
   Example: What change has Todd ("Meet Your Patient") experienced in the 3 days before admission to the ED? Is there any developmental or situational explanation for his decreased sensation and mobility? No. It is an unhealthy response: a cue.

3. Indications of delayed growth and development.
   Example: A 17-year-old girl has not yet experienced menses, her breasts are just barely developed, and she has very scant pubic and underarm hair.

4. Changes in usual behaviors in roles or relationships.
   Example: During her first year at college, a previously successful student begins to skip classes. She stays up late partying and sleeps most of the day. She no longer keeps in contact with her friends, and despite a previous close relationship with her parents, she barely talks to them when they telephone.

5. Nonproductive or dysfunctional behavior.
   This may or may not be a change in behavior. It could be a long-standing dysfunctional behavior. *Example:* A man has been drinking heavily for many years, even though it is causing many problems with his family and job and has begun to damage his liver.

Source: Gordon, M. (1994). *Nursing diagnosis: Process and application* (3rd ed.). St Louis: C V Mosby.

2. Cluster Cues

A **cluster** is a group of cues that are related to each other in some way. The cluster may suggest a health problem. To help ensure accuracy, you should always derive a nursing diagnosis from data clusters rather than from a single cue. Consider this example. Alma was transferred to the hospital from a long-term care facility. Because of a CVA (cerebrovascular accident, or stroke), Alma can make sounds but cannot speak; and because of joint contractures, she cannot use her hands and arms. Alma is frequently incontinent of urine, so the nurses have diagnosed Total Urinary Incontinence and are resigned to the idea that Alma will not be able to control her urine. Because Alma makes loud vocal noises, they have placed her in a room near the nurses' station. When Alma is assigned to the care of a nursing student, the student looks for cues in addition to urinary incontinence. The student notices that urinary incontinence often occurs after loud vocalizing by Alma. She sees a pattern in these cues: urinary incontinence, cannot use hands and arms, and cannot communicate verbally. The student changes the nursing diagnosis to Self-Care Deficit: Toileting related to immobility and inability to communicate the need to void. After the student provides a call device that fits under Alma's arm, Alma is able to press the device and call the nurse when she needs to void. She is no longer incontinent of urine.

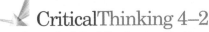 CriticalThinking 4–2

For each of the following cue clusters, decide whether the cues represent a pattern; that is, are all the cues related in some way? If so, explain how they are related. If not, state which cue does not fit. If you do not have enough theoretical knowledge to know for sure, draw on your past experiences and discuss the clusters with other students.

a. Dry skin, abnormal return of skin turgor (more than 4 seconds), thirst, and scanty, dark yellow urine
b. Pain and limited range of motion in knees, uses walker, medical diagnosis of osteoarthritis
c. Has hard, painful bowel movement about every 3 days; does not exercise regularly; eats very little dietary fiber; dry skin

Clustering data forces you to think about the relationships between the cues. For item (c) in the preceding example, you would think, "What might cause hard, painful BMs? I know that dietary fiber promotes peristalsis, so lack of fiber might contribute to constipation. And I remember that lack of exercise is associated with constipation. I don't see how dry skin would be related to constipation."

3. Identify Data Gaps and Inconsistencies

As you cluster and think about relationships among the cues, you will identify the need for data that was not apparent before. In the preceding constipation example (c), you have enough data to support a diagnosis of Constipation. However, you still need to identify factors contributing to the problem. You have two: lack of dietary fiber and lack of exercise. But you should also ask about other causes of Constipation. How much fluid does the client drink? Does he postpone defecation? Does he have a history of relying on laxatives?

As another example, look again at Todd's data ("Meet Your Patient"). Except for medical diagnoses, there is really very little data. The following data gaps exist:

- His admitting diagnosis, chronic renal failure, suggests the possibility of fluid imbalance; however, there is no other data to support that. What is his

intake? His output? His skin turgor? The appearance of his urine? Does he have edema? Does he complain of thirst? What are his hemoglobin and hematocrit levels?

- Admission to the ED could cause Anxiety. If you wish to pursue that line of thinking, you will need to observe for physical and verbal symptoms of Anxiety.

- Decreased sensation in his lower extremities might create mobility or safety problems. However, you would need to know the degree of sensation loss and the exact meaning of "slight loss of mobility" to determine whether to focus on the mobility or the safety issue.

- The effect of diabetes on the circulation and the skin certainly places Todd at risk for skin problems. However, you need more data to determine whether he has any actual skin problems (e.g., presence or history of sores on his feet).

In addition to missing data, look for inconsistencies in the data. Suppose a client tells you, "I really don't eat much. Three meals a day, and I don't snack between meals." However, she is 5 ft tall and weighs 190 lb. This seems inconsistent because your theoretical knowledge tells you that obesity is usually caused by excessive intake of calories. It is hard to imagine how someone could be so much overweight without "eating much." In this case, you would need more specific data about what the client actually eats; consider having her keep a food diary of everything she eats for a week or two. What else would you want to know? For example, does she have any medical problems that might cause obesity (e.g., hypothyroidism)? Is there any reason she might not want to tell you the truth about her eating pattern? Does she know the number of calories in various foods?

Drawing Conclusions About Health Status

After clustering cues and collecting any missing data, the next step is to begin drawing conclusions about the patient's health status—strengths as well as problems. Possible conclusions are that the cluster represents:

- *A patient strength.* If data seems to meet standards and norms, you can conclude that the patient has a strength in that area. Using Todd as an example, his strengths might include his marital status, family involvement, and employment status.

- *No problem or a wellness diagnosis.* If data seems to meet standards and norms and no nursing interventions are needed, you can conclude that no problem exists in that area. If, in addition, the patient expresses the wish to achieve a higher level of wellness, you would make a wellness diagnosis.

- *A possible problem.* This means that there are cues that suggest a problem, but ongoing monitoring will be needed to confirm or rule out the problem.

- *An actual nursing diagnosis.* You reach this conclusion when a cue cluster contains the signs and symptoms (defining characteristics) of a problem that you can treat independently.

- *A risk (potential) nursing diagnosis.* You reach this conclusion when a cue cluster contains risk factors that make nursing interventions necessary to keep a problem from developing.

- *A collaborative problem.* The client's medical diagnosis or treatment indicates the need to monitor for development of complications and to take some measures to prevent the complication.

- *A medical diagnosis.* Nurses are not licensed to make medical diagnoses. If you recognize signs and symptoms suggestive of a medical diagnosis, refer them to a physician for diagnosis and treatment.

4. Make Inferences

Making inferences is a critical thinking skill. Recall that cues are facts (or data), whereas inferences are conclusions (judgments, interpretations) that are based on the data. An inference is not a fact, because you cannot directly check its truth or accuracy. For example:

Fact: Patient is crying. (You can observe that directly.)
             Patient is trembling. (You can observe that directly.)
Inference: Patient is anxious. (You cannot observe anxiety, but you know that crying and trembling may be signs of anxiety.)

Even though you cannot ever be completely sure that an inference is accurate, clearly some inferences are supported by more data than others. In the preceding example, suppose you said to the patient, "You seem upset. Can you tell me what's going on?" Suppose the patient replied, "I've never been in the hospital before, and so much has been happening, I guess I'm just anxious about everything." Now you have enough data to support your inference, and you can be reasonably sure that it is accurate (valid). But remember, you cannot be absolutely certain. For example, although it is unlikely, the patient might not be telling you the truth. Perhaps she is crying because her husband said cruel things to her, and she is too embarrassed to share that with you. Or perhaps she is a spy and is trying to divert your attention while an accomplice finds the hospital's hidden secrets. Yes, that is ridiculous; but this exaggerated example should convince you that an inference—even one that appears to be more valid than this one—is not a *fact*.

This is an important point in diagnosing. Nursing diagnoses, because they are inferences, are only your reasoned judgment about a patient's health status. So try not to think of a diagnosis as right or wrong, but

instead as more or less accurate. Realize that you can never write a "perfect" diagnosis, but strive to make your diagnostic statements as accurate as possible. Inaccurate diagnoses result in ineffective care.

KnowledgeCheck 4–5

- What are the possible conclusions you can draw about a client's health status (e.g., that no problem exists)?
- What is the difference between a cue and an inference?
- How can you be satisfied that you have made a valid inference?

 Go to Chapter 4, **Knowledge Check Response Sheet and Answers,** on the Electronic Study Guide.

5. Identify Problem Etiologies

A problem **etiology** consists of the factors that you believe are causing or contributing to the problem. Etiologies may be pathophysiological, treatment related, situational, social, spiritual, maturational, or environmental. It is important to identify the etiology correctly because it directs the nursing interventions. For example, for a diagnosis of Constipation related to inadequate intake of dietary fiber, the etiology suggests that you encourage the client to eat more high-fiber foods. You might also teach the client about foods that are high in fiber. But what if that etiology is incomplete? What if you overlooked the fact that the client does not drink enough fluids? And what if you didn't realize that he often postpones defecation when he feels the urge because he is a kindergarten teacher in a crowded, bustling classroom, and he simply cannot leave the children unattended except at scheduled times. In that case, your efforts to increase intake of high-fiber foods would probably not help relieve the person's constipation.

To identify the etiology of a health problem, use your theoretical knowledge (e.g., of psychology, physiology, disease processes) and the patient data to answer questions such as the following:

- What factors are known to cause this problem?
- What patient cues are present that may be contributing to this problem?
- How likely is it that these factors are contributing to the problem?
- What past experiences do I have that support my judgment that these factors are linked to the problem?
- Are these cues *causing* the problem, or are they merely *symptoms* of the problem?

An etiology is always an inference because you can never actually observe the "link" between etiology and problem. You can often be certain that the etiological factors are present. For example, in the nursing diagnosis "Constipation related to inadequate intake of dietary fiber," you could measure (observe) the person's fiber intake. You could also observe infrequent, hard

stools (Constipation). But you cannot observe that the lack of fiber is the cause of the Constipation. You have to infer that link based on your knowledge of normal elimination and your experiences with other patients.

CriticalThinking 4–3

- How would your nursing interventions be different for the following?
  a. Constipation related to lack of knowledge about laxative use
  b. Constipation related to weakened abdominal muscles secondary to long-term immobility
- How would your nursing interventions be different for the following?
  a. Ineffective Breastfeeding related to lack of knowledge about breastfeeding techniques
  b. Ineffective Breastfeeding related to inability of infant to latch on to the breast and to coordinate sucking and swallowing, secondary to prematurity

Verifying Problems with the Patient

After identifying problems and etiologies, verify them with the patient to help ensure that your conclusions are accurate. A diagnostic statement is an interpretation of the data, and the patient's interpretations may differ from yours. For example, if you have diagnosed Ineffective Breastfeeding related to lack of knowledge about breastfeeding techniques, you might verify it by saying, "It seems to me that you are having difficulty breastfeeding the baby because you are not sure how to position him and get him to latch onto your breast. Does this seem accurate to you?" The woman might confirm your diagnosis, or she might say, "No. I *do* know how to do it; I am just tired and a little nervous with you watching me." Think of nursing diagnoses as tentative, and remain open to changing them based on new data or insights from the patient.

Prioritizing Problems

Up to this point, the diagnostic process has focused on identifying and validating health problems. However, clients often have more than one problem, so you must use nursing judgment to decide which ones to address initially and which can wait until later. This is **prioritizing.** Prioritizing places the problems in order of importance, but it does not mean that you must resolve one problem before attending to another. Problem priority is largely determined by the theoretical framework you use—for example, whether your criteria are human needs, problem urgency, future consequences, or patient preference.

Maslow's Hierarchy of Human Needs

Even though it is not a nursing framework, many nurses use Maslow's hierarchy to prioritize nursing

diagnoses. In Maslow's model, basic needs must be met before a person can focus on higher needs. Maslow (1970) ranks human needs on the following five levels, beginning with the most basic needs:

1. *Physiological.* Survival needs such as food, air, water, shelter, sleep and rest, elimination, activity, and temperature regulation. Examples: Imbalanced Nutrition: Less Than Body Requirements, Impaired Gas Exchange
2. *Safety and security.* This includes both physical and psychologic safety and security. Examples: Risk for Falls, Fear, Risk for Self-Directed Violence
3. *Love and belonging.* This includes roles and relationships, the need to give and receive affection, and the feeling of belonging. Examples: Impaired Social Interaction, Ineffective Sexuality Pattern, Risk for Impaired Parent/Infant/Child Attachment
4. *Self-esteem.* The person needs to feel good about himself or herself, that is, to feel confident, capable and independent. The person also needs respect, recognition, and appreciation from others. Examples: Chronic Low Self-Esteem, Social Isolation
5. *Self-actualization.* This is the need to develop one's abilities and qualities to the full extent possible, to achieve one's maximum potential. It would be rare for a nursing diagnosis to fall into this category; however, perhaps some wellness diagnoses might.

Kalish (1983) divides Maslow's physiological needs into the need for survival and stimulation, with survival being the most basic:

Survival. Food, air, water, temperature, elimination, rest, pain avoidance (e.g., Chronic Pain)
Stimulation. Activity, sex, exploration, manipulation, novelty (e.g., Impaired Walking)

For further information on the Maslow theory, see Chapter 8.

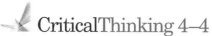

CriticalThinking 4–4

Prioritize the following nursing diagnosis labels (problems) based on the Kalish-Maslow framework. (1) First assign each diagnosis a high, medium, or low priority. Some may have the same priority. (2) Next rank them in order of importance, with 1 being most important and 5 being least important; use each number only once.

Ineffective Airway Clearance
Ineffective Breathing Pattern
Diarrhea
Risk for Falls
Impaired Memory

Problem Urgency

If you use problem urgency as your ranking criteria, you would rank the problems according to the degree of threat they pose to the patient's life or to the immediacy with which treatment is needed. Assign:

High priority to problems that are life-threatening (e.g., Ineffective Airway Clearance) or that could have a destructive effect on the client (e.g., substance abuse)
Medium priority to problems that do not pose a direct threat to life, but which may cause destructive physical or emotional changes (e.g., Ineffective Denial, Unilateral Neglect)
Low priority to problems that require minimal supportive nursing intervention (e.g., Risk for Delayed Development, Interrupted Breastfeeding, mild Anxiety)

Future Consequences

When assigning priorities, also consider the possible future effects of a problem. Even if a problem is not life-threatening, and even if the patient does not see the problem as a priority, it may result in harmful future consequences for the patient. For example, suppose that Todd ("Meet Your Patient") is hospitalized for 5 days and undergoes inpatient dialysis. His physician prescribes a renal diet and insulin (instead of his previous oral medications) for his DM. Todd announces that he would like to go home as soon as possible. "I need to get back to my job and my family," he tells you. He resists learning about his medicines and how to administer his insulin. "Just give me a list of my medicines, and I'll take them when I get home," he says. You are aware that his renal failure is secondary to uncontrolled DM and that he was very erratic about taking his medicines in the past. You suspect that he has not been taking his medicines because he is in denial about his health problems. Clearly his Ineffective Denial may lead to further problems with his treatment plan. You would assign high priority to this problem and address this problem before attempting to provide teaching for his nursing diagnosis of Deficient Knowledge (insulin).

Patient Preference

Give high priority to problems the patient thinks are most important, provided that this does not conflict with basic/survival needs or medical treatments. Patients cooperate more fully with interventions they consider important. In addition, they may be more motivated to work on other problems after their perceived priorities are addressed.

Consider this example. Mr. Amani has had a major surgery within the past 24 hours. His main concern is to obtain pain relief. He refuses to turn, cough and deep-breathe (TCDB) because it causes pain. However, as his nurse, you realize that these activities are essential for preventing Ineffective Airway Clearance, so you cannot safely agree with Mr. Amani's priorities. You should of

course, provide pain medication prior to helping him TCDB, but it may be impossible for him to be entirely pain-free during these activities. You would explain your actions and continue to emphasize the importance of TCDB. Often when you explain the importance of your priorities, patients come to agree with them.

Documenting Priorities

You will usually prioritize problems as you are recording them. You can indicate the priority by designating each problem as high, medium, or low priority or by ranking all the problems in order from highest to lowest (i.e., 1, 2, 3, and so on). For example:

Labeling Each Problem	Ranking the Problems
Pain (high)	1—Risk for Falls
Risk for Falls (high)	2—Pain
Chronic Low Self-Esteem (low)	3—Imbalanced Nutrition
Imbalanced Nutrition (medium)	4—Chronic Low Self-Esteem

Notice that risk problems can have a higher priority than actual problems. In this case, it is more urgent to prevent falls than to treat low self-esteem.

 CriticalThinking 4–5

Suppose that upon his transfer from the ED, you made the following nursing diagnoses for Todd ("Meet Your Patient"):

Risk for Imbalanced Fluid Volume secondary to renal failure
Risk for Falls related to decreased sensation and mobility in legs
Anxiety r/t unknown prognosis of renal failure and ED environment
Deficient Knowledge (renal disease process) r/t new diagnosis of renal involvement secondary to type II DM

Using problem urgency as your criterion, assign each of these diagnoses a low, medium, or high priority. You may not have much theoretical knowledge about type II DM and chronic renal disease, but use the information provided in the scenario and in the etiologies to prioritize as well as you can. Discuss the situation with your classmates and your instructor.

Computer-Assisted Diagnosing

Many nurses use computers for planning and documenting patient care. Some expert (knowledge-based) systems allow you to enter assessment data, and the computer program will generate a list of possible problems. After you choose a problem label, the computer will then provide a screen with the definition and defining characteristics of the problem so you can compare them to the actual patient data. After you "accept" the diagnostic label, you complete the problem statement by choosing etiologies from the next computer screen. To see examples of such computer screens,

 Go to Chapter 4, **Tables, Boxes, Figures: ESG Figures 4–1 and 4–2,** on the Electronic Study Guide.

KnowledgeCheck 4–6

List the steps in the diagnostic process.

 Go to Chapter 4, **Knowledge Check Response Sheet and Answers,** on the Electronic Study Guide.

REFLECTING CRITICALLY ON YOUR DIAGNOSTIC REASONING PROCESS

An inaccurate diagnosis is useless and can even be harmful. Diagnostic reasoning is complex and vulnerable to error, so after you have your prioritized list of problems, you need to evaluate the list for accuracy. When diagnosing, you apply critical thinking to your theoretical and personal knowledge and to the patient data (recall the full-spectrum nursing model in Chapter 2).

Critical thinking + Knowledge + Data
= Statement of health status

Think About Your Theoretical Knowledge

The better your knowledge base, the better your diagnostic reasoning. Ask yourself the following questions:

• Is my diagnosis based on sound knowledge (e.g., of pathophysiology, psychology, nutrition, and other related disciplines)?

• Do I have sound knowledge about the defining characteristics associated with various nursing diagnoses?

• Do I feel reasonably sure I have interpreted the data correctly?

• Have I identified the problem type correctly—that is, can this problem be treated primarily by nursing interventions?

• Am I qualified to make this diagnosis, or should I ask for consultation (e.g., from a more experienced nurse or a physician)?

To avoid diagnostic error, build a good knowledge base and learn from your clinical experiences. If you lack knowledge in an area, review the literature. A good knowledge base will help you to (1) recognize cues and patterns, (2) associate patterns with the correct problem, (3) give you confidence in your ability to reason, and (4) keep you from relying too much on authority figures (Wilkinson, 2001).

Think About Your Self Knowledge

Realize that your beliefs, values, and experiences affect your thinking and can be misleading. For example,

imagine that a nurse in a labor and delivery unit believes it is important to be strong and uncomplaining, even when experiencing severe pain. When this nurse cares for a woman in early labor who cries out and complains of pain, the nurse sees it as a problem of either Anxiety or Ineffective Coping, not as a problem of Pain. Can you see how that changes the focus of the nurse's care? Ask yourself the following questions (Wilkinson, 2001).

- *What biases and stereotypes may have influenced my interpretation of the data?* A **bias** is the tendency to slant your judgment, as the nurse did in the preceding example. **Stereotypes** are judgments and expectations about an individual based on the beliefs you have about his group (e.g., men are unemotional, Asians are smart, fat people are lazy, teenagers are irresponsible). Referring to patients by their diagnosis or developmental group is a form of stereotyping (e.g., "the elderly man in room 110"; "the broken hip in 288"). You form stereotypes by making assumptions when you have little or no actual experience with a person or group.

- *Did I rely too much on past experiences?* This is like stereotyping in that you draw conclusions about an individual based on what you know about people in similar situations. Consider, for example, a nurse who has cared for many first-time mothers (primiparas) during labor. Most of these women experienced moderate anxiety even during early labor. Now each time the nurse cares for a primipara, she expects to see anxiety, and she tends to identify cue clusters as Anxiety, failing to check for other explanations such as Pain or Deficient Knowledge.

- *Did I rely too much on the client's medical diagnosis, the setting, or what others say about the client (e.g., "He's angry and uncooperative") instead of on the data?* Medical diagnoses and statements from others can help you to think of possible explanations for your data, but they can also bias your thinking and prevent you from gathering your own data. For example, Ms Grayson has cancer. She arrived back on the unit last evening after undergoing a total colectomy and colostomy (removal of the colon and creation of an artificial opening for removal of stool). She had expected to have only an exploratory laparotomy surgery to evaluate abdominal symptoms. This morning in report, the night shift nurse stated, "Ms Grayson is aware of her cancer and is coping well." While providing a bedbath for Ms Grayson, you begin to tell her about her colostomy. She seems shocked. "I didn't know they did that! What's wrong with me?" As you answer her questions, you realize that she has been very groggy from the anesthesia and pain medication and does not recall being told about her surgery and cancer.

Think About Your Analysis and Conclusions

After reflecting on your knowledge, think about how you used the diagnostic process. Be sure that your analysis of the data was thorough, that you have accurately identified the patient's problems, and that they are logically linked to the etiologies. Review your interactions with the patient: Do the diagnostic statements reflect his perceptions and priorities, or did he just give you the answers he thought you wanted? Box 4–3 provides questions to use in critiquing your diagnostic process.

KnowledgeCheck 4–7

To help you fix them in your mind, list at least 10 questions to ask yourself when evaluating your diagnostic reasoning. Refer to Box 4–3 if you need help answering this question.

 Go to Chapter 4, **Knowledge Check Response Sheet and Answers,** on the Electronic Study Guide.

Practical Knowledge
knowing how

After you have completed the diagnostic reasoning process, the final activity in diagnosis is to record the strengths and problem statements (nursing diagnoses or collaborative problems). Practical knowledge regarding nursing diagnosis involves selecting the correct standardized problem labels and writing the diagnostic statements.

HOW ARE DIAGNOSTIC STATEMENTS WRITTEN?

This section explains the need for standardized languages, describes the NANDA standardized terminology for nursing diagnoses, explains how to choose the correct label, and describes formats for nursing diagnosis and collaborative problem statements.

Standardized Nursing Languages

In order to communicate, people need a shared language. A **standardized language** is one in which the terms are carefully defined and mean the same thing to all who use them. One example is the periodic table for chemical elements. When a chemist in New York writes Fe or Zn, all other chemists in the world know that she means iron or zinc. Moreover, they know exactly what is meant by iron and zinc, because each is defined by its own atomic number, atomic mass, number of protons, number of neutrons, and so on. There is no confusion. **Standardized nursing languages** are a

BOX 4-3   Critiquing Your Diagnostic Reasoning Process

Data Analysis

Did you:

- Identify all the significant data (cues)?
- Omit any important cues from the cluster?
- Include unnecessary cues that may have confused your interpretation?
- Try more than one way of grouping the cues?
- Consider the patient's social, cultural, and spiritual beliefs and needs?
- Identify all the data gaps and inconsistencies?

Drawing Inferences and Interpretations of the Data

- Did you consider all the possible explanations for the cue cluster?
- Is this the best explanation for the cue cluster? *Remember that a variety of explanations may be possible. Look for the best one based on your knowledge and the data.*
- Did you have enough data to make that inference? *When the data are insufficient, you should suspend judgment until you gather more data.*
- Did you look at patterns, not single cues?
- Did you look at behavior over time, not just isolated incidents?
- Did you jump to conclusions? *Always take the time to carefully analyze and synthesize the data.*

Critiquing the Diagnostic Statement (Problem + Etiology)

- Is the diagnosis relevant, and does it reflect the data?
- Does the diagnostic statement give a clear and accurate picture of the patient's problem or strength?
- When identifying the problem and etiology, did you look beyond medical diagnoses and consider human responses?
- Did you consider strengths and wellness diagnoses?
- Can you explain how the etiology relates to the problem—that is, how it would produce the problem response?
- Does the complete list of problems fully describe the patient's overall health status?

Verifying the Diagnosis

- Did the patient verify this diagnosis?
- When you verified the diagnosis, did you explain clearly enough? Are you certain that the patient understood your description of his health status?
- Did you obtain feedback from the patient, or did you just assume that the patient agreed?
- Did you keep an open mind, realizing that all diagnoses are tentative and subject to change as you acquire more data?

Prioritizing

- Considering the whole situation, what are the most important problems?
- What aspects of the situation require immediate attention?
- Did you consider patient preferences when setting priorities? If not, was there a good reason?

---

comparatively recent attempt to bring clarity to communication about nursing knowledge and nursing thinking.

Nurses need clear, precise, consistent terminology when referring to the same clinical problems and treatments. A uniform language can do the following:

- Support computerized patient records
- Define and communicate nursing knowledge
- Expand nursing knowledge
- Facilitate research to demonstrate the contribution of nurses to health care
- Facilitate research to influence health policy decisions
- Improve patient care by facilitating the testing of nursing interventions

For a full discussion of the benefits of a uniform nursing language

 Go to Chapter 4, **Supplemental Materials: Why Do We Need a Standardized Nursing Language?,** on the Electronic Study Guide.

What Is a Taxonomy?

A **taxonomy** is a system for classifying ideas or objects based on characteristics they have in common. Classifications are created and used for various reasons. The periodic table classifies elements according to their atomic mass, number of protons, and so on. Medications are classified in various ways; one way is to classify them according to their use (e.g., analgesics, antibiotics). The following classification systems are widely used in health care:

- The American Psychiatric Association (APA) *Diagnostic and Statistical Manual (DSM-IV)* describes mental disorders (e.g., bipolar disorder, schizoaffective disorder).
- The *International Classification of Disease (ICD-10)* names and classifies medical conditions (World Health Organization, 1992)

- The *Current Procedural Terminology (CPT)*, used for reimbursement of physician services, names and defines medical services and procedures (American Medical Association, 2006).

The following are classification systems that the American Nurses Association (ANA) has recognized for describing nursing diagnoses (some describe outcomes and interventions as well):

- *NANDA.* The first use of standardized nursing language began in the 1970s, with the NANDA classification of nursing diagnoses. This taxonomy includes over 170 diagnostic labels with etiologies, risk factors, and defining characteristics. Most chapters of this textbook will use NANDA terminology.

- *Clinical Care Classification (CCC).* Similar to the NANDA system. Contains interventions as well as nursing diagnoses. The CCC is primarily for home health use.

- *Omaha System.* Contains 42 nursing diagnoses (also interventions and outcomes). The Omaha system is primarily for community health use.

- *Perioperative Nursing Data Set (PNDS).* For use in perioperative nursing only. Consists of 64 nursing diagnoses (also includes nursing interventions and patient outcomes). This was the first nursing language developed by a nursing specialty.

- *International Classification for Nursing Practice (ICNP).* Includes diagnoses, outcomes, and nursing actions. The ICNP intends to provide a common language for nurses in various clinical settings worldwide.

NANDA Taxonomy of Diagnostic Terminology

Which of the following could you group together? In what ways are the grouped objects similar?

a five-dollar bill	a penny
weeds (still growing)	new grass
an iron skillet	a needle

You could group: A $5 bill and a penny (because they are both money). You could group: A penny, an iron skillet, and a needle (because they are all metal). You could group: A $5 bill, grass, and weeds (because they are all green). Maybe you even thought of other groupings. Any number of principles can be used to classify things and to organize a taxonomy.

The first NANDA taxonomy was simply an alphabetical list. To see that taxonomy,

Go to Chapter 4, **Supplemental Materials: Alphabetical List of NANDA Diagnostic Labels,** on the Electronic Study Guide.

NANDA's *Taxonomy II* (NANDA International, 2003) categorizes nursing diagnoses into 13 domains and 46 classes. A **domain** is an area of activity, study, or interest (e.g., health promotion, nutrition). A **class**

is a subdivision of a domain (e.g., health awareness is a class under health promotion; digestion is a class under nutrition).

 Go to Chapter 4, **NANDA Taxonomy II: Domains, Classes, and Diagnoses (Labels),** in Volume 2.

A strength of the NANDA taxonomy is that it has been developed by nurses from administration, education, practice, and research, and from all specialty areas (e.g., maternity, mental health, medical-surgical, community). Because they represent the thinking of a broad spectrum of nurses, the diagnostic labels can be used in any setting or specialty.

What Are the Components of a NANDA Nursing Diagnosis?

Each nursing diagnosis in the NANDA taxonomy has four parts: label, definition, defining characteristics, and related or risk factors. You must consider all four parts when formulating a nursing diagnosis.

- The **diagnostic label** (**title** or **name**) is a word or phrase that represents a pattern of related cues and describes a problem or wellness response, such as Disturbed Body Image or Readiness for Enhanced Nutrition. Some labels include descriptors for time, age, and other factors (e.g., acute, deficient, delayed). For the complete list of "Descriptors for NANDA Nursing Diagnoses,"

 Go to Chapter 4, **Descriptors for NANDA Nursing Diagnoses,** in Volume 2.

- The **definition** explains the meaning of the label and distinguishes it from similar nursing diagnoses. For example, for a patient with a sleep problem, would you label the problem Sleep Deprivation or Disturbed Sleep Pattern? The following definitions can help you to decide:

  Sleep Deprivation: Prolonged periods of time without sleep

  Disturbed Sleep Pattern: Time limited disruption of sleep amount and quality

- **Defining characteristics** are the cues (signs and symptoms) that allow you to identify a problem or wellness diagnosis. For you to use a problem label appropriately, a cluster of defining characteristics must be present in the patient data. For example, you cannot decide to use the label Sleep Deprivation merely by reading the definition. You must be sure that the patient actually has some of the defining characteristics for Sleep Deprivation.

- **Related factors** are the cues, conditions, or circumstances that cause, precede, influence, contribute to, or are in some way associated with the problem (label). They can be pathophysiological, psychological,

social, treatment-related, situational, maturational, and so on. NANDA lists the related factors that are most often associated with each problem label, but keep in mind that:

1. *The list is not exhaustive.* Factors other than those listed by NANDA could also be associated with the problem. For example, imagine the variety of factors that might cause someone to have Chronic Low Self-Esteem.

2. *The problem may have more than one related factor.* Human beings are complex, and their problems rarely have one single cause. Nursing diagnoses may have multiple factors as their etiology.

3. *An individual patient will not have all the factors on the list* in his problem etiology.

- **Risk factors** are events, circumstances, or conditions that increase the vulnerability of a person or group to a health problem. They can be environmental, physiological, psychological, genetic, or chemical. For example, ignoring the urge to defecate and being pregnant increase the risk that a person will become constipated. The diagnostic statement would be: Risk for Constipation r/t pregnancy and habitually ignoring the urge to defecate.

    For potential (risk) nursing diagnoses, risk factors function as the defining characteristics. They must be present in order to make the diagnosis, and they almost always form at least a part of the etiology of the diagnostic statement. If **related factors** are present, an actual, rather than potential, problem exists. To help you remember, as a rule:

    Related factors are similar to signs and symptoms (of actual problems)

    Risk factors are similar to etiologies (of potential problems)

KnowledgeCheck 4–8

- What are the four parts of a NANDA nursing diagnosis?
- What purpose does each part of the nursing diagnosis serve for directing the care of the client?

 Go to Chapter 4, **Knowledge Check Response Sheet and Answers,** on the Electronic Study Guide.

How Do I Know Which Label to Use?

During the diagnostic process, you will already have determined the general topic of the problem and perhaps even have some tentative problem labels in mind.

1. *First, identify the broad topic (or domain) that seems to fit the cue cluster.* You can look at the NANDA taxonomy to see which domain the problem seems to fit. For example, suppose that after further assessment, you find that Todd ("Meet Your Patient") has the following defining characteristics:

    Intake exceeds output
    Oliguria (scanty urine)
    Generalized edema
    Recent rapid weight gain

    Which of the following NANDA domains are suggested by those cues?

Health Promotion	Role Relationships
Nutrition	Self Perception
Elimination	Activity/Rest

    The most logical guesses would be Nutrition and Elimination. However, you would need to read the domain definitions in the NANDA list (in Volume 2) and look at the classes to be sure.

2. *Narrow your search (to the class or most likely labels).* In the NANDA list, read the definitions for the Nutrition and Elimination domains. Then look at the classes in each. Under Elimination, you will find that Class 1 is Urinary System. Because Todd has renal failure, you may think that his nursing diagnosis will be found in this class. However, remember that renal failure is a pathology or pathological condition; you are looking for Todd's *responses* to renal failure. On examining the diagnosis labels in the Urinary System class, you will see that none of those really represents Todd's defining characteristics.

    Now look at the Nutrition domain. You will see the classes Ingestion, Digestion, Absorption, Metabolism, and Hydration. Look at the diagnostic labels listed for the class Hydration. All five of those labels describe fluid balance. You can easily eliminate both "risk" labels because Todd has an actual problem (he has symptoms). You can eliminate Readiness for Enhanced Fluid Balance because it is a wellness diagnosis. So, you must choose between Deficient Fluid Volume and Excess Fluid Volume. From this point, you simply compare Todd's cue cluster to the defining characteristics and definitions of those two labels and choose the best match.

3. *Using a nursing diagnosis handbook, compare definitions and defining characteristics of the diagnostic labels to your cue cluster.* A brief look at the NANDA list should convince you that you cannot know exactly what a diagnostic label means from the label name alone. For example, suppose you have a patient who is not sleeping well at night. As a result, she is too tired to concentrate during the day. Which label would you use to describe this problem: Activity Intolerance, Fatigue, Acute Confusion, or Impaired Thought Processes? You can answer that question only if you know the definition and defining characteristics of those nursing diagnosis labels.

Not all of the defining characteristics need to be present, but recall that the more data you have when you make an inference, the more certain you can be that your inference is correct.

Example: NANDA lists 14 defining characteristics for Ineffective Thermoregulation, including the following:

1. Fluctuations in body temperature above and below normal range
2. Cyanotic nail beds
3. Pallor
4. Slow capillary refill
5. Tachycardia

You could diagnose Ineffective Thermoregulation on the basis of the first defining characteristic alone, but you might be more certain of your diagnosis if the other cues were also present.

 CriticalThinking 4–6

- In the preceding example, what if defining characteristic 1 were not present and you had only 2, 3, and 4 as cues? Could you conclude that Ineffective Thermoregulation is causing those signs? What other explanations might there be for cyanotic nail beds, pallor, and slow capillary refill?
- What if defining characteristic 5 were present without 1? What could cause tachycardia? Do you see the importance of using clusters rather than individual cues?

Formats for Diagnostic Statements

A diagnostic statement consists of a problem and an etiology linked by a connecting phrase.

- *Problem.* The problem describes the client's health status (or a human response to a health problem) and identifies a response that needs to be changed. Use a NANDA label when possible. As noted earlier, many NANDA labels include a descriptor such as *acute, impaired,* or *deficient.* You will see them arranged in alphabetical lists with the descriptor after the main word (e.g., Physical Mobility, Impaired). However, you should record them as you would say them; for example:

  Incorrect: Physical Mobility, Impaired r/t pain in left knee

  Correct: Impaired Physical Mobility r/t pain in left knee

- *Etiology.* As discussed earlier, the etiology contains the factors that cause, contribute to, or create a risk for the problem. The etiology may include a NANDA label, defining characteristics, related factors, risk factors, or other factors. Remember that an etiology may consist of several factors. The etiology will help you to individualize nursing care because etiologies

are unique to the individual. For example, suppose two patients have the following nursing diagnoses:

John: Anxiety r/t lack of knowledge of the treatment procedure

Janet: Anxiety r/t prior negative experiences and lack of trust in health professionals

The problem, Anxiety, is defined the same for both patients. They probably share some of the same defining characteristics, and you would use some of the same interventions for both John and Janet. For example, for all anxious patients, regardless of etiology, a calm, reassuring approach is important. However, to prevent the anxiety from recurring, you would need to treat its cause. To relieve John's anxiety, you would teach him what to expect from the impending procedure. But teaching would do nothing to relieve Janet's anxiety. For her, you would need to spend time building a trusting relationship and demonstrating that you can be trusted. You would also encourage her to talk about her fears and feelings.

Because the etiology directs the nursing interventions, include only factors that are influenced by nursing interventions. For example, it is inappropriate to use a medical diagnosis or a medical treatment as an etiology, because you cannot write nursing orders to change it. For example, there are no independent nursing actions that would change the etiologies in the following diagnosis: Deficient Fluid Volume related to medical order of NPO (nothing by mouth).

Most NANDA related factors are listed in non-specific terms, so you will usually need to individualize them to reflect each person's unique problem etiology. For example, one of the related factors for Impaired Skin Integrity is "extremes in age." In order to plan care, you need to know whether this means very old or very young; even better, you should specify the exact age. You would write the diagnostic statement as Impaired Skin Integrity r/t very young age (2 days).

- *Connecting phrase (related to).* Most nurses use *related to (r/t)* to connect the problem and etiology, believing that the phrase *due to* implies a direct causal relationship. Because human beings are complex, there are usually many factors that combine to "cause" a problem, so it is nearly impossible to prove an exact cause. In fact, even if you eliminate the etiological factors, the problem might remain. For example, even if Janet begins to trust health professionals, she may become anxious for another reason.

A diagnostic statement should describe the client's health status as specifically as possible. The format will vary depending on the type of problem you are describing. Refer to Table 4–3 for examples of different formats.

TABLE 4-3 Examples of Diagnostic Statements

Format	Problem Type	Problem (Client Response; NANDA Label)	Etiology	Defining Characteristics or "Secondary"
Basic One-Part	Wellness diagnosis	Health-Seeking Behaviors (salt-restricted diet)		
	Syndrome diagnosis	Disuse Syndrome		
	Very specific label	Death Anxiety		
Basic Two-Part	Actual problem	Impaired Social Interaction	r/t self-consciousness following amputation of bilateral lower extremities	
	Potential problem	Risk for Impaired Parent/ Infant/Child Attachment	r/t separation from infant at birth because of mother's illness	
	Possible problem	Possible Impaired Parent/ Infant/Child Attachment	r/t separation from infant at birth because of mother's illness	
Basic Three-Part	Actual Problem	Impaired Social Interaction	r/t self-consciousness following amputation of bilateral lower extremities	AEB avoidance of others, social isolation, blaming others for current condition
	Possible Problem	Impaired Social Interaction	r/t self-consciousness following amputation of bilateral lower extremities	AEB blaming others for current condition
Variations	(specify)	Decisional Conflict (whether to accept chemotherapy)	r/t desire to protect family from financial hardship of a lingering illness	
	secondary to	Decisional Conflict (whether to accept chemotherapy)	r/t desire to protect family from financial hardship of a lingering illness	secondary to diagnosis of terminal cancer
	two-part NANDA label	Imbalanced Nutrition: Less Than Body Requirements	r/t loss of appetite from nausea	secondary to side effects of chemotherapy
	adding words to the label	Impaired Physical Mobility: inability to turn self in bed	r/t generalized weakness	secondary to residual effects of stroke
	Unknown etiology	Parental Role Conflict	r/t unknown etiology or possibly r/t recent divorce	
	Complex etiology	Chronic Low Self-Esteem	r/t complex etiology	
Collaborative Problems	Potential complications of disease, test, or treatment	Potential Complication of preeclampsia: renal failure		

Basic Two-Part Statement

The two-part statement is used for actual, risk, and possible diagnoses. The format is:

> *Problem*   *r/t*   *etiology*
> or
> *NANDA label*   *r/t*   *related factors*

For actual diagnoses, the etiology consists of related factors; for risk diagnoses, it consists of risk factors. For example, for a client with excessive vomiting you might write Risk for Deficient Fluid Volume r/t excessive losses through vomiting.

Basic Three-Part Statement

The three-part statement is also called the **PES format** (problem, etiology, and symptom). Some nurses use *AEB (as evidenced by,)* whereas others use *AMB (as manifested by)*. The format is:

> *Problem r/t etiology as manifested by (AMB) signs or symptoms*

This format adds the patient signs or symptoms that led you to make the diagnosis. For example: Constipation r/t inadequate intake of fluids and fiber-rich foods AMB painful, hard stool; BM every 3 or 4 days. This is a good method for students because it helps to ensure that you have enough data to support the problem you have identified.

Although ideally the problem and etiology should thoroughly describe the patient's health status, you can sometimes make the description more clear and useful by including the cues in the statement. However, this method can create a long, unwieldy statement. For example:

> Decisional Conflict (whether to accept chemotherapy) r/t desire to protect family from financial hardship of a lingering illness AMB verbalizing uncertainty about what to do and feelings of distress; vacillation between having and not having chemo; exhibiting physical signs of anxiety (increased heart rate, restlessness); questioning personal values and beliefs ("I'm not sure what to do. I hate to leave them any sooner than I have to, but I don't want to ruin them financially, either").

For such situations, you can record the cues in the nurses' notes. Another alternative is to list the signs and symptoms below the nursing diagnosis on the care plan instead of including it as part of the statement. For example:

> Decisional Conflict (whether to accept chemotherapy) r/t desire to protect family from financial hardship of a lingering illness
>   *Subjective cues:* Verbalizes uncertainty about what to do and feelings of distress; vacillates

between having and not having chemo; questions personal values and beliefs ("I'm not sure what to do. I hate to leave them any sooner than I have to, but I don't want to ruin them financially, either").
>   *Objective cues:* Exhibits physical signs of anxiety (increased heart rate, restlessness)

Obviously you cannot use the PES format for risk nursing diagnoses, because symptoms are not present with risk diagnoses.

One-Part Statement

You can omit the etiology from certain kinds of diagnostic statements:

- *Syndrome diagnoses.* Recall that a syndrome diagnosis is a label that represents a collection of several nursing diagnoses. A syndrome diagnosis usually does not need an etiology.

- *Wellness diagnoses.* As a rule, NANDA wellness diagnoses are one-part statements beginning with the phrase Readiness for Enhanced (e.g., Readiness for Enhanced Parenting, Readiness for Enhanced Nutrition). However, some of the older labels are stated differently (e.g., Effective Breastfeeding, Health-Seeking Behaviors). Because the wellness label does not represent a problem, no etiology ("cause") is needed.

- *Very specific labels.* A few NANDA labels are so specific that they imply the etiology, or the only possible etiology is a medical diagnosis (e.g., Death Anxiety, Latex Allergy Response). For Latex Allergy Response, it would be redundant to write Latex Allergy Response r/t allergic reaction to latex. The etiology adds nothing to your understanding of the problem, nor does it suggest interventions different from those suggested by the problem label. The same is true for Death Anxiety.

Format Variations

The following are some variations of the basic two- and three-part formats.

"Specify"

You will see the word *specify* in some NANDA labels, for example, Decisional Conflict (specify). This means that the label is useful only if you describe the problem more specifically; for example, Decisional Conflict (whether to accept chemotherapy) r/t desire to protect family from financial hardship of a lingering illness.

"Secondary To"

When the defining characteristics are vague (e.g., Chronic Pain r/t chronic physical disability) you may need to add a second part to the etiology following the

words *secondary to (2°)*. This second part is usually a pathophysiology or disease process (e.g., Chronic Pain r/t chronic physical disability secondary to rheumatoid arthritis). As a rule, you should avoid using pathophysiology or medical diagnoses in the etiology because they cannot be addressed by independent nursing interventions. The words *secondary to* make it clear that the nurse is not ultimately responsible for that part of the etiology. Do not use this phrase routinely. Use it only if it adds to the understanding of your diagnostic statement.

Two-Part NANDA Label

Some NANDA labels have two parts. The first part describes a general response; the second part, following a colon, makes it more specific, for example, Imbalanced Nutrition: Less Than Body Requirements.

Adding Words to the NANDA Label

The problem label must describe the client's health status precisely because general categories are not useful for planning nursing care. For example, what do you think a problem label of Impaired Physical Mobility means? Does it mean that the patient cannot grasp objects with her hands, or that she cannot walk, or that she cannot move at all? For such labels, you will need to add your own words to the label to make it more descriptive, for example, Impaired Physical mobility: inability to turn self in bed r/t generalized weakness secondary to residual effects of stroke.

Other labels that often need to be clarified include: Acute Pain, Chronic Pain, Risk for Infection, and Risk for Injury. Think carefully about whether the clarifying words belong in the problem or the etiology. For example, you may see a pain diagnosis written as: Acute Pain r/t surgical incision. However, surgical incision is a medical treatment and should not be used as the etiology. It would be better to write: Acute Pain (abdominal incision) r/t turning and moving secondary to abdominal surgery. The "rule" for adding words is to first try to make the statement specific or descriptive by writing a good etiology, using the PES format, or adding *secondary to*. If that does not fully describe the health status, add descriptive words to the problem label.

Unknown Etiology

Sometimes you will be able to identify the patient's problem but not know the etiology. For example, your patient might have defining characteristics for Parental Role Conflict, but you may need more information in order to determine the cause. Perhaps there is an impending divorce, perhaps she has just had to take on the care of an elderly parent, and so on. In this case you could write Parental Role Conflict r/t unknown etiology. Later, when you obtain more data, you

will be able to complete the etiology. A similar situation exists when you have some, but not enough, information about the etiology. In this case you would write Parental Role Conflict possibly r/t recent divorce.

Complex Etiology

Some problems have too many etiological factors to list, or the etiology is too complex to explain in a brief diagnostic statement. For example, imagine the number of factors that might contribute to problems such as Chronic Low Self-Esteem, Disabled Family Coping, and Adult Failure to Thrive. For such problems you can replace the etiology with the phrase "complex factors" (for example, Disabled Family Coping r/t complex factors).

Collaborative Problems

A collaborative problem is always a potential problem—a complication of a disease, test, or medical treatment. The disease, test, or treatment is actually the etiology of the problem. Because you cannot treat the etiology with independent nursing interventions, you should not use the "problem + etiology" format. The focus of your interventions is monitoring for and preventing the complication. The format is:

> Potential Complication of thrombophlebitis: pulmonary embolism

As you can see, the word(s) following the colon represent the problem you are monitoring and trying to prevent.

In actual practice, you would not write an etiology for a collaborative problem. However, as a student, you may wish to do so when it clarifies your diagnostic statement or when it helps to suggest nursing interventions (Wilkinson, 2001). For example, a student statement might be:

> Potential Complication of magnesium sulfate therapy: Respiratory depression r/t increased blood levels of magnesium (Mg^{++}) because of decreased kidney function secondary to preeclampsia (a pregnancy-related disorder with hypertension as a major pathology).

In addition to alerting you to monitor for respiratory depression, this statement might help remind you to monitor the serum magnesium level, assess for other data related to kidney function, and monitor blood pressure. Again, as a professional nurse, you would *not* write an etiology.

KnowledgeCheck 4–9

Write an example of each of the following diagnostic statement formats, using the following listed components—mix and match:

> *Problem labels:* Anxiety, Pain (lower back)
> *Etiologies:* unknown outcome of surgery; muscle strain and
>   tissue inflammation;

Cues: exhibits physical manifestations of anxiety (e.g., hands shaking); states pain is 9 on a scale of 1 to 10;

- Basic two-part statement
- Basic three-part statement
- Basic two-part statement, using "secondary to" (create your own disease/pathology)
- Statement with unknown etiology
- Possible nursing diagnosis
- Risk nursing diagnosis

 Go to Chapter 4, **Knowledge Check Response Sheet and Answers,** on the Electronic Study Guide.

How Does the Nursing Diagnosis Relate to Outcomes and Interventions?

Keeping in mind that there are exceptions, as a general rule: The problem suggests goals, and the etiology suggests interventions.

The Problem Suggests Goals

The problem describes an unhealthy response—a health status that needs to be changed. From the problem, you can determine the patient outcomes for measuring this change. Consider the following diagnostic statement: Risk for Impaired Skin Integrity r/t complete immobility 2° spinal cord injury. The goal, or outcome, is the opposite of the unhealthy response: Skin will remain intact and healthy.

The problem also suggests assessments, which are nursing interventions. The diagnosis Risk for Impaired Skin Integrity tells you to monitor the patient's skin condition. If the problem is not an accurate statement of health status, then your assessments and evaluation of patient health status will be wrong. If you wrongly identified the previous problem as Impaired Physical Mobility 2° spinal cord injury, then you would monitor the patient's mobility—which would not improve—and might miss a developing skin problem.

The Etiology Suggests Interventions

The aim of the nursing interventions is to alter the factors contributing to the problem. In the preceding mobility example, you could not cure the spinal cord injury or restore the patient's ability to move about. However, you could restore some mobility by turning and repositioning the patient frequently. This would help prevent Impaired Skin Integrity.

If the etiology is incorrect or incomplete, you might omit important nursing interventions. Suppose there are missing etiological factors in the preceding skin diagnosis and that it should have read: Risk for Impaired Skin Integrity r/t poor nutritional status and complete immobility 2° spinal cord injury. You can see that interventions to support mobility would not be adequate to prevent Impaired Skin Integrity.

REFLECTING CRITICALLY ABOUT DIAGNOSTIC STATEMENTS

Just as you critiqued your diagnostic reasoning process, (see pages 68–69), you must reflect on the content, format, and meaning of your diagnostic statements.

Guidelines for Judging the Quality of Diagnostic Statements

After you have written your diagnostic statements, use the following criteria to judge their quality (Wilkinson, 2001).

1. *In choosing a NANDA label, do not rely on the label definition alone.* Always compare patient data to the defining characteristics of the label as well as to the definition.

   Example: The definition for Parental Role Conflict is "parent experience of role confusion and conflict in response to crisis." You cannot actually observe role confusion and conflict in a patient; however, the defining characteristics for this label include more specific cues, such as "Reluctant to participate in usual caretaking activities."

2. *Include both problem and etiology, with "cause and effect" stated correctly.* A quick check of this is to read your statement backwards: "Etiology causes problem," and see if it makes sense.

   Correct example:
   Diagnostic statement: Ineffective Breastfeeding r/t Deficient Knowledge (positioning infant at breast)
   Read backwards: This statement says that deficient knowledge about positioning the infant at breast "causes" Ineffective Breastfeeding. This makes sense.

   Incorrect example:
   Diagnostic statement: Deficient Knowledge r/t Ineffective Breastfeeding (incorrect positioning infant at breast)
   Read backwards: This statement says that Ineffective Breastfeeding causes deficient knowledge. This does not make sense.

3. *Be sure that the etiology does not merely restate the problem.*

   Incorrect example: Impaired Physical Mobility r/t inability to walk

   Correct example: Impaired Physical Mobility: Inability to walk r/t weakness and pain in legs

In the incorrect example, inability to walk *is* the specific impaired physical mobility. The etiology should state the factors that are causing the inability to walk.

4. *Avoid using medical diagnoses and treatments as etiological factors.* Recall that nursing interventions are directed at changing or removing the etiological factors. What could the nurse do to change the following etiology?

Incorrect example: Risk for Impaired Skin Integrity (ulcers, infection) r/t diabetes mellitus

The answer, of course, is that the nurse can do nothing to change or get rid of the DM. Try to reword the etiology in terms of something the nurse *can* change, for example:

Correct example: Risk for Impaired Skin Integrity (ulcers, infection) r/t lack of knowledge of self-care measures for inspecting feet and trimming toenails

If you cannot reword the etiology in terms of something the nurse can change, you may have identified the problem incorrectly; perhaps it is merely the stimulus for another patient problem that you can address independently. In the following example, Risk for Impaired Skin Integrity is one possible "response" to the stimulus, Impaired Physical Mobility.

Incorrect example: Impaired Physical Mobility (total) r/t paralysis secondary to high spinal injury

Correct example: Risk for Impaired Skin Integrity (pressure ulcers) r/t Impaired Physical Mobility (total) secondary to high spinal injury

If none of these seem to work, you can resort to using "secondary to" instead of "related to," as in the following example:

Risk for Deficient Fluid Volume secondary to prescribed NPO

5. *Write the statement clearly.* The statement should give a clear picture of the client's health status, and other health professionals should be able to understand it readily. Avoid abbreviations and jargon as much as possible. For example, do you know what the first statement means?

Incorrect example: Imp. Phys. Mobility (inability to get OOB w/o assist.) r/t muscle weakness and pain in LL

Correct example: Impaired Physical Mobility (inability to get out of bed without assistance) r/t muscle weakness and pain in left leg

6. *Write the statement concisely.* A wordy statement is likely to be unclear. The following will help limit statement length:
   a. Use "complex etiology" instead of listing numerous etiological factors.

   b. If there are numerous signs and symptoms, either do not use PES format, or describe the signs and symptoms in the nurses notes.

   Incorrect example: Constipation r/t habitually ignoring the urge to defecate, insufficient exercise, weak abdominal muscles, side effects of iron medications, insufficient intake of fluids and fibers, and long-standing reliance on laxatives

   Correct example: Constipation r/t complex factors (see nurses notes)

7. *Be sure the statement is descriptive and specific.* A vaguely stated problem and/or etiology cannot provide guidance for formulating goals and nursing interventions. Follow this guideline even if it means the statement is not as concise as you'd like. You can make the NANDA labels more specific by:
   a. Being sure to include all appropriate etiological factors.
   b. Reviewing the label definition. (Do not write the definition, but when you know the meaning of the label, you may find that it is descriptive enough.)
   c. Using PES format to add the patient's signs and symptoms.
   d. Adding qualifying words (e.g., "mild," "severe," "occasional," or "constant") to the label.

      Example: Severe Neck Pain r/t muscle spasms 2° herniated intervertebral disc
   e. Adding "secondary to" to the etiology.

      Example: Severe Neck Pain r/t muscle spasms 2° herniated intervertebral disc
   f. Adding a colon and descriptors to the label.

      Example: Impaired Physical Mobility: Inability to walk r/t weakness and pain in legs

8. *State the problem as a patient response.*
   a. A problem is not a patient need. As a rule, avoid using the word "need" in a problem statement. A need may cause a problem, but it is not a human response.

      Incorrect example: Needs increased fluids related to . . .

      Correct example: Risk for Deficient Fluid Volume, or Deficient Fluid Volume related to . . .
   b. A problem is not a medical test, treatment, diagnosis, or equipment.

Incorrect examples	Correct examples
Starting on diabetic diet	Deficient Knowledge, Ineffective Denial
Foley catheter in place	Risk for Infection, Urinary Retention
Risk for pneumonia	Risk for Ineffective Airway Clearance

Traction to left leg — Impaired Physical Mobility

c. A problem is not a nursing goal, a nursing problem, or a nursing action.

Incorrect examples	*Correct examples*
Prevent urinary tract infection (nursing goal)	Risk for Urinary Tract Infection
Combative, hits caregivers (nursing problem)	Risk for Other-Directed Violence Ineffective Coping; Acute Confusion
Provide emotional support	Anxiety, Decisional Conflict, Anticipatory Grieving

9. *Use nonjudgmental language.* If you examined your biases during the diagnostic process, your statements will probably be neutral. Look for phrases that may imply criticism of a patient, for example:

Incorrect: Risk for Infection r/t poor hygiene and housekeeping

Better: Risk for Infection r/t lack of information about sanitation and hand washing

10. *Avoid legally questionable language.* Be alert for legal implications. Look for phrases that seem to blame caregivers or patients or that refer negatively to patient care. For example, do not write:

Impaired Skin Integrity (excoriated perineum) r/t need for more frequent changes of clothing and linen after incontinence

Risk for Falls r/t lack of staff to adequately supervise ambulation

 CriticalThinking 4–7

Rewrite the two preceding diagnostic statements so they contain no legally questionable language. Use imaginary etiological factors if you need to.

Critiquing the NANDA System

Despite its potential benefits, some nurses have criticized the NANDA labels. Critics have pointed out that some labels are too abstract to be useful (e.g., Impaired Adjustment), other labels are merely reworded medical diagnoses (e.g., Decreased Cardiac Output), and no one outside nursing knows what the labels mean (e.g., "Why not just say 'tooth decay' or 'missing teeth' instead of 'Impaired Dentition'?") These are legitimate concerns, but as you have learned, when you know the label definition, the term

is more meaningful. Also, you can make the labels more specific and useful by adding descriptors, etiological factors, and defining characteristics to the diagnostic statement.

Another criticism is that the NANDA diagnosis labels have not been researched. Historically, this has been true. However, an elected diagnostic review committee evaluates each submitted diagnosis to determine whether it complies with the criteria for inclusion in the taxonomy. Moreover, research on the labels has been conducted and is continuing. In 1994, a research team at the University of Iowa (the Nursing Diagnosis Extension Classification [NDEC]) began collaborating with NANDA to extend and refine the NANDA work. They intend to address some of the difficulties with the labels, such as specificity, clinical usefulness, and clinical testing.

Compared to the terminology for describing medical diagnoses, the NANDA system is relatively new (recall that the first NANDA diagnoses were created just over 30 years ago). For example, 30 years ago AIDS was not a medical diagnosis. All classification systems evolve and change, so many of the difficulties with individual labels will be corrected as the terminology is refined. Meanwhile, try not to reject the idea of standardized language just because of a few problematic labels. You do not need to use the official NANDA labels exclusively. If you are uncomfortable with a label, change the wording to make it more useful, or write a completely new label.

The most serious criticisms are leveled by those who say that nurses should not use any standardized languages to describe nursing knowledge and nursing work. They contend, for example, that using a NANDA label to describe health status is "labeling"—that it dehumanizes and stereotypes the person. If this is true, then medical diagnoses would meet the same objection. This objection ignores the fact that we must name objects and ideas in order to communicate them to other people.

Many of the criticisms flow from disillusionment. It may be that nurses expect too much from nursing diagnosis. Although it is important, it is, after all, merely a process for identifying, naming, and communicating patient health status. We should not expect it to be the "magic bullet" that single-handedly cures all problems of the nursing profession and the patients. For a more comprehensive critique of standardized nursing language, and the NANDA system in particular,

 Go to Chapter 4, **Supplemental Materials: Critique of Standardized Nursing Language,** on the Electronic Study Guide.

| toward evidence-based practice |

Read about the following two studies, and then answer the questions at the end of the box.

Thoroddsen, A. & Thorsteinsson, H. (2002). Nursing diagnosis taxonomy across the Atlantic Ocean: Congruence between nurses' charting and the NANDA taxonomy. *Journal of Advanced Nursing, 37*(4), 372–381.

Researchers in Iceland reviewed patient charts to analyze terminology nurses use to describe client problems. The setting was a 400-bed acute care hospital. A total of 1217 charts were retrieved from two 6-month periods in two separate years. Researchers analyzed 2171 nursing diagnoses statements.

The study found that nurses in Iceland did use NANDA nursing diagnoses in documenting patients' problems. The results demonstrated a lack of agreement between what nurses record as psychological or emotional problems and what the NANDA taxonomy presents. A principal conclusion ensuing from this study is that nursing diagnoses cultivated in one culture may not function the same in other cultures.

Welton, J., & Halloran, E. (1999). A comparison of nursing and medical diagnoses in predicting hospital outcomes. *Proceedings of the American Medical Informatics Association Symposium*, pp. 171–173.

Researchers analyzed a large data set from a Midwestern university hospital. The data set included 75,765 patients. Researchers took nursing diagnoses, the patient's diagnostic related group (DRG), and the All Payer Refined DRG (APR-DRG) from the hospital discharge abstracts. They compared their ability to predict these outcomes: hospital days, ICU days, and total charges. (*Note:* the DRG and the APR-DRG are medical terminologies for describing health status). Results showed that nursing diagnoses are a significant predictor of hospital days, ICU days, and total charges. Results also showed that using nursing diagnoses along with DRG or APR-DRG improves the ability to predict hospital days, ICU days, and total charges. The results of the study support the argument that nursing data should be included with physician diagnoses when evaluating care and assessing patient outcomes.

---

1. Imagine that your hospital is changing to completely computerized patient records. All patient records will include the patient's medical diagnosis. Which study would you use to support your suggestion that patient records should also include the patient's nursing diagnoses? Why?

2. Suppose that a nurse says to you, "Each country needs its own set of nursing diagnosis labels because the labels have a different meaning in each culture." Which study would the nurse probably cite? Why?

3. Before accepting the Thoroddsen and Thorsteinsson study as "proof" that each country needs its own set of nursing diagnosis, what other studies would you like to see? That is, what else would you like to know?

 Go to Chapter 4, **Toward Evidence-Based Practice Suggested Responses,** on the Electronic Study Guide.

 Go to Chapter 4, **Resources for Caregivers and Health Professionals,** on the Electronic Study Guide.

 Suggested Readings: Go to Chapter 4, **Reading More About Diagnosis,** on the Electronic Study Guide.

 Bibliography: Go to Volume 2, Bibliography.

Nursing Process:
Planning Outcomes

Learning Outcomes

After completing this chapter, you should be able to:

* Define the following terms: *formal planning, informal planning, initial planning, ongoing planning,* and *discharge planning.*

* Identify patients who need a comprehensive, formal discharge plan.

* Explain the importance of a written plan of care.

* Describe the information contained in a comprehensive nursing care plan, regardless of format or approach.

* Compare critical pathways to integrated plans of care (IPOCs) and other standardized care-planning documents.

* Discuss the advantages and disadvantages of computerized care planning.

* Describe a process for writing an individualized care plan, making use of available standardized care-planning documents.

* Define the following terms: *goal, outcome, expected outcome, nursing-sensitive outcome.*

* Differentiate between short-term and long-term goals.

* List and give examples of the components of a goal statement.

* Recognize action (active) verbs.

* Explain how a goal is derived from a nursing diagnosis.

* Differentiate between essential and nonessential goals.

* Write appropriate goals for actual, risk, and possible nursing diagnoses.

* Use standardized terminology to state patient goals.

* Write realistic specific, concrete, and observable goals that do not conflict with the medical plan of care and are stated in terms of patient responses/behaviors.

MEET Your Patient

Ben Ivanos has just been admitted to an orthopedic unit after a motorcycle accident. Mr. Ivanos is 24 years old, normally healthy, and on no medications. He has casts and traction on both legs and a cast on one arm. He is receiving meperidine (Demerol) intravenously via patient-controlled analgesia (PCA) pump. Imagine that you are an orthopedic nurse and must plan care for Mr. Ivanos. You rank the following nursing diagnoses as highest priority:

1. Acute Pain secondary to musculoskeletal trauma (arms, legs, body) and muscle spasms
2. Risk for Peripheral Neurovascular Dysfunction secondary to casts/traction

You write the following desired outcomes (goals) on the care plan:

Goals for diagnosis 1
Demonstrates correct use of PCA pump

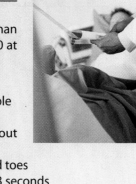

Rates pain not higher than 4 on a scale of 1 to 10 at all times

Goals for diagnosis 2
Peripheral pulses palpable
Fingers and toes warm
Fingers and toes without pallor or cyanosis
No edema of fingers and toes
Capillary refill less than 3 seconds

These goals will guide you in choosing nursing interventions for relieving Mr. Ivanos's pain and preventing peripheral neurovascular dysfunction. When the nursing shift changes, the written care plan will provide directions for the new caregivers so that they will continue to focus on Mr. Ivanos's most important needs.

WHAT IS PLANNING?

As a professional nurse, care planning is your responsibility. You cannot delegate it. Box 5–1 lists ANA and CNA standards that specifically identify planning as the role of the registered nurse.

Planning can be formal or informal. **Formal planning** "is a conscious, deliberate activity involving decision making, critical thinking, and creativity" (Wilkinson, 2001, p. 252). During the planning phases of the nursing process, you will work with the patient and family to derive desired outcomes from identified patient problems (e.g., nursing diagnoses) and then to identify nursing interventions to help achieve those outcomes. The end product of formal planning is a holistic plan of care that addresses the patient's unique problems and strengths.

Not all plans are written. You may do **informal planning** while performing other nursing process steps. For example, while performing neurovascular checks for Ben Ivanos, you might discover that he is not obtaining adequate pain relief. Reflect on this situation. What would you do?

Any response in that scenario would require some mental planning. For example, you might make a mental note (plan) to notify the physician and obtain an order for an increase in the analgesic dose.

This text separates the process of planning outcomes from the process of planning interventions because, although related, they are distinctly different activities. This chapter (1) describes planning as a general process, (2) explains how to create a nursing care plan, and (3) discusses how to write patient goals/expected outcomes. Chapter 6 explains how to plan nursing interventions and write nursing orders.

How Is Planning Related to Other Steps of the Nursing Process?

All nursing process steps are overlapping and interdependent. To develop a plan of care with realistic goals and effective nursing orders, you must have accurate, complete *assessment* data and correctly identified and prioritized *nursing diagnoses*. The goals/desired outcomes flow logically from the nursing diagnoses. By stating what is to be achieved, the goals then suggest nursing interventions (which are written as nursing orders in the *planning interventions* phase). The plan of care is carried out in the *implementation* phase. In addition, in the *evaluation* step the goals/desired

BOX 5-1 Professional Standards for Planning Outcomes

American Nurses Association Standards of Nursing Practice

Standard 3. Outcomes Identification

The registered nurse identifies expected outcomes for a plan individualized to the patient or the situation.

Measurement Criteria:

The registered nurse:

Involves the patient, family, and other healthcare providers in formulating expected outcomes when possible and appropriate.

Derives culturally appropriate expected outcomes from the diagnoses.

Considers associated risks, benefits, costs, current scientific evidence, and clinical expertise when formulating expected outcomes.

Defines expected outcomes in terms of the patient, patient values, ethical considerations, environment, or situation with such considerations as associated risks, benefits and costs, and current scientific evidence.

Includes a time estimate for attainment of expected outcomes.

Develops expected outcomes that provide direction for continuity of care.

Modifies expected outcomes based on changes in the status of the patient or evaluation of the situation.

Documents expected outcomes as measurable goals.

Note: There are additional standards for advanced practice nurses.

Source: Reprinted with permission from American Nurses Association, *Nursing: Scope and standards of practice* (3rd ed.). © 2004. American Nurses Publishing, American Nurses Foundation/American Nurses Association, 600 Maryland Ave., SW, Suite 100 W, Washington, DC 20024–2571.

Canadian Provincial Standards of Practice (Examples)

In Canada, practice standards are set by each province. The following are examples that apply to planning outcomes.

Province of Alberta

The registered nurse continually strives to acquire knowledge and skills to provide competent, evidence-based nursing practice.

Accesses appropriate information and resources that enhance patient care and achievement of desired patient outcomes.

Demonstrates critical thinking in collecting and interpreting data, planning, implementing, and evaluating all aspects of nursing care.

Source: Alberta Association of Registered Nurses. (1999). *Nursing practice: Professional conduct: Nursing practice standards.* Retrieved January 17, 2003, from http://nurses.ab.ca/profconduct/npa.html

Province of Nova Scotia

The registered nurse demonstrates competencies relevant to own area of nursing practice. Each registered nurse

Applies appropriate knowledge and skills to assess, plan, intervene and evaluate services, and revises plan as needed.

Source: Registered Nurses' Association of Nova Scotia. (1997). *Standards for nursing practice.* Retrieved January 17, 2003, from http://www.rnans.ns.ca

outcomes serve as criteria for evaluating whether the nursing care has been effective. Figure 5–1 illustrates the relationship of planning outcomes to the other stages of the nursing process.

Initial and Ongoing Planning

Initial planning begins with the first patient contact. It refers to the development of the initial comprehensive care plan, which should be written as soon as possible after the initial assessment. Because the nurse who performs the admission assessment has the benefit of personal contact (rather than relying completely on the written database), that nurse has the best information about the patient and, ideally, is the one who should initiate the care plan.

You may sometimes need to begin care planning even though the initial database is incomplete. For example, the patient may require emergency care before assessment is complete. Or you may have a different patient who requires your immediate attention. In such situations, develop a preliminary plan with whatever information you have. You can complete and refine the plan when you are able to perform a more detailed assessment.

Ongoing planning refers to changes made in the plan as you evaluate the patient's responses to care or as you obtain new data and make new nursing diagnoses. For example, after Ben Ivanos's first night on the hospital unit, the nurses discovered that he had not slept well. They identified a new nursing diagnosis for him: Disturbed Sleep Pattern related to unfamiliar environment

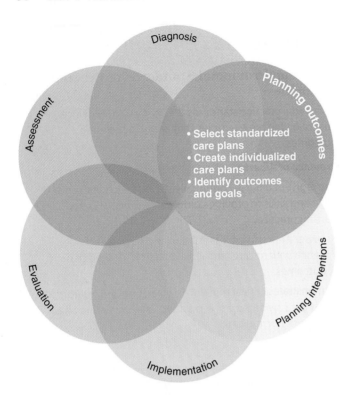

FIGURE 5–1   Nursing process phases: planning outcomes.

and pain. They then developed a plan for addressing this problem. Ongoing assessment allows you to decide which problems to focus on each day that you care for the patient.

Discharge Planning

In the hospital where Ben Ivanos is being treated, the recommended length of stay for patients with surgical reduction of fractures is 2 days. He will still have casts on his arm and both legs when he leaves the hospital. Obviously he will not be able to manage his own activities of daily living (shopping, cooking, bathing, and so forth). What questions come to your mind when you think about how he will manage after he leaves the hospital? It is important to stretch your mind, so take a moment now to jot down your ideas.

You may have thought of questions such as the following: Is there anyone who can help Mr. Ivanos with his personal care? Does he live in a house or an apartment? Will he need to go up and down stairs? Who will drive him home from the hospital? Can he be discharged home or will he need to go to a rehabilitation facility? How soon does he need to see his physician again? How will he get to the doctor's office? How will he manage his pain at home; what will he use in place of the PCA narcotics?

Discharge planning is the process of planning for self care and continuity of care after the patient leaves a healthcare setting. Ben Ivanos's case is not unusual. In the United States, outpatient surgeries and short

hospital stays are the norm. Many patients are discharged in spite of ongoing need for nursing care and complex treatments. If appropriate services are not provided or if family members perform care incorrectly, the patient may experience delayed recovery or complications that require further treatment or hospital admission. This means that nurses must prepare family members to perform tasks such as bathing, changing sterile dressings, and monitoring intravenously administered medications. If family members are not available or if skilled nursing care is needed, arrangements must be made for home health care or transfer to a skilled nursing or rehabilitation facility. Sometimes a case manager is assigned, but often staff nurses must plan and coordinate services.

Discharge Planning Begins at Assessment

Because patients are in the surgery center or hospital for such a short time, discharge planning must begin at the initial assessment, which should include the following patient data:

- Physical condition and functional and self-care limitations
- Emotional stability and ability to learn
- Financial resources (e.g., personal finances, insurance, community resources such as food stamps, Medicaid)
- Family or other caregivers available
- Environment, both home and community (e.g., stairs, space for supplies and equipment, availability of transportation to healthcare services)

Written Discharge Plans

All patients need at least some discharge planning, but you will not always need a separate, written discharge plan. It may be enough to include discharge assessments and teaching as nursing orders on the patient's comprehensive care plan. For example, a middle-aged patient who has been hospitalized for deep vein thrombosis (a blood clot in a major vein, usually the lower leg) will be able to care for herself independently when she goes home. For this patient, you could simply write a nursing order to teach her about the side effects of the warfarin (Coumadin, an anticoagulant) she will be taking at home. In contrast, you will probably need a comprehensive, formal discharge plan if the patient has complex needs or one or more of the following:

- Difficulty learning or a memory deficit
- A terminal illness
- A complicated major surgery
- No family or significant others to help provide care
- A complex treatment regimen to continue at home

- Self-care deficits (e.g., dressing, feeding, bathing, toileting)
- An illness with an expected long period of recovery
- Inadequate financial resources
- A newly diagnosed chronic disease (e.g., diabetes)
- Emotional or mental illness
- Inadequate services available in the community

For an example of a discharge planning form,

 Go to Chapter 5, **Discharge Planning Form,** in Volume 2.

Discharge Planning Requires Collaboration

Comprehensive discharge planning involves significant collaboration. Ideally, it is done *with,* not *for,* the patient—patient involvement is important for achieving desired outcomes. Additionally, a patient's post-discharge needs often call for services from a multidisciplinary team, which may include home care service personnel; private-duty nurses; physical therapists; social service professionals; speech, occupational, and hearing therapists; physicians; and members of the patient's family.

KnowledgeCheck 5–1

- What does the nurse do in the planning phases of the nursing process?
- What is the purpose of initial planning? Ongoing planning? Discharge planning?

 Go to Chapter 5, **Knowledge Check Response Sheet and Answers,** on the Electronic Study Guide.

NURSING CARE PLANS

The **comprehensive nursing care plan** (also called *patient care plan*) is a document—usually several documents— that is the central source of information needed to guide holistic, goal-oriented care to address each patient's unique needs. It specifies dependent, interdependent, and independent nursing functions necessary for care of a specific patient and usually uses both standardized and individualized approaches to care.

Why Is a Written Nursing Care Plan Important?

A well-written comprehensive care plan benefits the patient and the healthcare institution by:

- *Ensuring that care is complete.* If specific directions are written (e.g., "Turn patient hourly"), they are less likely to be overlooked by busy caregivers.
- *Providing continuity of care.* This helps ensure that when an effective intervention is found, all caregivers

will use the same approach with the patient. For example, suppose a child who is dehydrated refuses to drink any liquids offered. The day nurse discovers that the child will eat red, and only red, popsicles. If he fails to note that on the care plan, the night nurse may be unable to persuade the child to take liquids orally and may have to administer fluids intravenously to prevent further dehydration.

- *Promoting efficient use of nursing efforts.* Specific, written instructions help to ensure that nurses do not waste time on ineffective approaches. In the preceding example, the night nurse may waste a great deal of time trying to persuade the child to drink liquids.
- *Providing a guide for assessments and charting.* The nursing orders and goals/expected outcomes on the care plan can help you recall what occurred and ensure that nothing is omitted from your documentation.
- *Meeting the requirements of accrediting agencies.* The Joint Commission on Accreditation of Healthcare Organizations (JCAHO) and professional standards review organizations (PSROs) require a patient-specific plan of care.

What Information Does a Comprehensive Nursing Care Plan Contain?

Regardless of their format, comprehensive care plans include directions for four different kinds of care and include both medical and nursing interventions:

1. *Basic needs and ADLs.* Regardless of the patient's diagnoses, nurses need to know what routine assistance the patient needs with hygiene, nutrition, elimination, and so on.
2. *Medical/multidisciplinary treatment.* Nurses need to know the medical orders for each patient (e.g., orders for intravenously administered fluids and medications) and the nursing activities necessary for carrying out those orders.
3. *Nursing diagnoses and collaborative problems.* This section may be referred to as the *nursing diagnosis care plan.* It contains goals and nursing orders for the patient's nursing diagnoses and collaborative problems.
4. *Special discharge needs or teaching needs.* Finally, nurses need to know patients' needs, if any, for formal discharge planning and for special teaching. For example, the client may require teaching in how to self-administer injections or how to follow a prescribed diet.

What Documents Make Up a Comprehensive Nursing Care Plan?

You will use a variety of documents to create a care plan. Care plans vary widely in format, appearance,

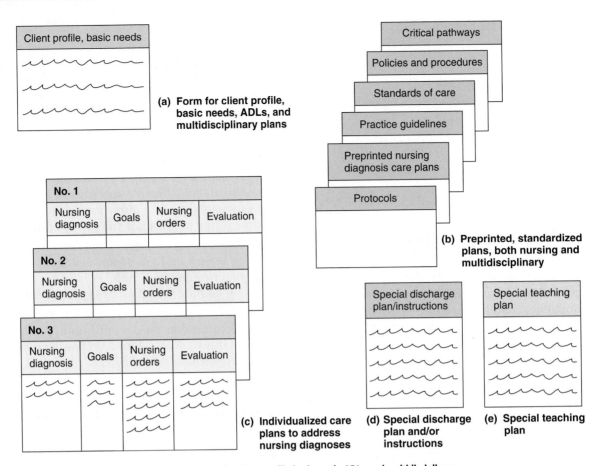

FIGURE 5–2   Components of a nursing care plan. *A,* Form for client profile, basic needs, ADLs, and multidisciplinary plans. *B,* Preprinted, standardized plans, both nursing and multidisciplinary. *C,* Individualized care plans to address nursing diagnoses. *D,* Special discharge plan and/or instructions. *E,* Special teaching plan.

and use. In most healthcare organizations, caregivers use preprinted, standardized plans that can be adapted to meet individual needs. Figure 5–2 shows the documents that are most commonly included in a comprehensive nursing care plan.

Form for Client Profile and Basic Needs

Care providers need quick and easy access to essential client data (1) that does not change, and (2) that is used or updated often. This includes the client's profile (age, physicians, drug allergies, and so on), basic needs (e.g., for hygiene, nutrition, and elimination), and diagnostic tests and treatments (e.g., laboratory tests, radiology procedures, and respiratory therapy). This information is usually recorded on a durable, standardized form and not organized according to medical or nursing diagnoses (see Figure 5–2a). One example is a Kardex, which is printed on cardstock and kept in a central location easily accessible to all care providers. To see a Kardex,

 Go to Chapter 5, **Tables, Boxes, Figures: ESG Figure 5-1,** on the Electronic Study Guide.

For clients who need more than routine attention to their basic needs, you may wish to write a nursing diagnosis care plan. Examples include a client with no appetite and the nursing diagnosis Imbalanced Nutrition: Less Than Body Requirements, or an immobile client with the diagnosis Risk for Impaired Skin Integrity.

Preprinted, Standardized Plans

As shown in Figure 5–2b, a comprehensive care plan usually includes one or more preprinted, standardized documents. It would be too time-consuming to handwrite a complete care plan for every patient. Standardized plans save nursing time, promote consistency of care, and help ensure that nurses do not overlook important interventions. You will find standardized instructions for patient care in a variety of documents within an organization. A document may (1) contain nursing or multidisciplinary interventions and (2) prescribe care for one or more nursing diagnoses (e.g., Impaired Skin Integrity) or a disease or medical condition (e.g., pneumonia). The following are examples of standardized, preprinted instructions for care.

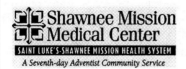

Patient Care Protocol

Title: Fall or Injury/Disruption of Care, Care of the Patient at Risk for **Effective Date:** 1/9/06

Expected Outcome: The patient at risk for falls will be identified and preventive measures initiated. The patient will not pull out indwelling devices.

Relevant Information: Initiate this protocol for adult patients who have a Conley Fall Scale score of ≥3.

Assessment: 1. The Conley Fall Scale will be administered on admission to adult inpatients. Further assessment will be based on patient population and identified patient need.

Interventions: Make alterations in environment, such as:
- Avoiding clutter in room.
- Moving patient closer to Nursing Station if indicated.
- Making sure call light, telephone and other personal items are within reach

Educate patient and family about:
- The possibility that family and friends may be called upon to stay with patient with high risk for fall or injury or who attempts to pull out indwelling devices.
- The possibility that, if the above measures are not successful in reducing the patient's fall risk or preventing attempts to pull out indwelling devices, alternative measures such as the use of restraints may have to be considered.

Evaluation: 1. Evaluate frequently to determine if expected outcome is being met. Change strategies as needed to reduce fall risks or to prevent disruption of indwelling devices.
2. **Criteria for initiation of Restraint Protocol:**
- If interventions have been implemented and patient continues to be at risk of falling or disrupting medical treatment, the protocol Care of the Patient in Restraint for Medical/Surgical Management is initiated.
- The CRN/Supervisor is notified at the time the restraint is initiated for med/surg management and reviews the need for restraint.

FIGURE 5–3 **Portion of Patient Care Protocol for patient at risk for falls.** *Source:* Courtesy of Shawnee Mission Health System, Shawnee Mission, KS 66204.

Policies and Procedures

Policies and **procedures** are similar to rules and regulations. When a situation occurs frequently or requires a consistent response regardless of who handles it, management develops a policy to govern how it is to be handled. For example, hospitals have policies about visiting hours and about the number of visitors permitted in a room. You should consider individual needs and use critical thinking to interpret policies in a caring manner. For example, in some critical care units a patient is allowed one visitor for 10 minutes each hour. Imagine, though, that a patient is expected to die soon, and that his daughter has brought her three children from a distant state for one last visit. Would you tell the daughter to take the children in to see their grandfather? Would you insist that she follow the rule and send them in without her, one at a time over a period of 3 hours?

Protocols

Protocols cover specific therapeutic actions usually required for a clinical problem unique to a subgroup of patients. For example, not every patient on a medical-surgical unit is at risk for falls, but many are. So for a patient in that subgroup (i.e., a patient at risk for falls), the nurse would add a falls protocol, such as in Figure 5–3, to that patient's care plan. Protocols may be written for a particular medical diagnosis (e.g., seizure), treatments (e.g., administration of oxytocin to induce labor), or diagnostic tests (e.g., barium enema). They may include both medical and nursing orders. Some include definitions and rationales for interventions.

Unit Standards of Care

Unit standards of care describe the care that nurses are expected to provide for all patients in defined

PATIENT PLAN OF CARE - GENESIS MEDICAL CENTER - Davenport, Iowa

PAIN, ACUTE: Experience of an unpleasant sensory and emotional sensation for a duration of less than 6 months.
SIGNS & SYMPTOMS: Observed or reported (select at least 2)

- [ ] Change in BP
- [ ] Patients self report of pain
- [ ] Change in respiratory pattern
- [ ] Restlessness
- [ ] Diaphoresis
- [ ] Whimpering
- [ ] Grimacing
- [ ] Increased muscle tension
- [ ] Whining
- [ ] Crying
- [ ] Change in pulse rate

OUTCOME SCORING

RELATED FACTORS	OUTCOMES	ADM				DC	INTERVENTIONS
[ ] Physical injuring agent [ ] Psychological injuring agent	[4] Pain control behavior – Recognizes causal factors – Uses non-analgesic relief measures – Uses analgesics appropriately – Reports pain controlled [3] Pain level – Oral/facial expressions of pain – Change in respiratory rate, heart rate BP – Restlessness – Reported pain [3] Comfort level – Reported satisfaction with symptom control – Expressed satisfaction with pain control – Reported physical well-being						[ ] Pain management [ ] Analgesic administration [ ] Patient-controlled analgesic (PCA) assistance [ ] Analgesic administration: Intraspinal [ ] Environmental management: comfort [ ] Anxiety reduction [ ] Transcutaneous electrical nerve stimulation (TENS) [ ] Heat/cold application [ ] Distraction [ ] Simple relaxation therapy [ ] Simple massage [ ] Developmental care [ ] Preparatory sensory information [ ] Positioning

Definition of scoring scales	1	2	3	4	5
Pain control — Personal actions to control pain	Never demonstrated	Rarely demonstrated	Sometimes demonstrated	Often demonstrated	Consistently demonstrated
Pain level — Severity of reported pain	Severe	Substantial	Moderate	Slight	None
Comfort level — Extent of physical and psychological ease	None	Limited	Moderate	Substantial	Extensive

Diagnosis _____

Date Initiated _____ RN Initials _____

Date Resolved _____

FIGURE 5–4 **Computer printout of standardized care plan for a single nursing diagnosis using standardized language.** *Source:* Adapted from Genesis Medical Center, Davenport, IA 52804. Used with permission.

situations (e.g., all women admitted to a labor unit or all patients admitted to the critical care unit). In this way, they are similar to protocols. Unlike protocols, however, they (1) apply to every patient in the defined situation, rather than a subgroup; (2) do not become part of the patient's care plan but are kept on file on the unit; and (3) do not usually include specific medical orders. Instead of describing ideal care, standards of care describe the minimum level of care the nurses are expected to achieve given the institution's resources and the client population. Unit standards of care are usually not organized according to nursing diagnoses and usually resemble a list of "things to do" (e.g., complete comprehensive assessment within 2 hours of admission) rather than detailed instructions for care.

Standardized Nursing Care Plans

Standardized (model) nursing care plans are guides that detail the nursing care that is usually needed for a particular nursing diagnosis or for all nursing diagnoses that commonly occur with a medical condition. Figure 5–4 is a standardized care plan for a single nursing diagnosis. Although similar to unit standards of care, model care plans are different in that they:

- Provide more detailed interventions. They may add to or delete from unit standards of care.
- Are usually organized by nursing diagnosis and include specific patient goals and nursing orders.
- Are kept as a part of the patient's total care plan and become a permanent part of the medical record.
- Usually describe ideal nursing care.
- Allow you to include addendum care plans and include checklists, blank lines, or empty spaces so that you can individualize goals and interventions.

Many books of model care plans are available. You can use them as guides, but be aware that they do not address the client's individual needs. For this reason, they may lead you to focus on the common, predictable problems and overlook an unusual problem the person is experiencing. Beginning with the standardized plan may stifle your creativity. When using a standardized plan, first use the process for writing a nursing care plan (see "What Is the Process for Writing an Individualized Nursing Care Plan?" p. 92). Then consult the model plan to see whether you have missed anything.

Critical Pathways

Critical pathways are often used in managed care systems. They are outcomes-based, interdisciplinary plans that sequence patient care according to case type. They specify predicted patient outcomes and broad interventions for each day, or in some situations, for each hour (Figure 5–5). They describe the minimal

standard of care required to meet the recommended length of stay for patients with a particular condition or *diagnosis-related group (DRG)* (e.g., postpartum, myocardial infarction, or total hip replacement). An agency usually develops critical pathways for its most frequent case types or for situations in which standardized care can produce predictable outcomes. Although they are developed by a multidisciplinary team, critical pathways tend to emphasize medical problems and interventions.

Integrated Plans of Care

Integrated plans of care (IPOCs) are standardized plans that function as care plans as well as documentation forms. Therefore, there is a different form for each day of care. Many critical pathways are designed as IPOCs; however, IPOCs do not necessarily (1) organize care according to diagnosis, (2) describe minimal standards of care, or (3) specify a timeline for interventions and outcomes. For an example of an IPOC,

 Go to Chapter 5, **Tables, Boxes, Figures: ESG Figure 5–2,** on the Electronic Study Guide.

Individualized Nursing Care Plans

Individualized nursing care plans are used to address nursing diagnoses unique to a particular client (see Figure 5–2c). These care plans reflect the independent component of nursing practice and, therefore, best demonstrate the nurse's critical thinking and clinical expertise. In addition to including goals and nursing orders that you write specifically for a patient, a complete individualized care plan may contain standardized single-problem care plans, such as the one shown in Figure 5–4.

As already mentioned, standardized plans focus on the common, predictable problems and the interventions needed by most patients. However, they do not address unusual problems and may not meet a patient's individual needs. You should always adapt standardized plans to add the necessary nursing diagnoses, goals/outcomes, and nursing orders not included in the standardized documents. For example, a standardized care plan for a client with a myocardial infarction (heart attack) would undoubtedly prescribe care for the nursing diagnosis Pain and the potential complication of heart failure. However, it might not address the needs of a person who is not complying with treatments because he is in denial about his illness (nursing diagnosis: Ineffective Denial). An individualized plan for resolving the patient's denial would improve the likelihood that the rest of the plan will be successful.

You may sometimes include medical orders in a nursing diagnosis or collaborative problem care plan, especially in a student care plan. For example, for a

HOSPITAL OF THE UNIVERSITY OF PENNSYLVANIA

TOTAL LOWER JOINT (HIP/KNEE)
CLINICAL PATHWAY

ELIGIBILITY CRITERIA: All primary unilateral total hip or total knee
replacements .

ADDRESSOGRAPH

EXPECTED LOS: 3 Days

CLINICAL KEYS:

1.   Pain managed ≤ midpoint on painscale
2.   Transfer to chair/commode with assistance POD 1; Ambulate in room, bathroom POD2
3.   DVT precautions
4.   Discharge plan completed by POD2
5.   Patient verbalizes knowledge of hip or knee precautions
6.   Knee motion 10° to 70° or better (TKA patients only)

	PACU	IMMED. POST-OP	POD 1	POD 2	POD 3-4
ASSESSMENTS	• NV checks with VS q1h × 4 • Pain • Effects of narcotics/ tolerance • 1 & 0 × 24hr • Pulse Ox q8 if on O2	• NV check / VS q 4hr → → • S/S DVT →	→ → → → • Pulse Ox × 1 on RA • Dsg/wound status q4	• NV check / VS q 8hr → → → • D/C pulse ox if O2 D/C • Dsg/wound status q8	→ → → → →
CONSULTS		• PT • PMR	→ (If not done already) → (If not done already)		
TESTS	• A/P hip X-ray (THA) • A/P knee X-ray (TKA)		• CBC	→ • INR (if on warfarin)	• A/P hip X-ray →
TREATMENTS	• O2	• D/C O2 if sat ≥ 94% • Incentive spirometry • Order walker (hip chair, elevated commode if needed) • Pneumatic compression device (ankle for knees, calf for hips)	→ → • D/C foley • Dressing change (1st dsg change by MD) →	→ → • Dressing change q day and pm →	 → → →
MEDICATIONS	• PCA or epidural	→ • Anticoagulation	• IV heplock → • Consider conversion to oral pain meds	• D/C heplock → • D/C PCA/PCEA • PO pain meds	→
ACTIVITY	• Bedrest • Hip precautions if THA • CPM for total knee	→ → →	• OOB to chair BID → → • Weight bear per order • Ambulate with assistive device	• OOB TID → → → → • PT ×2	→ → → → → →
NUTRITION	• NPO	• NPO → ice → advance to full as tolerated	• Regular	→	→
EDUCATION / D/C PLANNING	• Deep breathing exercises	• Pain management • Initiate d/c plan	→ • Home vs rehab decision • Anticoagulation if indicated	→ • S/S wound infection • Medications • Activity level • D/C plan in place	→ → → • Car transfer

Transfer to rehab when:
1. Able to participate in care
2. Tolerating 2 physical therapy sessions
3. Not requiring IV pain medicine
4. Blood values are stable
5. Motivation is commensurate with projected functional status

Discharge to home when:
1. Mobility and ADL's appropriate for degree of assistance at home and home environment
2. Appropriate assistive device and necessary adaptive equipment is used
3. Independent with hip/knee precautions
4. Independent with home exercise program or ongoing PT in the home or outpatient
**IF D/C TO HOME, ENSURE APPROPRIATE CONSULTS TO ARRANGE HOME CARE FOLLOW-UP AND EQUIPMENT

FIGURE 5–5   Portion of a critical pathway. *Source:* Hospital of the University of Pennsylvania, Philadelphia, PA. Used with permission.

client with a nursing diagnosis of Deficient Fluid Volume, you might list the medical order for intravenously administered fluids in the "Nursing Orders" column.

Nursing diagnosis	*Nursing orders*
Deficient Fluid Volume related to vomiting and diarrhea	1. Check skin turgor q4hr
	2. Medical order: IV normal saline, 150 mL/hr

Special Discharge or Teaching Plans

The nursing care plan may also include one or more discharge or client teaching plans (see Figure 5–2d). These are sometimes referred to as *special-purpose* or *addendum* care plans. You can address routine discharge planning and teaching needs by using standardized plans, or by using nursing diagnosis care plans in which you include teaching as part of the nursing orders. For example, a care plan for the diagnosis Acute Pain might include a nursing order, "Teach patient to splint incision when turning in bed." Chapter 24 includes an example of a special teaching plan for the diagnosis Deficient Knowledge (see p. 541).

Computerized Care Plans

More healthcare organizations are using *computerized care plans*. The computer stores standardized plans (e.g., for nursing diagnoses, medical diagnoses, or DRGs). When you enter a diagnosis or a desired outcome, the computer generates a list of suggested interventions. You then choose appropriate interventions from the list, individualize by choosing from checklists, or type in your own interventions and strategies.

 Go to Chapter 5, **Tables, Boxes, Figures: ESG Figure 5–3,** on the Electronic Study Guide.

ESG Figure 5–3 shows a computer screen displaying a care plan for the nursing diagnosis Pain. It lists a patient goal and broadly stated interventions, including assessments and patient education. Most computer programs allow you to print the plan.

Computer prompts help ensure that you consider a wide variety of actions and keep you from overlooking common and important interventions. After the initial learning curve, they also reduce the time spent on paperwork. However, computerized planning requires constant use of a step-by-step thinking process, which may cause a decrease in intuition, insight, ability to care, and nursing expertise (Harris, 1990). You must resist the temptation to accept "one size fits all" solutions. Always look for creative approaches that might be more effective for a particular individual. Think, "What would work for *this* person?"

Student Care Plans

You may have already noticed that the care plans you see in clinical settings look different from the ones you create as a part of your clinical preparation. This is because student care plans are a learning activity as well as a plan of care. They are designed to help you learn and apply concepts from the nursing process, physiology, and psychopathology. For this reason, they contain longer and more detailed nursing orders as well as other information the instructor may require (e.g., information about lab tests, medications, and assessment data to support the nursing diagnoses). Some instructors may ask you to write rationales and cite references to support them. **Rationales** state the scientific principles or research basis you used to select a nursing intervention. Writing rationales helps demonstrate that you understand the reasons for the interventions—understanding *why* you do *what* you do is one aspect of functioning as a professional. For an example of a student care plan,

 Go to Chapter 5, **Student Care Plan,** on the Electronic Study Guide.

Mind-Mapping Student Care Plans

Mind-mapping is a technique for showing relationships among ideas and concepts in a graphical, or pictorial, way. Mind-mapping is thought to stimulate "whole-brain" and critical thinking, and to foster the development of holistic plans of care (Mueller, Johnston, & Bligh, 2002). A mind-mapped care plan uses shapes and pictures to represent the parts of the nursing process (i.e., assessment data, nursing diagnoses, patient goals, interventions, and evaluation), as well as the patient's pathophysiology, medications, and

other pertinent information. For complete information about mind-mapping,

 Go to Chapter 5, **Supplemental Materials: Mind-Mapping,** on the Electronic Study Guide.

What Is the Process for Writing an Individualized Nursing Care Plan?

Writing an individualized nursing care plan follows in natural sequence from the assessment and diagnosis phases of the nursing process:

- *Make a working problem list.* Earlier in the nursing process, you will already have developed and prioritized a list of the patient's nursing diagnoses, collaborative problems, and strengths. Suppose that, after assessment, you prioritized Ben Ivanos's problems as follows:

  1. Acute Pain secondary to musculoskeletal trauma (arms, legs, body) and muscle spasms
  2. Risk for Peripheral Neurovascular Dysfunction secondary to casts/traction
  3. Self-Care Deficit (Total) related to immobility secondary to casts, especially cast on dominant right arm
  4. Potential Complication of fracture: delayed, union, malunion, or nonunion of bone

- *Decide which problems can be managed with standardized care plans or critical pathways.* What institutional documents are available? Suppose that, for Ben Ivanos, there is a critical pathway for "Patients With Casts and/or Traction." This critical pathway would contain goals and interventions to guide the care for problems 2 and 4. It would specify regular neurovascular assessments and management of the traction apparatus, for example.

- *Individualize the standardized plan as needed.* Mark off any instructions that do not apply to your patient, and add or adapt nursing orders as appropriate. Many standardized plans provide space for individualizing the goals and interventions. For example, the plan might say "Perform neurovascular checks q_____." You would fill in the frequency of the assessment according to the patient's needs.

- *Transcribe medical orders to appropriate documents.* For example, you might write orders for pain medications on a special medication sheet. Details about the traction would probably go on a Kardex or special section of the critical pathway.

- *Write ADLs and basic care needs in special sections of the Kardex, care plan, or computer.* For Ben Ivanos, you might note on the Kardex that he requires a complete bedbath and help with eating.

- *Develop individualized care plans for problems not addressed by standardized documents.* For Ben Ivanos, you would need to write a plan for problems 1 and 3.

The critical pathway probably contains some expected outcomes and basic interventions for problem 1, Pain, but you might need to individualize them to make them more effective. If your unit had a Pain protocol, similar to the Falls protocol in Figure 5–3, you would add it to Mr. Ivanos's care plan. If not, you would hand-write goals and interventions for the Pain diagnosis.

Problem 3, Self-Care Deficit, would be partially addressed in the basic care section of the Kardex on file for Mr. Ivanos. But he has special needs—for example, he will need teaching and therapy to increase his ability to care for himself. So you would need to hand-write a plan for this nursing diagnosis.

KnowledgeCheck 5–3

Briefly describe a process for creating a comprehensive, individualized care plan that incorporates collaborative care and standardized planning documents.

 Go to Chapter 5, **Knowledge Check Response Sheet and Answers,** on the Electronic Study Guide.

PLANNING PATIENT GOALS/OUTCOMES

After assessment and diagnosis, the next step in individualized care planning is to formulate goals for improving or maintaining the patient's health status. **Goals** (also called **expected outcomes, desired outcomes,** or **predicted outcomes**) describe the changes in patient health status that you hope to achieve. **Nursing-sensitive outcomes** are those that can be influenced by nursing interventions. Although critical pathways describe the expected outcomes of multidisciplinary care, they do not provide a way to judge *nursing* effectiveness. The rest of this chapter discusses individualized care planning and nursing-sensitive outcomes.

Goal/expected outcome formulation is the responsibility of the professional nurse (see Box 5–1). You should involve the client as much as possible in goal setting, because goal achievement is more likely if the client believes the goals are important and realistic. Of course the client must be alert and independent enough to participate. If physical or mental impairments prevent active participation, the nursing team acts on the client's behalf to develop client-centered goals.

What Do the Terms *Goal* and *Outcome* Mean?

Many nurses use the terms *goal* and *outcome* interchangeably. In this text, we usually use the Nursing Outcomes Classification (NOC) terminology: the word *outcome,* used alone, means *any* patient response (positive or negative) to interventions (e.g., the pain could become better or worse; both are outcomes). When referring to desired (positive) patient responses,

we use *goals, expected outcomes, desired outcomes,* or *predicted outcomes.* For example:

Outcome	Decision Making
Goals/expected outcomes	Participates in decisions about own care. Chooses between two or more alternatives.

Some nurses use the term *goal* to mean a broad, nonspecific statement about the desired results of nursing activities. They use *outcomes* (and other outcome terms such as *expected outcomes*) to mean the more specific, observable responses you would use to judge whether the goal has been met. When goals are defined in this way, you must include both goals and expected outcomes on the care plan because a broad goal does not provide enough guidance for evaluating patient responses to care. You can combine the broad goal and specific expected outcome into a single statement by writing, "as evidenced by," as in the following example:

Broad statement (goal)	Relieve constipation
Specific expected outcome (evaluation criteria)	Will have soft, formed bowel movement within 24 hours
Combined statement (goal + outcome)	Constipation will be relieved *as evidenced by* soft, formed bowel movement within 24 hours

Use of broad goals on the care plan is optional; however, expected outcomes are not optional. You must include them on the care plan.

What Is the Purpose of Goal/Outcome Statements?

Goals are important for planning, implementation, and evaluation. Precise, descriptive, clearly stated goals/expected outcomes:

- Form the criteria you will use in the evaluation phase of the nursing process.
- Provide a guide for selecting nursing interventions by describing what you wish to achieve.
- Motivate the client and the nurse by providing a sense of achievement when the goals are met. This is especially important when the client must make difficult lifestyle changes.

How Do I Distinguish Between Short-Term and Long-Term Goals?

Long-term goals are changes in health status that you wish to achieve over a longer period—a week, a month, or more. They describe the optimum level of functioning

you expect the patient to achieve, given health status and available resources. Ideally this is a return to normal functioning, but that is not always possible.

Short-term goals are those you expect the patient to achieve within a few hours or days. They are important:

- In situations in which the patient may be discharged before you can evaluate progress toward long-term goals (e.g., as in a day surgery).
- For providing positive reinforcement to clients who are working toward long-term goals.

See Table 5–1 for a comparison of short-term and long-term goals.

KnowledgeCheck 5–4

Refer to "Meet Your Patient," on page 82. State whether each of Mr. Ivanos's goals was a short-term or long-term goal.

 Go to Chapter 5, **Knowledge Check Response Sheet and Answers,** on the Electronic Study Guide.

What Are the Components of a Goal Statement?

Every expected outcome/goal statement must have the following parts:

1. *Subject.* The subject is understood to be the client, but it can also be a function or part of the client. For example:

   [Mrs. Johnson] Will walk to the doorway with the help of one person by 12/13/06.
   Lung sounds will be clear to auscultation within 2 days after receiving antibiotics.

   Assume that the subject is the client unless otherwise stated. Think, "Client will . . ." to help you phrase the goal statement correctly, but do not write it. For example, in the first goal, you should not write "Mrs. Johnson."

2. *Action verb.* Use an action verb to indicate the action the client will perform: what the client will learn, do, or say (e.g., Will *walk* to the doorway). Use concrete verbs (i.e., describing actions that you can see, hear, smell, feel, or measure), such as the following:

apply	explain	report
choose	eat	select
demonstrate	list	transfer
describe	measure	turn
drink	prepare	verbalize

3. *Performance criteria.* These are the standards for evaluating the client's performance. They describe the extent to which you expect to see the action or behavior. Write them in concrete, observable terms because they indicate what you need to

TABLE 5-1   Comparison of Short-Term and Long-Term Goals

	Definition	Situations for Use	Example
Short-Term Goals	• Can be achieved in a few hours or a few days	• Acute care • Day surgery • Clinics • Focus on immediate needs • Students • Evaluation of progress toward long-term goals	• Describes pain as < 3 on a 1–10 scale *within 30 min* after receiving analgesic. • Limits food intake to 1500 calories *per day*.
Long-Term Goals	• Expected changes that occur over a week, a month, or more • Optimum level of functioning given health status and resources	• Home health care • Extended-care facilities • Rehabilitation centers • Chronic illness • Conditions that are managed, not cured	• Infant will double birth weight within 5 months. • Within 3 months after physical therapy treatments, will dress self except for buttons.

measure in order to evaluate outcomes. Performance criteria specify:

How, what, when, or where something is to be done

Amount, quality, accuracy, speed, distance, and so forth

The following example specifies the distance the client is expected to walk.

[Client] Will walk *to the doorway* with the help of one person by 12/13/06.

4. *Target time.* The realistic date or time by which the performance/behavior should be achieved. The target time is the "when" part of the performance criterion.

[Client] will walk to the doorway with the help of one person *by 12/13/06.*

Other examples of target times are *by discharge, within 24 hours, at the next visit, each hour, at all times.* For risk (potential) nursing diagnoses, the desired outcome is that the problem never will occur. You assume that the desired response should occur "at all times," but you may wish to schedule times for evaluating the outcome. For example:

Nursing diagnosis: Risk for Constipation r/t inadequate fluid intake

Expected outcome: Bowel movements will be of normal frequency and consistency

(*Target time:* At all times)

(*Evaluate:* Daily)

5. *Special conditions.* Describe the amount of assistance or resources needed or the experiences/

treatments the client should have to perform the behavior. Include special conditions when it is important for other nurses to know them. For example:

[Client] Will walk to the doorway *with the help of one person* by 12/13/06.

After two teaching sessions, [client] will be able to identify foods to avoid on a low-fat diet by 3/1/06.

KnowledgeCheck 5–5

In the following predicted outcomes, identify the subject, action verb, performance criterion, target time, and special conditions (if any). State which components are assumed, if any.

- Will walk to the doorway with the help of one person by 12/13/06.
- After two teaching sessions, (client) will be able to identify foods to avoid on a low-fat diet by 3/1/06.
- Bowel movements will be soft and formed and of his usual frequency.
- Lungs clear to auscultation at all times.

 Go to Chapter 5, **Knowledge Check Response Sheet and Answers,** on the Electronic Study Guide.

How Do Goals Relate to Nursing Diagnoses?

Expected outcomes are derived directly from the nursing diagnosis. Therefore, they are appropriate only if you identify the nursing diagnosis correctly. The problem clause (the clause at the left) of a nursing diagnosis describes the response or health status that you wish to change. A desired outcome states the *opposite* of the

TABLE 5-2 Comparison of Nursing Diagnoses and Goals

Nursing Diagnosis (Problem Side)	Goal/Expected Outcome
Problem response	Opposite of problem response
Present health status	Desired health status
Response that you hope to change	Response that you hope to achieve
Example:	*Examples:*
Ineffective Airway Clearance ⟶	Lungs clear to auscultation
r/t ineffective cough secondary to incision pain ⟶	Coughs productively

problem and implies that this response is what the interventions are intended to achieve, as in Table 5–2.

CriticalThinking 5–2

Answer the following questions for Ben Ivanos's nursing diagnosis of Acute Pain secondary to musculoskeletal trauma (arms, legs, body) and muscle spasms:

- What would be the opposite, healthy response to his problem?
- What changes should you see in appearance, body functions, symptoms, knowledge, and emotions?
- If the problem is prevented or solved, how will Mr. Ivanos look or behave? What will you be able to observe (e.g., see, hear, smell, taste, or touch)?
- What should Mr. Ivanos be able to do to demonstrate a positive change? How well, or how soon, should he be able to do it?

Take a few minutes to think about and write the answers to those questions.

You might have said that the opposite response to pain would be absence of (or relief from) pain, but you couldn't really observe that. "Absence of pain" might

serve as a broad goal statement. But how about more specific, observable expected outcomes? How would you know that Mr. Ivanos's pain was relieved?

Specific, observable behaviors that demonstrate absence of pain include the following:

Relaxed body posture
Relaxed facial expression
Does not complain of pain
States that his pain is relieved (or manageable, or gone)
Rates pain as less than 3 on a scale of 1 to 10

Essential versus Nonessential Goals

In general, the problem side of the nursing diagnosis suggests the goals, and the etiology suggests nursing interventions. Some goals can also be derived from the etiology; however, the **essential patient goals** flow from the problem side of the nursing diagnosis (see the bold print in Table 5–3) because the problem side describes the unhealthy response that you intend to change.

Notice in Table 5–3 that the goals derived from the etiology may help resolve the problem, but they could

TABLE 5-3 Deriving Goals and Interventions from Nursing Diagnoses

Nursing diagnosis	Goals/Expected Outcomes	Nursing Activities
Problem: *Ineffective Airway Clearance* r/t	⟶ **Lungs clear to auscultation** **Coughs productively** **Respirations 12–20/min** **No dyspnea or shortness of breath (SOB)** **No pallor or cyanosis**	⟶ Teach deep breathing and coughing Auscultate lungs q4hr Assess respiratory rate, breathing, and skin color q4hr
Etiology: *Ineffective cough secondary to incisional pain*	⟶ Coughs forcefully/effectively Rates pain as <3 on 1–10 scale Splints incision while coughing	⟶ Teach to splint incision while coughing Turn, cough, and deep-breathe (TCDB) hourly Medicate for pain 30 min before TCDB

TABLE

5-4 Expected Outcomes for Various Problem Types

Type of Problem	Example of Diagnosis	Explanation of Diagnosis	Focus of Nursing Interventions	Example of Expected Patient Outcome
Actual Nursing Diagnosis	Constipation r/t inadequate dietary fiber and fluids	Symptoms of constipation present (e.g., no BM)	Resolution or reduction of problem; prevention of complications	Will have normal, formed BM within 24 hr after receiving stool softener
Risk (Potential) Nursing Diagnosis	Risk for Constipation r/t inadequate dietary fiber and fluids	Risk factors present (e.g., not drinking enough or eating adequate fiber)	Prevention and early detection problem	Will have bowel function within normal limits for patient (e.g., daily bowel movement with no need for stool softener or laxative)
Possible Nursing Diagnosis	Possible Constipation r/t suspected inadequate intake of dietary fiber and fluids	Not enough data (e.g., no BM for 2 days, but no data on intake or on his usual bowel habits)	Confirm or rule out problem	No patient goal. The nursing goal is "Confirm or rule out the problem"
Collaborative Problem	Potential Complication of abdominal surgery: ileus	Medical treatment creates risk for complication that is prevented by collaborative care	Primarily detection; prevention is collaborative	None. Patient responses depend on collaborative care. The broad *nursing* goal is early identification of the problem
Wellness Diagnosis	Readiness for Enhanced Nutrition	Bowel habits and dietary intake within normal limits, but can be improved	Maintain or promote higher level of health	Reports increased intake of dietary fiber and fluids; reports bowel functioning within normal limits

also be achieved without resolution of the problem. Suppose that you had written only the goals in regular type for a patient with Ineffective Airway Clearance. If the patient coughs forcefully and effectively, rates pain as less than 3, and splints his incision while coughing, you might discontinue the interventions for Ineffective Airway Clearance. However, the problem might still exist. Even a client who demonstrates all three of those responses might not be coughing productively enough to clear the airways and might still not have clear lung sounds. This means that you should follow this rule:

For every nursing diagnosis, you must state one goal that, if achieved, would demonstrate resolution or improvement of the problem.

Goals for Actual, Risk, and Possible Nursing Diagnoses

You will develop expected outcomes to promote, maintain, or restore health, depending on the status of the nursing diagnosis. See Table 5–4 for explanations and examples. Review Chapter 4 as needed.

Goals for Collaborative Problems

Recall that collaborative problems are physiological complications of diseases (e.g., diabetes) or medical treatments (e.g., cardiac catheterization) that nurses monitor to detect onset or changes in status. Always,

the desired outcome is that the complication will not develop. However, unlike outcomes for nursing diagnoses, these outcomes are not nurse-sensitive; that is, they do not result primarily from nursing interventions. They occur as a result of interventions by several disciplines. Consider the following example:

Collaborative problem: Potential Complication of abdominal surgery: paralytic ileus (paralysis of the ileum of the small intestine)
Goal: Patient will not develop paralytic ileus

Suppose that 36 hours after the surgery, the patient's bowel sounds are absent, his abdomen is distended and painful, and he begins vomiting. What could the nurse have done to prevent this situation? What can the nurse do to relieve the ileus and bring about return of peristalsis? Very little, actually. The primary interventions are medical and, if there is obstruction, probably surgical. Therefore, it would not be appropriate to include a goal for this problem on a nursing care plan, because that would imply that nurses are primarily accountable for the outcome. All goals on a nursing care plan should be nursing-sensitive goals. Instead of a patient outcome, you might wish to write a nursing goal such as: "Early detection of complication, should it occur." See Table 5–4.

On student care plans, to aid your learning, you can write the symptoms of the complication or the normal physiological response you hope to observe (e.g., Bowel sounds present within 24 hours; no abdominal distention; no vomiting), but these are not appropriate on an institutional care plan. However, collaborative goals are appropriate on multidisciplinary care plans and critical pathways.

How Do I Use Standardized Terminology for Outcomes?

In Chapter 4, you learned about the NANDA standardized terminology for nursing diagnoses. The ANA has also approved several standardized vocabularies for describing client outcomes. The one used throughout most of this book is the Nursing Outcomes Classification (NOC) (Moorhead, Johnson, & Maas, 2004).

What Is the Nursing Outcomes Classification (NOC)?

The NOC is a standardized vocabulary of more than 260 nursing-sensitive outcomes developed by a research team at the University of Iowa. In the NOC vocabulary, an **outcome** is "an individual, family, or community state, behavior, or perception that is measured along a continuum in response to nursing interventions" (Moorhead et al., 2004, p. 20). Thus, the NOC is versatile because it is appropriate for use in all specialty and practice areas.

BOX 5–2 Outcomes Linked to NANDA Diagnosis

Nursing Diagnosis: Situational Low Self-Esteem
Definition: Negative self-evaluation/feelings about self that develop in response to a loss or change in an individual who previously had a positive self-evaluation

Suggested Outcomes:
Decision Making
Grief Resolution
Psychosocial Adjustment: Life Change
Self-Esteem

Source: Johnson, M., Bulechek, G. M., McCloskey Dochterman, J., Maas, M., & Moorhead, S. (2001). *Nursing diagnoses, outcomes, & interventions: NANDA, NOC, and NIC linkages.* St Louis: Mosby, pp. 284–285.

Additional Associated Outcomes:
Abuse Recovery Status
Abuse Recovery: Emotional
Abuse Recovery: Physical
Abuse Recovery: Sexual
Anxiety Level
Coping
Fear Level
Fear Level: Child
Neglect Recovery
Personal Autonomy
Role Performance
Stress Level

Source: Moorhead, S., Johnson, M., & Maas, M. (Eds.). (2004). *Nursing outcomes classification (NOC).* (3rd ed). St Louis: Mosby, p. 637.

Components of a NOC Outcome

Each NOC outcome consists of an outcome label, indicators, and a measurement scale. The *outcome label* (usually referred to as "the outcome") is broadly stated (e.g., Decision Making, Mobility Level, Concentration). It is a neutral label (a variable), to allow for positive, negative, or no change in patient health status. Because NOC outcomes are linked to NANDA nursing diagnoses, you can look up a nursing diagnosis to see the list of outcomes suggested for it. See Box 5–2 for an example of NOC outcomes suggested for one NANDA diagnosis. You can find suggested outcomes for each NANDA diagnosis in the NANDA/NIC/NOC "linkages" book (Johnson, Bulechek, McCloskey Dochterman, &

TABLE 5–5 Example of a NOC Outcome

Decision Making (0906)
Domain—Physiologic Health (II)
Class—Neurocognitive (J)
Scale(s)—Severely compromised to Not compromised
Definition: Ability to make judgments and choose between two or more alternatives

Decision Making	Severely Compromised	Substantially Compromised	Moderately Compromised	Mildly Compromised	Not Compromised
Overall Rating	*1*	*2*	*3*	*4*	*5*
Identifies relevant information	1	2	3	4	5
Identifies alternatives	1	2	3	4	5
Identifies potential consequences of each alternative	1	2	3	4	5
Identifies resources necessary to support each alternative	1	2	3	4	5
Recognizes contradiction with others' desires	1	2	3	4	5
Acknowledges social context of the situation	1	2	3	4	5
Acknowledges relevant legal implications	1	2	3	4	5
Weighs alternatives	1	2	3	4	5
Chooses among alternatives	1	2	3	4	5

Source: Moorhead, S., Johnson, M., & Maas, M. (Eds). (2004). *Nursing outcomes classification (NOC)* (3rd ed.). St Louis: Mosby, p. 251.

Moorhead, 2002). You can find "Additional Associated Outcomes" for each diagnosis in Part IV of the *Nursing Outcomes Classification (NOC)* (Moorhead et al., 2004).

The *indicators* are the observable behaviors and states that you can use to evaluate patient status. In Table 5–5 the indicators are in the first (left) column. The first one is "Identifies relevant information." This indicator is one way you could know that Decision Making (the broad outcome) was being achieved. For each outcome, you select the indicators that are appropriate to the patient. You can add to the list of indicators if necessary.

For each outcome, NOC has a 5-point *measurement scale* (the numbers in Table 5–5) that is used to describe patient status for each indicator. As a rule, 1 is least desirable and 5 is most desirable. If you are using NOC, you do not need to write traditional goal statements. You simply write the label, choose the appropriate indicators, and assign a number from the measurement scale. In your initial assessment, you assign the number that represents the patient's present

health status. To form the "goal," you assign the scale number that the patient can realistically achieve after the interventions. Using Table 5–5, for example, you might assign the following numbers:

(NOC Outcome) **Decision Making**
Goals (Indicators + measurement scale)
Identifies relevant information (4, often demonstrated)
Identifies alternatives (4, often demonstrated)
Identifies potential consequences of each alternative (5, often demonstrated)

For a list of the NOC measurement scales,

VOL 2 Go to Chapter 5, **Standardized Language,** in Volume 2.

KnowledgeCheck 5–6

Figure 5–5, a patient plan of care for Acute Pain, uses NOC language.
• What outcomes did the nurse choose for this patient?

- List two indicators for each of the outcomes.
- For which outcome does the nurse expect the highest level of functioning to occur after interventions? (Note that in this care plan the measuring scale has been applied to the outcomes rather than to the indicators.)

 Go to Chapter 5, **Knowledge Check Response Sheet and Answers,** on the Electronic Study Guide.

 CriticalThinking 5–3

In Figure 5–4, what do you think the nurse expects to happen? Why do you think she ranked the outcomes this way?

Using NOC with Computerized Care Plans

Standardized language (e.g., NOC) is especially useful in computerized care systems. To see computer screens for locating and choosing NOC *outcomes* and for choosing NOC *indicators,* respectively,

 Go to Chapter 5, **Tables, Boxes, Figures: ESG Figures 5–4 and 5–5,** on the Electronic Study Guide.

In that figure, the nurse has chosen Circulation Status as a patient outcome, and the program has provided the definition and the NOC indicators for that outcome. The nurse would then check the indicators that apply to the patient.

Remember that the computer does not think for you. You are responsible for deciding which outcomes and indicators to use for each patient, and for identifying a target time. Most computer programs have a screen that allows you to type in your own goals.

How Do I Write Goals for Groups?

Home and community health nurses are especially likely to write goals for aggregates (groups), such as families and communities. **Community health goals (public health goals)** are those you would use to specify and evaluate the health of groups, aggregates, or populations. They tend to emphasize health promotion, health maintenance, and disease prevention outcomes. For example, the U.S. Public Health Service (USPHS) has developed two group goals—the following broad, overarching goals for improving the health of the nation by a target date of 2010 (*Healthy People 2010,* p. 2, Vol. I):

1. Increase quality and years of healthy life
2. Eliminate health disparities

NOC currently includes nine outcomes targeted to Community Health, which they define as "outcomes that describe the health, well-being, and functioning of a community or population" (Moorhead et al., 2004, p. 105). Two examples are Community Competence and Community Risk Control: Lead Exposure. NOC also has ten outcomes that describe the health of a family as a unit. Two examples are

Family Coping and Family Health Status. NOC outcomes can be used in all settings, including home and community nursing. For further explanation, see Chapters 42 and 43. Also,

 Go to the **NOC web site** at **http://www.nursing.uiowa.edu/ centers/cncce**

However, the following taxonomies were created specifically for describing family and community outcomes.

- **The Clinical Care Classification (CCC).** The CCC system was developed by Virginia Saba, a nurse researcher from Georgetown University, for use in home health nursing. In the CCC, formerly the Home Health Care Classification, you form goals by adding modifiers to the nursing diagnoses. This system has four nursing diagnoses that are clearly for family units:

   Family Coping Impairment
   Compromised Family Coping
   Disabled Family Coping
   Family Processes Alteration

The CCC includes one diagnosis specifically for communities: Community Coping Impairment.

For a complete description of the CCC system,

 Go to the **CCC web site** at **http://www.sabacare.com**

- **The Omaha System.** The Omaha System was developed specifically for community health nursing. In that system, you must label all nursing diagnoses as either *individual, family,* or *group.* You can write aggregate outcomes by specifying a *family* or *group* diagnosis and then creating a goal from it, as in the following example.

   Omaha Nursing Diagnosis: Personal Hygiene. Family. Deficit (Actual Problem)

Present status	*Expected outcome*
Minimal knowledge of family personal hygiene	Adequate knowledge of family personal hygiene

For a complete description,

 Go to the **Omaha System web site** at **http://www.omahasystem.org**

 KnowledgeCheck 5–7

- Which standardized classification system was designed specifically for community health nursing?
- Which standardized classification system was designed specifically for home health care?
- Which standardized classification system was designed for use in all areas and specialties of nursing?

 Go to Chapter 5, **Knowledge Check Response Sheet and Answers,** on the Electronic Study Guide.

How Do I Write Goals for Wellness Diagnoses?

Whether standardized or individualized, expected outcomes for wellness diagnoses describe behaviors or responses that demonstrate health maintenance or achievement of an even higher level of health. For example: Over the next year, [Mr. Needham] will continue to eat a balanced diet, with more emphasis on including whole grains and fiber. By using the highest number (5) on the rating scale, you can use the NOC to write wellness outcomes. For example:

> *Nursing diagnosis:*
> Readiness for Enhanced Nutrition
> *Expected outcome:*
> Nutritional Status: (5) Not compromised

In addition, many NOC outcomes can be used to measure health (e.g., Activity Tolerance, Child Development, Growth, Nutritional Status). See Chapter 41 or go to the NOC web site for a complete list of wellness outcomes.

Outcomes for Special Teaching Plans

As discussed earlier, some patients need a special teaching plan to address learning needs. Expected outcomes are written in the same way as for any other care plan, but they are usually called teaching objectives. **Teaching objectives** describe what the patient is to learn and the observable behaviors that will demonstrate learning, and they should state whether learning is to be cognitive, psychomotor, or affective. An example of a cognitive objective is: "By May 1, will list four foods to avoid on a low-fat diet." An example of an affective objective is: "By May 1, will verbalize feeling less anger about diet limitations." An example of a psychomotor goal is: "By May 1, will demonstrate how to use grasp extender to obtain food from the top shelf." For further information about teaching objectives, see Chapter 24.

REFLECTING CRITICALLY ABOUT EXPECTED OUTCOMES/GOALS

After writing the expected outcomes for a client in your care, use the full-spectrum nursing model to help you evaluate their quality. You can use the following questions to guide your final evaluation of your goals/outcomes.

For each nursing diagnosis:
1. *Is there at least one goal that, when met, would demonstrate problem resolution; that is, does at least one goal flow from the problem clause?* (See "Essential versus Nonessential Goals" pp. 95–96.)
2. *Are the predicted outcomes adequate to completely address the nursing diagnosis?* If you have written outcomes in very specific, measurable terms, you may need several for a single nursing diagnosis. Notice in Table 5–3, that none of the outcomes, alone, would demonstrate that the problem of

Ineffective Airway Clearance had been resolved. All of those outcomes are important; the ones in bold print are essential.

For each expected outcome:
3. *Is the outcome appropriate for the nursing diagnosis?* In Table 5–3, for example, "Obtains 8 hrs sleep at night" would not be an appropriate outcome for the nursing diagnosis Ineffective Airway Clearance, because it does not flow from either the problem or etiology clause. It may seem related because Ineffective Airway Clearance would probably cause Disturbed Sleep Pattern. If so, a new nursing diagnosis should be written rather than adding a not-quite-related goal to the existing plan.
4. *Is each outcome derived from only one nursing diagnosis?* That is, does it describe only one patient response? Notice that in the following incorrect example, even though diarrhea may cause excoriation of perianal skin, obtaining a good skin outcome would not tell you anything about the status of the Diarrhea diagnosis.

   Incorrect:
   For a diagnosis of Diarrhea: Will have no diarrhea in the next 12 hours, and skin will be intact and without redness in the perianal area.
   Correct:
   For a diagnosis of Diarrhea: Will have no diarrhea in the next 12 hours.
   For a diagnosis of Impaired Skin Integrity: Skin will remain intact and without redness in the perianal area.

5. *Does each outcome describe only one patient response or behavior?* Look at the "correct" example in (4), for the Impaired Skin Integrity diagnosis. How many patient responses does it contain? (It has two responses: skin will remain intact, and skin will not be red.) So our "correct" example meets criteria for (4) but not for (5).

 CriticalThinking 5–4

Why is it a problem to write the Skin Integrity outcome as shown in #4?

6. *Is the outcome stated as a patient behavior, not a nurse activity?*

   Incorrect (nurse activity): Prevent skin irritation
   Correct (patient response): Skin will not show signs of irritation

7. *Is the outcome stated in positive terms?* When possible, state what you hope will occur, not what you hope will not occur. For example:

Positive wording:	Incision edges approximated
	Incision dry
Negative wording:	No incision drainage
	No redness of incision

| toward evidence-based practice |

Daly, J. M., Buckwalter, K., & Maas, M. (2002). Written and computerized care plans. Organizational processes and effect on patient outcomes. *Journal of Gerontological Nursing, 28*(9), 14–23.

This study, done in a long-term care facility, used an experimental design to compare the use of standardized terminology for nursing diagnoses and interventions on (1) paper care plans and (2) computerized care plans. The study variables were patient outcomes, specifically: level of care, activities of daily living, perception

of pain, cognitive abilities, number of medications, number of bowel medications, number of constipation episodes, weight, percent of meals eaten, and incidence of altered skin integrity. "Level of care" was measured by the number of nursing activities and interventions documented.

No significant difference was found for any of the patient outcomes. There were significantly more nursing interventions and activities on the computerized care plan; however, the computerized care plans took longer to develop than did paper care plans.

1. If you had to decide on the basis of this study alone, would you be for or against using computerized care plans in your organization?

2. Use the results of the study to justify your choice. What benefits of computerized care plans does the study suggest? What disadvantages?

 Go to Chapter 5, **Toward Evidence-Based Practice Suggested Responses,** on the Electronic Study Guide.

This is not always possible, especially for potential problems. It is better, for example, to write "No redness" (even though it is negative) than to write "Skin color normal," because "normal" is too vague. For potential problems, a negatively worded outcome is actually a list of the patient responses you are trying to prevent.

8. *Is the outcome measurable or observable?*

Correct: Explains the actions and side effects of Coumadin, by 8/11
Incorrect: Understands the actions and side effects of Coumadin, by 8/11

There is no way to observe someone's understanding, so you could not use the second (incorrect) goal to evaluate client progress. Use action verbs; think, "What do I want to see, hear, feel, or smell?"

9. *Are the performance criteria specific and concrete?* Avoid words such as *normal, sufficient, enough, more, less, adequate, increased.* Vague words can be interpreted differently by different people. Does "Will receive *adequate* sleep" mean that the patient will sleep 8 hours per night, will fall asleep within an hour of going to bed, will feel rested in the morning, or will not become sleepy during the day?

10. *Does each goal include all the necessary parts?* Is there a subject (implied or actual), action verb, performance criterion, target time, and special condition (when needed)?

11. *Is the expected outcome realistic and achievable by this patient, given the available resources?* The

outcome "Will rest for an hour twice a day" may not be realistic for a single mother with several small children and no help at home. People usually will not work to achieve goals unless they believe they are possible to achieve.

Be sure to consider the patient's support system, financial status, available community services, and physical and mental status. Also consider whether institutional resources are adequate. For example, there is no point in writing, "Will express anxieties and questions freely to the nurse" if staffing is inadequate to allow the nurse to spend enough time with the patient to develop a relationship.

12. *Does the outcome conflict with the medical or other collaborative treatment plan?* For example, an outcome of "Will attempt to breastfeed the newborn within the first 2 hours after birth" would not be compatible with the medical treatment plan for a new mother with severe preeclampsia, who is sleepy and lethargic from the side effects of medications.

13. *Does the patient, family, or community value the outcome?* The care plan is more likely to be effective if the goal is important to the client. You may, for example, believe that smoking cessation is an important goal for the patient. However, a patient who has been smoking for 50 years and is having only moderate breathing difficulties might not be motivated to achieve this goal, even when given all the related information. When your goals conflict with the patient's, explore the patient's

reasoning. Explain your reasoning and try to find a compromise or an alternative approach.

14. *Does the goal conflict with any religious or cultural values?* You may know that early ambulation (e.g., "Ambulates to bathroom within 4 hours after birth of the baby") promotes circulation and helps to prevent thrombophlebitis. However, in some cultures, childbirth is viewed as an illness, and the mother expects to remain in bed for several days with family members taking care of her needs. When the mother is "noncompliant," the reason may be that she is complying with her cultural beliefs rather than the caregiver's plan of care.

KnowledgeCheck 5–8

List at least eight questions you could use to critically evaluate the quality of your goal/outcome statements.

 Go to Chapter 5, **Knowledge Check Response Sheet and Answers,** on the Electronic Study Guide.

 Go to Chapter 5, **Resources for Caregivers and Health Professionals,** on the Electronic Study Guide.

 Suggested Readings: Go to Chapter 5, **Reading More About Planning Outcomes,** on the Electronic Study Guide.

 Bibliography: Go to Volume 2, Bibliography.

Nursing Process:
Planning Interventions

Learning Outcomes

After completing this chapter, you should be able to:

✳ Define the term *nursing intervention*.

✳ Compare and contrast independent, dependent, and interdependent (collaborative) nursing interventions.

✳ Explain how theories and research influence the choice of nursing interventions.

✳ Explain how nursing interventions are determined by problem status (i.e., actual or potential problem).

✳ Describe a process for generating nursing interventions for a client.

✳ Explain how to use a standardized vocabulary to choose nursing interventions and activities.

✳ Name the standardized vocabulary developed especially for family and home health interventions.

✳ Name the standardized vocabulary developed specifically for community health nursing.

✳ Give one example of a standardized wellness (health promotion) intervention and one individualized nursing order for performing that intervention.

✳ Give one example of a standardized spirituality intervention and one individualized nursing order for performing that intervention.

✳ Write complete, detailed nursing orders, in correct format, for patients.

✳ Give examples of some questions to ask yourself when reflecting critically about nursing orders you have written.

MEET Your Patient

Ben Ivanos, whom you met in Chapter 5, is confined to bed after a motorcycle accident. He has casts and traction on both legs and a cast on one arm. Since admission to the hospital 3 days ago, he has been receiving narcotic analgesics for severe pain. He has a new nursing diagnosis today: Constipation related to immobility and decreased gastrointestinal (GI) motility secondary to narcotic analgesics. The nurse enters the diagnosis into a care-planning program. In addition to a list of suggested assessments, the computer suggests the following treatment interventions:

1. Institute a program to establish a regular pattern of bowel movements.
2. Administer laxative or stool softener, as ordered.
3. Administer enema.
4. Remove stool manually.
5. Encourage increased fluid intake.
6. Instruct on and encourage a high-fiber diet.
7. Encourage regular program of activity and exercise.
8. Perform manual reduction of rectal prolapse.

Which interventions should the nurse choose? Which can he eliminate, based on the information provided? (You may not yet have enough nursing knowledge to be sure about your answers to these questions, but before reading on, try to think it through with the information and life experience available to you.)

The nurse eliminated interventions 1, 3, 4, 7, and 8. Take a few moments to see if you can explain the nurse's reasons for deleting these interventions.

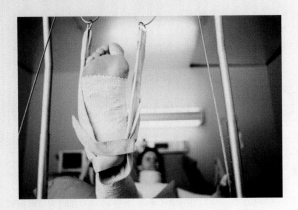

Compare your explanations to the following reasons given by the nurse. The nurse eliminated intervention:

• 1 because it is useful for patients who are constipated as a result of irregular bowel habits, whereas Mr. Ivanos's problem is caused by immobility and narcotic side effects.

• 3 and 4 because Mr. Ivanos's symptoms did not seem severe enough to warrant an enema or manual removal of stool.

• 7 because it is not practical: Mr. Ivanos cannot exercise in his present condition.

• 8 because it is not relevant: Mr. Ivanos does not have rectal prolapse.

The nurse chose the following interventions to include in the care plan:

• 2 because it directly addresses the problem, Constipation.

• 5 and 6 because they address the etiology of the problem—fluid and fiber soften the stool and help to stimulate bowel activity.

The nurse also reasoned that because narcotics cause constipation, it would be good to administer them less frequently to Mr. Ivanos—if other satisfactory pain-relief measures could be found. So he added the following nursing orders to the care plan:

Assist to change position q1–2hr.
Encourage distraction (e.g., watching TV, reading, listening to music).
Assist with relaxation and visualization techniques.
Obtain medical order for non-narcotic analgesics to enhance nonpharmacological pain-relief measures.
Assess effectiveness of nonpharmacological interventions for pain.
Give prescribed narcotic analgesics if other measures are ineffective.

The nurse recalled that people are often self-conscious or embarrassed about using a bedpan, especially in the presence of others. So he also added to the care plan:

> Encourage Mr. Ivanos to summon the nurse when he feels the urge to defecate (place call light within reach). If he does not, then ask at least q4hr whether he needs the bedpan.
>
> Warm the bedpan and provide privacy: pull the bed curtain, turn on the TV or radio if he has a roommate, explain that you will leave the room and that he should call when he is ready for you to return, and shut the door.

As you can see, to develop interventions to meet Mr. Ivanos's needs, the nurse needed to do more than just look at a list and follow physician orders. He drew on (1) his theoretical knowledge (about narcotics, bowel elimination, and psychological needs), (2) his past experiences with similar patients, and (3) the data about Mr. Ivanos and the factors contributing to his problem (knowledge of the patient situation). By thinking of interventions to meet the client's specific needs, this nurse may prevent Mr. Ivanos's constipation from worsening. A nurse with less knowledge and experience might have used only those interventions in the computer database, failing to effectively meet the desired outcomes (goals) for Mr. Ivanos.

WHAT ARE NURSING INTERVENTIONS?

Nursing interventions are actions based on clinical judgment and nursing knowledge that nurses perform to achieve client outcomes. (Figure 6–1 shows how planning interventions relates to the other phases of the nursing process.) Interventions are also referred to as *nursing actions, measures, strategies,* and *activities.* This chapter will use those terms interchangeably except when referring to the Nursing Interventions Classification (NIC) standardized labels (discussed later in the chapter), which are always called *interventions.*

Nursing Interventions Reflect Direct and Indirect Care

No matter what term is used, nursing interventions include a broad range of activities. A **direct-care intervention** is one performed through interaction with the client(s). Direct-care activities include physical care, emotional support, and patient teaching. An **indirect-care intervention** is an activity performed away from the client but on behalf of a client or group of clients. Indirect care activities include advocacy, managing the environment, consulting with other members of the healthcare team, and making referrals.

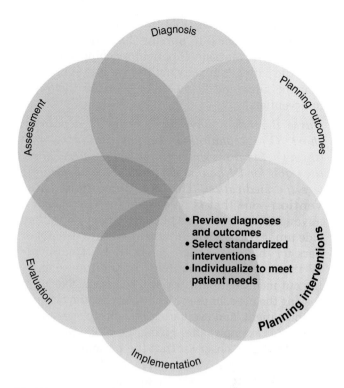

• Review diagnoses and outcomes
• Select standardized interventions
• Individualize to meet patient needs

FIGURE 6–1   Nursing process phase: planning interventions.

CriticalThinking 6–1
• Can you think of an example of a direct-care intervention?
• Can you think of an example of an indirect-care intervention?

Nursing Interventions Include Independent, Dependent, and Collaborative Actions

Nurses work collaboratively with other healthcare providers. Some things you do for patients will require a physician's order; many will not. Sometimes the activities of care providers overlap. For example, physicians, nurses, and respiratory therapists may all measure a client's blood pressure, and both a nurse and a dietitian may teach the client about a diet to help manage hypertension. Consider the following scenarios:

• *Nurse A makes a nursing diagnosis of* Anxiety *related to deficient knowledge about barium enema; she writes a nursing order to teach the patient what to expect from the upcoming diagnostic test, a barium enema.* This is an **independent intervention**—one that nurses are licensed to prescribe, perform, or delegate based on their knowledge and skills. It does not require a physician's order. Knowing how, when, and why to perform an activity makes the action **autonomous** (independent). As a rule, nurses prescribe and perform independent interventions in response to a nursing diagnosis. Understand that you are

accountable (answerable) for your decisions and actions with regard to nursing diagnoses and independent interventions. If patient teaching did not relieve the patient's anxiety in this example, it might be that the nurse misdiagnosed or chose an ineffective intervention.

- *Nurse B reads a physician's order in a patient's chart: Give cephalothin sodium (Keflin) 1 g IV (through the intravenous line) before surgery, and then q6h for 24 hours. She prepares and administers the medication.* This is a **dependent intervention**—one that is prescribed by a physician or advanced practice nurse but carried out by the bedside nurse. Dependent interventions are usually orders for diagnostic tests, medications, treatments, IV therapy, diet, and activity. In addition to carrying out medical orders, you will be responsible for assessing the need for the order, explaining the activities to the patient, and evaluating the effectiveness of the order. For example, after giving the Keflin (an antibiotic), the nurse observes that the patient has developed a severe rash. Suspecting an allergic reaction, she contacts the physician so that the medication order can be changed and antibiotic prophylaxis can be continued after surgery without danger to the patient.

  In addition, you may write nursing orders to individualize a medical order, based on the client's condition. For example, the physician may order, "Force oral fluids up to 3000 mL per 24 hours." You might individualize the order to give 1500 mL on the day shift, 1000 mL on the evening shift, and 500 mL during the night, so that the patient will not have to be awakened frequently during the night.

- *Nurse C notes that a client newly diagnosed with diabetes has been seen by a dietitian, who taught and provided materials about a diabetic diet. The nurse observes the client's menu choices. She notes that the client is eating candy brought by visitors. She explains to the patient how concentrated sugar affects his diabetes; she also communicates her assessments and teaching to the dietitian.* This is an **interdependent (collaborative) intervention**—one that is carried out in collaboration with other health team members (e.g., physical therapists, dietitians, and physicians). Because nurses care for the whole person, their responsibilities often overlap with those of other team members.

CriticalThinking 6–2

- What are some other examples of independent interventions?
- What are some other examples of dependent interventions?
- What are some other examples of interdependent interventions?

HOW DO I DECIDE WHICH INTERVENTIONS TO USE?

Box 6–1 identifies professional standards of care related to planning interventions. Use these standards to guide you in selecting interventions appropriate for the client's nursing diagnoses (or collaborative problems) and the desired outcomes. In addition to these standards, a variety of theories, nursing research, and the patient's problem status will all influence your choice of interventions.

As a nurse, you will be responsible for choosing nursing interventions. You cannot delegate this responsibility to unlicensed assistive personnel. For more information about delegation, see "What Should I Know About Delegation and Supervision?" on pages 126–128.

How Do Theories Influence My Choice of Interventions?

A **theory** is a set of interrelated concepts (ideas) that describes or explains something—nursing, for example. Theories influence your perspective: What you notice, what you consider to be a problem, and how you define a problem more or less determine what you choose to do about it. For example, suppose a patient is pale and fidgeting and has sweaty palms and a rapid pulse. If you viewed this person through the lens of psychological theory, your first thought might be that the patient is anxious. Your first intervention, then, would probably be to assess for the cause of his anxiety. If you were using a physiological lens, you might suspect pain. Your first intervention, then, might be to ask the patient if he is having pain. For more information about nursing theories, see Chapter 8.

How Does Nursing Research Influence My Choice of Interventions?

Although much nursing and medical practice is still based on tradition, experience, and professional opinion, this is not ideal. Ideally a nurse would choose an intervention on the basis of firm evidence that it is the best possible approach for the patient. It stands to reason that such interventions would be those that were developed from a sound body of research. ANA Standards of Nursing Practice (ANA, 2004, p. 40) state that the registered nurse:

- Utilizes best available evidence, including research findings, to guide practice decisions.
- Actively participates in research activities . . . [which] may include: Critically analyzing and interpreting research for application to practice.

Research-based support for an intervention includes single studies, critical pathways and protocols, clinical practice guidelines, and evidence reports.

BOX 6-1 Professional Standards for Planning Interventions

American Nurses Association Standards of Nursing Practice

Standard 4. Planning

The registered nurse develops a plan that prescribes strategies and alternatives to attain expected outcomes.

Measurement Criteria:

The registered nurse:

Develops an individualized plan considering patient characteristics or the situation (e.g., age and culturally appropriate, environmentally sensitive).

Develops the plan in conjunction with the patient, family, and others, as appropriate.

Includes strategies within the plan that address each of the identified diagnoses or issues, which may include strategies for promotion and restoration of health and prevention of illness, injury, and disease.

Provides for continuity within the plan.

Incorporates an implementation pathway or timeline within the plan.

Establishes the plan priorities with the patient, family, and others as appropriate.

Utilizes the plan to provide direction to other members of the healthcare team.

Defines the plan to reflect current statutes, rules and regulations, and standards.

Integrates current trends and research affecting care in the planning process.

Considers the economic impact of the plan.

Uses standardized language or recognized terminology to document the plan.

Note: There are additional standards for advanced practice registered nurses.

Source: Reprinted with permission from American Nurses Association, *Nursing: Scope and standards of practice* (3rd ed.). 2004. American Nurses Publishing, American Nurses Foundation/American Nurses Association, 600 Maryland Ave, SW, Suite 100 W, Washington, DC 20024-2571.

Canadian Provincial Standards of Practice

In Canada, practice standards are set by each province. The following are examples that apply to planning interventions.

Province of Alberta

The registered nurse:

Demonstrates critical thinking in collecting and interpreting data, planning, implementing, and evaluating all aspects of nursing care.

Sets justifiable priorities when giving care.

Source: Alberta Association of Registered Nurses. (1999). *Nursing practice: Professional conduct: Nursing practice standards.* Retrieved August 27, 2002, from http://nurses.ab.ca/profconduct/npa.html

Province of British Columbia

Competent Application of Knowledge: Determines client status and responses to actual or potential health problems, plans interventions, performs planned interventions, and evaluates client outcomes.

Indicators: Designs plans of care which include data about assessments, planned interventions, and evaluation criteria of client outcomes to address client status.

Source: Registered Nurses Association of British Columbia. (2000). *Standards for nursing practice in British Columbia.* Retrieved November 1, 2002, from http://www.rnabc.bc.ca/stndrds/stan2000.htm

Single Studies

You can usually find individual studies that give you an idea of the effectiveness of an intervention. Research reports are available in research journals, and they are often interpreted and published in such widely circulated journals as the *American Journal of Nursing (AJN), Nursing,* and *RN,* as well as online sites. Unfortunately, there may be only one or two studies of an intervention, and they may have included only a small number of patients. Thus, single studies may not be reliable. To see several examples of single intervention studies,

 Go to Chapter 6, **Reading More About the Nursing Process: Planning Interventions,** on the Electronic Study Guide.

Critical Pathways and Protocols

Critical pathways (also called *clinical pathways* and *collaborative care plans*) are standardized plans of care for frequently occurring conditions (e.g., total hip replacement) for which similar outcomes and interventions are appropriate for all patients with the condition. They are tools developed by an agency or organization for its own use and are intended to guide best practice at the local level—to ensure consistency and efficiency of care and improve patient and family education about the plan of care. However, they may not be based on research if the agency's practitioners who develop them are reluctant to change traditional practices that they believe to be effective. Furthermore, issues of cost to the organization influence the decision to include an intervention in the plan of care. Nevertheless, critical pathways provide a guide for nursing interventions in that, at the very least, they have been developed on the basis of expert opinion. See Chapter 5 for discussion and examples of critical pathways and protocols.

Evidence-Based Practice

You can feel more confident about an intervention if several studies have supported it. **Evidence-based medicine** (and by implication, evidence-based nursing) is a term that has been coined to mean the use of firm data rather than anecdote, tradition, intuition, or belief in making decisions about medical and nursing practice (Venes & Thomas, *Taber's Cyclopedic Medical Dictionary,* 2005). The goal of evidence-based practice is to identify the most effective and cost-efficient treatments for a particular disease or condition. A number of healthcare organizations and groups are devoted to compiling study results that provide evidence to use in formulating guidelines for medical and nursing practice. You will find such compiled information in clinical practice guidelines, evidence reports, and sometimes in local healthcare agency tools (e.g., clinical pathways and protocols). One example of a compilation of research is found in the March 2003 supplement to the *American Journal of Nursing,* titled "State of the Science on Urinary Incontinence," which is a report from a recent symposium on incontinence (Newman & Palmer, 2003). For full discussion on the importance of research and evidence-based nursing practice, see Chapter 8.

Clinical Practice Guidelines

Clinical practice guidelines are systematically developed statements to assist practitioners and patients in making decisions about appropriate health care for a particular disease or procedure (Institute of Medicine, 1992). Clinical practice guidelines are usually developed by clinicians, patients, and advocacy groups and are published by specialty organizations, universities, and government agencies. The following are examples:

- The Association of Women's Health, Obstetric and Neonatal Nursing (AWHONN) guidelines on *Neonatal Skin Care* (2001a) and *Promotion of Emotional Well-Being During Midlife* (2001b).
- University of Iowa research-based guidelines for care of the elderly (Titler, Mentes, Rakel, Abbott, & Baumler, 1999).

Not all organizational standards of care are research based, though; many are based on the experience and opinion of experts in the field.

Evidence Reports

Evidence reports are state-of-the-art, systematic reviews on clinical topics for the purpose of providing evidence for guidelines, quality improvement, quality measures, and insurance coverage decisions (Cronenwett, 2002). Evidence reports are usually developed by scientists rather than clinicians, patients, and advocacy groups. One source of such reports is the Evidence-Based Practice Center (EPC) Program of the federal Agency for Healthcare Research and Quality (AHRQ). The EPC uses explicit grading systems to review studies and rank the strength of their evidence. For free access to online reviews,

 Go to the **AHRQ web site** at **http://www.ahrq.gov/**

Clinical practice guidelines are also developed from some of the evidence reports—for example, the guidelines on pressure ulcer formation in Box 6–2 form the basis for nursing interventions. For years, relying on conventional wisdom and word of mouth, nurses tried to prevent pressure ulcers by writing on care plans: "Massage skin over bony prominences." They reasoned that because poor circulation can contribute to the formation of pressure ulcers, improving circulation to the area would prevent them. As you can see in item D of the box, however, research-based practice guidelines show that massage may actually be harmful. This report would certainly motivate you, as a full-spectrum nurse, to remove this "standard" intervention from your practice.

KnowledgeCheck 6–1

- Explain how theory influences your choice of nursing interventions.
- Why does a clinical practice guideline provide better support for an intervention than does a single study?
- Why does a clinical practice guideline provide better support for an intervention than does an agency's critical pathway?

 Go to Chapter 6, **Knowledge Check Response Sheet and Answers,** on the Electronic Study Guide.

How Does Problem Status Influence Nursing Interventions?

Nursing interventions include activities for observation/assessment, prevention, treatment, and health promotion. The status of the problem (i.e., whether it is a collaborative problem or an actual, potential, possible, or wellness nursing diagnosis) determines which types of activities are required (for a review of problem status, see Chapter 4).

- *Observation/assessment interventions* are used for:
  —Actual nursing diagnoses, to detect change in status (improvement, exacerbation of problem).
  —Potential (risk) nursing diagnoses, to detect (1) progression to an actual problem or (2) an increase or decrease in risk factors.
  —Possible nursing diagnoses, to obtain more data to confirm or rule out a suspected nursing diagnosis.
  —Collaborative problems, to detect onset of a complication.
  —Wellness diagnoses, to assess a client's wellness practices.
- *Prevention interventions* are used for:
  —Actual nursing diagnoses, to help keep the problem from becoming worse.
  —Potential (risk) nursing diagnoses, to remove or reduce risk factors in an effort to keep the problem from developing.
  —Collaborative problems, to help prevent development of a complication.
  —Wellness diagnoses, to prevent specific diseases (e.g., giving immunizations).
- *Treatment interventions* are used for:
  —Actual nursing diagnoses, to (a) relieve symptoms and (b) treat etiologies (contributing factors).
  —Collaborative problems, to implement nursing medical orders for relieving or eliminating the problem.
- *Health promotion interventions* are used for wellness diagnoses in order to support a client's health promotion efforts and achieve a higher level of wellness.

A nursing strategy can be a preventive measure in one situation and a treatment in another. For example, you might write the nursing order, "Refer to La Leche League for breastfeeding assistance," to treat a woman with an actual diagnosis of Ineffective Breastfeeding or to help prevent the problem for a woman with a diagnosis of Risk for Ineffective Breastfeeding.

KnowledgeCheck 6–2

Review problem status (actual, potential, or possible nursing diagnosis; collaborative problem; or wellness diagnosis) in Chapter 4. For which type(s) of problem(s) would you write:

BOX 6–2 Portion of a Clinical Practice Guideline on Pressure Ulcer Formation

Skin Care and Early Treatment*

Note: This portion of the practice guideline addresses only the interventions related to skin care and early treatment. Other portions of the guideline address positioning, mattresses, education, and other factors contributing to pressure ulcer formation.

Goal: Maintain and improve tissue tolerance to pressure in order to prevent injury.

A. All individuals at risk should have a systematic skin inspection at least once a day, paying particular attention to the bony prominences. Results of skin inspection should be documented. (Strength of evidence = C)

B. Skin should be cleansed at the time of soiling and at routine intervals.… Avoid hot water.… [and] minimize the force and friction applied to the skin. (Strength of evidence = C)

C. Minimize environmental factors leading to skin drying, such as low humidity (less than 40 percent) and exposure to cold. Dry skin should be treated with moisturizers. (Strength of evidence = B)

D. Avoid massage over bony prominences. Current evidence suggests that massage over bony prominences may be harmful. (Strength of evidence = B)

*Note: "Strength of evidence" is an AHRQ ranking of the amount and quality of research supporting the guideline. The best ranking is A.

Source: Agency for Healthcare Research and Quality, National Institutes for Health. (2002). Clinical practice guideline. Pressure ulcer formation: Skin care and early treatment. Retrieved August 30, 2002, from http://hstat.nlm.nih.gov/hq/Hquest/screen/TextBrowse/t/1030737344857/s/58838 Also available from http://www.ahrq.gov

---

- Nursing orders for observation/assessments?
- Nursing orders for treatments?
- Nursing orders for health promotion interventions?
- Preventive nursing orders?

 Go to Chapter 6, **Knowledge Check Response Sheet and Answers,** on the Electronic Study Guide.

What Process Can I Use for Generating and Selecting Interventions?

As you can see from the case of Ben Ivanos, there are usually several nursing measures that might be effective for any one problem. The idea, of course, is to select

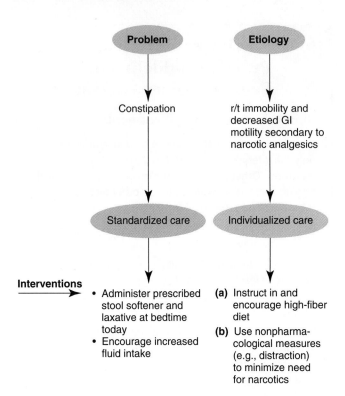

FIGURE 6–2 **Nursing interventions flow from the nursing diagnosis.**

those most likely to achieve the desired goals. In doing that, you must consider the patient's abilities and preferences; the education, experience, and capabilities of the nursing staff; the resources available (e.g., time, equipment); medical orders; and institutional policies and procedures. When generating interventions, you will use critical thinking skills. For example, imagine that you are caring for a hospice patient who has cancer and is dying. She has told you that she is experiencing significant pain, but also that she wants to spend her last hours with her husband and two daughters, who are staying with her. Critical-thinking skills you might use include the following:

- Making interdisciplinary connections (e.g., "What did I learn in psychology class that might help me here?")
- Predicting (e.g., "If I give morphine to the patient, it should relieve her pain, but she will probably become drowsy.")
- Generalizing (e.g., "I have used touch to relieve anxiety many times in similar situations; perhaps it will also help for this patient.")
- Explaining (e.g., "The morphine causes drowsiness by depressing the central nervous system.")
- Therapeutic judgment (e.g., "The patient wants to spend quality time with her family before she dies. Because the morphine will make her drowsy, I should find out if she wants me to give a smaller dose, even though it will not provide good pain relief, along with some nonpharmacological measures.")

You must always rethink an intervention for each patient. You cannot assume that a strategy that was useful in the past will be effective in every situation. In the "Meet Your Patient" scenario, Mr. Ivanos's nurse may have used distraction to successfully relieve the pain of other patients he has cared for. However, if Mr. Ivanos has severe pain, or if he has difficulty concentrating, then distraction may not be effective. A full-spectrum nurse takes such details into account before choosing an intervention. The following process will help you to select the best interventions (Wilkinson, 2001):

1. Review the nursing diagnosis.
2. Review the desired patient outcomes.
3. Identify several interventions or actions.
4. Choose the best interventions for the patient.
5. Individualize standardized interventions to meet the patient's unique needs.

Review the Nursing Diagnosis

Choose strategies that you expect will reduce or remove the etiological factors of actual problems, or that will reduce or remove risk factors for potential problems. Knowledge of the etiology (the "related to" clause of a nursing diagnosis) enables you to individualize the nursing interventions. The etiology describes the factors that contribute to the unhealthy response, so you will choose nursing strategies to target those factors.

1. When it is not possible to change the etiology, choose strategies to treat the patient's symptoms (these may be found in the NANDA "defining characteristics"). For example, if the cause of pain is a surgical incision, you cannot suddenly "cure" the incision. Your nursing actions should focus on measures to relieve the pain.
2. Also, you may not always know the etiology of the problem. Some interventions may relieve a problem regardless of its cause. For example, when you have a client with Anxiety, regardless of its cause, it is helpful to approach the patient calmly; and when you have a client with Constipation, regardless of its cause, it is always appropriate to assess the frequency of the bowel movements and the characteristics of the stool. Consider the nursing diagnosis and interventions for Mr. Ivanos in Figure 6–2.

You can see that nonpharmacological pain strategies would not be needed for all patients. Obviously, some people with constipation do not have pain. The pain-relief nursing order, which flows from the etiology of the problem, is specific to Mr. Ivanos's needs. Administering a stool softener and laxative, however, is a common strategy for constipation, whatever its cause. As a rule, standardized interventions (care common to all patients with a condition) flow from the

6-1 Interventions Flow from Desired Outcomes

Goals/Outcomes	Strategies Suggested by Goals
1. Will have bowel movement within 12 hours after receiving stool softener and laxative.	**A. Administer prescribed stool softener and laxative at bedtime today.**
2. Will have daily soft, formed bowel movement during rest of hospital stay.	B. Instruct in and encourage high-fiber diet.
	C. Encourage increased fluid intake.
3. <u>Within 24 hours, will need narcotics to manage pain < 2×/day.</u>	D. <u>Use nonpharmacological measures (e.g., distraction) to minimize need for narcotics.</u>
4. *Calls nurse when urge to defecate is felt; does not delay defecation.*	E. *Encourage Mr. Ivanos to summon the nurse when he feels the urge to defecate.*
	F. *Provide privacy (e.g., pull the bed curtain, turn on the TV, leave room).*

Note: Dotted lines indicate indirect contribution to goal.

problem side of a nursing diagnosis; individualized interventions, from the etiology.

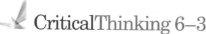

CriticalThinking 6–3

For the following nursing diagnoses, write one intervention to address the problem and one for the etiology of the problem.

- Ineffective Airway Clearance r/t thick secretions and decreased chest expansion secondary to dehydration and pain
- Self-Care Deficit: Bathing/Hygiene and Dressing/Grooming r/t fatigue secondary to disturbed sleep pattern

Review the Desired Patient Outcomes

Desired outcomes (goals) suggest nursing strategies that are specific to the individual patient. For example, Table 6–1 shows some goals and outcomes for Mr. Ivanos's Constipation diagnosis. For each goal on the care plan, ask "What intervention(s) will help to produce this patient response?"

Strategy A in Table 6–1 would help to achieve goal 1; but because the effects of these medications are short-lived, it would do nothing to achieve goals 2 through 4.

Strategies B and C both help to achieve goal 2.

Strategy D (minimize narcotics), in contrast, directly addresses goal 3 and indirectly helps to achieve goal 2.

Strategies E and F both directly address goal 4 and indirectly address goal 2.

As you can see, there may be one or more interventions for each goal, and a single intervention may help to achieve more than one goal. There is no strict one-to-one correspondence between goals and interventions.

Identify Several Interventions or Actions

The next step in choosing interventions is to think of several nursing activities that might achieve the desired outcomes. Don't try to narrow down your list at this point; include unusual and creative ideas. You can refer to a standardized list of interventions (e.g., the Nursing Interventions Classification list on your Electronic Study Guide) or choose interventions from standardized care plans and agency protocols. Alternatively, you can generate the interventions yourself, based on your knowledge, experience, and use of nursing texts, journal articles, and professional nurses. To get started, ask yourself: For this nursing diagnosis, (1) What assessments/observations do I need to make? (2) What do I need to do for the patient? Include both dependent and independent activities as appropriate.

Choose the Best Interventions for the Patient

The best interventions are those you expect to be most effective in helping to achieve client goals. When possible, choose interventions based on research and scientific principles. Use the following critical-thinking questions from the full-spectrum nursing model to help you determine the best actions.

Contextual awareness

- Is this intervention acceptable to the client (e.g., congruent with the patient's values and wishes)?
- Is this intervention culturally sensitive?
- What is going on in the patient's life outside the hospital (e.g., family, work situation, financial status) that may enhance or interfere with the effectiveness of the intervention?

TABLE 6-2   Individualizing Nursing Actions for Ben Ivanos

Standardized Interventions	Individualized Nursing Orders
1. Encourage increased fluid intake.	1. Remind patient to drink a glass of water every hour; keep ice and tea available at bedside.
2. Instruct on and encourage a high-fiber diet.	2. Assist with menu choices to obtain more fiber; encourage family to bring salads and fruits from home for snacks.
3. Encourage distraction (e.g., watching TV, reading, listening to music).	3. Provide books from hospital library (he does not enjoy TV); have family bring radio or CD player and headphones from home.
4. Give prescribed narcotic analgesics if other measures are ineffective.	4. Give Tylenol #3 q4hr if relaxation, visualization, and distraction are ineffective. If orally administered Tylenol #3 is not effective, advise patient to administer IV morphine via patient-controlled analgesia pump.

- What is going on in the patient's health status (e.g., knowledge, abilities, resources, severity of illness) that may enhance or interfere with the effectiveness of the intervention?
- How is this like situations I have seen before? How is it different?

Credible sources

- Have I used valid, reliable sources of information to identify this intervention (e.g., patient, other professionals, references)?
- Did I consider professional, ethical, and legal standards?
- What is the research basis for this intervention, if any?

Considering alternatives

- Is there adequate rationale for this intervention (e.g., principles, theory, facts)?
- Which action(s) is (are) most reasonable? Why are the others not as reasonable?
- Which action(s) is (are) most likely to achieve stated goals?

Analyzing assumptions

- Which beliefs or values are shaping my choice of actions?
- What biases do I have that may affect my thinking and my choice of interventions?
- Do I feel any discomfort with this intervention?

Reflecting skeptically

- Are there other interventions I have overlooked?
- What might be the consequences of this intervention
  —"What will happen if . . .?"
  —Does it have any potential ill effects?
  —If so, how will we manage them?

- Is this intervention feasible (e.g., is it cost-effective, are the time and personnel available for it, can the patient or family manage it at home?)
- How will the intervention interact with medical orders (e.g., you cannot order "elevate head of bed" to facilitate breathing if there is a medical order to keep the patient flat to improve circulation to the neck and head.)
- In priority order, what should I do in this situation and why?
- Do I have the knowledge and skills needed for the intervention, or do I need to consult with another nurse more qualified in this area?
- What might I delegate in this situation?

Individualize Standardized Interventions

Practice guidelines, protocols, critical pathways, and even textbooks describe interventions that are appropriate to most people or the average person. However, they cannot take into account all the individual factors that contribute to a problem or that might affect the effectiveness of an intervention. You must always consider how an intervention can be used with a particular person. For example, after Ben Ivanos's nurse decided which of the computer-generated list of interventions to use, he adapted them to fit Ben's unique needs and preferences. Table 6–2 provides examples of standardized and individualized interventions for Mr. Ivanos.

KnowledgeCheck 6–3

Describe a five-step process for generating and choosing nursing interventions.

 Go to Chapter 6, **Knowledge Check Response Sheet and Answers,** on the Electronic Study Guide.

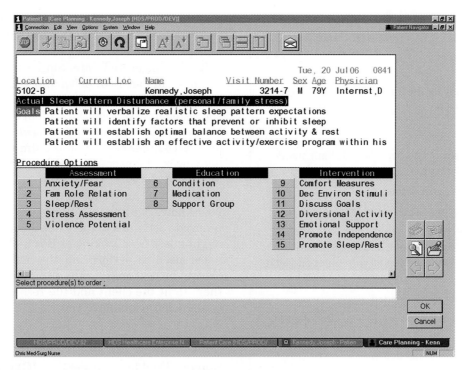

FIGURE 6–3 Computer care planning: When the nurse selects a nursing diagnosis of Sleep Pattern Disturbance, the computer suggests goals and "procedure options" (interventions); the nurse then chooses those best suited for the patient. *Source:* Copyright © Ergo Partners, L.C. All rights reserved. Used with permission.

Computer-Generated Interventions

Most computerized care planning programs will generate a list of suggested interventions when you enter either a problem (nursing diagnosis, medical, collaborative) or an outcome (Figure 6–3). You then choose the interventions appropriate for the patient (as in the case of Ben Ivanos) or type in nursing actions of your own. Computer prompts provide a wide range of interventions for your consideration. However, you must resist the temptation to "settle for" the ready-made solutions. You should always look for other, perhaps more effective, strategies based on the patient data. Always ask, "Are there other interventions I have overlooked? How should I adapt this for *this* patient?"

To see a computer screen showing how an intervention (Pain Control Techniques Education) is converted to nursing orders,

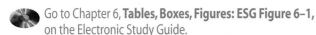 Go to Chapter 6, **Tables, Boxes, Figures: ESG Figure 6–1,** on the Electronic Study Guide.

HOW CAN I USE STANDARDIZED LANGUAGE IN PLANNING INTERVENTIONS?

As a review before reading this section, you may wish to do the following:

• See Chapter 4 for a discussion of standardized language to describe nursing diagnoses (NANDA).

• See Chapter 5 for a discussion of standardized language to describe patient outcomes (NOC).

Recall that standardized nursing terminologies are important for computerized record systems, for research, and for clear, precise, consistent communication among nurses and with other disciplines. The American Nurses Association (ANA) has recognized 12 standardized vocabularies for recording and tracking the clinical care process (American Nurses Association/Nursing Information & Data Set Evaluation Center [ANA/NIDSEC], 2002). Those most commonly used for describing nursing interventions are the Nursing Interventions Classification (NIC), the Clinical Care Classification (CCC), and the Omaha System. NIC classifies only interventions. The CCC and the Omaha System include nursing diagnoses, outcomes, and interventions.

What Is the Nursing Interventions Classification (NIC)?

Developed by a research team at the University of Iowa, NIC was the first comprehensive standardized classification of nursing interventions (McCloskey & Bulechek, 1992). The fourth edition NIC (2004) describes 514 direct and indirect-care activities performed by nurses. The NIC is versatile—appropriate for use in all specialty and practice areas, including home health and community nursing.

BOX 6-3 NIC Intervention: Bathing

Definition

Cleaning of the body for the purposes of relaxation, cleanliness, and healing

Activities

Assist with chair shower, tub bath, bedside bath, standing shower, or sitz bath, as appropriate or desired

Wash hair, as needed and desired

Bathe patient in water of a comfortable temperature

Use fun bathing techniques with children (e.g., wash dolls or toys; pretend a boat is a submarine; punch holes in bottom of plastic cup, fill with water, and let it "rain" on child)

Assist with perineal care, as needed

Assist with hygiene measures (e.g., use of deodorant or perfume)

Administer foot soaks, as needed

Shave patient, as indicated

Apply lubricating ointment and cream to dry skin areas

Offer hand washing after toileting and before meals

Apply drying powders to deep skin folds

Monitor skin condition while bathing

Monitor functional ability while bathing

Source: Dochterman, J. M., & Bulechek, G. M. (Eds.). (2004). Nursing interventions classification (NIC) (4th ed). St Louis: Mosby, p. 183. Used with permission from Elsevier Science.

Each NIC intervention consists of a label, a definition, and a list of the specific **activities** nurses perform in carrying out the intervention (see Box 6–3 for an example). The **label,** usually consisting of two or three words, is the standardized terminology. The **definition** explains the meaning of the label. You are free to word the activities any way you choose in a care plan or client record. For a complete list of NIC intervention labels and definitions,

 Go to **NIC Interventions** on the Electronic Study Guide.

Locating Appropriate NIC Interventions and Activities

NIC interventions are linked to NANDA nursing diagnoses and NOC outcome labels, so you can look up either a nursing diagnosis or a desired outcome to see the list of interventions suggested for it. Refer to Table 6–3 for an example of interventions linked to the nursing diagnosis Risk for Aspiration. Notice that there are 16 "suggested" interventions and 8 "additional optional"

interventions from which to choose. The three shaded interventions are "priority" interventions—in NIC terminology, those most likely to resolve the diagnosis. You will find suggested interventions for each NANDA diagnosis in Part Four of *Nursing Interventions Classification* (Dochterman & Bulechek, 2004); you will find suggested interventions for patient outcomes in *Nursing Diagnoses, Outcomes, and Interventions: NANDA, NOC, and NIC Linkages,* or, more simply, the NNN linkages book (Johnson, Bulechek, Dochterman, Maas, & Moorhead, 2002).

Once you have chosen the interventions (based on your knowledge and judgment), you then choose the appropriate activities to carry out the intervention. As you might guess from looking at Box 6–3, you will probably never need to perform all the activities for a client; choose the best ones for the situation, and individualize them to fit the client and the resources (e.g., supplies, equipment) available to you.

Using NIC in Computerized Care Plans

Standardized language (e.g., NIC) is especially useful in computerized care systems. For a computer screen with NIC suggested interventions for a NANDA nursing diagnosis,

 Go to Chapter 6, **Tables, Boxes, Figures: ESG Figure 6–2,** on the Electronic Study Guide.

For any NIC intervention, the program will also list the more specific nursing activities, which you can individualize as nursing orders.

 Go to Chapter 6, **Tables, Boxes, Figures: ESG Figure 6–3,** on the Electronic Study Guide.

Remember that you are responsible for choosing which interventions to use for each patient, when to use them, and which activities to write as specific nursing orders. You can reject *all* of the suggested interventions if they do not fit the individual patient's needs. Most computer programs have a screen that allows you to type in your own interventions and activities.

Standardized Languages for Home Health and Community Care

The NIC includes interventions applicable in all settings, including home health and community nursing. For further explanation,

 Go to the **NIC web site** at **http://www.nursing.uiowa.edu/ centers/cncce/**

However, the following taxonomies were created specifically for those uses:

- **The Clinical Care Classification (CCC).** Previously called the *Home Health Care Classification,*

TABLE 6-3

NIC Interventions Linked to NANDA Diagnosis, Risk for Aspiration

Aspiration, Risk for: The state in which an individual is at risk for entry of gastrointestinal secretions, oropharyngeal secretions, or solids or fluids into tracheobronchial passages.

Suggested Nursing Interventions for Problem Resolution

Airway Suctioning	Positioning
Amnioinfusion	Postanesthesia Care
Artificial Airway Management	Respiratory Monitoring
Aspiration Precautions	Resuscitation: Neonate
Cough Enhancement	Sedation Management
Neurologic Monitoring	Surveillance
	Swallowing Therapy
	Teaching: Infant Safety
	Teaching: Toddler Safety
	Vomiting Management

Additional Optional Interventions

Asthma Management	Mechanical Ventilation
Enteral Tube Feeding	Mechanical Ventilatory Weaning
Feeding	Medication Administration: Enteral
Gastrointestinal Intubation	Vital Signs Monitoring

Note: Shaded interventions are NIC Priority Interventions.

Source: Dochterman, J. M., & Bulechek, G. M. (Eds.). (2004). *Nursing interventions classification (NIC)* (4th ed). St Louis: Mosby, p. 789. Used with permission from Elsevier Science.

the CCC was developed for use in home health care (Saba, 1995). In addition to terminology for nursing diagnoses and outcomes, the CCC has 198 interventions. For a complete description of the CCC system, see the nursing process section of Chapter 43.

 Go to the **CCC web site** at **http://www.sabacare.com**

• **The Omaha system.** The Omaha system was developed for community health nurses to use in caring for individuals, families, and **aggregates** (community groups or entire communities) (Martin & Scheet, 1992). It includes terminology for diagnoses, outcomes, and interventions. For a complete description of the Omaha system, and for NIC community interventions, see the nursing process section of Chapter 43.

 Go to the **Omaha system web site** at
http://www.omahasystem.org

KnowledgeCheck 6–4
• Name and describe three standardized intervention vocabularies recognized by the ANA.
• In the NIC system, what is the difference between interventions and activities?

 Go to Chapter 6, **Knowledge Check Response Sheet and Answers,** on the Electronic Study Guide.

Does Standardized Language Interfere with Holistic Care?

Some nurses have criticized standardized terminologies for focusing on illness and physical interventions. However NIC, Omaha, and CCC do include interventions to address health promotion, cultural, and spiritual needs. If you have a holistic attitude, you will give holistic care. Using a common language should help rather than hinder your choice of interventions. See Chapter 40 for further discussion of holistic nursing

care. The following bulleted items identify interventions focused on wellness, spiritual needs, and culturally sensitive care.

- *Wellness interventions.* When you are caring for a healthy client, the client is the primary decision maker. You will function mainly as a teacher and health counselor. You can write nursing orders in terms of nurse behaviors or client behaviors. Frequently, the nursing orders outline lifestyle modification or behavior changes the client wants to make, along with self rewards to reinforce the behaviors. For example:

  Specific behavior change: I will consume under 1400 calories per day for the next week.

  Self reward: I will reward myself with an evening out to hear my favorite band.

  The NIC contains most of the wellness interventions you will need. However, they are not all grouped together in one class. Some examples are Decision-Making Support, Exercise Promotion, and Health Screening. For more information on using the NIC, Omaha, and CCC standardized languages to describe wellness interventions, see Chapter 41.

- *Spiritual care interventions.* People frequently have spiritual needs related to their illness. NIC, CCC, and the Omaha system all include terminology to describe spiritual interventions. The following are just a few examples:

NIC:	Spiritual Growth Facilitation, Religious Ritual Enhancement
CCC:	Spiritual Care, Coping Skills
Omaha:	Spiritual Support, Bereavement Support

  Chapter 14 provides full discussion of standardized nursing interventions to address spiritual needs. As you will see, you could also use most of the interventions (e.g., Coping Skills) for other than spiritual problems.

- *Culturally sensitive care.* Except for the NIC Culture Brokerage intervention, there are no standardized interventions that are unique to culturally based needs. All standardized interventions will result in culturally sensitive care if they are delivered by a culturally competent nurse. See Chapter 13 for further discussion.

WHAT ARE NURSING ORDERS, AND HOW DO I WRITE THEM?

Nursing orders are instructions, usually written on a nursing care plan, that describe how and when nursing interventions are to be implemented. Other nurses and unlicensed assistive personnel are responsible and accountable for implementing nursing orders.

complementary and alternative modalities (CAM)

Because nursing is a holistic discipline, many nurses are enthusiastic about the techniques and modalities of complementary and alternative care. They believe that such interventions as acupressure, aromatherapy, biofeedback, guided imagery, humor, journaling, music therapy, promotion of meditation and relaxation, and therapeutic touch help them to address the physical, mental, emotional, and spiritual dimensions of care.

Nursing theories and conceptual models of practice (see Chapter 8) and the current standardized language taxonomies support the use of CAM by nurses.

- CAM performed from within a context of a nursing theory or model takes on meaning as the interventions become part of the purposeful action to achieve goals of care that evolve from the theory.

- CAM performed and documented according to one of the standard taxonomies makes clear that the techniques are appropriate as nursing interventions.

Source: Frisch, N. C. (2001, May 31). Nursing as a context for alternative/complementary modalities. *Online Journal of Issues in Nursing, 6*(2), Manuscript 2, p. 2. Retrieved August 30, 2002, from http://www.nursing world.org/ojin/topic15/tpc15_2.htm

 CriticalThinking 6–4

Suppose you are caring for a patient 24 hours after a major surgery. You see the following order on the nursing care plan: Ambulate 24 hr postoperatively

- When you care for the patient, how will you go about implementing this nursing order?
- What else do you need to know to effectively carry out this order?

Components of a Nursing Order

Did you have trouble answering the questions just posed? Even experienced nurses would, because this nursing order is incomplete. As you see from this example, nursing orders must be specific and detailed because many caregivers will use the care plan, and they need to be able to interpret the orders correctly. A well-written nursing order, whether on a paper or computer care plan, contains the following components:

- *Date.* The date the order was written. The date will change each time you review or revise the order. Why do you think it is important to have the date?

- *Subject.* Nursing orders are instructions to nurses, so they are written in terms of *nurse* behaviors. Therefore, the subject of the order is "the nurse." Because anyone reading the care plan should understand this, you do not actually need to write "the nurse" in your orders. For each order, think, but do not write, "The nurse will . . ." or "The nurse should . . ." This will help you to state the order properly so that it doesn't sound like a goal statement. Goals state patient behaviors; nursing orders state nurse behaviors. For example:

  Goal/expected outcome
  (Patient) Drinks 100 mL
      fluids per hour on
      day shift

  Nursing order
  (Nurse will) Offer 100 mL
      water or juice per hour

- *Action verb.* This tells the nurse what action to take—what to do. Examples of action verbs are *assist, assess, auscultate, bathe, change, demonstrate, explain, give, teach,* and *turn.* The following nursing orders show the action verbs in italics:

  Teach the components of a healthy diet, 9/13, day shift

  Offer 100 mL water every hour

  Administer acetaminophen 500 mg orally at least 30 min before dressing change

- *Times and limits.* State when (e.g., which shift, what day), how often, and how long the activity is to be done. Consider the unit routines (e.g., visiting hours, mealtimes), the patient's usual rest times, scheduled tests and procedures (e.g., x-ray studies), and treatments (e.g., physical therapy). The following nursing orders show times and limits in italics:

  Teach the components of a healthy diet *on 9/13, day shift*

  Offer 100 mL water *every hour between 0700 and 1900*

  Administer acetaminophen 500 mg orally *at least 30 min before dressing change*

  If you omit specific times, such as "day shift," the order may not be followed. It is easy to for a nurse to think, "Perhaps someone else will do it (or has done it)."

- *Signature.* The nurse writing the order should sign it. A signature indicates that you accept legal and

| toward evidence-based practice |

Read about the following two studies, and then answer the questions at the end of the box.

Hartford, K., Wong, C., & Zakaria, D. (2002). Randomized controlled trial of a telephone intervention by nurses to provide information and support to patients and their partners after elective coronary artery bypass graft surgery: Effects of anxiety. *Heart and Lung: The Journal of Acute and Critical Care, 31*(3), 199–206.

In this study, six telephone calls were made to 131 patients and their partners to provide information and support after coronary artery bypass graft surgery (CABG). The calls were made over the 7 weeks following discharge, when patients' anxiety was rated as moderate to severe. Results, which the researchers obtained by using a structured tool to rate the patients' anxiety, indicated that this intervention significantly lowered the patients' anxiety during the early period after discharge (day 2 at home).

Moore, S. M., & Dolansky, M. A. (2001). Randomized trial of a home recovery intervention following coronary artery bypass surgery. *Research in Nursing and Health, 24*(2), 93–104.

This study tested a discharge information intervention on 180 patients who had had CABG surgery. The

intervention, titled the Cardiac Home Information Program (CHIP), consisted of providing a 15-minute audiotape for patients and family members to use at home during the first month after discharge. Results indicated that the CHIP produced positive effects on physical functioning in women and on psychological distress, vigor, and fatigue in men. This suggests that the CHIP intervention aids home recovery of patients having CABG.

---

1. How are these two studies similar? (Ignore the results.)

2. Now think about the interventions tested in the two studies. What are their differences?

3. Using these two studies, write two nursing orders for a client, Dave Hamilton, who will be discharged tomorrow after having CABG. Your nursing agency does not have an audiotape such as CHIP, but it does have a pamphlet containing similar information.

4. For what nursing diagnosis would these two nursing orders be appropriate? Write the nursing diagnosis as you would write it on Mr. Hamilton's care plan.

 Go to Chapter 6, **Toward Evidence-Based Practice Suggested Responses,** on the Electronic Study Guide.

ethical accountability for your orders and allows others to know whom to contact if they have questions or comments about the order.

KnowledgeCheck 6–5

List the five components of a nursing order.

 Go to Chapter 6, **Knowledge Check Response Sheet and Answers,** on the Electronic Study Guide.

Reflecting Critically About Nursing Orders

After writing the nursing orders, reflect on the interventions you have chosen. If you followed the process on pages 109–112, you will already have thought critically and made some considered decisions as you were choosing the interventions and activities. The following are questions to guide your final judgments about the plan of care.

1. *Is the set of orders complete?* That is, do they address all aspects of the problem?

   —Do they address the etiology of the problem?

   —If the etiology cannot be changed, do they focus on the symptoms of the problem?

   —Have I considered physical, emotional, interpersonal, spiritual, and cultural needs?

2. *Is each order technically complete?* That is, does it contain all the required components?

3. *Are the orders clear, specific, and precise?* If you have included all the required components, the orders will usually provide specific enough directions (e.g., when, how often, and so on) to be useful to other nurses. However, you must avoid vague language. For example, an order to "Offer emotional support" is too general to offer direction for care. One nurse might think this means to ask the client about his family, another might sit quietly with the patient, and still another might use a therapeutic statement such as, "This must be difficult for you." Ask yourself, "Would all nurses interpret this order in the same way? Would they all do the same thing after reading it?"

4. *Is the order individualized for this particular patient?* For example, even if you have written an order, "Offer 100 mL fluids q hr," it is even better if you make a note of the kinds of fluids the patient likes or can tolerate.

5. *Are the orders concise?* Long, complex statements may be unclear. Keep the orders as brief as possible without sacrificing clarity and specificity. If the patient requires complex procedures (e.g., wet-to-dry dressing changes), don't write the details of the procedure on the care plan. Simply refer to the source of instructions for the procedure: perhaps an agency procedure manual, or a list of instructions to be found at the bedside. Do write in the care plan any modifications to a procedure (e.g., "Do not use alcohol; client's skin is very dry.")

6. *Which orders have priority?* Which nursing orders must be implemented immediately? Which must be done on this shift? Which must be done today? If possible, write them in priority order.

If you have followed the recommended processes and reflected critically on your interventions, you should have a holistic plan of care individualized to meet the client's needs.

 Go to Chapter 6, **Resources for Caregivers and Health Professionals,** on the Electronic Study Guide.

 Suggested Readings: Go to Chapter 6, **Reading More About the Nursing Process: Planning Interventions,** on the Electronic Study Guide.

 Bibliography: Go to Volume 2, Bibliography.

Nursing Process:
Implementation
& Evaluation

Learning Outcomes

After completing this chapter, you should be able to:

✳ Define *implementation*.

✳ Explain how to prepare the nurse, the patient, and supplies or equipment before implementing nursing orders.

✳ Describe nursing activities that occur in the implementation phase of the nursing process.

✳ Define the terms *delegation* and *supervision*.

✳ Identify and describe the "five rights" of delegation.

✳ Define *evaluation*.

✳ Explain how standards and criteria are used in evaluation.

✳ Explain how structure, process, and outcomes evaluation are related.

✳ Distinguish among ongoing, intermittent, and terminal evaluation.

✳ Describe a process for evaluating client health status (outcomes).

✳ Describe a process for evaluating the effectiveness of the nursing care plan.

✳ List variables that may influence the effectiveness of a nursing intervention; state which ones the nurse can and cannot control.

✳ Discuss the importance of nurses' involvement in evaluating the quality of care in an organization.

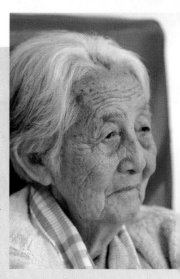

MEET Your Patients

Patient #1

Jeannette Wu is a very thin 80-year-old woman who has just been admitted to a skilled nursing facility after fracturing her hip 5 days ago. Her hip was surgically repaired 4 days ago, but because of her overall fragile health and some postsurgery confusion, her recovery is slower than usual. One of her nursing diagnoses is Self-Care Deficit (Bathing/Hygiene, Dressing/Grooming, and Toileting) related to weakness, pain, confusion, and decreased mobility. Her nursing orders include (NIC) Bathing and Self-Care: Activities of Daily Living (ADLs). As the nurse is helping a newly hired aide (unlicensed assistive personnel, or UAP) with Mrs. Wu's bath, she notices a reddened area on Mrs. Wu's sacrum. Realizing that this may be the beginning of a pressure ulcer, she observes carefully and notes a small skin excoriation (abrasion) in the area. She repositions Mrs. Wu to prevent further pressure on her sacrum. After finishing the bath, the nurse charts her findings and enters on Mrs. Wu's care plan a nursing diagnosis of Impaired Skin Integrity related to impaired bed mobility and minimal subcutaneous tissue. She writes appropriate nursing orders, including an order to observe skin over bony prominences every 4 hours, and then delegates to the UAP the task of turning and repositioning Mrs. Wu every 2 hours.

Patient #2

Patsy Jiminez is a healthy 25-year-old woman with no medical problems. She eats a balanced diet but does not exercise much ("I really hate to exercise!"). She and the nurse have created a plan to help her increase her physical activity. Ms. Jiminez will try to walk for 30 minutes at least 5 days a week. Each week she is successful, she plans to reward herself with a movie or a milkshake, which she usually avoids because of the fat content. The nurse would prefer that Ms. Jiminez not reward herself with food, but respects the patient's decision and realizes that if it is to serve as motivation, the reward must be something that Ms. Jiminez values.

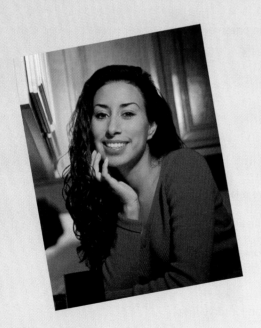

CriticalThinking 7–1

- For Jeannette Wu, which parts of the scenario illustrate *doing* by the nurse?
- For Jeannette Wu, which parts of the scenario illustrate *thinking* by the nurse?
- For Patsy Jiminez, who will be implementing (carrying out) the plan of care?

IMPLEMENTATION: THE ACTION PHASE OF THE NURSING PROCESS

Think of implementation as the action phase of the nursing process. Of course, implementation involves both thinking and doing, but the emphasis is on doing. During **implementation,** you will perform or delegate planned interventions—that is, carry out the care plan. The implementation phase ends when you record the nursing actions on the chart; it evolves into evaluation as you record the resulting client responses (Figure 7–1).

As in all phases of the nursing process, encourage the client and family to participate as much as possible in the implementation of their care. When Mrs. Wu is less confused and better able to move about, for example, the nurse will encourage her to help bathe herself. Be aware that clients vary in their ability and desire to participate. In the opening scenarios, Mrs. Wu was able to participate very little, but Patsy Jiminez participated fully. Typically, the client implements health-promotion interventions, with little or no involvement by the nurse.

As with other steps of the nursing process, professional nursing organizations have developed standards relating to implementation. These are identified in Box 7–1.

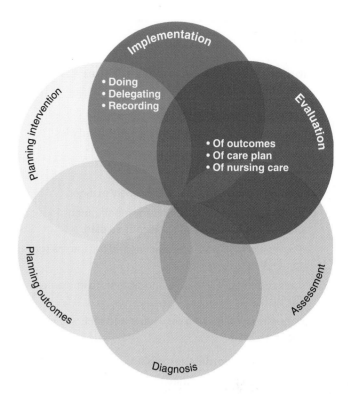

FIGURE 7–1 **Nursing process phases: implementation and evaluation.**

How Is Implementation Related to Other Steps of the Nursing Process?

Nursing process phases are interdependent (Figure 7–1). Each affects and is affected by others. Without the assessment, diagnosis, and planning steps, implementation would reflect only dependent functions, such as carrying out policies, protocols, and medical orders. The autonomous nursing activities performed during implementation are built on the nurse's reasoning in the previous three steps. Implementation overlaps in some way with every other phase of the nursing process.

Implementation overlaps with assessment. Nurses use assessment data to individualize interventions for a specific person rather than just giving "routine care." For example, a nursing order may read, "Offer clear liquids hourly; patient likes tea." When taking the tea to the patient, you may discover that she likes sugar in her tea and prefers it without ice. This allows you to further individualize the intervention.

Implementation also provides you the opportunity to assess your patients at every contact. In "Meet Your Patients," what assessments did the nurse make while bathing Mrs. Wu?

Some nursing orders specifically direct ongoing, focused assessments. When performing an ordered ongoing assessment, you are both implementing and assessing. What ongoing assessment was ordered for Mrs. Wu?

Implementation overlaps with diagnosis. Nurses use data discovered during implementation to identify new diagnoses or to revise existing ones. What new nursing diagnosis did the nurse make for Mrs. Wu after bathing her?

Implementation overlaps with planning outcomes and interventions. When you implement a nursing intervention it produces patient responses. Patient responses provide the data you need for revising the original goals and nursing orders. As you care for a client, you begin to know her better, and her unique needs become more apparent.

Implementation overlaps with evaluation. You will compare the responses you observe during implementation to the existing goals (which were written in the planning outcomes phase) to evaluate patient health status and progress toward goals.

How Should I Prepare for Implementation?

In addition to "doing, delegating, and recording," implementation also involves some preparation. Although the care plan will already have been developed in the planning stages of the nursing process, you should do some more planning just before implementing the plan—as explained in the following sections.

BOX 7-1   Professional Standards for Implementation

American Nurses Association Standards of Practice

Standard 5. Implementation

The registered nurse implements the identified plan.

Measurement Criteria:

The registered nurse:

Implements the plan in a safe and timely manner.

Documents implementation and any modifications, including changes or omissions, of the identified plan.

Utilizes evidence-based interventions and treatments specific to the diagnosis or problem.

Utilizes community resources and systems to implement the plan.

Collaborates with nursing colleagues and others to implement the plan.

Standard 5A: Coordination of Care

The registered nurse coordinates care delivery.

Measurement Criteria:

The registered nurse:

Coordinates implementation of the plan.

Documents the coordination of the care.

Standard 5B: Health Teaching and Health Promotion

The registered nurse employs strategies to promote health and a safe environment.

Measurement Criteria:

The registered nurse:

Provides health teaching that addresses such topics as healthy lifestyles, risk-reducing behaviors, developmental needs, activities of daily living, and preventive self-care

Uses health promotion and health teaching methods appropriate to the situation and the patient's developmental level, learning needs, readiness, ability to learn, language preference, and culture.

Seeks opportunities for feedback and evaluation of the effectiveness of the strategies used.

Note: There are additional measurement criteria for advanced practice nurses.

Source: Reprinted with permission from American Nurses Association, Standards of Practice, in *Nursing scope and standards of practice* (3rd ed.). © 2004 American Nurses Publishing, American Nurses Foundation/American Nurses Association, 600 Maryland Ave., SW, Suite 100 W, Washington, DC 20024-2571.

Canadian Provincial Standards of Practice

In Canada, practice standards are set by each province. The following are examples that apply to implementation.

Province of Alberta

Knowledge-Based Practice

The registered nurse:

Demonstrates critical thinking in collecting and interpreting data, planning, implementing, and evaluating all aspects of nursing care.

Documents timely, accurate reports of data collection, interpretation, planning, implementing, and evaluating care.

Provision of Service to the Public

The registered nurse is accountable for her/his delegation of care to other health team members.

Source: Alberta Association of Registered Nurses (1999). *Nursing practice: Professional conduct: Nursing practice standards.* Retrieved August 27, 2002, from http://nurses.ab.ca/profconduct/npa.html

Check Your Knowledge and Abilities

Before beginning a nursing activity, review the care plan and reflect critically on the nursing and medical orders. As a professional nurse, you will be obligated ethically and legally to clarify or question orders that you believe to be unclear, incorrect, or inappropriate. At the same time, you must decide whether you are qualified to carry out the orders. You should ask for help when:

- You do not have the knowledge or skill needed to implement an order. For example, you may be unfamiliar with a medication, or you may not ever have performed an ordered procedure such as a urinary catheterization.

- You cannot perform the activity safely alone (e.g., helping a heavy, weak patient to ambulate). As another example, when catheterizing Ms. Wu, if she is very weak, the nurse will need someone to help her maintain the desired position during the catheterization.

- Performing the activity alone would cause undue stress for the patient (e.g., giving back care to a patient with multiple fractures).

Organize Your Work

Because you will be providing care for more than one patient on each shift, you will need to make a time-sequenced work plan ("worksheet") to prioritize your patient care for the day. With the current organizational emphasis on cost and efficiency, you may have a great deal of work to accomplish, so you must make the most of every patient contact. Think ahead which interventions you can perform together. Mrs. Wu's nurse performed a skin assessment while she was giving a bedbath. As another example, you might do patient teaching while assisting with breathing exercises. Or while changing a dressing, you might also use that time to show interest and concern for an anxious patient. Many institutions have forms for this type of scheduling; or you may need to write your own list of "things to do" in the order you need to do them.

Establish Feedback Points

Establishing feedback points is a part of organizing your work. You cannot assume you will be able to carry out a nursing order in exactly the way it was written. For example, suppose the nursing order states, "Help to ambulate in the hall b.i.d." When you help the patient to stand, he becomes pale, dizzy, diaphoretic, and short of breath. Would you still carry out the nursing order? Of course not. You must always be ready to alter the activity on the spot as the patient's responses demand. This means that you must look for **feedback** (patient responses to the activity) as you perform care.

When organizing your work, identify points in each intervention where you want to pause for feedback. For example, if you are assisting with range-of-motion exercises, you might plan to assess for pain during movement of each joint and to assess for activity intolerance after exercising both arms and again after exercising the legs. Feedback is not always verbal. For example, it could be a change in vital signs, skin color, or level of consciousness.

Prepare Supplies and Equipment

Preparing supplies and equipment is another aspect of organization. Gather all the supplies and equipment you need before you go to the patient's room. This allows you to work efficiently by eliminating the need to go to the supply room for items you have overlooked. Also, it prevents the stress to your patient that occurs when you interrupt a procedure to go get a needed item.

Suppose you are working alone to insert an intravenous (IV) catheter—a sterile procedure. You have donned your gloves, applied the tourniquet, and done all the steps prior to inserting the IV catheter. When you insert the catheter, you "blow" the vein and are unable to use it to start the IV fluid. Reaching in the IV kit for another IV catheter, you discover that there is not another one there; you have used the last one.

What are your options at this point? Are there any *good* options?

The answer is that there are no good options. You might call another busy caregiver (provided that one is available) to bring you a sterile IV catheter. Or you could interrupt the procedure and get it yourself, making it necessary to leave the patient, don another pair of gloves, and prep another site. Either way, time and money would be lost, as might your patient's confidence in you. You cannot prevent "blowing" an IV; however, by preparing ahead, you can prevent inefficiency and waste.

Prepare the Patient

Before performing a nursing activity, reassess the patient to make sure that the activity is still necessary and that the patient is physically and psychologically ready for the intervention.

- *Check your assumptions.* This is just good critical thinking. Don't assume that an intervention is still needed simply because it is written on the care plan. For example, a few days after Jeannette Wu's transfer to the skilled care facility, the nursing assistant is preparing to give her a bedbath, as instructed on the care plan (Table 7–1, entry for December 18). However, Mrs. Wu has regained some of her strength and is able to sit in a chair. So the nurse and the assistant agree that, with help, Mrs. Wu can bathe at the sink instead of requiring a complete bedbath.

- *Assess the patient's readiness.* To obtain the most benefit from an intervention, a client must be physically and psychologically ready. The hospital's critical pathway for hip fractures recommended a "help bath" on post-operative day 3. However, Mrs. Wu's age and physical condition indicated that she needed a complete bedbath. The nurse did not assume that Mrs. Wu was ready to progress just because the critical pathway dictated it. The following are more examples of assuring readiness:

  - Because her patient was anxious about his test results, a nurse postponed a teaching session until the man was feeling more calm.

  - While preparing to perform a painful dressing change, a nurse discovered that the patient had visitors. The nurse waited until the visitors had gone to do the procedure.

- *Explain what you will do and what the patient will feel.* Clients are not passive recipients of your care. Many interventions require their participation or cooperation.

  - Explaining the reasons for the action helps to motivate the person to participate.

  - Explaining what the person is expected to do gives the person the information she needs to participate.

TABLE 7-1 Portions of the Care Plan for Jeanette Wu

Date: 12/16/06 Care Plan Prior to Implementation on Day 4 Post-Op

Nursing Diagnosis	Desired Outcomes	Nursing Orders	Evaluation
12/16 Self-Care Deficit (Bathing/ Hygiene, Dressing/ Grooming, and Toileting) related to weakness, pain, confusion, and decreased mobility	By day 7 post-op (12/19) will assist with bath and oral hygiene	• Complete bedbath daily in A.M. • Give prescribed analgesic 1/2 hr before bath • Assist with range-of-motion exercises	

Date: 12/16/06 Care Plan After Implementation on Day 4 Post-Op

Nursing Diagnosis	Desired Outcomes	Nursing Orders	Evaluation
12/16 Self-Care Deficit (Bathing/ Hygiene, Dressing/ Grooming, and Toileting) related to weakness, pain, confusion, and decreased mobility	By day 7 post-op (12/19) will assist with bath and oral hygiene	• Complete bedbath daily in A.M. (UAP) • Give Tylenol #3, tabs i by mouth, 1/2 hr before bath • Assist with range-of-motion exercises t.i.d. (RN)	12/16 Too soon to evaluate.
12/16 Impaired skin integrity (sacrum) r/t pressure 2° immobility	*By 12/23, skin healed over sacrum; skin intact and normal color over all bony prominences*	• *Turn and reposition q2hr; do not place supine (UAP)* • *Observe skin over bony prominences q4hr (RN)*	

Date: 12/18/06 Care Plan After Implementation on Day 6 Post-Op

Nursing Diagnosis	Desired Outcomes	Nursing Orders	Evaluation
12/16 Self-Care Deficit (Bathing/ Hygiene, Dressing/ Grooming, and Toileting) related to weakness, pain, confusion, and decreased mobility	By day 7 post-op (12/19) will assist with bath and oral hygiene	• ~~Complete bedbath daily in A.M.~~ *12/18 UAP help with bath at sink daily in A.M. Patient can wash upper body and perform oral hygiene* • Give prescribed analgesic 1/2 hr before bath • Assist with range-of-motion exercises t.i.d. (RN)	*12/18 Goal met. Sat in chair for help bath. Performed oral hygiene and upper body bath.*
12/16 Impaired skin integrity (sacrum) r/t pressure 2° immobility	By 12/23, skin healed over sacrum; skin intact and normal color over all bony prominences	• Turn and reposition q2hr; do not place supine (UAP) • Observe skin over bony prominences q4hr (RN) • *12/18 Requested foam and fatty mattress pad* • *12/18 Refer to nutritionist for evaluation*	*12/18 Skin excoriation over sacrum is larger: now 2 cm x 2 cm, and about 1/2 cm deep.*

- Explaining what sensations the person can expect helps to relieve anxiety, enables the person to cope with unpleasant or painful sensations, and promotes a trusting relationship.
- *Provide privacy.* This helps to assure psychological readiness.

KnowledgeCheck 7–1

- Why is it important to organize your work before implementing care?
- In addition to organizing your work, what other preparations should you make before implementing care?

 Go to Chapter 7, **Knowledge Check Response Sheet and Answers,** on the Electronic Study Guide.

 CriticalThinking 7–2

Suppose your patient, Jeannette Wu, has become incontinent of bowel and bladder. Because she already has Impaired Skin Integrity, the physician has written a new order to insert an indwelling urinary catheter (a drainage tube inserted through her urinary meatus into her bladder). Urinary catheterization is a sterile technique. You have practiced this procedure in the skills lab, but you have never actually performed it on a patient.

- As a student, what should you do?
- If you were an RN, what are some things you could do to ensure that both you and the patient are prepared for the procedure?

Implementing the Plan: Doing or Delegating

After both you and the patient are prepared, it is time to act. Nursing actions include both those you do yourself and those you delegate to others; and they may be collaborative, independent, or dependent (see Chapter 6 if you do not recall the meaning of these terms). During implementation you will coordinate and carry out both the nursing orders on the nursing care plan and the medical orders that relate to the patient's medical treatment.

What Knowledge and Skills Do I Need?

There is almost no limit to the number and kinds of nursing interventions you might perform. The *Nursing Interventions Classification* (2004), for example, lists 514 broad interventions (e.g., Hypothermia Treatment), each of which includes approximately 15 to 20 specific activities. For example, one activity for Hypothermia Treatment is "Remove cold, wet clothing and replace with warm, dry clothing" (p. 430). During implementation, then, you can expect to use all the types of knowledge presented in Chapter 2: theoretical, practical, personal, and ethical knowledge, as well as knowledge about the patient situation.

You will use various combinations of cognitive, interpersonal, and psychomotor skills to perform nursing activities. For example, when you are inserting an IV catheter, you need cognitive knowledge of sterile procedure, interpersonal skills to reassure the patient, and psychomotor skills to apply the tourniquet and insert the IV catheter.

 CriticalThinking 7–3

Use the examples provided in the preceding paragraph to help you write a definition for each of the following terms:

- Cognitive skills
- Interpersonal skills
- Psychomotor skills

How Can I Promote Client Participation and Adherence?

Different interventions require differing levels of participation. However, even a nurse-initiated intervention, such as inserting a urinary catheter, goes more smoothly if the patient participates at least to the extent of holding still while you perform the procedure. Many interventions (for example, instituting a low-calorie diet) depend almost entirely on the patient's adhering to the therapy. In the case of Ms. Jiminez, implementation of the intervention, walking for 30 minutes five times a week, depends entirely on the client.

People fail to follow therapeutic regimens for various reasons. They may not understand the routine or the reasons for it; there may be cultural objections to the therapy; their lifestyle may make adherence difficult (e.g., no time to exercise); they may be afraid of failing; they may be reluctant to ask questions, either from embarrassment at their lack of knowledge or from hesitance to "bother" a busy nurse or physician. You can promote cooperation with treatments and therapies by:

- *Assessing the client's knowledge* about his illness and the treatments and providing the necessary information.
- *Assessing the client's supports and resources.* You cannot assume that every patient owns a car or even has other transportation to the clinic. Even if they wish to follow the therapy, some people do not have enough money for food or medicine, some people cannot read printed instructions; some do not have family or friends to help with their care at home, and so on.
- *Being sensitive to the client's cultural, spiritual, and other needs and viewpoints.* For example, regardless of the need for dietary protein, some people do not like the taste of meat, poultry, or fish; others might have religious or cultural objections to eating these foods. You will need to alter your recommendations to reflect client preferences and beliefs.

• *Realizing and accepting that some attitudes cannot be changed.* For example, regardless of the effects of obesity on blood pressure, a client will not lose weight simply because you tell him it is important. The client must *want* to lose weight. Information alone will not change a person's behavior.

• *Determining the client's main concerns.* For example, you may be concerned that lack of exercise makes it difficult to regulate a client's blood sugar; the client's main concern may be that exercise makes her joints hurt.

• *Helping the client to set realistic goals.* Clients usually more readily accept small, rather than drastic, behavioral or lifestyle changes. Perhaps a client with a child who has asthma cannot even imagine that she could stop smoking. But you may be able to convince her that it would be better for her child if she would smoke outdoors rather than in the house or in the car (London, 1998).

What Should I Know About Coordinating Care?

For successful implementation, you need the skills of collaboration and coordination. As discussed in Chapter 6, *collaboration* simply means working with other caregivers (e.g., physicians, respiratory therapists) to plan, make decisions, or perform interventions. Unlike delegated activities (discussed in the following section) true collaboration requires shared decision making.

Coordination of care includes scheduling treatments and activities with other departments (e.g., laboratory, physical therapy, radiology department), but it is more than that. In the hospital, nurses are the professionals who have the most frequent and continuous contact with the patient, so they have the most complete picture of the person. Unlike nurses, most other caregivers focus on only a very specific aspect of the patient (e.g., breathing, eating, surgical incision). You will be expected to put together the bits and pieces of information (e.g., the patient's response to physical therapy, dietary intake, emotional status, and vital signs) to provide a holistic view of the person. You will need to read the reports of other professionals, help interpret the results for the patient and family, and make rounds with other professionals to be sure that everyone sees the whole picture.

Outside the hospital, the health professional who has the most contact with the client usually assumes the coordination role. For example, if a client is receiving episodic care for ongoing health problems, the primary care provider (e.g., physician or advanced practice nurse) may coordinate care. For a client discharged home after a hip fracture, the physical therapist may coordinate care.

KnowledgeCheck 7–2

• What are some reasons that a client may not follow a recommended treatment regimen?
• List at least four things you can do to promote client participation in care or adherence to recommendations for treatment.

 Go to Chapter 7, **Knowledge Check Response Sheet and Answers,** on the Electronic Study Guide.

What Should I Know About Delegation and Supervision?

Delegation is the transfer to another person of the authority to perform a task in a selected situation—the person delegating retains accountability for the outcome of the activity (ANA 1996; National Council of State Boards of Nursing [NCSBN], 1995a). As a registered nurse, you will frequently delegate patient care activities to licensed vocational (or practical) nurses (LVN/LPNs) and unlicensed assistive personnel (UAPs). You may also (for example, as a nurse in charge of making unit assignments for the day) *assign* tasks to other RNs; however, this is not delegation because those RNs are accountable for the outcome of their activities. Remember, you can only delegate *down* in the chain of command.

Understand that you cannot delegate nursing care decisions. You can delegate only the responsibility for performing a defined activity in a particular situation. So, even though the nurse has delegated to the UAP the task of turning Mrs. Wu ("Meet Your Patient") every 2 hours, it is *the nurse* who must assess her skin condition and take action if it does not improve.

The ANA is concerned that in many healthcare settings UAPs are used inappropriately to perform functions that are legally nursing functions (e.g., administering medications). The ANA believes this inappropriate delegation is a threat to patient safety and that it violates state nursing practice acts. According to the ANA, any nursing intervention that requires independent, specialized, nursing knowledge, skill, or judgment cannot be delegated (1992a, 1992b, 1996).

When deciding whether to delegate tasks, you should think critically about the task, the circumstance, the person, the direction or communication, and the supervision. For a checklist to help you consider these five critical elements, or "five rights" of delegating,

 Go to Chapter 7, **Delegation and Evaluation Checklists, The Five Rights of Delegation,** in Volume 2.

Right Task?

The first question to ask is, "Can I delegate this task?" As a rule, you should delegate an activity

only if it meets *all* of the following criteria. The activity:

- Is within your scope of practice to perform and delegate, as defined by your state nurse practice act.
- Is within the LVN/LPN or UAP's scope of practice.
- Is in accordance with agency policies, if they exist.
- Does not require complex observations or critical decisions.
- Is performed according to a set procedure and requires little innovation.
- Does not require repeated nursing assessments.
- Occurs frequently in the daily care of patients on the unit
- Has reasonably predictable results.
- Is *not* one that requires independent, specialized nursing knowledge, skills, or judgment (ANA, 1996).
- Is *not* health teaching or counseling.

Remember that you are assigning the UAP to a *task,* not to a patient. You cannot assign a UAP the responsibility for total patient care; and you cannot allow a UAP to delegate care to other UAPs. Only a professional nurse can evaluate a UAP's ability to perform a nursing task.

Right Circumstance?

UAPs are being used in settings where acuity and technology have increased while length of stay has decreased. This means that they are caring for sicker patients. We often think of bathing, feeding, and turning patients as tasks appropriate for the UAP; however, such tasks may not be appropriate if the patient is seriously ill. Before deciding to delegate, assess your patient to be certain that her needs match the abilities of the UAP. It is best if the patient is relatively stable (e.g., with a chronic rather than an acute condition) and does not need extensive help with self-care activities. If the client is very ill or if the results of the task are unpredictable, the task should probably not be delegated. For a tool to help you make appropriate delegation decisions,

 Go to Chapter 7, **Delegation Decision-Making Grid,** in Volume 2.

Right Person?

You must also be sure that the UAP is competent to perform the task and that his workload allows time to do the task properly. The following are evidence of competence:

- The facility has documented proof that the person has demonstrated competence.
- The UAP has performed the task often or has worked with patients with similar diagnoses.

If evidence is lacking, you need to establish the UAP's competence. For example, you might observe and evaluate his performance, or you might ask the UAP, "How many times have you done this procedure?" or "Will you need help with this procedure?" (Also see the next section, "Right Direction/Communication.")

"Right person" also refers to:

1. The nurse who is delegating the task; this means that the task must be something that the nurse is competent to delegate (see the preceding section, "Right Task").
2. The patient receiving the care (see the preceding section, "Right Circumstance").

Right Direction/Communication?

Right direction/communication means that when you delegate, you should communicate clearly and specifically about each task. You can communicate orally or in writing, but leave no room for misinterpretation.

- *Explain exactly what the task is,* including what to do and what not to do. For example, "Empty the catheter bag, and measure the amount of urine using the clear, marked plastic container"—not just, "Measure the urine."
- *Include specific times and methods for reporting.* For example, "Come tell me her temperature every hour."
- *Explain the purpose or objective of the task.* For example, "Change Mrs. Wu's position every 2 hours to prevent bedsores; she is not able to turn by herself."
- *Describe the expected results or potential complications to expect.* For example, "She will probably cry out when you turn her, but that is more from fear than from pain," or "I have given her medications, so her temperature should be below 100°F by 9 A.M. If not, let me know immediately."
- *Be specific in your instructions.* For example, "Let me know if Mrs. Wu has any red spots or broken skin areas when you turn her"—not "Tell me what her skin looks like."

Right Supervision?

The last item in the checklist involves **supervision,** which has been defined by professional nursing groups as:

- The active process of directing, guiding, and influencing the outcome of an individual's performance of an activity or task (ANA, 1996).
- The provision of guidance or direction, evaluation, and follow-up by the licensed nurse for accomplishing a nursing task delegated to UAP (NCSBN, 1995a).

When you delegate tasks to a UAP or LVN/LPN, you or another RN should be available to answer questions and provide help, if necessary. You are also

responsible for providing supervision and evaluating the outcomes. This includes:

- *Monitoring the UAP/LVN/LPN's work* to be sure it complies with agency policies and procedures and standards of practice. For example, after the UAP bathes a patient, you might check to see whether the patient is clean; or you might choose to observe for a few minutes while the UAP is working.

- *Intervening, if necessary.* Many UAPs receive little training, so you may need to demonstrate some caregiving activities.

- *Obtaining and providing feedback* from the worker. Give positive, as well as negative, feedback often. If performance is not acceptable, talk privately with the UAP to explain the specific mistakes that were made. Listen to the UAP's view of the situation. For example, there may have been too many tasks to complete in the time allowed.

- *Evaluating client outcomes,* both the physical response and the relationship with the UAP. Ask the client for input after the care is given.

- *Ensuring proper documentation.* Some agencies permit UAPs to record vital signs and other patient data. You are responsible for seeing that all necessary data are recorded and that they are accurate.

KnowledgeCheck 7–3

- List the "five rights" of delegation.
- List at least four characteristics of a "right task"—that is, a task that would be acceptable to delegate.
- As an RN, how could you establish that a UAP is competent to perform a task?
- List at least three ways to help assure that the UAP will understand clearly when you delegate a task.
- List at least three things you should do when providing supervision to an unlicensed caregiver.

 Go to Chapter 7, **Knowledge Check Response Sheet and Answers,** on the Electronic Study Guide.

 CriticalThinking 7–4

For your patient, Jeannette Wu:

- Which activity did the nurse delegate to someone else?
- What collaborative activities should the nurse consider?

Documenting: The Final Step of Implementation

After giving care, you will record the nursing activities and the patient's responses. Documentation is a mode of communication among the members of the health team, and it provides the information you need to evaluate the patient's health status and the nursing care plan. For a thorough discussion of documenting, refer to Chapter 16.

Reflecting Critically About Implementation

During the implementation phase, perhaps more than at any other time, nurses combine thinking and doing. You should always be prepared to modify the activity based on the patient's responses. Afterward, when you have some time to reflect, you can think critically about what happened (good or bad) and why. Use the following questions, or refer to the critical thinking model (See Table 2–2 for other ideas.)

1. What was done? Why was it done? What were the patient's responses?
2. Did I forget to do anything?
3. What was going on in the situation that may have influenced the outcome?
4. What factors influenced my behavior (or others' behavior) in this situation?
5. Would the activity have been more successful if I had had more knowledge or skill? If so, why did I not realize that ahead of time, and how can I avoid this in the future?
6. What assumptions or biases (mine or the patient's) contributed to the problem in this situation?
7. Did I communicate clearly to the patient?
8. Did I convey respect and caring?
9. What could I have delegated? What did I delegate that I should *not* have? Why?
10. After reflecting on it, what would I do differently in this situation?

Refer to Table 7–2 for examples that demonstrate how the reflection questions might be used in a clinical situation.

EVALUATION: THE FINAL STEP OF THE NURSING PROCESS

Evaluation, the final step of the nursing process, is a planned, ongoing, systematic activity in which you will make judgments about:

- The client's progress toward desired health outcomes
- The effectiveness of the nursing care plan
- The quality of nursing care in the healthcare setting

Why Is Evaluation Essential to Full-Spectrum Nursing?

Evaluation is an essential part of full-spectrum nursing for the following reasons:

- *The patient is the nurse's first priority.* The aim of all nursing activity is to achieve positive outcomes for patients. Evaluation lets you know whether your interventions are helping the patient as intended. No matter how carefully and conscientiously you perform a procedure, if it does not help the patient achieve desired outcomes, it has "missed the point."

TABLE 7-2 Examples of Reflecting Critically About Implementation

Situation	Question for Reflection	What Might Have Happened?
The nursing order read, "Assist to ambulate to the end of the hall …" However, the patient was able to walk only about half that distance before becoming too weak to stand.	What was going on in the situation that may have influenced the outcome?	Perhaps the patient was weak because he had not slept well the night before; or perhaps he had just had a long, tiring session of physical therapy.
When the patient became too weak to walk, the nurse called for help. Why did she do that instead of helping the patient to sit where he was, or instead of helping him back to the room by herself?	What factors influenced the nurse's behavior in this situation?	Perhaps the patient was very large and the nurse realized she was not strong enough to provide support. Can you think of other reasons the nurse might have chosen that action?

- *Evaluation helps nurses to conserve scarce resources.* Nurses are in short supply. Therefore, nursing time is precious and must be used wisely. Evaluation allows you to discard interventions that are not working well and focus on more effective ones. In addition to saving time, there may be cost savings as well.

- *Professional standards of practice require evaluation.* See Box 7–2.

- *The ANA code of ethics requires evaluation.* "The nurse's primary commitment is to the recipient of nursing and health care services—the patient—whether the recipient is an individual, a family, a group, or a community. . . . The nurse has a responsibility to implement and maintain standards of professional nursing practice. The nurse should participate in planning, establishing, implementing, and evaluating review mechanisms designed to safeguard patients and nurses, such as peer review processes or committees, credentialing processes, quality improvement initiatives, and ethics committees" (ANA, 2001, Section 2.1 and Standard 3.4).

- *The Joint Commission on Accreditation of Healthcare Organizations (JCAHO) and professional standards review organizations (PSROs) require evaluation.* These organizations use outcomes and performance measures to evaluate the quality of care in healthcare institutions. They conceptualize quality of care as the degree to which health services increase the likelihood of desired health outcomes.

- *Evaluation helps ensure nursing's survival.* Linking nursing interventions to achievement of client outcomes demonstrates the value of nursing. In today's competitive healthcare market, that is essential for ensuring continued funding for nursing services, education, and research.

- *Evaluation demonstrates caring and responsibility.* Without evaluation, you would not know whether your care was effective. Examining outcomes implies that you care about how your activities affect your clients.

How Are Standards and Criteria Used in Evaluation?

In a broad sense, evaluation is the systematic process of judging the quality or value of something by comparing it to one or more standards or criteria. In our daily lives, we evaluate many things: for example, a meal, a TV program, an insurance policy we are thinking of buying. However, for formal evaluation, you must decide *in advance* which standards and criteria you will use. As you learned in Chapter 1, standards represent expected or accepted levels of performance; they provide a model for what ought to be done. They are established by authority, custom, or consensus. In nursing, standards are used to describe quality nursing care. The American Nurses Association's standards of practice are a good example of broadly written standards (see Boxes 7–1 and 7–2).

Notice that each of the ANA standards includes a set of criteria to help describe the standard. **Criteria** are measurable or observable characteristics, properties, attributes, or qualities. They describe the specific skills, knowledge, behaviors, and attitudes that are desired or expected. Judges at a diving competition, for example, might evaluate a dive by using criteria for difficulty, technique, and style.

The patient goals and outcomes discussed in Chapter 5 are also examples of criteria. As you learned there, these criteria should be concrete and specific enough to serve as guides for collecting evaluation data. In addition, they should be reliable and valid. A

BOX 7-2 Professional Standards of Care: Evaluation

American Nurses Association Standards of Practice

Standard 6. Evaluation

The registered nurse evaluates progress towards attainment of outcomes.

Measurement Criteria:

The registered nurse:

Conducts a systematic, ongoing, and criterion-based evaluation of the outcomes in relation to the structures and processes prescribed by the plan and the indicated timeline.

Includes the patient and others involved in the care or situation in the evaluative process.

Evaluates the effectiveness of the planned strategies in relation to patient responses and the attainment of the expected outcomes.

Documents the results of the evaluation.

Uses ongoing assessment data to revise the diagnoses, outcomes, the plan, and the implementation, as needed.

Disseminates the results to the patient and others involved in the care or situation, as appropriate, in accordance with state and federal laws and regulations.

Note: There are additional measurement criteria for advanced practice nurses.

Source: Reprinted with permission from American Nurses Association, Standards of Practice, in *Nursing scope and standards of practice* (3rd ed.). © 2004 American Nurses Publishing, American Nurses Foundation/American Nurses Association, 600 Maryland Avenue, SW, Suite 100W, Washington, DC 20024-2571.

Canadian Provincial Standards of Practice

In Canada, practice standards are set at the provincial level. The following are excerpts from provincial standards that apply to evaluation.

- The registered nurse demonstrates critical thinking in collecting and interpreting data, planning, implementing, *and evaluating all aspects of nursing care.*
- The registered nurse documents timely, accurate reports of data collection, interpretation, planning, implementing, and *evaluating care.*
- (Indicator) Perform interventions safely and accurately, *evaluates outcomes and modify interventions according to evaluation*
- (Indicator) Articulate and carry out the role of registered nurses in planning, development, implementation and *evaluation of health care*
- Each registered nurse applies problem-solving processes in decision making, and *evaluates these processes.*
- Each registered nurse applies appropriate knowledge and skills to assess, plan, intervene and *evaluate services, and revises plan as needed*

Sources: Alberta Association of Registered Nurses. (1999). *Nursing practice: Professional conduct: Nursing practice standards.* Retrieved August 27, 2002, from http://nurses.ab.ca/profconduct/npa.html; Registered Nurses' Association of Nova Scotia. (1997). Standards for nursing practice. Retrieved December 11, 2002, from http://www.crnns.ca/; College of Registered Nurses of Manitoba. (2001). *Standards of practice for registered nurses.* Retrieved December 11, 2002, from http://222.crnm.mb.ca/standards.htm

criterion is **reliable** if it yields consistent results—that is, the same results every time, regardless of who uses it. For example, suppose you and another nurse measure a patient's temperature by (1) using an oral thermometer and (2) placing the back of your hand on the patient's forehead. Which method would probably give the same (or nearly same) results? As you probably concluded, the oral thermometer is more reliable.

A criterion is **valid** if it is really measuring what it was intended to measure. For example, fever is often used as a criterion for concluding that a person has an infection. However, if used alone, it is not a valid indicator because (1) other conditions, such as dehydration, can cause a fever, and (2) elevated temperature is not present in all infections. However, validity of that criterion is increased when you use additional criteria (e.g., elevated white blood cell count, presence of signs of infection such as redness and pus).

 CriticalThinking 7–5

- The outcome "Patient will not complain of pain" by itself is not a valid criterion for measuring pain. Why? What would be a more valid criterion for pain?
- A criterion reads, "Measures client vital signs once per shift, or as ordered." For which of the following standards would it be valid (that is, which conclusion could you draw if you knew that a nurse measured the vital signs once per shift, or as ordered)?

  Follows unit policies
  Performs skills accurately

Types of Evaluation

Evaluation is categorized according to (1) what is being evaluated (structures, processes, or outcomes) and (2) frequency and time of evaluation.

Evaluation of Structures, Processes, and Outcomes

Structures, processes and outcomes all work together to affect care; however, each requires different criteria and methods of evaluation. **Structure evaluation** focuses on the setting in which care is provided. It explores the effect of organizational characteristics on the quality of care. It requires standards and data about policies, procedures, fiscal resources, physical facilities and equipment, and number and qualification of personnel. Examples of criteria for structure evaluation include the following:

> At least one registered nurse is present on each unit at all times.
>
> A resuscitation cart is available on each floor.

Process evaluation focuses on the manner in which care is given—the activities performed by nurses (and other personnel). It explores whether the care was relevant to patient needs, appropriate, complete, and timely. Your instructor uses process evaluation to evaluate your clinical performance. Your clinical evaluation describes what you did and how well you did it. As a rule, it does not describe the *results* of your activities. Examples of criteria for process evaluation include the following:

> Protects patient's privacy when performing procedures.
>
> Washes hands before each patient contact.

Outcomes evaluation focuses on demonstrable (measurable) changes in the patient's health status that result from the care given. Although structure and process are important to quality, the most important aspect is improvement in patient health status. The evaluation step of the nursing process uses outcomes evaluation. Examples of outcomes criteria include the following:

> Patient will walk, assisted, to end of hall by day 5 post-op.
>
> Patient reports pain less than 4 on a 1–10 scale within 1 hour after analgesic administration.

Outcomes evaluation is also used when evaluating quality of care in an organization. In organizational use, the criteria also state the percentage of clients expected to have the outcome when care is satisfactory. For example:

> Post-catheterization urinary tract infection does not occur.
>
> *Expected compliance: 98%*

This means that the criterion would be met if no more than 2% of the patients developed a urinary tract infection after being catheterized.

Ongoing, Intermittent, and Terminal Evaluation

Evaluation begins as soon as you have performed the first nursing activity and continues during each client contact until all goals are achieved or the client is discharged from nursing care. The client's status determines how often you evaluate. A critically ill patient may need a nurse constantly at the bedside; after a client undergoes surgery, you may measure vital signs every 15 minutes; as the client nears discharge, you may evaluate once a day. In long-term care settings, in contrast, clients often have chronic health problems that require evaluation over an extended period of time. Most care is provided by LVN/LPNs and UAPs, and the RN may participate in weekly care conferences to evaluate the client's response to the current plan of care.

You will perform **ongoing evaluation** while implementing, immediately after an intervention, or at each patient contact. In contrast, **intermittent evaluation** is performed at specified times. It enables you to judge the progress toward goal achievement and to modify the care plan as needed. Goals and expected outcomes should designate times for collecting evaluation data. For example:

1. Will rate pain as < 3 on 1–10 scale within *1 hr after medication*.
2. Will lose 1 lb *per week* until weight of 125 lb is achieved.
3. *By the second home visit,* mother will demonstrate proper techniques for breastfeeding.

Terminal evaluation describes the client's health status and progress toward goals at the time of discharge. Most institutions have special discharge forms for terminal evaluation that also include instructions about medications, treatments, and follow-up care.

As in all phases of the nursing process, you should involve the patient and family in evaluation to the extent they are able. As the nurse, you are responsible for drawing evaluative conclusions; however, you should use input from the patient, the family, UAPs and other caregivers (see Box 7–2).

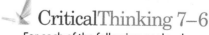

CriticalThinking 7–6

For each of the following goals, when or how often should the nurse collect evaluation data?

- Will rate pain as < 3 on scale of 1 to 10 within *1 hr after medication*.
- Will lose 1 lb *per week* until weight of 125 lb is achieved.
- *By the second home visit,* mother will demonstrate proper techniques for breastfeeding.

Edit Outcome Progress   ☒

Outcome Definition

Name

Acceptance: Health Status

Initial Scale   On Date

Limited ▼   06/24/2006   ...

Expected Scale   On Date

Substantial ▼   07/24/2006   ...

Outcome progress

Outcome Scale   Encounter Date   Save

Substantial ▼   07/30/2006   ...   Close

Explanation of Figure

Computer field	Nursing process terminology	Represents	Status recorded on computer
Initial scale	Initial assessment	*Actual* status *before* intervention	Limited acceptance of health status
Expected scale	Goal	*Desired* status *after* intervention	Substantial acceptance of health status
Outcome scale	Evaluative statement	*Actual* status *after* intervention	Substantial acceptance of health status

FIGURE 7–2   Computer screen showing outcome progress, using NOC.

Using standardized language from NOC, you might write a goal (*desired* status) of:

> *Goal:* Circulation Status: 5 (5 means "not compromised" in the NOC scale).

Each of the indicators could also be made into a goal by adding the desired scale numbers, as follows:

> Systolic BP in expected range: 5
>
> Diastolic BP in expected range: 5
>
> Mean BP in expected range: 5
>
> Orthostatic hypotension not present: 5 (meaning "none")

Evaluation statements are written exactly the same as goals, but the scale number describes the patient's *actual* status. So, if on reassessment the patient's blood pressure is quite low and he has orthostatic hypotension, the evaluative statement might be:

> *Evaluative Statement:* Circulation Status: 3 (3 means "moderately compromised" on this NOC scale)

Figure 7–2 is a computer screen showing the NOC outcome of Acceptance: Health Status. The "Initial Scale" shows the initial assessment; the "Expected Scale" is the goal; and the "Outcome Scale" is the evaluative

statement after intervention and reassessment. Did the interventions achieve the desired effect, or not? For a computer screen showing a NOC outcome definition and indicators,

 Go to Chapter 7, **Tables, Boxes, Figures: ESG Figure 7-1,** on the Electronic Study Guide.

KnowledgeCheck 7–5

Using the following outcomes and reassessment data, determine whether each goal has been met, partially met, or not met.

Goal: By 8/24, will walk, unassisted, to the end of the hall without pallor or shortness of breath.
Reassessment data: 8/24. Walked, unassisted, to end of hall; states no shortness of breath, but skin color was noticeably pale.

Goal: By 8/24, will walk, unassisted, to the end of the hall without pallor or shortness of breath.
Reassessment data: 8/23. Walked, unassisted, to end of hall. Skin color pink; respirations 14/min; no dyspnea observed; states no shortness of breath.

Goal: By 8/24, will walk, unassisted, to the end of the hall without pallor or shortness of breath.
Reassessment data: 8/25. Walked halfway to end of hall before becoming pale and short of breath.

 Go to Chapter 7, **Knowledge Check Response Sheet and Answers,** on the Electronic Study Guide.

How Do I Evaluate Collaborative Problems?

For collaborative problems, you will collect reassessment data the same as for nursing diagnoses. However, nurses share the responsibility for preventing complications that occur with collaborative problems with the physician and other members of the health team. The desired outcome for all collaborative problems is that no complication will occur. For example, if a patient's collaborative problem is Potential Complication of myocardial infarction: congestive heart failure (CHF), the logical goal is "CHF will not occur." Clearly, nursing actions alone cannot prevent CHF. It requires collaborative efforts.

For collaborative problems, compare the reassessment data to established norms (e.g., normal temperature, normal electrocardiogram pattern, normal blood glucose) and determine whether data are within an acceptable range. If the data indicate that the client's condition is worsening (that the complication may be occurring), notify the physician. For example, if a patient with the collaborative problem Potential Complication of myocardial infarction: CHF develops fatigue, dyspnea, a productive cough, or abnormal lab results (e.g., elevated blood urea nitrogen [BUN] and creatinine levels), you would suspect CHF and notify the physician. See Chapter 4 if you need to review collaborative problems.

Evaluating and Revising the Care Plan

After evaluating patient progress, you will use your conclusions about goal achievement to decide whether to continue, modify, or discontinue the care plan.

Relate Outcomes to Interventions

Even when goals have been met, you cannot assume that the nursing interventions caused the patient outcomes. You need to use critical reflection to identify factors that might have supported or interfered with the effectiveness of an intervention. Recall that organizational structures and processes can also affect patient care. The following are variables that can affect the ability of an intervention to produce the desired outcome:

- The client's ability and motivation to follow directions for treatment
- Availability and support from family and significant others
- Treatments and therapies performed by other healthcare team members
- Client failure to provide complete information during assessment
- Client's lack of experience, knowledge, or ability
- Staffing in the institution (ratio of licensed to unlicensed caregivers; number of patients for whom a nurse is responsible)
- Nurse's physical and mental well-being

Identifying these factors allows you to reinforce or change them. For example, if Jeannette Wu does not achieve a goal of "Intact skin over sacrum" even after being turned q2hr by the UAP, you may discover that Ms. Wu's skin is more fragile than normal because her hydration and nutrition are not adequate. You could then take measures to support her intake of food and fluids, increasing the effectiveness of the turning intervention. Notice, though, that you cannot control all the variables that might affect the success of an intervention (e.g., the client's lack of experience, staffing in your institution).

Draw Conclusions About Problem Status

Whether you retain or remove a nursing diagnosis from the care plan depends on whether or not goals were met, as follows:

Goals met: If all goals for a nursing diagnosis have been met, you can discontinue the care plan for that diagnosis.

Goals partially met: If some outcomes are met and others not, you may revise the care plan for that problem; or you may continue with the same plan but allow more time for goal achievement.

Goals not met: If goals are not met, you should examine the entire plan and review all steps of the nursing process to decide whether to revise the care plan.

For an example of computerized evaluation of problem status for a client with multiple nursing care needs,

 Go to Chapter 7, **Tables, Boxes, Figures: ESG Figure 7–2,** on the Electronic Study Guide.

Notice that all the problems on this figure are "active."

Revise the Care Plan

To decide how to revise the care plan, you must review each step of the nursing process. You cannot just discontinue the "ineffective" interventions and try new ones. The interventions may not need to be changed at all. When goals have not been met, errors in other steps of the nursing process may be the reason. You will find a checklist you can use to evaluate the care plan and the process by which it was developed (Wilkinson, 2001) in

 Go to Chapter 7, **Delegation and Evaluation Checklists,** in Volume 2.

1. *Review of assessment.* Review all initial and ongoing assessment data. All steps of the nursing process depend on complete and accurate data. So if there are errors or omissions, you may need to revise any or all sections of the care plan (i.e., nursing diagnosis, outcomes, nursing orders).

Also, the data may have changed since the care plan was written: the client's condition may have changed, or new data may have been identified.

2. *Review of diagnosis.* Even if there were no errors of assessment, you may need to revise or add new nursing diagnoses. Perhaps the nurse who wrote the diagnostic statement did not communicate the patient's condition clearly. This might have caused an incorrect focus for outcomes and interventions.

3. *Review of planning outcomes.* You will probably need to revise the outcomes if you have added data or revised the nursing diagnosis. If assessment and diagnosis are satisfactory, perhaps the outcomes were unrealistic, written too broadly, or had unrealistic target times.

4. *Review of planning interventions.* If you have revised nursing diagnoses or outcomes, you will probably need to modify nursing orders. You may need to revise them or add new ones anyway if you determine that they were not effective in achieving the desired outcomes.

5. *Review of implementation.* It could be that goals were not met because of a failure to implement the nursing orders or because of the manner in which they were implemented. Get input from the client, significant others, other caregivers, and the client records to find out what went wrong. For example, the person implementing care may have been tired, in a hurry, or abrupt with the client. Or perhaps they did not have the necessary skills. See "Delegating and Supervising Care," pages 126–128.

Reflecting Critically About Evaluation

After evaluating the patient's health status and the nursing care plan, you should think critically about your thinking during the evaluation process. That's right: Think about your thinking, not just about your actions. The critical thinking model from Chapter 2 suggests some questions you might use for reflection.

Inquiring
Is my evaluation statement clearly stated (goal met or not met, plus supporting data)?
Were my information sources reliable (e.g., was the patient being honest or merely trying to please me)?
Did I jump to conclusions about goal achievement? Do I need any other data to validate my conclusion?

Noticing context
What was going on either before or during evaluation that might have influenced my ability to gather data or draw conclusions (e.g., Was I in a hurry? Did the patient have visitors?)
What emotional responses influenced my conclusions about goal achievement (e.g., Would I feel as though I had failed if the goal was not met?)

Analyzing assumptions
What biases do I have that may have affected my ability to reassess or evaluate goal achievement?

Reflecting skeptically
Did I make evaluating a priority? Did I schedule time for it, the same as I do for interventions? Could I have done it better? What would I do differently next time?

The most common errors of evaluation are failing to (1) evaluate systematically, (2) record the results, or (3) use the reassessment data to examine and modify the care plan. Because nurses are action-oriented, it is easy for most to make a plan and take action. And most nurses regularly observe the patient's responses to the actions. But you will need determined effort to make time to observe *regularly and systematically* and *document the patient's responses* to your actions. Only in that way can you be sure that the care has met the client's needs.

Evaluating the Quality of Care in a Healthcare Setting

As a nurse, you may be involved in evaluating and improving the overall quality of nursing care in an organization or a geographical area. At a minimum, your documentation will provide data that regulatory agencies (e.g., JCAHO, state boards of nursing) use to determine whether nursing care meets nursing standards.

Quality assurance (QA) programs are specially designed programs to promote excellence in nursing. Variations of quality assurance are quality improvement (QI), continuous quality improvement (CQI), total quality management (TQM), and persistent quality improvement (PQI). Whatever the approach, the goal is to evaluate and improve the care provided in an agency or for a group of patients.

This chapter has described (1) outcomes evaluation of *client progress* and (2) process evaluation of the *effectiveness of the nursing care plan.* Quality assurance involves evaluation of structures, as well as outcomes and processes. All are important because structures and processes affect patient outcomes. Adequate structures (e.g., staffing, money) and processes (e.g., policies and procedures) do not guarantee desired patient outcomes; however, without them, it is very difficult to obtain good outcomes. For example, a unit could be well staffed (structure) and follow infection-control procedures carefully (process), yet have a higher-than-average rate of urinary tract infections (outcome). The reason may be that most of the patients treated have compromised immune systems, making them especially susceptible to infection. For a full discussion of QA/QI evaluation, see Chapter 1 and

 Go to Chapter 1, **Supplemental Materials,** on the Electronic Study Guide.

| toward evidence-based practice |

Read about the following studies, and then answer the questions at the end of the box.

Standing, T., Anthony, M., & Hertz, J. (2001). Nurses' narratives of outcomes after delegation to unlicensed assistive personnel. *Outcomes Management for Nursing Practice, 5*(1). 18–23.

This qualitative study analyzed questionnaires and open-ended responses from 148 licensed nurses. Nurses were asked to write two narratives: one to describe a situation in which delegation of a task to a UAP had a positive outcome, and another that had a negative outcome. In addition, phone interviews were conducted with 27 nurses to expand on those findings. The following results were reported:

- Negative outcomes occurred most often because the UAP (1) did not follow directions or agency procedures, or (2) was overconfident (e.g., carried out activities that had not been delegated).
- With regard to the Five Rights of Delegation, deficiencies were most often related to the right communication or right supervision.

Thomas, S., Barter, M., & McLaughlin, F. (2000). State and territorial boards of nursing approaches to the use of unlicensed assistive personnel. *JONA'S Healthcare Law, Ethics and Regulation, 2*(1), 13–21.

This survey, administered to 53 state and territorial boards of nursing in 1998, found that:

- Most states had guidelines or regulations for RNs who supervised UAPs
- Few states used the ANA or NCSBN definitions for delegation, supervision, or assignment; most formulated their own definitions.
- Most states reported that they had no standardized curriculum for UAPs employed in acute care hospitals— and no plans for developing a curriculum.

Parsons, L. (1999). Building RN confidence for delegation decision-making skills in practice. *Journal of Nurses Staff Development, 15*(6), 263–269.

This study evaluated the effects of a structured teaching intervention on (1) RN delegation decision making and

(2) RN knowledge and confidence in delegating to team members. Researchers reported that the teaching intervention significantly increased RN delegation knowledge and overall confidence in decision making.

Badonivac, C., Wilson, S., & Woodhouse, D. (1999). The use of unlicensed assistive personnel and selected outcome indications. *Nursing Economics, 17*(4), 194–200.

This 2-month study gathered data regarding the implementation of a patient care delivery system using UAPs as nurse extenders. Based on a sample of 40 patients, 15 RNs, and 9 UAPs, the study compared the current data to risk management statistics from a comparable period 2 years prior. Results were as follows:

- There was no significant difference in the number of patient falls before and after patient care was delegated to UAPs.
- Patient satisfaction scores were higher after the institution began delegating tasks to UAPs.

Imagine that a study similar to study 1, with similar results, was done in your agency. There is concern in your organization because the rate of errors and incidents for delegated tasks is unusually high. You are a member of a task force of nurses who are charged with making a plan to decrease the number of errors and incidents in delegated tasks.

1. One nurse says, "The best approach would be to not use UAPs at all and go back to an all-licensed, professional staff." Imagine that you disagree with this nurse. Which of the studies (2, 3, or 4) could you cite to support your view?

2. What information from study 1 (as done in your agency) would also support your view when disagreeing with this nurse?

3. What idea for a solution could you get from study 2?

4. What idea does study 3 suggest for your institution?

5. Which idea from the studies seems most directly related to your institution's problem (as described in study 1)?

 Go to Chapter 7, **Toward Evidence-Based Practice Suggested Responses,** on the Electronic Study Guide.

 Go to Chapter 7, **Resources for Caregivers and Health Professionals,** on the Electronic Study Guide.

 Bibliography: Go to Volume 2, Bibliography.

CHAPTER 8

Nursing Theory
& Research

Learning Outcomes

After completing this chapter, you should be able to:

* Define nursing theory.

* List four components of a theory.

* Describe how a nursing theory is developed.

* List the four essential concepts in a nursing theory.

* List three ways nurses can use nursing theory.

* Discuss the relevance of Florence Nightingale's nursing theory to contemporary nursing practice.

* Name three predominant thinkers who proposed theories of caring.

* Describe three non-nursing theories and their contributions to nursing.

* Define nursing research.

* Describe the significance of evidence-based nursing practice.

* Describe the history of nursing research in the United States.

* Compare and contrast quantitative and qualitative nursing research.

* List three components of the research process, and explain their importance.

* Name three priorities in the process of protecting research participants, and explain the significance of these to the nursing research process.

* List at least four steps in the process of analytic reading of research reports, and explain their significance to the critique.

* Describe how to use nursing research in nursing practice.

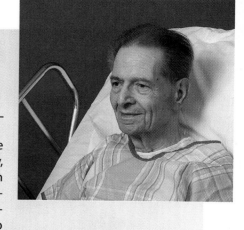

MEET Your Patient

Imagine you are the charge nurse on the night shift at a long-term care facility. You hear the certified nursing assistant (CNA) and another voice talking loudly down the hall. You immediately go to see what has happened. You are surprised and shocked by what you see. An older patient, Mr. Wilkey, is naked and in bed with another patient, Mrs. Fredrickson, who is crying and shouting, "Get out! Get out!" Mr. Wilkey is tearful and looks frightened. He keeps repeating, "Where is Momma? Where is Momma?" The CNA is visibly upset and is grabbing at Mr. Wilkey in an effort to get him out of the bed.

What are you going to do, and why do you think it will help? Don't be concerned if you don't think you know enough to answer this question. Before you read on, try to answer it based on the knowledge and experience that you *do* have.

There are two general ways to approach this problem. One way is to be upset with Mr. Wilkey and remove him from the room immediately, reprimanding him sternly for his behavior. Another possibility is to ask the CNA to calm Mrs. Fredrickson while you gently dress Mr. Wilkey and take him out of the room. You would talk to him in a quiet manner and not rush him. While you are talking to him, you might ask, "Who is Momma? What does she look like? Do you miss her?" By the time you lead him to his room, you might realize he is exhibiting stage II dementia. You infer that he probably woke up scared and confused and began looking for his long-dead mother. Seeing Mrs. Fredrickson, Mr. Wilkey thought he had found his mother and crawled into her bed.

If you chose the first approach in the scenario, you were demonstrating **mechanistic nursing,** which is based on getting the tasks done. If you chose the second solution, you based your behavior on **holistic nursing,** which requires meeting the needs of the whole person. This scenario demonstrates the powerful impact of nursing theory and research on your daily practice as a nurse. Although there are several theories that guide nursing practice, this chapter draws heavily on theories of caring to illustrate key points. We believe that caring is central to nursing and informs all the actions that nurses take. You will find other theories that pertain to specific aspects of practice in later chapters. For example, developmental theories are discussed in Chapter 9, theories of self-concept in Chapter 11, and family theories in Chapter 12.

THE IMPORTANCE OF NURSING THEORY AND RESEARCH

This chapter introduces you to nursing theory and research. You will learn how nursing theories and nursing research guide and form the foundations for your daily practice. Following are three examples that demonstrate how important theory and research are to you in your career as a nurse.

The Framingham Study is a longitudinal, multidisciplinary research project (*longitudinal* means done over a long period of time) carried out over 50 years (from 1948 to 1998) to identify the health and health care practices of one specific community: Framingham, Massachusetts. The results of the various Framingham studies influenced health care practices for diabetes mellitus, breast cancer, heart disease, osteoarthritis in older adults, and other disease entities. For example, one commonly accepted practice that came out of the Framingham study is the use of mammography to screen for breast cancer. There was a time when mammography was considered unreliable and unimportant. The Framingham project changed that attitude and, as a result, improved the health care of women.

Dr. Jean Watson (Figure 8–1) developed a nursing theory called the **Science of Human Caring** (1988). This theory describes what *caring* means from a nursing perspective. It may not seem that nurses need to be taught how to care, but Dr. Watson and other nursing theorists found that they did. Prior to the "caring

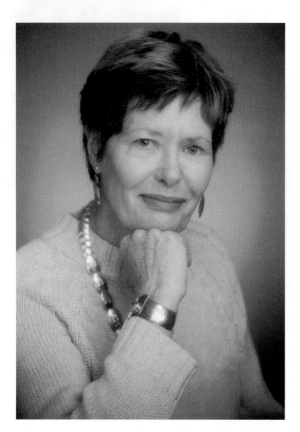

FIGURE 8–1 Dr. Jean Watson, distinguished professor and nursing theorist.

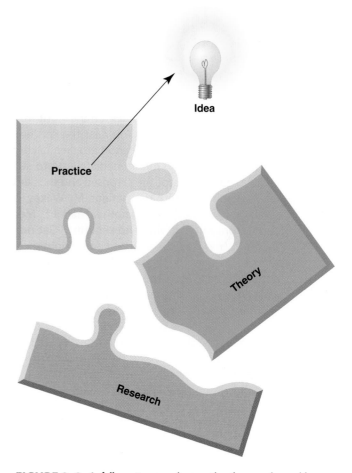

FIGURE 8–2 In full-spectrum nursing practice, the nurse has an idea, conducts nursing research to test the idea, and finally develops a theory.

theorists," nurses were somewhat mechanistic in the work they did (much like the first alternative for dealing with Mr. Wilkey). For example, a nurse has a list of things to do; the nurse completes the list and does nothing more. The "something more" behaviors often are the caring behaviors, such as singing to a frightened child or taking the time to teach a new mother for the second time how to bathe her baby.

This is not to say that nurses didn't care about their patients before Watson. The point is that a *theory* of caring (such as Watson's) changes the *focus* of nursing. Certainly Nightingale must have cared about the soldiers who were her patients. But what she wrote about and what she taught the nurses was a set of "things to do." Nurses were valued for the tasks they performed in patient care. Caring theories demonstrate the value of the non-task-oriented aspects of nursing.

Dr. Patricia Benner, in the book *From Novice to Expert* (1984), proposed a theory that should be of special interest to you. This theory, which was explained in Chapter 1, describes the progression of a beginning nurse to increasing levels of expertise. You are a **novice,** or a beginning nurse, simply because you are new to the nursing profession. Benner's theory provides the information necessary to understand how you learn and perform your nursing responsibilities.

Benner's theory of caring is discussed later in the chapter.

Think of full-spectrum nursing as a jigsaw puzzle (Figure 8–2). Initially, a nurse has an idea, which usually comes out of experiences in *practice* (the first puzzle piece). Perhaps the idea is something simple like: "Why don't I slow down and spend more time with the patients' families? It would really help them if I took more time."

After seriously considering the new idea, the nurse may decide the idea is worth investigating with *research* (the second puzzle piece). The research question might be: "How does spending more time with family members affect the quality of care the patient receives?" If the research supported the nurse's idea, she could then use the research findings to develop a *theory* (the third puzzle piece). The nurse could even take the research results to nursing administrators to determine whether the theory could be put into practice in the organization—perhaps as a policy or in a standardized care plan. That would be the beginning of what is called a ***clinical practice theory,*** a theory that is immediately applicable in the clinical setting.

KnowledgeCheck 8–1

- Compare mechanistic and holistic nursing. Select one of these concepts and describe a scenario where it is being used.
- Briefly describe the Framingham Study, and list three diseases for which this study influenced care.

 Go to Chapter 8, **Knowledge Check Response Sheet and Answers,** on the Electronic Study Guide.

NURSING THEORIES

Theoretical Knowledge
knowing why

Florence Nightingale (1859/1992) stated that nursing theories describe and explain what is and what is not nursing. That makes them critical to learn in the beginning of your nursing education. Before focusing on nursing theory, though, you need to learn a little more about theory in general. Exactly what *is* a theory? And how is a theory created?

A **theory** is an organized set of related ideas and concepts that helps us find meaning in our experiences (such as nursing), organize our thinking around an idea (such as caring), and develop new ideas and insights into the work we do. Put simply, a theory answers the questions: What is this? And how does it work? Although a theory is based on observations of facts, the theory itself is *not* a fact. A theory is a way of viewing phenomena (reality); it defines and illustrates concepts and explains how they are related or linked. Theories can be, and are, changed.

What Are the Components of a Theory?

Theories are made up of phenomena, concepts, assumptions, definitions, and statements (or propositions). You can think of these as the building blocks of a theory.

Phenomena

Phenomena are aspects of reality that you can observe and experience. Phenomena are the subject matter of a discipline (when used in this sense, they are often called *phenomena of concern*). Think of phenomena as marking the boundaries (*domain*) of a discipline—making one discipline unique from another. For example, for cartographers (map makers) the phenomena of concern are land formations and land use. For pharmacists, the phenomena of concern are medications: their chemical composition and their effects on the body. For nurses, the phenomena of concern are human beings and, more specifically, their body-mind-spirit responses to illness and injuries. It may seem a subtle difference, but Watson's theory of caring gave us the words and ideas for describing the nursing phenomena of concern in terms of *human beings in their environments.*

Assumptions

Assumptions are ideas that we take for granted. In a theory, they are the ideas that the theorist or researcher presumes to be true and does not intend to test with research. They are statements about concepts or relationships between concepts. For example, Watson assumed that nursing had its own professional concepts and that one of them was caring. Assumptions may or may not be stated. For example, most nursing theorists assume but do not state that human beings are complex. One exception is Martha Rogers (1970), who states outright that human beings are unified wholes that are more than and different from the sum of their parts.

Concepts

A **concept** is a mental image of a phenomenon. It is formed by generalizing an abstract idea from your experiences and observations of events, objects, and properties, and it exists as a symbol (e.g., a word or picture) in the mind. For example, what does the word *fever* bring to mind? From your own experience with fever, you know the subjective feeling that fever produces. You have the theoretical knowledge that it is an elevated body temperature; you know the physiology of temperature regulation, so you know what is going on in the body. You may have the visual image of a thermometer or someone who is red-faced and perspiring. The word *fever* is a symbol for all of those ideas and images.

Concepts range from simple to complex and from fairly concrete to very abstract. Simple, concrete concepts are those you can observe directly (e.g., height, weight, gender, body type). More abstract and complex concepts are those you observe indirectly (e.g., hematocrit level, brain activity, nutritional status). Very abstract concepts are those you must infer from many direct and indirect observations (e.g., self esteem, wellness).

A theory usually contains several concepts. For example, Watson includes ten "caring processes" in her theory (Box 8–1). Each of those is a complex concept.

Definitions

A **definition** is a statement of the meaning of a term or concept that sets forth the concept's characteristics or indicators. A definition may be general or specific. A *theoretical definition* refers to the conceptual meaning of a term, whereas an *operational definition* specifies how you would observe or measure the concept (e.g., when doing research). For example, for pain:

Theoretical definition: Pain is an unpleasant sensory and emotional experience associated with actual or potential tissue damage.

BOX 8–1 Watson's Ten Caring Processes

1. Forming a humanistic-altruistic system of values
2. Instilling faith and hope
3. Cultivating sensitivity to self and others
4. Forming helping and trusting relationships
5. Conveying and accepting the expression of positive and negative feelings
6. Systematic use of the scientific problem-solving method that involves caring process
7. Promoting transpersonal teaching-learning
8. Providing for supportive, protective, and corrective mental, physical, sociocultural, and spiritual environment
9. Assisting with gratification of human needs
10. Sensitivity to existential-phenomenological forces

Source: Watson, J. (1988). *Nursing: Human science and human care. A theory of nursing.* Publication No. 15-2236. New York: National League for Nursing Press.

Operational definition: Pain is the patient's verbal statement that he is in pain.

Statements/Propositions

Statements systematically describe the linkages and interactions among the concepts of a theory. The statements, taken as a whole, make up the theory. In Maslow's theory, for example, two concepts are *physiologic needs* and *self-esteem needs*. An example of a statement in that theory would be: "*Physiologic needs* must be met to an acceptable degree before a person can attempt to meet his *self-esteem needs*" or perhaps, "*Physiologic needs* are more basic (lower level) than *self-esteem needs*." Maslow's theory is explained fully on pages 150–151.

Theory, Framework, Model, or Paradigm?

In any discussion of nursing knowledge, you may hear the terms *theory, framework, model,* or *paradigm*. It may be difficult for you to differentiate between these terms because (1) they are so abstract, (2) they are defined differently by theorists, and (3) you may hear them used interchangeably in general conversation among nurses. As you progress in your career and education, you will need to pay more careful attention to the similarities and differences among these terms. For now, you can use the following definitions (*theory* was defined earlier):

A **paradigm** is the worldview or ideology of a discipline. It is the broadest, most global conceptual framework of a discipline. It includes and guides the values, philosophy, knowledge, theories, and research processes of the discipline. It is a way of thinking that is shared by a community of scholars who are studying and working on the same phenomena. For example, the medical paradigm views a person through a lens that focuses on identifying and treating disease. This lens causes you to look in depth at the person's "parts" (e.g., cells, organs). The nursing paradigm views the person through a lens that focuses more broadly on the entire person and how he responds to isolated changes in his cells and organs. Again, paradigms are not theories; they are just "how we see things."

A **conceptual framework** (also referred to as a *theoretical framework*) is a set of concepts that are related to form a whole or pattern. As a rule, frameworks are not developed using research processes and have not been tested in practice. The relationships among the concepts are described in less detail than in a theory, and assumptions are not stated. Frameworks (and models) tend to be broader and more philosophical than theories. Don't be alarmed if you can't tell the difference between a theory and a theoretical framework. The experts don't always agree, either. Many theorists, for example, classify the early nursing theories (e.g., Orem's self-care deficit theory and others presented in this chapter) as conceptual frameworks; others (Chinn & Kramer, 1999) classify them as theories.

A **model** is a symbolic representation of a framework or concepts—a diagram, graph, picture, drawing, or physical model. The plastic body parts you have seen in anatomy class are models of the real human body. Models are developed to promote understanding of concepts. Figure 8–2 is a model of the relationships between nursing practice, theory, and research, for example. Some models are more complex. A **conceptual model** (often used interchangeably with *conceptual framework*) is a model that is expressed in language—the symbols are words. In one sense, all models are "conceptual" because they all represent ideas. For now, it is enough to remember that:

1. The terms *theory, model,* and *framework* all refer to a group of related concepts, and
2. The terms differ in meaning, depending on the extent to which the set of concepts has been used and tested in practice and on the level of detail and organization of the concepts.

 Critical**Thinking** 8–1

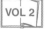 Go to Chapter 4, **NANDA Taxonomy II: Domains, Classes, and Diagnoses (Labels),** in Volume 2.

Do you think this is a theory, a conceptual framework, or a model?

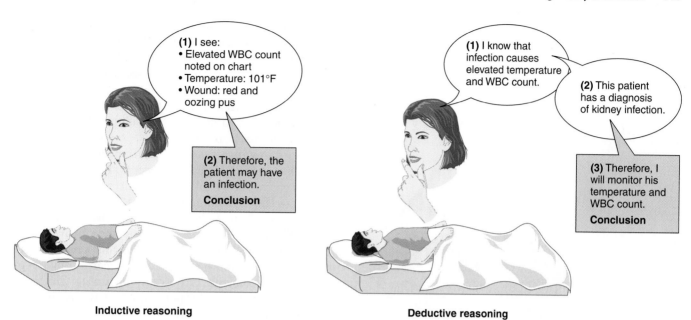

FIGURE 8–3   A comparison of inductive and deductive reasoning. Theorists and nurses in practice use both types of reasoning.

KnowledgeCheck 8–2

- Name the five "building blocks" of a theory.
- How is a paradigm different from a theory?

 Go to Chapter 8, **Knowledge Check Response Sheet and Answers,** on the Electronic Study Guide.

How Are Theories Developed?

To begin developing a theory, a nurse has an idea that seems worth exploring through research. As an example, Dr. Jean Watson had an idea about caring behaviors toward patients. Once the idea was clear in her mind, she performed research to see whether her ideas made sense. She used the validated ideas to develop her theory. Once she had a research-based theory, she shared it with others, and it changed nursing practice.

Theories are developed through a specific way of thinking called logical reasoning (Marriner-Tomey & Raile-Alligood, 2002). Generally, you can think of **reasoning** as connecting ideas in a way that makes sense. The purpose of **logical reasoning** is to develop an argument or statement based on evidence that will result in a logical conclusion. Nursing theories cannot be based on guesswork; they must be developed on a solid foundation of logical reasoning. The most commonly used types of logical reasoning are inductive and deductive reasoning.

Inductive reasoning is often used in the nursing process. If you walk into a person's room and note that the patient has a temperature of 101°F (38°C), a pulse of 104, and respirations of 20 per minute, you could reasonably *induce* (conclude) that the person is ill. Induction moves from the specific to the general.

You gathered separate pieces of information, recognized a pattern, and formed a generalization. You could not say that the person had a *specific* infection (e.g., measles), but you could induce that the person is ill. Remember induction by thinking, "I have specific data 'out there,' and I bring it 'in' to make the generalization. Refer to Figure 8–3.

Deductive reasoning is the opposite of inductive reasoning. Deduction starts with a *general premise* and moves to a *specific deduction*. Suppose you receive a call from the emergency department stating you will be admitting a new patient with acute pyelonephritis (kidney infection). Because you know what is involved in the general premise (pyelonephritis), you deduce that the patient will probably have an elevated temperature and back pain. You have the "big picture" about what is true in general, and from that you can figure out logically what is likely to be true for a particular individual.

Understanding logical thinking, even on this basic level, will help you understand the thinking that goes into both nursing theory and nursing research. ***Caution:*** *Induced and deduced conclusions are not facts. They may or may not accurately reflect reality.*

CriticalThinking 8–2

- Your patient is grimacing, groaning, and holding his hands over his abdominal incision. You induce that the patient is having incision pain. How could you be sure that your induction is factual (true)?
- Earlier you deduced that your emergency department patient with pyelonephritis will have a temperature and back pain. How confident are you that this is actually so? How could you be more certain that your deduction is correct?

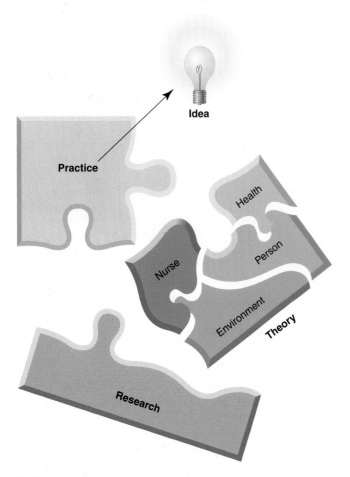

FIGURE 8–4   The four components of a nursing theory are person, nurse, health, and environment.

The preceding Critical Thinking exercise should demonstrate that inductions and deductions are not "facts" or "truth," but rather that they point you in the direction to go in seeking truth (reality). And they allow you to make connections between ideas when you are developing a theory. The more information you have to support your conclusions, the more confident you can be that they are correct.

What Are the Essential Concepts of a *Nursing* Theory?

There are four basic concepts that represent phenomena of concern for nursing and that should be addressed by any nursing theory (Flaskerud & Halloran, 1980): **person, environment, health,** and **nursing.** Notice that this further divides the puzzle piece for nursing theory into four more pieces (Figure 8–4).

As Watson, Benner, and other theorists considered their questions, research design, and possible outcomes, they undoubtedly kept these four concepts in mind. A meaningful nursing theory defines these four puzzle pieces and explains how they are related to each other. Consider a theory that does not include

the concept of person. Such a theory would describe the needs of the nurse and the condition of the environment, as well as the health of the person. However, it would not deal with the person's reaction to her health or lack of health. As a result, the person's learning needs, fears, family concerns or discharge arrangements would not be considered. That sounds quite mechanistic, doesn't it?

The following is an illustration of how Watson (1988) views the four basic concepts. In her science of human caring, she explores the concept of *caring* as it relates to the person, environment, health, and nursing. Watson focuses heavily on the *person* and the *nurse*. She talks about the "transpersonal" caring moments that exist between the two. She presents the *environment* as another way to show caring: by keeping it clean, colorful, or quiet or including whatever promotes health for the person. All of the caring behaviors (see Box 8–1) listed in Watson's theory focus on improving the *health* of the person.

 ## CriticalThinking 8–3

Think of an experience you have had in clinical. Perhaps it was taking vital signs or bathing a confused patient. Describe how each of the four components of a nursing theory occurred in your clinical situation. Share your thinking with a classmate or co-worker.

- Who was the *person(s)* involved (*person* refers to the patient or resident or the family and support persons)?
- What was the *environment*? A community center? A bathing room in a nursing home? The person's bedside in a hospital?
- What was the *health* condition of the person? For example, was the person seeking information for self care? Critical? In pain? Ready for discharge?
- How was *nursing* involved? For example, was the nurse compassionate? Angry? Efficient? A novice or an expert?

Observing nursing situations within the framework of the four components of nursing theory will help you understand the importance of each. This is very important because the finished puzzle reflects excellent (full-spectrum) nursing care.

KnowledgeCheck 8–3
- What are the four essential concepts in a nursing theory?
- What is the title of Dr. Watson's theory?
- Caring processes are critical to her theory. What is the purpose of the caring processes?

Go to Chapter 8, **Knowledge Check Response Sheet and Answers,** on the Electronic Study Guide.

How Do Nurses Use Theories?

Nursing theories try to describe, explain, and predict human behavior. You have already seen in the case of Mr. Wilkey ("Meet Your Patient") how the use of a

certain theory could guide the nurse to more compassionate care. Think of a theory as a lens. You can see the stars more clearly if you look at them through a telescope than you can by using binoculars. As another metaphor, the lens of your sunglasses removes glare, allowing you to see more clearly in bright sunlight but decreasing your ability to see in dim light. Theories offer a way of looking at nursing, and in this way they affect your entire perspective. The theory you use influences what you look for, what you notice, what you perceive as a problem, what outcomes you hope to achieve, and what interventions you will choose.

In Practice

Nursing theories serve as a guide for assessment, problem identification, and choosing nursing interventions. They help nurses communicate to other members of the health team what it is that makes nurses unique and important to the interdisciplinary team.

Clinical practice theories very specifically guide what you do each day. They are limited in scope—that is, they do not attempt to explain all of nursing. A theory on human interaction directs nurse-client communication; another theory provides a guide for teaching people how to be self reliant. The following are other examples:

1. Nightingale's theory emphasized the importance of the environment in the care of patients. Her work affected the design and building of hospitals for decades.
2. Dr. Imogene Rigdon (Rigdon, Clayton, & Dimond, 1987) developed a theory about bereavement of older women after noticing (and having an idea!) that older women handled grief differently from men and younger women. Hospice organizations all over the country now use this theory to work with older women who have lost a significant other.
3. Nola Pender's theory (2001) on health promotion (see Chapter 41) is the basis for most health promotion teaching done by nurses.
4. Dr. Katharine Kolcaba (1994) developed a theory of holistic comfort in nursing, which provides a more holistic view than earlier theories of pain and anxiety.

In Education

Schools of nursing use theories to guide curriculum planning, programs, and projects. These are frequently grand theories, such as Watson's theory of caring or Rogers's science of unitary human beings. A **grand theory** covers broad areas of concern within a discipline. A grand theory is usually abstract and does not outline specific nursing interventions. Instead, it tends to deal with the relationships among nurse, person, health, and environment.

A school using Watson's theory, for example, would include aspects of her theory in each class. A course might even be organized around the caring factors listed in Box 8–1. As another example, an inservice education director in a nursing home may choose a narrower and more specific theory (*mid-range* or *practice theory*) of comfort, using it to devise policies and procedures and design educational programs.

In Research

Theories help generate new knowledge by suggesting questions for researchers to study. Researchers also use theories and models as a framework for structuring a study. They provide a systematic way to define the questions for study, identify the variables to measure, and interpret the findings. For example, Kolcaba tested her statement that comfort interventions, as defined in her theory, would improve the health of the whole person.

Who Are Some Important Nurse Theorists?

You will need to thoroughly understand the theories you use in practice and the one (or more) used by your school of nursing. As an educated nurse, you should also have at least a nodding acquaintance with the nurse theorists who have influenced nursing practice. The following three theorists are presented in detail because of their historical significance. The description of their theories is simple and applicable to what you do every day as a nurse.

Florence Nightingale

As you learned in Chapter 1, Florence Nightingale revolutionized nursing. When she went to the Scutari Hospital during the Crimean War, the soldiers slept on mats on the floor, where rats scampered and raw sewage flowed. Nightingale's "idea" was that *more men would survive if they had a clean and healthy environment and nutritious food (so that the body could heal itself)*. That may not seem remarkable to you, but consider that the germ theory of infectious disease had not yet been identified.

Nightingale also was an outstanding researcher. She stayed awake late at night to keep records of what was happening at Scutari hospital before and after she introduced her ideas (research). By changing the environment, she dramatically reduced the death rate of the soldiers (Dossey, 1999). She used her research to develop her theory that a clean environment would improve the health of patients. Because of her theory and research, Nightingale changed the way the entire British Army hospital system was managed. For more information about Nightingale,

Go to **http://www.valdosta.edu/nursing/history_theory/ florence.html**

Virginia Henderson's List of Basic Needs

1. Breathe normally.
2. Eat and drink adequately.
3. Eliminate body wastes.
4. Move and maintain desirable posture.
5. Sleep and rest.
6. Select suitable clothes—dress and undress.
7. Maintain body temperature within normal range by adjusting clothing and modifying the environment.
8. Keep the body clean and well groomed, and protect the integument.
9. Avoid dangers in the environment and avoid injuring others.
10. Communicate with others in expressing emotions, needs, fears, or opinions.
11. Worship according to one's faith.
12. Work in such a way that there is a sense of accomplishment.
13. Play or participate in various forms of recreation.
14. Learn, discover, or satisfy the curiosity that leads to normal development and health and use of the available health facilities.

Source: Marriner-Tomey, A., & Raile-Alligood, M. (2002). *Nursing theorists and their work* (5th ed.). St. Louis: Mosby, p. 101.

Virginia Henderson

Virginia Henderson was born in 1897. She began her career as a U.S. Army nurse in 1918. She also was a visiting nurse in New York City and then a teacher of nursing. Her pamphlet, *Basic Principles of Nursing Care,* was published in 1960 by the International Council of Nursing. It was published in 20 languages.

While a nursing student at Walter Reed Army Hospital, Henderson began to question the mechanistic nursing care she was taught to give, as well as the fact she was expected to be the physicians' handmaiden. As a teacher of nursing, she came to recognize that there was no clear description of the purpose and function of nursing. She was the first nurse to identify that as a concern. Her "idea" was that *nurses deserve to know what it means to be a nurse.*

Henderson's 1966 book, *The Nature of Nursing,* described her theory of nursing's primary, unique function. She identified 14 basic needs that are addressed by nursing care (Box 8–2). Although the simple things on that list are commonplace today, they had not been identified as components of nursing care until Virginia

Henderson did so. Henderson's (1966, p. 3) definition of nursing states: "The unique function of the nurse is to assist the individual, sick or well, in the performance of those activities contributing to health or its recovery (or to a peaceful death) that he would perform unaided if he had the necessary strength, will or knowledge. And do this in such a way as to help him gain independence as rapidly as possible." Henderson defined what nursing was in the 20th century. For more information on Henderson,

Go to **http://www.angelfire.com/ut/virginiahenderson/index .html** or **http://www.enursescribe.com/ nurse_theorists.htm**

Hildegard Peplau

Hildegard E. Peplau was born in 1909 to immigrant parents in Pennsylvania. She was a psychiatric nurse and has contributed much to nursing in general. She influenced the advancement of standards in nursing education, promoted self-regulation in nursing through credentialing, and was a strong advocate for advanced nursing practice.

Dr. Peplau's "idea" was that *health could be improved for psychiatric patients if there were a more effective way to communicate with them.* Again, you may feel this is an unnecessary theory because nurses communicate with patients all the time. But remember that in the early 1900s, actually talking to and developing a personal relationship with psychiatric patients simply was not done. Psychiatric patients did not have the benefit of psychotropic drugs currently available to manage their symptoms. They were often agitated and extremely difficult to communicate with.

Peplau's research showed that developing a relationship with psychiatric patients does make their treatment more effective. She developed the theory of interpersonal relations, which focuses on the relationship a nurse has with the patient. This is a theory you use every day without even knowing it existed. For more information on Peplau's theory,

Go to **http://publish.uwo.ca/%7Ecforchuk/peplau/hpcb.html**

The Caring Theorists

The three leading caring theorists in nursing are Dr. Jean Watson, Dr. Patricia Benner, and Dr. Madeleine Leininger. We have been using Watson's ideas to illustrate principles and concepts of theory. In this section, we discuss Benner and Leininger.

Patricia Benner

Caring is the central concept in Benner and Wrubel's *primacy of caring model.* The nurse's caring helps the client cope. Moreover, it offers opportunity for the nurse

to connect with others and to receive as well as give help (Benner & Wrubel, 1989). Caring involves personal concern for persons, events, projects, and things. Therefore, it reveals what is stressful for a person (because if something does not matter to a person, it will not create stress) and provides motivation. Caring also makes the nurse notice which interventions are effective. This theory stresses that each person is unique, so that caring is always specific and relational for each nurse-person encounter.

In Chapter 1, we discussed another of Benner's theories. A critical care nurse, she wanted to find out *what makes an expert nurse.* In this case, the idea took the form of a question. An example of an expert nurse, for her, was an intensive care unit (ICU) nurse who "knew" intuitively when it was time to extubate a critical patient. Benner wanted to know what makes a nurse expert enough to know that and other critical information. She therefore interviewed ICU nurses and, from her research, identified five stages of knowledge development. As you may recall, the first level is that of a novice nurse (you). The others are advanced beginner, competent, proficient, and expert nurse (see Chapter 1).

Let's see whether this novice-to-expert theory addresses the four components of a nursing theory. *Person* and *nurse* are very clearly points of focus. Knowing the *nurse's* skill level (novice, advanced beginner, competent, proficient, or expert) provides for an intelligent way to match the nurse's skill with the patient's (*person*) acuity. This is the basis of the theory. The theory also indicates that the nurse contributes to the person's *health* according to her skill level. The *environment* is clearly stated as the ICU. Benner's theory does meet the criteria of the four components of a theory, although some are emphasized more than others. Differences in emphasis are typical of theories, by the way.

Madeleine Leininger

Leininger is the founder of transcultural nursing (Figure 8–5) and was the first nurse in the United States to earn a doctoral degree in cultural and social anthropology. Her theory focuses on caring as **cultural competence** (using knowledge of cultures and of nursing to provide culturally congruent and responsible care). Her "idea" came from working with children from diverse cultures who were under her care in a psychiatric hospital: *Would the psychotherapy for the children be more effective if delivered within the framework of the child's culture* (Marriner-Tomey & Raile-Alligood, 2002)? Leininger performed the research to confirm her idea that culturally competent care made a difference, and then she developed her theory. She followed the pattern of the puzzle pieces referred to throughout this chapter.

The *person* in Leininger's theory is an individual with cultural beliefs that are specific to herself and that may differ from the beliefs of others. Human

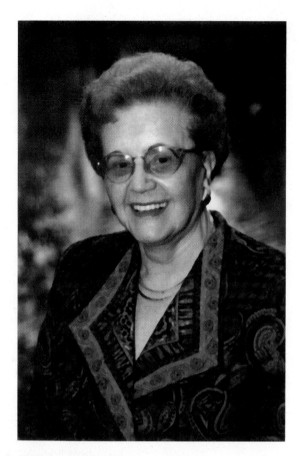

FIGURE 8–5 Leininger's theory on cultural competence calls for understanding of people of all cultures.

beings can feel concern for others, but ways of caring vary across cultures. The *nurse* is the professional who values the cultural diversity of the person and is willing to make cultural accommodations for the health benefit of the person. This requires specialized cultural knowledge. The *environment* is wherever the *nurse* and the *person* are together in the health care system. *Health* is defined by the *person* and may be culturally specific in its definition. For more about Leininger's theory, see Chapter 13.

You may be thinking, "This is all about culture; what does that have to do with caring?" Leininger's theory brings together the cultures of the *person,* the *nurse,* and the *healthcare system* (indeed, there is a culture of health care, as you will discover in Chapter 13) to improve healthcare delivery and its effectiveness. For example, as a nurse, you may need to welcome the Shaman from a Native American tribe who has been asked to perform a sacred dance in the hospital room. This is one way to demonstrate caring and respect for the person who is ill.

This is a true culture-care story: As a young nurse I was caring for a patient who was a monk from a local religious order. He had just had abdominal surgery, and he would not take any pain medication. He wanted to "offer the pain up to God." That was a serious values

TABLE 8-1   Selected Nurse Theorists

Theorist	Date	Theory	Additional Information
Peplau, Hildegard E.	1952	Interpersonal relations model: interpersonal communication can improve mental health.	http://publish.uwo.ca/%7Ecforchuk/peplau/hpcb.html
Henderson, Virginia	1955	14 basic needs addressed by nursing care; definition of nursing; do for the patient what he cannot do for himself.	http://www.angelfire.com/ut/virginiahenderson/index.html and http://www.enursescribe.com/nurse_theorists.htm
Abdellah, Faye G.	1960	21 nursing problems; deliver care to the whole person.	http://www.enursescribe.com/Faye_Abdellah.htm
Orlando, Ida Jean	1961	Interpersonal process; nursing process theory.	http://www.enursescribe.com/orlando.htm
Wiedenbach, Ernestine	1964	The purpose of nursing is to support and meet patients' needs for help. Nursing is a helping art.	Wiedenbach, E. (1964). *Clinical nursing: A helping art.* New York: Springer.
Levine, Myra	1967	Conservation model, published in 1973; designed to promote adaptation of the person while maintaining wholeness, or health.	Levine, M. E. (1967). The four conservation principles of nursing. *Nursing Forum, 6,* 45–59. Levine, M. E. (1969). *Introduction to clinical nursing.* Philadelphia: F. A. Davis Company.
Johnson, Dorothy	1968, 1980	The behavioral system model: incorporates five principles of systems thinking to establish a balance or equilibrium (adaptation) in the person. The patient is a behavioral system consisting of subsystems.	Johnson, D. E. (1968). Theory in nursing: Borrowed and unique. *Nursing Research, 11,* 206. Johnson, D. E. (1980). The behavioral system model for nuring. In J. P. Riehl & C. Roy (Eds.), *Conceptual models for nursing practice* (2nd ed.) (pp. 207–216). New York: Appleton-Century-Crofts.
Rogers, Martha	1970	The science of unitary human beings focuses on the betterment of human kind through new and innovative modalities. Maintaining an environment free of negative energy is important.	http://www.washburn.edu/sonu/rogers1.htm
Orem, Dorothea	1971	The self-care deficit nursing theory explains what nursing care is required when people are not able to care for themselves. Goal is to help client attain total self-care.	http://members.aol.com/annmrn/nursing_portfolio_l_index.html

clash for me because I believed the patient was jeopardizing his health, yet I did respect his right to live his cultural beliefs. We worked out a compromise. The monk agreed to take pain medication every 8 hours (instead of the prescribed q3–4hr), and I was vigilant in attending to ambulation, hygiene, and other needs during the times the medication was in effect. This is an example of applying a theory directly to the needs of the person who is ill.

Other Selected Nurse Theorists

You will find a list of selected nurse theorists and a brief description of their theories in Table 8–1. For a more complete discussion of those theories, see the web sites listed there, and

 Go to Chapter 8, **Supplemental Materials: Other Selected Nurse Theorists,** on the Electronic Study Guide.

TABLE 8-1	*(continued)*			
King, Imogene	1971	First of two theories was the interacting systems framework, designed to explain the organized wholes within which nurses are expected to function, i.e., society, groups, and individuals. The first theory led to the theory of goal attainment, which focuses on mutual goal setting between a nurse and patient and the process for meeting the goals.		http://www.enursescribe.com/imogene_king.htm
Neuman, Betty	1972	Neuman systems model is based on general systems theory (a non-nursing theory) and reflects the nature of living organisms as open systems.		http://www.neumann.edu/academics/undergrad/nursing/model.asp
Roy, Sr. Callista	1974	Adaptation model was inspired by the strength and resiliency of children. The model relates to the choices people make as they adapt to illness and wellness.		http://www2.bc.edu/%7Eroyca
Leininger, Madeleine M.	1978, 1984	Cultural care diversity and universality theory. Caring theory.		http://www.tcns.org/menu/menu22.shtml
Newman, Margaret	1979	Theory of health as expanding consciousness describes nursing intervention as nonintervention, where the nurse's presence helps patients recognize their own pattern of interacting with the environment.		http://www.healthasexpanding consciousness.org/
Watson, Jean	1979	Caring theory. Nursing is an inter-personal process.		http://www2.uchsc.edu/son/caring/content/
Parse, Rosemarie Rizzo	1981	Theory of human becoming focuses on the human-universe-health process and knowledge related to human becoming (or reaching one's potential).		http://www.humanbecoming.org/index.html
Benner, Patricia and Wrubel, J.	1989	Primacy of caring model. Caring is central to the model and helps the client cope with stressors of illness.		http://www.enursescribe.com/nurse_theorists.htm

KnowledgeCheck 8–4

Define in a brief conceptual form or title the nursing theory of each theorist listed below:

- Florence Nightingale
- Virginia Henderson
- Hildegard Peplau

 Go to Chapter 8, **Knowledge Check Response Sheet and Answers,** on the Electronic Study Guide.

How Do Nurses Use Theories from Other Disciplines?

Theory development is relatively new in nursing. Except for Nightingale (1859/1992), it was not until the mid-1950s that nursing leaders began to publish their theories about nursing. The profession relied heavily on the theories of other disciplines. Nurses still use knowledge from other disciplines as a part of their

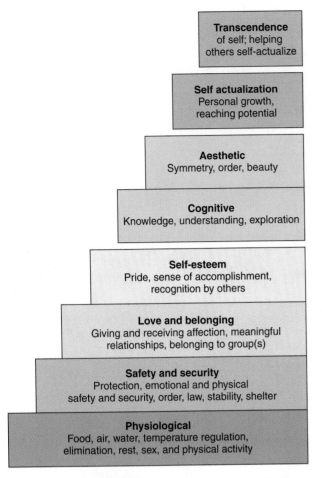

FIGURE 8–6   Maslow's hierarchy of human needs is a theory nurses use every day. *Sources:* Adapted from Maslow, A. (1971). *The farther reaches of human nature.* New York: Viking Press; and Maslow, A., & Lowery, R. (Eds.). (1998). *Toward a psychology of being* (3rd ed.). New York: Wiley & Sons.

scientific knowledge base. The following are a few of the many "borrowed" theories you will use in nursing.

Maslow's Hierarchy of Basic Human Needs

One of the classic theories still used in most nursing education and practice settings is Maslow's hierarchy of needs (1970). Maslow observed that certain human needs are common to all people, but some needs are "more basic" than others. The lower-level (e.g., physiological) needs must be met to some degree before the higher needs (e.g., self-esteem) can be achieved (Figure 8–6). For example, if you sit down to study but the room is cold, you will likely decide to put on a sweater or turn up the heat before opening your books. Nevertheless, a person may consciously choose to ignore a lower-level need in order to achieve a higher need. For example, the rescuers at the World Trade Center ignored their need for safety and security to help others (transcendence of self). In daily life, most people are partially satisfied and partially unsatisfied at each level.

Everyone has a dominant need, but it varies among individuals. For example, a teenager may have a (self-esteem) need to be accepted by a group. A heroin addict needs to satisfy her cravings for heroin and will not worry much about being accepted by others.

Physiological Needs

Physiological needs are those that must be met to maintain life. They include the needs for food, air, water, temperature regulation, elimination, rest, sex, and physical activity. Most healthy adults meet their physiologic needs through self care. However, many of your nursing interventions will support patients' physiologic needs.

Safety and Security Needs

The needs for safety and security are the next priority. Safety and security may refer to either physical or emotional needs. *Physical safety and security* mean protection from physical harm (e.g., falls, infection, and effects of medications) and having adequate shelter (e.g., housing). Many people in our society do not feel safe enough to go for a walk in their neighborhood.

Emotional safety and security involve freedom from fear and anxiety—feeling safe in the physical environment as well as in relationships. We need the security of a home and family. If there is an abusive husband, for example, the wife will be "stuck" at this level. She will spend an inordinate amount of time attempting to create a safe environment that does not trigger episodes of violence or abuse. This leaves little energy for meeting, for example, self-esteem needs.

Love and Belonging Needs

Needs for love and belonging are sometimes called social or affiliation needs. When they dominate, the person strives for meaningful relationships with others. Everyone has a basic need to love and be loved, give and receive affection, and have a feeling of "belonging," for example, in a family, peer group, or community. When these needs are not met, a person may feel isolated and lonely and may withdraw or become demanding and critical.

Self-Esteem Needs

People who have begun to satisfy the need to belong may begin to feel the need for self-esteem. Self-esteem comes through a sense of accomplishment and recognition from others and brings confidence and independence. As we discuss in Chapter 11, illness can affect self esteem by causing role changes (e.g., inability to perform one's job), or a change of body image (e.g., loss of a body part). When recognition cannot be obtained through positive behaviors, the person may resort to disruptive or irresponsible actions.

Self-Actualization Needs

The highest level on Maslow's original hierarchy, self actualization refers to the need to reach your full potential and to act unselfishly. At this level, a person develops wisdom and knows what to do in a variety of situations. Maslow studied self-actualized people to develop a list of their characteristics.

 Go to Chapter 8, **Tables, Boxes, Figures: ESG Box 8-1,** on the Electronic Study Guide.

In his later work, Maslow identified two growth needs that must be met prior to reaching self-actualization (Maslow & Lowery, 1998):

1. *Cognitive needs* to know, understand, and explore
2. *Aesthetic needs* for symmetry, order, and beauty

Transcendence of Self

Later research led Maslow to identify one higher need (Maslow, 1971): the need for *transcendence of self.* This is the drive to connect to something beyond oneself and to help others realize their potential. Some people include spirituality at this level, which is also the basis for acts of self-sacrifice (for example, donating a kidney so that another person can live).

Application of Maslow's Theory

The following example illustrates how you might use Maslow's theory when teaching patients. Suppose you have been assigned to teach Mrs. Gallegos about her colostomy prior to her discharge. You put a great deal of effort into obtaining materials in Spanish, Mrs. Gallegos's primary language, and you have arranged for an interpreter in case she has some questions you can't understand or answer. As you walk in the door to begin teaching, you immediately observe that Mrs. Gallegos seems to be in a great deal of pain. What will you do?

Maslow's hierarchy of needs tells you very clearly that until the pain (a physiological need) is managed successfully, Mrs. Gallegos cannot learn. (Maslow considers pursuit of knowledge a self-actualization need.) You arrange for pain medication to be administered and reschedule the teaching session. If you went ahead and taught, the experience would be for the sole purpose of "crossing it off your list" (remember mechanistic nursing?) rather than actually teaching Mrs. Gallegos.

Validation Theory

Validation theory (Feil, 1993) arises from social work and provides for a way to communicate with older people with dementia. The theory asks the caregiver to "go where the demented person is in his own mind." For example, if Mr. Wilkey ("Meet Your Patient") is talking about his mother, who has been dead for many years, you would ask questions about her rather than tell him that she is dead. Learning of his mother's death would be a shocking and horrible experience, which would be relived each time he heard the news. Instead, you would "go where the demented person is in his own mind" by asking him, for example, about the color of his mother's eyes, what songs she sings to him, or other questions that will stimulate conversation about the mother.

Stress and Adaptation Theory

Hans Selye (1993) developed the stress and adaptation theory. There are many theories about stress, but Selye's was the grandfather of them all. His theory states that a certain amount of stress is good for people; it keeps them motivated and alert. However, too much stress, called *distress,* results in physiological symptoms and eventual illness. Does that happen to you at the end of the semester when you are "distressed" over the number of papers due and the difficulty of the tests for which you are studying? Generally the human body will respond to distress with an illness, such as a cold, that will force the body to slow down or simply go to bed. For further discussion of Selye's theory, see Chapter 25.

Developmental Theories

Developmental theories look at stages that individuals, groups, families, and communities progress through over time. Several important examples include Erickson's psychosocial developmental theory (discussed in Chapter 9), theories of family development (discussed in Chapters 11 and 12), and Kohlberg's and Gilligan's theories of moral development (discussed in Chapters 9 and 44). These theories are useful in nursing practice because they identify norms and expectations at various stages in development and help you identify activities and interventions that are appropriate for your client.

System Theory

Ludwig von Bertalanffy was the creator of system theory in the 1940s (von Bertalanffy, 1976). He intended it to be abstract enough to use for theory and research in any discipline. Today the understanding of systems has evolved to the point that many of the concepts are a part of our everyday language (e.g., healthcare system, body systems, information systems, family systems).

One of the premises of systems theory is that all complex phenomena, regardless of their type, have some principles, laws, and organization in common. A **system** is made up of separate components (or **subsystems**), which constantly interact with each other and with other systems. For example, the cardiovascular

and renal systems are subsystems of the body; the cells are subsystems of those systems. All of those systems and subsystems exchange processes and information with each other and with systems outside the body.

A system maintains some organization even though it is constantly facing internal and external changes. All systems have some common elements. The goal (function) of any system is to process **input** (the energy, information, or materials that enter the system) for use within the system or in the **environment** (everything outside the system) or both. Other common elements include the following:

Output is the product or service that results from the system's throughput (processing of technical, social, financial, and human input). Examples of output are documents, money, nursing diagnoses, cars.

Throughput consists of the processes the system uses to convert input (raw materials) into output (products to be used by the system or environment). Examples are thinking, planning, sorting, meeting in groups, sterilizing, hammering, and cutting.

Feedback is information about some aspect of the processing that is used to monitor the system and make its performance more effective (e.g., evaluation in the nursing process: how the patient responded to the interventions)

Open systems exchange information and energy freely with the environment. Open systems are capable of growth, development, and adaptation. Examples of open systems include, people, body systems, hospitals, and businesses.

Closed systems have fixed, automatic relationships among their components and very little give and take with the environment. One example is a rock. A nursing example is a family that is isolated from the community and resists outside influences.

Several nursing theories have been built on system theory, for example, Johnson's (1968, 1980) behavioral system model, King's (1971) interacting systems framework, and the Neuman systems model (Neuman & Young, 1972), to name a few. For information about these theorists,

 Go to Chapter 8, **Supplemental Materials: Other Selected Nurse Theorists,** on the Electronic Study Guide.

KnowledgeCheck 8–5

- Name four theories nurses "borrow" from other disciplines.
- What are the five original levels of Maslow's basic human needs (not including cognitive needs, aesthetic needs, and transcendence)?

 Go to Chapter 8, **Knowledge Check Response Sheet and Answers,** on the Electronic Study Guide.

Practical Knowledge
knowing how

Practical knowledge about theory means using theories to guide you in your use of the nursing process. Recall the lens metaphor: A theory's concepts and principles determine what you look for and what you notice. In the assessment step of the nursing process, your theory tells you what to assess and provides the rationale for the assessments; its major concepts serve as categories for organizing the data. In the diagnosis step, your theory guides you in defining patient problems; in fact, it determines whether you will even recognize a cluster of cues as a problem. The theory helps you to generate appropriate, achievable client outcomes, to choose effective nursing interventions, and to provide rationale for your actions.

There is no reason to discuss theory in this book unless you can apply the information. To show you how, this section applies caring theory to the planning of nursing interventions. Of course you can use *any* theory for this purpose. We use caring theory because of the powerful and positive impact it can have on your nursing care. In reading this chapter, you should have become familiar with two well-known caring theories. Test your recall by writing the theorists' names and basic ideas. If you have difficulty, be sure to review the information about caring theorists before proceeding.

CriticalThinking 8–4

Write a paragraph describing a clinical experience in which you applied or observed one or both of the caring theories. Record your thinking on a piece of paper, and be prepared to share it with your classmates. You may title it "My Experience in Caring."

Planning Theory-Based Interventions/Implementation

The Nursing Interventions Classification, or NIC (Dochterman & Bulechek, 2004), introduced in Chapter 6, is theory development in its early stages. Each of the standardized intervention labels (e.g., Exercise Promotion, Infection Control) is a concept, and defining or describing concepts is an important step in theory development.

In this section, we use nine key concepts of Watson's caring theory to describe important nursing activities and approaches.

1. *Holistic nursing care.* The basis of modern nursing, holistic nursing care allows nurses to examine the entire person and the person's world when making healthcare decisions. It goes beyond "just" giving the medication or dressing a wound. These are important tasks, but try to see nursing as

giving care to the entire person and all that this entails (e.g., family, friends, fears, cultural beliefs).

2. *Honoring personhood.* None of the three caring theorists refers to the person in the healthcare system as a patient unless they need to for clarification. They firmly believe that the "patient" is someone who deserves to be honored for individuality in behavior as well as needs. If you accept the need to honor personhood, you will learn the names of the people in your care and will refer to them by name instead of "Room 331," or "the kidney infection down the hall." Honoring personhood takes time, because you need to look at, talk to, and touch the person to understand what their personhood is. It requires you to control the rush and fast pace of nursing and take time with your patients.

3. *Transpersonal caring moments.* Watson says the concept of transpersonal caring is a moral ideal rather than a task-oriented behavior (remember Mr. Wilkey?). Transpersonal caring moments occur when an actual caring occasion or authentic caring relationship exists between the nurse and the person. This can be a challenge! In the current healthcare environment, people are moved rapidly through the system. How can you find the time to develop authentic caring relationships? The first step is to make a commitment to be a caring nurse: to go to work with the thought, "Today I will be authentic with the people in my care." The word *authentic* simply means to be genuine or real. Or you might think, "I will focus on creating transpersonal caring moments instead of rushed and harried ones." Think back to Mr. Wilkey at the beginning of the chapter. Where did opportunities for transpersonal caring moments with him arise? As a student, you might think, "Today I will practice changing sterile dressings, starting intravenous solutions, or giving intramuscular injections." However, developing the ability to have transpersonal caring moments is just as important.

4. *Personal presence* is another phrase for being authentic and "in the moment." If the person in the bed is fearful, you should be fully present, recognize the fear, and support the person experiencing it. Your support may take the form of answering simple questions or providing more in-depth education. It may simply be staying with the person for 2 to 3 minutes while quietly listening and holding the person's hand. The concept denotes that you, the nurse, are emotionally and physically *with* the person for the time you are there. You are not thinking about a medication pass or medical orders you need to get. Developing the ability to provide presence is a process. As your psychomotor and nursing process skills become second

nature to you, you will find it easier to remain in the moment.

5. *Comfort.* Most nurses think of comfort as the relief of pain, but it is much more. In Kolcaba's (1994) theory, comfort occurs in four contexts: physical, psychospiritual, social, and environmental. For example, is the person comfortable with you as the caregiver? Some women, especially from Middle Eastern or Asian cultures, are uncomfortable with male nurses. Other questions to consider are whether the patient's modesty is being respected, whether there is too much or too little environmental stimuli, whether the room temperature is right, what cultural values must be respected, whether the patient needs more rest periods in order to heal, and whether the patient needs someone to spend a transpersonal caring moment with him so he can express fears and anxiety. This is the complex picture of comfort.

6. *Listening.* Listening requires you to quiet your mind and truly listen with your mind and heart. The caring theorists also talk about listening "from within yourself." Some call that type of listening *intuition.* Benner believes it is intuition that allows nurses to advance to expert level practice.

7. *Spiritual care* is a critical aspect of holistic nursing care (see Boxes 8–1 and 8–2). You need to know what an individual's spiritual needs are and make appropriate plans to meet them. If the person does not want to talk about or deal with her spirituality, you will listen and follow her instructions. However, generally the opposite is true. People who are ill often want to talk about their spiritual needs, but they may be uncomfortable doing so. Helping someone to meet spiritual needs may be as simple as offering to call a clergy member or praying with the person who is sick. Chapter 14 provides more information about spiritual care.

8. *Caring for the family.* All nurses who base their practice on caring theories recognize the importance of including the family of the person who is receiving care. Nontraditional family structure (e.g., a same-sex couple, a polygamist family) is not a reason to withdraw support. Sometimes in the rush of the day, this can be challenging. What about an older family member with dementia? This person deserves to know what is happening to his loved one even though he most likely will forget the information. If he does forget, patiently repeat what he needs to know. Following the principles of holistic nursing care, respect the need to include all of the family as part of your responsibility. You will find more information about family care in Chapter 12.

9. *Cultural competence.* This was discussed in the explanation of Leininger's cultural care theory. See the beginning of this section and Chapter 13.

Do you see the value of each of these nine abstract concepts? From them flow very real, concrete nursing actions that make a difference in the lives of patients. Theory is not just "pie in the sky." Understanding nursing theories and applying them throughout your career are essential to full-spectrum nursing care. To perform the essential clinical tasks of nursing within the framework of caring is the highest possible performance of the profession.

KnowledgeCheck 8–6

List and explain three ways to incorporate caring theory into your nursing care.

 Go to Chapter 8, **Knowledge Check Response Sheet and Answers,** on the Electronic Study Guide.

NURSING RESEARCH

You now have a good beginning (novice) background in nursing theory. Remember the puzzle pieces (Figure 8–2)? A nurse has an idea, does research to determine whether the idea is a valid one, and then develops a nursing theory. It is now time to study the research piece of the puzzle.

Theoretical Knowledge
knowing why

Many people, including some nurses, do not know that nurses do research. They see nurses as people who work in hospitals, wear scrubs, and hang stethoscopes around their necks. Were you aware of the work done in the field of caring prior to reading this chapter? Most novice nurses would not be. Remember the Framingham Study, which changed medical and nursing practice? Had you heard of that before? To be an effective professional nurse in the 21st century, you need to understand the basic principles of nursing research and their powerful impact on health care and the nursing profession. This section of the chapter is designed to show you what research is and how to incorporate it into your practice.

Although there are many definitions of nursing research, this chapter defines **nursing research** as the systematic, objective process of analyzing phenomena of importance to nursing (Nieswiadomy, 2002). By definition, then, nursing research encompasses all clinical practice arenas, nursing education, and nursing administration.

Nurse researchers currently are making important contributions to the evidence-based practice necessary for professional nursing. Consider this example: When you are in the clinical setting, you will notice that when a nurse discontinues an intravenous (IV) fluid infusion, she sometimes replaces it with a "lock" or "plug" to maintain a route for IV medications, even though the patient no longer needs the fluids. Not many years ago, she would periodically flush the plug with heparin to keep blood from clotting and blocking the IV catheter. But heparin is a drug, and it has side effects. Nurses and other professionals performed several studies to see whether saline (which has no side effects) would work just as well. Goode and others (1991) performed a **meta-analysis** of those studies, showing that saline was indeed just as effective; that is now the standard of care in most institutions.

Like theory, research affects you every day you are a nurse. Full-spectrum nurses participate in research by

- Identifying ideas that should be examined through the research process
- Assisting in, designing, and/or performing research
- Using research as a basis for their practice

What Is the History of Nursing Research?

The records Florence Nightingale kept while nursing soldiers in the Crimea were the beginning of formalized nursing research. As she developed schools of nursing throughout Britain and the United States, Nightingale urged her students to do clinical research. Yet because she had passed on to them the authoritarian tradition of her time, she found they were not prepared to perform it. Authority-based education does not promote intellectual inquiry or critical thinking, two characteristics essential for research. This is one reason why nursing research was slow to develop.

As baccalaureate, master's, and doctoral programs grew, so did the number and quality of research projects nurses performed. Nursing research is now supported by federal funds and private grants, and results are reported in a growing number of nursing (and other) research journals. Nurses present their research at national and international conferences and publish their results in national and international journals. The preparation of doctoral-level nurses with a strong background in research has enhanced the quality and diversity of nursing research.

How Are Priorities for Nursing Research Developed?

Nursing research provides evidence on which to base nursing care. Ideally, all nursing interventions should be validated through research to show their safety and effectiveness. Professional organizations, such as the American Nurses Association (ANA) and specialty organizations (e.g., the Oncology Nurses Association),

have established research priorities that will assist nursing to build a strong knowledge base in areas of importance to society. Brockopp and Tolsma (2003) state that nursing research will continue to be focused on clinical issues. The National Institute of Nursing Research (NINR), a federally funded agency that is a part of the National Institutes of Health (NIH), periodically identifies research themes and priorities for funding (NINR, 2003a). For more information about nursing research priorities,

 Go to Chapter 8, **Supplemental Materials: What Are the Priorities for Research in the 21st Century?,** on the Electronic Study Guide.

KnowledgeCheck 8–7
- Define nursing research.
- According to the text, why has nursing research been slow to develop?

 Go to Chapter 8, **Knowledge Check Response Sheet and Answers,** on the Electronic Study Guide.

What Educational Preparation Is Necessary to Do Nursing Research?

At each level of educational preparation, nurses function in different roles in the research process.

Associate degree and diploma nursing. At this educational level, there are three research roles you can fulfill. You can (1) be aware of the importance of research to evidence-based practice, (2) help identify problem areas in nursing, and (3) help collect data with a more experienced nurse researcher.

Baccalaureate degree in nursing. If you are a baccalaureate-prepared nurse, you should be able to (1) critique research for application to clinical practice, (2) identify nursing research problems and help implement research studies, and (3) apply research findings to establish sound, evidence-based clinical practice.

Master's degree in nursing. Nurses with graduate degrees should be able to (1) analyze problems so that appropriately designed research can be used to solve the problem, (2) through clinical expertise, apply research-based practice to nursing care situations, (3) provide support to ongoing research projects, and (4) conduct research for the purpose of assuring quality nursing care.

Doctoral degree in nursing or related field. Doctorally prepared nurses are specifically educated to be nurse researchers. Because of their background, they should be able to (1) conduct nursing research, (2) serve as leaders in applying research results to the clinical arena, and (3) develop ways

to monitor the quality of nursing care being administered by nurses (adapted from ANA, 1981). In addition, they should disseminate their research findings via publications and conferences.

Practical Knowledge
knowing how

No one expects you to have a sophisticated understanding of research at this point in your career. However, you do need some basic practical knowledge, including information about the scientific method, types of research design, the research process, how to find practice-related research articles, how to identify researchable problems, and how to critique research reports.

What Is the Scientific Method?

Recall that in Chapter 2 you learned the different kinds of nursing knowledge: theoretical, practical, personal, and ethical. There are also various ways to *gain* knowledge.

Trial and error plus common sense. Suppose a patient has been medicated but is still in pain. You might try repositioning him. If that doesn't help, you might try distraction or visualization techniques. And so on. If visualization provides some relief, you would probably try that technique first when a similar situation occurs with another patient.

Authority and tradition. This means to rely on an expert or to do "what has always been done." For the patient with unrelieved pain, this would mean that you might ask a more experienced nurse what to do. Or you could consult a procedure manual.

Intuition and inspiration. Intuition is a "feeling" about something—an inner sense. Nurses say, "I just had a feeling something was wrong with the patient, but I can't explain why." For the patient in pain, you might "have a feeling" that a complication was developing, that the pain was due to more than just ineffective pain medication. (However, as a novice, you should always check with a more experienced nurse before acting on your intuition.)

Logical reasoning. Using your knowledge and the facts available, you form conclusions (refer to "How Are Theories Developed?" on p. 143). For the patient in pain, you might think, "This man weighs 300 lb., but I gave him only the standard dose of medication. Probably he needs a higher dose."

TABLE 8-2 Characteristics of the Scientific Method

Begins with an identified problem or need to be studied.

Uses *theories,* models, and conceptual themes that have been empirically tested.

Uses systematic, orderly methods to acquire empirical evidence to test theories.

Uses methods of control for ruling out other variables that might affect the relationship between the variables they are studying.

Avoids explanations that cannot be empirically tested.

Prefers to generalize the findings (knowledge) so that it can be applied in cases other than those in the study.

Uses built-in mechanisms for self correction.

Source: Adapted from Wilson, H. S. (1993). *Introducing research in nursing* (2nd ed.). Redwood City, CA: Addison-Wesley Nursing.

Scientific method. Research is based on the scientific method (or scientific inquiry). **Scientific inquiry** is the process in which the researcher, through use of the senses, systematically collects observable, verifiable data to describe, explain, or predict events. The goals of scientific inquiry are to find solutions to problems and to develop explanations of the world (theories). The scientific method has two unique characteristics that the other ways of knowing do not:

1. *Objectivity,* or *self-correction.* This means that the researcher uses techniques to keep her personal beliefs, values, and attitudes separate from the research process.

2. *The use of empirical data.* Empirical data are gathered through observation rather than the researcher's subjective beliefs. It consists of information gathered through sight, hearing, taste, touch, or smell. The researcher attempts to verify the information gathered through a variety of methods so that the research conclusions are based in "reality" rather than on the researcher's beliefs or hunches (Wilson, 1993).

Table 8–2 summarizes the characteristics of the scientific method.

The scientific method makes use of a variety of procedures and study designs aimed to increase the chances that the data collected will be reliable, relevant, and unbiased. You should recognize the two major categories of research design: quantitative and qualitative. Each category has within it several specific types of research methodologies; however, for now you need to

understand only the basic differences (Table 8–3). For an expanded discussion,

Go to Chapter 8, **Supplemental Materials: Quantitative Research and Qualitative Research,** on the Electronic Study Guide.

Quantitative Research

The main purpose of **quantitative research** is to gather data from enough *subjects* (people being studied) to be able to generalize the results to a similar population. *Generalizing results* means that you say, "What I found to be so for this group of people will probably be the same for all people who are similar" (e.g., "My findings for *this* group of women over age 40 in the United States will probably be useful for *all* women over age 40 in the United States"). In quantitative research, researchers carefully control data collection and are careful to maintain the objectivity of the process. Quantitative data are reported as numbers. The Framingham Study is a classic example of a quantitative study—actually of several quantitative studies. To read more about this landmark research,

Go to **http://www.nhlbi.nih.gov/about/framingham/index.html**

Another classic example of quantitative nursing research is the Conduct and Utilization of Research in Nursing (CURN) project. Many of the protocols (procedures) developed from these studies are used today with some modification. The following are some CURN protocol examples:

Clean intermittent catheterization
Intravenous cannula change
Distress reduction through sensory preparation
Preventing decubitus ulcers

Qualitative Research

Qualitative research focuses on the lived experience of people. The purpose is not to generalize the data, but to share the experience of the person or persons in the study. There is no need for large numbers. A case study of one person can examine the lived experience, for example, of a 19-year-old single mother of triplets or a middle-aged woman with HIV. Qualitative research uses words, quotations from persons interviewed, observations, and other non-numeric sources of data. The Nun Study, a long-term, multidisciplinary project involving a convent of Catholic nuns in Minnesota, included some qualitative research (e.g., data obtained by interviews and reported in the nuns' own words, and samples of writing from the nuns' diaries, reports, and letters). For more information about the Nun Study,

Go to **http://www.nunstudy.org** and **http://www.centeredpendulum.org/Nun.htm**

TABLE 8-3 Comparison of Quantitative and Qualitative Research

	Quantitative Research	Qualitative Research
Data	Numerical data, e.g., questionnaires, number of incidents, or reactions to a medication	Non-numerical data; data may consist of words from interviews, observations, written documents, and even art or photos
Persons studied	Large numbers of *subjects* so it can be generalized to other similar populations	Small numbers of *participants;* is not designed to be generalized
Hypothesis	Has a hypothesis	No hypothesis, because it is the research of the "lived experience" of the person or persons being studied
Environment	Can be in a laboratory setting; needs to be a controlled environment	Is done in the "natural" setting, i.e., the person's home or work setting

KnowledgeCheck 8–8

- Define quantitative research. Name one study presented as an example in this chapter.
- Define qualitative research. Name one study presented as an example in this chapter.

 Go to Chapter 8, **Knowledge Check Response Sheet and Answers,** on the Electronic Study Guide.

What Are the Steps of the Research Process?

At the novice level, you will be using but not performing research. But in order to critique the research you read, you should have a general idea of the steps for conducting valid, reliable research. The research process is a problem-solving process, similar to but not the same as the nursing process. Different study designs require different steps, and you will find some variation in how different authors present the research process steps. However, in general, the steps include the following:

1. Identify and state the problem you wish to study (or question that you wish to answer).
2. Clarify the purpose of the study—the legitimate reason(s) for performing the research.
3. Review the related literature: Find out what is already known about the problem.
4. Develop a theoretical/conceptual framework. For example, if you wish to study diseases indigenous to Native Americans, you might use Leininger's cultural competence theory to guide your research.
5. Formulate the hypothesis or research question. The **hypothesis** is a statement of what the researcher expects the results of the study to be.

6. Define study variables/terms. **Variables** are those things that could "vary" (e.g., one group receives written teaching, the other group watches a video).
7. Select the population and sample. The **population** is the *group* (e.g., divorced fathers, rats, schools, persons who have had coronary bypass) being studied. The **sample** consists of the actual people (or other subjects) selected from the population from whom you will actually collect data.
8. Conduct a small pilot study and/or collect the data. **Pilot studies** help to weed out problems ahead of time so they do not occur in the actual study.
9. Analyze the data. Researchers usually use a computer program to analyze data.
10. Interpret the findings. This means to look at the research results and determine what they have to say about the problem or question you identify.
11. Communicate the findings (e.g., in professional journals and oral presentations).

KnowledgeCheck 8–9

- List at least four steps in the research process.
- What is the first step in the research process?
- What is the final step in the research process?

 Go to Chapter 8, **Knowledge Check Response Sheet and Answers,** on the Electronic Study Guide.

CriticalThinking 8–5

Take 10 minutes to sit quietly and think about nursing research. Do you have an idea or a problem you would like to see investigated with a research project? If nothing comes to mind quickly, then ponder for a few moments more. Complete the information on a sheet of paper. Take the time to do

your best thinking. Then share what you have written with your instructor and other students.

- Share your idea or problem. What would you like to have more information about in nursing? Explain why it is a problem or what brought about your idea.
- If you were the research assistant on a nursing research project on your topic, what one-sentence problem statement would you write regarding your research idea?
- What is the purpose of doing this research project? Why should it be done?

You may struggle with this assignment and wonder about its value to you, yet one of the most important things that nurses do is identify problems. Here is your chance to practice.

What Are the Rights of Research Participants?

Every nurse has a moral and legal responsibility to protect research participants* from being harmed during the research process. Although research is crucial to the development of the profession, it should never be held in higher regard than the rights of the individuals being studied.

The current ethical standards for research, from all disciplines, are a direct result of the atrocities committed in the name of research in the German prison camps during World War II. After the trials, for war crimes committed at that time, the Nuremberg Code (1947) was developed to protect research participants from unethical behavior. The Nuremberg Code prompted many other codes and standards for performing ethical research. The United States government, through the Department of Health and Human Services (DHHS), has a complex set of standards by which all persons conducting research must abide (Brockopp & Hastings-Tolsma, 2003).

Informed Consent

As a rule, **informed consent** must be obtained from every participant in a study. Consent is obtained by discussing what is expected of the participant, providing written information on the project to the participant, and obtaining the participant's written consent to be a subject. The following critical concepts are part of the informed consent.

- *Right to not be harmed.* The information given to the participant outlines the safety protocols of the study. If at any time preliminary data indicate potential harm to the participant, the study must be stopped immediately.

- *Right to full disclosure.* Participants have a right to answers to such questions as: What is the purpose of this research? What risks are there? Are there any benefits? Will I be paid? What happens if I get sick or feel worse? Who do I contact with questions and concerns?

- *Right to self-determination.* This refers to the right of a participant to say no. At any time in a study, the participant has the right to terminate her participation, for any reason. As the nurse, you are responsible to support a participant during the process of withdrawing from a study. Do not allow anyone to coerce the participant into remaining in the study.

- *Rights of privacy and confidentiality.* All research participants have the right to have their identity protected. Generally they are given a code number rather than being identified by name. Once the study is completed and the data are analyzed, the researcher has the responsibility for destroying the raw data (such as questionnaires, taped interviews).

Institutional Review Boards

The mechanism for overseeing the ethical standards established by the DHHS is the Institutional Review Board (IRB). Every hospital, university, and other healthcare facility where federal funds are involved has an IRB designed to protect the rights of research participants. It consists of healthcare professionals as well as people from the community who are willing to review and critique research proposals. The two main responsibilities of the IRB are to (1) protect the research participants from harm and (2) ensure that the research is of value.

How Can I Help Identify Clinical Nursing Problems?

Even as a novice nurse, you should be prepared to identify clinical problems for research. Identifying a clinical nursing problem comes from being alert and interested in what you are doing each day in your clinical setting. How do you think the tympanic thermometer came into being? Someone became frustrated with the discomfort patients experienced when temperatures were taken rectally. At the same time, there was a great deal of concern over the inaccuracy of axillary temperatures. Someone noticed the problem and wondered: "Is there a better way to do this?" Common sources of clinical problems are experience, social issues, theories, ideas from others, and the nursing literature (Polit & Beck, 2003).

Experience. As you go about your work, whether you are a novice or an expert, you will notice interventions that may not be working or that require a great deal of effort for the minimal good they do. You will wonder, "How could we do this better?" Or you may notice that for clients with a particular health

---

*Quantitative studies usually use the term *subjects*. Qualitative studies use the term *participants*.

problem, the outcomes are often not good. You will wonder, "How could we improve the care so that the patient's health improves?" Other questions might be, "Why do we do this thing this way? "What do I need to know in order to plan new interventions for patients with this health problem?" You will find plenty of problems if you are curious about why things are done as they are and about what might happen if changes were made. Problems might be related to staffing, equipment, nursing interventions, or coordination among health professionals.

Social issues. You may be concerned about broader social issues that affect or require nursing care, such as issues of gender equity, sexual harassment, and domestic violence. You may be concerned about patients who do not have access to health care or about the health problems of a particular group or subculture.

Theories. Recall that theories must be tested in order to be useful in nursing practice. You might want to suggest research to test a theory you are interested in. If the theory is accurate, what behaviors would you expect to find, or what evidence would you need to support the theory?

Ideas from others. Your instructor may suggest a research topic, or perhaps you might brainstorm with nurses or other students. Agencies and organizations that fund research often ask for research proposals on certain topics. Recall the ANA and NINR priorities on the Electronic Study Guide. Such a list of priorities could focus your attention on similar topics in your work.

Nursing literature. You may identify researchable problems by reading articles and research reports in nursing journals. This may occur as follows:

- An article may stimulate your imagination and interest in a topic.
- You may notice a discrepancy in what staff nurses are doing and what the literature recommends.
- You may notice inconsistencies in the findings of two different studies on the same topic.
- You may read a study on a topic of interest to you (e.g., a technique for measuring blood pressure) and wonder whether the results would be the same if the study had been done in a different setting (e.g., a clinic instead of a hospital) or with a different population (e.g., healthy instead of ill people).

Read widely in your field of interest. See Chapter 39 for information about nursing journal databases and literature searches. You will find the best research articles in refereed journals. **Refereed journals** are professional journals (not lay magazines, such as *Reader's Digest* or *Time*) in which a group of professionals with expertise in the topic reviews each article and then recommends that the article be published or not. The easiest way to identify a refereed journal is to see whether it has an extensive editorial board. The board will be listed in the front of the journal. Refereed journals meet a higher standard for publishing, which makes the information you read more credible (and therefore more useful to your work). Two examples of nursing research journals are *Advances in Nursing Science* and *Nursing Research.* Several others are listed on your Electronic Study Guide.

 Go to Chapter 8, **Supplemental Materials: Nursing Research Journals,** on the Electronic Study Guide.

How Do I Analyze the Research I Read?

You cannot expect to do a sophisticated critique of a research report at this stage of your education. However, you need to know enough to help you decide which articles are worthy of using in your practice. You will make that decision after you have examined the research to determine whether it is well done and meaningful to your work. You can do this by learning to read analytically. Wilson (1993, p. 25) says that **analytic reading** occurs when you "begin asking questions of what you are reading so that you can truly understand it." The questions are as follows:

1. *What is the book, journal, or article about as a whole?* That is, what is the theme of the article, and how is it developed?
2. *What is being said in detail, and how?* What are the author's main ideas, claims, and arguments?
3. *Is the book, journal, or article "true" in whole or part?* You must decide this for yourself. The strategies following in this section may help you to determine the truth of a research report.
4. *What of it?* Is it of any significance? Is there any way to use the information to improve patient care, education, or other areas of nursing?

Use your critical-thinking skills when you evaluate research presentations or publications. Not all research is good research. Some published studies contain serious flaws, and you need to be able to recognize them. An effective strategy for conducting a research critique is to read the entire article, using the four "analytic reading" questions above and making notes of questions you have. Then go back and evaluate the article section by section, using the following information (Wilson, 1993).

- *Researcher qualifications* are an easy place to start. Was the researcher qualified as an expert on the study topic? Try to determine whether the author's credentials and background "fit" with the topic.

- *The title* should be concise and clear. Key words in the title should provide clues to the research topic.

- *The abstract* is a brief (perhaps 500 words) summary of the study. It should be interesting and usually describes at least the purpose, methods, sample, and findings of the study.

- *The introduction* should catch your interest and set the stage for the rest of the report. The introduction may contain the *review of the literature, theoretical (conceptual) framework, assumptions, and limitations*. At this stage of your expertise, you should primarily check that these are present; however, some explanation follows.

- *Review of the literature* should be thorough and relevant. The references should logically pertain to the study topic and methods and consist primarily of research and theory articles. The references should support the researcher's variable definitions, methodology, and choices of data-collection tools; it should also present background work on the topic being studied.

- *Identify the study assumptions.* Assumptions are beliefs that you "take for granted" as true but that have not been proven. For example, you assume that when people are in bed, they sleep; and you assume that study participants answer truthfully to the researcher's questions. Assumptions should be clearly stated to avoid confusion regarding the study.

- *Limitations of the study.* Every study has limitations or weaknesses. Look for the author to admit the things that could not be controlled. For example, a study may test a population of people that would not generalize to other populations, (e.g., testing only Caucasian students instead of testing a variety of students who represent the ethnic diversity of the university).

- *The purpose* should be stated clearly. It should give the reasons for doing the study. Ask these three questions to help you judge it: Will the study (1) solve a problem relevant to nursing, (2) present facts that are useful to nursing, or (3) contribute to nursing knowledge?

- *The problem statement* should be presented early in the report, and it should be "researchable"; that is, it (1) is stated as a question, (2) involves the relationship between two or more variables, and (3) can be answered by collecting empirical data.

- *Definition of terms* is essential in a formal research report. However, it often is not included in a published article because of the lack of space.

- *The research design* indicates the plan for collecting data. As a novice, you probably cannot judge the adequacy of the design, but you should be sure that the researcher names and describes it and discusses its strengths and weakness. The researcher should include an explanation of what was done to enhance the validity and reliability of the study. To oversimplify,

validity means that the study actually measures the concept it claims to measure. **Reliability** refers to the accuracy, consistency, and precision of a measure; that is, if someone else repeated the study using the same design, would they obtain similar results? For example, if you weighed the same item on a scale each day and obtained the same *weight* each time, you could say that the scale is reliable. But a scale would not give you a valid measure of *body fat*.

- *Setting, population, and sample.* The researcher should identify the type of setting where the data was collected, describe the population and sample, and state the criteria that were used for choosing study participants. This section may also contain information about how informed consent was obtained.

- *Data-collection methods* answer the basic questions of what, how, who, where, and when. Data-collection instruments are the "tools" used to gather the data (e.g., questionnaires or a laboratory instrument). The researcher should provide evidence (pilot tests, literature) that the tools used were reliable and valid.

- *Data analysis.* A quantitative report would include statistical analyses of the data. A qualitative report would include quotes from the participants. The analyses of both types of data are very specific and beyond the scope of this textbook.

- *Discussion of findings and conclusion* are the sections of a research report that you may find most interesting. They are the "So what was learned?" sections. All findings should be presented in an objective manner, and compared with information found in the literature. The easiest errors for you to recognize with your present knowledge level are that the researcher:

1. Generalizes beyond the data or the sample. For example, the sample may have been young adult women in a clinic setting, but the researcher might have suggested that the same intervention be used for all women in the clinic, regardless of age.

2. Does not mention any limitations that might have influenced the results.

3. Does not present findings in a clear, logical manner (i.e., you have trouble figuring out what the findings actually are).

- *Implications and recommendations* are the final pieces of the research critique. The implications are the "shoulds" of the research. In essence, the researcher says, "Now we know this fact; therefore, nurses should . . ." For example, the research "should" be replicated with another population, or the instrument "should" be revised and retested, or that nurses "should" use the study intervention in their practice.

When you read a research article, examine it for each of the preceding items. Although you have limited knowledge and experience, every time you review

an article thoroughly, you will learn more about the research process. As you learn, you will be better able to determine the quality of research you will accept as a basis for changing your nursing practice.

How Do I Find Research Articles Related to My Practice?

If you are convinced that reading research articles is important, you are probably thinking, "How do I find research articles?" Obviously you need to go to a library or online and search an index for appropriate references. The best index for you, as a novice nurse, is the Cumulative Index to Nursing and Allied Health Literature (CINAHL). This is a comprehensive index that includes more than 1200 nursing and allied health journals. Generally, whatever you are looking for in clinical nursing will be available in CINAHL. For more information about indexes, see Chapter 39.

In the library you will find the printed version of CINAHL in a set of large red books in the reference section. Most university libraries have access to CINAHL and other indexes online. If you are an online user, it will be worth your time to get the information from the library about conducting online searches.

Once you have access to CINAHL in either format, you then select words that relate to your topic (e.g., dementia or nursing ethics). The index will list journal articles related to the key words. Sometimes, you will get a large number of articles (more than 1000) that carry that word. When that happens, you need to ask the librarian for assistance in narrowing your search. It is beyond the scope of this chapter to provide sophisticated instructions for literature searches.

It also is easy to search in a specific journal for articles. The title of a journal provides clues to the content. The critical care journals will have, obviously, articles on critical care information. Oncology, orthopedics, and other specialty journals carry information specific to their own specialty. Looking for such journals is another way to do a casual search for articles of interest.

How can you tell whether the article you retrieve is a research article? You identify a research article by looking for the steps in the research process described earlier in this chapter. Does the article have a problem statement and a purpose? Is there a section on the sample and site of the research? And so on.

If your focus is clinical practice, you should not overlook specialty journals, such as *Geriatric Nursing* or the *Journal of Gerontological Nursing,* if you really want information on, say, older adults with dementia. They

are not research journals, but they generally have one or two research articles in each issue. Most specialty organizations have a journal you can access. If you do not have a specialty interest, review the *American Journal of Nursing* or *RN* for articles of general interest. Again, remember that it is up to you to identify whether the article is research or another form of information sharing.

KnowledgeCheck 8–10

Where do you go to use CINAHL?

 Go to Chapter 8, **Knowledge Check Response Sheet and Answers,** on the Electronic Study Guide.

What Is Research Utilization?

Research is more than just an exercise that nurses engage in to earn master's and doctoral degrees. The ultimate reason for conducting research is to establish an evidence-based practice or to gain greater understanding of a phenomenon. This means that nurses in practice have a responsibility for finding and using the research that others do. Remember the discussion of authority-based practice during Florence Nightingale's era? Even in the 21st century, much nursing practice is still based on authority and tradition. That is not acceptable for full-spectrum professional nurses. You must have reasons for what you do. That is the purpose of research.

According to Nieswiadomy (2002), there are five reasons why nurses *do not* use research as the basis for their practice: (1) lack of knowledge of nursing research, (2) negative attitudes toward research, (3) inadequate forums for disseminating research, (4) lack of support from the employing institution, and (5) study findings that are not ready for the clinical environment.

You can utilize nursing research to enhance your practice by acting on the information in this chapter. Learn the content, and read and talk about research with your colleagues and instructors. Once you have a research-based idea clear in your mind, try it out in your clinical setting (with approval from the nurse manager or instructor). Then discuss it with others. You can learn to effectively use research, and then you can motivate others to do the same.

 Go to Chapter 8, **Resources for Caregivers and Health Professionals,** on the Electronic Study Guide.

 Suggested Readings: Go to Chapter 8, **Reading More About Nursing Theory and Research,** on the Electronic Study Guide.

 VOL 2 **Bibliography:** Go to Volume 2, Bibliography.

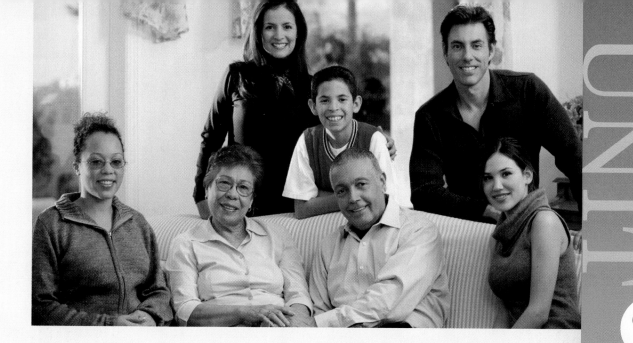

Factors Affecting
Health

9

Growth

& Development Through the Life Span

Learning Outcomes

After completing this chapter, you should be able to:

* Discuss the principles of growth and development.

* Compare and contrast developmental task theory, psychoanalytic theory, cognitive theory, and the psychosocial theory of growth and development.

* Outline the major principles involved in moral and spiritual development.

* Identify conditions that influence the growth and development of all ages.

* Discuss the cognitive and psychosocial challenges of each age group.

* Identify common health problems that occur in each stage of development.

* Describe special assessments unique to each age group.

* Discuss age-appropriate interventions for each age group.

* Incorporate growth and development principles into nursing care.

Go to **Chapter 9** on the Electronic Study Guide for the expanded chapter. This volume provides a brief introduction to growth and development.

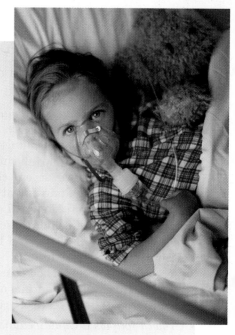

MEET Your Patients

Your roommate is currently in her pediatric rotation. At the end of her first clinical day, she tells you about the patients for whom she provided care. She was assigned to three children who were diagnosed with pneumonia:

- Tamika, a 3-year-old, lives with her grandparents. Her grandmother is present only during afternoon visiting hours because she must care for her husband, who suffers from numerous health problems.
- Miguel, a 2-month-old, lives with his mother. Since his admission yesterday, Miguel's mother has stayed at his bedside and provided most of her son's care.
- Carrie, a 13-year-old, lives with her parents. Both parents are able to visit only during evening visiting hours, when they leave work.

On your first clinical day, you were assigned to care for a patient with pneumonia, Ethel Higgenbotham, an 80-year-old woman who lives alone.

Each of these patients is unique. Although they share the same medical diagnosis, their needs and your nursing care will differ dramatically. These differences stem from a variety of factors, one of the most significant of which is each patient's stage of growth and development.

Theoretical Knowledge
knowing why

The Greek Philosopher Heraclitus said, "Nothing is permanent but change." We readily see this truth in the dramatic physical, cognitive, and emotional growth that children undergo from one month to another, but it is true also for adults. Throughout the life span, human beings are in a constant process of change, not always visible to the eye.

It is essential to consider a client's stage of growth and development when you plan and provide care. In this chapter, we present a very brief overview of some principles and theories of growth and development. For a thorough discussion of normal growth and development across the life span, including common health concerns, nursing assessments, and health promotion interventions,

 Go to **Chapter 9** on the Electronic Study Guide.

WHAT ARE GROWTH AND DEVELOPMENT?

Growth refers to physical changes that occur over time, such as changes in height, sexual development, or fluctuations in weight and muscle tone. **Development** refers to the process of adapting to one's environment over time. For example, a child comes to recognize right from wrong, an adolescent decides on a vocation, or an older adult recognizes the nearness of death.

What has been the most important force in your becoming the person you are now: characteristics that you inherited from your parents, or the environment in which you were raised?

For centuries, scientists have debated the effect of nature versus nurture on growth and development. **Nature** refers to genetic endowment, whereas **nurture** is the influence of the environment on the individual. The birth of a child can be compared to the planting of a tulip. The bulb has all the required factors to produce a beautiful plant, but whether it reaches its full potential is highly dependent on the environment. Is the soil rich in nutrients? Is the amount of sunshine adequate? Is there sufficient water? The bulb can grow into a beautiful flower only if it has these necessary ingredients supplied by the environment. A child is similar. The joining of ovum and sperm forms chromosomes that determine appearance, characteristics, and much about how the child will grow and develop. However, environmental factors, such as access to food, human contact, and education, also affect how the child will develop throughout the life span.

Principles of Growth and Development

Important principles of growth and development include the following:

- *Growth and development usually follow an orderly, predictable pattern. However, the timing, rate of change, and response to change are unique for each individual.* For example, all children learn to sit before they walk. However, one child may learn to sit at 6 months of age and walk at 10 months, whereas another child may first sit at 7 months and not walk until 13 months. Each of these children is developing in the same pattern, and both are progressing within a normal time frame. Similarly, menarche in girls follows a series of body changes associated with puberty. However, the normal onset of menstruation ranges from 9 to 15 years of age.

- *Growth follows a cephalocaudal pattern: beginning at the head and progressing down to the chest, trunk, and lower extremities.* When an infant is born, the head is the largest portion of the body. In the first year, the head, chest, and trunk gain in size, yet the legs remain short. Growth of the legs is readily apparent in the second year.

- *Development proceeds in a proximodistal pattern: beginning at the center of the body and moving outward.* For example, infants learn how to hold up their head before they develop the fine motor functions of the fingers and toes.

- *Simple skills develop separately and independently. Later they are integrated into more complex skills.* Many complex skills that we take for granted as adults actually represent a compilation of simple skills. Your ability to feed yourself is an example. This act requires the ability to find your mouth, swallow solid food, grasp an object, control movement of that object, and coordinate movement of the hand from the plate to the mouth. If you have ever tried to learn to play a musical instrument, you are familiar with this principle. You must master simple steps before you are able to play a tune.

- *Each body system grows at its own rate.* This principle is readily apparent in fetal development; however, it applies throughout life. Perhaps the most noticeable example is the onset of puberty. In the years leading up to puberty, the cardiovascular, respiratory, and nervous systems grow and develop dramatically, yet the reproductive system changes very little. Puberty is a constellation of changes that leads to full development of the reproductive system. The hormone changes that occur with puberty also trigger growth in the musculoskeletal system.

- *Body system functions become increasingly differentiated over time.* Have you ever seen a newborn respond to a loud noise? The newborn's startle response involves the whole body. With maturity, the response may be limited to covering the ears. An adult is often able to state the location of the sound and distinguish the origin of the sound.

Theories of Growth and Development

Theories of development across the life span attempt to explain and describe patterns of growth and development common to all people. These theories provide an organizing framework to help you understand and plan for the needs of the patients you will encounter, and they provide a basis for nursing interventions and clinical decision making. The needs of a 6-year-old differ greatly from those of a 25-year-old or a 65-year-old, even though they may have the same medical diagnosis or even the same nursing diagnosis.

Robert Havighurst, Sigmund Freud, Jean Piaget, Erik Erikson, and others have postulated theories to explain life span development. Each theorist has focused on a domain of human nature to examine how humans develop and has divided the life span into stages. Each stage represents a period of time that shares common characteristics. Most theorists have also identified tasks that are usually accomplished in each stage. As with the caring theories discussed in Chapter 8, an understanding of these key developmental theories is essential to full-spectrum nursing practice.

Developmental Task Theory

Robert Havighurst was an educator who theorized that learning was a lifelong process. He believed that a person moves through six life stages, each associated with a number of tasks that must be learned. Havighurst characterizes **developmental task** as follows: "A developmental task is midway between an individual need and societal demand. It assumes an active learner interacting with an active social environment" (1971, p. vi). Failure to master a task leads to unhappiness of the individual, difficulty mastering future tasks, and difficulty interacting with others.

Psychoanalytic Theory

Sigmund Freud was a pioneer in the science of human development. His psychoanalytic theory, which focuses on instincts that drive or motivate human behavior and personality development, became the dominant theoretical foundation of early 20th century psychotherapy. However, Freud developed his theory in the Victorian era, when societal norms were very strict. Sexual repression and male dominance over female behavior were the cultural standard. The relevance of many aspects of his theory to life in the 21st century has therefore been questioned by today's social scientists.

Freud identified several forces that influence the development of our personality. Each has a unique function.

- The **id** represents instinctual urges, pleasure, and gratification, such as hunger, procreation, pleasure, and aggression. It is dominant in infants and young children.
- The **ego** begins to develop around 4 to 6 months of age. It strives to balance what is wanted (id) and what is possible to obtain or achieve.
- The **superego** is sometimes referred to as our conscience. This force develops in early childhood (age 5 to 6).
- The **unconscious mind** is composed of thoughts and memories that are not readily recalled but unconsciously influence behavior.

In 1953, Freud's daughter, the psychologist Anna Freud, identified a number of **defense mechanisms,** which she described as thought patterns or behaviors that the ego employs in the face of threat to biological or psychological integrity (Townsend, 2003). In other words, defense mechanisms protect us from excess anxiety. See Chapter 25.

Freud believed that human development is perpetuated by instinctual drives, such as libido (sexual instinct), aggression, and survival (Sadock & Sadock, 2003). These drives have varying emphases, depending on the age of the individual.

Cognitive Development Theory

Jean Piaget studied his own children to understand how human beings develop cognitive abilities. According to Piaget, cognitive development requires three core competencies: adaptation, assimilation, and accommodation. **Adaptation** is the ability to adjust to and interact with one's environment. To be able to adapt, one must assimilate and accommodate. **Assimilation** is the integration of new experiences with one's own system of knowledge. **Accommodation** is the change in one's system of knowledge that results from processing new information. For example, an infant is born with an innate ability to suck. Presented with the mother's nipple, the infant is able to assimilate the nipple to the behavior of sucking. If given a bottle, the infant can learn to accommodate the artificial nipple. However, the baby may adapt by accepting the artificial nipple only from the father, crying and fussing if the mother offers a bottle instead of her breast.

According to Piaget, cognitive development occurs from birth through adolescence in a sequence of four stages: sensorimotor, preoperational thought, concrete operations, and formal operations. A child must complete each stage before moving to the next. The speed at which a child moves through the four stages is determined by inherited intellect and the influence of the environment. Piaget does not address cognitive development after adolescence.

Psychosocial Development Theory

In the 1950s Erik Erikson introduced his theory of psychosocial development. Erikson was strongly influenced by Freud but believed that personality continues to evolve throughout the life span as the individual interacts with the social world. He hypothesized that individuals must negotiate eight stages as they progress through the life span. Most individuals successfully move from stage to stage; however, a person can regress during times of stress to earlier stages or be forced to face tasks of later stages because of unforeseen life events, such as terminal illness. Failure to successfully negotiate a stage leads to maladjustment. Erikson's theory is widely used in nursing and health care. Below are Erikson's eight stages.

Stage 1: Trust versus mistrust (birth to about 18 months)
Stage 2: Autonomy versus shame and doubt (about 18 months to 3 years)
Stage 3: Initiative versus guilt (3 to 5 years)
Stage 4: Industry versus inferiority (6 to 11 years)
Stage 5: Identity versus role confusion (11 to 21 years)
Stage 6: Intimacy versus isolation (21 to 40 years)
Stage 7: Generativity versus stagnation (40 to 65 years)
Stage 8: Ego integrity versus despair (over 65 years)

Moral Development Theories

Lawrence Kohlberg developed his theory of moral development by studying the responses to moral dilemmas of 84 boys whose development he followed for a period of 20 years. In this theory, moral reasoning appears to be somewhat age related, with the most primitive reasoning based on a desire to avoid punishment. According to Kohlberg, moral development is based on one's ability to think at progressively higher levels. Increased maturity does provide some degree of higher-level thinking but does not guarantee the ability to function at the highest level. Kohlberg believed that not all people are able to achieve those levels.

As just noted, Kohlberg's research subjects were exclusively male. The validity of his theory for women has been sharply criticized, most prominently by Carol Gilligan (1982). To address the moral development of women, Gilligan proposed an alternative theory that incorporates the concepts of caring, interpersonal relationships, and responsibility. Gilligan describes a three-stage approach to moral development.

Stage 1: Caring for oneself
Stage 2: Caring for others
Stage 3: Caring for oneself and others

See Chapter 44 for a fuller discussion of moral development.

Spiritual Development Theory

James Fowler, a minister, defined faith as a universal human concern and as a process of growing in trust. He noticed that his congregants had very different approaches to faith and that the differences depended on their age. Basing his studies on the work of Piaget, Erikson, and Kohlberg, he developed a theory of faith development, which includes a pre-stage (Stage 0) and 6 stages of faith (Fowler, 1981).

APPLYING CONCEPTS OF GROWTH AND DEVELOPMENT

Recall the case of 3-year-old Tamika, who is being raised by her grandmother and has been hospitalized with pneumonia ("Meet Your Patient" scenario). Imagine that Tamika has been abandoned by her mother, who is addicted to heroin. If you observe that Tamika is small for her size and has not met developmental milestones appropriate for a 3-year-old, you could write the following *diagnostic statement:*

> Delayed Growth and Development r/t abandonment by mother and recent change in living status as evidenced by underweight status, short stature, limited verbal skills, and onset of walking at 36 months of age

To address Tamika's diagnosis you might use the following *outcomes:*

NOC outcome: Child Development: 3 Years
Individualized goal: Tamika will achieve growth between the 35th and 65th percentiles for her age group and be able to walk up steps, verbalize with two- to three-word sentences, and eat a variety of foods within 6 months.

Tamika will need care that helps her catch up developmentally and allows her to establish a strong relationship with her grandmother. Because the grandmother is also caring for an ailing spouse, you may need to refer this family to community support services for ongoing help. *NIC interventions* appropriate for Tamika are as follows:

Developmental Care
Teaching: Toddler Nutrition
Teaching: Toddler Safety

Specific interventions for Tamika might include therapeutic play with age-appropriate toys, reading stories, and engaging in conversation, as well as teaching the grandmother about these activities. This family may need counseling to assist with this transition.

Ethel Higgenbotham, the 80-year-old-woman introduced in the "Meet Your Patient" scenario, has also entered the hospital with pneumonia. Her son tells you that she began to lose weight rapidly, complains of no appetite, and became withdrawn after the death of her husband. At a recent visit he found his mother confused, with a productive cough, and with small open areas on her lower legs. These problems led to her hospitalization. You observe that she is very thin and frail and refuses to eat. "I just want to die," she tells you. An appropriate *nursing diagnosis* for Ms Higgenbotham might be Adult Failure to Thrive.

An appropriate *NOC outcome* would be Will to Live. You might develop the following *individualized goal:*

> Ms Higgenbotham will gain 1 pound and participate in at least one daily group activity by the first of next month.

Interventions depend on the diagnosis and its etiology. Ms Higgenbotham will need care that helps her adjust to widowhood, provides adequate nutrition, and offers activities that provide interaction with others. *NIC interventions* appropriate for Ms Higgenbotham are as follows:

Coping Enhancement
Hope Instillation
Self-Care Assistance
Spiritual Support

Individualized Interventions for Ms Higgenbotham include grief counseling, nutritional support, and working with her and her family to determine whether it is appropriate for her to continue to live independently.

SUMMARY

The examples of Tamika and Ms Higgenbotham illustrate the importance of theoretical knowledge of growth and development to your nursing care. We have provided a brief review of principles and theories of growth and development. To review information for specific age groups and for suggestions on how to adapt nursing care for various age groups, see Procedure 9–1, Assessing for Abuse, in Volume 2, and

 Go to **Chapter 9** on the Electronic Study Guide.

 Suggested Readings: Go to Chapter 9, **Reading More About Growth and Development Through the Life Span,** on the Electronic Study Guide.

 Bibliography: Go to Volume 2, Bibliography.

CHAPTER 10

Experiencing
Health & Illness

Learning Outcomes

After completing this chapter, you should be able to:

* Explore the concepts of health and illness from a holistic perspective.

* Compare and contrast three models of health and illness.

* Describe the various ways that people experience health and illness.

* Identify factors that disrupt health.

* Describe the five stages of illness behavior.

* Differentiate between acute and chronic illness.

* Identify factors that influence individuals' responses to illness.

* Apply the concepts presented in this chapter to a variety of patient care situations.

* Explain what the concepts in this chapter mean to you as you work toward becoming a full-spectrum nurse.

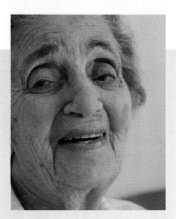

MEET Your Patient

Evelyn is 87 years old and has lived in a nursing home for the last 5 years. She suffers from congestive heart failure, hypertension, diabetes, macular degeneration resulting in near blindness, a severe hearing deficit, urinary incontinence, and immobility resulting from a hip fracture.

Evelyn was married nearly 60 years to Lloyd, who died 6 years ago. They had 5 children, 17 grandchildren, and 14 great-grandchildren. Evelyn never worked outside the home. In these last few years, she has experienced the loss of her husband, home, vision, hearing, mobility, and bladder control. Despite these limitations, she keeps current in the lives of all of her children, grandchildren, great-grandchildren, brothers and sisters and their families, and friends. She is very involved in the lives of the staff of the nursing home. She is their confidante

and knows about their children, their romances, and the gossip around the nursing home. She is an avid Minnesota Twins fan and also keeps track of the televised high school basketball tournaments. Whenever there is an election, she makes sure that she gets to vote. She "reads" every talking book she can get her hands on. Recently Evelyn was admitted to the hospital in severe congestive heart failure. She told her pastor, "I don't want to die yet. I'm having too much fun!"

Evelyn's situation is a far cry from what most people would picture as "good health." However, as you consider the ideas of health presented in this chapter, you might conclude that she is a reasonably healthy person from many standpoints.

Theoretical Knowledge
knowing why

Every day there is something in the news about health or illness. Politicians talk about their desire to improve their constituents' health and reorganize health care. Public schools want students to eat right, exercise, and receive regular immunizations. In an attempt to reduce health insurance claims, employers open on-site fitness centers and employ nurses and counselors. Everyone says they want to be healthy. As a nursing student, you have probably already cared for clients in various stages of health and illness. But have you ever considered what those terms mean?

Our understanding of health and illness is influenced by our family, culture, health history, and a host of other factors. As you evolve as a nurse, you'll find that your understanding of these concepts evolves, too. Here we examine some ways that you and your clients might define health and illness and some ways that full-spectrum nurses have come to understand these terms.

HOW DO WE UNDERSTAND HEALTH AND ILLNESS?

What is your image of **health**? Is it the "body beautiful"—an athlete's build, glistening hair, straight white teeth, and a glowing complexion? One drawback of this *perfect body view of health* is that being a "picture of health" depends on whether you were born in the right era—or in the right country, for that matter. Styles of beautiful bodies come and go. For instance, much Indian, African, Greek, and European art portrays ideal women as well-rounded creatures. The perfect body view of health also denies the possibility of health to people who use wheelchairs, prosthetics, or even eyeglasses and hearing aids. Yet many full-spectrum nurses working with disabled clients would indeed describe their clients as healthy.

In describing healthy people, would you disqualify someone with a cold, dandruff, or athlete's foot? What about diabetes, heart disease, or cancer? Doing so would reflect another view of health: that is *not having illness*. There is unfairness in this view, too, because it restricts health only to those who do not have some kind of physical impairment.

Another popular concept is that health is *something you can buy:* a weight-loss system, a treadmill, an exercise bike, membership in a health club, medicine, tummy tucks, coronary bypasses, and so on. In this view, health does not come from within. It's something "out there" that is available if you have enough money or insurance.

Health can also be described as *an ideal state of physical and mental well-being:* something to strive for, but never to attain. Good health is always around the corner but never actually reached, because there is always something more to be achieved. In this view, health is the goal itself, the end instead of one of the means to fulfilling life's purposes.

Theologian Jurgen Moltmann (1983) described health in a different way. He stated that "true health is the strength to live, the strength to suffer, and the strength to die. Health is not a condition of my body; it is *the power of my soul to cope with the varying condition of that body*" (p. 142). Similarly, novelist Robert Louis Stevenson wrote of health, "It is not a matter of holding good cards; *it's playing a poor hand well.*" For more traditional definitions of health, refer to Box 10–1.

Now that we've explored some definitions of health, let's consider a definition of illness. When you think of that term, what comes to mind? If you answered with a list of disorders such as heart disease, diabetes, or schizophrenia, you're not alone. Most people have a medical view of **illness** as disease, which is a pathology affecting an organ or body system. Traditional definitions would encompass traumatic injury and psychiatric disorders as well. But is illness merely the sum of these terms?

Nurses Understand Health and Illness as Individual Experiences

If you were the nurse caring for Evelyn in the "Meet Your Patient" scenario, would you understand health as a perfect body or the absence of disease? Probably not. Nurses understand health and illness as individual experiences, emerging from each patient's unique responses. The person with an illness rarely perceives the experience as a medical diagnosis. Instead, people typically describe their illness in terms of how it makes them *feel.* Think back to the last time you were ill. How did you feel? Did you feel pain, sadness, fatigue, loss? Did you feel overwhelmed? These responses are disruptions to health and, as such, constitute the lived experience of illness. This lived experience is *unique to each patient:* Just as Evelyn might describe herself as "raring to go," another patient who is 10 years younger and on half as many medications may describe herself as "exhausted all the time" and "just waiting to die." In short, nurses honor the client's understanding of his or her state of being.

BOX 10-1 What Do the Experts Say About Health?

- *The World Health Organization (WHO)* defines health as "a state of complete physical, mental and social well-being and not merely the absence of disease or infirmity" (WHO, 1948).

- *Traditional Chinese medicine* considers health to be a balance between yin and yang.

- *Ayurveda,* an ancient Indian medical system, describes health as the trinity of body, mind, and spiritual awareness (Gorin & Arnold, 1998).

- *Florence Nightingale* believed that health was prevention of disease through the use of fresh air, pure water, efficient drainage, cleanliness, and light (1859).

- *Nursing theorist Jean Watson (1979)* believes that health implies at least three elements: (1) a high level of overall physical, mental, and social functioning; (2) a general adaptive-maintenance level of daily functioning; and (3) the absence of illness (or the presence of efforts that lead to its absence). To Watson, health is a matter of perception. Even an individual with a terminal illness may be considered healthy if he has a high level of functioning, is coping with the diagnosis, and is actively making efforts to improve his status.

For many years, nurses have recognized that, like Evelyn, some clients strive to maintain a state of optimal health even when coping with chronic and even terminal disease. Many experience this state as **wellness:** "a way of life oriented toward optimal health and well-being in which body, mind, and spirit are integrated by the individual to live more fully within the human and natural community" (Myers, Sweeney, & Witmer, 2000, p. 252). This perspective acknowledges the influence of attitude and lifestyle choices on the client's state of being. It also implies that nursing interventions in support of wellness are important for healthy clients, those who are experiencing disease, and even those facing death.

 CriticalThinking 10–1

What qualities are essential to your own personal definition of health? How do you define illness?

KnowledgeCheck 10–1

- Provide at least two popular definitions of health.
- Explain how full-spectrum nurses define health and illness.
- Define wellness in your own words.

 Go to Chapter 10, **Knowledge Check Response Sheet and Answers,** on the Electronic Study Guide.

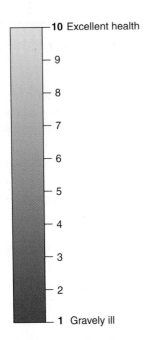

FIGURE 10–1 The health-illness continuum.

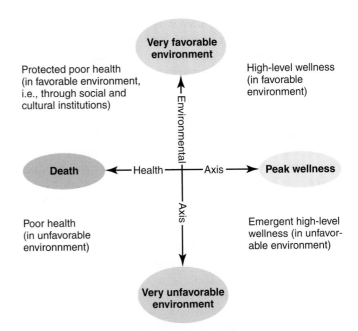

FIGURE 10–2   Dunn's health grid: Health is affected by an individual's status on the health-illness continuum as well as environmental conditions. *Source:* Dunn, H. L. (1959). High level wellness for man and society. *American Journal of Public Health, 49*(6), 786–788.

Nurses Use Conceptual Models to Understand Health and Illness

You can use a variety of models to understand health and illness. Each emphasizes somewhat different aspects of these complex experiences. Nurses have found the following models particularly useful.

The Health-Illness Continuum

Most of us recognize that our health status changes frequently. For example, although today I feel pretty good and yesterday I was exhausted, I believe I was healthy on both of those days. I know that my exhaustion was related to staying up late enjoying the company of good friends. My medical chart states that I have diabetes and hypertension, but I am well controlled with both diseases. I take multiple medications, read food labels, exercise aerobically 5 days a week, and lift weights 3 days a week. On the one hand, my mother used to tell me, "You do too much. Relax, take the medicines, and eat treats once in a while. You'll be happier." On the other hand, my father always said, "The more you take care of yourself, the less you rely on medicines, and the better off you are." Am I healthy, ill, or a health nut?

The above example illustrates the complex and dynamic nature of human health. In attempting to describe this complex state, many theorists speak of a *health-illness continuum;* that is, they see health and illness as a graduated spectrum that cannot be divided—except arbitrarily—into parts. For any individual person, the spectrum is constantly changing according to physiological changes, lifestyle choices, and the results of various therapies. As shown in Figure 10–1, the number 1 represents a state of being gravely ill, and

10 represents excellent health, a person in peak form. Notice, however, that a client like Evelyn in the "Meet Your Patient" scenario may view herself at various points on this continuum according to how she feels on any particular day. In other words, the continuum is personal and dynamic: Over the course of time, a client's health will move up and down along this gradient.

Dunn's Health Grid

Dunn (1959) created a health grid that plots a person's status on the health-illness continuum against environmental conditions (Figure 10–2). Many nurses use this grid to help them predict the likelihood that a client will experience a change in health status. For example, Evelyn ("Meet Your Patient") has several problems that are causing a decline in her health status. On a scale of 1 to 10, an independent observer might rate her health as a 3. However, Evelyn has a positive outlook and tells her pastor, "I don't want to die yet. I'm having too much fun!" She also has excellent support from her friends, family, and the nursing home staff. Clearly, Evelyn is in a favorable environment. This positive setting protects her from harm and provides a good quality of life. On Dunn's grid, Evelyn would probably fall in the area of "protected poor health."

Neuman's Continuum

Nursing theorist Betty Neuman (1995) views health as an expression of living energy available to an individual. The energy is displayed as a continuum

with high energy (wellness) at one end and low energy (illness) at the opposite end (Figure 10–3). The person is said to have varying levels of energy at various stages of life. When more energy is generated than expended, there is wellness. When more energy is expended than is generated, there is illness—possibly death. Although Evelyn ("Meet Your Patient") has several clearly identified health problems, she is engaged in life and active with her family, friends, and nursing home staff. We might not all agree on where to place her on Neuman's continuum, but certainly her activity and energy counterbalance her physical frailty.

HOW DO PEOPLE EXPERIENCE HEALTH AND ILLNESS?

In envisioning health and illness as a continuum, full-spectrum nurses promote wellness regardless of the circumstances that clients face now or in the future. This approach requires the holistic understanding that health is multidimensional. The following are some of the many dimensions of health that we experience along the health-illness continuum.

Biological Factors

Although biological factors are not entirely within our control, most people consider them when they describe themselves as "well" or "ill." A healthy genetic makeup and freedom from debilitating age-related changes are certainly desired states, and they tip the scale toward the wellness end of the health-illness continuum.

- *Genetic makeup.* For example, the risk of breast cancer increases dramatically in women who have a family history of a mother, sister, or daughter with breast cancer. Recently, a genetic marker for this type of breast cancer has been discovered. Some women with these genetic markers choose to have prophylactic mastectomies to decrease their risk.

- *Gender.* Many diseases occur more commonly in one gender than another. For example, rheumatoid arthritis, osteoporosis, and breast cancer are more common in women, whereas ulcers, color blindness, and bladder cancer are more common in men.

- *Age and developmental stage.* Age and developmental stage influence the likelihood of becoming ill. Certain health problems can be correlated to developmental stage. For example, over 75% of new breast cancer cases are diagnosed in women over age 50. As another example, adolescent boys have much higher rates of head injury and spinal cord injury than the general public because of their tendency toward risk-taking behaviors, which peaks during this stage. For further discussion of growth and development, see Chapter 9 in this book and

Go to **Chapter 9** on the Electronic Study Guide.

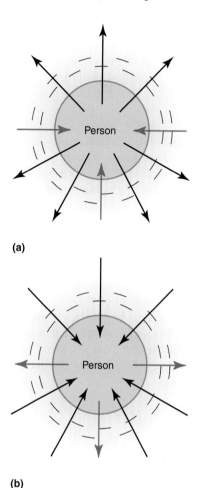

(a)

(b)

FIGURE 10–3 **Neuman's continuum: A balance of input and output. A, When energy output exceeds input, illness results. B, Wellness occurs when more energy is generated than expended.** *Source:* Neuman, B. (1995). The Neuman systems model. In B. Neuman, *The Neuman systems model* (3rd ed.) (pp. 3–61). Norwalk, CT: Appleton and Lange.

Developmental stage influences a person's ability to cope with stressors that tend to move him toward the illness end of the continuum. Infants or children who are ill, frightened, or hurt have a limited repertoire of experiences, communication ability, and understanding to help them in their responses. As we progress through the stages of development, we develop understanding and skills to help us deal with illness.

When disease, loss, or other disruptions occur at a younger age than expected, they change our perception of the event and may present a greater challenge to our coping skills than disruptions that are expected. For example, a child's death may seem more tragic than that of an older adult. It is important, though, not to discount the impact of disruptions that *do* occur during the period of an individual's life when they might be expected. For example, a client's advanced age does not necessarily make the death of a

spouse less traumatic than it would be for a young spouse. Losing someone with whom one has spent most of one's life is an incredible loss, whether or not it is "expected" at that stage of life.

Nutrition

Health requires nourishment, and the most obvious form of nourishment is food. The influence of diet on human health is undeniable: Nutrient-deficiency diseases, such as pellagra and night blindness, are unknown in people who consume a nutritious diet. In addition, many chronic diseases, such as type II diabetes mellitus and heart disease, are known to be influenced by our diets, and nutrition appears to play at least a moderate role in a variety of other diseases, such as osteoporosis and some forms of cancer (Thompson & Manore, 2004). As more studies look at the protective properties of some foods (e.g., phytochemicals, antioxidants) and the hazards of others (e.g., simple carbohydrates, trans fatty acids), the phrase "You are what you eat" seems more accurate each day. Chapter 26 discusses nutrition in greater detail.

Physical Activity

Healthy people are usually active people. When they are unable to maintain previous levels of activity, they may perceive themselves as less healthy. Studies support the benefit of moderate physical activity in reducing the risk of chronic disease and promoting longevity (Thompson & Manore, 2004). As little as 30 minutes of gardening or 15 minutes of jogging on most days of the week can lead to these benefits. In addition, certain types of exercise have been shown to reduce the risk of specific diseases, such as osteoporosis and heart disease. For example, weight training has been shown to increase bone density and reduce the risk of osteoporosis in women over 40, and aerobic activity, such as walking, decreases the risk of heart disease. Some studies even indicate that regular aerobic exercise helps preserve neurological function as we age.

Sleep and Rest

Sleep nourishes health. During sleep, our bodies release the majority of our growth hormone, which assists in tissue regeneration, synthesis of bone, and formation of red blood cells. Sleep is also important to mental health, because it provides time for the mind to slow down and rejuvenate. Perhaps that is why problems often look much smaller in the morning. In controlled studies, people kept awake for 24 hours experienced difficulty concentrating and performing routine tasks. With increasing levels of sleep deprivation, sensory deficits and mood disturbances occurred. Outside the laboratory, mild but chronic sleep deprivation is common, particularly among students, mothers of infants and young children, and people in pain. Sleep and rest are discussed in more detail in Chapter 33.

Meaningful Work

Many people find that work is a healthy way to cope with stressors. Psychologist Victor Frankl, who survived internment in a Nazi concentration camp, observed in *Man's Search for Meaning* (1959, 1962, 1984) that engaging in meaningful work promotes health and, even in the midst of horrific stressors, can defend against physical and mental breakdown. The definition of meaningful work varies, but many share the view offered by Morrie Schwartz in *Tuesdays with Morrie:* "You know what really gives you satisfaction? Offering others what you have to give. . . . [D]evote yourself to your community around you, and devote yourself to creating something that gives you purpose and meaning. You notice, there's nothing in there about a salary" (Albom, 1997).

People also experience meaningful work as a dimension of wellness. For many people, volunteering, pursuing hobbies, and engaging in pleasurable activities can be forms of meaningful work. For example, some find that singing, playing a musical instrument, or listening to music is particularly healing. For others, it may be literature, art, studying the intricacies of the human body, playing basketball, doing counted cross-stitch, gardening, hiking in the wilderness, or even shopping. Remember that being healthy is not all drudgery, such as denying yourself the pleasure of hot fudge sundaes and french fries. By supporting clients' life work, hobbies, and personal interests, you help them nourish their spirit in their unique way.

Lifestyle Choices

People who consider themselves healthy are usually those who make healthy lifestyle choices. They are aware of the threats to health created by cigarette smoking, alcohol consumption, drug abuse, unprotected sex, and other risky behaviors. Consider the following examples:

- A history of smoking increases recovery time from other illnesses, injuries, and surgery. Smoking also increases the risk of infertility, low-birth-weight and preterm babies, and perinatal death.

- Studies have indicated that drinking a glass of red wine each day can reduce the risk of heart disease and slow bone loss. In contrast, excessive alcohol consumption damages the brain, liver, pancreas, and intestines and can lead to malnutrition. It has also been implicated in several forms of cancer and in fetal alcohol syndrome in newborns. Finally, excessive alcohol consumption is implicated in about half of all motor vehicle accidents.

- Drug abuse is a deterioration in health, functioning, or social relationships as a result of injection or ingestion of drugs. Even prescription drugs can be abused. Drug abuse is a risk factor in many diseases. For example, people who inject illegal drugs are at increased risk of HIV infection, malnutrition, and hepatitis.

You can learn more about effects of lifestyle choices on wellness and safety in Chapter 9, Chapter 21, and Chapter 41.

Family Relationships

Living in a healthy family is an important dimension of wellness. Moreover, the family influences a person's view of himself as well or ill. For each of the following contrasting pairs of families, which one would help you to experience high-level wellness?

- Some families place a high priority on health promotion, whereas others tend to respond to health issues only in times of serious illness.
- Some encourage adventure and risk-taking, whereas others emphasize caution in new situations.
- Some families are very open about expressing feelings and disagreements, whereas others tend to squelch personal feelings to avoid conflict in the family.
- Some families view themselves as capable and successful, others as powerless victims.
- Some families teach good negotiation skills and build a network of family support and community while encouraging the development of independence. In contrast, some parents do not have a large repertoire of skills to share with their children.

Especially when clients are coping with life-threatening disease, family relationships can provide critical sustenance and preserve optimal wellness during the experience. Weeks before his death from amyotrophic lateral sclerosis (ALS), a neurological disease, sociologist Morrie Schwartz stated, "It's become quite clear to me as I've been sick. If you don't have the support and love and caring and concern that you get from a family, you don't have much at all. Love is so supremely important" (Albom, 1997). The role of family in human health is discussed in more detail in Chapter 12.

When illness occurs, some people prefer to be totally independent, priding themselves on never asking for or accepting help. But the reality is that during times of disruption, support from others is crucial. Families, friends, co-workers, healthcare workers, pastors, and counselors may be very effective in helping even rugged individualists deal with difficult life situations. Knowing that support is available, and being willing to accept the support, can greatly affect a person's response to disruptions.

Culture

Culture influences a person's healthcare decisions as well as her view of herself as well or ill. Individual and family health may be influenced by ethnic culture, the culture of a region or a neighborhood, the culture of a school or work environment, the culture of affluence or poverty, or the culture of a religious group. For example, the cultural group may share health-promoting values, such as a nutritious diet or regular physical activity. This is not to say that individuals can be "pegged" by their cultural background. Just as some clients respond in ways unlike their families, some make a conscious decision to break away from culturally conditioned responses.

Our response to illness is also partly determined by our culture. In *Grace and Grit,* philosopher Ken Wilber (1991) identifies 11 culturally determined responses to illness. For example, people who belong to fundamentalist faiths may interpret illness as a punishment from God for some sort of sin and bear symptoms stoically as retribution for their wrongs. People who identify themselves with the New Age movement may believe that illness is a lesson we give ourselves to teach us something we need to learn for our spiritual evolution. They may therefore try to identify the lesson of their illness—for example, "I need to slow down and be good to myself"—and then attempt to practice it. The culture of health care has traditionally responded to illness with specific therapies aimed at treating a biophysical disorder, whereas nursing, as part of the culture of holism, responds to the physical, emotional, mental, and spiritual dimensions of illness. For more information about the influence of culture on health and illness, see Chapter 13.

Religion and Spirituality

Religion and spirituality are closely tied to culture, and clients' religious beliefs and practices can influence their healthcare choices. For example, some people believe that spiritual beliefs influence the mind-body connection to promote wellness and healing. A dramatic example is seemingly spontaneous recovery following a religious rite, as when, for example, Native Americans visited by the "false faces" (shamans wearing masks depicting spirits) recover from an illness.

When healing is not possible because of terminal illness or external circumstances beyond our control, spiritual reserves can help maintain our view of ourselves as "well." Nien Cheng in *Life and Death in Shanghai* (1986) tells her story of surviving 7 years in solitary confinement during China's Cultural Revolution. One of the ways she nourished herself was through reciting scriptures she had memorized. She had nourished her mind during "good" times in her life. When her life became barren, she nourished her

mind and spirit through the reserves she had stored. Part of health is having the reserves when you need them, whether physical, mental, or spiritual. The influence of spirituality on health is discussed in more detail in Chapter 14.

Environmental Factors

The environment can also nourish wellness. For institutionalized clients, a little corner of the room that is uniquely "theirs," with photos and other mementos, can be healing. Other clients may be soothed by the quietness of a chapel, a walk in the country, or even a trip to a shopping mall! Spending time in any place where they feel harmony and peace and draw strength can promote clients' health.

On the other hand, environmental pollutants are a common cause of illness. For example, exposure to secondhand smoke causes an estimated 3000 deaths from lung cancer among American adults each year (CDC, 2003a), and carbon monoxide poisoning kills more than 500 (CDC, 2003b). Lead poisoning, molds, radon, and other pollutants also cause serious disease. Environmental safety is discussed in more detail in Chapter 21.

Finances

It is often said that money doesn't buy happiness. Certainly, this is true. However, money does buy access to health care and healthcare choices and thus nourishes wellness. In the United States, health insurance is often tied to employment or income level, and health insurance dictates which providers you have access to and what services are available to you. Even in countries with national health programs, such as Canada and European countries, the standard care available may not include the services or medications a person desires.

Sometimes healthcare providers wonder why people do not take advantage of services that are available to them. Why do they let things go so long before seeking help—or fail to follow up with recommended treatment plans? What may seem very reasonable to us as healthcare professionals may seem totally out of reach or unacceptable to those needing the help. A client's apparent lack of concern or lack of compliance to a treatment regimen may be, in reality, a problem regarding access to healthcare resources. Several factors influence access: proximity to the resources; knowledge of available resources; financial ability to access resources; financial ability to make lifestyle adjustments, such as diet or changes in employment; and trust in the resources that are available. Any one or combination of these factors may keep individuals and families from getting the help that they need.

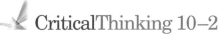

CriticalThinking 10–2

- In what ways could you improve your eating, exercise, and sleep habits?
- How might a hospitalized patient get away from the routine and find peace and harmony?

WHAT FACTORS DISRUPT HEALTH?

We spend much of our lives trying to maintain good health—eating, sleeping, keeping our bodies at a comfortable temperature—in general, tending to our high-maintenance bodily needs. It's a continual process because of the many disruptions to health we face. Not all of these disruptions are incapacitating, but all challenge our ability to function and enjoy our everyday lives, and they tend to move us toward the illness end of the health-illness continuum.

Physical Disease

Disease disrupts our lives in so many ways. It may reduce our ability to perform our life roles effectively or to engage in activities we used to enjoy. The diagnosis of a chronic or life-threatening disease may bring shock, fear, anxiety, anger, or grief: Will I become disabled? How will I support my family? What did I do to deserve this? How can I bear saying good-bye to the people I love? It may also cause clients to question the meaning and purpose of their lives, to become more inwardly focused, or to embrace life even more fully. When she first learned of her diagnosis of breast cancer at age 36, Treya Killam Wilber wrote, "Strange things happen to the mind when catastrophe strikes. It felt like the universe turned into a thin paper tissue, and then someone simply tore the tissue in half right in front of my eyes. I was so stunned that it was as if absolutely nothing had happened. A tremendous strength descended on me, the strength of being both totally jolted and totally stupefied. I was clear, present, and very determined" (Wilber, 1991).

Injury

Injury can cause the same symptoms and emotions as disease, but perhaps its most disruptive aspect is its suddenness. In *Still Me,* actor Christopher Reeve describes his thoughts in the first days after he recovered consciousness following his cervical spinal cord injury: "The thought that kept going through my mind was: I've ruined my life. I've ruined my life, and you only get one. You can't say, 'I've spoiled this one, so can I have another, please?' There's no counter you can go up to and say, 'I dropped my ice cream cone; could I please have another one?'. . . . Why isn't there a higher authority you can go to and say, 'Wait a minute, you didn't mean for this to happen to *me*'" (Reeve, 1998).

Mental Illness

Clients with mental illness and their families experience a level of pain, suffering, and chronic sorrow that is difficult for healthy people to fully appreciate (Glod, 1998). In addition, if the illness affects work ability, they experience loss of income and altered role relationships, accompanied by the costs of various therapies. Family members may also live in constant fear of their loved one's committing suicide.

Mental illness carries with it a stigma that has been described as the single most debilitating handicap for people with mental illness (Glod, 1998). This stigmatization can also disrupt the health of family members. For example, an adult sister, whose only sibling has had repeated hospitalizations from exacerbations of schizophrenia, reported overhearing a cousin at a family gathering ask her uncle, "So where is that crazy Dee? Is she in or out of the hospital again? I hope her sister doesn't catch her craziness." The sister stated, "I really feel labeled along with my sister" (Glod, 1998).

Pain

Whether mild or severe, temporary or long-lasting, pain is a disruption. It's not that we can't live with pain—many people do, every day of their lives. However, pain disrupts the smooth operation of our lives. It's hard to concentrate on what we are trying to accomplish when pain is competing for our attention.

Pain that is easily remedied with over-the-counter medications or that is short-lived serves only as a minor disruption in our lives. However, pain that is all-encompassing permeates a person's entire existence. Sometimes that pain is physical, sometimes psychological. One young mother of a profoundly mentally disabled 14-year-old girl spoke of "hurting so bad that my bones hurt."

As we discussed in Chapter 1, some of our nursing interventions inflict pain. We ask patients to turn, cough, and deep-breathe after surgery, even though it hurts—a *lot*! We put needles in them, catheterize them, and get them out of bed when they would rather sleep. We pull off tape. We invade their physical personal space. We ask them questions about personal things, such as their bowel movements. It is a challenge to be a comforting, healing presence when we have to do things that cause discomfort.

Loss

Whether the loss of a job, the end of a romantic relationship, the death of a loved one, or the loss of youth, beauty, functioning, or identity, loss cuts to the core of who we are. Most of us cling to a unique identity, which often does *not* include gaining weight or getting wrinkles and gray hair, let alone being a "patient" or losing major bodily functions. When such losses occur, people typically experience a period of significant disintegration that may continue until they either find a way to cope with the loss or succeed in reinterpreting the loss in a meaningful way. Toward the end of her battle with cancer, Treya Killam Wilber lost her near vision. One way she coped with this loss was by replacing her passion for reading with sitting at her window contemplating the mountains beyond (Wilber, 1991).

Many have written about the indignities people suffered in concentration camps (Frankl, 1959, 1962, 1984; Valladares, 1986; Bettelheim, 1979), including nakedness, exposure to human excrement, and being treated like children incapable of thoughtful judgment. The Nazi guards knew that those three indignities were crucial threats to their prisoners' sense of self. Sadly, patients in hospitals and other institutions may also suffer those three indignities. In situations of illness, think how patients feel who have to don a hospital gown and allow their body to be exposed for various tests or procedures or how it feels to lose control of urination and/or defecation. One woman who was paralyzed as the result of a metastatic lesion on her spine indicated that one of the toughest things she had to deal with was having her daughter give her enemas and clean her up as if she were a baby. As healthcare providers, we may easily forget how humiliating such "routine procedures" may be for the patient. As we have discussed, the disease or injury is a disruption in itself; you can prevent further disruption when you respect patients' dignity by providing for their privacy and allowing them to make choices regarding their care.

If temporary losses are difficult, what about those that are permanent? C. S. Lewis (1961) writes this about his response to the death of his wife: "I know that the thing I want is exactly the thing I can never get. The old life, the jokes, the drinks, the arguments, the lovemaking, the tiny, heartbreaking commonplace. On any view whatever, to say 'H. is dead,' is to say 'All that is gone.' It is a part of the past" (p. 22). As nurses, we would like to "fix" everything. Though we can't "fix" the holes that are left when a person suffers a loss, we can be open and sensitive to their heart's cry.

Impending Death

We all know that we have a 100% chance of dying; however, it is easy for most of us to ignore this finality and live as though death were only a remote possibility. Lifton and Olson (1974) state that during middle age, even without the presence of life-threatening illness, people tend to become more aware of the compelling reality of death: "One's life is suddenly felt to be limited, finite. It also becomes apparent that one cannot finish everything; there will not be time for all one's projects" (p. 63).

As a nurse, you will care for clients who are living in the shadow of death. Some may be aware of their condition; others may choose to deny it, ignore it, or "fight it to the end" by trying a series of conventional and alternative therapies. Caring for dying clients makes us painfully aware of our own frailty and is one of the most difficult experiences you will face as a nurse. Refer to Chapter 15 for further discussion of loss, grieving, and dying.

Competing Demands

Even in the normal flow of life, there are many competing demands. Taken independently, they may be easy to handle. Taken together, the cumulative effect wears us down. In times of illness, the other competing demands continue. Children need to be cared for. Aging parents may need care. Bills still need to be paid. Job responsibilities press in. One man with depression reported, "[T]he whole thing bundled together—one caused the other which caused more and it was just a degenerative loop. . . . [O]ne thing feeds another which feeds another and so forth until you just constantly go down" (Smith, 1992, p. 104).

Sometimes people ignore health issues because the competing demands are too great. Symptoms may even go unnoticed because attention is scattered in so many directions and there is not enough energy to focus on one more issue. Lack of time makes it difficult to research one's symptoms, schedule a doctor's appointment, or follow through with treatments.

When a loved one's illness is acute, such as a broken bone, the stress is usually bearable. It is surprising what people can deal with if they can mark off the days on a calendar, knowing how many days are left of a disruption. Bettleheim (1979) states: "The worst calamity becomes bearable if one believes its end is in sight" (pp. 3–4). But when the illness is chronic, the competing demands can take a heavy toll. One woman who took care of her husband who lived at home on a respirator recounted the overwhelming burden she felt when, after 2 years, he was "no better and no worse. This could go on forever!" Her life was consumed with his care. Although people came in to help, she felt she had to maintain constant alertness in case something went wrong with his respirator. But even in the face of her husband's unrelenting needs, she still had to meet many other demands and challenges each day.

As nurses, we sometimes find it easy to see how people ought to deal with their situations, even to criticize them. But it is so important to realize that the short amount of time that you spend with someone in a hospital or clinic or in a home visit is only one tiny fragment of the cumulative experience that patients and their families experience, sometimes unrelentingly for years on end.

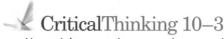

CriticalThinking 10–3
How might you assist your patient to maintain normalcy in spite of illness?

The Unknown

Even normal life changes present challenges. For example, most new parents bringing their first baby home from the hospital are in for plenty of surprises. Every new squeak, twitch, and rash raises concern. Think of the couple who adds to that equation serious health problems in their infant. They go from anticipating a "bundle of joy" to a new world perhaps involving surgery, breathing treatments, seizures, feeding tubes, clinic visits, and keeping track of numerous medications.

With some unknowns, there is time to do research and prepare. For example, if an expectant couple learn via amniocentesis (a prenatal test) that their child has a genetic defect, then during the remaining months of pregnancy they can read about the disorder and meet with other parents who have had children similarly affected. This can help prepare them to anticipate their child's needs. But as we noted earlier, injuries and illnesses can happen abruptly, with no chance to prepare ourselves for new realities. A woman described her experience of finding out she had cancer of the lung with metastasis: "It was on a . . . Friday— I got to feeling kind of bad—kind of like you had the flu or something, you know? And I got to throwing up, so I went to the doctor. . . . I didn't even call, I just went. And he sent me to the hospital. And I arrived there and they started doin' tests on me—all kinds of tests—and found out I had cancer" (Smith, 1992, p. 107).

Imbalance

Our sense of justice tells us that when we are good, good things should happen. When we are bad, bad things should happen. The Buddhist concept of karma suggests that there is an equitable balance between what one gives to life and what one receives. Thus, when we perceive that life has violated this rule, we experience the violation as a disruption. Our sense of balance is perhaps most dramatically disturbed by the death of children. Such deaths are sometimes referred to as "out of order" because children (of any age) "should" not die before their parents. Balance is also disrupted when patients, expecting that their painful and harrowing treatments "should" help them get better, do not get better. One young woman under treatment for advanced cancer described it like this: "It's just—you've been working hard, and it's not doin' a . . . bit of good. You know . . . you're workin' as hard as you can, and you're doin' what you're supposed to be doin' and focusing and all this and that—and your body is still not responding" (Smith, 1992, p. 111).

Have you seen the bumper sticker "Life is hard. And then you die"? Cynical perhaps, but we do not have to live long before we realize that as much as we would like for everything to be fair, it is not going to happen. Knowing this intellectually, however, does not necessarily reduce the disruptive effect of the imbalance.

Isolation

How many times have you thought, "No one knows what I'm going through!"? Despite the universality of suffering, a sense of isolation or aloneness seems to accompany it. C. S. Lewis (1961) states, "You can't really share someone else's weakness, or fear or pain" (p. 13). Vanauken (1977), in writing about the death of his young wife, reveals that it was not only suffering his loss, but having to go through the experience *without* her that made it so difficult: "Along with the emptiness . . . I kept wanting to *tell* her about it. We always told each other—that was what sharing was— and now this huge thing was happening to me, and I couldn't tell her" (p. 181).

The sense of aloneness reported by seriously ill clients is related in part to their actual physical separation from loved ones during treatments, hospitalizations, or clinic visits. But it also stems from their feeling that there is no one who is really "in their world." Having someone physically present does not necessarily remove the sense of aloneness. One woman in an advanced stage of cancer talks about others being there, yet not being there; and her being there, but not being part of the action:

> *When I lay here it's lonely—very, very lonely. Because [her daughter] can't just sit here and talk to me all the time. She's got wash to do, fold and all that stuff. And then the kids to worry about. . . . The worst thing I've found about this whole disease is the loneliness. . . . Because your family can be with you and if they don't come and sit down and talk to you about different things, you're lonely. It's the loneliness that makes you sad inside. . . . It's like everybody's afraid of you or something. They're afraid that maybe they're gonna catch what you got or something. (Smith, 1992)*

KnowledgeCheck 10–2
Identify at least four factors that disrupt health.

 Go to Chapter 10, **Knowledge Check Response Sheet and Answers,** on the Electronic Study Guide.

CriticalThinking 10–4
- What impact do disruptions have on your life?
- How could you apply the information about disruptions to the health of a community? To the health of a nation?

HOW DO PEOPLE EXPERIENCE ILLNESS?

Earlier in this chapter, we mentioned that people vary greatly in terms of their response to life situations. Why is this so? Why do some people react to seemingly insurmountable problems with calmness and grace, while others fall apart over seemingly "small" disruptions? The human experience is so complex and interactive that is impossible to make neat little categories that we might add up to determine a score predicting how a person will respond to a given situation. There are several factors, however, that may influence an individual's responses to illness.

Stages of Illness Behavior

Suchman (1972) identified five stages of illness behaviors that people move through as they cope with disruptions to health: experiencing symptoms, sick role behavior, seeking professional care, dependence on others, and recovery.

Experiencing symptoms is a signal that illness has begun. If the symptoms are recognizable, such as runny nose, sneezing, and a cough, you may identify the problem as a common cold and turn to previously used remedies. Common problems rarely progress beyond this stage. However, if the symptoms are unusual, severe, or overwhelming, you may progress to the next stage.

Sick role behavior is assumed when you have identified yourself as ill. This role relieves you from normal duties, such as work, school, or tasks at home. The severity of the symptoms and anticipated length of illness determine whether you will progress further along the stages of illness.

Seeking professional care is the next stage. To reach this stage, you must determine that you are ill and that professional care is required to treat the illness. Persons who seek professional care are asking for validation of their illness, explanations for their symptoms, appropriate treatment, and information about the anticipated length of illness. Health care professionals often bypass this stage, relying on themselves to identify and treat the problem. This is not always the best course of action because it is difficult to be objective when examining yourself.

Dependence on others begins when you accept the diagnosis and treatment of the health care provider. The severity of the illness and the type of treatment determine the extent of dependence. In some cases this may be limited to listening to the provider's instructions, filling the prescription, and following directions given in the office. However, illness that requires hospitalization is often associated with dependence on nursing staff and hospital personnel for activities of daily living, medications, and treatments. Some people easily make the transition to dependence; others

---

BOX 10–2   Examples of Chronic Illness

AIDS or AIDS-related problems	Chronic back pain	Hypertension
Alcohol abuse	Chronic obstructive pulmonary disease	Mental illness
Angina	Chronic pain syndrome	Peripheral vascular disease
Asthma	Coronary artery disease	Renal failure
Cancer	Dementia	Rheumatoid arthritis
Cerebral palsy	Diabetes mellitus	Substance abuse
Cerebral vascular accident (Stroke)	Epilepsy	

---

remain as independent as possible even in the face of severe illness. Personal characteristics and values play a large role in determining how each of us will respond to the challenges of being dependent.

Recovery is the final stage of illness. Dependence is given up, and there is a gradual return to normal roles and functioning. In minor illness, this is usually a return to the status quo. Severe illnesses may require a newly defined level of optimum function. The greater the change, the more difficult this transition will be.

The Nature of the Illness

The nature of the illness affects the way persons react to disruptions. An **acute illness** occurs suddenly and lasts for a limited amount of time. Acute illnesses, such as a cold, flu, or viral infection, may be minor and require no formal health care. Some acute illness, such as strep throat, may require a visit to a health provider for treatment or even hospitalization or surgery, as in cholecystitis (gallbladder inflammation secondary to gallstone formation) or pyelonephritis (infection of the kidney). Although hospitalization and surgery can be quite traumatic, in each case the person is expected to recover. In acute illness a person may experience the disruptions of pain, competing demands, and the unknown. However, an end is in sight. Relief is expected.

In contrast, **chronic illness** lasts for a long period of time, usually 6 months or more, often for a lifetime. Chronic illness requires the person to make life changes. These changes might be regular visits to the clinic or hospital, daily medications, or lifestyle modifications. Examples of chronic illness include AIDS, diabetes mellitus, rheumatoid arthritis, and hypertension. Because of the lengthy period of illness, people with chronic disease often experience periods of remission or exacerbation. A **remission** occurs when symptoms are minimal to none. An **exacerbation** occurs when symptoms intensify. Clients with chronic illness often complain about the unrelenting nature of their health problems.

A person with chronic illness may experience virtually all of the disruptions identified earlier. Box 10–2 identifies a number of chronic illnesses that you may encounter during your clinical rotations.

Hardiness

Why does one client who drinks, smokes, overeats, and avoids exercise live into his 90s, yet another client who "follows all the rules" dies of a sudden heart attack at age 39? Our bodies do not react to the same stressors in the same way. One factor that may contribute to this difference is the person's hardiness.

Hardiness has been described as *developing a very strong positive force to live*—and enjoying the fight! A man with heart problems said, "I guess everybody that's in the situation, who has to fight to live, and has learned the mental wizardry of it, you know, to make yourself want to live on. But if you want to, you develop this—this very, very strong positive force to make it go" (Smith, 1992, p. 131). Seigel (1977) reported a study by London researchers that revealed a 10-year survival rate of 75% "among cancer patients who reacted to the diagnosis with a 'fighting spirit,'" compared with a 22% survival rate "among those who responded with 'stoic acceptance' or feelings of helplessness or hopelessness" (p. 25).

A dramatic example is one woman in an advanced stage of cancer and receiving chemotherapy who got up and went to work every day. Even though it was extremely difficult to drag herself out of bed and get ready for work, she felt much better when she could carry on her normal activities instead of dwelling on her constant pain and the threat of impending death. Carrying on normally is not easy to do, however. It takes a concerted, determined effort to persevere.

Another aspect of hardiness is the willingness to draw on resources within oneself or from others to *break out of old patterns of living* when life situations change. Some people find it too difficult to make life changes, and they just give up. Hardy individuals are willing to seek out information and take initiative in

dealing with life situations rather than sitting back and letting someone else control their lives.

Some people don't have many resources to call on. When disruption hits, they lack the cognitive, communicative, creative, and spiritual resources that would support them during difficult times. Ironically, some people blossom during times of adversity. Those who see themselves as hardy tend to approach disruptions with an "I can deal with this" attitude.

The Intensity, Duration, and Multiplicity of the Disruption

Everyone has limits. For healthcare providers, too many demands over too long a period of time can lead to "burnout," a feeling of being overwhelmed and demoralized. For clients and their families, dealing with the cumulative effect of illness and other life disruptions can break down what might otherwise be excellent coping skills. Therefore, their responses may not be typical of what they usually have demonstrated.

KnowledgeCheck 10–3

Identify the factors that affect how a person responds to the disruptions of illness.

 Go to Chapter10, **Knowledge Check Response Sheet and Answers,** on the Electronic Study Guide.

Practical Knowledge
knowing how

In the preceding section, you have learned how people experience health, wellness, and illness. In this section, we will look at how this information can be applied to your nursing practice.

USING THE NURSING PROCESS TO PROMOTE HEALTH

Throughout this textbook, you will learn to use the nursing process to help clients deal with a variety of health problems. Using the nursing process in relationship to the broader aspects of health and illness described in this chapter involves helping clients to look within themselves to develop creative ways to deal with the realities they are facing.

Patients may fail to comply with a proposed health care regimen if healthcare providers fail to develop a plan of care that has cultural or personal relevance for the patient (or family). Perhaps the plan does not consider the knowledge level of the patient or caregiver; or perhaps it is not feasible in terms of available support, time, energy, finances, or location.

Patients may leave a hospital setting against medical advice (AMA), thereby endangering their chances of recovery. They may believe that the treatment offered them will not help or that the illness is preferable to the proposed treatment.

Remember that people do not necessarily refuse to carry out a plan of care simply out of stubbornness, hostility toward healthcare providers, or wanton disregard for their own welfare. The challenge for nurses is to develop an individualized plan of care in collaboration with patients, based on mutual goals and respect.

|Assessment|

In looking at an individual's health status, you might easily emphasize measurable aspects of physical status (to read about physical assessments, see Chapter 19). Physical needs obviously are crucial, but competing issues may be present and cause the client to view the therapeutic interventions as irrelevant or even disruptive. Obtaining data about the psychosocioal, emotional, and spiritual aspects of health requires a level of communication that goes beyond a neat list of skills. Communicating genuine care, concern, and sensitivity comes from who you are as a person, not from assuming a professional persona (putting on your "nurse's hat").

Your initial approach to a patient creates a climate that determines the level of communication that takes place. The patient is probably in a new environment, and your tone, words, and facial expressions can bring comfort and ease. Nurses can be in new situations too, and taking a few moments to **settle in** to the situation can be helpful in facilitating communication.

Attuning, being maximally attentive, is another key factor in facilitating communication. Most people are hungry for someone to listen to them. So often, listeners are so busy thinking about what they want to say that they fail to really listen. Try to focus on what the patient or family has to say instead of thinking ahead to what you want to ask next.

Another vital aspect of communicating is **acceptance**—acceptance of appearance, lifestyles, ways of coping, and values. You might ask, "How can I be accepting when there are aspects of this person that go against my entire value system?" Accepting is not the same as "agreeing with." You can accept people as valued, creative, unique individuals, despite their differences from your own ways of being. This view of acceptance does not mean that people will not be held accountable for their actions, for example, in cases of domestic violence and child abuse. It does mean, though, that in your role as a caregiver, you must convey an attitude of accepting the intrinsic value of life—in whatever form that life takes.

Perhaps even more difficult than accepting is **enjoying.** You will come into contact with a wide array

of individuals, many of whom are different from people you have grown up around and have come to know and enjoy. A challenge for you is to broaden your repertoire of people you enjoy: to see and enjoy commonalities among individuals seemingly so different and to recognize and appreciate the pathos of suffering, in whatever form it takes.

Settling in, attuning, respecting, and enjoying—certainly this is not a step-by-step process, but each is vital to creating a climate for the openness and communication needed for assessment. You might argue that the healthcare environment does not allow time for such a high level of attentiveness. Consider, though, how much time is spent in delivering nursing care. As a full-spectrum nurse, you will assess patients continually during the delivery of all this care. In fact, the physical contact involved in carrying out nursing procedures seems to break down barriers of communication. Nurses hold a unique opportunity in "being with" individuals during difficult life situations; indeed, Benner and Wrubel (1989) state that expert nurses call this the "privileged place of nursing" (p. xi).

One way to approach assessment, whether in outpatient, acute care, long-term care, or home settings, is to ask the patient, "What is the biggest concern you are dealing with today?" You may have a plan of care that addresses areas that you know to be important, but it may fall far short of meeting your patient's needs if you have not addressed the concern that is fundamental to your patient.

In addition to communicating, developing your observation skills will enable you to assess your patients more fully. Watching your patient's responses to you and your care, observing the presence or absence of visitors and the effect on your patients, and observing signs of religious or cultural practices that have significance all provide important information about your patient's strengths and needs.

| Diagnosis |

Several of the nursing diagnoses labels identified by NANDA International relate to health issues discussed in this chapter. Some examples are Anxiety, Caregiver Role Strain, Situational Low Self-esteem, and Spiritual Distress. The assessment data that you gather also provide the information needed to describe related causal factors, such as Spiritual Distress related to fear of impending death or Situational Low Self-esteem related to loss of job secondary to frequent absences for chemotherapy.

| Planning Outcomes/Evaluation |

Goals and outcomes should be both realistic and valued by the patient and family. When you set goals in the broader dimension of health and illness (as in this chapter), it is much harder to be specific in describing

expected outcomes and time frames. As a nurse, your role is to help the patient (or family member) envision acceptable outcomes and to set smaller, realistic goals so that the patient recognizes progress. For example, an older woman caring for a spouse with Alzheimer's disease may have a nursing diagnosis of Caregiver Role Strain related to care of spouse with dementia. Together you would establish acceptable goals and break them down into realistic steps. You also would identify outcomes to indicate that the caregiver actually experiences a reduction in strain, such as being able to sleep or having time to pursue meaningful activities.

| Planning Interventions/Implementation |

The ideal approach is to draw on patient and family strengths to help achieve the desired outcomes. In the preceding example of the older adult caregiver, you would discuss with her the options available to provide support, but she would identify which options were acceptable to her and her spouse. In the heat of the moment, patients and families may not recognize the strengths and creative abilities that they bring to a situation. Part of the art of nursing is to envision strengths and potential in patients and families, just as an artful teacher might recognize a "spark" in a child and encourage that child to learn and grow.

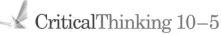 CriticalThinking 10–5

- How can you use the concepts of health when you are admitting a patient to a hospital setting? To a clinic? To an emergency department? To a rehabilitation or long-term care setting? In initiating home care?
- What questions can you ask or what observations can you make to help you gain information about individuals' health strategies, disruptions to health, and factors contributing to their responses to disruptions?
- How would you consider health concepts in planning for patients' discharge from healthcare settings?

HOW CAN I HONOR EACH CLIENT'S UNIQUE HEALTH/ILLNESS EXPERIENCE?

Choosing nursing as a profession means choosing to be an instrument of healing in a hurtful world. However, being an instrument of healing does not come automatically with the title of nurse. Nor does it allow you the luxury of learning just one approach and applying it to every client. It means cultivating a healing presence by listening, being maximally attentive, being aware of your own gifts and limitations of communication, being willing to learn from those in your care, recognizing and respecting others' ways of coping, and enjoying others for who they are.

Nursing care demands a high level of theoretical knowledge: of physiological, psychological, and social

principles, as well as savvy knowledge of highly technical equipment. Patients may be impressed, even amazed, by the healthcare technology used to diagnose and treat their illness. However, what they most often remember, perhaps through the rest of their lives, is that person who connected with them in a very special way. One man, quadriplegic for 26 years following a car accident in his teens, spoke of a senior nursing student who cared for him during his initial hospitalization. He said that after 26 years, he not only still remembered her, but also still could sense the warmth of her caring presence.

During times of vulnerability, people seem acutely attuned to those who are helpful to them and also to those who slight them in hurtful ways, whether intentionally or not. What a challenge for nurses this makes! In this section, we discuss steps you can take to prepare yourself for responding to your clients in ways that are meaningful and healing to them.

Examine Life's Uncertainties

Wellness is a balancing act between living in the mostly known present and the mostly unknown future. Encourage your clients to make active decisions that positively affect their future. You do not have control over a drunk driver who sails across the median and hits you head on, but you do have control over getting the brakes on your car fixed or wearing your seat belt. Likewise, you do not know whether you will develop cancer or heart disease, but you can take responsibility for learning and practicing prevention and detection of problems.

Making health-promoting lifestyle choices is important, but it cannot protect us from risk. Significant life experiences, such as getting married, having children, investing in friendships, venturing into business, and selecting a profession all involve risk. Making a commitment to *anything* is a risk. Each person has a different "risk-comfort range." Some are willing to risk little, have fewer disappointments, and less sparkling achievements. Their lives may not glitter, but they may be enjoyable. To others, security is not as important, and they are comfortable taking greater risks.

In *A Severe Mercy,* Sheldon Vanauken (1977) writes about finding and losing a great love. He reasons: "The joy would be worth the pain—if, indeed, they went together. If there were a choice . . . between, on the one hand, the heights and the depths and, on the other hand, some sort of safe, cautious middle way, he, for one, here and now chose the heights and the depths" (p. 9). He did, indeed, find a great love, and when he lost his wife at an early age, he was able to accept their time together as one of his life's greatest blessings. As a nurse, you will face many uncertainties and dilemmas. You will certainly face new experiences and challenges, situations you thought *you* never would have to deal with. You will observe

pain, suffering, and death. You may never understand the apparent inequity of it all. But often life brings new meaning when it takes a different direction from the one planned. For example, a teen who severs his spinal cord in a motor vehicle accident begins to speak at high schools about the dangers of drinking and driving. Or a couple formerly embittered over their third miscarriage finds joy in adopting two children with disabilities.

As a nurse, you will also be privileged to witness many joys. Some might even qualify as minor triumphs: a patient taking his first steps after major surgery, a pathology report that isn't as bad as feared, or even a peaceful death that brings closure to a grieving family. As you move from novice to expert, you may find that such witnessing causes you to stop questioning life's uncertainties and instead to start treasuring them.

 ## CriticalThinking 10–6
- What uncertainties have you struggled with?
- What approaches have proven effective for you in dealing with uncertainties?

Envision Wellness for Your Clients and Yourself

Wherever there is a dream, there is someone there to tell you it can't be done, or at least not by you. There is something to be said, however, for "envisioning" wellness for your clients and yourself. Remember Evelyn ("Meet Your Patient")? If her nurses had labeled her as debilitated and close to death, how would that have affected her? In contrast, their acceptance of her vision of herself as well and full of life supports her and aids her healing. In the same way, think of how you view your own health. Is the life you envision for yourself characterized by zest and vigor? What are your family relationships like? What are your values? Does your work give meaning and purpose to your life?

The wellness that you envision for yourself can be the blueprint for what you want to become. The skeptic in you might say, "What if I do everything that I know to do to maintain a healthy life and still have a heart attack at 45?" As we have seen, life is full of uncertainties. That does not mean that you have to stop envisioning. Instead, use *flexible envisioning,* adjusting your goals and dreams to each new reality. Health does not mean always getting your first choice. Part of health is being able to dream a new dream, starting over if you need to, but always envisioning that there is something worth striving for.

Establish Trust at Your First Patient Contact

When patients are admitted to a hospital or ambulatory care facility, you will need to support them in

their transition from wellness to illness, in dealing with the unknown, and in adjusting to a new environment. The relationship and trust you establish in your first contact with patients can go a long way toward relieving their anxiety and preserving the energy needed for healing. You can make the transition smoother for them if you are prepared. The following activities should be incorporated into your nursing care.

- *Greet the client.* Gather basic information ahead of time, such as name, diagnosis, and anticipated length of stay. Imagine how it might feel if you arrived on a gurney for admission and you heard the staff say, "Who's this? I didn't know we were getting an admission. How am I supposed to take care of this one, too?"

- *Introduce yourself to the client and family.* Explain who you are. Don't be afraid to tell a client that you are a nursing student. Many clients are aware that students have more time to spend with them.

- *Prepare the room.* A room that is prepared for the client conveys a message of acceptance. Room preparation depends on the type of unit or facility, the client's needs, and the anticipated treatment.

- *Orient the client to the room and the unit.* Make sure the client knows how to use the bed, the call light, and any equipment that you expect him to use. Show the client the location of the restroom. If you will be measuring the client's intake and output, tell him so during your orientation. If the client is alert, he may be able to assist you with these measures. Remember that one of the disruptions associated with illness is the disruption of the unknown. If you do not tell your client what to expect, his fears may increase.

- *Gather a health history.* In Chapter 3, you learned about assessment. Chapter 19 provides a step-by-step approach to physical assessment. Be sure to include in your health history the client's expectations and concerns.

- *Establish a relationship with the client.* Take time to get to know your client. Try to set a tone of caring, respect, and understanding.

| toward evidence-based practice |

Cohen, S., Doyle, W. J., Turner, R. B., Alper, C. M., & Skoner, D. P. (2003). Emotional style and susceptibility to the common cold. *Psychosomatic Medicine, 65*(4), 652–657.

Using a healthy population of 334 volunteers between the ages of 18 and 54, researchers explored the relationship between emotional style and the risk of common cold. Phase I of the study assessed volunteers for the tendency to experience positive and negative emotions. Positive emotions included such feelings as happy, pleased, and relaxed. Negative emotions included anxious, hostile, and depressed.

In Phase II, each volunteer was given nasal drops containing rhinovirus and monitored for the development of the common cold. After adjusting for age, sex, education, race, body mass, and season, researchers discovered that volunteers with positive emotional styles had greater resistance to infection from the common cold and reported fewer unfounded symptoms (not verifiable by objective examination). Negative emotional style was associated with greater infection and reporting more unfounded symptoms.

Barton, C., Clarke, D., Sulaiman, N., & Abramson, M. (2003). Coping as a mediator of psychosocial impediments to optimal management and control of asthma. *Respiratory Medicine, 97*(7), 747–761.

This meta-analysis examined published research indexed in the Medline and PsychInfo databases with search terms *asthma* and *coping*. Researchers concluded that patients with asthma used different strategies for coping with stress and illness compared to healthy subjects and subjects with other chronic illness. Denial and negative emotions were more commonly expressed by patients who did not fully comply with their medication regimen, who required emergency department visits for care, who were admitted to hospital for asthma, or who suffered near-fatal asthma attacks. The availability of coping resources and support systems positively influenced individuals' beliefs about their asthma and the likelihood of adhering to the medication regimen.

1. How do the results of these studies apply to the concept of health as presented in this chapter?

2. Can you identify ways in which the methods and findings could be applied to other populations?

 Go to Chapter 10, **Toward Evidence-Based Practice Suggested Responses,** on the Electronic Study Guide.

critical aspects of procedure 10–1

Admitting a Patient to a Nursing Unit

 For steps to follow in *all* procedures, refer to the inside back cover of Volume 2.

- Orient patient and family to hospital environment.
- Answer patient's and family's questions.
- Complete nursing admission paperwork according to agency policy.
- Institute nursing care plan or clinical pathway.

For detailed directions on how to admit a client to a hospital unit,

 Go to Chapter 10, **Procedure 10–1: Admitting a Patient to a Nursing Unit,** in Volume 2.

The accompanying box, Critical Aspects of Procedure 10–1, provides the highlights of this procedure.

Provide a Healing Presence

Part of what you do as a healing presence will never show up in a written care plan. However, your healing presence may be the most important aspect of care that you have to offer. A statement by a young woman undergoing chemotherapy illustrates the difference the healing presence of a nurse made:

The nursing care I got was in response to the physical symptoms I showed. If I was not feeling good, they were sympathetic with me, you know. If I was feeling good, they were cheerful with me, and things like that. But it was nothing further than that. There was no exploration of feelings or anything like that.

Some of them were—seemed to be very caring. I remember [one nurse] up there, but she was just a really nice *person. And I remember one time that I was throwing up dreadfully for some reason. . . . And I rang for her and I said, 'I'm sorry,' and she was almost crying and she said, 'No, I'm sorry you have to do this—you must feel* awful.' *And she was just very empathetic with it, and I felt like, you know, I wasn't infringing upon her to make her empty my emesis basin or anything like that. (Smith, 1992, pp. 233–234)*

Is a Healthy Life Attainable?

The themes suggested in this chapter as ways to live a healthy life did not come from people who had easy lives. These themes were teased from literature, autobiographies, and interviews with people who were dealing with life situations that would be viewed as difficult from anyone's standpoint. However, in the midst of their circumstances, they were very much involved in *living.* Ripples or even waves of disruption or despair came into their lives, but through it all evolved an overriding sense of life worth pursuing. This can be true for you as a nurse and also for those privileged to be under your care.

As a nurse, you offer your personal health and strength to your patients and their families every day. If you barely have enough physical, emotional, and spiritual strength to manage your own stressors, you will not have much available to offer others who are depleted. This is why it is so important for you to nurture yourself in all aspects of your life, to balance learning how to care for others with caring for yourself, to develop yourself as a healing presence in this world.

 Go to Chapter 10, **Resources for Caregivers and Health Professionals,** on the Electronic Study Guide.

 Suggested Readings: Go to Chapter 10, **Reading More About Experiencing Health and Illness,** on the Electronic Study Guide.

 Bibliography: Go to Volume 2, Bibliography.

11 Psychosocial
Health & Illness

CHAPTER

Learning Outcomes

After completing this chapter, you should be able to:

✳ Explain the relationship of psychosocial factors to overall health and development.

✳ Identify the factors that influence the development and stability of self-concept.

✳ List the four interrelated components of self-concept.

✳ Identify ten general categories to include in a comprehensive psychosocial assessment.

✳ Perform a self-concept assessment using the domains of self-concept, self-esteem, self-identity, and body image.

✳ Develop a nursing care plan for patients exhibiting disturbances in self-concept and self-esteem.

✳ Describe nursing diagnoses, outcomes, and interventions specific to body image disturbance.

✳ Describe interventions for preventing depersonalization.

✳ Describe the anxiety continuum.

✳ List the psychological and physiological effects of anxiety.

✳ Identify the levels and symptoms of anxiety that are severe enough to merit referral to a mental health professional.

✳ Devise a nursing care plan for the nursing diagnosis of Anxiety.

✳ Identify several ways in which clients manifest depression.

✳ Differentiate between mild depression and that which should be referred to a mental health professional.

✳ Describe how to communicate effectively with someone who is depressed.

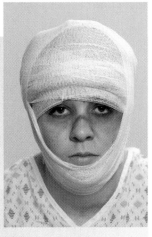

MEET **Your Patient**

You are caring for a 16-year-old patient named Karli who is suffering from fractures to both arms and several ribs, as well as extensive first- and second-degree burns to 30% of her body, following a motor vehicle accident. Karli had recently received her driver's license. She was driving her parents' car home from her part-time job when she lost control of the car and crashed into a containment wall. The car exploded into flames. A passerby quickly reported the accident, and fast action by the emergency response team saved Karli's life.

Karli is suffering from a moderate amount of shock and pain. She alternates between outbursts of anger, self-directed sarcasm, and despondence. She tells you that she cannot understand how the accident happened, that one moment she was adjusting the car radio, and the next moment she awoke in the hospital. Then suddenly she explodes. "It's not fair! I just took my eyes off the road for a second; that's all!" She bursts into tears. Picking at her bandages, she sobs that no one will love her looking as she will, that her life is over, and that she hates herself. You take her hand. "I used to be pretty," she says, "but now I'll look like a freak! What did I do to deserve this? I know plenty of kids who drive drunk or high all the time. I wasn't doing anything wrong! Why did this happen to me?"

Before reading on, jot down a list of the multiple physical, psychological, and social issues that you would need to consider in developing a comprehensive care plan for Karli. You can revisit your list throughout this chapter to compare your answers.

 CriticalThinking 11–1

 Go to **Chapter 9** on the Electronic Study Guide.

- What theoretical knowledge about Karli's developmental stage will assist you in determining nursing diagnoses, interventions, and outcomes?
- Considering that Karli will need a significant amount of assistance for activities of daily living (ADLs) because of her fractures and burns, how might you use the time to develop your therapeutic relationship?

This chapter will introduce you to the concepts of psychosocial health, self-concept, anxiety, and depression. It is designed to help you provide basic psychosocial care for patients in general practice settings.

PSYCHOSOCIAL HEALTH

Have you ever wondered why some health and life crises are easy to manage whereas others seem like the very last straw? The interactions of the mind and body are continuous and complex. One of the strengths of nursing is that we can go beyond a *biomedical* (disease-oriented) focus to care for the whole person. Nurses recognize that patient responses to illness are influenced not only by the physical pathology but also by the person's psychosocial health and its relationship to her overall wellness.

Theoretical Knowledge
knowing why

The term **psychosocial** encompasses both psychological and social factors: A person's psychological state interacts with his social development and position within society to contribute to his overall—or **biopsychosocial**—well-being (Figure 11–1). Figure 11–2 illustrates the interlocking psychosocial influences on health and personal development.

Keep in mind that any human dimension may dominate health needs at a given time. For example, a patient suffering from a severe flare-up of psoriasis (a skin disease characterized by red, scaly patches) may require physiologic interventions during the acute stage. He may not be ready to deal with body image issues until his skin lesions are better. Remember, though, that your patients' psychosocial needs are just

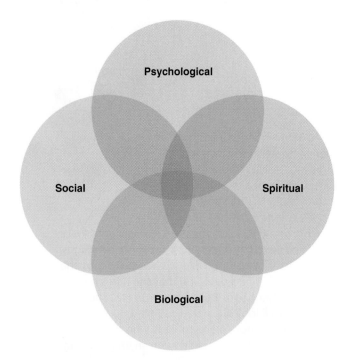

FIGURE 11–1 In the biopsychosocial view of health, biological, psychological, and social factors, as well as spirituality, all interact to contribute to a client's health.

as important as, for example, their dietary requirements or their level of pain.

You can think of **psychosocial theory** as a method of understanding people as a combination of psychologic and social events. For more information,

Go to Chapter 11, **Supplemental Materials: Psychosocial Theory,** on the Electronic Study Guide.

Of the many theories of *psychosocial development,* the works of the German psychologist Erik Erikson (1902–1994) are foremost. Using Erikson's theory, you can assess for successful completion of developmental

tasks. Refer to Chapter 9 for more information about Erikson's theory. For a summary of developmental tasks,

Go to Chapter 11, **Tables, Boxes, Figures: ESG Table 11–1,** on the Electronic Study Guide.

Chapter 8 presents another important psychosocial theory that is relevant for healthcare providers: psychologist Abraham Maslow's theory of self-actualization and self-transcendence. Maslow (1968) developed a widely accepted hierarchy of human needs and motivations, in which essential needs (e.g., air, water, and food) must be met before higher needs (e.g, learning, creating, understanding, and self-fulfillment). Recall that, in order from most basic to highest need, Maslow's hierarchy includes physiological, safety and security, love and belonging, self-esteem, and self-actualization needs.

KnowledgeCheck 11–1

- Why is psychosocial theory relevant to health care?
- What does the term *biopsychosocial* mean?
- Explain the implication of Maslow's hierarchy of human needs for working with a homeless man with gangrene.

Go to Chapter 11, **Knowledge Check Response Sheet and Answers,** on the Electronic Study Guide.

What Is Self-Concept?

A critical aspect of psychosocial health is **self-concept,** that is, one's overall view of oneself. Self-concept is your complete and unique answer to the question, "Who do you think you are?" (e.g., "I am a student"; "I am successful and competent"). Self-concept forms out of a person's evaluation of his physical appearance, sexual performance, intellectual abilities, success in the workplace, friendship and approval from others,

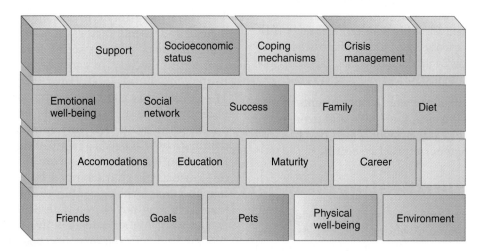

FIGURE 11–2 Interlocking psychosocial influences.

problem-solving and coping abilities, unique talents, and so on.

Self-concept both influences and is influenced by social functioning. For example, if it continues, Karli's perception that she is no longer pretty and that she "looks like a freak" (her self-concept) may cause her to withdraw from social interaction and make it difficult to form new relationships (social functioning). Equally, if others—for example, prospective employers—*do* see her as hideously ugly, she may have difficulty finding a place in society.

The "Dynamic Self"

Throughout the ages, mystics, philosophers, anthropologists, and psychologists have observed that the self forms and changes in response to our environment. Thousands of years ago, spiritual texts such as the Hindu *Bhagavad Gita* (or *Song of God*) distinguished between a higher Self, seen as eternal and immutable, and a lower self that is constantly changing as old ideas are discarded "like worn-out clothes." Centuries later, the Roman Catholic concepts of the soul and body would also reflect this theme.

Anthropologist Margaret Mead's (1934) theory states that discovering who we are is a lifelong process of differentiating from and comparing our self to others. As we experience life events, we continually reconstruct and develop an understanding of our self. Dickstein (1977) called this idea the **dynamic self,** meaning that who we are is subject to change through social and environmental influence.

If our concept or our self is changeable, how does it first develop? What factors cause it to change? Can it be harmed, and how? These questions are explored next.

How Is Self-Concept Formed?

Human beings are not born with a concept of self; rather, it develops during infancy and childhood as the child interacts with family members, peers, and others. The broad steps of self-concept formation are as follows:

1. (Infant) Learning that the physical self is different from the environment: "me; not me"
2. (Child) Internalizing others' attitudes about the self, primarily parents and peers: "Who do *they* say that I am?"
3. (Child and adult) Internalizing standards of society: "How do I compare to others?"
4. (Adult) Self-actualization and self-adjustment: "This *is* who I am and who I will continue to be."

ESG Table 11–2 summarizes the growth of self-concept through the various developmental stages. Change occurs gradually, and the stages overlap. Also,

the age at which the stages occur varies widely among individuals.

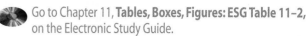
Go to Chapter 11, **Tables, Boxes, Figures: ESG Table 11–2,** on the Electronic Study Guide.

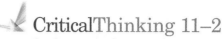

CriticalThinking 11–2

- Explain how each of Maslow's five basic needs is related to psychosocial development; that is, how might each of the needs affect psychosocial health if met or not met?
- To what extent do social relationships help or hinder a person in meeting each need?

What Factors Affect a Person's Self-Concept?

Of the factors affecting a person's self-concept, we begin with those that are fixed, such as gender, developmental level, and socioeconomic status. Understanding that such factors are not within a patient's control may help you provide more sensitive, compassionate care to patients experiencing impaired self concept.

Gender and Developmental Level

Certain aspects of self-concept differ by gender. For instance, girls typically rate teamwork and cooperation as important to their sense of self, whereas most boys place a higher value on individual achievement. In elementary and high school, boys have a higher self-concept for mathematical and physical dimensions, and girls have a higher self-concept for verbal and social skills (Bracken, 1996; Hattie, 1992). Incidentally, these differences appear to be related to the role expectations of boys and girls rather than any true difference in ability. Physical appearance seems more important to girls, and they may be less satisfied and more self-conscious throughout life because of this. As role expectations and career choices for both men and women expand, these gender-based differences in self-concept may fade.

As we mature, our self-concept becomes more objective; that is, our ideas about who we are are less influenced by others (e.g., friends, the media). We become less likely to view our failures and shortcomings as evidence of worthlessness and more likely to see them as challenges common to human beings everywhere. A few weeks before his death from a degenerative neurologic disease, sociologist Morrie Schwartz reminded his friend Mitch, "We all have the same beginning—birth—and we all have the same end—death. So how different can we be?" (Albom, 1997).

Socioeconomic Status

In the past, Caucasians in the United States were believed to have a higher self-concept than members of minority groups. However, recent research indicates that **socioeconomic status** (social class) is a greater

predictor of high or low self-concept than race (Crain, as cited in Bracken, 1996). In a country where material goods have a high social value, it seems logical that socioeconomic factors, such as income level and the ability to support oneself, would influence self concept.

Family and Peer Relationships

The family strongly influences a child's developing self-concept. As an infant's sense of self permanence develops and becomes stable, categories of self begin to emerge (Feiring & Taska, as cited in Bracken, 1996). These include notions of gender, values, and a sense of having a distinct "place" among family members. **Self-identity** develops as children become familiar with those who consistently interact with them. **Social identity** is first fostered by interactions between infants and their parents and broadens in toddlerhood through relationships with siblings, grandparents, and extended family members. For older children, peers become more important than family in this respect.

Internal Influences

Whereas the preceding external influences contribute to the *formation* of our self-concept, internal influences help us to *moderate* it. People who allow their inner "voice" to influence their self-concept have what is called an **internal locus of control.** Such people feel they can exert control over their lives. They take appropriate responsibility for their life experiences and for their responses to them. This enables them to interpret unexpected adverse events (e.g., injuries and illnesses) in a more positive light. For example, consider a new mother who wanted a natural birth but consented to an emergency cesarean. With an internal locus of control, she might say, "Well, I wanted a natural birth like my sister and my best friend had, but when the midwife told me that my baby wasn't breathing right, the type of birth suddenly didn't seem important. I chose a cesarean, and now I have a beautiful, healthy baby. That's what really matters."

In contrast, when people have an **external locus of control,** they attribute control of their situation to external factors, including other people, institutions, and God. Given the same set of circumstances, a mother with an external locus of control might report: "I wanted a natural birth, but I knew as soon as I walked into the hospital I'd be forced to do things their way. Sure enough, the midwife told me that I had to have a cesarean."

KnowledgeCheck 11–2

- When does self concept become stable?
- What factors have been determined to have an impact on our self concept?

 Go to Chapter 11, **Knowledge Check Response Sheet and Answers,** on the Electronic Study Guide.

What Are the Components of Self-Concept?

To sociologists and psychologists, self-concept is a form of shorthand that embraces four interrelated components: body image, role performance, personal identity, and self-esteem.

Body Image

How often do you hear someone say something like the following?

> "Look at the muscles on that man. He looks good!"
>
> "I shouldn't eat this cookie, it probably has 200 calories."
>
> "Look at her pigging out. She needs that candy like I need a hole in my head."

As a child, you probably grew up overhearing similar statements. Such preoccupations with food, weight, and appearance have led to a prejudice against people who do not have perfect bodies. No wonder that people engage in unhealthy behaviors in order to be thin or that patients like Karli have difficulty coping with disfiguring accidents or with surgeries such as limb amputation and mastectomy.

Body image is your mental image of your physical self, including physical appearance and physical functioning. Both cognitive understanding and sensory input influence body image. For instance, if you understand that darkly tanned skin can indicate harmful exposure to the sun, then you might perceive your own untanned skin as positive, despite media messages to the contrary. Our cognitive understanding is in turn influenced by family, social, and cultural norms; education; and exposure to alternative values. The American media portray the ideal male as a young, tall, and muscular; nevertheless, many older, short, slender men maintain a positive body image because their cognitive understanding indicates that they are in good health, are attractive to their partners, and so on.

Ideal Versus Perceived and Actual Body Image

People do not always see their own bodies as objectively as others see them. Some psychological disorders interfere with the ability to interpret sensory data objectively. For example, people with the eating disorders **anorexia nervosa** and **bulimia nervosa** see themselves as fat even when their mirror reflects, and other people see, an emaciated body. The closer the match between a person's **ideal body image** and sensory input about his or her body (**perceived body image),** the more positive the person's body image is likely to be.

Example: For Janalee, thick, luxurious hair is an important component of her ideal body image. Amy

hardly thinks about her hair at all; she keeps it very short so that it is easy to care for. Both women have been receiving chemotherapy to treat their cancer, and both are experiencing severe hair loss. Which person do you think will be more likely to experience body image disturbance because of this?

Influence of Appearance and Function on Body Image

Not surprisingly, a physical handicap such as blindness, deafness, or paraplegia can interfere with the development of a positive body image. Children born with a physical handicap have a high incidence of poor self-concept and depression. This is partially due to the physically handicapped child's inability to form adequate social relationships, but it may also relate to the person's perception that he has low social value.

In contrast, an attractive appearance and superior functioning, whether in a career, sports, or academics, contribute to a positive body image. But again, cognitive understanding can increase self-concept even in people who are average in appearance or achievement. For instance, adolescents of average appearance who learn to value integrity, honesty, teamwork, and other social values more than physical attractiveness or success in sports are less likely to suffer from body image disturbance.

Gradual Versus Sudden Body Changes

Gradual changes in physical appearance occur naturally throughout life as the body matures and grows old. Most people adapt to such changes relatively easily, especially because their friends and colleagues are aging, too. In contrast, when changes in appearance or functioning occur abruptly (e.g., following an acute illness or an accident, as happened to your patient, Karli), they are much more difficult to accept. Denial, anger, self-hatred, and despair are a few of many reactions that can follow such an abrupt change in body image. In *Still Me,* actor Christopher Reeve describes the "demons" that haunted him in the first weeks after his cervical spinal cord injury. "I'd try to go back to sleep, but it wouldn't work, and I'd start to think again, the same tormenting thoughts. It always began with: This can't be me. . . ." (Reeve, 1998).

Influence of Body Image on Health

Body image influences health and health behaviors. A negative body image has been associated with depression (Walker, Timmerman, Kim, & Sterling, 2002), with initiation of smoking among adolescents (Winter, de Guia, Ferrence, & Cohen, 2002; Stice & Shaw, 2003) and to increased risk for unintended pregnancy, sexually transmitted diseases, and HIV infection (Wingood, DiClemente, Harrington, & Davies, 2002). In contrast, a positive body image was found to be a major contributor to overall life happiness in adult women (Stokes &

Frederick-Recascino, 2003). There is not yet enough evidence to determine how much of the effects is due to body image alone and how much to body image in combination with other psychological issues.

Role Performance

Before you began your nursing program, what were your expectations? What activities did you imagine yourself engaged in, and what behaviors did you think would be expected of you? Together, these expectations make up your conception of the *role* of nursing student. In addition to being a student, you probably play several roles, such as parent, sibling, friend, breadwinner, caregiver, volunteer, and so on.

Role performance can be defined as the actions a person takes and the behaviors he demonstrates in fulfilling a role. Instead of expectations, role performance is the reality. If you expected that you would sail through your nursing program and instead you find yourself so overwhelmed that lately you have begun to skip classes, then you are experiencing **role strain,** a mismatch between role expectations and role performance. Additionally, your ideas about how to perform the nursing student role may be very different from those of your instructors. When such a mismatch occurs, you are experiencing an **interpersonal role conflict.** Other types of role conflict are also common. For instance, what if you are a single parent and your child's sudden illness causes you to miss a week of classes and clinicals? When two roles make competing demands on an individual, **interrole conflict** occurs.

Personal Identity

How would you describe yourself to others? Make a list of ten labels or short phrases that describe who you are (e.g., student, motorcycle rider, woman). Then list them in order, with the most important one first. Are you happy with your list? Are you satisfied with who you are? Compare your list with a friend's list. Could you identify her based on her list of identifying labels? Could she identify you?

Your **personal identity** is your view of yourself as a unique human being, different and separate from all others. Unlike body image, which is expected to change over time, personal identity is relatively constant and consistent. It is culturally determined and learned through socialization. Identity develops over time, beginning in childhood when you identified with your parents, and then later with teachers, peers, and others.

People with a strong sense of personal identity are less likely to compare themselves to, or be unduly influenced by, others. They tend to appreciate the unique perspective and contributions of others and value their own perspectives and contributions. In contrast, people with a weak sense of personal identity have difficulty distinguishing their boundaries

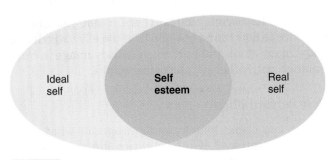

Ideal self: expectations and aspirations; "what I ought to be," "what I wish I were"

Real self: current skills, attributes, and successes; "what I really am"

FIGURE 11–3 Self esteem is determined by the relationship between an individual's ideal self and real self.

from those of others. They may interpret events in the environment personally, or they may interpret their personal experiences as belonging to everyone. For example, a patient with a weak personal identity may insist that a breakdown in the hospital's air conditioning system is a punishment for his complaint that his room was too cold.

Patients may experience an impaired sense of identity when they are challenged by a serious or chronic illness (e.g., cancer, AIDS, or rheumatoid arthritis). They then place too many limitations on their activities or interpret the responses of others in light of their illness. For instance, a woman with osteoporosis (loss of bone density) might say, "I used to enjoy going bird watching, but I don't go anymore because I might trip and fall."

 ### CriticalThinking 11–3

Think about Karli in the "Meet Your Patient" scenario. If you asked Karli to list ten labels to identify herself, what do you think they would be? (You may not have enough information to come up with ten, but think of as many as you can.)

Self-Esteem

Self-esteem is, in the simplest terms, how well a person likes himself. It is the difference between the "ideal self" and "actual self," that is, between "what I think I ought (or want) to be" and "what I really am." The area of overlap in Figure 11–3 illustrates the extent of self-esteem. The more overlap, the higher the self-esteem.

The balance between our self-expectations and our true abilities can be precarious to maintain. When we succeed beyond our ambitions, then we experience a high sense of self-esteem; but when we aim for an ideal self beyond our capabilities, then we risk loss of self-esteem. For example, if as a nursing student you find that you are more successful than you expected to be when you enrolled in your nursing program, that is a boost to your self-esteem. If, however, your expectations

of being a skillful nurse outweigh your current abilities, then low self-esteem is likely.

It is not difficult to imagine how a sudden, disfiguring accident such as Karli's might provoke a crisis in self esteem, but even mild illnesses and minor setbacks can cause some people to question their self worth. This is especially true if the problem is interpreted as one incident in a continuing pattern. Consider, for instance, a couple hoping to become parents who experience a third miscarriage, or a man who aspires to be a full professor at a leading university who is laid off from his fourth teaching job at a community college.

 ### CriticalThinking 11–4

• What if a person does not have any aspirations to success, but is content to meet each day as a learner, vitalized by her daily discoveries? How do you think a high score on an exam would affect her self-esteem? How do you think a poor score on a clinical skills test would affect her self-esteem?

KnowledgeCheck 11–3

• What four components contribute to an individual's self-concept?
• What is self-esteem?

 Go to Chapter 11, **Knowledge Check Response Sheet and Answers,** on the Electronic Study Guide.

Practical Knowledge
knowing how

Physical illness may be particularly stressful when it occurs in combination with psychosocial issues. For example, think of Karli ("Meet Your Patient"). Might her condition have been less complicated if (1) she had no disfiguring injuries or (2) if she were an older adult at a developmental stage when appearance is less crucial?

| Assessment |

No matter what the patient's medical diagnosis, you need to perform accurate and ongoing psychosocial assessments in order to develop holistic nursing diagnoses and interventions.

Psychosocial Assessments

A comprehensive psychosocial assessment should include the following categories (Newell & Gournay, 2000, p.107):

• Biological, psychological, and social details
• Functional abilities (behavioral performance)
• Self-efficacy (the belief that you can influence your own behaviors and outcomes)

- Family relationships
- Relationships with the wider social environment
- Interpersonal communication
- Social resources and networks
- Understanding about current illness
- Usual coping mechanisms
- Health priorities

For an example of a psychosocial assessment tool,

 Go to Chapter 11, **Tables, Boxes, Figures: ESG Figure 11–1,** on the Electronic Study Guide.

Psychosocial information is personal and sometimes sensitive. To encourage patients to share this information, you will need to use your developing communication skills. For example:

- Use active listening through eye contact and verbal response.
- Proceed from general details ("How do you get along with your parents?") to the specific ("Does your mother ever hit you?").
- Use an open and positive voice tone, facial expression, and body language.
- Be respectful and sensitive to cultural and gender-specific details.
- Use open-ended questions (questions that cannot be answered with a yes or no).
- Follow the patient's cues by using reflection and restating.
- Be flexible and use humor as appropriate.
- Provide empathetic feedback and touch as appropriate.

See Chapter 18 for more information about communication skills.

 Critical Thinking 11–5

Psychologically, Karli is worried about the unfairness of her situation, and is probably struggling with body image issues. In addition, what do you think her *social* concerns might be?

Assessing Self-Concept and Self-Esteem

If you were working in a mental health agency, you would probably collect in-depth information regarding self-concept by using a psychological measurement tool. However, for an all-purpose nursing assessment that you might use in any setting,

 Go to Chapter 11, **Technique 11–1: Assessing Self-Concept Problems,** in Volume 2.

Also observe for behaviors and comments specifically associated with low self esteem. People with low self-esteem tend to avoid eye contact and have a

stooped posture. They may move slowly and have poor grooming. Their verbal behaviors include speaking hesitantly, being overly critical of others and of self ("I never do anything right"), not accepting positive comments about self ("Oh, anybody could have done it"), apologizing frequently, and verbalizing feelings of powerlessness ("Whatever you say is fine with me"; "It doesn't matter what I do; it won't change anything"). To assess specifically for the self-esteem dimension of a person's self-concept,

 Go to Chapter 11, **Technique 11–2: Performing a Self-Esteem Inventory,** in Volume 2.

When assessing self-concept, keep an open mind—do not automatically assume on the basis of a patient's psychosocial history or physical handicaps that she suffers from low self-concept. If you suspect serious problems with self-concept, document the patient's responses in your nursing notes and refer the patient for appropriate psychological testing.

 Critical Thinking 11–6

In the "Meet Your Patient" scenario, Karli perceives herself as unlovable "looking this way." You should not assume that you know exactly what Karli means by this.

- Which of her words do you need to clarify with her?
- What might you say to her to get her to provide more information about the psychosocial meaning of her statement?

| Nursing Diagnosis |

Psychosocial and self-concept issues can be a problem, a symptom of a problem, or the etiology of a problem. It is important for you to determine what is cause and what is effect, although this can be hard to unravel at times. As you can see in Table 11–1, what you identify significantly affects your choice of goals and nursing activities.

Psychosocial Diagnoses

Psychosocial issues involve nearly all areas of patient functioning, so there is some overlap between what we are calling "psychosocial" diagnoses and those used in the rest of the chapter to describe the more specific problems of self-concept, anxiety, and depression. That is, you may use some of these psychosocial diagnoses for clients who have problems of self-concept, anxiety, and depression. It would be impossible to list every possible psychosocial diagnosis; the following are but a few.

- *Interrupted Family Processes.* Use when there has been a change in family relationships and/or functioning that is significantly affecting the patient's health.
- *Family Coping [Compromised and/or Disabled].* Use when support (comfort and assistance) from a usual family member or significant other is either

TABLE 11-1 Implications of Identifying a Psychosocial Issue as Problem, Etiology, or Symptom

Note the differences in the goals and interventions for each nursing diagnosis.

Nursing Diagnosis	As Problem	As Etiology	As Symptom
	Interrupted Family Processes r/t tumult from parental divorce	Delayed Development r/t lack of stimulation **secondary to Interrupted Family Processes** (parental divorce)	Ineffective Individual Coping (Mother) r/t poor judgment and impaired reality perception, **as manifested by Interrupted Family Processes** and risk-taking behaviors
Sample Goals (based on problem)	*NOC Outcome* Family Functioning	*NOC Outcome* Child Development: 4 Years	*NOC Outcomes* Coping, Decision Making, Role Performance, Social Support, Impulse Control
	Goals Members perform expected family roles Family cares for dependent members	*Goals* Child demonstrates age-appropriate motor activities Child uses four- and five-word sentences	*Goals* Identifies coping strategies that have been effective in the past Discusses the implications of decision alternatives with family
Sample Interventions and Activities (based on etiology)	*NIC Interventions* Family Integrity Promotion Family Process Maintenance Normalization Promotion	*NIC Interventions* Developmental Enhancement: Child Parent Education Health Screening	*NIC Interventions* Coping Enhancement Decision-Making Support Impulse Control Training Family Involvement Promotion Support Group Support System Enhancement
	Specific Activities Promote parental involvement in health care. Assist the family with skills and education of conflict resolution, coping skills, and problem solving. Link the individual and family to the appropriate support and education services.	*Specific Activities* Establish time for one-on-one care. Provide for creative play (e.g., clay, blocks, painting). Teach parents appropriate stimulation. Teach parents about developmental milestones and expected behaviors. Assess changes in family processes.	*Specific Activities* Identify and discuss alternative behaviors. Encourage to delay decision making when under stress. Help the mother solve problems constructively. Assist her to evaluate her own behavior. Identify and discuss past successful coping behaviors she has used.

compromised (insufficient or withdrawn) or disabled (competing or maladapted), causing a significant health challenge.

- *Parental Role Conflict.* Use when you assess significant role confusion and/or conflict by a parent in response to crises.
- *Ineffective Individual Coping.* Use when the patient fails to comprehend and effectively judge stressors, when he perceives incorrect or dangerous life choices as normal, and when there is an inability

to use available resources. Inability to identify strengths and resources may be secondary to low self esteem.

- *Post Trauma Syndrome* applies where there is a maladaptive learned response to a traumatic and distressing event.
- *Risk for Loneliness* exists when there is separation from persons, culture, objects, or environments to which a person may have ongoing attachments.

• *Social Isolation* applies when the person experiences significant aloneness that has a negative impact on health, or when the isolation is perceived as a threat to health.

• *Risk for Violence: Directed at Others* can be used in situations in which a person threatens or uses aggression or violence to harm others. The intention of harm may not be limited to physical harm.

• *Impaired Social Interaction.* Use for patients who show significant difficulties in social exchange due to an inability to use social skills.

Self-Concept Diagnoses

When analyzing data for self-concept problems, keep the following two guidelines in mind:

• *Avoid seeking simplistic cause-and-effect relationships.* Instead, recognize the complexity of human responses. For example:

> Molly, a 19-year-old student, has just been admitted to your unit and is presenting with clinical depression and low self-esteem. Is Molly depressed because she has low self-esteem? Or is longstanding low self-esteem causing her to feel depressed? Or are the two interrelated?

• *Avoid confusing low self-concept with clinical emotional and/or behavioral psychiatric diagnoses.* There is no recognized diagnosis, describing self-concept disorder in the American Psychiatric Association's current *Diagnostic and Statistical Manual of Mental Disorders* (DSM-IV-TR, 2000). Self-concept (particularly self-esteem) plays a secondary role in a number of disorders but is not a primary disorder itself (Prout & Prout, in Bracken, 1996).

As is true of most conditions, a self-concept issue may be described by a NANDA problem label, or it may be the etiology (cause) of other problems.

Self-Concept or Body Image as a Problem

A problem with body image or self-concept occurs when the problem is the result of a condition and might not exist if not for the condition (e.g., a profoundly deaf adolescent develops self-worth problems). The following nursing diagnoses may be useful for patients with either low overall self concept or difficulties in specific domains of self-concept (e.g., self-esteem):

• *Chronic Low Self-Esteem.* The person expresses ongoing (longstanding) overall self-dissatisfaction and negative self-appraisal (i.e., wide differences between "ideal" and "actual" or "perceived" self). *Etiologies* include but are not limited to depression, mismatch in ideal and perceived self, dysfunctional family, anxiety, or failure to adapt to a change in physical appearance or functioning.

• *Situational Low Self-Esteem.* An individual exhibits self-disapproval and negative self-evaluations as a specific reaction to loss or change. *Etiologies:* See Chronic Low Self-Esteem, preceding.

• *Disturbed Personal Identity.* Negative and incorrect assessment of self-identity and inability to determine boundaries between self and others. *Etiologies* include but are not limited to distorted perceptions of self, such as occur in certain mental illnesses; loss of health, limb, physical appearance, or functioning; dysfunctional family.

• *Ineffective Role Performance.* A person experiences or perceives difficulty in fulfilling a usual role, or there is a mismatch between role expectations and role performance (either perceived or societal expectations). *Etiologies* include but are not limited to job demands exceeding abilities, inadequate resources or support system, family conflicts, domestic violence, unrealistic role expectations, lack of a role model, substance abuse, cognitive deficits, illness or disease, low self-esteem, pain, fatigue, cognitive deficits.

• *Disturbed Body Image.* An individual has a confused image of his physical self or negatively evaluates his body or an aspect of it. *Etiologies* include but are not limited to loss of functioning or appearance (e.g., acne, scars, breast removal, amputation), eating disorder, gender conflict, or personality disorder.

CriticalThinking 11–7

• Refer to Karli in "Meet Your Patient." Look at the preceding five NANDA labels for self-concept problems (Chronic Low Self-Esteem, Situational Low Self-Esteem, Disturbed Personal Identity, Ineffective Role Performance, Disturbed Body Image). Which one most clearly applies to Karli? Explain your thinking.

• How would you write the nursing diagnosis (problem r/t etiology)?

Self-Concept or Body Image as Etiology

Self-concept problems are an etiology when they precede a condition such as depression and play a central role in the condition (e.g., low self-esteem causing and maintaining depression or leading to an anxiety disorder). The following are examples of nursing diagnoses with self-concept (e.g., self-esteem) as the etiology:

• *Impaired Adjustment* should be used where a patient experiences difficulties adapting perception and evaluation of self after changes in health status.

• *Anticipatory* or *Dysfunctional Grieving* may develop in anticipation of or following body changes (e.g., hysterectomy) or loss of key roles (e.g., death of a spouse).

• *Deficient Knowledge* of healthcare situation may occur because of low self-esteem and lack of confidence in ability to learn or to manage care. Low self-esteem diminishes motivation to learn.

| Planning Interventions/Implementation |

Interventions for anxious clients will depend on the cause of the anxiety; however, for *all* anxious clients, regardless of the etiology, the nursing goals in most situations are to help the client:

1. *Recognize that he is anxious.* Because the symptoms may be varied, subtle, and physical, a person may demonstrate anxious behaviors without even realizing why he is doing so. Or he may attribute his symptoms to a physical illness.
2. *Identify the source of his anxiety.* This may sometimes require a more extended relationship than you might have with a hospitalized client, because it involves the uncovering of emotional conflicts. Nevertheless, a more permanent relief can be obtained once the client recognizes the conflict and can use his conscious, rational mind to deal with it.
3. *Deal with the symptoms of his anxiety,* for example, with massage, relaxation techniques, and so forth.

NIC standardized interventions and selected activities for anxiety-related diagnoses are listed in Volume 2.

 Go to Chapter 11, **Tables, Selected Standardized Outcomes and Interventions for Anxiety-Related Diagnoses,** in Volume 2.

Specific nursing activities for reducing anxiety include the following:

- Provide a calm and safe environment, including a quiet, reassuring approach to communication and nursing activities. This will help the person remain centered and focused.
- Establish a relationship of trust, caring, and unconditional positive regard (i.e., don't make promises you can't keep; don't make any "judgment" statements, such as, "You ought to . . ." or "You shouldn't . . .").
- Be present and stay with the individual to help allay fears, create trust, and promote safety.
- Help the person identify triggers and situations that create anxiety.
- Use clear and factual knowledge that is tailored to the individual's circumstances.
- Explain and, if necessary, explore details of all health-care procedures.
- Develop coping strategies and behavior modification techniques.
- Encourage enjoyable, nonstressful activities to give the person opportunity to think about something other than the anxiety-producing situation.
- Advise regular physical exercise unless contraindicated by a physical condition.
- Control the environment by removing anxiety-provoking equipment and people.

- Administer and monitor antianxiety medication when required.
- Assist the individual in relaxation methods, such as biofeedback, meditation, and therapeutic touch. See Chapter 40 for specific information about these methods.
- In addition, specific interventions for Death Anxiety include the following (also refer to Chapter 15):

   Stay physically close to the patient when he is fearful.
   Obtain spiritual support for the patient and family, as needed.
   Inquire about the patient's and family's specific requests for care.

Nursing Care for Depression

The nurse-patient relationship is vital when you work with people who are depressed. Whereas an anxious patient may actively seek your assistance, a depressed person is likely to avoid your approach and may even feel unworthy of your time and effort. Establishing a nurse-patient bond requires a specific, empathetic approach involving warmth, acceptance, and understanding (unconditional positive regard) even in the face of an unresponsive, even angry, reaction.

| Assessment |

When assessing for depression you should observe for symptoms in the following areas:

- *Affective:* Denial of feelings, anger, anxiety, guilt, helplessness, hopelessness, sadness
- *Behavioral:* Tearfulness, regression, restlessness, agitation, withdrawal, past or current alcohol or substance abuse, past history of suicide attempts
- *Cognitive:* Preoccupation with loss (e.g., of job, of function), self blame, ambivalence, blaming others
- *Physiological:* Anorexia or overeating, insomnia or hypersomnia, headache, backache, chest pain, constipation

Because depression is so common, many of the patients you see in other areas (e.g., medical-surgical, maternity, clinics) will have at least some degree of depression. It will be important for you to differentiate between temporary, situational sadness, low energy, and a psychiatric diagnosis (clinical depression). Figure 11–5 illustrates the continuum of mild to severe depression incorporating aspects of mood, behavior, thoughts, and physical symptoms. For two alternative methods you can use for identifying patients who should be referred to a mental health specialist for evaluation and/or treatment of depression,

 Go to Chapter 11, **Technique 11–3: Identifying Depressed Patients Who Should Be Referred for Evaluation,** in Volume 2.

If you suspect severe depression, document the patient's responses in your nursing notes, and refer the patient to a mental health specialist. If you believe there is a risk of suicide, refer immediately. Presence of any of the following should alert you to make a referral (U.S. Preventive Services Task Force, 2005):

- Personal history of recurrent depression or bipolar disorder
- Family history of recurrent depression or bipolar disorder
- Personal history of recurrence of depression within 1 year after stopping effective treatment
- Episode of major depression before age 20
- Severe, sudden, or life-threatening depressive episode (i.e., suicide attempt)

Nursing Diagnosis

Depression is a psychiatric diagnosis, so you will not make that diagnosis. Nevertheless, you will need to describe associated problems that are appropriate for nursing intervention. The NANDA taxonomy does not have a specific diagnosis that uses the term *depression;* however, the following nursing diagnoses may be useful in describing the feelings and mood of patients who are depressed:

- *Hopelessness* may apply to an individual who is unable to seek or comprehend opportunities, options, and alternatives because of distressed emotional and unmotivated state. Note that research shows hopelessness to be highly correlated with suicide (Ghosh & Victor, 1994; Beck, Brown, & Berchick, 1990).
- *Powerlessness* may be diagnosed when an individual's perception of control over situations and life events is significantly impaired and externally based.
- *Risk for Suicide* must always be considered when a patient is depressed, especially when the person has a history of prior attempts or is verbalizing the desire to die or the intent to kill himself.

Remember that depression can cause a variety of physical and behavioral problems, such as the following:

Sleep Pattern Disturbance	Imbalanced Nutrition: More than Body Requirements
Adult Failure to Thrive	
Activity Intolerance	Ineffective Health Maintenance
Constipation	
Disturbed Thought Processes	Ineffective Therapeutic Regimen Management
Disturbed Sleep Pattern	Impaired Social Interaction
Fatigue	
Imbalanced Nutrition: Less than Body Requirements	Noncompliance
	Self-Care Deficit (Bathing/Hygiene, Dressing/Grooming)

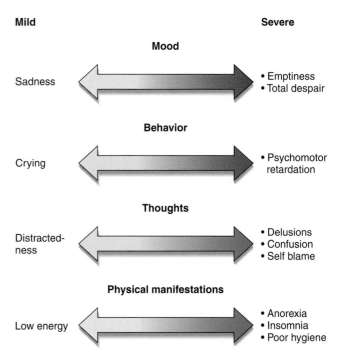

FIGURE 11–5   Assessment continuum incorporating mood, behavior, thoughts, and physical state.

The NANDA diagnoses of Situational and Chronic Low Self-Esteem are also useful because depressed clients often experience low self-esteem. These diagnoses were presented in the preceding "Self-Concept Diagnoses" section (see pp. 195–196).

Planning Outcomes/Evaluation

You will use outcomes developed in the planning stage as criteria for evaluating the patient's progress and the success of your nursing interventions.

For *selected NOC standardized outcomes and indicators* for depression-related diagnoses,

 Go to Chapter 11, **Tables, Selected Standardized Outcomes and Interventions for Depression-Related Diagnoses,** in Volume 2.

Individualized goal/outcome statements should relate to the patient's specific nursing diagnosis, stating behaviors that will indicate that the problem is resolving. The following are some examples:

For Depressed Mood:
  Affect is appropriate to the situation.
  Refrains from negative self-talk.
  Engages in positive self-talk.
  Reports feeling less sadness and depression.
  Interacts willingly and appropriately with others.
  Eats a well-balanced diet to prevent weight loss.
  Sleeps 6 to 8 hours per night and reports feeling rested.

Bathes, washes and combs hair, dresses—
maintains grooming and hygiene.

For Hopelessness:
Expresses positive belief in self, others, and
meaning of life.
Demonstrates interest in life/activity.
Displays stabilization and control of mood.
Maintains spiritual belief system or religious
affiliation.

For Powerlessness:
Participates in group activities (e.g., church,
sports, book group).
Participates in heathcare decisions to the extent
possible.
Assumes responsibility for engaging in healthy
behaviors.
Sets realistic goals for self.

For Risk for Suicide:
Verbalizes any suicidal ideas to staff.
Trusts staff enough to disclose any specific plans
for suicide.
Does not attempt suicide.

| Planning Interventions/Implementation |

For *NIC standardized interventions and selected activities* for depression-related diagnoses,

Go to Chapter 11, **Tables, Selected Standardized
Outcomes and Interventions for Depression-Related
Diagnoses,** in Volume 2.

Individualized nursing activities for depression-
related diagnoses focus on altering the problem etiologies and relieving symptoms of depression. In general,
care of the depressed person involves (1) developing a
therapeutic relationship through effective communi-

cation and (2) promoting nutrition, exercise, and personal hygiene.

- Use therapeutic communication:

  Be honest and open.
  Be patient.
  Be consistent.
  Do not use false reassurance ("You'll feel better
  soon").
  Avoid phrases such as, "Cheer up," or, "Think how
  lucky you are to have a good family."
  Do make comments such as, "I like the way you
  look in that dress."
  Do not be overly cheerful.
  Encourage the client to express feelings, including
  anger.
  Be accepting and nonjudgmental when the client
  expresses feelings.
  Encourage communication that explores reality,
  grief, and personal loss.

- Promote activity. Activities in small groups can help
  build self-esteem.

- Promote and teach good nutrition and hydration.

- Provide support as needed for self-care and decision
  making, while promoting as much independence as
  possible.

- Assess for and provide information about use of
  complementary and alternative therapies for depression (see accompanying box).

- Monitor for suicide risk. Ask directly: "Have you
  thought about harming yourself? If so, what do you
  plan to do?"

- Institute measures to build self-esteem (see "Promoting Self-Esteem and Self-Concept" on page 197).

- Provide information on support and educational
  groups.

- Encourage the person to maintain his religious affil-
  iations.

Many people use herbal therapies to relieve symptoms of anxiety and depression. Patients may self-treat, or herbal therapies may be prescribed by CAM practitioners. You should assess for CAM to be sure the method is not contraindicated and that the patient has informed the primary care provider about its use.

Depression

CAM	Active Ingredients	Side Effects	Contraindications	Patient Teaching
Ginkgo biloba	Ginkgentin, ginkgolic acid, zascorbic acid, flavonols, sterols	Nausea Vomiting Diarrhea Headache	Pregnant or breast-feeding Children Patients using anti-coagulants (use with caution)	Can take 6–8 weeks for patient to feel any better. Mixing with some fruits and nuts could produce poison ivy–like reaction.
Ginseng	Ginsenosides, beta-elemine, sterols, flavonoids, peptides, vitamins B_1, B_2, B_{12}, nicotinic acid, fats, minerals, enzymes	(many) Nausea Vomiting Diarrhea Chest pain Headache Nosebleeds Palpitations Nervousness Insomnia	Cardiovascular disease Hypertension Hypotension Diabetes Pregnancy or breast-feeding	There are many kinds of ginseng; patient should look up the specific type he is using.
Kava	Kavapyrones, pypermethystine	Visual disturbances Changes in reflexes and judgment Decreased platelet and lymphocyte counts	Pregnancy Breastfeeding Use of alcohol, alprazolam, or CNS depressants	May experience symptom relief within 1 week. Significant adverse reactions may occur. Kava enhances effects of alcohol and CNS medications.
St. John's wort	Tannin, naphthodi-anthrones, flavonoids, bio-flavonoids, phloroglucinols	Dry mouth Constipation GI upset Sleep disturbances Restlessness	Pregnancy or lactation Children Use of MAOIs, alcohol, or OTC cold and flu medications	Teach contraindications and side effects.
SAMe	Amino acid and ATP, which are pro-duced naturally in the body and are now being reproduced artificially as well	Few side effects Gastric upset Hypomania (in patients with bipolar disorder) Anxiety (in patients with depression) Headache		Patients with bipolar disorder should not use this supplement unless under direct supervision of their physician. Use enteric-coated forms to decrease gastric irritation.

Anxiety

Kava	See "Depression," preceding.

Source: Adapted from Neeb, K. (2001). *Fundamentals of mental health nursing* (2nd ed.). Philadelphia: F. A. Davis Company, pp. 365–378.

| toward evidence-based practice |

The following nursing research article demonstrates an example of how research can be used to formulate strategies to help patients with their psychosocial health.

Dewar, A. (2003). Boosting strategies: Enhancing the self-esteem of individuals with catastrophic illnesses and injuries. *Journal of Psychosocial Nursing and Mental Health* Services, *41*(3), 24–32, 42–43.

This study investigated the psychological endurance of chronically ill persons who had suffered severe, life-threatening changes in their health (such as cancer, spinal cord injuries, renal disease, severe heart disease, massive burns, or multiple sclerosis). The author used a qualitative research method on a sample of 28 people. Results revealed that the participants were able to improve self-esteem and psychosocial health with the strategy of "boosting communication" through "social and temporal downward comparisons." *Downward comparison* refers to the patient's comparison of himself to others in worse condition. *Temporal comparison* refers to the patient's comparison of his present situation to the situation (better or worse) at a different time (past or future).

Boosting. Patients used three principal strategies—protecting, modifying, and boosting—to make adaptations and adjustments that maintained and enhanced their physical and psychosocial well-being. *Boosting* consists of comparing self to others or to worsening situations (upward and downward social comparisons).

Selective Evaluation. Patients became very distressed when health professionals made comparisons about them. When patients made such comparisons themselves, they were *selective*—meaning that they chose specific cases at certain times, not to minimize their situation but to focus on the positives.

---

1. If selective self-evaluation led to downward comparison and temporal comparison, what effect do you think this had on the patients' self esteem?

2. How might you encourage patients to use boosting strategies?

3. Based on study findings, what would you be careful *not* to do as you encouraged patients to use boosting strategies?

 Go to Chapter 11, **Toward Evidence-Based Practice Suggestion Responses,** on the Electronic Study Guide.

 Go to Chapter 11, **Resources for Caregivers and Health Professionals,** on the Electronic Study Guide.

 Suggested Readings: Go to Chapter 11, **Reading More About Psychosocial Health and Illness,** on the Electronic Study Guide.

 Bibliography: Go to Volume 2, Bibliography.

The Family

Learning Outcomes

After completing this chapter, you should be able to:

* Distinguish among different family structures.

* Describe approaches to working with various types of families to provide optimal care to both well and ill clients.

* Explain how family theories provide a framework to understand family functioning.

* Identify family risk factors in five different stages of the family life span.

* Discuss ways in which economic factors influence nursing practice, family care, and access to services.

* State how HIV/AIDS can affect families.

* Identify populations most at risk for homelessness.

* Demonstrate an understanding of family violence.

* Conduct a family assessment.

* Identify common health beliefs and communication patterns among families.

* Identify nursing interventions appropriate when a family member is ill.

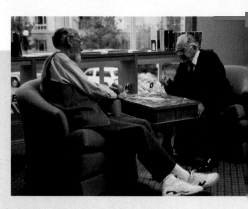

Your Patient

J.B. is an 80-year-old man who is hospitalized for end-stage renal disease. His wife died 4 years ago. His remaining family includes two married daughters and four grandchildren. J.B. has several siblings, but they live far away and phone or visit only rarely.

J.B. has lived in the same neighborhood for over 55 years. When he and his wife, Pamela, first moved into the neighborhood, they lived across the street from Mike and Lena. The two couples socialized, raised their children, and enjoyed many holidays and festivities together. After the children were grown, the two couples sold their homes and each moved into a townhouse near the center of town. They lived next door to each other and continued to spend time together. A year after Pamela died, Mike's wife, Lena, died from liver cancer.

J.B. and Mike now spend every day together. J.B. subscribes to the local paper, and Mike gets a national paper. They read both papers together over breakfast before they start the events of the day. They have season tickets to the baseball games and watch sports together on the TV. "Thank goodness we have each other," says Mike. Mike comes to the hospital every morning. He brings both papers and breakfast muffins for J.B., himself, and the staff. He spends the day at the hospital and leaves shortly after dinner.

Theoretical Knowledge
knowing why

WHAT IS A FAMILY?

Traditionally, people have thought of a family as consisting of a husband, wife, and their children. However, as lifestyles have changed, the concept of family has become broader. We define **family** as a group of individuals who provide physical, emotional, and economic support and assistance to each other (Figure 12–1). They may or may not be blood relatives. Most often, people who consider themselves to be family live in the same household; however, adult children living apart from their parents may still define themselves as belonging to one family, which may also include siblings, aunts and uncles, and cousins. In short, families come in many forms.

Family Structures

A husband who is in the labor force, a wife who is not, and one or more children living together constitute a *traditional nuclear family*. Such families now represent only 13% of all married-couple families in the United States. In contrast, *dual-earner families* with children now represent 31% of married-couple families (Population Reference Bureau, 2003).

Single-parent families result from divorce, from the death of a partner, or when partners choose not to marry or live together. They make up about 25% of all families with children. Most single-parent families are headed by women; however, the number of father-only families has increased. Single parents often remarry to form new structures, such as *stepfamilies* (in which a single parent marries someone who may or may not have children), and *blended families* (in which two single parents marry and raise their children together).

Adults who are *married but have no children* account for 13% of American families (Population Reference Bureau, 2003). *Cohabiting adults* choose to live together but not marry or live together as a "trial run" prior to marriage. Cohabiting couples who marry have a higher rate of separation than their counterparts who do not live together prior to marriage.

In many cultural groups, it is common for *extended family* members (e.g., grandparents, aunts, uncles, cousins) to live within a single dwelling and be considered immediate family. Although J.B.'s siblings are members of his extended family, they do not live with him, and he would not consider them part of his immediate family. The growing number of older adults has created the "sandwiched generation" (Schwartz, 1979), in which middle-aged adults who still have children at home must care for aging parents and often share their household with them as well. It is also becoming more common for grandparents to raise their grandchildren

when the parents become unable to do so (e.g., because of unemployment, divorce, or illness) or have been legally declared unfit to care for the children.

In addition to blood and marriage relations, other family types exist. These include *single individuals* who may reside in a common household, *gay and lesbian couples,* and *individuals or couples who adopt children.* Recall that family is a group of individuals who provide support and assistance to each other. Although J.B. and Mike are not blood relatives and do not live together, they provide strong support for each other. Many refer to this type of bond as **kith,** persons with a kinship bond. For some people, this bond is stronger than blood-line bonds.

Approaches to Family Nursing

Family nursing refers to nursing care that is holistically directed toward the whole family as well as to individual members. It is a philosophy of care that supports family involvement by encouraging family visiting, liberal visiting hours, and family participation in decision making and even physical care. For J.B., for instance, the nurses would support Mike's daily visits. The staff would involve Mike and J.B.'s adult children in his care, discharge planning, and follow-up care at home. They would also teach Mike about J.B.'s medications and treatments so that he can assist J.B. in his activities of daily living.

Three perspectives on family nursing include the family as (1) context, (2) unit of care, and (3) system. Family nursing is a specialty; for you to work with the family as a unit of care or as a system, you may need additional preparation. However, as a new graduate, you should be prepared to work, at least, with the *family as the context* for care of an individual person. Your focus in this approach is on one individual (the one who is ill); from this perspective, you view the family as either a resource or a stressor to your patient. Using this approach, you might ask J.B., "Will your daughters be able to help you when you go home?" You would also recognize the importance of J.B.'s friend, Mike, who is a daily presence and who may be his most important source of support.

A slightly more complex approach views the *family as the unit of care.* Wellness of each member is critical to promoting family health. In this approach, you would view the family as the sum of all individual members and provide assessment and care for all family members; however, you might direct interventions to individual family members rather than the family as a whole. For example, you might provide teaching on nutrition and physical activity to all family members to promote their health. Or, to use our earlier example, you might check Mike's blood pressure when he visits J.B.

The third perspective is the *family as a system.* In this approach, you focus on the family as a whole and

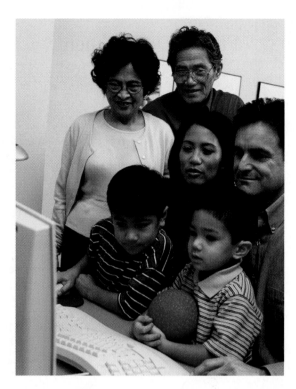

FIGURE 12–1 Family nursing refers to nursing care that is holistically directed toward the whole family as well as to individual members.

as an interactional system. Using this perspective, you direct your assessment and intervention to communications and interactions between family members. The systems approach sees the family as embedded in and interacting with a larger community. Using this approach, you might ask, for example, "How has your family's relationship with the school community changed since your illness?"

KnowledgeCheck 12–1

- Name at least three types of family structure.
- What are two topics that the nurse can discuss with the family as a unit?

 Go to Chapter 12, **Knowledge Check Response Sheet and Answers,** on the Electronic Study Guide.

CriticalThinking 12–1

How can you promote family cohesion for a family whose members live great distances from each other?

WHAT THEORIES ARE USEFUL FOR FAMILY CARE?

Several theories have been proposed to help us understand family functioning. Three such theories are general systems theory, structural-functional theories, and developmental theory.

TABLE 12-1 Family Development

Stages	Tasks	Children's Age (Approximate)
Beginning family	• Making marriage work • Deciding whether to have children	None
Childbearing family	• Achieving pregnancy and birth • Adjusting to life changes following birth and to the infant's needs • Determining ways to meet all members needs • Renegotiating marriage • Increasing contact with extended family	Newborn to 2 years
Family with preschool children	• Adjusting to increased costs associated with family life • Socializing the preschoolers • Coping with loss of parental energy and privacy	3–5 years
Family with school-age children	• Adjusting to the needs and demands of growing children • Promoting joint decision making among parents and children • Encouraging and supporting educational and school-related activities	6–12 years
Family with teenagers and young adults	• Maintaining open communication among family members • Reinforcing ethical and moral values • For teens, balancing independence with parental rules	13–20 years
Family launching young adults	• Maintaining support to young adults as they leave the security of family • Rediscovering marriage	21–30 years
Postparental family	• Preparing for retirement • Adjusting to children's moving into new phases of adulthood, marriage, and childbearing and to becoming a grandparent	Adult
Aging family	• Adjusting to retirement and changes associated with aging • Adjusting to the loss of a spouse and friendships	Adult

Sources: Friedman, M. M. (1992). *Family nursing: Theory and practice* (3rd ed.). Norwalk, CT: Appleton & Lange; Friedman, M. M., Bowden, V. R., & Jones, E. G. (2003). *Family nursing: Research, theory, and practice* (5th ed.). Upper Saddle River, NJ: Prentice Hall; Hanson, S. M. (2001). *Family health care nursing: Theory, practice, and research* (2nd ed). Philadelphia: F. A. Davis Company; Leahy, J. M., & Kizilay, P. A. (Eds.). (1998). *Foundations of nursing practice: A nursing process approach.* Philadelphia: W. B. Saunders; and McGoldrick, M., & Carter, E. (1985). The stages of the family life cycle. In J. Henslin (Ed.), *Marriage and family in a changing society.* New York: Free Press.

General Systems Theory

General systems theory (see Chapter 8) focuses on interactions between systems and the changes that result from these interactions. In the case of the family, interaction can occur between members of the family or between multiple families. Changes in the behaviors or attitudes of an individual member affect the family unit, and changes in family structure and functioning affect individual members. It may help to think of a system as a mobile: If one piece of the mobile is moved, that movement sets the whole mobile in motion.

Other systems surround the family unit (e.g., the community, the city, the state, the healthcare system).

Because these systems are broader than the family, they are referred to as **suprasystems.** Smaller components that fit within the family system (e.g., the mother, the marital couple) may be viewed as **subsystems.** Each system has a particular function. For example, one family member might be viewed as the decision maker, another as the peacekeeper, and another as the disciplinarian for the children.

Structural-Functional Theories

Structural-functional family theories are based on the developmental theories of Freud, Erikson, and Havighurst (see Chapter 9 for review) and include the

concepts of family roles and interactions. According to Parsons and Bales (1955), the structural-functional approach includes the following assumptions:

1. A family is a social system with functional requirements.
2. A family is a small group possessing certain features common to small groups.
3. The family accomplishes functions that serve both the individual and society.
4. Individuals act according to internalized norms that are learned through socialization.

Although they view the family as a social system, structural-functional theories, unlike systems theory, focus on *outcome* rather than process; that is, you would use this theory to assess how well the family functions, both internally among family members and externally with outside systems. Examples of family functions include socialization of children, meeting the physical, financial, and emotional needs of family members, caring for older members, and being productive members of society.

Developmental Theories

Developmental theories focus on the stage of family development. As shown in Table 12–1, there are typically eight stages in the family life cycle. Generally these stages follow one another in a linear progression; however, some families may simultaneously be in more than one stage or may revert to previous stages. This overlap or reversion is most common in families that have children spaced far apart, in blended families, and in stepfamilies. See Chapter 9 for developmental theories applicable to individual family members.

KnowledgeCheck 12–2
- Which type of theory focuses on interactions between families, family members, and groups in the environment?
- What is the name of the theory that views families as a social system with a focus on outcomes?
- What are some examples of family functions as defined by structural-functional theories?

 Go to Chapter 12, **Knowledge Check Response Sheet and Answers,** on the Electronic Study Guide.

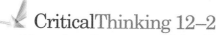 CriticalThinking 12–2
- Using systems theory, you could view J.B., his siblings, his children, and his grandchildren as a system. Refer to the section on family structures—how would you categorize this family structurally?
- Again using systems theory, what or who are the subsystems in the family system described in the preceding question?
- Considering J.B. alone, at what developmental stage is his "family"?

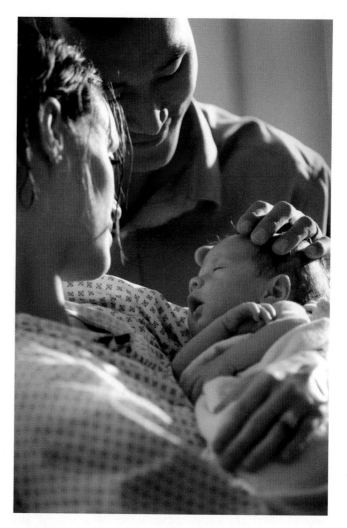

FIGURE 12–2 Newly married couples, couples who are trying to become pregnant, and new parents are vulnerable to stress as they adapt to new roles.

WHAT ARE SOME FAMILY HEALTH RISK FACTORS?

Many health risk factors are the same for families as for individuals, and they are similar across age groups and family types. Basically, destructive behaviors remain destructive behaviors, regardless of developmental stage and regardless of whether they are group or individual. For a more complete discussion of this topic,

 Go to Chapter 12, **Supplemental Materials: What Are Some Family Health Risk Factors?,** on the Electronic Study Guide.

Also see Chapter 9 on growth and development, Chapter 18 on communicating, Chapter 24 on teaching clients, and Chapter 25 on stress and adaptation.

Childless and Childbearing Couples

Adapting to new roles creates stress for newly married couples, couples who are trying to become pregnant, and new parents (Figure 12–2). Use of maladaptive

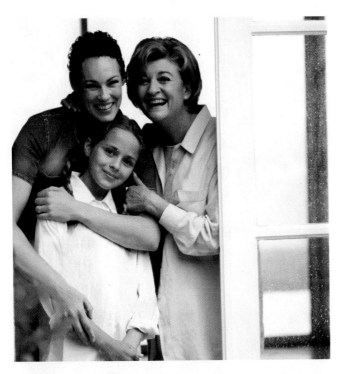

FIGURE 12–3 In families with adolescents or young adults, the parents may become "sandwiched" between the needs of the growing adolescents and the needs of their own parents.

coping mechanisms can lead to health problems. For example, someone who smokes to deal with stress is at risk for lung and other types of cancers, and their family members are at risk for the negative effects of second-hand smoke. Additional health risks for the childbearing couple include the risk for miscarriage, congenital malformations and genetic defects, and concern for the health and safety of the mother and fetus during the labor and birth process.

Families with Young Children

Families with young children often experience financial difficulties. For example, dual-earner couples struggle to pay for the costs of child care. Finding safe, nurturing, and affordable day care can be a huge source of stress for working parents. Parenting concerns include the child's development, socialization, education, discipline, nutrition, sleeping, toileting, and safety. In addition, the demands of work and child-rearing mean less time is available to nurture the couple's relationship, leaving them at increased risk for marital discord.

Injuries and illness create risks to family health. For example, children in day care and school are exposed to other children with minor infectious diseases (such as colds and "flu"), which may spread to other family members. To reduce the risk for serious infectious diseases (e.g., polio), parents need to be aware of the importance of adhering to the recommended childhood immunization schedule. For families who

must cope with a chronic illness, such as asthma, or a developmental or learning disability, such as attention deficit hyperactivity disorder (ADHD), the stress of health problems, educational concerns, and even day-to-day living can become overwhelming.

Families with Adolescents

Families with adolescents are concerned about their risk-taking behaviors. Adolescents may participate in risky behaviors to belong to the "popular" group or to impress others in their environment. They do not seem to appreciate the risks involved. Specific risk-taking behaviors include experimenting with tobacco, alcohol, and other drugs; daredevil stunts or dares; rebelling against authority; and sexual experimentation.

At the same time, these families may be dealing with aging grandparents (Figure 12–3). In this stage, it is common for the adolescent's grandparents to need assistance from other family members. Families may become "sandwiched" between the needs of the growing adolescents and the needs of grandparents. Women are particularly at risk for stress in these situations because it is most frequently the woman who assumes the additional care that is needed for older relatives.

Families with Middle-Aged Adults

Midlife changes create stressors for middle-adult families whose adult children are establishing or have just established their own households. Parents worry when their newly independent children confront new life experiences and encounter such problems as financial struggles, unrealistic expectations for meaningful work and personal relationships, travel, and the responsibility for maintaining property. At the same time, the parental unit experiences a new sense of freedom and need for adjustment. The additional time on their hands may be welcomed, or it may be stressful, causing the couple to become bored and worry about how to spend their time.

The effects of long-standing unhealthy behaviors often become apparent in middle-adulthood. For example, individuals who have been smokers for many years may now begin to notice an increase in cough and chest congestion; and those who have consumed high-fat diets may develop high blood pressure or elevated cholesterol levels. Remember, individual health affects family health.

Families with Older Adults

Falls and trauma are a common health risk for families of older adults. For more information about this, see Chapter 9 and Chapter 21.

Older adults are at risk for social isolation and loneliness because of the loss of relationships that occurs with aging. Family dynamics change as the older person copes with the death of a spouse, sibling, or other loved ones. At the same time, retirement brings the loss of daily contact with work colleagues. Friends can be a significant source of support (Figure 12–4), but functional losses may cause the person to curtail volunteer work, churchgoing, and other social activities.

Maintaining good nutrition becomes more difficult as a person ages. Some older adults who live alone experience malnutrition because they forget to eat. The risk of malnutrition increases if they do not have adequate transportation to shop for food. Nutrition may also be compromised by lack of money to buy food, physical changes (e.g., in the tastebuds) that change the taste of food, and poorly fitting dentures and painful gums. For more information about nutrition, see Chapter 26.

It is easy to understand from the above scenarios the cascading effect that one deficit, such as lack of transportation, can have on the health of an older adult and her family. Many families are not aware of community resources that can provide help. A crucial aspect of your role in caring for the family with older adults is to educate them about the availability of community resources, such as Meals on Wheels and home health aides.

 CriticalThinking 12–3

• What developmental stage is your family in? How do you know?
• What health risks do J.B. and Mike ("Meet Your Patient") face?

WHAT ARE SOME CHALLENGES TO FAMILY HEALTH?

We have already mentioned the effect of some demographic changes, such as an aging population, on families. This section examines other regional and national trends that affect families.

Poverty and Unemployment

When the economy takes a downturn, families may struggle to provide for basic needs (e.g., food and shelter) and health care. Nearly 43.6 million Americans do not have health insurance (AMA, 2002). In 1997, about 16% of pregnant women in the United States did not receive early prenatal care. Nearly half of these women gave as their reason lack of money or insurance to pay for the visits (CDC, 2000).

Single-parent and low-income families are hardest hit. Most workers who are living at or below the federal poverty level work in minimum-wage jobs. In a sluggish economy these "disposable" jobs are the

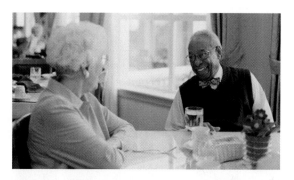
FIGURE 12–4 Friends play an important role in the support system of older people.

first to be eliminated, and it may be difficult to find another such job. Furthermore, when economic problems are severe, state budgets may be cut. Aid to families is often one of the first programs targeted. Although people find some creative solutions to such problems (e.g., a woman who is laid off assumes child care for another family whose members remain employed), many families experience extreme hardships when the economy is slow.

Middle-income families are also affected because companies may also eliminate middle-management positions. Even families who were living well may not have adequate reserves to cover a period of unemployment. Many people have significant credit card debt, a mortgage, two car payments, a variety of insurance premiums, and perhaps school loans or other loans to pay.

KnowledgeCheck 12–3

• Which financial group of families is hardest hit during poor economic periods?
• How are middle-income families affected by poor economic times?

 Go to Chapter 12, **Knowledge Check Response Sheet and Answers,** on the Electronic Study Guide.

Infectious Diseases

Family health may be affected by any number of new or resistant pathogens. For example, severe acute respiratory syndrome (SARS), a viral respiratory illness, was first reported in Asia in 2003, and the global outbreak spread to include North America. The West Nile virus was not documented in the Western Hemisphere before 1999. One of the most devastating pathogens, human immunodeficiency virus (HIV), is the virus that causes acquired immunodeficiency syndrome (AIDS). AIDS was first reported in 1981 and has since become a global epidemic. In the United States, women and children are among the fastest-growing groups of HIV-positive individuals.

HIV infection is a devastating event that significantly impacts the family. In addition to the obvious

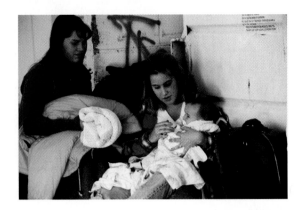

FIGURE 12–5 Homelessness is a growing stressor for families.

physicial and financial stressors, women who inadvertently infect their infants with HIV bear a tremendous burden of guilt. Some families keep the diagnosis a secret and blame each other, whereas other families support each other and manage the illness the best they can. Advances have been made in treating the infection and preventing its spread. Advances have also been made in developing a vaccine. However, we are likely still years away from a cure or a successful vaccine that can be administered to the general public.

Even "old" diseases can return to threaten health. For example, the decreased levels of vaccinations in the U.S. increase the risk for diseases such as polio and even smallpox (which is thought to have been eradicated). And tuberculosis, which has been cured by antibiotics for over 50 years, has returned in a highly contagious and fatal, multidrug-resistant form.

KnowledgeCheck 12–4

- What age and gender groups are experiencing the fastest rate of growth in new HIV cases?
- Name two previously eradicated diseases that have become a threat again.

 Go to Chapter 12, **Knowledge Check Response Sheet and Answers,** on the Electronic Study Guide.

Homelessness

Homelessness is a growing stressor (Figure 12–5). Homelessness can result from financial problems, unemployment, lack of job skills, mental illness, excessive healthcare expenses not covered by insurance, or the inability or lack of desire to live within the socially accepted norms of society. Many homeless people literally sleep on the streets, although others live temporarily with relatives or in mission shelters. Homeless families are likely to be socially isolated and therefore vulnerable to disabilities and deprivation in all aspects of life. Merely finding food and shelter requires most of the family's time and energy, threatening family relationships and the long-term physical and emotional health of family members. At least half of homeless children cannot attend school, and those who do tend to perform poorly. Family assistance is critical to those who may "fall through the cracks" in the healthcare system.

Single women, members of minority groups, and single-parent families are particularly vulnerable to homelessness. Many divorced women end up with far less income than their ex-husbands. In addition, women also tend to have sole custody of their children, which creates additional expenses for them. In many states, social service departments are so overwhelmed that they cannot follow up on fathers who do not pay child support.

Violence and Neglect Within Families

Violence—including physical, emotional, and sexual abuse—is widespread in our society, affecting all racial, social, and economic groups. Youth violence is on the rise, and gang violence causes a substantial number of deaths each year among both gang members and innocent bystanders.

Abuse within the family (e.g., spouse abuse, child abuse, and elder abuse) is a specific type of violence. As many as one in every four women will be a victim of violence during her lifetime, and over 3 million children each year are reported to child protective services agencies as alleged abuse victims. It is estimated that over 500,000 children in the United States are seriously injured each year by all forms of maltreatment. Such reports have maintained a steady growth over the past 10 years, increasing by 45% since 1987 (International Child Abuse Network, 2003).

Any type of violence is likely to have long-lasting effects on the victims and on the family. It may result in the disintegration of the family (e.g., sending the children to foster care, escaping to a battered women's shelter). And even though the emotional and physical pain may end when the victim leaves the family environment, often there are long-term effects. To learn more about abuse and violence,

 Go to **Chapter 9** on the Electronic Study Guide.

KnowledgeCheck 12–5

- Name two causes of homelessness.
- Name two groups of individuals who are vulnerable to homelessness.
- Name two types of violence.
- True or false: Effects of violence generally are minimal after the physical injury has healed.

 Go to Chapter 12, **Knowledge Check Response Sheet and Answers,** on the Electronic Study Guide.

Practical Knowledge
knowing how

A holistic view of family health includes the biological, social, cultural, and spiritual aspects of life and refers to individual members as well as the whole family.

| Assessment |

Health assessment for the family is similar to that for individuals. Gather all essential assessment information for each family member. (See Chapter 19 for additional information on physical assessment.) In addition to the individual factors, assess the health of the family unit. For an example of a family assessment form used by a community health agency,

 Go to Chapter 12, **Tables, Boxes, Figures: ESG Figure 12–1,** on the Electronic Study Guide.

In general, a family assessment should include the following.

- Identifying data
- Family composition
- Family history and developmental stage (see Table 12–1)
- Environmental data
- Family structure, including communication patterns and power and role structures
- Family functions
- Health beliefs, values, and behaviors
- Family stressors and coping
- Abuse and violence within the family

 Go to Chapter 9, **Procedure 9–1: Assessing for Abuse,** in Volume 2.

For a more complete description of the context of a family assessment,

 Go to Chapter 12, **Technique 12–1: Conducting a Family Assessment,** in Volume 2.

The following sections discuss in more detail the assessment of family health beliefs, communication patterns, and coping processes.

Assessing the Family's Health Beliefs

Health beliefs can vary widely among families and among individuals within families. The differences can be especially great among different generations of a family (e.g., between grandparents and their grandchildren). Some common health beliefs are expressed in such adages as "Doctor knows best," and "Feed a cold, starve a fever." Some families may have an intense distrust of medical care and hospitals and may seek treatment only when absolutely necessary (e.g., when the pain becomes unbearable). Many of these beliefs are passed on from generation to generation.

Even if an individual client does not share all of the beliefs of the family, you need to be aware of the family's beliefs because they may influence the individual's decision making. Also, when family members provide care after the acute event, their beliefs influence whether, when, and how prescribed therapies are completed. For example, a wife who does not believe in modern medicine may not give her recovering husband's medications on the prescribed schedule or may even avoid giving them at all. For more information on health beliefs, see Chapter 41.

 CriticalThinking 12–4

- As a nurse, how can you promote wellness in a family with a critically ill member?
- What health beliefs would you want to ask J.B.'s family about?

Assessing the Family's Communication Patterns

To assess family communication patterns, you will need to interview the family and also make astute observations of interactions between family members. Try to uncover the following information:

- Who is the primary decision maker in the family?
- How are family decisions made: by one individual or by family conference?
- What is the most frequent means of communication among family members: visits to the home, telephone, e-mail, social situations (e.g., family get-togethers, going out to dinner), religious activities, church attendance?

Do not rely solely on the information provided by the family members during the interview process. Family members who participate in dysfunctional communication patterns may not come to scheduled family meetings and may not be present during the initial interview. Families usually also want to "put on the best face" for healthcare providers, so they may be careful to give socially desirable responses. Carefully observe both verbal and nonverbal communication with, and especially *among,* family members.

Assessing the Family's Coping Processes

The physiological manifestations of stress (e.g., anxiety, increased pulse rate) may decrease the effectiveness

BOX 12-1 Characteristics of a Healthy Family

Health is more than merely the absence of family dysfunction or disease in an individual member. Health includes the following:

- A state of family well-being
- A sense of belonging and connectedness
- Shared responsibility
- A sense of trust and respect
- Spending time together, sharing rituals and traditions
- Flexibility: adaptability and ability to deal with stress, openness to change
- Commitment: working together to maintain the family
- Spiritual well-being
- Respect for privacy of individual members
- Positive, effective communication
- Ability to compromise and disagree
- Appreciation and affection for each other
- Responding to the needs and interests of all members
- Egalitarian distribution of power
- Health-promoting lifestyle of individual members

of interventions and negatively affect a client's clinical course. Family members who are not coping effectively may cause the client to become stressed or anxious or to have problems sleeping. Assessing family coping is a first step to helping the family develop more effective coping patterns. Observe for the following:

- Signs of stress, anxiety, or loss of sleep in the client. Help the client identify their causes.
- Visitors and the client's reaction to them. Family members who are not coping well may avoid coming to the hospital. Thus, who is visiting and who is not are indicators of family coping.
- Whether family members are irritable and "snap at" (speak harshly or curtly to) one another.

KnowledgeCheck 12–6

- Why is it important for you to ask about family health beliefs?
- What factors may impede a family's ability to cope with an individual's illness?

 Go to Chapter 12, **Knowledge Check Response Sheet and Answers,** on the Electronic Study Guide.

| Nursing Diagnosis |

Recall that in the diagnostic process you must analyze the data for cues (data that deviate from norms).

Therefore, you should be familiar with the characteristics of a healthy family (refer to Box 12–1) so that you can use them as your basis for comparison.

For individual family members, of course, any NANDA diagnosis may be appropriate for describing a client's health status. *Family diagnoses,* however, are meant to describe the health status of the family as a whole. The following are examples:

Caregiver Role Strain (actual and risk for)
Family Coping: Compromised
Family Coping: Disabled
Dysfunctional Family Processes: Alcoholism
Impaired Home Maintenance
Impaired Parenting (actual and risk for)
Ineffective Family Therapeutic Regimen Management
Interrupted Family Processes
Readiness for Enhanced Family Coping
Readiness for Enhanced Parenting
Risk for Impaired Parent/Infant/Child Attachment
Social Isolation

| Planning Outcomes and Evaluation |

NOC outcomes specifically for families as units are found in the NOC domain "Family Health", which includes the classes Family Caregiver Status, Family Member Health Status, Family Well-Being, and Parenting. Outcomes from other domains may apply as well, depending on the nursing diagnosis you have made. For a list of NOC outcomes in the Family Health domain,

 Go to Chapter 12, **Standardized Outcomes and Interventions,** in Volume 2.

Individualized goals/outcome statements you might write for a family include the following examples, which represent some of the traits of healthy families in Box 12–1. The family:

Affirms and supports each member.
Teaches respect for others within and outside the family.
Demonstrates a sense of humor and plays together.
Observes rituals and traditions (e.g., celebrates birthdays).
Respects the privacy of each member.
Communicates effectively and openly.

Remember that the outcomes you develop for the care plan serve as the criteria for evaluating your patient's responses to nursing interventions.

| Planning Interventions/Implementation |

NIC interventions for families as units are found in the NIC domain "Family," which include the classes Childbearing Care, Childrearing Care, and Life-Span Care. Interventions from other domains may apply as well,

depending on the nursing diagnosis you have made. For NIC family interventions,

 Go to Chapter 12, **Standardized Outcomes and Interventions,** in Volume 2.

Individualized nursing actions you might use with families include the following examples. (Other interventions are described in succeeding sections):

- Help families access community agencies, for example, for job skills training, home health services, and counseling services.
- Refer the family to federal programs to help meet basic needs for women with young children.
- Assess and monitor family relationships.
- Assist with communication and conflict resolution.
- Encourage and role-model open expressions of affection.
- Establish trusting relationship with family members.
- Encourage the family to be assertive in seeking healthcare information.
- Arrange for respite care, as needed.

Promoting Family Wellness

Encouraging families to value and incorporate health promotion into their lifestyles will also affect the health of individual members. Health-promotion behaviors are, after all, learned within the family. You can promote family wellness by addressing both individual and family needs. It is important to identify both strengths and weaknesses of the family to adequately meet healthcare needs.

Involving the family in each phase of the nursing process promotes positive health outcomes and helps establish trust between the family and the nurse. Wellness interventions may include contracting, health teaching, anticipatory guidance, and promoting family cohesion during a crisis (e.g., hospitalization of a family member). For specific health promotion activities, see Chapter 41.

Interventions When a Family Member Is Ill

When a family member is ill or hospitalized, the other family members experience a range of emotions—especially when the illness is severe or of sudden onset. Family members may display signs of stress in a variety of ways, for example, by arguing with each other or with healthcare providers, by insisting on immediate care for their loved one, by avoiding the client's room, or by frequently asking that information be repeated. These are normal reactions; do not take them personally.

The patient and family need to understand their medical diagnosis, the plan of care, and what the recovery process will be like. In addition, it is often the nurse who provides extensive discharge instructions to the client and family before they leave the hospital. Specific interventions to help the family cope with the hospitalization of their loved one and manage stress include the following:

- Provide written materials explaining the client's diagnosis or condition.
- Actively involve the family in team meetings.
- Promptly follow up with family concerns or questions.
- Encourage the family to go home and rest.
- Encourage the family to call for updates when they cannot be present.
- Suggest ideas for stress-reducing activities (e.g., walking, meditating).
- Inform the family about on-site availability of a chaplain or chapel.
- Encourage the family to participate in care activities as appropriate.
- Keep the family informed of the client's progress.
- Provide anticipatory guidance regarding outcome and expectations for discharge.

Interventions When There Is a Death in the Family

Death of a close family member is one of the most devastating life experiences. A family needs sensitive and compassionate care during this time, and such care is an appropriate focus for family-centered nursing. Interventions include facilitating the grieving process, encouraging communication, providing spiritual support, and providing compassionate care of the body after death. For more in-depth information about care of the family of a dying patient, see Chapter 15.

| toward evidence-based practice |

Gerdner, L. A., Buckwalter, K. C., & Reed, D. (2002). Impact of a psychoeducational intervention on caregiver response to behavioral problems. *Nursing Research, (51)*6, 363–374.

In this study, families caring for loved ones with Alzheimer's disease were taught how to manage behavioral problems (which are common among persons with this disorder because of brain deterioration and memory loss). Many family caregivers do not have adequate knowledge about how to care for their loved one, and many lack the support of others for the work that they do. The authors conducted this study to help these family members provide better care to their loved ones and to cope more effectively with some of the difficulties that

they encounter. Caregivers who received the assistance from the research team had lower levels of stress and responded more effectively to the patients' needs. Some participants reported fewer memory and behavioral problems with their loved ones. There were no differences in how well the person with Alzheimer's disease was able to function.

---

1. Based on this research, if you were the nurse, what kinds of information would you want to gather from families caring for a loved one with Alzheimer's disease?

 Go to Chapter 12, **Toward Evidence-Based Practice Suggested Responses,** on the Electronic Study Guide.

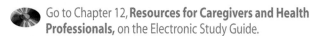 Go to Chapter 12, **Resources for Caregivers and Health Professionals,** on the Electronic Study Guide.

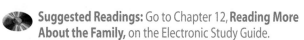 **Suggested Readings:** Go to Chapter 12, **Reading More About the Family,** on the Electronic Study Guide.

 Bibliography: Go to Volume 2, Bibliography.

Culture
& Ethnicity

Learning Outcomes

After completing this chapter you should be able to:

* Identify concepts pertaining to cultural diversity in nursing.

* Discuss patterns of behavior that can reflect cultural and ethnic influences.

* Identify the characteristics of culture, including their relationship to acculturation.

* Define and give an example of culture universals and of culture specifics.

* Describe types of healthcare practices—including folk beliefs that influence wellness, illness, and health-seeking behaviors—in culturally diverse populations.

* Identify the phenomena of culture, including how they can affect the nursing care needs of clients and families.

* Describe ways to overcome the cultural barriers to health care.

* Relate the differing views of culturally diverse clients, including biomedical, holistic, and alternative health systems, such as folk medicine.

* Discuss the definitions, theories, and models relating to the provision of culturally competent care.

* Explain guidelines for performing a transcultural assessment, including a cultural assessment model.

* Describe nursing strategies that promote delivery of culturally competent care to clients and their families.

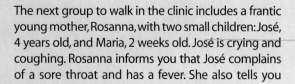

MEET Your Patients

Your instructor has given you a clinical assignment. You are to spend the day in a walk-in clinic with a primary care provider and other students from your program. Your initial job is to greet the new clients and help them complete a health history form. The first client that you greet is Romano Salvatore, a middle-aged man. He points to his head and moans. When you ask him what is wrong, he makes a gesture to convey to you that he does not understand what you are saying. He speaks a foreign language that sounds to you like Italian.

The next group to walk in the clinic includes a frantic young mother, Rosanna, with two small children: José, 4 years old, and Maria, 2 weeks old. José is crying and coughing. Rosanna informs you that José complains of a sore throat and has a fever. She also tells you that she has been to her *curandero,* but José is not getting any better. You also notice that both children have on heavy coats and knit hats although it is quite warm outside. When you question Rosanna about the children's clothing, she says that José is "cold."

Lee Chan, an elderly Chinese American man enters the clinic. Mr. Chan is accompanied by eight family members. Because the waiting area is small, all except his daughter Kim are asked to wait outside. Mr. Chan is quiet and does not make eye contact with you. His daughter Kim explains that her father has stomach cancer and is in a lot of pain because of disharmony. When you ask him to rate his pain, he just shakes his head and looks away. Would you wonder what *disharmony* means?

Theoretical Knowledge
knowing why

Try to answer the following questions about the patients you have just met. You may not have the theoretical knowledge to answer them all—you will acquire that in this chapter—but do your best based on the background you now have.

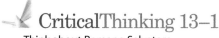 CriticalThinking 13–1

Think about Romano Salvatore.

- If you could speak Italian, what would you ask him?

  Think about Rosanna and her children.

- One question that might spring immediately to your mind is, "What is a curandero?" How could you find out this information?
- Why do you think that the children are dressed more warmly than you would expect for the weather?

Think about Mr. Chan and his family.

- How would you feel about so many of his family members coming with Mr. Chan to the clinic?
- Why do you think he is not looking at or speaking to you?
- How could you communicate with Mr. Chan? Would you assume that he does not speak your language? Explain your reasoning.

One important reason to learn about culture and ethnicity is that you will almost certainly care for patients who are not from your culture. The United States and Canada are multicultural societies. The past decade has seen increasing immigration from Asian and Spanish-speaking nations, coupled with a higher growth rate among African Americans. The result is that what were previously referred to as minority groups, when taken together, will soon make up a majority. Current U.S. census data (U.S. Census, 2003b) also show an increase in the number of cultural and ethnic groups. Similarly, population statistics in Canada reveal more than 200 different ethnic groups and a threefold increase in

minority populations since 1981, with Chinese Canadians comprising the largest minority group (Canadian Census, 2003). Figure 13–1 illustrates the change in racial and ethnic makeup that is expected to occur in the United States by 2050. For recent U.S. Census data,

 Go to Chapter 13, **Tables, Boxes, Figures: ESG Table 13–1,** on the Electronic Study Guide.

 CriticalThinking 13–2
- With what cultural groups do you identify?
- In the neighborhood where you live, identify the cultural or ethnic groups that are different from your own. How many are there?
- In the school you are now attending, how many different cultural or ethnic groups are represented? What are they?

Providing care to a culturally diverse population has become a challenge for nurses. In North America most nurses are white, and the healthcare culture reflects their culture. However, as you saw in the "Meet Your Patient" scenarios, nurses care for patients from many different races and cultures. Nursing care that is appropriate for the dominant cultural group may be ineffective and inappropriate for people with a different cultural heritage.

Of course it is impossible to know about every culture, but it is important to learn about the ones you will encounter most often in your practice. In addition, you will need to delegate and supervise others, ensuring that all clients have equal access to culturally appropriate care. You need a good understanding of culture and ethnicity not only for providing direct care, but also for teaching and role-modeling culturally competent care for other care providers.

KnowledgeCheck 13–1
- What do recent demographic trends in North America indicate?
- Why should nurses know more about the culture and ethnicity of clients?

 Go to Chapter 13, **Knowledge Check Response Sheet and Answers,** on the Electronic Study Guide.

WHAT CONCEPTS ARE RELATED TO CULTURE?

To provide care in a culturally diverse population, you will need to understand concepts related to culture. Start at the beginning by learning what the word *culture* means. Rooted in sociology and more specifically anthropology, we know that culture is both *universal* (everyone has it) and *dynamic* (active). Put simply, **culture** is what people in a group have in common, but it changes over time.

Purnell and Paulanka (2003) define *culture* as "the totality of socially transmitted behavior patterns, arts,

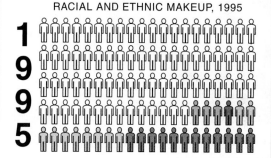

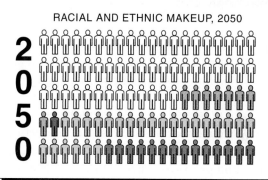

FIGURE 13–1 Racial and ethnic makeup in the United States: 1995 and 2050. *Source:* Hanson, S. (2001). *Family health care nursing: Theory, practice, and research* (2nd ed.). Philadelphia: F. A. Davis Company, p. 39.

beliefs, values, customs, lifeways, and all other products of human work and thought characteristic of a population of people that guide their worldview and decision making" (p. 3). For other definitions of culture,

 Go to Chapter 13, **Supplemental Materials: Definitions of Culture,** on the Electronic Study Guide.

When you are trying to determine what is meant by *culture* or *cultural,* keep in mind the following characteristics:

- *Culture is learned.* Learning occurs through life experiences shared with other members of the culture.

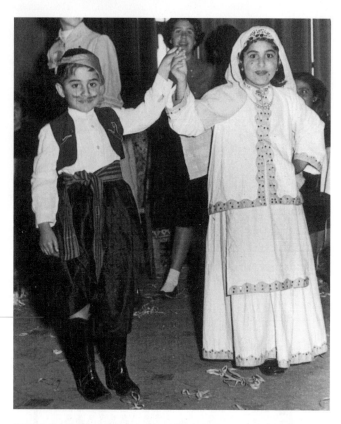

FIGURE 13–2 Children dancing the Kalamatiano, a Greek dance representing village tradition.

- *Culture is taught.* Cultural values, beliefs, and traditions are passed down from generation to generation, either formally (e.g., in schools) or informally (e.g., in families).
- *Culture is shared by its members.* Cultural norms are shared through teachings and social interactions.
- *Culture is dynamic and adaptive.* Cultural customs, beliefs, and practices are not static, but change over time and at different rates. Cultural change occurs with adaptation in response to the environment.
- *Culture is complex.* Reread the Purnell and Paulanka (2003) definition to review the many aspects of culture. Cultural assumptions and habits are unconscious and thus may be difficult for members of the culture to explain to others.
- *Culture is diverse.* Culture demonstrates the variety that exists among groups and among members of a particular group.
- *Culture exists at many levels.* Culture exists in both the material (art, writings, dress, or artifacts) and the nonmaterial (customs, traditions, language, beliefs and practices).
- *Culture has common beliefs and practices.* Members of the culture share the same beliefs, traditions, customs, and practices as long as they continue to be adaptive and satisfy the members' needs. Some

members of the group may deviate from cultural norms, but for a norm to be considered cultural, many members must follow it.
- *Culture is all-encompassing.* Culture can influence everything its members think and do.
- *Culture provides identity.* Cultural beliefs provide identity for its members as long as they do not conflict with the dominant culture and continue to gratify its members.

CriticalThinking 13–3

Figure 13–2 depicts an example of ways members of particular cultural groups express their cultural uniqueness in dance. Can you think of other ways that people express their culture?

Bicultural is a term that describes a person who identifies with two cultures and maintains some of the values and lifestyles of each (Giger & Davidhizar, 2004). Consider a Jewish man who marries an Italian Catholic woman. Their bicultural children may choose to follow Jewish tradition while still holding some of the values and beliefs of their Italian heritage. A bicultural person may experience divided loyalties.

In this chapter, **multicultural** refers to many cultures and is used to describe groups rather than individuals. Many regions of the United States are multicultural, meaning that the region is populated by individuals from many different cultural groups. The same can be said about workplace settings. Remember that culture does not always refer to the ethnicity of a group. Think of a hospital: Caregivers may be members of various ethnic and religious groups, and the nurses, physicians, physical therapists, and students each comprise a different subculture. A hospital is thus a multicultural setting.

Dominant Cultures, Subcultures, and Minority Groups

If you are white (e.g., European American) and someone asks you, "What is your culture?" you may reply, "I don't know; I don't think I have one." But that is because you are from what has historically been the mainstream. Because the white culture has been dominant in North America, most white people have been around others similar to themselves. They have not been aware of their culture because they did not see it in contrast to other ways of being. Or, if they did see differences, they assumed their ways were the norm and that everyone else was culturally different. **Ethnocentrism** is the tendency to think that your own group (cultural, professional, ethnic, or social) is superior to others and to view behaviors and beliefs that differ greatly from your own as somehow wrong, strange, or unenlightened. The tendency to ethnocentrism exists in all groups, not just in the dominant culture.

What do you think is the dominant culture of the United States and Canada? If you said white or Caucasian or European American, you would be only partially correct. The ancestors of most white Americans emigrated from Europe, and many were of Protestant or other Christian religions. We can then say that the dominant culture in the United States and Canada is white Anglo-Saxon Christian of European descent. A **dominant culture** is the group that has the most authority or power to control values and reward or punish behaviors. It is usually, but not always, the largest group.

Subcultures are groups within a larger culture or social system that have some characteristics (e.g., values, behaviors, ancestry) that are different from those of the dominant culture. People in subcultures have had different experiences from those in the dominant group because of status, residence, gender, sexual orientation, ethnic background, education, or other factors that unify the group (Purnell & Paulanka, 2003). You may be able to recognize subcultures by their speech patterns, dress, gestures, eating habits, lifestyles, and so on. Some examples of subcultures are street gangs, physicians, nurses, women, older adults, persons with disabilities, gays and lesbians, people of Appalachian heritage, rural Midwesterners, and people who abuse certain drugs.

Minority groups are also made up of individuals who share race, religion, or ethnic heritage; however, a minority group has fewer members than the majority group. Depending on the type of group, they may or may not share beliefs, practices, or physical characteristics. The term *minority* is sometimes used to refer to a group of people who receive different and unequal treatment from others in society. Some consider it an offensive term because it suggests inferiority and marginalization.

Vulnerable Populations as Subcultures

Vulnerable populations are those groups who are more likely to develop health problems and experience poorer outcomes because of limited access to care, high-risk behaviors, and/or multiple and cumulative stressors. Examples include people who are homeless, poor, or mentally ill, people with physical disabilities, the young, older adults, and some ethnic and racial minority groups. Vulnerable populations can be considered subcultures of all of the major cultural groups.

Socioeconomic vulnerability is particularly important. There is probably more variation among people of the same ethnic group but of different social classes than there is among people of different ethnic groups but of the same social class. The subculture of poverty can be found throughout the world. Figure 13–3, for example, shows children earning money by dancing for tourists.

The public health initiative *Healthy People 2010* (2002) addresses the care of vulnerable populations and includes an objective to eliminate health inequities. Nursing research is beginning to address these inequities, such as in the treatment of the mentally ill

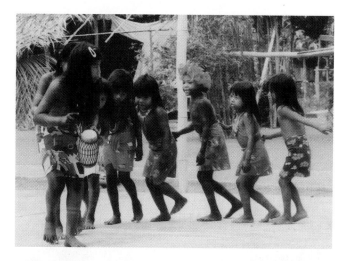

FIGURE 13–3 Children of the Panamanian Embera Indians dance for money for local tourists.

(George, 2000), and in the diagnosis and treatment of heart disease in women of color (Graham-Garcia, Raines, Andrews, & Mensah, 2001).

When caring for patients from vulnerable populations, it is important that you focus on their strengths and resources, not exclusively on their difficulties and risks.

Gender as a Subculture

It should come as no surprise that some behaviors are considered acceptable for men but not for women, and vice versa; and that there are values and responses considered more typical of one sex than of the other. For example, in the dominant culture it is more acceptable for women to cry out in pain than for men, who are supposed to "be strong." As another example, the U.S. and Canadian cultures tend to view caring and nurturing as the province of women, not of men. Only 5.4% of registered nurses in the United States are men, although the percentage has doubled from 2.7% in 1980 (U.S. Department of Health and Human Services [USDHHS], 2000).

Ethnicity, Race, and Religion

People sometimes use the terms *culture, ethnicity* and *race* interchangeably, but in fact they have separate, specific meanings.

Ethnicity

Ethnicity is similar to *culture* in that it refers to groups whose members share a common social and cultural heritage that is passed down from generation to generation (Giger & Davidhizar, 2004). However, ethnicity is also similar to *subculture,* in that the members of an **ethnic group** have some characteristics in common (e.g., race, ancestry, physical characteristics,

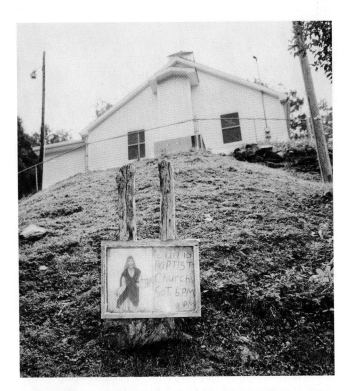

FIGURE 13–4 Even in this tiny community of rural Appalachia, people have built a place for worship.

geographic region, lifestyle, religion) that are not shared or understood by outsiders. Examples of ethnic groups include French Canadians, Roman Catholics, people of Appalachian heritage, and Latinos.

Ethnicity may include race, but it is not the same as race. To demonstrate this statement, the U.S. Census Bureau has six categories for race (see the next section). In addition, it identifies two categories describing ethnicity: (1) Hispanic or Latino and (2) *Not* Hispanic or Latino. Hispanics and Latinos may be of any race. **Hispanic Americans** are people who originally came from any Spanish-speaking country (e.g., Mexico, Spain, and countries in Central and South America). **Latino,** strictly speaking, refers only to people from Latin America (Central or South America). If you know a client's country of origin, it is more accurate to use it when referring to the client's ethnic origin—for example, Mexican American, Colombian American, and so on—than to use either the term *Hispanic* or *Latino*.

Race

Unlike ethnicity, **race** is strictly related to biology. *Race* refers to the grouping of people based on biological similarities. Members of a particular race share distinguishing physical characteristics, such as skin color, blood type, or bone structure (Giger & Davidhizar, 2004). The terms *race* and *ethnicity* overlap somewhat, because race can be a characteristic of a specific ethnic group. The U.S. Census Bureau divides the population into the following six racial categories. Remember, these are Census Bureau terms; if you are culturally

sensitive, you will ask people what race they identify with and what name they prefer to use for it.

- American Indians and Alaskan Natives
- Asian Americans
- Black or African Americans
- Native Hawaiians or Other Pacific Islanders
- White
- Some Other Race (This allows people to select more than one race in identifying themselves or to write in a race if they cannot identify with those listed.)

For definitions of these categories,

 Go to Chapter 13, **Supplemental Materials: Race,** on the Electronic Study Guide.

Can you determine a person's race by his appearance? Frequently not. So, then, is race determined by heredity? What race is someone whose father is black and whose mother is white? Most North Americans would say that the person is black. In some other countries (e.g., most of South America), though, that same person would be categorized as white. Although we usually think of race as being based on biological characteristics, anthropologists prefer to think of it as human variation or diversity. Many believe that race is socially rather than biologically determined. For more information on race as a social construct,

 Go to **http://www.gazette.net/200018/frederickcty/state/10106-1.html**

We all tend to group and categorize data to make it meaningful and useful, but we must be careful to avoid using these categories as the basis for interacting with people or providing care. For example, there are hundreds of subcultures under the broad category of white. When you need to designate a name for a group, be as specific as possible; that is, when you know the client's country of heritage, say, for example, Syrian American instead of white.

Religion

Religion may be confused with ethnicity because people within an ethnic group may share the same religion. **Religion** refers to an ordered system of beliefs regarding the cause, nature, and purpose of the universe, especially the beliefs related to the worship of a God or gods (Andrews & Boyle, 2003). In many cultures, religion is a high priority (Figure 13–4).

These distinctions between culture, ethnicity, race, and religion might seem confusing, but think of it this way: You are a member of the subculture of nursing, but you are also a member of an ethnic group (e.g., Portugese Americans from the Azores), a racial group (e.g., white), and a religion (e.g., Roman Catholicism), each with its own sets of beliefs and values. So, your culture is a blend of all of those.

Socialization, Acculturation and Assimilation

Socialization is the process of learning to become a member of a society or a group. A person becomes socialized by learning social rules and roles, by learning the behaviors, norms, values, and perceptions of others in the same group or role. Families, schools, churches, peer groups, and the media are agents of socialization and foster the development of a culture and its members' identification with it.

Immigrants (new members of a group or country) assume the characteristics of that culture through a learning process called **acculturation.** A person who is acculturated accepts both their own and the new culture, adopting elements of each. Acculturation is the outgrowth of the minority group's need to survive and flourish in the new culture. Many experts theorize that it takes three generations for an immigrant group to become acculturated.

Cultural assimilation occurs when the new members gradually learn and take on the dominant culture's essential values, beliefs, and behaviors. Assimilation is complete when the newcomer is fully merged into the dominant cultural group. A person becomes assimilated by, for example, learning to speak the dominant language, marrying a member from the new (host) culture, and making close, personal relationships with members of the new group. For example, if you emigrated to Mexico, you would take with you your own language and food preferences. But over time, you would gradually begin to eat more of the local foods and learn to speak Spanish.

KnowledgeCheck 13–2

- Define culture.
- Give an example of each: ethnic group, race, religion.
- How does culture provide identity for an individual?
- Give an example of acculturation.

 Go to Chapter 13, **Knowledge Check Response Sheet and Answers,** on the Electronic Study Guide.

HOW DO CULTURAL VALUES, BELIEFS, AND PRACTICES AFFECT HEALTH?

Values are important because they help shape health-related beliefs and practices. Do you know what values are? Think for a minute about what you "value" in your own life. What are the five ideals, principles, or things that are most important to you?

You may name, for example, learning, family, independence, faith, and cleanliness. Or you may have said something entirely different. Simply put, a **personal value** is a principle or standard that has meaning or worth to an individual (Purnell & Paulanka, 2003). An example is cleanliness. In contrast, a **belief** is something that one accepts as true (e.g., "I believe that germs cause disease"), and a **practice** is a set of behaviors that one follows (e.g., "I always wash my hands before preparing food"). Do you see how values, beliefs, and practices are related?

Cultural values, beliefs, and practices are the principles, standards, ideas, and behaviors that members of a cultural group share. An example of a cultural value is the European-American obsession with bodily cleanliness. Other values of the dominant U.S. culture include youth, beauty, success, independence, and material belongings. You should not assume that clients share your values, beliefs, and practices—nor those of the dominant culture. Instead, become familiar with the specific values, beliefs, and practices of clients from the different cultural and ethnic (**ethnocultural**) groups in your community. Remember, though, that individuals within an ethnocultural group vary widely and that *learning commonalities is no substitute for careful assessment of each person.*

What Are Culture Specifics?

Culture universals are the values, beliefs, and practices that people from *all* cultures share. In contrast, **culture specifics** are those values, beliefs, and practices that are special or unique to a culture. Let's look at an example. All cultures celebrate the birth of a new baby in some way (a culture universal), but different cultures celebrate "birth rites" in different ways (a culture specific). In Belize, a baby is christened before visitors are allowed, a practice carried out to prevent the *evil eye* (bad spells cast by others); in Greece, *amulets* (objects or charms worn to protect from evil spirits) may be placed on the baby; and in Israel, Jewish male infants are circumcised on the eighth day of life (Spector, 2004). Similarly, people from all cultures practice marriage rituals. In India, a groom is prepared for the wedding ceremony in an elaborate ritual that is culture-specific (Figure 13–5).

Acknowledging that there are commonalities within a group is not the same as saying that *all* people in the group have those characteristics. Bear in mind there is probably more variation among people *within* an ethnic or cultural group than there is *between* the groups and that much variation stems from socioeconomic differences or regional origin. Each person must be seen as unique—as *influenced* by his heritage, but not *defined* by it. The ANA emphasizes, "It is important that the nurse consider specific cultural factors impacting on individual clients and recognize that intracultural variation means that each client must be assessed for individual cultural differences" (1997, p. 1).

How Do Culture Specifics Affect Health?

Just as they influence our celebrations of births and weddings, culture specifics affect our health beliefs and behaviors. Thus, knowledge of the culture specifics of groups in your community will enhance your ability

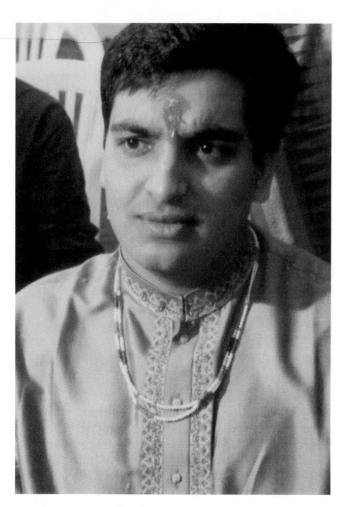

FIGURE 13–5 In India, the groom is prepared for his wedding in an elaborate ritual.

to understand clients' behaviors. It will help explain why clients from different cultures have different expectations of health care. And ultimately, it will help you to provide culturally competent care.

Now let's look at six culture specifics that influence health (Giger & Davidhizar, 2004): communication, space, time orientation, social organization, environmental control, and biological variations. We will also discuss several other culture specifics: religion and philosophy, politics and the law, the economy, and education. For more information about each of these dimensions of culture,

 Go to Chapter 13, **Tables, Boxes, Figures: ESG Table 13–2,** on the Electronic Study Guide.

Communication

Communication includes verbal and nonverbal language (i.e., spoken language, gestures, and even silences). Think how difficult it would be if you became ill in a foreign country. How would you tell the caregivers your symptoms? How would you know what they were going to do to treat your illness? Language differences present one of the most difficult obstacles to providing

care. Even when you and the client speak the same language, culture influences how feelings and thoughts are expressed and which verbal and nonverbal expressions are appropriate to use (Giger & Davidhizar, 2002). For example, Arabs keep steady eye contact when talking, but not between men and women; Asians and Native Americans usually do not make eye contact. You will learn more about communication strategies when we discuss culturally competent care. Also see Chapter 18 for communication strategies.

Space

Space refers to a person's personal space, or how the person relates toward the space around him. Another similar word, **territoriality,** means the behavior and attitude that people exhibit about the area around them they have claimed (Spector, 2004). Both of these ideas are influenced by culture. A person's comfort level is related to space. When an individual's personal space is protected, he feels secure and safe, less anxious, and in control. The following are some examples of culturally influenced attitudes toward personal space:

- Americans, Canadians of Northern European ancestry, and the British keep at least 18 inches of space between themselves and the person with whom they are conversing.

- Arabs and others from the Middle East typically stand quite close when talking.

- Germans usually require a great deal of space, and they consider even looking into a room an invasion of privacy.

Within all cultural groups, personal space varies depending on the relationship between the people speaking: intimates versus acquaintances, people of the same versus opposite sex, and people of a different position within the social hierarchy.

Time Orientation

Time orientation (past, present, and future) varies among people of different cultures. Some persons tend to be present- or future-oriented, whereas others are more rooted in the past. As an example, European Americans tend to be future-oriented. In contrast, Native Americans and Latinos may be more present-oriented. Differences in time orientation can be important as you plan nursing interventions for your clients. For example, for clients who are present-oriented and may tend to show up late (or not at all) for follow-up appointments, you should provide a written or telephone reminder of their appointment.

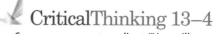 CriticalThinking 13–4

- Suppose you say to a client, "You will need to exercise and follow a low-calorie diet to lose weight and control your

diabetes." What kind of time orientation would a client most likely have in order to follow your directions?

- Suppose a client says, "I know I need to lose weight, but I work so much, and the children take so much time. I just don't have time to shop and cook for the right foods or to exercise." What time orientation does this illustrate?

Social Organization

Social organization includes the family unit (e.g., nuclear, single-parent, or extended family) and the wider organizations (e.g., community, religious, ethnic) with which the individual or family identifies (Spector, 2004). A close social organization can be found in all cultures; however, the specifics vary. For example, in Middle Eastern and Latino cultures, the man is likely to be the dominant family member and the woman the homemaker. But many African American families are matriarchal; that is, the decision maker and family leader is a woman.

The social organization of your clients' cultures can provide clues as to how they will act during such life events, as birth, death, illness, grieving, and mourning. For example, imagine a patient who must depend on Medicaid to pay for her health care, but who does not trust large institutions or government agencies. She is likely to use home remedies and to delay seeing a conventional medical physician.

Kinship and social ties also determine who receives health care, and in what priority. In the United States, for example, someone of high status (e.g., a celebrity or political figure) is likely to receive better care than a poor person who is unknown in the community. In some cultures, men receive care before women and children.

Environmental Control

Environmental control refers to a person's perception of his ability to plan activities that control nature or direct environmental factors (Giger & Davidhizar, 2004; Spector, 2004). Included in this phenomenon are health and illness beliefs and practices. For example, if a person does not believe he can do anything to "change things," how would this attitude affect his decision to seek medical care? To take medications? To exercise and eat properly? Perception and tolerance of pain is an example of the effect of environmental control. Some people, especially Asian Americans, tend to accept pain stoically, and not demand relief. They do not view circumstances as something to be "controlled." Think again about Mr. Chan ("Meet Your Patient"). Why do you think he just shakes his head and looks away when asked to rate his pain?

Biological Variations

Biological variations include ways in which people are different genetically and physiologically. They create susceptibility to certain diseases and injuries. Biological variations include body build and structure, skin color, vital signs, enzymatic and genetic variations, and drug metabolism (Spector, 2004, p. 23; Andrews & Boyle, 2003). Most drug studies in the past were based on European American subjects, so "variations" refers to differences from those norms (e.g., African Americans metabolize antihypertensives differently from European Americans). For more information about assessing biological variations,

 VOL 2 Go to Chapter 13, **Technique 13–1: Assessing for Biological Variations,** in Volume 2.

To read more about biological susceptibility to diseases,

Go to Chapter 13, **Supplemental Materials: Disease Risks for Each of the Major Cultural Groups of the United States,** on the Electronic Study Guide.

Other Culture Specifics

The following may also be culture specifics. The first two, religion/philosophy and education, vary among subcultures in the United States. The other three (technology, politics/law, and the economy) exert broader effects that can be seen among different countries, but less so among subcultures within a country.

- **Religion and philosophy.** A person's religion may determine what health care is acceptable to him. For example, some religions (e.g., Jehovah's Witnesses) do not accept blood transfusions, and many religions forbid abortion.

- **Education.** Education influences the perception of wellness and illness and the knowledge of options that are available for health care. These, in turn, affect the person's expectations for care (Leininger, 1991, 1995, 2002a; Leininger & McFarland, 2002; Reynolds & Leininger, 1993).

- **Technology.** The availability of supplies and equipment determines what is used in the healthcare setting and what comes to be culturally expected. Nurses in most of North America, for example, assume they will have bed linens, water, electricity, necessary medications, and technology such as electrocardiography and x-ray imaging. In many parts of the world, however, these items are not available.

- **Politics and the law.** Governmental policies affect health care. They determine what practitioners will be available and what programs will be funded; for example, the federal government helps fund Medicare, which provides basic medical insurance for people age 65 and above. The legal system defines roles, functions, and standards of health professionals.

TABLE 13-1   Folk Healers and Practices

Cultural Group	Folk Healers	Folk Practices
White, European American	Nurse Physician Chiropractor Acupuncturist Massage therapist Physical therapist Occupational therapist Respiratory therapist	Medicines (OTC and prescribed) Therapeutic or modified diets Exercise Religious healing rituals (including prayer) Sleep Cleanliness Amulets
Hispanic	Curandero Espiritualista (spiritualist) Yerbero (herbalist) Sabador	Hot and cold therapies Medals and amulets Prayers Herbs and herbal teas Massage Jewelry to ward off the "evil eye"
African American	"Old lady" healers Spiritualist Hougan, or voodoo priest or priestess	Herbs and roots Oils and poultices Talismans and amulets (worn or carried to ward off evil) Religious rituals ("laying on of hands")
Native American, Eskimo, and Aleut	Shaman Crystal gazer hand trembler (diagnostician) Medicine woman or man	Herbs and plants Incantations and prayers Rituals and healing ceremonies Blessed medicine bundles or other dried plants or flowers, or burning of dried plants Stargazing and sandpainting
Asian and Pacific Islander	Herbalist Acupuncturist Physician	Hot and cold foods Herbs and roots Meditation Acupuncture (inserting needles into meridians or life energy pathways) Acupressure Energy to restore yin, yang balance

Sources: Adapted from Andrews, M. M., & Boyle, J. S. (2003). *Transcultural concepts in nursing care* (4th ed.). Philadelphia: Lippincott; Giger, J., & Davidhizar, R. (1999). *Transcultural nursing: Assessment and intervention* (3rd ed.). St Louis: Mosby; Purnell, L., & Paulanka, B. (2003). *Transcultural health care: A culturally competent approach* (2nd ed.). Philadelphia: F. A. Davis Company; and Spector, R. (2004). *Cultural diversity in health and illness* (6th ed.). Upper Saddle River, NJ: Prentice Hall.

• ***Economy.*** The condition of the economy directly affects the availability of funds for publicly funded services. It also affects the individual's ability to pay for health care.

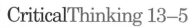

CriticalThinking 13–5

Consider this example: Mrs. Lin, a Japanese American, has been admitted to your care on a medical-surgical unit from the post-anesthesia care unit (PACU), having undergone a major surgical procedure. She refuses pain medicine, although she appears to you to be in pain. As the hours pass, Mrs. Lin continues to refuse the pain medication, so eventually the nurses stop asking.

• Do you assume that she is experiencing no pain?
• Are you or the other nurses stereotyping her for her cultural response to pain?
• What would you do?

KnowledgeCheck 13–3

- Identify at least six culture specifics affecting health.
- How could you use this information about culture specifics to provide better care to your clients?

 Go to Chapter 13, **Knowledge Check Response Sheet and Answers,** on the Electronic Study Guide.

WHAT IS THE "CULTURE OF HEALTH CARE"?

In any culture, two healthcare systems usually exist side by side: indigenous healthcare systems and professional healthcare systems (Leininger, 1995). Each has its own culture. The **indigenous health care system** consists of *folk medicine* and *traditional healing methods,* which may also include over-the-counter (OTC) and self-treatment remedies. Different groups have different folk practices (Table 13–1).

In contrast, the **professional healthcare system** is run by a set of professional healthcare providers who have been formally educated and trained for their appropriate roles and responsibilities. In North America, professional healthcare is dominated by the **biomedical healthcare system,** which combines Western biomedical beliefs with traditional North American values of self-reliance, individualism, and aggressive action. The professional healthcare system also includes practitioners formally trained in **alternative health care,** such as diet therapy, mind-body control methods, therapeutic touch, accupressure, reflexology, naturopathy, kinesiology, and chiropractic. All cultural groups probably use the professional healthcare system to at least some degree.

Many professional healthcare providers do not understand the beliefs and practices of the indigenous health care systems and traditional healers. For this reason, conflicts arise: The professional health care provider views the indigenous beliefs and practices as uncivilized and based on the supernatural, and believers in indigenous methods view the professional healthcare culture with distrust. This type of thinking benefits no one. As a nurse, you should become aware of and understand a variety of health beliefs and practices so that you can meet the needs of your clients and families.

What Are Health and Illness Beliefs?

To provide culturally competent care, you need to know how people in various cultural groups understand life processes, how they define health and illness, and what they believe to be the causes of illness (ANA, 1997). Generally speaking, people follow one of three major health belief systems: scientific, magico-religious, or holistic (Andrews & Boyle, 2003). You are probably familiar with the **scientific** or **biomedical health system.** Belief in supernatural forces dominates the **magico-religious system,** which is

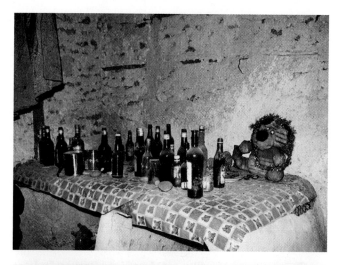

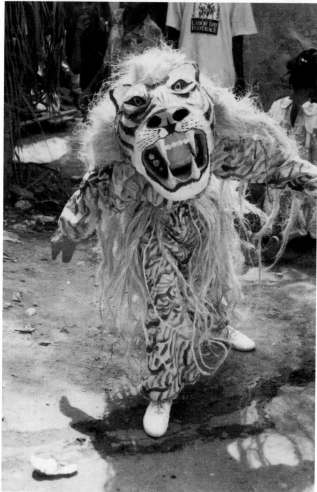

FIGURE 13–6 Voodoo is an example of a magico-religious belief system. Top, A Haitian voodoo shrine (notice the lion). Bottom, A Haitian man costumed for Carnival as the spirit of the lion.

considered "alternative" or "indigenous" in the United States and Canada. One example is voodoo, which is practiced in some developing nations in Africa, Latin America, and the Caribbean, and which considers the lion a spiritual symbol (Figure 13–6). The **holistic**

belief system can be similar to magico-religious, but it focuses more on the need for harmony and balance of the body with nature.

What Are Health and Illness Practices?

In addition to knowing the values and beliefs of different cultures, you need to know what people in various cultural groups do to maintain wellness (ANA, 1997).

CriticalThinking 13–6

- What do you do to keep yourself healthy?
- What do you do to treat minor illnesses when you do not want to see a physician?

Think about Mr. Chan ("Meet Your Patient"). If he or his daughter asked for a Chinese priest to come to his room and perform a ceremony to restore his harmony, do you think this ceremony would be harmful or helpful to him? Would you support or discourage this? What about Rosanna's dressing the children in heavy coats and knit hats although it is quite warm outside? Is this harmful or helpful to them? Would you support or discourage this? As you think about those questions, keep in mind that cultural health practices can be any of the following (Giger & Davidhizar, 2004):

- Efficacious (helpful)
- Neutral (neither helpful nor causing harm)
- Dysfunctional (harmful)
- Uncertain (not known)

You should encourage practices that could be helpful and discourage those that may cause harm. There should be no harm in allowing a patient to continue a neutral health practice. For example, some Irish methods to prevent illness and protect health include eating porridge at night before bed and avoiding going to bed with wet hair (Giger & Davidhizar, 2002). You would not want to interfere with these neutral practices. However, you should discourage dysfunctional activities, such as taking herbal remedies along with prescribed drugs without informing the healthcare provider.

KnowledgeCheck 13–4

- List three types of alternative health care that are delivered by formally trained practitioners as a part of the professional healthcare system.
- What are magico-religious belief systems?
- As a nurse, in which of the following cultural health practices would you support your client: efficacious, neutral, dysfunctional, uncertain? Why?
- Refer to the "Meet Your Patient" feature. Identify an efficacious practice.

 Go to Chapter 13, **Knowledge Check Response Sheet and Answers,** on the Electronic Study Guide.

CriticalThinking 13–7

What aspects of the indigenous and professional systems have you used for yourself or your family? Give examples.

What Is the Culture of the North American Healthcare System?

Members of the biomedical healthcare system in the United States and Canada belong to a culture with its own set of norms. That culture can be further divided into subcultures, such as those of physicians, nurses, respiratory therapists, and so on. Some of the norms found in these overlapping subcultures include the following (Leppa, 2000):

- Belief in and reliance on the biomedical system
- Valuing of technology
- Desire to conquer disease
- Definition of health as the absence or minimization of disease
- Adherence to a set of ethical standards and codes of conduct

Table 13–2 summarizes the norms of the North American healthcare system.

Nursing and Other Professional Subcultures

Nursing is the largest subculture within the healthcare culture. Leininger (1978) defines the **culture of nursing** as the learned and transmitted lifeways, values, symbols, patterns, and normative practices of members of the nursing profession that are not the same as those of the mainstream culture. The nursing subculture's beliefs and values have been formed in part by the society at large, which historically has been dominated by white Anglo-Saxon Protestants. Nursing values include, in addition to those listed in Table 13–2, the following:

- Silent suffering as a response to pain
- Objective reporting and description of pain, but not an emotional response
- Use of the nursing process
- Nursing autonomy
- Caring

In this book, we add *knowledge* and *critical thinking* to the list of nursing values. Although these values are not consistently rewarded in practice, we believe that a steadily increasing number of nurses realize their importance—that nursing is "knowledge work" and that the nurse's knowledge and thinking are of paramount importance to the well-being of patients.

As you become more socialized into the nursing culture, you should continue to examine professional

values to see how strongly you identify with them and how they affect your work with patients. For example, if you value silent suffering in response to pain, how might that cause you to respond to a woman in very early labor who is screaming and crying even though her contractions are very weak? Would you dismiss her for being a "whiner"? Or scold her ("You can't be hurting that bad this early in labor")? You must be careful not to lose the ability to understand health and illness from the patient's point of view.

Review the case of Rosanna and José ("Meet Your Patient"). The primary care provider prescribes an antibiotic for José's fever and sore throat. You observe that Anna does not seem to be happy with the medicine, so you stress to her the importance of buying the medicine right away to make him better. On her way out of the clinic, Anna throws the prescription in the trash. Why do you think she threw away the prescription?

If you had difficulty thinking of possible answers to the question, refer to the Hispanic health beliefs in ESG Table 13–2 on the Electronic Study Guide and Table 13–3 in this chapter. Some people of Mexican heritage believe that illness is caused by the body's imbalance of "hot" and "cold" (not related to temperature). The scenario doesn't tell you for sure, but it could be that Anna did not believe the medication would help her son, so she decided not to spend money on it. Could this problem have been prevented? The answer is yes. You or the primary care provider should have assessed Anna's health beliefs and practices and involved her in José's care by discussing treatment options with her. The provider should have asked Anna whether the medication was acceptable to her, and if not, asked her to explain her ideas about José's illness. For example, if she considered his ear infection to be "hot," then a "cold" herb or medication would be needed. The provider might have been able to explain that the ordered medication would get rid of the heat and pain that José is experiencing from the infection or find another medication that Anna would consider to be "cold."

 Go to Chapter 13, **Tables, Boxes, Figures: ESG Table 13–2,** on the Electronic Study Guide.

This is an example of what can happen when healthcare providers are so rigidly grounded in the beliefs of the professional healthcare culture that they fail to recognize and understand the health beliefs and practices of their clients. As you may guess, this way of practicing is a barrier to culturally competent care.

KnowledgeCheck 13–5

How do the cultural norms of the North American healthcare system differ from those of other cultural groups? Refer to ESG Table 13–2 on the Electronic Study Guide and Tables 13–2 and 13–3 in this chapter as needed.

 Go to Chapter 13, **Knowledge Check Response Sheet and Answers,** on the Electronic Study Guide.

TABLE 13–2 Summary of Cultural Norms of the North American Healthcare System

Norm	Examples
Beliefs	Standardized definitions of health and illness Significance of technology
Practices	Maintaining health and preventing disease through such practices as immunizations and avoidance of stress Annual physical examinations and diagnostic tests
Habits	Handwashing Use of jargon (e.g., giving "meds") Use of problem-solving methods Documentation
Likes	Punctuality Neatness and organization Compliance (e.g., with medical "orders")
Dislikes	Tardiness Disorganization Messiness, lack of cleanliness
Customs	Use of procedures (e.g., circumcision) surrounding birth and death Professional respect and observance of hierarchy found in autocratic and bureaucratic systems
Rituals	Annual physical examination The surgical procedure

Sources: Adapted from Giger, J., & Davidhizar, R. (2004). *Transcultural nursing: Assessment and intervention* (4th ed.). St. Louis: Mosby; Luckmann, J. (2000). *Transcultural communication in health care.* Albany, NY: Delmar; Purnell, L., & Paulanka, B. (2003). *Transcultural health care: A culturally competent approach* (2nd ed.). Philadelphia: F. A. Davis Company; and Spector, R. (2004). *Cultural diversity in health and illness* (6th ed.). Upper Saddle River, NJ: Prentice Hall.

Traditional and Alternative Healing

You need to know how healers from various cultures cure and care for members of their group (ANA, 1997). All cultures think of their healthcare system and beliefs as "traditional"; however, we use *traditional* in this chapter to refer to alternative beliefs, not to those of the Western, North American, biomedical, or professional healthcare systems. You have already learned about different healthcare beliefs and practices clients may have (e.g., biomedical or scientific, holistic, magico-religious). The following section focuses on the types of healing systems that are used in different cultures.

Values and Health and Illness Beliefs and Practices for Selected Ethnocultural Groups in North America

TABLE 13-3

Group	Dominant Values	Health and Illness Beliefs	Health and Illness Practices
Native American	Bonding to family or group Acceptance of nature (Mother Earth) Tradition Sharing Belief in a spiritual power Respect of elders	Health means living in harmony with nature Surviving under difficult circumstances Body treated with respect Illness is associated with disharmony or evil spirits Illness is caused by an action that should not have been performed	Rituals and ceremonies Chanting Purification Meditation Herbs
Asian and Pacific Islander	Extended family Respect for elders Group orientation Subordination to authority Conformity Self respect and self control Love of the land	Health is a state of physical and spiritual harmony Illness is disharmony of basic world principles: yin and yang	Acupuncture Amulets Moxibustion Herbs
Black or African American	Family bonding Matrifocal Spiritual orientation Present-oriented	Health is harmony with nature (mind, body, and spirit) Illness is due to disharmony or failure to eat proper foods	Prayer Laying on of hands Magic rituals Voodoo Herbs
Hispanic or Latino	Extended family Group emphasis Fatalistic Faith and spirituality	Health is good luck or a reward for good behavior; a gift from God Illness is body imbalance (hot or cold, wet or dry) or punishment	Prayer Belief in miracles Wearing of religious metals or amulets Religious relics in home Herbs and spices Rituals Hot & cold therapy
White or European American	Independence Individuality Wealth Comfort Cleanliness Achievement Youth and beauty	Health is a state of physical and emotional well-being Illness is contagion or contamination that is hereditary, psychosomatic, or super natural	Biomedical care Home remedies Religious traditions Diet and exercise

Note: Most people in North America use a combination of biomedical and traditional (specific to their culture) healthcare practices.

Sources: Adapted from Giger, J., & Davidhizar, R. (2004). *Transcultural nursing: Assessment and intervention* (4th ed.). St Louis: Mosby; Luckmann, J. (2000). *Transcultural communication in health care*. Albany, NY: Delmar; Spector, R. (2004). *Cultural diversity in health and illness* (6th ed.). Upper Saddle River, NJ: Prentice Hall; Andrews, M., & Boyle, J. (1999). *Transcultural concepts in nursing care* (3rd ed.). Philadelphia: Lippincott; and Purnell, L., & Paulanka, B. (2003). *Transcultural health care: A culturally competent approach* (2nd ed.). Philadelphia: F. A. Davis Company.

Folk Medicine

When you feel as if you're getting a cold or the flu, what do you do? If you said that you take aspirin or vitamin C or eat chicken soup, then you are practicing folk medicine. You most likely do what your mother or some other relative did for you in similar situations. In North America there is a pill for almost everything, and virtually everyone self-medicates with over-the-counter medicines. For many cultures, folk medicine involves natural medicines, such as herbs, plants, minerals, and animal substances. Magico-religious folk medicine involves the use of charms, holy words, rituals, and holy actions for preventing and treating illnesses (Spector, 2004).

Folk medicine is defined as the beliefs and practices that the members of a cultural group follow when they are ill, as opposed to more conventional (i.e., biomedical or professional) standards (Andrews & Boyle, 2003). Leininger (1995) observes that all cultures throughout the world use folk medicine. These treatments have lasted over time, and knowledge of them is passed down from generation to generation by oral tradition (Andrews & Boyle, 2003). Folk medicine includes both self treatment and use of folk healers.

Why would someone want to see a folk healer rather than a professional healthcare provider? In the dominant North American culture, the folk healer *is* the professional healthcare provider (i.e., the nurse practitioner, physician, certified nurse midwife, and so on). In other cultures, people may seek out folk healers because they speak their native language, share their values and beliefs, charge less money, are readily available, or make house calls. If people perceive that the professional healing system cannot meet their needs, they are likely to seek care from the folk healers within their cultures and avoid the professional system. Table 13–1 identifies folk healers of various cultures and their practices.

Many folk healing traditions are guided not only by cultural practices but also by religious beliefs and rituals. Religious rituals are often associated with births (e.g., circumcision) and death (e.g., who is allowed to wash the body and prepare it for burial). It can be almost impossible to separate cultural from religious beliefs. Nevertheless, you cannot assume that because your patient is a member of a certain culture that he will also be of a certain religion. It is safer to ask.

Complementary and Alternative Medicine

Complementary medicine is the use of rigorously tested therapies *to complement* those of conventional medicine (Andrews & Boyle, 2003). Examples include chiropractic care, biofeedback, and the use of certain supplements. In contrast, **alternative medicine** is defined as therapies used *instead of* conventional (i.e., biomedical) medicine, and whose reliability has not been validated through clinical testing in the United States. Examples of alternative therapies include iridology, aromatherapy, and magnet therapy. Some complementary and alternative modalities (CAM) are derived from the ancient and indigenous healthcare systems of people of other countries, such as traditional Chinese medicine (TCM), and **ayurveda,** the traditional healthcare system of India. As mentioned previously, certain therapies require a healer specially trained in their use (e.g., chiropractic, reflexology, massage therapy). Some alternative and CAM healers (e.g., massage therapists) are licensed by the state. The National Institutes of Health's National Center for Complementary and Alternative Medicine is currently conducting and funding research on a number of CAM therapies.

Always ask clients about their use of alternative and folk medicine. Many people use them, but they may be reluctant to tell you so. The client may fear ridicule or at least disapproval. Some nurses may perceive alternative or folk practices to be odd or useless, but this attitude may be due to a lack of knowledge. You will probably not consider these practices to be so "strange" once you become familiar with them.

KnowledgeCheck 13–6

- What is folk medicine?
- What are some common folk medicine practices?
- Why might members of some cultural groups seek out the local folk healer rather than the conventional healthcare provider?

 Go to Chapter 13, **Knowledge Check Response Sheet and Answers,** on the Electronic Study Guide.

WHAT IS CULTURALLY COMPETENT CARE?

The terms *cultural awareness, cultural sensitivity,* and *cultural competence* are often used interchangeably; however, they are different. **Cultural awareness** refers to an appreciation of the external signs of diversity, whereas **cultural sensitivity** has more to do with personal attitudes and being careful not to say or do something that might be offensive to someone from a different culture (Purnell & Paulanka, 2003, p. 3).

The American Nurses Association supports the need for nurses to understand cultural diversity and to become culturally competent. However, there is no consensus as to *how* the nurse's knowledge, skills, and attitudes will best serve the diverse populations. Cultural competence is attained on a continuum ranging from cultural destructiveness (most negative) to cultural proficiency (most positive) (Cross, Bazron, Dennis, & Isaac, 1989). You cannot achieve cultural competence overnight because it is a developmental process. As you become more aware of and sensitive to the needs of individuals from various ethnocultural groups, you

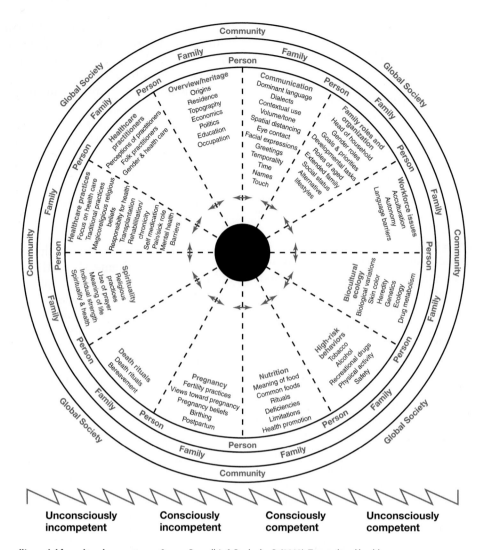

FIGURE 13–7 **Purnell's model for cultural competence.** *Source:* Purnell, L. & Paulanka, B. (2003). *Transcultural health care: A culturally competent approach* (2nd ed.). Philadelphia: F. A. Davis Company, p. 10. Reprinted with permission.

will move forward on the journey toward cultural competence: being able to use knowledge and sensitivity in practice. The following are some ideas about **cultural competence.**

Purnell and Paulanka

The Purnell model for cultural competence stresses teamwork in providing culturally sensitive and competent care to improve outcomes for individuals, families, and communities (Purnell, 2000, 2002; Purnell & Paulanka, 2003). The pie-shaped wedges in Figure 13–7 depict the issues that all societies and humans share (e.g., pregnancy, nutrition, high-risk behavior, family organization, and death) but that are expressed in ways specific to the culture. These domains provide the organizing framework for the model. The center of the model is empty and represents that which is unknown about a cultural group.

Defined in the context of nursing, Purnell's model (Purnell & Paulanka, 2003, pp. 3–4) describes cultural competence as:

- Developing an awareness of one's own existence, sensations, thoughts, and environment without letting it have undue influence on those from other backgrounds
- Demonstrating knowledge and understanding of the client's health-related needs and concepts of health and illness
- Accepting and respecting cultural differences
- Realizing that the values and beliefs of healthcare providers may be different from the client's
- Resisting judgmental attitudes, such as "different is not as good"
- Being open to cultural encounters

- Adapting care to make it congruent with the client's culture

- Recognizing culture as a conscious and nonlinear process

Leininger

Although Madeline Leininger does not use the specific term *cultural competence,* her (2002a) theory fits with that concept. The goal of her theory is "to use research findings to provide culturally congruent, safe, and meaningful care to clients of diverse or similar cultures" (p. 190). Nurses can obtain this goal by:

1. Discovering cultural care and caring beliefs, values, and practices
2. Analyzing the similarities and differences of these beliefs among the different cultures

For more information on Leininger's theory of culture care diversity and universality,

 Go to Chapter 13, **Supplemental Materials: Madeline Leininger,** on the Electronic Study Guide.

Campinha-Bacote

The culturally competent model of care (Campinha-Bacote, 2002) views cultural competence as a process, not an end point. The model identifies five components of cultural competence, using the mnemonic ASKED:

Awareness (cultural sensitivity, cultural biases)
Skills (cultural assessment tools)
Knowledge (cultural worldviews, theoretical frameworks)
Encounters (cultural exposure, cultural practice)
Desire (to be culturally competent)

 CriticalThinking 13–8

What kind of knowledge do you need to become culturally competent (theoretical, practical, personal, ethical)? Explain your answer. See Chapter 2 to review types of knowledge, if necessary.

What Are Some Barriers to Culturally Competent Care?

Your ability to provide culturally competent care may be hampered by the following barriers:

- *Lack of knowledge* about the cultural and ethnic values, beliefs, and behaviors of people within their community is not unusual among healthcare providers. It can cause them to misinterpret a client's behaviors.

- *Emotional responses* such as fear and distrust—both yours and the client's—can arise any time members of different cultural groups meet. If you are aware that this may happen, you may be able to avoid this barrier and communicate with your clients effectively.

- *Ethnocentrism* (discussed earlier) may negatively affect care. People have a tendency to be **biased** toward their own culture, believing that their own beliefs and values are right and that those of other cultures are wrong (or at least bizarre). If you take this attitude, your patient may feel that you disapprove of him or, at the least, that you don't understand or respect him.

- A **cultural stereotype** is the unsubstantiated belief that all people of a certain racial or ethnic group are alike in certain respects. A stereotype may be positive or negative.

- Similar to a stereotype, **prejudice** refers to negative attitudes toward other people that are based on faulty and rigid stereotypes about race, gender, sexual orientation, and so on.

- Whereas prejudice refers to people's attitudes, the term **discrimination** refers to the behavioral manifestations of that prejudice. For example, prior to the 1960s many U.S. hospitals refused treatment to African Americans. Slightly more subtle discrimination against minority groups still exists in housing, banking, and the job market. It is, in some places, more difficult for a woman, someone who is openly homosexual, or an African American to obtain a loan or to be hired for certain jobs.

- **Racism** is a form of prejudice and discrimination based on the belief that race is the principal determining factor of human traits and capabilities and that racial differences produce an inherent superiority (or inferiority). The word *race* alone evokes powerful emotional responses for people who feel that they or their ancestors have been oppressed or exploited, and equally for those who deny such a responsibility. In the United States, the history of discrimination against non-whites, and especially against African Americans, has created a focus on differences and racial divisiveness. As a nurse, you must recognize that unconscious racism can play a major role in your ability to communicate with people of other races.

- **Sexism,** widespread throughout history, is the assumption that members of one sex are superior to those of the other sex. For example, women have been viewed as more emotional and less rational than men, and assertiveness, considered a positive trait in men, may be seen as "pushiness" or aggressiveness in women. On the other hand, men who are nurses must combat the kind of sexism that asserts that it is "unnatural" for men to engage in caring behaviors. Some female nurses may not accept their male colleagues, and some patients—both male and female—may object to their care, at least initially.

Male chauvinism (assumption of male superiority) is common in many cultures and in healthcare settings. It may be overt or subtle. In the wider society, for example, men may receive higher pay for performing the same work as a woman. In the healthcare setting, you might, even now, hear a male physician calling female nurses or patients "dear," or using a voice tone more appropriate to addressing a child. When you have the opportunity to do so, observe a conversation between a male nurse and a male physician. You may note that the male nurse communicates more directly and uses more eye contact than female nurses do with this same physician. We are not assuming that all physicians (or nurses) are chauvinistic; we are simply stating that you will probably be able to observe this kind of interchange among some professionals. As in other settings, the assumption of equality—by either party—changes the way people communicate.

- A *language barrier* will obviously affect your ability to communicate with clients. Language barriers can involve foreign languages, dialects, regionalisms (words or pronunciation particular to a specific region), street talk, and jargon (words or expressions used by a subculture, including medicine).

  For example, recall Mr. Salvatore, in "Meet Your Patient." Suppose it is found that he has a brain tumor and needs immediate surgery. You would need to get his consent for surgery even though he and his family do not speak English. You might call the telephone language line to which your hospital subscribes. But suppose that the interpreter has difficulty understanding Mr. Salvatore completely because he uses a different dialect or slang.

  This is not an unusual situation. In such a case, you would need to explore the resources and policies of your healthcare facility. If there were no other options for translation help, you would have to resort to nonverbal language and pictures to communicate until further resources could be found. It's not the best option, but it may be the only one, at least temporarily. However, if a consent issue is involved, the hospital will almost certainly have a policy to handle the situation.

- *Street talk, slang, and jargon* can be as challenging as a foreign language. For example, the word *bad* can mean bad or good; the meaning changes, and not everyone has the same interpretations. Ebonics (also called African American Vernacular English, or AAVE) is a type of English that has, in the past, been spoken primarily by African Americans, but many white youth enamored with hip-hop culture now embrace Ebonics as a way to connect with the street culture.

  Health care jargon can often be distressing to clients. In the healthcare field, we have our own terminology, including abbreviations, which we use so often we may forget that our clients don't understand them. For example, you may frighten some clients if you say to them, "I'm going to take your vitals" before assessing their blood pressure. You may be surprised to learn that many patients will not know what you mean if you ask, "Have you voided today?" Even worse, patients may hesitate to ask for clarification because they don't like admitting that they don't understand a certain word. What other examples of nursing or medical jargon can you think of that might be confusing to clients?

KnowledgeCheck 13–7

- Define *cultural competence*.
- How do the barriers of ethnocentrism and language impede nursing care of diverse populations?

 Go to Chapter 13, **Knowledge Check Response Sheet and Answers,** on the Electronic Study Guide.

Practical Knowledge
knowing how

Each phase of the nursing process presents an opportunity to provide culturally sensitive, congruent, and competent care. Regardless of the patient's cultural group, it is important for you to establish rapport before beginning data collection—especially for sensitive or personal information.

| Assessment |

Cultural assessment, as does any assessment, consists of an interview and a physical assessment (both subjective and objective data). When you perform a cultural assessment, you should gather data directly from your client, but if this is not possible, you may ask for help from a friend or family member. When you need to use an interpreter—even if it must be a family member—be aware of confidentiality (private information) issues.

The Health History

The **health history** is an important component of assessment. To encourage clients to talk about themselves, you must convey empathy, show respect, build rapport, establish trust, listen actively, and provide appropriate feedback (Luckmann, 2000). Ask open-ended questions when beginning a cultural assessment.

You will not need to perform an in-depth cultural assessment on every patient, but you will need to recognize situations in which this is needed. Lipson and

Meleis (1985) suggest that the following minimum information is important:

Language(s) spoken; proficiency in language of the host

Length of time client has been in the host country

Where client was raised

Ethnic affiliation and identity

Usual religious practices

Nonverbal communication style

Family roles and primary decision-maker about your health care

Social support in the host country

For a list of questions to help you obtain this information,

 Go to Chapter 13, **Technique 13–2: Obtaining Minimal Cultural Information,** in Volume 2.

Physical Assessment

Physical assessment may reveal biocultural variations. To assess and evaluate clients accurately, you need to know the normal physiological variations among healthy members of selected populations, for example, body proportions, vital signs, general appearance, skin, the musculoskeletal system, illness, and laboratory values (Andrews & Boyle, 2003). For example, knowledge of biocultural variations in skin is important because of the importance of assessing for pallor, cyanosis, jaundice, erythema, and petechiae, which may be more difficult to evaluate in darkly pigmented persons. For more information about assessing the skin, see Chapter 19, and

 Go to Chapter 13, **Technique 13–1: Assessing for Biological Variations,** in Volume 2.

Assessing for Pain

Culture influences the patient's illness behaviors, including responses to pain (Mechanic, 1963; Suchman, 1964, 1965; Zborowski, 1952, 1969; and Zola, 1966). Because pain and comfort are subjective responses, you will need to quantify your client's pain as objectively as possible, for example, by using a pain measurement scale. For some descriptions of some cultural responses to pain,

 Go to Chapter 13, **Technique 13–3: Assessing Pain Perception in Selected Cultural Groups,** in Volume 2.

Regardless of the literature descriptions of cultural responses, it is essential to investigate the meaning of pain to each individual.

Cultural Assessment Models and Tools

Some agencies have special tools for in-depth cultural assessments. If yours does not, you can structure your assessments using any culture model, such as the following examples. For more information on these assessment models,

 Go to Chapter 13, **Tables, Boxes, Figures: ESG Figures 13–2 and 13–3, and ESG Boxes 13–1 and 13–2,** on the Electronic Study Guide.

1. *Giger and Davidhizar's transcultural assessment model* (2002). See ESG Figure 13–2.

 Also go to Chapter 13, **Technique 13–4: Performing a Cultural Assessment,** in Volume 2.

2. *Spector's heritage assessment model* (2000, 2002, 2004). See ESG Figure 13–3. Instead of assessing culture specifics, this tool assesses **heritage consistency:** the degree to which a person's lifestyle reflects his traditional culture (country of origin, race, or ethnic group). This assessment tool also reveals the degree to which the client still identifies with his cultural origins.

3. *Purnell model for cultural competence* (2003). See ESG Box 13–1.

4. *Andrews and Boyle transcultural nursing assessment guide* (2003). See ESG Box 13–2.

| Nursing Diagnosis |

There are no NANDA diagnoses that specifically address culture. However, cultural factors can be the etiology of various problems. Any of the NANDA diagnostic labels can be used for clients of any culture, provided that the defining characteristics are present. Some possible examples include the following:

- *Risk for Imbalanced Nutrition: Less Than Body Requirements* might apply to a client who is hospitalized and cannot obtain foods prepared in the traditional way of his ethnic group.

- *Impaired Parenting* could occur if the patient's traditional methods of discipline are not acceptable or appropriate in the dominant culture.

- *Spiritual Distress* might occur because a necessary treatment is not congruent with a client's religious beliefs.

- *Powerlessness* might occur when the patient is unable to make healthcare personnel understand the importance of his religious and dietary beliefs.

- *Impaired Verbal Communication* can apply to clients who do not speak or understand your language. However, this diagnosis is of questionable value in such circumstances. In a classic study, Geissler (1991) found that Impaired Verbal Communication related

BOX 13-1

NANDA Nursing Diagnoses with Potential for Cultural Bias

Imbalanced Nutrition: Less Than Body Requirements

Imbalanced Nutrition: More Than Body Requirements

Ineffective Role Performance

Anxiety

Decisional Conflict

Disturbed Thought Processes

Effective Breastfeeding

Ineffective Breastfeeding

Impaired Social Interaction

Social Isolation

Impaired Verbal Communication

Ineffective Denial

Ineffective Coping

Disabled Family Coping

Deficient Knowledge

Noncompliance

Acute Pain

Chronic Pain

Powerlessness

more to cultural differences between the client and healthcare provider than to the inability to communicate. So if the client is verbally "impaired," the nurse is *equally* "impaired"; that is, communication is as much a "problem" for the nurse as for the client.

- *Risk for Noncompliance* can be used for clients and/or caregivers who do not follow a health-promoting or therapeutic plan the healthcare provider believes they agreed to. For example, the plan may not "fit" with the client's perception of the cause of his illness. But again, you must use this diagnostic label with care. The Geissler (1991) study also found that additional defining characteristics are needed before Noncompliance can be appropriately applied to clients not of the dominant U.S. culture.

The preceding examples illustrate the concern that standardized nursing diagnoses are not always culturally sensitive; that is, they may not apply accurately to patients who are not from the dominant culture. Nursing diagnoses should describe responses that *patients* see as problematic. A nurse and patient who are from different cultures will likely have different perceptions of health and illness. This can lead to misdiagnosis. The nurse may either diagnose a problem that doesn't exist for the patient or diagnose a "real" problem but fail to describe it accurately (Wilkinson, 2001).

Suppose that a 60-year-old woman who works as a hotel maid is repeatedly admitted to your hospital for uncontrolled hypertension. You know that uncontrolled hypertension can lead to strokes. You determine that she does not take her medication, and you diagnose Noncompliance (failure to take prescribed medication). But do you know that an antihypertensive medication can cost more than $100 for a month's supply? Perhaps your patient is raising her grandchildren and that paying for shelter, utilities, food, and clothing uses up her entire income.

Box 13–1 lists some NANDA nursing diagnoses that could be interpreted differently by people from different cultures. Undoubtedly there are others. The point is to use all labels carefully and to validate nursing diagnoses with the patient to be sure that the statement describes her health status as *she* sees it.

Planning Outcomes/Evaluation

The outcomes you choose (whether standardized or individualized) depend on the nursing diagnoses you have identified. If the diagnoses are culturally sensitive, the outcomes should be as well. However, you must involve the client in order to be certain. For example, suppose your patient is dying. Both you and the patient agree that her diagnosis is Acute Pain, but your goals may be different. You might want the patient to be free from pain. However, the patient's goal may be to stay alert enough to interact with her family, even if it means she will have to endure some pain. When cultures are different, it is even more important to validate the goals with the patient. Some individualized goal/outcome statements associated with cultural differences might include the following:

- Agrees to take prescribed analgesic (pain medication) before bedtime and after family leaves for the evening.
- Talks to her spiritual adviser about the possibility of surgery that conflicts with her religious beliefs.
- Freely shares information about folk practices and over-the-counter medications with the primary care provider.
- Asks for clarification from healthcare professional when she does not understand clearly what was said.

Planning Interventions/Implementation

When planning care for your clients, you need to include information about their cultural values, beliefs, and practices to identify interventions that will support these practices and incorporate them into their care as much as possible (Wilkinson, 2001). For example, when you are teaching about a specific treatment regimen ordered by the primary care provider, you should find out whether it conflicts with any of the patient's folk beliefs or alternative treatments so that you can suggest any necessary modifications. Remember also to identify

educational methods that are most appropriate for your client's needs (translated materials and/or diagrams) and to make community referrals as necessary.

Although nursing care depends on the client's specific problems and their etiologies, some nursing interventions and activities can be especially appropriate for providing culturally competent care. *NIC standardized interventions* related to culture include the following:

Active Listening (for Impaired Verbal Communication)
Family Involvement Promotion (for Readiness for Enhanced Family Coping)
Self-Responsibility Facilitation (for Powerlessness)
Culture Brokerage (for Noncompliance)

Individualized nursing activities and focused assessments are important for all clients. However, clients from different cultural and ethnic groups may have unique needs. According to Dochterman and Bulechek (2004), **Culture Brokerage,** a Nursing Intervention Classification (NIC) intervention, is defined as "the deliberate use of culturally competent strategies to bridge or mediate between the patient's culture and the biomedical health care system" (p. 271). Many of these activities are included in the discussion that follows regarding the provision of culturally competent care.

KnowledgeCheck 13–8

- Describe, in general, how the nursing process can help you provide culturally competent care.
- How can nursing diagnoses cause bias in the planning of care for clients from different cultures?

 Go to Chapter 13, **Knowledge Check Response Sheet and Answers,** on the Electronic Study Guide.

Nursing Strategies for Providing Culturally Competent Care

You should become familiar with the cultural groups you are most likely to encounter. Choose one of the transcultural models to help you to use critical thinking and the nursing process to provide the holistic care your clients deserve. Leininger's theory describes the following three "modes" of nursing decisions and actions (Leininger, 1991; Leininger, 2002a; Leininger & McFarland, 2002; Reynolds & Leininger, 1993):

1. *Cultural care preservation/maintenance,* which sustains clients' cultural lifestyles in meaningful ways. These are actions that help the client retain or preserve cultural values related to health.

   Example: Encouraging the family to bring ethnic foods that are appropriate for the patient's prescribed diet.

2. *Cultural care accommodation/negotiation,* which adapts clients' lifestyles or nurses' actions. The nurse supports and enables the client to adapt to therapies or to negotiate with professionals to achieve satisfying health outcomes. **Negotiation** acknowledges the gap between the nurse's and client's perspectives. You must negotiate when folk or traditional practices might be harmful to the client.

   Example: Negotiating with the client to continue seeing the *curandero,* but to come to the clinic every 6 weeks to have his blood pressure checked. If the client refuses all biomedical or nursing interventions, the only avenue still open is to continue monitoring the client to identify changes in his health status. If a health crisis occurs, it may be possible to renegotiate the care.

3. *Cultural care repatterning/restructuring,* which changes nurses' actions or clients' lifestyles into different patterns. The nurse supports and encourages the client to greatly modify his behaviors and to adopt new, different, and beneficial health behaviors, while still respecting the client's cultural values and beliefs.

   Example 1: When the client absolutely refuses to take the prescribed pain medication, the nurse uses massage, distraction, and other nonpharmacological techniques to help relieve his pain (change in nurse's actions).

   Example 2: A client refuses to see a biomedical doctor for her family's needs. However, when the folk healer is unsuccessful in treating her child's illness and the child becomes critically ill, the nurse convinces the client to bring the child to the emergency department (modification of the client's behaviors).

There are several specific strategies for you to consider and many resources to help you develop strategies specific to various cultural groups. Consider the following as you move forward on your journey toward cultural competence (also see Table 13–4):

- Consider each client as a unique individual, influenced but not defined by his culture.
- Understand your own cultural values and practices and appreciate how they may differ from those held by people of other cultures.
- Recognize your own biases about people and groups, and consider how they may affect the care you provide.
- Learn as much as you can about the cultural groups in your community and work area.
- Make an effort to incorporate beliefs and practices from various cultures into your nursing care and teaching materials.
- Encourage helpful or neutral cultural practices, and discourage those that are dysfunctional (harmful).
- Suggest alternatives to harmful practices.

TABLE 13-4 Cultural Phenomena Affecting Cultural Care Etiquette

Cultural Phenomenon	Behaviors	Nursing Interventions/Etiquette
Time	Visiting Being on time	• Inform clients when you are coming. • Avoid surprises. • Explain your expectations about time. • Ask clients from other religions and cultures what they expect.
	Taboo times	• Be familiar with times and meanings of client's ethnic and religious holidays.
Space	Body language and distancing	• Know cultural and/or religious customs regarding contact and touch with others.
Communication	Greetings	• Know proper forms of addresses for people from a given culture and the ways by which people welcome one another. • Know when touch (e.g., handshake) is expected and when touch is prohibited.
	Gestures	• Be aware that gestures do not have universal meaning—what is accepted in one culture may be taboo in another.
	Smiling	• Be aware smiles may indicate friendliness to some, but to others may be forbidden.
	Eye contact	• Be aware that avoiding eye contact may be a sign of respect.
Social organization	Holidays	• Know what dates are important and why, whether or not to give gifts, what to wear to special events, and what the customs and beliefs are.
	Special events: Births Weddings Funerals	• Know how the event is celebrated, meaning of colors for gifts, and expected rituals at home or at religious services.
Biological variations	Food customs	• Know what can be eaten for certain events, what foods may be eaten together or are forbidden, and what and how utensils are used.
Environmental control	Health practices and remedies	• Know the general health traditions for a given client, and ask questions to verify that your observations are valid.

Source: Spector, R. E. (2000). *Cultural care guides to heritage assessment and health traditions* (2nd ed.). Upper Saddle River, NJ: Prentice Hall, pp. 14–16. Used with permission.

• Accommodate cultural dietary practices when possible. For inpatients, some dietary departments can make special foods, and you can encourage families to bring food from home. In all situations, help patients and families adapt cultural foods to therapeutic diets.

• Become familiar with appropriate verbal and nonverbal communication patterns within the cultural groups, and use them selectively in your communication approaches.

• Respect your clients regardless of cultural background, and never force, pressure, manipulate, or coerce them to participate in care that conflicts with their values and beliefs.

• Advocate for all of your clients, but especially for those not from the dominant culture.

• Consider the cultural role of the family member who makes the primary decisions. To ignore this person is to doom your interventions to failure.

- Work with the folk medicine practitioner in the interest of the patient.
- Learn from your mistakes, and don't make them again.

This is by no means an exhaustive list. Most likely, you can think of other strategies. It may help you to "take a trip to BALI":

Be aware of your own cultural heritage
Appreciate that the client is unique: influenced, but not defined by his culture
Learn about the client's cultural group
Incorporate the client's cultural values/behaviors into the care plan.

How Do I Communicate with Clients from Other Cultures?

One of your major considerations as you become more culturally competent is your ability to communicate with clients from different cultures. Giger and Davidhizar (2004) encourage the following guidelines:

- Assess personal beliefs of persons from different cultures.
- Assess communication variables from a cultural perspective.
- Consider both verbal and nonverbal communication in the techniques you use with your clients.

| toward evidence-based practice |

Health practices and perceptions of wellness and illness vary between and within cultures. Although we have learned much about these beliefs and practices from transcultural texts and nursing research studies, more data needs to be collected to help healthcare providers provide culturally competent care.

Higgins, P. G., & Learn, C. D. (1999). Health practices of adult Hispanic women. *Journal of Advanced Nursing, 29*(5), 1105–1112.

This ethnographic study was conducted to determine the patterns and variability of health practices among seven Hispanic American women. These women described their health as good, were somewhat aware of current health-promotion practices (such as good nutrition and exercise), and practiced safety for themselves and their families. The researchers found that the women took better care of their families than of themselves. The women did not report any information on specific cultural disease-prevention behaviors and described only a few practices related to their own culture. The importance of spirituality was prominent in the findings.

Mendelson, C. (2002). Health perceptions of Mexican American women. *Journal of Transcultural Nursing, 13*(3), 210–217.

Using an ethnographic design to describe health perceptions, this researcher selected a sample of 13 highly acculturated Mexican women. Findings indicated that they perceived good health as being well physically and mentally, with a socially and spiritually satisfying life. Illness was not necessarily considered to be the opposite from health. Family, a belief in God, and finding balance

were important to health. The researchers found that many of the sample's perceptions differed from the traditional portrayal of Mexican American women in the literature.

Purnell, L. (2001). Guatemalans' practices for health promotion and the meaning of respect afforded them by health care providers. *Journal of Transcultural Nursing, 12*(1), 40–47.

Using the Purnell model for cultural competence, this study described Guatemalan practices for health promotion and wellness and for disease and illness prevention using a sample of 51 participants (the majority were female). Spirituality findings indicated that religion and prayer were very important. The researcher determined that many of the people in the sample followed good nutritional habits, but no one mentioned the hot-cold food balance that has been commonly cited in the literature as a key component to dietary health promotion in this culture. A balanced diet, exercise, and sleep were the most frequently reported healthcare practices. Maintaining hot-cold balances in the body was also mentioned as a common health practice, although not specifically in relation to nutrition.

---

1. Based on the preceding studies, what would you consider to be the most common health beliefs and practices of the adult Hispanic woman?

2. What assumptions must you make to use these studies to answer your question?

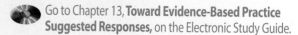 Go to Chapter 13, **Toward Evidence-Based Practice Suggested Responses,** on the Electronic Study Guide.

- Plan care based on the client's communicated needs and cultural background.
- Modify communication approaches to meet cultural needs.
- Understand that respect for the client and communicated needs are central to the therapeutic relationship.
- Communicate in a nonthreatening manner.
- Use validating techniques in communication.
- Be considerate of a client's reluctance to talk when the subject involves sexual matters.
- Adopt special approaches when the client speaks a different language.
- Use interpreters to improve communication.

How Do I Communicate with Clients Who Speak a Different Language?

Communicating with clients who do not speak your language can be especially challenging. The best way to provide culturally competent care to such patients is to use a professional medical interpreter. Largely in response to the changing population composition of the United States, the Office of Minority Health (OMH) developed the National Standards for Culturally and Linguistically Appropriate Services (CLAS) in health care. These guidelines require healthcare organizations receiving federal funding to provide language assistance services, including bilingual staff and interpreter services, at no cost to the patient. They must also provide materials and signs in the languages of the commonly encountered groups in their service area (U.S. Department of Health and Human Services, Office of Minority Health 2001). For a complete listing of the CLAS standards,

 Go to Chapter 13, **Supplemental Materials: CLAS Standards,** on the Electronic Study Guide.

An **interpreter** is specially trained to provide the meaning behind the words, whereas a **translator** just restates the words from one language to another. An interpreter can serve as a cultural broker by conveying the client's responses to questions and by providing general information about the client's culture (Luckmann, 2000). For guidelines when using any type of interpreter,

 Go to Chapter 13, **Technique 13–5: Communicating with Clients Who Speak a Different Language,** in Volume 2.

KnowledgeCheck 13–9

- List five factors to consider when communicating with clients from different cultures.
- List five factors to consider when communicating with a client using an interpreter.
- List five factors to consider when communicating with a client who does not speak your language, when an interpreter is not available.

 Go to Chapter 13, **Knowledge Check Response Sheet and Answers,** on the Electronic Study Guide.

How Can I Become Culturally Competent?

Of course you can't become culturally competent just by reading. Theoretical knowledge can increase your awareness and appreciation of cultural differences. But you can achieve cultural competence only if you are motivated to do so, and even then only by interacting with people from cultures different from your own. Carballeira (1997) sums up this process with the LIVE and LEARN model for culturally competent family services:

Like		**L**isten
Inquire		**E**valuate
Visit	and	**A**cknowledge
Experience		**R**ecommend
		Negotiate

 Go to Chapter 13, **Resources for Caregivers and Health Professionals,** on the Electronic Study Guide.

 Suggested Readings: Go to Chapter 13, **Reading More About Culture and Ethnicity,** on the Electronic Study Guide.

 Bibliography: Go to Volume 2, Bibliography.

Spirituality

Learning Outcomes

After completing this chapter, you should be able to:

* Describe the differences and similarities between religion and spirituality.

* Identify a model of spirituality that explains its concepts in terms of everyday life and living.

* For each of the religions briefly covered in this chapter, describe its major beliefs and their implications for nursing care.

* Identify five barriers to spiritual care.

* Perform a spiritual assessment.

* Plan nursing interventions based on the data obtained in a spiritual assessment.

* Distinguish the differences between spiritual care diagnoses and those that may serve as etiologies of other nursing diagnoses.

* Describe various spiritual interventions and examine your own level of comfort in terms of performing the interventions.

* Describe collaborative efforts to ensure the spiritual care of the patient or family.

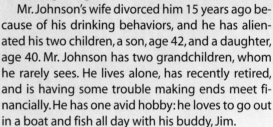

MEET Your Patient

Charles Johnson is a 65-year-old African American man with newly diagnosed cancer of the lung. He began smoking at age 15. His physicians want to start chemotherapy to try to increase his life span. He is unsure whether he wants to have chemotherapy.

Mr. Johnson was brought up in the Baptist Church but has fallen away from practicing his faith over the years. He has been a heavy drinker all of his adult life and, as a young man, became alienated from churchgoing. He explains: "Church folk are all a bunch of hypocrites, if you ask me. I choose not to be a part of any of that." Nevertheless, he says that he tries to be kind to and tolerant of others. "I've messed up my life, so I figure I don't have any business telling other people how to live. I guess I just figure that how a person lives is between themselves and God."

Mr. Johnson has one surviving relative, a sister, who is concerned about him. His sister is a devout Jehovah's Witness, and she has tried several times to talk to Mr. Johnson about how important Jehovah is in her life. She continually leaves religious pamphlets and materials in his mailbox to encourage him to think about religion again.

Mr. Johnson's wife divorced him 15 years ago because of his drinking behaviors, and he has alienated his two children, a son, age 42, and a daughter, age 40. Mr. Johnson has two grandchildren, whom he rarely sees. He lives alone, has recently retired, and is having some trouble making ends meet financially. He has one avid hobby: he loves to go out in a boat and fish all day with his buddy, Jim.

- Mr. Johnson clearly has some physical and psychosocial difficulties. Can you identify them?
- Assess Mr. Johnson's support system. Who can he rely on for help?
- How might you help Mr. Johnson to add some spiritual supports to his available resources?

Theoretical Knowledge
knowing why

Spirituality in nursing has multiple layers. Each nurse has her own spirituality that (overtly or covertly) serves as a guiding framework for her practice. You will encounter a variety of ways that patients and families understand spirituality. Their spirituality may be deeply ingrained in religious practices and understandings, or it may be separate from formal religion. Many schools of nursing teach spiritual care interventions while emphasizing a philosophy of "not imposing" one's religious beliefs on patients. In addition, nursing practice settings provide multiple levels of care, which impose time constraints on what you can address in day-to-day activities. These layers of competing concerns can lead to great confusion and frustration in providing spiritual care.

This chapter presents a holistic interpretation of spirituality—one that views spirituality as a component of every human being's life. It also encourages you to engage your own spirituality to improve your patients' health and wholeness. It should help you to answer some of the questions posed for Mr. Johnson.

HISTORY OF SPIRITUALITY IN NURSING

Through the ages, nurses and other caregivers have demonstrated deep concern for the spiritual as well as the physical and psychological needs of those who are sick and infirm. In the *pre-Christian era,* caring for the sick was an expression of the values of hospitality and charity. In addition, people prayed to the god(s) for healing and as an adjunct for primitive medical procedures. In the *early Christian era,* nursing the sick was honored and respected because it was one of Jesus' primary teachings. Caring for the sick was a vital component of loving one's neighbor. Gradually, religious communities of women and men in the 4th through 12th centuries provided models for combining the healing arts with religious care.

In Europe during the *post-Reformation* period, nursing orders continued to flourish, among them the Daughters of Charity, the Sisters of Mercy, and the Kaiserswerth Deaconesses (Donahue, 1985). Florence

TABLE 14-1 Comparison of Religion and Spirituality

Religion (the Map)	Spirituality (the Journey)
A "roadmap" that defines: • Beliefs • Values • Code(s) of conduct and ethics	One's journey through life A personal quest to define meaning, fulfillment, and satisfaction in life A will to live A belief in self
A tradition or system of worship that provides: • Rituals • Answers • Norms • Connection with God	A dynamic relationship with that which transcends A capacity to know and be known (a sense of openness, expectation) Connectedness with self, others, nature, and a higher power (Cavendish, Konecny, et al., 2003)
The roadmap and tradition define: • What is to be believed • How beliefs affect life • Self image and identity	A lifelong process of growth (which may involve joy and/or struggle) A constant process of taking in "truth" and then adding individual insight to arrive at a way of perceiving and acting in the world
Issues: faith, belief, trust, the nature of good and evil, the meaning of suffering, judgment, or enlightenment	Issues: faith, hope, love

Nightingale trained under Pastor Fliedner at his Deaconess School in Kaiserswerth, as well as under the Daughters of Charity of St. Vincent de Paul in France. For Nightingale, spirituality was at the very heart of human nature and thus was fundamental to healing. Nightingale instilled this idea in her nurses, particularly in their missions to the Crimea where "the lady with the lamp" brought comfort and relief to the sick and the dying (Macrae, 1995).

By the middle of the 20th century, nursing in the United States had begun to see spiritual care as less important. As science continued to develop and expand, and as more nurses studied in university settings, nursing joined ranks with the scientific disciplines: Its spiritual underpinnings were replaced by what could be "seen and tested" by the scientific method (Donahue, 1985). Only recently has nursing (and the greater health community) reclaimed the spiritual dimension as a vital part of its identity and recognized its power to influence health.

Today, professional standards of care make clear that patients' spiritual needs are a nursing concern. The Joint Commission on Accreditation of Health Care Organizations (2002) has established standards for spiritual care. In addition, the American Nurses Association *Code for Nurses* (2004) states that nurses should consider each patient's lifestyle, value system, and religious beliefs in planning care; and that nursing care measures should enable the patient to live with as much physical, emotional, social, and spiritual well-being as possible.

WHAT ARE RELIGION AND SPIRITUALITY?

Although there is overlap, spirituality and religion differ in several important ways (Table 14–1). One way to distinguish religion from spirituality is to think of religion as a map and spirituality as a journey. We begin by exploring the map.

What Is Religion?

Many people use a map to get to a certain location. The "map" of religion tells you what to believe and what values are essential. It provides codes of conduct that integrate beliefs and values into a way of living. The map itself may be in the form of a religious tradition (e.g., Christianity) or denomination (e.g., Baptist), which provides an identity and a "lens" for reading the world. The rituals, symbols, sacraments, and holy writings associated with religions serve as bases of authority and provide diverse ways to transcend the physical and access the divine (Figure 14–1). Regardless of their differences, many of the world religions have the following in common:

- **Theology**—that is, discussions and theories related to God and God's relation to the world
- Sacred writings that are regarded as authoritative and/or reveal the nature of the divine (e.g., God) in some way
- A notion of created order and purpose
- A definition of *human being* that includes important life events

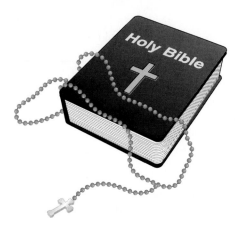

FIGURE 14–1 Associated with religion are symbols and holy writings, such as this cross and Bible representing Christianity.

- A notion of sin (primarily in Western religions)
- An explanation of the origin of evil and the nature of suffering
- A conception of either salvation (in Judaic religions) or enlightenment (in Eastern religions)
- A view toward **eschatology,** or doctrines about the human soul and its relation to death, judgment, and eternal life (primarily a Western concept)
- An explanation of the nature of reality, the higher Self or soul, the relationship between human beings and the divine, and the purpose of human existence

What Is Spirituality?

If religion serves as the map, spirituality is the day-to-day, moment-by-moment journey in life and living. Like a journey, spirituality takes place over time and involves the accumulation of life experiences combined with the understandings gained (i.e., in terms of finding meaning, value, and purpose in life). Many life events that prompt spiritual growth are fulfilling and joyful, but growth often results from painful life events that cause great internal upheaval, struggle, and challenge.

You can also think of spirituality as an accumulation of life experiences and insights. They may agree or conflict with traditional religious values and cultural teachings. For example, an American raised in the Episcopal Church, after studying a variety of religions and traveling in Asia for several years, may develop a spirituality that is both universal and highly individual and may feel "at home" in any place of worship in the world.

Like religion, spirituality also allows various ways and means to access the divine in our daily lives, to transcend the physical world, or simply to be still and introspective. For centuries, Eastern traditions have emphasized that spirituality is awareness, paying attention, and being "sensitive to reality" (Krishnamurti, 1989). One Western model of spirituality is found in Frederic and Mary Ann Broussat's (1996) *Spiritual*

Literacy: Reading the Sacred in Everyday Life. The authors assert that we learn "to read" the spiritual in everyday events only when we attain a new "level of literacy." Such "literacy" enables us to recognize that each day is filled with signs that point to an active Spirit in the world. Life is a process of recognizing this Spirit and understanding its meaning. Being literate in this way allows us to learn about ourselves and others in new and profound ways. The Broussats state that we can engage this Spirit through such sources as nature, animals, leisure, creativity, and service.

It is critical for a nurse to recognize and respect the different ways that patients understand religion and spirituality. You need to understand that most people are comfortable with their beliefs (or lack thereof) and that, in providing spiritual care, your primary goal is to support their healing, not convert them to a different view. You must also be able to recognize situations when patients may be experiencing spiritual distress and may need referral to professionals with more specialized training. These aspects of spiritual care are discussed later in this chapter.

KnowledgeCheck 14–1

- Regardless of their differences, what do many world religions have in common?
- Which can be compared to a journey: religion or spirituality?
- True or false? Both religion and spirituality allow a person various ways to access the divine.
- What is Mr. Johnson's religion ("Meet Your Patient")?
- What is his sister's religion?

 Go to Chapter 14, **Knowledge Check Response Sheet and Answers,** on the Electronic Study Guide.

 CriticalThinking 14–1
What do you know, or what can you speculate, about Mr. Johnson's ("Meet Your Patient") spirituality?

Core Issues of Spirituality

As just discussed, spirituality has many dimensions. We will limit discussion here to three "core" issues. In his first letter to the Corinthians in the New Testament of the Bible, Saint Paul identified "three things that last": namely, faith, hope, and love. Following in this tradition, a contemporary manual for nursing care of the dying (Aspen Publishers, 2002) identifies this same trio as the three core "issues" of spirituality.

Faith

Faith is our ongoing effort to make sense of our life and purpose for being. Like spirituality itself, faith represents a set of beliefs developed over time, through events that cause us to suffer and those that enable us to rejoice. *Faith struggles* are common among people

who experience illness and significant loss. People experiencing faith struggles might feel anger, guilt, self judgment, and worthlessness. C. S. Lewis, a devout Christian, following the death of his wife, reveals that his grief caused him to doubt whether God exists at all, or if so, whether He is perhaps a "Cosmic Sadist" (1961, p. 35) who deliberately tortures us. Finally, Lewis came to understand that such shattering experiences are "one of the marks of His presence" (Lewis, 1961, p. 76).

People who are experiencing the *joys of faith* exhibit a sense of self, as well as insights into their gifts and talents. In his book *Callings,* Gregg Levoy (1997, p. 65) observes that our joy and our enthusiasm move us "toward a kind of divine presence because, through our passions, we are utterly present. . . . We hitch ourselves to something bigger."

Implicit in faith is the idea of *trust:* Trust contributes to a certain confidence in our faith despite the questions that arise along life's way. Trust is so fundamental to faith that a seeming crisis of faith may in truth be a crisis of trust. A patient dying of cancer may claim that she has lost her faith in God, yet still rail at God for "betraying her" by giving her a terminal illness.

Hope

Hope includes our basic human needs to achieve, create, and to shape something of our life that will endure. If faith is expressed in terms of belief, then hope is rooted in purpose—who am I, what is my purpose, and why have I been created. People who are confronting a debilitating or terminal illness often lose hope. After suffering from a near-fatal spinal cord injury, actor Christopher Reeve experienced such a struggle, yet he concludes his second book, *Nothing Is Impossible,* with an essay on hope: "Hope must be as real. . . . in that way it is different from optimism or wishful thinking. When we have hope, we discover powers within ourselves we may have never known—the power to make sacrifices, to endure, to heal, and to love. Once we choose hope, everything is possible" (Reeve, 2002, p. 176).

Love

Many people think of **love** as a trade: We extend our love because we hope to find that love returned in some way. But relationships can be a source of pain. We want to be loved as we are, yet we fear what our loved ones think of us, and we compare ourselves with others. Worse, we encounter disappointments, outright rejection, and feelings of abandonment. Even when our love is shared, we must inevitably face separation at our death or the death of our loved ones. Thus, while active loving in human relationships opens us up to joy, it also carries with it the certainty of heartbreak.

Illness and sudden injury commonly prompt such "struggles with love." For example, when a man with a debilitating disease loses his ability to work and requires increasing levels of caregiving, he may experience himself as a "burden" and wonder whether his loved ones would be "better off" if he were to die. When patients question the presence of unconditional love in their lives, family members may be invaluable in reminding them of their inner integrity and worth. Reeve states that the most powerful words his wife spoke to him in the first days after his injury, "the words that saved my life," were, "You're still you. And I love you" (Reeve, 1998, p. 32).

Forgiveness is one aspect of love. People have a spiritual need to forgive others and to be forgiven. When a person cannot forgive others, it separates him from them and interferes with giving and receiving love. When a person cannot forgive himself, he may feel the pain of shame, guilt, and anger. Or the person may be hurting because he wants forgiveness from someone he has wronged or from God. Many people interpret their illness as punishment for sins. Some find it difficult to seek forgiveness and to believe that they have been forgiven, but this is important to achieving spiritual peace.

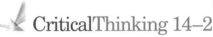 CriticalThinking 14–2

Faith is a constant search for comprehension and meaning. What are some of your struggles with faith, and what are some of the "joys" of your faith?

HOW MIGHT SPIRITUAL BELIEFS AFFECT HEALTH?

Although the preceding sections discussed religion and spirituality as two separate constructs, current research into their influence on health tend to combine the two into one: namely, religion. For whatever reasons (and they are numerous) most studies have measured both religion and spirituality in terms of *religious involvement.* Examples of such broad measures include the subjective reporting of one's own religiousness, denominational affiliation, church attendance or membership, membership in the clergy, and dietary and social habits (e.g., "On a scale of 1 to 5, how religious are you?" "How often do you attend church?") Despite such limitations, findings have been surprisingly positive in terms of predicting health outcomes.

Current research suggests that there are many ways that religion affects physical and mental health (George, Ellison, & Larson, 2002; Koenig, McCullough, & Larson, 2001; Seybold & Hill 2001; Larson, Swyers, & McCollough, 1998; Larson, Pattison, Blazer, Omran, & Kaplan, 1986; Plante & Sherman, 2001). For example:

- One study found that people who score higher on measures of religious involvement have longer lives than those with lower religious involvement (McCollough, Hoyt, Larson, Koenig, & Thoresen, 2000).

- Likewise, the literature also suggests that even simplistic measures regarding religion and spirituality (e.g., religious affiliation or church attendance) are significant predictors of health outcomes (Koenig, et al., 2001).
- There is a growing body of literature that investigates the possible effects of religion on heart disease, cholesterol, hypertension, cancer, mortality, and health behaviors.

In all of these, the variables studied tend to be broadly stated and nonspecific and thus do not allow for researchers to examine whether there might be potential harmful effects of religion.

Although the research suggests that religion has a positive influence on healthcare outcomes, it does not yet answer *how* or *why* religion has this effect. However, there is growing awareness that religion and spirituality are complex variables involving cognitive, emotional, behavioral, interpersonal, and physiological dimensions. Recent research into how religion may affect health can be grouped around the following promising areas:

Perceived closeness to God
Religion and spirituality as motivating factors (e.g., to live a healthy lifestyle)
Religious support (e.g., relationships with other religious people)
Religious struggles (e.g., doubt, loss of hope)

For a more complete description of those four research areas,

 Go to Chapter 14, **Supplemental Materials: Religion and Health: Recent Research,** on the Electronic Study Guide.

KnowledgeCheck 14–2
- What are some of the ways that religion might positively influence health?

 Go to Chapter 14, **Knowledge Check Response Sheet and Answers,** on the Electronic Study Guide.

CriticalThinking 14–3
- How might religion "negatively" influence health?
- Has there been a pivotal moment in your life, a moment of crisis or despair that eventually provided an opportunity for spiritual growth?

MAJOR RELIGIONS: WHAT SHOULD I KNOW?

The more you know about the differences between and similarities among the world's major religions, the more you will be able to offer comprehensive and compassionate care to patients. Of course, learning about other religions requires you to be open and nonjudgmental.

When you care for a patient from a known religious background, you will need to think about how the person's beliefs affect her ideas of health, healing, hospitalization, and the experience of dying. To help you make these connections, the following brief descriptions of several of the world's major religious traditions provide you with several different "worldviews." For more detailed information about each religion,

 Go to Chapter 14, **Supplemental Materials: Major Religions: What Should I Know?,** and **Reading More About Spirituality,** on the Electronic Study Guide.

To learn about the influence of various religions on end-of-life care, see Chapter 15.

Judaism

Judaism is one of the western world's oldest religions and the foundation on which Christianity and Islam were built. The Jewish Law is set down in the collective writings of the Torah. Judaism is based on the worship of one God **(monotheism),** carrying out the Ten Commandments, and practicing charity and tolerance toward others. The degree to which Jews celebrate rituals and holy days depends on whether the person identifies with the Orthodox, Liberal, Conservative, or Reconstructionist (Pawlikowski, 1990) beliefs.

Jews celebrate the Sabbath from sunset on Friday to sunset Saturday evening. For orthodox Jews, "work" is prohibited on the Sabbath. This includes writing, traveling, and switching on lights and appliances. During Passover (in March or April), some Jewish patients may require special foods. The Day of Atonement, or Yom Kippur (in September or October), is the holiest day of the Jewish calendar. It is a special day of fasting, but fasting is not required if it would be a danger to the patient. A Jewish patient will normally wish to keep that day to pray and be quiet. For Orthodox patients, you must offer alternatives to oral medication (e.g., injections or suppositories).

Conservative Jews observe strict dietary laws: Only kosher foods are accepted. **Kosher foods** have been prepared under strict guidelines for how animals are slaughtered and do not contain pork, certain types of seafood, or combinations of dairy and meat. If possible, consult a rabbi or dietitian who is knowledgeable about Jewish dietary laws for assistance in planning dietary and activity modifications.

Orthodox Jewish women prefer to have their bodies and limbs covered. They may also prefer to keep their hair covered with a scarf. Orthodox men keep their head covered with a hat or skull cap (*Kappel*). Some Orthodox Jews forbid contraception unless the woman's health is at risk. Nearly all Jewish boys are circumcised, usually 8 days after birth. Orthodox Judaism usually forbids organ transplants, but opinions vary and decisions may rest with the rabbinic authority.

Christianity

Although rituals and practices vary among denominations, Christians are collectively known for their worship of Jesus Christ and their use of the same sacred text, the **Bible,** which includes the Judaic Old Testament and the New Testament on the life of Christ. However, there are many denominations within Christianity, including Roman Catholicism (with allegiance to the pope in Rome), Orthodoxy (with allegiance to the patriarch of Constantinople), Protestant denominations (for example, Lutheran, Baptist, United Methodist), and others (e.g., Jehovah's Witnesses, Christian Science). For the most part, Christians hold that Jesus' death atoned for the sins of men and women, providing a way to experience the forgiveness of God and to gain eternal life.

In Roman Catholicism, the **sacraments** are a means to obtain grace. A Roman Catholic who is seriously ill might wish to receive the sacrament of *anointing the sick*. This sacrament, once known as the last rites, can be repeated if the person recovers and then becomes ill at a later time. Only a priest can hear the *sacrament of reconciliation* (confession), during which God, through the agency of the priest, grants forgiveness for past sins. The *eucharist* (communion bread), consecrated at the *mass* (a religious service), may be brought to hospitalized patients by a priest, deacon, or designated lay eucharistic minister. Other denominations within Christianity (e.g., Episcopalians and Lutherans) observe certain sacraments as well, although the meaning and details of the ritual may vary.

Many denominations practice baptism, so when babies or children are very ill, baptism should be offered. Christians usually have no special dietary requirements, although some do abstain from eating meat on Fridays. Some Christians may wish to abstain from food (fast) before receiving Holy Communion. Some (depending on the denomination) abstain from alcohol.

Family planning varies from religion to religion within Christianity. Some denominations allow birth control methods; others do not. There are no religious objections to blood transfusion or organ transplantation.

Christian Science

The Christian Science faith is a unique form of Christianity. Established in the United States in 1879, Christian Science teaches a reliance on God for healing rather than on medicine or surgery. Therefore, you might encounter believers as patients only following accidents or because of family or legal pressures.

Christian Scientists do not use alcohol and tobacco; strict Christian Scientists may not drink tea or coffee. Adults will probably not accept a blood transfusion, but parents usually consent to transfusion and other medical care for their child if doctors consider it essential or the law requires them to do so. Adults will not usually consent to donate or receive organs.

Jehovah's Witnesses

Jehovah's Witnesses try to live according to the commands of God as written in both the Old and New Testaments of the Bible. They will accept most medical treatments, but they believe that "taking blood into one's body" is morally wrong. This means that they will not allow transfusions of whole blood or its components. The Jehovah's Witness faith also does not permit donation or receipt of an organ through which blood flows. If blood is not involved (e.g., corneal transplants) they may accept transplantation.

Mormonism

The Mormon Church is also known as the Church of Jesus Christ of Latter-Day Saints. Mormons believe in Jesus and one God; however, they adhere to a more recently revealed sacred writing, the Book of Mormon (which they believe an angel gave to Joseph Smith in the 19th century). Mormons follow a strict health code, known as the Word of Wisdom, which advises healthful living and prohibits the use of tea, coffee, alcohol, and tobacco. Some Mormons (both men and women) wear a sacred undergarment that they remove only for hygiene purposes. Nurses may also remove it before surgery, but it must at all times be considered intensely private and be treated with respect.

Islam

The word *Islam* means submission. In particular, a Muslim is one who submits to Allah (God). The principal book of authority in Islam, the **Koran (Qu'ran),** is the result of a vision received by Muhammad, the founder of Islam, in the early 7th century A.D. Islam teaches that all faiths have essentially one common message: There is a Supreme Being whose sovereignty is acknowledged in worship and whose teaching and commandments must be obeyed.

Muslims are forbidden to eat any pork. They may eat other meat, but it has to be *halal* meat, that is, killed in a special manner stated in Islamic law. Fish and eggs are allowed, but not if they are cooked near pork or non-halal meat. During the month of Ramadan, a Muslim fasts between sunrise and sunset; however, those who are sick are not expected to fast. Essential drugs and medicines are allowed at all hours during Ramadan.

Muslims always wash their hands before eating. Patients prefer to wash in free-flowing water, so tub baths are considered unhygienic. If a shower is not available, provide a jug to use in the bath.

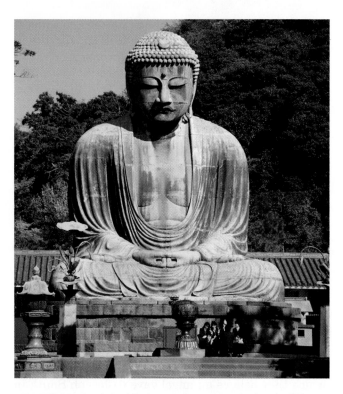

FIGURE 14–2 The Buddha is revered as an example of a way of life.

Women prefer to be treated by female staff. Some women may refuse vaginal examination by a male nurse or physician because they are forbidden to expose their bodies to or be touched by any man other than their husband. Women may wear a locket containing religious writing around the neck in a small leather bag. These are kept for protection and strength, so you should never remove them.

There is no specific religious rule prohibiting blood transfusion or organ transplantation; however, strict Muslims will not usually agree to organ transplants. Orthodox Muslims do not approve of contraception; however, individuals vary widely in their practices. Abortion is frowned on but may be tolerated for medical reasons.

Baha'i

The Baha'i faith was established in 1863 in Persia and has its roots in Babism, a reformist outgrowth of Islam. A Baha'i patient in the hospital will accept usual routines and treatment. Alcohol, including that used in cooking, is not permitted.

Hinduism

Hinduism, which many religious scholars believe is the oldest major religion still practiced today, does not embrace a single body of beliefs and practices. Nor does it maintain the existence of a single god, believing that no one manifestation of God can possibly capture the limitless nature of God. Thus, Hindus may worship several or even hundreds of gods and goddesses. Even elements in the natural world, such as rivers, fire, and so forth, are considered aspects of God. Sacred Hindu texts include the **Vedas,** the **Bhagavad Gita** (Song of the Blessed One), and the **Ramayana,** the story of the life of the god Rama. Despite commonly held beliefs and texts, Hindu religious practices vary a great deal, depending on areas of origin.

Hindus practice **ayurvedic medicine,** which encompasses all aspects of life, including diet, sleep, elimination, and hygiene. Some believe in the medicinal properties of "hot" and "cold" foods—"hot" and "cold" having nothing to do with either temperature or spicy qualities. Although some Hindus will eat eggs and even chicken, most are lactovegetarians, consuming milk but no eggs. Fasting, which may mean eating only "pure" foods such as fruit or yogurt, is common during major festivals but is not expected of the sick. Tobacco and alcohol may or may not be accepted.

Hindus prefer to wash in free-flowing water (e.g., a shower instead of a tub bath). If a shower is not available, provide a jug of water for the person to use in the bath. Women are modest and usually prefer to be treated by female medical staff. Jewelry often has a religious or cultural significance. Some Hindus wear "sacred thread" around the body or wrist. Do not remove or cut this thread without permission from the patient or next of kin. There is no religious objection to contraception, blood transfusion, or organ donation, as a rule.

Sikhism

Sikhism combines the teachings of Hinduism and Islamic Sufism, which is the mystical branch of Islam. Tenets of the religion include monotheism and the realization of God through religious exercises and meditation. Many Sikhs are completely vegetarian. Alcohol and tobacco are forbidden. Sikhs may use contraception but do not speak openly about it. They do not generally object to blood transfusions or organ transplantation.

Buddhism

The Buddha, or the "Awakened One," is revered not as a god, but as an example of a way of life (Figure 14–2). He was born into a royal family in 624 B.C. in a part of northern India that is now in Nepal, gained **enlightenment** at the age of 35, and then began to teach others how to attain liberation from suffering, not only for themselves, but for others.

One of the Buddha's core teachings is that suffering can be ended by following the eightfold path: right understanding, right intention, right speech, right action, right livelihood, right effort, right mindfulness, and right contemplation (Borelli, 1990). **Nirvana,** similar

to the Christian concept of heaven, can only be attained through an absence of desire, the achievement of perfection, and the lack of a unique identity (Borelli, 1990).

Many Buddhists follow a vegetarian diet; in some cases, the diet may include both milk and eggs. Fasting customs vary by tradition. Buddhists accept contraception but typically condemn abortion and active euthanasia. They will usually accept blood transfusion and organ transplantation.

Native American Religions

Although each Native American nation or tribe (and there are over 400 federally recognized nations) has its own traditions and cultural heritage, some general beliefs underlie the more specific tribal ideas. The Earth is considered to be a living organism, the body of a higher individual, and humankind has an intimate relation with this organism through nature. When the Earth is harmed, humankind is harmed, and vice versa. The land belongs to life, life belongs to the land, and the land belongs to itself (Boyd, 1974).

Health is a state of harmony with nature. Whenever disharmony exists, disease or illness can occur. The traditional healer is the medicine man or woman who is wise in the interrelationships of land, humankind, and the universe. Many Native Americans believe that the treatments they receive from medicine men and women and traditional healers are far better than those rendered by the dominant health care establishment, which often treats Native Americans with scorn or disrespect. You should know that note-taking by the professional is forbidden; when you take a history or perform an exam, you must rely on your memory to record findings later. Native Americans tend to converse in a very low tone of voice and may maintain long periods of silence. Be sure that the setting is quiet enough to allow you to hear the patient, because it is impolite to indicate that you did not hear the communications.

Rastafarianism

The Rastafarian movement began in the 1930s in the West Indies. It emphasizes personal dignity and a deep love of God. Rastafarians use the Old and New Testaments of the Bible as their authoritative writings, but they do not consider themselves to be Christian. There are no churches, services, or official clergy.

Rastafarians do not eat pork and shellfish, some are completely vegetarian, and some do not drink milk or coffee. Wearing second-hand clothing is forbidden, so the patient may be unwilling to wear hospital gowns that have been worn by others. You may need to provide a disposable gown or allow the person to wear her own personal nightclothes. Patients may be anxious about accepting blood transfusion (because of concern

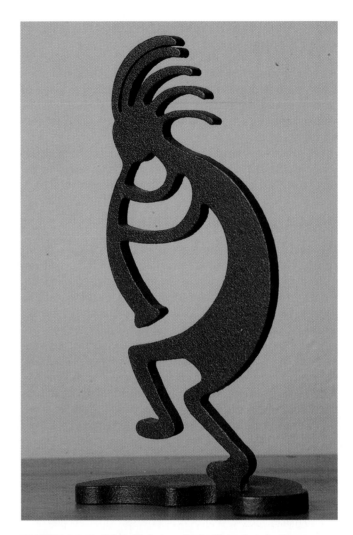

FIGURE 14–3 Kokopelli, the humpbacked flute player, has been a sacred figure to Native Americans of the Southwest for thousands of years. He is a legendary symbol of fertility who brought well-being to the people.

about contamination); however, many Rastafarians will accept transfusions after being reassured.

KnowledgeCheck 14–3

- Which major religion believes in the anointing of the sick or dying?
- Which denomination or religion does not believe in blood transfusions?
- In terms of Native American beliefs and health care, who is the traditional healer or the person to be consulted in the event of "illness"?
- True or false: Most Hindus are vegetarian.

 Go to Chapter 14, **Knowledge Check Response Sheet and Answers,** on the Electronic Study Guide.

CriticalThinking 14–4

What are some of the ways that world religions might influence nursing care?

SELF-KNOWLEDGE: WHAT EVERY NURSE SHOULD KNOW

As you have seen, your patients' spiritual and religious backgrounds may be diverse and may involve ways of thinking and doing that seem strange to you or that you do not fully understand. Before trying to understand the many varieties of religious experience, you must give considerable thought to your own spiritual journey. Recall that attaining self knowledge is an important aspect of becoming a full-spectrum nurse.

What Are Your Personal Biases?

We each carry our own perspectives with us at all times. We tend to view the world through lenses we acquired in childhood, adolescence, and early adulthood. Additionally, our religious education is often taught with a certain flavor of "upmanship"; that is, we are taught that our religious beliefs and practices are superior to all others. When you view your own experience as the norm or as the preferred way of organizing the world, you tend to limit the range of care you provide to the patient who believes differently. Spiritual care demands nonjudgmental attitudes and an open manner of thinking that invites rather than excludes.

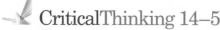 CriticalThinking 14–5

Consider the following examples. For each person, what moral judgments must the nurse be careful *not* to make?

- A nurse is caring for a gay man who is hospitalized with end-stage AIDS.
- A woman has come to the clinic to be treated for gonorrhea (a sexually transmitted disease). She says she has had at least six sexual partners this year.
- A man comes to the emergency department (ED) at least once a month to ask for morphine to treat his back pain. He is known to abuse drugs and to visit other EDs for the same purpose.

If you are aware of your biases, it will be easier to avoid abuses of spiritual care, such as attempting to convert others to your beliefs. For example, if a patient is near death, he and his family might be offended if their nurse inquires whether they are "saved" Christians. By remaining focused on the need of the *patient* to talk about meaning, salvation, or other end-of-life issues, you provide full-spectrum spiritual care. As another example, notice that Mr. Johnson's sister (in "Meet Your Patient") seems very close to imposing her religion on him. She may alienate him further if he perceives that he is being "pushed."

Another form of abuse is to believe that you can be all things to all people, regardless of the person's background or the extent of spiritual care needed. Clearly, there are times when you should refer to others with more knowledge and experience in religion and spirituality, with the patient's permission, of course. In addition, whenever a patient requests the services of a rabbi, priest, or other spiritual adviser, you should relay that request to the agency's chaplain so that communication and planning are multidisciplinary and all disciplines remain informed throughout the care delivery process.

In summary, to work effectively with a diverse population of people, you must first obtain a greater degree of self knowledge by (1) being open to the many possibilities for diverse thinking, (2) welcoming challenging experiences that allow for personal growth, and (3) taking the time necessary to contemplate how your actions and biases might affect the care of others. The more you know about yourself, the more effectively you care for others.

What Are Some Barriers to Spiritual Care?

Although most nurses would acknowledge that patients have a spiritual dimension, few actually identify spiritual problems or provide spiritual interventions. This may be a result of economic constraints, poor staffing, and high-tech care, which force nurses to focus on physical needs to the exclusion of spiritual needs (Cavendish et. al., 2003). You may judge these nurses less harshly after you understand more about the barriers to spiritual interventions by nurses.

Lack of Awareness of Spirituality in General

One study of oncology nurses found that over half incorrectly identified the patient's religion and that only 16% incorporated any kind of spiritual assessment into their care (Sodestrom & Martin, 1987). Highfield's (1992) study confirms the incidence of inaccurate spiritual assessment by nurses of patients in their care. A greater awareness of spirituality in general will help you tune into the spiritual needs of patients (Highfield, 1992) and improve your comfort in communicating about spiritual matters.

Lack of Awareness of Your Own Spiritual Belief System

To feel comfortable making spiritual interventions, you will need more than just theoretical knowledge. Introspection and an awareness of your own spiritual journey are required to integrate the spiritual domain into patient care. Lane (1987) identifies three steps in the spiritual growth of nurses:

1. Developing a "greater awareness of the spirit within self" in order to be a better listener for the patient
2. Opening the self by being totally present with the patient
3. Allowing the patient to share his feelings and emotions without reserve

You must find ways to take care of and nurture your own spiritual needs; otherwise, providing this aspect of care can be emotionally draining.

Differences in Spirituality Between Nurse and Patient

Patients and nurses can be at different levels in terms of spirituality. When a patient's spiritual beliefs are very different from your own, you must be careful not to impose your beliefs on the patient or discount the importance of the patient's beliefs and rituals. When the patient's views or beliefs are similar to yours, you must be careful not to make false assumptions about his spiritual needs. Just because you agree on some things does not mean you will have the same views or needs in all areas of spirituality or religion.

 CriticalThinking 14–6

- How does your religion or spirituality differ from Mr. Johnson's?
- How is it similar?
- Can you think of problems these differences and similarities could cause you in caring for him?

Fear That Your Knowledge Base Is Insufficient

Nurses sometimes avoid giving spiritual care because they believe they lack knowledge of spirituality or of the patient's religion. This is a realistic concern. In several studies, nurses were found to be unsure of what constituted spiritual problems and spiritual interventions (Sodestrom & Martin, 1987; Highfield & Cason, 1983; Ryan, 1992). In some cases they did not identify the spiritual dimension of care, or they took religious aspects into account but did not place them into a broader spiritual perspective. Highfield and Cason (1983) found that oncology nurses placed greater emphasis on physical and psychosocial nursing care and that they frequently did not identify the patient's spiritual needs. The good news is that spiritual care has never been more welcomed by patients. You can provide truly holistic care for the patient when you address spiritual needs in a plan of care.

Fear of Where Spiritual Discussions May Lead

Many nurses fear that inquiring into the spiritual domain might cause harm to the patient. For example, what if a patient asks you, "Do you think active euthanasia is morally wrong? Would it jeopardize my salvation?" Here are some fears that may arise:

- You may not feel prepared to answer the questions.
- You might have an answer based on your personal religious beliefs but fear that the patient may think you are imposing your beliefs on him.

- You might wonder whether communicating your own beliefs (for example, if you favor active euthanasia) might jeopardize the patient's spiritual life if your ideas turn out to be "wrong."

The following are some ideas that may help counter your fears. First and foremost, keep in mind the fact that the patient is addressing this concern with you indicates that you are open to the spiritual domain of care. Second, the patient in this example is concerned with issues related to euthanasia. This could lead to discussions about the patient's fears of pain, dependence, being a burden on family members, and dying alone. Third, this is an area for which you should seek collaboration with a chaplain, who is more prepared to deal with specific religious issues. You should realize that being open to the spiritual realm and assessing the patient's need for spiritual intervention does not mean that you must be a chaplain or have the extraordinary ability to deal with all spiritual or religious questions or requests. The following section will provide a more detailed understanding of your role in spiritual care.

KnowledgeCheck 14–4

- What qualities can you demonstrate that may help you improve the quality of spiritual care you provide?
- What common barriers to spiritual interventions do nurses encounter?
- True or false: No matter how nonjudgmental and open we may think ourselves to be, we all carry our own unique biases and prejudices that have the potential to affect patient care.

 Go to Chapter 14, **Knowledge Check Response Sheet and Answers,** on the Electronic Study Guide.

 CriticalThinking 14–7

- What are some of the possible abuses of spiritual care provided by nurses?
- What are some ways that you can develop a greater awareness of the "spirit within the self"?
- Discuss ways that nurses (and patients, for that matter) can nurture their own spiritual needs.

Practical Knowledge
knowing how

Most hospital admission forms include a place to record the patient's "religious preferences," and most nursing assessment forms even include questions such as, "What religious rituals do you practice?" Unfortunately, some nurses believe that in completing such forms, they have addressed the patient's spiritual needs. They may be relieved because they don't feel competent to deal any further with spirituality or

because they are afraid to be perceived as imposing their own religion on the patient. However, armed with your basic theoretical knowledge of spirituality and your growing spiritual self knowledge, you should be able to provide a level of support that extends beyond paperwork to compassion and caring. To see a care plan for a client with Spiritual Distress,

 Go to Chapter 14, **Care Plan,** on the Electronic Study Guide.

| Assessment |

People of the same religion often vary greatly in the degree to which they follow religious practices. It is not enough to "fill in the religion blank" on an assessment form; you must assess each person individually to determine religious needs and practices.

Spiritual Assessment Tools

One easy-to-use screening tool, the JAREL spiritual well-being scale, was developed and is commonly used by nurses (Hungelmann, Kenkel-Rossi, Klassen, & Stollenwerk, 1996). Cutting across religious and atheistic belief systems, it assesses three key dimensions: (1) faith/belief, (2) life/self-responsibility, and (3) life-satisfaction/self-actualization. For the JAREL tool,

 Go to Chapter 14, **Tables, Boxes, Figures: ESG Figure 14–1,** on the Electronic Study Guide.

Highfield (2000) has proposed a comprehensive method of spiritual assessment. It involves an interview that is concerned with six key areas designated by the acronym SPIRIT: spiritual/religious belief system, integration with a spiritual community, ritualized practices and restrictions, implications for medical care, and terminal events planning. To see a copy of a spiritual assessment based on this model,

 Go to Chapter 14, **Assessment Guidelines and Tools, Spiritual Assessment,** in Volume 2.

You can combine the SPIRIT model with the JAREL tool presented in ESG Figure 14–1 and with the combined assessment tool and plan of care presented in ESG Figure 14–2.

 Go to Chapter 14, **Tables, Boxes, Figures: ESG Figure 14–2,** on the Electronic Study Guide.

And, of course, you can design assessment tools tailored to your particular healthcare setting.

KnowledgeCheck 14–5

What are the six areas for spiritual assessment summarized in Highfield's (2000) acronym SPIRIT?

 Go to Chapter 14, **Knowledge Check Response Sheet and Answers,** on the Electronic Study Guide.

 ## CriticalThinking 14–8

Complete the SPIRIT assessment on yourself. Discuss it with your classmates.

 Go to Chapter 14, **Assessment Guidelines and Tools, Spiritual Assessment,** in Volume 2.

Levels of Spiritual Assessment

Given the time constraints of the patient admission process (for inpatient facilities), stresses involved with the patient's introduction to a healthcare setting, and the multiple people involved, it is difficult to obtain meaningful information on initial assessment. For this reason, initial data is often limited to the patient's church preference, name of clergy, whom to call in case of emergency, dietary requirements, and any religious implications for medical care (e.g., refusal of organs or blood transfusion). Over time, as you have more contact with the patient and family, trust will develop, and you will be able to obtain more sensitive, complex, and meaningful information.

| Nursing Diagnosis |

When analyzing spiritual assessment data, consider the person's developmental stage. People progress through stages of spiritual development in much the same way as they develop physically and cognitively. Spiritual behaviors that seem problematic in one stage may not be so in an earlier stage. To review spiritual development,

 Go to **Chapter 9** on the Electronic Study Guide.

Spirituality Diagnoses

The following are three NANDA diagnostic labels that specifically deal with spirituality.

- *Spiritual Distress* is "impaired ability to experience and integrate meaning and purpose in life through a person's connectedness with self, others, art, music, literature, nature, or a power greater than oneself" (NANDA International, 2005, p. 186). Defining characteristics (signs and symptoms) of this diagnosis include the following.

  Connections with self: Expressing a lack of hope, love, courage, acceptance, or peace; a lack of meaning and purpose in life; inability to forgive self; feelings of anger or guilt

  Connections with others: Refusing to see clergy; refusing to interact with family or friends; reporting lack of support system; expressions of alienation

  Connections with art, music, literature, nature: No interest in nature, decrease in previous interest in music, writing, art, no interest in spiritual reading

Connections with power greater than self: Inability to pray, inability or refusal to participate in religious activities, feelings of abandonment by God, expressions of anger toward God, requests to see a religious leader, sudden changes in spiritual practices (increased or decreased)

- *Risk for Spiritual Distress* exists when the patient experiences energy-consuming anxiety, low self esteem, mental illness, physical illness, blocks to self love, poor relationships, physical or psychological stress, substance abuse, loss of loved one, natural disasters, situational losses, maturational losses, or inability to forgive. Illness creates countless risk factors for spiritual distress.

- *Readiness for Enhanced Spiritual Well-Being* describes healthy spirituality. NANDA defines it as the "ability to experience and integrate meaning and purpose through connectedness with self, others, art, music, literature, nature, or a power greater than oneself" (2005, p. 189). It is the opposite of Spiritual Distress, so you will see positive expressions of faith, hope, love, courage, acceptance, and peace; healthy connections with others and with art, music, literature, and nature; and prayer and other expressions of a connection with a power higher than oneself.

Three other diagnostic labels approved for inclusion in the 2005 edition of the NANDA taxonomy are:

- Impaired Religiosity
- Readiness for Enhanced Religiosity
- Risk for Impaired Religiosity

The following are examples of full diagnostic statements for spiritual problems:

> *Spiritual Distress* related to overwhelming anxiety associated with the need to have a surgical procedure that is not accepted by her religion

> *Risk for Spiritual Distress* related to unremitting pain and loss of hope for relief, as manifested by patient's question about the usefulness of prayer ("God has forgotten about me.")

 ## CriticalThinking 14–9

Which of the first three preceding nursing diagnoses would you use for Mr. Johnson ("Meet Your Patient"): Spiritual Distress, Risk for Spiritual Distress, or Readiness for Enhanced Spiritual Well-Being? Why?

Other Diagnoses Related to Spirituality

In the spiritual realm, it is difficult sometimes to determine what is the problem and what is the etiology. Does the patient experience Spiritual Distress because of pain and hopelessness? Or did the patient first lose faith in God, which led to hopelessness and anxiety? Either way, spiritual support is needed.

Spiritual Care

Spiritual interventions, especially prayer, are a frequently used CAM:

- A recent study found that 63% of adult patients with cancer used at least one CAM therapy, which they all believed helped to improve their quality of life by helping them to cope with stress, obtain a sense of control, decrease the discomforts of treatments and illness (Sparber, et al., 2000).

- In this same study, the CAMs most often used were spiritual, relaxation, imagery, exercise, lifestyle, diet, and nutritional supplementation (Sparber, et al., 2000).

- Keegan (2000) found prayer to be the CAM most frequently practiced by both Mexican and Anglo Americans.

- Dunn and Horgas (2000) found that 96% of community-dwelling elders use prayer to cope with stress and that it was the most frequently reported CAM.

- At least one study (le Gallez, Dimmock, & Bird, 2000) found spiritual healing to be ineffective in achieving improved laboratory parameters or clinical symptoms (e.g., pain) in patients having rheumatoid arthritis.

complementary and alternative modalities (CAM)

NANDA diagnoses related to spirituality as either problem, etiology, or symptom include Anxiety, Death Anxiety, Fear, Social Isolation, Hopelessness, Powerlessness, Dysfunctional Grieving, Ineffective Denial, and Disturbed Personal Identity. Non-NANDA problems include anger or resentment; feelings of guilt, shame, inadequacy, abandonment, or distrust; depression or sadness; and the inability to find meaning in life. The following are examples of diagnostic statements with spiritual etiologies:

Anxiety related to inability to reconcile decision to use birth control with religious proscriptions

Chronic Sorrow related to loss of faith in spiritual power outside self

Death Anxiety related to feeling unprepared for death and concern about the afterlife

Decisional Conflict related to confusion about the religious implications of the decision to forego heroic treatment measures

Hopelessness related to lack of belief in a power outside self, combined with overwhelming lack of energy

Impaired Adjustment related to inability to find meaning in illness

Interrupted Family Processes related to conflicts among family members about the type of spiritual support needed by the patient

Noncompliance (with treatment regimen) related to the belief that the illness is "God's will" and that healing will occur (without treatment) for the same reason

Powerlessness related to perceiving that prayers have not been answered and that God is either not hearing him or is punishing him

KnowledgeCheck 14–6

Consider the following statement: A nursing diagnosis that reflects either an actual or a potential problem may reflect religious and/or spiritual dimensions of the human condition.

- Is this statement true?
- Would it be true for a *physical* diagnosis (e.g., Disturbed Sleep Pattern)? Explain your thinking.

 Go to Chapter 14, **Knowledge Check Response Sheet and Answers,** on the Electronic Study Guide.

| Planning Outcomes/Evaluation |

The outcomes you establish in the planning stage of the nursing process serve as the criteria for your evaluation of the patient's progress and the success of the nursing interventions.

NOC standardized outcomes associated with spirituality diagnoses include, but are not limited to, the following: Dignified Life Closure, Hope, Quality of Life, Spiritual Health, and Will to Live (Moorhead, Johnson, & Maas, 2004).

Individualized goals/outcome statements you might write for spiritual diagnoses include the following:

Risk for Spiritual Distress
1. Potential spiritual issues are assessed, identified, and explored.
2. Exhibits no signs or symptoms of Spiritual Distress (e.g., finds meaning in life, expresses hope and faith, follows usual religious practices).

Spiritual Distress
1. Returns to previous state of spiritual well-being and comfort (e.g., expresses a sense of peace, asks to see religious adviser).
2. Shares spiritual and religious concerns.

Readiness for Enhanced Spiritual Well-Being
1. Experiences a higher level of connectedness with self, others, higher power, and/or nature.
2. Experiences a nonjudgmental environment in which he feels free to express all questions and concerns.
3. Establishes relationship with care provider that promotes the exploration of spiritual issues and their impact on health care.

| Planning Interventions/Implementation |

You will, of course, base your nursing activities on the patient's symptoms and the problem etiologies. However, there are some nursing interventions that, in general, address spiritual problems.

NIC standardized interventions linked to the spirituality diagnoses include the following (Dochterman & Bulechek, 2004):

- For Spiritual Distress and Risk for Spiritual Distress: Dying Care, Forgiveness Facilitation, Hope Instillation, Presence, Spiritual Growth Facilitation, and Spiritual Support.
- For Potential for Enhanced Spiritual Well-Being: NIC interventions for this diagnosis do *not* include Dying Care. In addition to the preceding list, they include Self-Awareness Enhancement, Self-Esteem Enhancement, and Values Clarification.

Technique 14–1 includes NIC activities for each of the preceding interventions. These should give you an idea about how to carry out each of the interventions.

Specific nursing activities, to be individualized to each client's needs, include those discussed in the following sections. Spiritual care involves you in relationships with people who have come face to face with a significant life event that calls forth a new sense of meaning and purpose. Stiles (1990) describes this kind of care as being "fully present to patients and families" and as accompanied by excellent nursing care. To provide excellent spiritual care, you will need to adopt a supportive approach to the patient; a sense of **benevolence** (a wish to benefit) toward the patient; awareness of the patient, yourself, and the impact of family and significant others; empathy; and nonjudgmental understanding (Dickenson, 1975).

What Are Spiritual Interventions?

Spiritual interventions are interventions to treat and prevent spiritual problems related to the patient's illness. You will direct some nursing activities to resolving the problem, others at removing the etiology, and still others at relieving symptoms. Three diagnoses related to the spiritual realm have been previously discussed (Readiness for Enhanced Spiritual Well-Being, Risk for Spiritual Distress, and Spiritual Distress). Any of the following interventions may be used with any of the given nursing diagnoses as they seem appropriate. For a more complete list of interventions,

 Go to Chapter 14, **Tables, Boxes, Figures: ESG Figure 14–2,** on the Electronic Study Guide.

- Be present with patient and family. This requires not only your actual presence at the bedside, but also your being open to issues and concerns of the

patient; allowing the patient to lead discussions rather than setting the agenda or controlling the conversation.

- Encourage expression of feelings. The best way to do this is simply to ask the patient how he is feeling or what he thinks about a particular situation.

- Help the patient identify feelings of guilt. You might ask the following after a patient has voiced a concern: "How do you feel about that?" or "You seem to feel bad about saying/doing that."

- Help significant others understand the patient's feelings and needs. Encourage family members to talk with the patient or simply to have a seat at the bedside. Periods of silence often lead into the most therapeutic of discussions.

- Maximize the patient's comfort and relief from pain. This is one of the most important spiritual activities a nurse can perform. A patient cannot think about spiritual issues when plagued with physical pain or discomfort.

- Listen to the patient's "stories" (life history) surrounding illness.

- Provide sources of prayer materials, music, or literature as needed.

- Assess the patient's needs for reconciliation with self, others, and God. If, like Mr. Johnson ("Meet Your Patient"), the patient has lost contact with family members because of disagreements related to past events, you could collaborate with the social worker and chaplain about ways to facilitate a meeting.

- Explore with the client the possible meanings of healing, miracle, and cure. Refer to the discussion at the end of this chapter.

- Collaborate with the dietary department to provide foods compatible with the person's religious needs. Encourage family to bring foods from home, as appropriate.

- Respect the patient's dress requirements as determined by his religion. This may include wearing religious icons, jewelry, or special clothes.

Making Referrals

As already mentioned, there are times when you should refer a patient to others with more knowledge and experience in religion and spirituality. For example, a patient may be experiencing Spiritual Distress because he believes he needs forgiveness for a past act, or a patient may refuse medical treatment because she thinks her church would not approve. For hospitalized and hospice patients, you can usually ask the chaplain's office to refer the patient and family to clergy or religious counselors in the community. If you are working in a home or community setting, look in the telephone or other directory for local churches.

Intercessory Prayer

complementary and alternative modalities (CAM)

Many people pray when they are ill, and prayer seems to have positive effects. But what about the effects of *intercessory prayer*—the prayers of people for *others* who are ill? How useful is intercessory prayer?

- *Matthews, Conti, & Sireci, S. (2001).* For 95 adult hemodialysis subjects with end-stage renal disease, this study found no appreciable improvement in physiological and psychological well-being.

- *Walker, Tonigan, Miller, Corner, & Kahlich (1997).* Intercessory prayer did not demonstrate clinical benefit in the treatment of alcohol abuse and dependence (although prayer by the participants themselves was associated with less drinking).

- *Roberts, Ahmed, & Hall (2000).* In a study performed in the United Kingdom, no evidence was found that intercessory prayer affected the numbers of people dying from leukemia or heart disease. Nor did it decrease the odds of a poor outcome for people with heart problems.

- *Harris et al. (1999).* Remote, intercessory prayer was associated with reduced overall adverse events and shorter length of stay for hospitalized cardiac patients when used as an adjunct to standard medical care.

- *Matthews, Marlowe, & MacNutt (2000).* In patients with rheumatoid arthritis, 6 hours of direct-contact intercessory prayer produced overall improvement during a 1-year follow-up. However there were no additional effects from the supplemental, distant intercessory prayers.

These studies, except for Matthews, Marlowe and MacNutt (2000), do not provide much support for the use of intercessory prayer as a CAM. This is not an exhaustive list of studies of intercessory prayer.

Priests, ministers, rabbis, and other spiritual advisers are all resources for you and the patient.

Prayer

Prayer is an integral component of almost every religion. A Time/CNN poll found that 82% of Americans believe that prayer can cure serious illness (as cited in Ameling, 2000). So, it is likely that a patient or a family member may ask you to pray *for* him or *with* him. This distinction is important. If the patient asks you to pray *with* him, you must determine whether he simply

wants you to be present while he or another person leads the prayer. Ask whether he wants you to begin the prayer or whether he wants to begin the prayer. If a patient asks you to pray *for* him, assess what it is that he wants you to pray for. Often the patient is merely asking you to pray for him on your own time, as frequently as your schedule allows.

Regardless of the situation, if you feel comfortable doing so, then you should enter the experience of prayer with confidence; after all, the patient or family member has asked you to be present because they feel comfortable with you and trust in your abilities. However, if you feel at all uncomfortable about offering prayer, then you should state those feelings and offer to find someone who is comfortable with prayer. For example, you might say either of the following to the patient or family, "Thank you for asking me to pray with you; there is another nurse on the floor who is more comfortable and better at this than I am. May I have your permission to seek that person out for you?" Or, you might reply as follows: "I am confident that the chaplain can help you in many ways with your request. May I make a referral to the chaplain for you?"

If you *do* wish to pray with patients, understanding the different types of prayer may help. **Prayer** consists of those ways that we respond to and interact with God, whether by words, thoughts, or actions. People tend to think of prayer in its narrowest sense as being requests *for* something. And though this is a very important and useful type of prayer, there are actually at least seven types of prayer (Book of Common Prayer, 1979):

Adoration is the directing of our focus and our thoughts to God, asking nothing but to enjoy the presence of God in our lives. This might take the form of meditation.

Praise involves the belief that the love of God draws our praises forth, not to obtain anything, but simply to offer words of praise.

Thanksgiving is offered to God for all the blessings of life and living and whatever draws our attention to God's presence in our lives.

Penitence is the desire to confess one's sins, with an intention to change.

Offering is the offering of all that we have (our life, our work, our hopes and dreams) to God for the purposes that God envisions for us.

Intercession is praying for the needs of others.

Petition is prayer that presents our own needs to God.

You can see that prayers exhibit a variety of form and use for those who believe in their power and influence. For many people, prayer provides for periods of intimacy with God, reveals the presence and love of God, and serves as a powerful source of comfort and hope. Symbolically, a nurse engaged in prayer manifests

the reality of God's presence with that patient. It is a reminder that God never abandons us.

If you wish to pray with a patient and would like some helpful guidelines,

 Go to **Technique 14–2: Praying with Patients,** in Volume 2.

Prayer has a variety of purposes, expressions, and meanings to patients and their families, as well as to nurses themselves. The effects of prayer may not be immediately apparent. But the act of engaging in prayer supports patients' spiritual journeys and may help them experience forgiveness, love, hope, trust, and meaning.

KnowledgeCheck 14–7

- What is prayer?
- Name seven different types of prayer.
- What are the "uses" of prayer by its believers?
- When a patient asks you to pray for him, what might be your most effective first response?

 Go to Chapter 14, **Knowledge Check Response Sheet and Answers,** on the Electronic Study Guide.

Cures, Miracles, and Spiritual Healing

Often, the patient, a family member, or a caregiver will ask for a prayer petitioning God for a cure when your expertise tells you that all curative measures have been exhausted. Certainly you should avoid saying that anything is impossible where prayer is concerned. But it is equally important to avoid exposing the patient and family to false hope. In such cases, it may be possible for you, as care provider and companion on the spiritual journey, to offer a way to reframe the situation for the patient or family. Perhaps healing does not necessarily have to imply the elimination of all types of suffering or of the disease. Rather, it may mean a transformation in a patient's thinking or feeling when that patient has become receptive to the workings of the spirit. In such instances, healing does indeed take place, and the person may experience a miracle.

A **miracle** is anything that allows for the presence of the transcendent (e.g., God, a Higher Being, the experience of one's angel, or any brush with the divine). It is an event that excites wonder and in which we see God at work in our ordinary day-to-day lives (Macquarrie, 1977), but it does not necessarily involve a physical cure. We typically think of miracles as events that break with the natural order of things (e.g., a blind person suddenly can see, with no treatment or explanation); however, miracles more commonly proceed according to natural law. What makes events miracles is the fact that they far exceed our expectations; for instance, an elderly woman, bitter for

| toward evidence-based practice |

Consider the results and/or conclusions from the following studies.

Westlake, C., & Dracup, K. (2001). Role of spirituality in adjustment of patients with advanced heart failure. *Progress in Cardiovascular Nursing, 16*(3), 119–125.

Patients described a process wherein spirituality contributed to their adjustment to advanced heart failure. The process involved regret over past behaviors, the search for meaning in the illness, and the search for hope for the future.

Thomson, J. E. (2000). The place of spiritual well-being in hospice patients' overall quality of life. *Hospital Journal, 15*(2), 13–27.

This study found spiritual well-being to be an important contributor to overall quality of life for hospice patients.

Beery, T., Baas, L., Fowler, C., & Allen G. (2002). Spirituality in persons with heart failure.

The combined spirituality scores predicted 24% of the variance in total quality of life for people with heart failure being treated medically or by transplant.

Tuck, I., McCain, N., & Elswick, R. (2001). Spirituality and psychosocial factors in persons livind with HIV. *Journal of Advanced Nursing, 33*(6), 776–783.

Studying patients with HIV, researchers found spirituality (as measured by a subscale called "existential well-being") was positively related to the patients' quality of life, social support, and effective coping strategies. It was negatively related to perceived stress, uncertainty, psychological distress, and emotional-focused coping.

Bradley, D. (1995). Religious involvement and social resources: Evidence from the data set "Americans' Changing Live." *Journal for the Scientific Study of Religion, 34*(2), 259–267. (Abstract obtained from International Center for the Integration of Health and Spirituality.)

This research found that frequent attendance of religious services was strongly associated with the size of a person's social support network.

Touhy, T. A. (2001). Nurturing hope and spirituality in the nursing home. *Holistic Nursing Practice, 15*(4), 45–56.

This study found that spirituality was the only factor, of those studied, that contributed significantly to hope in institutionalized elders.

Oxman, T., Freeman, D., & Mannheimer, E. (1995). Lack of social participation or religious strength or comfort as risk factors for death after cardiac surgery in the elderly. *Psychosomatic Medicine, 57*, 5–15. (Abstract obtained from International Center for the Integration of Health and Spirituality.)

Researchers found that religious faith was the most consistent indicator of survival after heart surgery in older patients. Those without religious faith had almost three times the risk of death; moreover, the more religious the patient, the greater the protective effect, the study found.

Koenig, H. G., et al. (1998). The relationship between religious activities and blood pressure in older adults. *International Journal of Psychology in Medicine, 28*(2), 189–213.

This study found that older adults who both attended religious services at least once a week *and* prayed or studied the Bible at least daily had consistently lower blood pressure. The study also found that people who tuned in to religious TV or radio shows regularly had higher blood pressure than those who were less frequent viewers or listeners.

---

1. For which of the following do these studies, taken as a whole, provide the stronger support? Explain your reasoning.
   a. Spirituality has a positive effect on physical factors.
   b. Spirituality has a positive effect on psychosocial or emotional factors.

2. Suppose you are a nursing home administrator in an institution where the focus is almost entirely on physical care. You are thinking about a program to teach and encourage your staff to integrate spiritual interventions into their care. Evaluate each of the studies to see how useful it would be in supporting your idea. Explain your thinking.

 Go to Chapter 14, **Toward Evidence-Based Practice Suggested Responses,** on the Electronic Study Guide.

decades over the death of her daughter during child-hood, "feels" her daughter's presence and dies in peace. Miracles are spiritual phenomena. As such, they are mysterious; they are neither entirely defin-able nor comprehensible. In one sense, they can be viewed as perfectly ordinary events; in another, they are extraordinary, for they allow the patient to see and know that God is present despite illness or other adversity (Macquarrie, 1977).

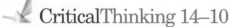 CriticalThinking 14–10

A patient dying of lung cancer asks you to pray with him early one morning. You agree and ask him what he would like you to pray for. He responds: "That I may be cured of my cancer and go back home." He is on oxygen therapy, has pain medications given as ordered, and is in a room by himself. Construct a prayer that might be meaningful and helpful.

Return to the scenario for Charles Johnson ("Meet Your Patient"). See whether you can answer the three questions more completely now than when you began reading the chapter.

 Go to Chapter 14, **Resources for Caregivers and Health Professionals,** on the Electronic Study Guide.

 Suggested Readings: Go to Chapter 14, **Reading More About Spirituality,** on the Electronic Study Guide.

 Bibliography: Go to Volume 2, Bibliography.

Loss, Grief,
& Dying

Learning Outcomes

After completing this chapter, you should be able to:

✳ Differentiate between loss and grief.

✳ Name and describe at least four types of loss.

✳ Identify the stages of grief as described by Worden, Rando, and Bowlby.

✳ Compare and contrast four different types of grief.

✳ List and discuss at least five factors that affect grieving.

✳ Define *death* according to the Uniform Determination of Death Act.

✳ Give a definition of *higher-brain death*.

✳ Create a timeline of the dying process, indicating the physiological signs and symptoms common to each stage.

✳ List and describe the Kübler-Ross stages of dying and grief.

✳ Define *end-of-life care, hospice care,* and *palliative care.*

✳ Identify the legal issues involved in death and dying.

✳ Assess, diagnose, plan, and implement care of dying patients and their families.

✳ Describe the responsibilities of the nurse regarding postmortem care.

✳ Identify nursing interventions to help clients who are grieving.

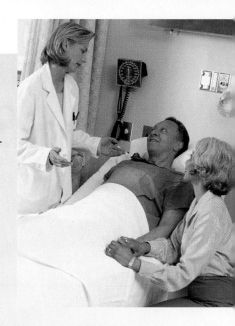

MEET Your Patient

Thomas Manning is a 47-year-old man who is in the oncology unit with end-stage cancer of the pancreas. He is married and has three children, ages 18, 15, and 13. His oldest daughter has been away at college for only 6 months. Mr. Manning's father died 3 months ago from complications of alcoholism, and his mother has been withdrawn and grieving. His wife, Mary, tells you that Thomas "just wants to die" and does not want anyone trying to revive him or "jumping on his chest" if he dies. Mary is distressed and wants him to "keep fighting."

Theoretical Knowledge
knowing why

LOSS AND GRIEF

Throughout your nursing career, you will care for patients coping with loss—of youth, beauty, previous health, functioning, or quality of life. Many of your patients, like Thomas Manning, will be confronting their own approaching death, while family members will be facing loss of their loved one. As their nurse, you can help these people cope with their losses and grieve in a way that is healing, even transformative. But to do so, you need to know how to assess each patient's response to loss, plan appropriate outcomes, and intervene with skill and compassion. As a foundation, you must understand your own feelings and attitudes about loss, grief, and dying. We encourage you to increase your self-knowledge as you work through this chapter.

What Is Loss?

What is the first thing that comes to mind when you think of *loss*? Many people think of losing a loved one through death. Loss, however, is a daily occurrence. Our losses begin at birth (i.e., having to leave the warmth and security of the womb) and end with the ultimate loss, the death of self. **Loss** can be defined as the undesired change or removal of a valued object, person, or situation.

Whenever there is change, there is loss, and because we experience many changes throughout our lives, we also experience much loss. Can you think of the first time that you experienced a loss and what that felt like? What subsequent losses have you undergone as you matured? For losses that are common at different developmental stages,

 Go to Chapter 15, **Tables, Boxes, Figures: ESG Table 15–1,** on the Electronic Study Guide.

For example, losses related to changing schools are common in childhood and adolescence, whereas losses related to retirement or changing jobs are common in middle and older adulthood. Loss may be categorized in the following ways:

• *Actual versus perceived loss.* **Actual loss** includes the death of a loved one (or relationship), theft, deterioration, destruction, and natural disaster. Actual loss can be identified by others, not just by the person experiencing it (e.g., hair loss during chemotherapy). In contrast, **perceived loss** is internal; it is identified only by the person experiencing it (e.g., a woman diagnosed with a sexually transmitted disease may perceive herself as having lost her purity).

• *Physical loss versus psychological loss.* **Physical loss** includes (1) injuries (e.g., when a limb is amputated), (2) removal of a bodily organ (e.g., hysterectomy), and (3) loss of function (e.g., loss of mobility). **Psychological losses** challenge our belief system. They are commonly seen in the areas of sexuality, control, fairness, meaning, and trust. An example is the loss of sexuality that some men feel after the removal of a cancerous prostate gland.

• *External versus internal loss.* **External losses** are actual losses of objects that are important to the person because of their cost or sentimental value (e.g., jewelry, pets, a home). These losses can be brought

about by theft, destruction, or disasters such as floods and fire. **Internal loss** is another term for perceived or psychological loss.

- *Loss of aspects of self* includes physical losses such as body organs, limbs, body functions, and/or body disfigurement. Psychological and perceived losses in this category include aspects of one's personality, developmental change (as in the aging process), loss of hopes and dreams, and loss of faith.

- *Environmental loss* involves a change in the familiar, even if the change is perceived as positive. Examples include moving to a new home, getting a new job and going to college. These losses can be perceived or actual.

- *Loss of significant relationships* is actual loss that includes, but is not limited to, loss of spouses, siblings, family members, or significant others through death, divorce, or separation (e.g., during war, a move to a foreign country).

 ## CriticalThinking 15–1

- Which kinds of loss do you think Thomas Manning is experiencing?
- Why is it important to recognize loss?

What Is Grief?

Whenever there is loss, there is grieving. Grieving requires energy, so it can interfere with health and delay healing. However, grieving is positive in the sense that it is essential to psychological healing following a loss. Consider the following losses and the different reactions of the women involved.

Both Mrs. Smith and Mrs. Jones have lost a dog. Mrs. Smith's son left his dog with her when he went away to college last year. It has died of old age. Mrs. Jones's dog has been with her for 10 years and has been her only companion since her husband died 5 years ago. Her dog was killed by a car today as they were on their morning walk. Which woman do you think will grieve her loss more? Why? Discuss this situation with a classmate. Do you both have the same opinion about this?

This exercise demonstrates that it is really impossible to decide who would feel "more" grief. The intensity of the grief depends on the *meaning* the person attaches to the loss. Both women probably felt sad. However, the meaning of and attachment to the dog are different for each one. You might have thought that Mrs. Smith's loss was minor; however, her dog was owned by her son and may have represented him in her mind. Mrs. Jones's dog was a companion and a protector and may have represented security and friendship. Each woman must grieve what the loss represents to her. This is true for everyone, whether the losses are actual or perceived, physical or psychological.

Grief is the physical, psychological, and spiritual responses to a loss. **Mourning** consists of actions associated with grief (e.g., wailing, wearing black clothing). These processes are normal and natural responses to a loss. The mourning and adjustment time following a loss is the period of **bereavement.** Although each person may express grief differently, some aspects of grief are shared by almost everyone.

KnowledgeCheck 15–1

What types of losses commonly occur in our lives?

Go to Chapter 15, **Knowledge Check Response Sheet and Answers,** on the Electronic Study Guide.

Stages of Grief

Many authors have focused on the stages or steps people experience in grieving. Remember that there is no single, correct way to grieve, nor do people move neatly from one stage or step of grief to the next. Rather, grieving is a fluid, ongoing process. There is constant movement between and among stages, including recurrences of phases the bereaved person thought were resolved. The following are three major theorists in the field (see Table 15–1 for a comparison of their theories).

William Worden

William Worden's (2002) theory describes the tasks a grieving person must achieve. These include the following:

- *Realizing that the loved one (or object) is gone.* In the hours and days after a significant loss, the grieving person typically feels numb and unable to accept the fact of the loss. This numbness is thought to be a helpful form of denial, which allows the person to "take in" only what the psyche is capable of handling at that time. So, the task of realizing that the loved one or object is gone may take several days or, in the case of a sudden death, weeks to achieve.

- *Experiencing the pain.* Once the grieving person has accepted the reality of the loss, the feelings and emotions that surface are intense and can change rapidly. This makes the person feel "out of control." People in this stage may say they feel as if they are "going crazy." This is usually the longest phase for two reasons. First, because none of us likes to be in pain, we become expert at finding ways not to feel it. We overeat, overmedicate, overwork, and drink to excess to avoid feeling the pain, and we thereby prolong the process of grief. Second, caring people do not like to see their loved ones in pain. Therefore, family and friends make attempts to remove the pain (e.g., by distraction) rather than letting the person experience it. Like avoidance, this well-meaning behavior also prolongs the process.

TABLE 15–1 Theories of Grief: A Comparison

Worden: Four Tasks of Grieving	Rando: Six R's of grieving	Bowlby Phases of Grief
Accepting the reality of the loss	**R**ecognizing the loss (awareness)	Shock and numbness
Working through the pain and grief	**R**eacting to the separation (feel the emotions)	Yearning and searching
Adjusting to an environment in which the deceased is missing	**R**ecollecting memories of the deceased (remembering, reliving)	Disorganization and despair
Emotionally relocating the deceased and moving on with life	**R**elinquishing the old attachment (new ways of living without the deceased)	Reorganization
	Readjusting to the new environment (new coping skills)	
	Reinvesting self (energy once turned inward on grief begins to be focused outward again)	

Sources: Worden, J. W. (2002). *Grief counseling and grief therapy: A handbook for the mental health practitioner* (3rd ed.). New York: Springer; Rando, T. (1984). *Grief, dying and death: Clinical interventions for caregivers.* Champaign, IL: Research Press; and Bowlby, J. (1982). *Attachment and loss.* 3 vols. New York: Basic Books.

- *Adjusting to the environment without the deceased.* This may mean performing alone activities and tasks, such as going for walks or shopping, that were once shared. Or it may include taking on roles and responsibilities that the deceased previously held. Such experiences can be extremely sad, frustrating and challenging, or very rewarding. However, once the person has established the new pattern, he or she typically feels satisfaction and increased self-esteem.

- *Investing emotional energy.* Initially all energy is focused on the deceased: thinking about the person, talking about him/her, reliving memories, and so on. It is nearly impossible to think of anything else. Concentration is difficult, so the grieving person finds it hard to engage in activities such as reading. When the person's energy begins to flow toward others or to different or former interests (e.g., working, socializing), the healing process is in progress.

Theresa Rando

Theresa Rando (1984, 1986, 1993, 2000) has identified three phases of grieving. *Avoidance* includes responses such as shock, disbelief, denial, anger, and bargaining. *Confrontation,* the phase during which the person actually faces the loss, is a very emotional and upsetting time. This is when the person feels the grief most acutely. In the *accommodation* phase, the person begins to live with the loss, feel better, and resume some routine activities. Rando's (1984) stages are commonly known as the six R's of grieving (see Table 15–1).

John Bowlby

Drawing on attachment theory, John Bowlby (1982) suggests that grief occurs when the bereaved observe that the object of their attachment is lost. Some experts assert that Bowlby's theory does not take into account the individual nature of grief and that it implies that loved ones can be replaced. Nevertheless, our understanding of grief is broadened by his idea that grief is a mature way of dealing with loss of attachment. He also provides a slightly different perspective on the stages of grief:

Shock and numbness: disorientation, feeling helpless
Yearning and searching: wanting to be reconnected with the deceased
Disorganization and despair: feeling the pain and emotions of grief
Reorganization: adjusting to life with out the deceased, developing new coping skills

 CriticalThinking 15–2

What are some of the similarities you see in the three theories mentioned?

Factors Affecting Grief

To begin thinking about factors affecting grieving, consider the following Critical Thinking exercise.

CriticalThinking 15–3

Mr. Klein is an 86-year-old man whose wife died of heart disease 2 months ago. He has two grown children who both visit him regularly. He also has a very supportive pastor, Mr. Owens, who meets him in the park to share stories. Mr. Owens is 30 years old and has been raising his 5-year-old daughter alone for the last 6 months since his wife died suddenly in an automobile accident. His parents and siblings live out of state. Both of these men are missing their wives very much.

- What factors do you think play a role in each man's grief?
- Who do you think will "get over it" faster?
- What are some issues that may make each man's grief uniquely difficult?

No two people ever grieve in the same manner because there are so many factors that play a role in the grieving process. They include the following.

Significance of the loss. The meaning the person has attached to the person or object lost will be different for each person. The more attachment to the relationship or object, the more difficult the grieving.

Amount of support for the bereaved. People with more emotional and psychosocial support typically have less complicated grief.

Conflicts existing at the time of death. A conflict left unresolved may cause prolonged grief. For example, if a couple had an argument just before one partner died suddenly, the remaining partner's grief may be complicated by guilt.

Circumstances of the loss. For example, was this a sudden, unexpected death, or had the person been suffering from a chronic illness? Specifically, was there an opportunity to prepare for it? Was the death a suicide or homicide? Was the death in any sense avoidable? Was the person in pain? If the circumstances of the loss leave the bereaved feeling guilty or responsible, his healing process may be impeded. This can result from losses other than death as well (e.g., loss of valued property by theft or disaster, loss of a relationship, loss of a job, rejection from college).

Previous loss. If the person has sustained more than one loss in a short period of time, the grieving process can become more complicated. In the hospital you will frequently care for patients experiencing multiple losses. For example, consider a patient who has suffered a stroke and loss of mobility and then has to move out of his home of many years to a nursing home. The patient's loss of health and functioning is compounded by the loss of his independence and familiar surroundings.

Developmental stages. Based on Erik Erikson's stages of psychological growth, we all must achieve certain psychological milestones during a lifetime. If you need to review Erikson's theory,

 Go to **Chapter 9** on the Electronic Study Guide.

Grief can affect the healthy development of these stages, and in turn, the person's stage of development affects the grieving process.

- *Childhood.* Because cognitive development is not yet complete, preschool children do not understand that death is final. The belief that death is temporary and reversible is reinforced by cartoon characters who "die" and then "come to life" again. Between ages 5 and 9, children begin to understand that death is permanent, but they believe it will never happen to them or anyone they know. During the weeks after a death, a child may feel immediate grief or may continue to believe that the person is still alive. Both are normal reactions. A child may display feelings of sadness on and off over a long period of time and often at unexpected moments.

  Young children believe they are the cause of what happens around them, so a death may cause them to feel guilt. Other responses include regressing to a previous developmental stage: "acting like a baby," demanding food and attention, becoming incontinent, and talking "baby talk."

- *Adolescence.* Adolescence is typically a time for dealing with confusion between one's identity and one's role. The adolescent struggles to learn who he is as a person as he breaks away from parental control. An adolescent who experiences the loss of a parent while "pushing the parent away," may feel a sense of guilt and "unfinished business."

  At the same time, the bereaved teen also faces psychological, physiological, social, and academic pressures. Although teens may look mature, they may lack emotional maturity. Teens are often expected to be "grown up" and support a surviving parent or younger siblings. When they feel this responsibility, they do not have the opportunity, or the permission, to mourn. Coping may be even more difficult for teens because the death may have come suddenly and unexpectedly. For example, a relatively young parent may die of a heart attack, or a brother may die in an auto accident.

- *Adulthood.* Adults are cognitively able to understand the nature of death, and they have usually experienced other types of loss by this time. Over time, they perceive loss as a normal part of living. How they respond to loss depends on factors such as the person's self-esteem and the availability of supports. The rest of this section refers primarily to factors that affect the adult grieving process.

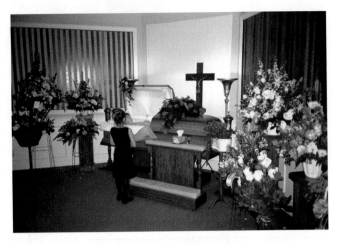

FIGURE 15–1 Rituals are used to facilitate grieving.

A special difficulty for *older adults* is that they experience so many losses. Most deaths occur among older adults, so they are likely to lose friends and siblings in rapid succession. Add to those losses the physical and functional losses and the loss of independence, and the cumulative effects may be devastating.

Spiritual/cultural. Spirituality and religious beliefs can help or hinder the grieving process. One person might believe the deceased is in a place of contentment and happiness, where all suffering is over. Another may believe that the deceased will soon be reborn, possibly into the same extended family. Another may believe that death is final and there is no longer any life after death. How do you think these beliefs might influence the grieving process?

Most cultures engage in rituals (e.g., funerals, as shown in Figure 15–1) that help the bereaved begin the grieving process by openly expressing their emotions and pain. Some cultures may emphasize keeping emotions more subdued and limiting expressions of grief to private settings.

Timeliness of the death. The death of a child or a young person is almost universally more difficult to accept than the death of an older person. In addition to loss of the person, there is a sense of unfairness because of the loss of *potential*—of what the person might have become or achieved. You may hear someone ask, "Why was her life cut short?" or state, "He had so much going for him, but God didn't give him a chance."

KnowledgeCheck 15–2

- What are the main tasks of the grieving process?
- What factors affect the grieving process?

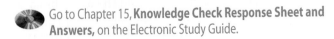

Go to Chapter 15, **Knowledge Check Response Sheet and Answers,** on the Electronic Study Guide.

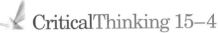

CriticalThinking 15–4

Refer to Thomas Manning and his wife ("Meet Your Patient"). Apply each of the preceding factors affecting grief to Thomas and to Mary (they may be different for each spouse). If the scenario does not provide enough information for you to comment, say so and then describe how you would obtain the data you need.

Types of Grief

Grief can be categorized in several ways, most of which have to do with timing and intensity.

Uncomplicated grief (normal grief) is the natural response to a loss. The bereaved person experiences the feelings, behaviors, and cognitions that are expected in light of his culture, social status, and relationship to the lost person or object (Table 15–2). The emotions are intense but gradually diminish over time (several months to several years). Some emotions will always be present, but the intensity will change.

Complicated grief is distinguished from uncomplicated grief by *length of time* and *intensity of emotion.* The person's responses are maladaptive, unusually prolonged, or overwhelming. For example, the bereaved may become severely depressed, violent, or suicidal; become a "workaholic"; or demonstrate addictive behavior. Or, after several years, the person may still be experiencing as much pain and disruption as in the first months after the loss. Typically, complicated grief results when the grieving process has been impeded for some reason (e.g., something keeps the person "stuck" in the grief process). Usually the bereaved benefits from the assistance of a grief counselor to help establish and work through the problem areas. Chronic, masked, and delayed grief are all examples of complicated grief:

- **Chronic grief** begins as normal grief but continues long term, with little resolution of feelings and inability to rejoin normal life.

- **Masked grief** occurs when the person is grieving but expressing the grief through other types of behavior. For example, a man whose wife has died may begin drinking heavily, or a couple whose child has died may find themselves engaging in violent arguments with each other. This change in behavior is part of their grief response, but they don't recognize it as such.

- **Delayed grief** is grief that is put off until a later time (e.g., "I'll think about it later. Right now, I'm busy trying to keep a roof over our heads and care for my children.").

Disenfranchised grief is experienced in connection with a loss that is not socially supported or

TABLE 15-2 Common Grief Reactions

Physical	Emotional	Behaviors	Cognitions
Loss of appetite	Anger	Forgetfulness	Decreased concentration
Weight loss or gain	Sadness	Being withdrawn	Forgetfulness
Fatigue	Guilt	Insomnia or too much sleep	Impaired judgment
Decreased libido	Relief	Dreaming of deceased	Obsessive thoughts of the deceased or lost object
Decreased immune system response	Shock	Verbalizing the loss	Preoccupation
Decreased energy	Numbness	Crying	Confusion
Possible physical symptoms, such as headache or stomach pain	Loneliness	Loss of productivity at work or school	Questioning spiritual beliefs
	Fear		Searching for understanding
	Anxiety		Searching for purpose and meaning
	Powerlessness		
	Helplessness		

acknowledged by the usual rites or ceremonies (Corr, Nabe & Corr, 2003). Disenfranchised grief may be experienced by a man whose wife has had a miscarriage, a mistress whose lover dies, or a bereaved partner in a homosexual relationship not recognized by the families. In each of these instances, the bereaved person lacks the communal support that is helpful in grieving.

Anticipatory grief is experienced before a loss occurs. A wife caring for her husband through a long illness may grieve as she sees the vibrant man she once knew change before her eyes and as she anticipates his death. Family members caring for a loved one with Alzheimer's disease commonly experience anticipatory grief, realizing that as mental capacity diminishes, the person they once knew will become ever more removed from them.

CriticalThinking 15–5

Thomas Manning ("Meet Your Patient") had a strained relationship with his father for most of his life. His father was alcoholic and constantly fought with his mother while Thomas was growing up. A few months ago, his father was hospitalized for the third time for complications of alcoholism, and Thomas visited him. He confronted his father regarding his drinking and the problems and pain it had caused him and the family. The confrontation ended in an argument. That night, Thomas' father slipped into a coma, and a few days later, without recovering consciousness, he died.

- What issues does Thomas have to deal with?
- Why might this be a complicated grief process?

DEATH AND DYING

Death is the ultimate loss. The dying person faces the loss of physical control and function, independence, relationships, possibilities, and ultimately life itself. In mainstream North American culture, death is not seen as a natural part of life, but rather as something to avoid at all costs. People even avoid talking or thinking about it.

How Is Death Defined?

The legal definition of death has evolved over the years. Historically, *death* was defined as the cessation of the flow of vital bodily fluids. This evolved into the traditional definition of **heart-lung death:** the irreversible cessation of spontaneous respirations and circulation. This criterion was used to define death until the 1960s, when it was replaced by **whole-brain death:** the irreversible cessation of all functions of the brain, including the brain stem. Spontaneous respirations cannot continue once the brain stem stops functioning; the heart, however, may continue to beat until it becomes oxygen starved from cessation of respirations.

In the 1970s, many practitioners began using the term **higher-brain death,** which defines death as the irreversible cessation of all "higher" brain functions (e.g., cognitive functioning, consciousness, memory, reasoning, and so on). By this definition, the brain stem can still be functioning, so both respiratory and cardiac activity may continue even though the person does not make purposive responses to external stimuli, cephalic reflexes are absent, and the electroencephalogram shows no activity.

BOX 15–1 Uniform Determination of Death Act

1. [Determination of Death] An individual who has sustained either (1) irreversible cessation of circulatory and respiratory functions, or (2) irreversible cessation of all functions of the entire brain, including the brain stem, is dead. A determination of death must be made in accordance with accepted medical standards.

2. [Uniformity of Construction and Application] This act shall be applied and construed to effectuate its general purpose to make uniform the law with respect to the subject of this Act among states enacting it.

Source: President's Commission for the Study of Ethical Problems in Medicine and Biomedical and Behavioral Research. (1981). *Defining death: A report on the medical, legal, and ethical issues in the determination of death.* Washington, DC: Government Printing Office, p. 73.

Based on the two preceding definitions of brain death, it is technically possible to keep a person "alive" indefinitely by using a mechanical ventilator. In 1981 the President's Commission for the Study of Ethical Problems in Medicine proposed the **Uniform Determination of Death Act** (Box 15–1). This definition, which includes the loss of brain stem function, provides a highly reliable means of declaring death for respirator-maintained bodies (DeSpelder & Strickland, 1996, p. 328). For criteria for assessing brain stem functioning,

 Go to Chapter 15, **Supplemental Materials: Some Criteria for Assessing Brain Stem Functioning,** on the Electronic Study Guide.

A **coma** is a prolonged, deep state of unconsciousness lasting days or even years. The patient cannot be aroused and may or may not have decreased brain stem reflexes. In a **persistent vegetative state (PVS),** which sometimes follows a coma, the person does not respond to stimuli, is unaware of the environment, and has no cognition or affective mental functions. However, the person has lost only the higher cerebral functions (see the definition of *higher-brain death*) and so continues to have a sleep-wake cycle, may have some spontaneous movements, and may open her eyes in response to external stimuli. However, the person cannot speak or obey commands. PVS sometimes follows a coma but can also occur after any event that affects cerebrovascular flow. Patients in a PVS may look somewhat normal and may occasionally grimace, cry, or laugh. The family may believe that the patient is responding to the environment and thus not want to give up hope for recovery. Because they cannot work through the grieving process, they continue to grieve each day.

What Are the Stages of Dying?

To help dying patients and their families understand the dying process, your theoretical knowledge base must include information on both physiological and psychological processes.

Physiological Stages

The following timeline describes the physiological responses of the body to impending death (Dworkind & Karnes, 2003). Obviously, except for the last bulleted item, this timeline does not apply to a person who dies suddenly and unexpectedly, as in an accident or massive heart attack.

- *One to three months prior to death.* The dying person begins to withdraw from the world and people. Sleep increases, and appetite decreases. It becomes difficult for the body to digest food, especially meats. Liquids are preferred.

- *One to two weeks prior to death.* A host of physical changes indicates that the body is beginning to lose its ability to maintain itself. Cardiovascular deterioration brings reduced blood pressure, changes in pulse and skin color (e.g., a yellowish pallor), and extreme pallor of the extremities. Temperature fluctuates and perspiration is increased. Respiratory rate may increase or decrease; during sleep, the dying person may experience brief periods of apnea. Congestion may cause a rattling sound and/or a nonproductive cough.

- *Days to hours prior to death.* Often a surge of energy brings mental clarity and a desire to eat and talk with family members. However, as death approaches, patients tend to become dehydrated and have difficulty swallowing, which results in decreased blood volume. The tissues of the tongue and soft palate sag, and the gag reflex declines, so secretions accumulate in the oropharynx and/or bronchi.

   Breathing may be shallow, rapid, or irregular: periods of apnea may lengthen to 10 to 30 seconds before breathing resumes. Congestion causes a "death rattle" that can be quite loud. **Cheyne-Stokes respirations** may occur. This is a cyclic pattern consisting of a 10- to 60-second period of apnea and then a gradual increase in depth and rate of respirations. Respirations gradually become slow and shallow, and then the cycle begins again with apnea.

   Peripheral circulation decreases, and the person perspires and feels "clammy." The blood pressure decreases, and the pulse may be hard to detect. The extremities become cool and mottled, and the underside of the body may be much darker. Decreased circulation

also results in reduced kidney function and decreased urinary output.

Muscles throughout the body relax, causing slack facial muscles. As peristalsis slows, the patient may retain feces. Sphincters relax, and bowel and bladder incontinence can occur. Vision blurs; the eyes may be open or partially open, but unseeing. Instead, the patient may see things that are not visible to others.

In the final hours of life, many patients become restless and agitated. This response may be caused by medications, liver failure, cerebral hypoxia, renal failure, stool impaction, distended bladder, increased pain, or unresolved emotional or spiritual issues. However, many patients become less communicative, quiet, and withdrawn (Pitorak, 2003).

- *Moments prior to death.* The dying person does not respond to touch or sound and cannot be awakened. Typically, there is a short series of long-spaced breaths before breathing ceases entirely and the heart stops beating (Dworkind & Karnes, 2003).

Psychological Stages

Perhaps the best known author on the psychology of dying is Dr. Elisabeth Kübler-Ross (1969). She felt that if people understood what dying patients are experiencing, they would be more competent in caring for them. From her research with dying patients, she observed that people tend to experience one or more of five psychological stages during the period from the terminal diagnosis to the actual death (Box 15–2). Her theory has become a classic for professional and lay readers alike; however, it has been criticized by people who misinterpreted it or attempted to apply it in the wrong way. When you study the Kübler-Ross stages, it is important to understand that dying people:

1. May not go through *every* stage.
2. May not go through the stages in a linear fashion, but rather in random order.
3. Do not necessarily complete one stage and move on to the next.
4. May experience two or three stages simultaneously.

Bear in mind that it is not the nurse's responsibility to move people on to the next stage so that everyone dies accepting death. It *is* our responsibility to accept and support people "where they are" and help them to verbalize their feelings. We need to understand patients, not change them.

What Is End-of-Life Care?

In an effort to humanize health care, organizations such as the Institute of Medicine, the American Association of Colleges of Nursing, and the Robert Wood Johnson Foundation have identified competencies for

---

BOX 15-2   Kübler-Ross: Stages of Dying and Grief

Stage	Defining Characteristics
• *Denial.*	"Not me." "This cannot be happening." I don't believe it." Usually the person is in a state of shock. Denial is not necessarily negative; it gives the person a chance to prepare psychologically for accepting the news.
• *Anger.*	"Why me?" "Why is this happening?" Anger can be obvious or subtle. It is the person's response to the feeling that the situation is unfair. The person may take his anger out on people who are "safe" (e.g., family, spouse) or from whom there will be no reprisals (e.g., nurses, physician).
• *Bargaining.*	"If only I can live until …" "Yes me, but …" Usually this takes the form of a bargain with God or a Higher Power, in which the person asks to live to see a birth, graduation, wedding, and so forth.
• *Depression.*	A withdrawn sadness, not to be confused with clinical depression. This is a response to the current loss as well as to any accumulated and/or future losses.
• *Acceptance.*	Not necessarily *wanting* death (or the loss), but coming to terms with it and ceasing to fight it. The person may seem almost void of feelings.

Source: Kübler-Ross, E. (1969). *On death and dying.* New York: MacMillan.

---

nurses that stress compassion, sensitivity, and technical skills during end-of-life care (Ferrell, Grant, & Virani, 1999). Some of these competencies include the following (Bednash & Ferrell, 2000):

- Holistic assessment of patients and families (i.e., physical, psychological, social, and spiritual)
- Acknowledging diversity in patients' beliefs and customs
- Using both traditional and complementary approaches
- Applying legal and ethical principles to end-of-life care
- Demonstrating respect for the patients' views and wishes during end-of-life care
- Assessing patient, family, colleagues, and one's own success in coping with suffering, grief, loss, and bereavement at the end of life

complementary and alternative modalities (CAM)

End-of-Life Care

- In Australia, Sloman (2002) found that *progressive muscle relaxation training* and guided imagery significantly improved depression and quality of life for people with advanced cancer. However, there was no improvement in depression.

- Johnstone, Polston, Niemtzow, and Martin (2002) studied the use of *acupuncture* to provide palliative symptom relief to patients in an oncology (cancer) clinic. The major symptoms treated were pain, xerostomia, hot flashes, and nausea and loss of appetite. The 89 patients received from one to nine treatments. Most patients (60%) showed at least 30% improvement in symptoms (taken as a whole).

- Thompson and Reilly (2002) explored the impact of the *homeopathic approach* on symptom control, mood disturbance, and quality of life for 100 patients attending a cancer clinic. The most common symptoms were pain, fatigue, and hot flushes. The symptoms of fatigue and hot flushes improved significantly, but there was no appreciable pain relief.

- In England, Gambles, Crooke, and Wilkinson (2002) studied the effects of four to six sessions of *reflexology* on the symptoms of 34 patients receiving palliative care. Patients comments were generally positive. They reported relief from tension and anxiety relief, as well as improved comfort and well-being.

For end-of-life nursing care competencies recommended by the American Association of Colleges of Nursing (AACN),

 Go to Chapter 15, **Tables, Boxes, Figures: ESG Box 15–1,** on the Electronic Study Guide.

End-of-life care includes palliative care and hospice care, which are similar in that both may involve caring for dying patients, and neither focuses on cure. Some people use the terms interchangeably; however, there are subtle differences.

Palliative Care

When patients reach a stage in their illness in which cure is no longer possible, or when they refuse further treatment, they may be eligible to receive "comfort care"—meaning that no further efforts will be made to stop the disease process or prevent the patient from dying, although certain symptoms (e.g., nausea, pain) will be treated. The correct interpretation of the term *comfort care* is, "Nothing more *can* be done to cure your loved one." However, family members sometimes interpret it to mean "Nothing more *will* be done." In this situation, the term *palliative care* may be more acceptable.

Palliative care is actually aggressively planned, holistic comfort care. It focuses on managing the symptoms of patients whose disease process no longer responds to treatment. A patient does not necessarily have to be "actively dying" to receive palliative care. It is also provided over a long period of time for those who have slowly progressive diseases. As a specialty, palliative care is provided by a holistic team of professionals. However, many patients receive palliative care from their general practice provider, especially if staff are comfortable with pain management and end-of-life care.

Hospice Care

The hospice movement was set in motion in England by Dame Cicely Sanders, who founded the first modern-day hospice within a London hospital in 1968. Currently there are over 3000 hospice programs in the United States alone (Family Hospice Association, 2003). **Hospice care** focuses on holistic care of patients who are dying or debilitated and not expected to improve. For a patient to be eligible for hospice insurance benefits, a physician must certify that the patient is likely to die within 6 months. It is in this way that hospice differs most from palliative care.

Hospice care is based on two key premises: (1) the quality of life is as important as the length of life, and (2) those who are terminally ill should be allowed to face death with dignity and surrounded by the comfort of their home and family. Thus, hospice providers consider helping family members an essential part of their role (Family Hospice Association, 2003).

Treatment is holistic, addressing the patient's emotional, spiritual, and physical needs. Physical care is primarily palliative, involving symptom management. For example, pain management is considered crucial, because patients must be relatively free from pain to make the most of the time remaining to them.

An interdisciplinary team plans care with the patient and family. Family members are encouraged to be an active part of the team as much as they are able. Nursing support is available 24 hours a day, and families are taught what to expect as the disease progresses. Psychosocial and spiritual care have high priority. After the patient dies, there is follow-up bereavement care for the families.

Although you may think of hospice as "home" care, hospice is a *way* of caring rather than a setting. Some hospitals are able to devote some inpatient beds to hospice care, and freestanding hospices also exist. The purpose of admitting a patient is to provide a family with some respite for a period of time or to stabilize

a patient who requires symptom management, or to care for a patient who is in the end stage of a disease (e.g., AIDS or cancer) and needs a level of expert care that family members cannot provide at home.

What Are Some Legal and Ethical Considerations?

The technology of life support makes it possible to prolong body functions almost indefinitely, leaving patients and families struggling to decide whether prolonging life is appropriate. More and more of these clients depend on nurses for education regarding patient rights and choices surrounding end-of-life care. Each situation is unique, and you should be able to explore with clients the various options available. See Chapter 44 and Chapter 45, for more information about the ethical and legal aspects of each of the following topics.

Advance Directives

An **advance directive** is a group of instructions (written or oral) stating a person's wishes relative to his health care if he were incapacitated or unable to make that decision. The Patient Self-Determination Act (PSDA), passed by Congress in 1990, requires that all healthcare providers who receive Medicare funds (e.g., hospitals, home care agencies, hospices, nursing homes) must educate staff and patients and provide opportunity for all patients to complete an advance directive. Laws regarding advance directives vary from state to state. It is important for you to understand the regulations of your own state as well as federal laws and the policies of your institution. Advance directives are of different types and serve different purposes.

- A **living will** is a document prepared by a competent person giving instructions regarding medical care if that person becomes unable to make decisions. The document provides specific instructions about the kinds of health care the person would wish or would wish *not* to have in particular situations. For example, it might specify that no artificial food or fluids be administered.

- A **durable power of attorney (healthcare proxy)** exists when a competent person names another individual to make decisions regarding his healthcare choices under certain conditions (e.g., irreversible coma, terminal illness) when he is unable to do so. These instructions are usually written and should include specific instructions about the patient's wishes regarding hydration, feeding tubes, medication, resuscitation, and mechanical ventilation. The document must be witnessed by two persons and can be changed or canceled at any time by the patient.

For an example of an advance directive,

 Go to Chapter 15, **Tables, Boxes, Figures: ESG Figure 15-1,** on the Electronic Study Guide.

For details of the Patient Self-Determination Act,

 Go to Chapter 15, **Supplemental Materials: Patient Self-Determination Act,** on the Electronic Study Guide.

Some people fear that once an advance directive is signed, no further care will be provided. Explain to families and patients that this is not the case; instead, the directive is to make sure that they will get however much or little care *they* wish. Remind people that everyone should have an advance directive and that they should not wait until they become ill to prepare one. Such explanations are independent nursing activities, for which you are responsible.

Orders for DNAR

A **DNAR order** is an order *not* to attempt resuscitation of the patient in the event of a cardiac or respiratory failure. The American Heart Association (AHA) is now using the term *DNAR (do not attempt resuscitation)* instead of *DNR (do not resuscitate).* For an example of a DNAR (DNR) order, see Figure 15–2. You must pay careful attention to these policies, as well as to any advance directives, to be prepared should one of your patients suffer a cardiac arrest.

Cardiopulmonary resuscitation (CPR) is performed almost automatically in many healthcare settings. This practice may be slowly changing, however. It is interesting that the AHA, which has for so long focused on preserving life, has in its most recent publications begun to point out that it is not always appropriate to use CPR. For example, some of their instructor's materials stress that asystole (cardiac standstill) is usually a confirmation of death rather than a rhythm to be treated.

Carefully explain to patients and families what CPR involves and what their options are. The patient and/or family has the ultimate say. They have the right to refuse CPR and may request DNAR orders; the physician cannot legally write a DNAR order if the patient and/or family do not wish it. The American Nurses Association (ANA) recommendations regarding DNAR are summarized in Box 15–3. For a complete list of the ANA recommendations,

 Go to Chapter 15, **Tables, Boxes, Figures: ESG Box 15-2,** on the Electronic Study Guide.

Assisted Suicide

Assisted suicide means making available that which is needed for the patient to end his own life (e.g., pharmacological agents or weapons). The patient is

DO NOT RESUSCITATE ORDERS

Physician: Complete Part I & II to initiate order. Part III is to be
completed every seven days.

☐ **DNR forms completed on previous admission. Verified by:** _____.
Date of original order: _____.   Signature   Date

NOTE: Words that appear in the directions in all capital letters are listed in the DNR definitions.

PART I: ☐ If this patient suffers a cardiac or respiratory arrest, a Cart is not to be called and no resuscitation measures are to be carried out.

PART II: ☐ This order is to be transcribed and instituted immediately. All required documentation is complete.

or

☐ This order is to be transcribed and instituted only after the CONCURRING PHYSICIAN'S statements have been completed.
I have requested Dr. _____ to be the CONCURRING PHYSICIAN.

_____, M.D.   _____, R.N.
Signature of ATTENDING PHYSICIAN   Signature of Transcribing Nurse

_____   _____   _____   _____
Date   Time   Date   Time

PART III: Review of DNR ORDER
This is to verify that review and determination of continued appropriateness of the DNR ORDER and the conditions under which it was obtained was done: (to be documented at least every 7 days)

Date	By	Date	By
			Continued on reverse side

PART IV: Wavier to DNR ORDER
I, the undersigned, have previously consented to a DO NOT RESUSCITATE ORDER. During the procedure and until I am returned to my room, I hereby waive my consent to the DO NOT RESUSCITATE ORDER and authorize my ATTENDING PHYSICIAN to write such an order.

_____   _____   _____   _____
Signature of patient or SURROGATE or PROXY   Date   Signature of WITNESS   Date
(or parent or legal guardian for minor)

☐ DNR ORDER suspended during the peri-operative period, as noted above.

_____, M.D.   _____, R.N.
Signature of ATTENDING PHYSICIAN   Signature of Transcribing Nurse

_____   _____   _____   _____
Date   Time   Date   Time

PART V: Revocation of DNR ORDER
I, the undersigned, hereby revoke the DO NOT RESUSCITATE ORDER previously consented to by me.

_____   _____   _____   _____
Signature of patient or SURROGATE or PROXY   Date   Signature of WITNESS   Date
(or parent or legal guardian for minor)

☐ DNR ORDER revoked.

_____, M.D.   _____, R.N.
Signature of ATTENDING PHYSICIAN   Signature of Transcribing Nurse

_____   _____   _____   _____
Date   Time   Date   Time

13610 3/01 side 1 of 2

FIGURE 15–2 **Do Not Attempt Resuscitation (DNAR) orders such as this are written after consultation with the patient and family members.**
Source: St Joseph's Hospital Health Center, 301 Prospect Ave, Syracuse, New York, 13203. Used by permission.

BOX 15-3 Highlights of ANA Recommendations Concerning DNAR

1. The competent patient's choices have highest priority when there is conflict.

2. When the patient is not competent, give highest priority to advance directives or the surrogate decision makers.

3. DNAR orders should be discussed explicitly with the patient and significant others.

4. DNAR orders must be documented, reviewed, and updated.

5. DNAR does *not* mean "discontinue care"!

6. If the DNAR order compromises your moral integrity, transfer the patient's care to another nurse.

Source: Adapted from American Nurses Association. (1992). *Position statement: Nursing care and do-not-resuscitate decisions.* Retrieved September 12, 2003, from www.nursingworld.org/readroom/position/ethics/etdnr.htm

Organ/Tissue Donor Card

I wish to donate my organs and tissues. I wish to give:

☐ any needed organs and tissues ☐ only the following organs and tissues:

_____

Donor
Signature _____ Date _____
Witness _____
Witness _____

FIGURE 15–3 Example of an organ donor card. *Source:* U.S. Department of Health and Human Services. Retrieved September 20, 2003, from *http://www.organdonor.gov*

physically capable of ending his own life, has expressed the intention to do so, and has turned to the health-care provider merely to supply the means. The ANA (1994) believes that "the nurse should not participate in active euthanasia (and assisted suicide) because such an act is in direct violation of the Code for Nurses and the ethical traditions of the profession. Nurses have an obligation to provide timely, humane, comprehensive and compassionate end-of-life care."

Euthanasia

The term **euthanasia** comes from the Greek word *euthanatos,* which means "good death." It refers to the deliberate ending of a life of someone suffering from a terminal or incurable illness. **Active euthanasia** occurs as a result of a direct action (e.g., giving an overdose of medication). Active euthanasia can be *voluntary* (patient consents); *involuntary* (patient refuses); or *nonvoluntary* (patient is unable to consent, or someone else makes the decision and the patient is unaware of it). Active euthanasia goes a step further than assisted suicide. In assisted suicide, the "assistant" makes available the means for the person to take his own life; in euthanasia, the "assistant" also serves as the direct agent of death (e.g., administers the medication).

Passive euthanasia occurs as a result of a *lack* of action (e.g., withholding medications or food necessary to sustain life). Honoring the refusal of treatments that a patient does not desire, that are burdensome, or that will not benefit the patient is not generally considered passive euthanasia and can be ethically and legally permissible. For more information about the ethical and legal issues surrounding euthanasia, see Chapter 44 and Chapter 45, respectively.

CriticalThinking 15–6

What are your feelings about assisted suicide and euthanasia? Focus on your feelings, not on principles, explanation, and rationale.

Autopsy

An **autopsy** is a medical examination of the body to determine the cause of death. Autopsies have also provided relevant data about disease processes and causes. The pathologist performs a detailed internal and external evaluation of the body, removes body organs, and extracts sample tissues for further examination. The organs are then replaced in the body, and the body cavities are closed with sutures. An autopsy requires signed permission from the next of kin, except in cases in which autopsy is required by law (e.g., deaths that are suspicious or unwitnessed).

Organ Donation

People sometimes wish to donate their organs to someone else when they die. Currently all 50 states have adopted the Uniform Anatomical Gift Act for organ donation. This document was revised in 1987 to eliminate the requirement of a witness signature and consent from next of kin. (See Box 15–4 for provisions of the document.) However, even though donor cards (Figure 15–3) are legal in all states many institutions will not procure organs from the deceased if there is strong family objection. Therefore, if a patient is planning to

BOX 15–4 Major Provisions of the Uniform Anatomical Gift Act

1. Any person over 18 may donate all or part of his or her body for education, research, therapeutic, or transplantation purposes.

2. If the person has not made a donation before death, the next of kin can make it unless there was a known objection by the deceased.

3. If the person has made such a gift the act says it cannot be revoked by his or her relatives. However, in actual practice this sometimes happens.

4. If there is more than one person of the same degree of kinship, the gift from relatives shall not be accepted if there is a known objection by one of them.

5. The gift can be authorized by a card carried by the individual or by written or recorded verbal communication from a relative.

6. The gift can be amended or revoked at any time before the death of the donor.

7. The time of death must be determined by a physician who is not involved in any transplantation.

Source: DeSpelder, L., & Strickland, A. (1996). *The last dance.* Mountain View, CA: Mayfield.

donate organs or tissues, be sure that he discusses these wishes with family members.

The list of persons waiting for organ donations continues to increase. If death is imminent, a healthcare team member (physician or nurse) should ask whether the patient has agreed to be an organ donor. In many institutions, a transplant coordinator contacts the family and makes the request for organ and tissue donation.

KnowledgeCheck 15–3

• What are advance directives?
• What is the ANA position on assisted suicide?

 Go to Chapter 15, **Knowledge Check Response Sheet and Answers,** on the Electronic Study Guide.

Practical Knowledge
knowing how

| Assessment |

When a patient is dying or has experienced a loss, you must carefully assess the patient and significant others for the common grief reactions listed in Table

15–2. Other important areas to assess include knowledge base, history of loss, coping patterns and abilities, meaning of the loss or illness, and support systems. For dying patients, you should also make the following assessments:

• When the client and family are ready, encourage them to talk about the client's wishes for burial or cremation or tasks that the client would like taken care of (e.g., giving away valuables, calling family members).

• Determine whether the dying client has a living will or advance directives.

• Discuss with client and family the possibility of organ donation, if appropriate for the client's circumstances.

For guidelines to follow when assessing dying and grieving patients,

 Go to Chapter 15, **Assessment Guidelines and Tools,** in Volume 2.

KnowledgeCheck 15–4

What assessments should you make for your terminally ill patient and his or her family?

 Go to Chapter 15, **Knowledge Check Response Sheet and Answers,** on the Electronic Study Guide.

| Diagnosis |

Keep in mind that most grief is normal, not dysfunctional. Do not use a Dysfunctional Grieving diagnosis for every person who is grieving a loss. **Dysfunctional grieving** is unusual in some way and is characterized by its *duration* and *intensity of emotion.* The person experiences disabling pain and grief, or the grieving continues over a very long time (perhaps several years). The person may deny or have difficulty expressing feelings of loss or may experience physical symptoms as a result of suppressing feelings.

Loss and Grieving as Problem

Several nursing diagnoses may be appropriate for a person who is dying or grieving. You must determine whether loss and grieving are the *problem* or the *etiology,* because (as you learned in Chapters 4 and 6) the answer will influence your interventions. Diagnoses related to death and dying and grief and loss overlap, so they are discussed together below. The nursing diagnoses in the table in Volume 2 (see the link below) focus on the emotional responses to loss or impending death—that is, loss and grieving *are* the problem.

 Go to Chapter 15, **Standardized Outcomes and Interventions for Loss and Grieving Diagnoses,** in Volume 2.

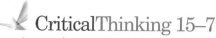 CriticalThinking 15–7

Answer the questions in the Standardized Outcomes and Interventions table in Chapter 15 of Volume 2 (see preceding reference).

Loss and Grieving as Etiology

Loss, grief, and dying are the etiology when they create problems in other areas of patient or family function, for example:

- Acute or Chronic Low Self-Esteem related to inability to change the event for self or significant other; or related to dying while having "unfinished business"
- Anxiety related to possible inability to cope with the loss; or related to unknown outcome of situation
- Death Anxiety (or Fear) related to impending death
- Decisional Conflict related to end-of-life treatment measures (e.g., concern about the expense of "useless" procedures or their effect on the family; knowledge that the treatment may lengthen life but decrease the quality of life)
- Deficient Knowledge related to the new experience of caring for a terminally ill person
- Fatigue related to demands of caring for a dying loved one
- Imbalanced Nutrition: Less Than Body Requirements related to inability to eat or drink secondary to grieving; or secondary to body system changes from approaching death
- Spiritual Distress related to loss of trust in a loving God

| Planning Outcomes/Evaluation |

Encourage the patient and family to play an active role in planning care. Involving family members helps facilitate their acceptance of the diagnosis and may put the patient more at ease. Questions such as the following will help to elicit the patient's goals for end of life (Matzo, Sherman, Sheehan, Ferrell, & Penn, 2003):

- "What do you still want to accomplish or do?"
- "What are the things you wish you could still do?"
- "If you have pain, what would be an acceptable level for you, on a 0 to 10 scale?"
- "Where do you want to spend the rest of your life? Where are you most comfortable?"
- "If spiritual peace is important to you, what would help you achieve it?"

NOC standardized outcomes are determined by the diagnostic label you use. For examples,

 Go to Chapter 15, **Standardized Outcomes and Interventions for Loss and Grieving Diagnoses,** in Volume 2.

Individualized goals/outcome statements you might write for a grieving or dying person include the following examples. The patient and/or family will:

- Communicate openly among themselves and healthcare providers (e.g., express fear, concerns, pain).
- Obtain satisfactory pain relief and symptom management.
- Make use of all resources available to assist with coping.
- Exercise control in the management of care to the extent possible.

As always, you will use the goals set in the planning stage as criteria for evaluating the patient's or family's health status.

KnowledgeCheck 15–5

- List three nursing diagnosis labels you might consider when dying or grieving is the primary problem.
- List three nursing diagnoses labels that might occur as a result of dying or grieving.

 Go to Chapter 15, **Knowledge Check Response Sheet and Answers,** on the Electronic Study Guide.

| Planning Interventions/Implementation |

NIC standardized interventions associated with death, dying, and bereavement appear in Volume 2.

Go to Chapter 15, **Standardized Outcomes and Interventions for Loss and Grieving Diagnoses,** in Volume 2.

Specific nursing activities are determined by the nursing diagnosis, especially by the etiology. Our ability to help someone who is grieving or dying is largely determined by our attitude. A compassionate approach is essential but challenging. Watching patients struggle with pain, loss, grief, and death may stir our own deepest doubts and fears, and we may reject the challenge to respond from the heart. We may be aware that employers usually reward nurses for what they *do* rather than who they *are* as people, so it is easy to rationalize that we have other tasks to accomplish that may be equally important. When we do that, we ignore the real gift we may have to offer the suffering patient: our willingness to "walk the walk" with them, if even for a short time. Full-spectrum nurses combine their psychomotor and thinking skills with compassion in ministering to those who are suffering.

Some important nursing interventions, including therapeutic communication, facilitating grief work, helping families, and specific activities involved in care of the dying person are discussed in the following sections. Also see the Nursing Care Plan and Care Map for Anticipatory Grieving.

Nursing Care Plan

Client Data

Wilma Peterson is caring for her son, Henry, who has AIDS. Henry is 20 years old; his older brother, William, died at home of AIDS-related pneumonia 2 years earlier at age 24. William had left home at 18 to live in Miami and returned to his home in rural Alabama when he became too ill to manage on his own. Henry stayed home to help his mother care for William and learned he was HIV-positive just before his brother died. Henry did not tell his mother of his diagnosis until he was hospitalized for the first time with cytomegalovirus infection. Since then, he has not followed nutritional and medical advice and has continued to stay out late and party when he feels well enough. His health has steadily declined.

You are participating in a special "caring for the caregiver" program set up by the public health nurse in your community. In this program, registered nurses visit primary caregivers to assess their needs and offer support services as needed. Thus, your client is Wilma Peterson.

Ms Peterson is initially cordial when you visit but tells you, "This is a mother's responsibility. I don't stop being his mother because he's grown up. I'm always his mama." As your discussion continues, Ms Peterson wistfully talks about when William and Henry were boys playing in the backyard. She says, "I didn't really understand this awful disease until William got so sick. Now, I look at Henry and I know what's waiting for him. I know we are going to lose him. Sad . . . just so sad . . ." Her voice trails off as tears well in her eyes.

Nursing Diagnosis

Anticipatory Grieving related to the client's anticipating the loss of a second son, as evidenced by her previous experience caring for her other son who died at home of AIDS and by the client's stating, "I know what's waiting for him."

NOC Outcomes	Individualized Goals / Expected Outcomes
Family Coping (NOC 2600) Psychosocial Adjustment: Life Change (NOC 1305)	(Short-term goals) At the end of the initial home visit, Ms Peterson will: 1. Identify community resources available to help her care for Henry at home during acute illnesses. 2. Begin to feel comfortable discussing her concerns with the nurse. (Long-term goals) Within 6 weeks, Ms Peterson will: 1. Explore activities she would like to participate in once she is no longer caring for Henry. 2. Talk with Henry to learn what type of funeral he would like.

Nursing Interventions and Activities*	Rationales
NIC Interventions Anticipatory Guidance (NIC 5210) Coping Enhancement (NIC 5230) Grief Work Facilitation (NIC 5290) **Nursing Activities** 1. Encourage Ms Peterson to talk about her experiences caring for William before he died.	Anticipatory Grieving often occurs in the context of repeated caregiving (Boyle, Bunting, Hodnicki, & Ferrell, 2001) or in situations in which the caregiver has other types of previous experience with the same or a similar terminal illness.
2. Ask her to relate similarities and differences between care for William and care for Henry.	Asking the client to discuss previous experiences allows the nurse to validate the nursing diagnosis (O'Connor & Lunney, 1998).
3. Ask Ms Peterson to describe the elements of Henry's care and to identify which she considers to be the most important.	Clients are holistic and consider more than just medical treatment in the care of a family member; their actions are often based on cultural and religious beliefs and their own previous experiences instead of a medically based care plan. Clients may operate on a different, parallel track from that of the health care providers (Boyle et al., 2001). By asking what Ms Peterson does and how she prioritizes Henry's care, the nurse can learn from the client rather than making assumptions based on the healthcare perspective. By showing respect for her experience as a caregiver, the nurse can build a stronger relationship with Ms Peterson, which will facilitate future nursing interventions and anticipatory guidance.
4. Talk with Ms Peterson to find out what community resources she used when she cared for William and whether she has accessed them now that she is caring for Henry.	Isolation and loneliness are risk factors for sole caregivers at home. By assessing community resources, the nurse can determine whether Ms Peterson is "connected" or isolating herself. Isolation puts her at risk for Dysfunctional Grieving (O'Connor & Lunney, 1998). Many community resources provide a sense of belonging and enhance and support coping strategies as well.
5. Promote shared decision making if this is acceptable to Henry Peterson.	Informing both Ms Peterson and Henry about the disease, prognosis, treatment, and comfort options allow them to retain some control over their lives together (Teno, Casey, Welch, & Edgman-Levitan, 2001). Henry's permission must be obtained to preserve his autonomy.
6. Provide nonjudgmental emotional support to Ms Peterson, and support healthy coping activities she is using.	Establishing a comfortable and emotionally safe environment will allow Ms Peterson to share her concerns without fear of being judged because of her son's diagnosis (Boyle et al., 2001).

➤

*Interventions are only a sample of those linked to this diagnosis by *NIC*. Activities should be individualized for each client.

Nursing Care Plan *(continued)*

Evaluation

Review the initial short-term outcomes and goals. Reassess your client to determine whether the goals are achieved in the stated time frame. In this case, long-term goals will fluctuate based on the progression of Henry's illness.

In this case, the following occurred as the care plan was implemented:

- Ms Peterson cried as she described the deterioration in William's health before he died. She worries that Henry will suffer and does not want him to lose his dignity the way she believes William did.

- Ms Peterson's greatest concern is that Henry is not eating enough. Much of her self-value as a mother arises from her ability to prepare homemade meals to feed her family, and Henry doesn't have much appetite. This is very distressing to her.

- She has not contacted community agencies. She is holding off, hoping that Henry will not be "so sick for so long. With these new drugs, he can get better."

- She remains involved in her church, which is the same one she attended as a little girl. However, she will not tell her church group that Henry has AIDS. "They talk too much," she says. Instead, she says he has leukemia.

Only one short-term goal is met at this visit—establishing a comfort level between the client and the nurse. Ms Peterson has not identified community resources related to caring for Henry at this time.

Plan for Further Evaluation

Additional supportive visits will be needed to help Ms Peterson understand that contacting community agencies does not mean Henry will die sooner; at this time, denying the need for community help is an important coping mechanism for Ms Peterson and is not affecting her ability to care for her son. If his condition worsens, this issue will need to be addressed promptly.

References

Boyle, J. S., Bunting, S. M., Hodnicki, D. R., & Ferrell, J. A. (2001). Critical thinking in African American mothers who care for adult children with HIV: A cultural analysis. *Journal of Transcultural Nursing, 12*(3), 193–202.

Dochterman, J. M., & Bulechek, G. M. (Eds.). (2004). *Nursing interventions classification (NIC)* (4th ed.). St Louis: Mosby.

Johnson, M., Bulechek, G., Dochterman, J., & Moorhead, S. (2001). *Nursing diagnoses, outcomes, and interventions: NANDA, NOC, and NIC linkages.* St Louis: Mosby.

Moorhead, S., Johnson, M., & Maas, M. (Eds.). (2004). *Nursing outcomes classification (NOC)* (3rd ed.). St Louis: Mosby.

O'Connor, L., & Lunney, M. (1998). Care of the caregiver—Family member with a chronic illness. *Nursing Diagnosis, 9*(4), 152; and

Teno, J. M., Casey, V. A., Welch, L. C., & Edgman-Levitan, S. (2001). Patient-focused, family-centered end-of-life medical care: Views of the guidelines and bereaved family members. *Journal of Pain and Symptom Management, 22*, 738–751.

Care Map

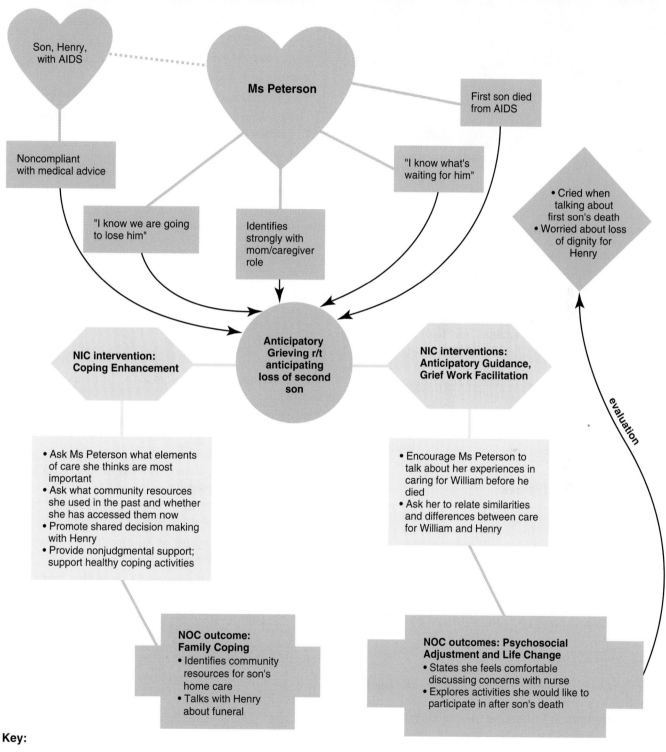

Son, Henry, with AIDS

Ms Peterson

First son died from AIDS

Noncompliant with medical advice

"I know what's waiting for him"

• Cried when talking about first son's death
• Worried about loss of dignity for Henry

"I know we are going to lose him"

Identifies strongly with mom/caregiver role

Anticipatory Grieving r/t anticipating loss of second son

NIC intervention: Coping Enhancement

NIC interventions: Anticipatory Guidance, Grief Work Facilitation

evaluation

• Ask Ms Peterson what elements of care she thinks are most important
• Ask what community resources she used in the past and whether she has accessed them now
• Promote shared decision making with Henry
• Provide nonjudgmental support; support healthy coping activities

• Encourage Ms Peterson to talk about her experiences in caring for William before he died
• Ask her to relate similarities and differences between care for William and Henry

NOC outcome: Family Coping
• Identifies community resources for son's home care
• Talks with Henry about funeral

NOC outcomes: Psychosocial Adjustment and Life Change
• States she feels comfortable discussing concerns with nurse
• Explores activities she would like to participate in after son's death

Key:

Data

Nursing diagnosis

NIC interventions

Nursing actions

NOC outcomes

Evaluation

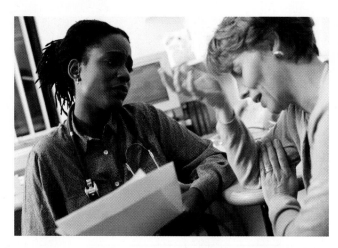

FIGURE 15–4 The nurse encourages and accepts expression of feelings.

Therapeutic Communication

Building a trusting relationship with the dying or grieving patient and family or significant others is especially critical (Figure 15–4). Perhaps most important is to listen to the dying patient and to be alert for and respond to nonverbal cues. Encourage patients and family members to express their feelings, and reassure them that their feelings are normal and not "wrong." See Box 15–5 for some barriers to end-of-life communication. For tips on communicating with people who are dying or bereaved,

 Go to Chapter 15, **Technique 15–1: Communicating with People Who Are Grieving,** in Volume 2.

Facilitating Grief Work

Whether grief results from a loss of health, from an impending death, or from some other loss, you can help patients and families work through their grief by helping them express their feelings, recall memories, and find meaning in their lives. Later in this chapter, we discuss interventions for helping families after the death of a loved one. This section focuses more generally on grieving *any* loss.

Expressing Feelings

Your theoretical knowledge already includes the fact that it is the family, not just an individual patient, who is grieving, whether because of death or some other loss. And you also know that for people to deal with grief in a healthy way, they need to communicate their feelings. Sometimes people are uncomfortable with expressing their feelings and hold them in. This reserve will interfere with their grief resolution, so you may have to facilitate the process. This is where therapeutic communication will be helpful (see Chapter 18).

BOX 15-5 **Barriers to End-of-Life Communication**

Fear of one's own mortality

Unresolved personal grief issues (e.g., the loss of one's own parent)

Lack of experience with death and dying

Fear of expressing emotion (i.e., crying)

Fear of not knowing the answer to a question

Not knowing whether to give an honest (and possibly unwelcome) answer to a question

Not understanding the family's culture

Keeping physical distance (e.g., standing away from the person or avoiding eye contact)

Insensitivity: interrupting communication, patronizing, giving false reassurance.

Source: Matzo, M., Shermann, D., Sheehan, D., Ferrell, B., & Penn, B. (2003). Teaching strategies from the ELNEC curriculum. *Nursing Education Perspectives, (21)*1,176–183.

The following are some ways to facilitate expression of feelings:

- Encourage questions, and respond to them within a reasonable time.
- When you observe the patient or family member expressing feelings, either verbally or nonverbally, encourage them to continue.
- Ask, "How can I help?" "What do you need?" "What would you like for me to do?"
- Be sure that everyone on the healthcare team understands and follows the care plan.
- Ask yourself what you would do if this were your family member.
- Do not compare another person's loss to your own experience. For example, avoid comments such as, "I know how you feel." Instead, say, "Tell me how you feel."

Recalling Memories

Grieving patients and family members may need to recall memories, both good and difficult. One way to encourage recall is to go through photo albums with them and ask questions about the people in the pictures. Also look for objects of sentiment (e.g., a family heirloom) in the environment and ask the dying or bereaved person to share their significance.

Finding Meaning

Another way to facilitate grief work is to help the patient or family find meaning in their lives or in their past. Talking through this meaning is a healthy way to cope. Facilitating life review is one technique to help the patient and/or family recognize the unique contributions this person has made to family, friends, and society. You can begin by asking about the various aspects of the patient's life, commenting on pictures in the room, or picking up on verbal cues that are expressed.

 CriticalThinking 15–8

- What would you say to Mrs. Manning ("Meet Your Patient") if you walked into a room and found her sitting in a chair and softly weeping while Mr. Manning sleeps?
- What response would you make when Mr. Manning waves his hand in the air and says, "I'm not taking any more of those damn pills" as you bring him his medications?
- A young woman approaches you in the hall and says, "I want to visit Mom and stay with her, but I just can't stand to see her like that. I feel guilty for wanting to leave." What would be your therapeutic response?

Helping Families of Dying Patients

When a patient is dying, it is especially important to view the family as your unit of care. If the patient is unresponsive, you may find yourself spending most of your care time with the family. This time should be spent providing education, support, and a listening ear. Watching their loved one dying can leave family members feeling confused, angry, helpless, and even devastated; thus, sensitive and compassionate care during this time is essential. You can make good use of the interventions in the preceding sections, "Therapeutic Communication" and "Facilitating Grief Work". For more specific interventions for helping families of dying patients,

 Go to Chapter 15, **Technique 15–2: Helping Families of Dying Patients,** in Volume 2.

KnowledgeCheck 15–6

- Describe four ways to facilitate the grief work of a grieving or dying person.
- List two specific interventions for helping grieving families.

 Go to Chapter 15, **Knowledge Check Response Sheet and Answers,** on the Electronic Study Guide.

Caring for the Dying Person

To effectively care for terminally ill patients, you must use a holistic model. This means meeting physiological, psychological, social, sexual, and spiritual needs. Most hospitals have an interdisciplinary team to provide holistic care to dying patients and their families. This team may be made up of a physician, nurse, social

---

| toward evidence-based practice |

The following are two studies of end-of-life care.

Maida, V. (2002). Factors that promote success in home palliative care: A study of a large suburban palliative care practice. *Journal of Palliative Care, 18*(4), 282–286.

This study examined the medical and nursing charts of 402 cancer patients who wished to die at home and had been referred to a palliative care service. It found the following factors to be significantly associated with home death:

- The presence of more than one caregiver
- An increased length of time between diagnosis and referral to palliative care
- An increased length of time under the referring physician's care
- Older age at referral to palliative care
- Home ownership
- Race

Casarett, D., Hirschman, K., Coffey, J., & Pierre, L. (2002). Does a palliative care clinic have a role in improving end-of-life care? Results of a pilot program. *Journal of Palliative Medicine, 5*(3), 387–396.

This study administered standardized assessment tools to 100 patients in a large urban clinic. They found the following factors to be significantly associated with enrollment in hospice care:

- White ethnicity
- A need for help around the home
- Insufficient money left at the end of the month

---

1. Based on these two studies, describe the typical user of hospice and palliative services.

2. Why do you think people who do not fit this profile are not using the service?

 Go to Chapter 15, **Toward Evidence-Based Practice Suggested Responses,** on the Electronic Study Guide.

worker, pastoral care worker, dietitian, physical therapist (and sometimes occupational and speech therapists), and volunteers.

Meeting Physiological Needs

Active dying usually occurs over a period of 10 to 14 days (although it can take as little as 24 hours). The "final hours" refers to the last 4 to 48 hours of life, in which failure of body systems results in death (Pitorak, 2003). See the discussion of the physiological stages of dying on page 270 for information on signs of impending death. Physiological needs during this time include mobility, oxygenation, safety, nutrition, fluids, elimination, personal hygiene and control of pain and symptoms (nausea, vomiting). For specific interventions and guidelines to use when caring for a dying patient,

 Go to Chapter 15, **Technique 15–3: Caring for the Dying Person,** in Volume 2.

Meeting Psychological Needs

When a patient is terminally ill, the physician is usually responsible for deciding what and how much to tell the person. Ideally, other health team members and the family should be involved in this decision. Everyone involved with the patient should know exactly what he and the family have been told. Most patients want to know their prognosis as soon as possible so that they can put personal affairs in order, share their feelings with family members, and come to terms with their life and death. Recent research (e.g., Fallowfield, Jenkins, & Beveridge, 2002) suggests that rather than protecting patients, efforts to shield patients from the reality of their situation usually creates greater difficulties for them. A "conspiracy of silence" causes fear, anxiety, and confusion, and it denies people the opportunity to make needed life adaptations. However, be aware that culture may determine which family members are to be informed and how much, if any, information is given to the patient. Also, many patients realize without being told that they are dying. For specific interventions to help meet the psychological needs of dying patients,

 Go to Chapter 15, **Technique 15–3: Caring for the Dying Person,** in Volume 2.

KnowledgeCheck 15–7

- Describe six nursing interventions to use in meeting the physiological needs of a dying person.
- Describe six nursing interventions to use in meeting the psychological needs of a dying person.
- What should be the focus of your interventions when the patient is very near death?

 Go to Chapter 15, **Knowledge Check Response Sheet and Answers,** on the Electronic Study Guide.

Addressing Spiritual Needs

When a person is terminally ill, his spirituality may become very important as he searches for meaning in the illness and suffering. The person may be looking for forgiveness and/or acceptance or be reaching out to feel connected. Ways to address this need include (but are not limited to) empathetic listening, contacting pastoral care or clergy if the patient asks for this service, special rituals, praying with the patient, music, meditation, or special readings.

Information about specific religious practices may help you provide appropriate interventions at end of life. For example, after the death of an Orthodox Jewish patient, you should handle the body as little as possible if you are not Jewish, but most Christian denominations will not object to your washing and preparing the body. Remember, though, that there are wide individual differences and that you must assess each patient and family to determine how closely they adhere to the rituals of their religion and culture. Review Chapters 13 and 14, as needed. For detailed information about a variety of religious practices surrounding death,

 Go to Chapter 15, **Supplemental Materials: Addressing Spiritual Needs,** on the Electronic Study Guide.

Addressing Cultural Needs

There is some overlap between religious and cultural practices. For example, most cultural groups engage in some type of religious ceremony that helps the bereaved begin the grieving process. Nevertheless, some death rituals and expressions of grief may be culture based but not necessarily involve religion. For example, some cultures may emphasize keeping emotions more subdued and limiting expressions of grief to private settings, whereas others gauge the value of the deceased by the amount of wailing and crying. As with spiritual care, remember that you cannot assume that a person follows the practices of her cultural group; you must assess to be sure.

To provide culturally sensitive care at end of life, you will need some information about specific cultural practices surrounding death. For this information,

 Go to Chapter 15, **Supplemental Materials: Addressing Cultural Needs,** on the Electronic Study Guide.

CriticalThinking 15–9

Reflect on this reading by Theresa Rando in *The Gift of Presence:*

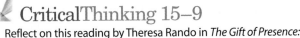

It is one of the most difficult things in the world to do to sit and listen while another's heart is breaking with grief, to hold the hand of a dying patient who cries silently while staring into space. The gift of presence, the gift of being with those in pain, is the only gift we can give. It is the sole armor patients have against the anguish. The very most we can do for dying patients is to make it better, with our presence and concern, than it would be if we were

not there....we cannot "do" anything that can get rid of the psychic pain of impending loss and death. (Rando, 1984, p. 272)

Close your eyes and visualize yourself sitting quietly beside a dying patient and holding her hand. Visualize the patient crying silently. Can you still your mind and remain silent, or do you feel you must say something to make the patient "feel better"?

Providing Postmortem Care

Postmortem care includes care of the patient's body after death and fulfilling any legal obligations. You will follow agency policies and respect cultural and spiritual preferences, along with the care that is commonly provided. In most states and provinces, the physician must pronounce death; in some areas, however, a coroner or a nurse may also perform this task.

Rigor mortis (the stiffening of the body) is caused by contraction of the muscles from a lack of adenosine triphosphate (ATP). It occurs about 2 to 4 hours after death. Rigor mortis begins in the involuntary muscles (e.g., the heart). It appears next in the head, neck, and trunk, and finally in the extremities. It disappears about 96 hours after death. **Algor mortis** occurs when the blood stops circulating. The body temperature drops about 1.8°F (1°C) per hour until it reaches room temperature. The dependent parts of the body appear bluish and mottled because when the blood stops circulating, the red blood cells break down, releasing hemoglobin. This is called **livor mortis.**

If the family wishes to be alone with the body, straighten the bedcovers and make the patient look as natural as possible. Give family members whatever time they need before you prepare the body. Ideally, you will have already established a relationship with the family and will have begun to facilitate their grieving during the patient's dying period. And you will have prepared them as the death becomes imminent. For specific guidelines for care of the body and other immediate postmortem interventions to support family members,

 Go to Chapter 15, **Technique 15–4: Providing Postmortem Care,** in Volume 2.

KnowledgeCheck 15–8

- Why is it important to position the body with a pillow under the head and shoulders soon after death?
- Why is it important to close the eyes and mouth of the deceased and position the body within at least 2 to 4 hours after death?

Go to Chapter 15, **Knowledge Check Response Sheet and Answers,** on the Electronic Study Guide.

Providing Grief Education

Sometime after the immediate postmortem period, explain the stages of grief and point out that it takes months or even years to resolve. Explain that grief may become more intense on the anniversary of the

death (or other loss) and on significant dates (e.g., birthdays).

Recall that once the bereaved person accepts that the loss is real, his feelings may be so intense that he may wonder if he is losing his sanity. The grieving person may be fatigued from not sleeping, may be disoriented or unable to concentrate, and so on; he may be concerned about what such symptoms mean. Reassure the person that such responses are expected and that there is no single "right" way to grieve (Egan & Arnold, 2003). Also assure him that although the grief process takes time, the symptoms won't last forever.

Helping Children Deal with Loss

Some families may need information about helping children deal with grief, especially when there is a death in the family. You may need to explain that children perceive death differently from adults. See the accompanying Self-Care box for teaching surviving relatives how to help children deal with grief.

---

self-care

Helping Children Deal with Loss

Teach surviving relatives the following:

- If a child is frightened about attending a funeral, the family should not force him to go. It is important, however, to include the child in some service or observance, such as lighting a candle, saying a prayer, or visiting the grave site, at a later time.

- The surviving relatives should spend as much time as possible with the child, making it clear that the child has permission to show her feelings openly or freely.

- Be prepared for intermittent expressions of sadness and anger from the child, over a long period of time.

- Be prepared for the possibility of regression to earlier developmental stages (e.g., talking "baby talk").

- Assure the child that he was in no way responsible for the death.

- The following are warning signs that may indicate the need for professional help, especially if they are prolonged: an extended period in which the child loses interest in daily activities and events, inability to sleep, loss of appetite, fear of being alone, extended regression, repeated statements about wanting to join the dead person, withdrawal from friends, refusal to attend school, or sharp drop in school performance.

Taking Care of Yourself

When caring for dying patients, you will confront your own feelings of mortality. It is important to understand your own attitudes, fears, and beliefs concerning death, so you should think about these in advance: before you encounter dying patients. This will enable you to deal in a more healthy way with patients and their families.

You will probably experience feelings of grief and loss. When you become involved with dying persons and their families at such an intimate time in their lives, you become connected to them. There is nothing wrong with this emotional involvement; it helps you to be effective in your work. But just as you care for these families, you need also to care for yourself during these times.

- Recognize that feelings of grief and loss are normal.

- Talk with other colleagues about your feelings. Nurses are known for being able to take care of everyone but themselves! Don't be afraid to ask for what you need.

- Do not be afraid to confront grief. Some nurses feel they have to be strong and tend to deny their feelings. They overwork and take care of others. If you use this approach, the feelings will accumulate and begin to wear you down physically and emotionally.

- If you wish, it is appropriate for you to attend calling hours and/or funeral services when one of your patients dies. This helps you diffuse some of your feelings of loss. It also is very meaningful to family members to know that you took the time to remember them and their loved one.

- Learn how to get support for yourself and how to support your colleagues when they experience the death of a patient. One idea is a nurses' support group that meets regularly to talk about the feelings and to remember those who have died. If you need or want a facilitator, pastoral care workers and social workers may be available for these services.

- Do some nice things for yourself on a regular basis (e.g., facial, massage, quiet bubble bath, aromatherapy). Try to set aside a special spot in your home that is only for relaxation; decorate it with items that help you focus on peaceful thoughts (e.g., candles, pictures, religious objects).

Caring for the dying can be very rewarding but is also emotionally draining. To be effective in your practice, learn to care for yourself as well.

 Go to Chapter 15, **Resources for Caregivers and Health Professionals,** on the Electronic Study Guide.

 Suggested Readings: Go to Chapter 15, **Reading More About Loss, Grief, & Dying,** on the Electronic Study Guide.

 Bibliography: Go to Volume 2, Bibliography.

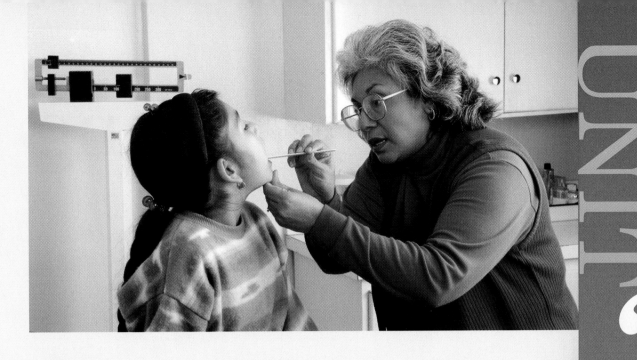

Essential Nursing

Interventions

UNIT 3

16 CHAPTER

Documenting
& Reporting

Learning Outcomes

After completing this chapter, you should be able to:

✳ Explain the purposes of documentation.

✳ Compare and contrast different types of documentation.

✳ Identify a variety of charting forms and their purposes.

✳ Use documentation forms in the clinical setting.

✳ Discuss the key elements to include when giving an oral report about a patient.

✳ Describe guidelines for documentation.

✳ Identify abbreviations for charting.

✳ Explain the process for verifying or questioning a medical order.

✳ Critique samples of charting.

✳ Follow documentation guidelines to accurately record patient health status, nursing interventions, and patient responses.

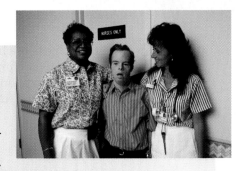

Your Patient

Steven Stellanski is a 16-year-old who has just been released from the post-anesthesia care unit (PACU) after an emergency appendectomy. You are to admit him to your unit. Steven is groggy but moaning in pain. "Help me, help me," he whispers. He is holding his abdomen and grimacing. The PACU nurse tells you that Steven has Down syndrome and functions at a school-age level.

Steven's vital signs are as follows: blood pressure, 104/68 mm Hg; pulse, 104; respirations, 24; and tympanic membrane temperature 99.9°F. An IV bag of lactated Ringer's solution is infusing at 125 mL per hour.

The abdominal dressing in the right lower quadrant of Steven's abdomen is dry and intact. A Foley catheter is draining pale yellow urine.

Steven's postoperative orders call for starting a patient-controlled analgesia pump that will deliver morphine sulfate at 1 mg intervals up to 4 mg per hour. He is to remain NPO (nothing by mouth) until bowel sounds have resumed. The surgeon has ordered the dressing to be changed tomorrow morning and for Steven to get out of bed in the A.M.

Theoretical Knowledge
knowing why

When you imagine yourself working as a nurse, what do you think of? Most people picture themselves at the bedside working with patients. When you look at ads for nursing jobs, the picture usually shows a nurse whisking a gurney down the hall, or hanging an IV bag, or perhaps teaching a patient. Photos rarely show the nurse charting or reporting care. Yet healthcare professionals rely on these two methods of communication to coordinate patient care. In this chapter we will discuss written and oral communication in patient care.

DOCUMENTATION

Documentation is the act of recording patient status and care in written form. Oral communication about a patient's status, called *reporting,* is discussed later in this chapter.

Why Do Healthcare Providers Use Written Communication?

The most common type of written communication in health care is the client record. The **client record** is a collection of materials that serves as a legal record of the client's healthcare experience. The written record serves the following purposes:

- *Communication.* Healthcare professionals use the client record to communicate about the client's status and care. For example, if you were unable to speak directly with the physician when she made rounds because you were providing care to another client, you could read her progress notes. If she writes that she is concerned that the patient may develop an infection, you would write a nursing diagnosis of Risk for Infection on the care plan, with nursing orders for regular observations for signs of infection.

- *Education.* As a student, you are well aware of this use of the client record. The record provides a snapshot of what is going on with the client so that you can prepare to give safe care.

- *Legal documentation.* The client record is scrutinized by attorneys whenever a dispute about a patient's care arises. In court, the record is legal evidence of the quality of care given to a client.

- *Quality assurance.* Healthcare agencies perform **chart audits** (reviews of client records) to identify ways to improve patient care, decrease length of stay, control costs, and design inservice education programs. Accrediting agencies, such as the Joint Commission on the Accreditation of Healthcare Organizations (JCAHO), review records to ensure delivery of quality care and public safety.

- *Reimbursement.* Insurance companies, budget managers, and facility billing staff use client records to determine the cost of care.

- *Research.* The client record is used to gather data for clinical research. For example, a researcher studying the care of clients with congestive heart failure

(CHF) may gather all charts of clients admitted in the last 6 months with CHF as a principal diagnosis. She could then compare treatment plans with outcomes, length of stay, and other variables.

What Are the Two Main Documentation Systems?

Each institution determines the documentation system in use. Most hospitals and long-term care facilities use source-oriented records; however, specialized units may require problem-oriented records.

Source-Oriented Records

Because patients in hospitals and long-term care facilities receive care from a variety of disciplines, these institutions commonly use **source-oriented records.** In this documentation system, members of each discipline record their findings in a separately labeled section of the chart. Nurses chart in the nurses notes section as well as in the graphic data section. A typical source-oriented record includes the following sections:

- *Admission data*—demographic information, insurance data, contact information
- *Advance directive*—information on client's wishes for intensity of care and actions that should be taken in the event of an emergency
- *History and physical*—a detailed summary of the current problem, past medical and social history, medications taken, review of systems, and physical examination data
- *Physician's orders*—orders for medications, treatments, and activities
- *Progress notes*—chronological charting by physicians on the patient's response to treatment
- *Diagnostic studies*—reports detailing the findings of tests that have been performed, such as x-ray, ultrasound, or other imaging studies, or pulmonary function tests
- *Laboratory data*—a compilation of results from laboratory studies
- *Nurses' notes*—chronological charting by nurses on the patient's response to treatment
- *Graphic data*—intake and output records, vital sign flowsheets, and often checklists regarding patient activity, dietary intake, and ADL tasks
- *Rehabilitation and therapy notes*—chronological charting by therapists on the patient's response to treatment; usually includes physical therapy, occupational therapy, and respiratory therapy
- *Discharge planning*—includes data from utilization review, case managers, or discharge planners on anticipated client needs after discharge

In source-oriented records, you can easily find the contribution of each discipline. However, a distinct drawback of this system is that data may be fragmented and scattered throughout the chart. You will need to review all sections of the chart to get a complete understanding of the client's condition and care. It is especially difficult with source-oriented records to track the treatments and patient outcomes associated with a particular problem. For example, suppose that as a result of fluid retention secondary to congestive heart failure, a client has shortness of breath on exertion. To find the interventions for this problem, you would need to look (1) in the physician's orders to see whether cardiac drugs or diuretics were ordered (to help with the fluid retention), (2) in the respiratory therapist's notes for breathing treatments, and (3) in the nurse's notes to see whether the client is being maintained in a therapeutic position for breathing. To see whether the medications were effective, you would need to read the nurse's notes about the client's responses to activity, the physician's progress notes, and the respiratory therapist's notes.

Problem-Oriented Records (POR)

Problem-oriented records are organized around the patient's problems. There are no separate sections for each discipline. The POR consists of four components: database, problem list, plan of care, and progress notes.

- The **database** consists of many parts: demographic data, the history and physical, nursing assessment data, and pertinent family and social history. As the patient's condition changes, the database is updated to reflect the patient's current status.
- The **problem list** is a concise listing of problems that have been identified from the database. Once a problem is resolved it is noted on the problem list. If a problem changes or is redefined, the problem list is updated to reflect the change. See Figure 16–1 for an example of a problem list.
- The **plan of care** includes physician's orders and the nursing care plan for addressing the identified problems. Other disciplines may also contribute to the plan.
- **Progress notes** are organized according to the problem list. Each discipline charts on shared notes. Charting is labeled according to problem number.

The POR system has several advantages. First, there is a common problem list that includes input from all disciplines. Second, it is easy to monitor the patient's progress because each problem is readily identified in the notes. Third, each discipline has ready access to the findings of the other members of the health team. This may encourage greater collaboration. The POR system requires a cooperative spirit among health providers as well as diligence in maintaining a current database and problem list.

KnowledgeCheck 16-1

- Identify the purposes of the client record.
- What are the key differences between source-oriented and problem-oriented records?

 Go to Chapter 16, **Knowledge Check Response Sheet and Answers,** on the Electronic Study Guide.

What Are Some Common Types of Charting?

The goal of all charting is a clear, concise representation of the client's healthcare experience. Nurses' notes can take many forms. The most common types are discussed here.

Narrative Charting

Narrative charting is used with both source-oriented and problem-oriented charts. The narrative chart entry tells the story of the patient's experience in a chronological format. The goal is to track the client's changing health status and progress toward goals. Narrative charting is especially useful when attempting to construct a timeline of events, such as a cardiac arrest or other emergency situations.

Narrative charting requires you to spend a good bit of time writing out all the details of the patient's care in sequence. Patient status, activities, nursing interventions, and response to treatment may all need to be included. One disadvantage of narrative charting is that it can allow you to ramble on without organizing the data. Although subjective and objective data may safely be grouped together, the entry can become difficult to understand if interventions and client responses are also clustered.

Recall the case of Steven Stellanski ("Meet Your Patient"). Below is a brief admission note using the narrative charting format. Underline any words or entries that you do not know the meaning of:

> 04/11/06 1600 Pt recd on unit from PACU. BP 104/68, P 104, RR 24, and TM temp 99.9 F. Arouses to call of name but quickly drifts off to sleep. Moaning, grimacing, holding abd, whispers "Help me. Help me." LR@125 mL/hr infusing in R forearm. Foley in place, draining pale yellow urine. Drsg dry & intact. Morphine PCA ordered. Will initiate. *R. Bradsby, RN*

You can see from this entry that nurses use many abbreviations in their charting. For a list of commonly used abbreviations in health care,

 Go to Chapter 16, **Abbreviations Commonly Used in Health Care,** in Volume 2.

Additional abbreviations that pertain to medication administration are included in Chapter 23. However,

Problem number	Date entered	Date resolved	Client problem
1	4/10/06	4/11/06	Abdominal pain (unknown etiology) Redefined 4/11/06
1A	4/11/06		Appendicitis resulting in emergency appendectomy
1B	4/11/06		Acute pain r/t abdominal incision 2° appendectomy
2	4/10/06		Down syndrome — functions at school-age level
3	4/11/06		Risk for constipation r/t opioid use for pain control and h/o appendicitis

FIGURE 16-1 A problem list for Steven Stellanski. Note that problem 1 has been redefined now that the cause of Steven's pain has been determined. Note also that the list contains both medical and nursing diagnoses.

each institution has a list of approved abbreviations that may be used. Consult your facility's list before you chart. The JCAHO Patient Safety Goals for 2003 recommend that abbreviations, acronyms, and symbols be standardized throughout the organization and that a list of acceptable abbreviations, acronyms, and symbols be developed (JCAHO, 2002). They have recently published a list of terms that they require organizations to add to their "do not use" list (JCAHO, 2004).

SOAP Charting

SOAP charting is also used in source-oriented and problem-oriented records. SOAP is an acronym for *subjective data, objective data, assessment,* and *plan.* This format may be used to address single problems or to write summative patient notes. Variations on this format include SOAPIE and SOAPIER. The additions to the acronym represent *intervention, evaluation,* and *revision.*

Below is an example of SOAP charting using the admission data of Steven Stellanski. In the previous section, this same data was used to create a narrative note. Notice that the data are identical; however, the narrative note is organized by data source.

04/11/06	**S:** "Help me. Help me."
1600	**O:** BP 104/68, P 104, RR 24, and TM temp 99.9 F. Arouses to call of name but quickly drifts off to sleep. Moaning, grimacing, holding abd. LR@ 125 mL/hr infusing in R forearm. Drsg dry & intact.
	A: Postoperative pain.
	P: Orders for morphine PCA rec'd. Will initiate. ————— *R. Bradsby, RN*

If the SOAPIER acronym is used, this note would continue as follows:

04/11/06 1615	**I:** Morphine PCA initiated. Pt instructed in use. 1st dose (1 mg) administered as demonstration. ———— *R. Bradsby, RN*
1625	**E:** Pt still moaning & grimacing. Has not initiated additional dose via PCA. 2nd dose given as additional demo. Will re-evaluate in 1 hour. May need continuous infusion. ———— *R. Bradsby, RN*
1645	**R:** Pt moaning & calling out in pain. Has not used PCA independently. Discussed c̄ Dr. Jadu. Continuous infusion begun at 2 mg/hr. Will supplement up to 4 mg/hr PRN. ———— *R. Bradsby, RN*

PIE Charting

PIE charting—an acronym for *problem, interventions,* and *evaluation*—originated from the POR system. Problems are identified at the admission assessment. Subsequent entries begin with identification of the problem number. This type of charting establishes an ongoing care plan. Critics complain that this style of charting focuses only on the listed problems and not the patient as a whole.

A PIE charting entry for Steven Stellanski might look like this:

4/11/06   1630

Problem: 1B

I: Pt c̄ PCA c̄ 1 mg doses up to 4 mg morphine/hr. Pt groggy yet c/o pain. Has not triggered PCA independently. Rates pain as 8 on scale of 1–10. PCA use reviewed with pt. Demonstrated use c̄ 1st dose at 1615.

E: Pt still moaning & grimacing. Has not initiated another dose via PCA. 2nd dose given as additional demo. Will reevaluate in 1 hour. May need continuous infusion if pt unable to use to control pain. ———— *R. Bradsby, RN*

Focus Charting ®

Instead of charting about problems (as do SOAP and PIE), **Focus charting**® highlights the client's concerns, problems, or strengths (Lampe, 1985). Charting is done in three columns. The first column contains the time and date. The second column identifies the focus or problem addressed in the note. The third column contains charting in a DAR format. DAR is an acronym for *data, action,* and *response.*

- *Data.* Document subjective and objective information that supports the focus. This aspect reflects the assessment phase of the nursing process.

- *Action.* Describe interventions performed, such as administering medications or making calls to the physician. This aspect reflects the planning and implementation phases of the nursing process.
- *Response.* Describe the patient's response to your interventions. This aspect reflects the evaluation phase of the nursing process.

Focus charting® has been praised for its ability to address the client's concerns holistically. Critics complain, however, that lack of a common problem list leads to inconsistency in labeling the focus of notes and may cause difficulty in tracking patient progress. The following is an example of a Focus® note.

| 4/11/06 1800 | Focus: Developmental delay | **D:** 16 yo rec'd on unit @ 1600 from PACU s/p appendectomy. Pt c̄ Down syndrome. Morphine PCA initiated. Pt unable to use to control pain. Continuous infusion @ 2 mg/hr begun @ 1745. Pt alert, drifting in & out of sleep. PACU RN reports pt functions @ school-age level. **A:** Will discuss pt status c̄ parents and adjust plan of care accordingly. |
| 1830 | | **R:** Met c̄ parents. Pt c̄ significant developmental delays, needs supervision c̄ all ADLs. Pt comfortable on 2 mg/hr infusion of morphine. Use of PCA for supplementary pain control reviewed c̄ pt and parents. Parents to assist pt c̄ PCA if addl meds needed. ———— *R. Bradsby, RN* |

Charting by Exception

Charting by exception (CBE) is a unique charting system designed to streamline documentation. CBE uses preprinted flowsheets to document most aspects of care. CBE assumes that unless a separate entry is made—an exception—all standards have been met and the patient has responded normally. Normal responses for various assessments (e.g., neurological, respiratory, gastrointestinal, emotional) are defined on the form. CBE flowsheets vary by specialty and, in some cases, even by diagnosis. Each flowsheet has entries for expected aspects of care.

CBE reduces the time required to chart, reduces repetitive charting of routine care, provides a record that is easily read and understood, and clearly highlights any variations from the expected plan of care. In many institutions, CBE records are kept at the bedside; this practice promotes timely documentation.

Inadvertent omissions are the biggest problem associated with CBE. Omissions may result from disagreement over what constitutes a significant variation. Critics of CBE believe that it deemphasizes the skilled judgment of nurses, reduces care to "routines," allows for greater replacement of RNs by fragmenting care into tasks, and potentially creates false documentation by assuming that care has been done (Dumple, James, & Phillips, 1999).

Which Charting Format Is Best?

Any charting format that adequately describes the patient's condition, care given, and response to care is adequate and will withstand review in a court of law. No charting format stands out as superior to another. Familiarize yourself with the charting you will use on the unit you are assigned. Review notes written by other nurses to become acquainted with different styles and approaches. You will also want to consult your clinical instructor or unit nurses if you have specific questions about charting formats. Many facilities have handouts or classes that provide additional information on charting. Take advantage of opportunities to build your knowledge when they arise.

KnowledgeCheck 16–2

Summarize the characteristics of narrative, SOAP, PIE, Focus, and CBE charting.

 Go to Chapter 16, **Knowledge Check Response Sheet and Answers,** on the Electronic Study Guide.

CriticalThinking 16–1

Compare the charting examples above. If you have had experience with charting in the clinical setting, apply this experience as well. Which charting format do you feel most comfortable with?

What Forms Do Nurses Use to Document Care?

The American Nurses Association *Standards of Nursing Practice* (2004) includes documentation in many of its standards. By the ANA standards, the registered nurse:

- Documents relevant data in a retrievable format. (Standard 1, Assessment)
- Documents diagnoses or issues in a manner that facilitates the determination of the expected outcomes and plan. (Standard 2, Diagnosis)

- Documents expected outcomes as measurable goals. (Standard 3, Outcomes Identification)
- Uses standardized language or recognized terminology to document the [care] plan. (Standard 4, Planning)
- Documents implementation and any modifications, including changes or omissions, of the identified plan. (Standard 5, Implementation)
- Documents the coordination of the care. (Standard 5a, Coordination of Care)
- Documents the results of the evaluation. (Standard 6, Evaluation)
- Collaborates in creating a documented plan focused on outcomes . . . (Standard 11, Collaboration)
- Documents referrals, including provisions for continuity of care. (Standard 11, Collaboration)

Documentation forms vary by purpose, institution, and unit. However, regardless of the system or forms used, nursing documentation reflects the nursing process: You record assessments, diagnoses, planning, implementation (what you actually did), and evaluation of client responses. This section discusses the most commonly used forms.

Admission Nursing Database

An admission nursing database is completed at the time of admission. As discussed in Chapter 3, creating a baseline assessment is vital for several reasons. (1) It may be used as a benchmark to monitor change; (2) it provides information about the support system of the client and helps forecast future needs; (3) it contains critical information: chief complaint or reason for admission, vital signs, allergy information, current medications, ADL status, physical assessment data, and discharge planning information. See pages 27–30 in Volume 2, and the Electronic Study Guide for examples of admission databases.

 Go to Chapter 3, **Nursing Admission Data Form,** in Volume 2.

 Go to Chapter 16, **Supplemental Materials: Admission Databases,** on the Electronic Study Guide.

Discharge needs should be evaluated when the patient first enters a healthcare facility. Acute hospital stays are very limited, and planning takes time. Ask yourself what this patient will need if he were to go home today. For example, would he need help with food preparation? Does he understand how to use his medicines? Discharge data is a part of the admission nursing database, but it is sometimes recorded on a separate form.

You will use admission forms in all settings, for example, in ambulatory clinics and long-term care

facilities. An ambulatory care admission form includes demographic data, allergy information, current medications, family health data, social history, and the patient's past medical history. The form completed by Joe Garcia (in Volume 2) at his first clinic visit is an example of an ambulatory care admission form. To see Mr. Garcia's completed form,

Go to **Meet the Garcias** in Volume 2.

Admission forms for long-term care are similar to hospital admission forms. Patients may stay in long-term care facilities for rehabilitation purposes after a hospital stay or may have extended stays for ongoing care. Whenever possible, this plan is identified on the patient's admission.

Flowsheets and Graphic Records

You will use flowsheets and graphic records to document assessments and care that are performed frequently, on a recurring schedule, or as a part of unit routines. For example, most hospital units require that vital signs be taken "routinely" every 8 hours. How often you chart (or perform the activities) depends on the unit policy and the patient's condition. In the first hour after surgery, for example, you would probably take the vital signs every 15 minutes.

The simplest forms are organized with time on one axis and the activities or patient assessment parameters on the other axis. Flowsheets and graphic records allow you to see patterns of change. For instance, you may view a steady increase in the line representing a patient's blood pressure. Or you may scan across a row of the form and see that your patient has not had a bowel movement for several days. Other types of information recorded on flowsheets include intake and output, weight, hygiene measures, ADLs, and medications administered. For an example of a graphic record, see Figure 3–4. To see an example of a flowsheet used in long-term care,

Go to Chapter 16, **Charting Forms, Flowsheet Used in Long-Term Care,** in Volume 2.

Checklists

Assessments and care may also be recorded on checklists. Common normal and abnormal findings are organized according to body systems. The nurse checks the box that reflects the current assessment findings. Some checklists include nursing actions, such as wound care, treatments, or IV fluid administration. Essentially these forms are comprehensive charting documents. Exceptions, patient care activities, and patient responses are recorded in the narrative note

section of the form. Figure 16–2 is an example of a checklist. To see a nursing assessment flowsheet,

Go to Chapter 16, **Charting Forms, Nursing Assessment Flowsheet,** in Volume 2.

Intake and Output Records

You will sometimes use separate intake and output (I&O) records to record data about the patient's fluid status. These records are especially important for clients with possible fluid overload or deficit (e.g., clients who have kidney disease or who have undergone major surgery). Usually they contain data from a 24-hour period. For an example of an I&O form,

Go to Chapter 16, **Charting Forms, Intake and Output Record,** in Volume 2.

When you are delegating care, be sure to alert all personnel when a client has fluid restrictions or is on I&O monitoring. I&O sheets may be kept at the bedside for convenient recording. Patients are increasingly active in their own care. If your patient is able to assist with measuring his I&O, teach him how to record data. Supply him with a list of common measures so that he can record his intake. Also show him how to collect his urine output. Chapter 27 provides detailed information about monitoring urine output.

Medication Records

Medication records contain detailed information about the medications that have been prescribed for the client. The information varies by setting, with significant differences between outpatient and inpatient facilities. For an example of a medication record, see Figure 23–7.

Outpatient Facilities

Outpatient facilities include clinics, primary care offices, and treatment facilities. Because patients do not stay at the facility, the medication record primarily contains information about how the patient is to use the medicines ordered. Patients retain responsibility for administering their own medications either independently or with the help of family or caregivers. Medication records at outpatient facilities contain the following items:

- Drug name
- Dosage
- Route of administration
- Number of pills, patches, and so on, to be dispensed at each filling of the prescription
- Number of refills ordered

DATE   /   /

TETON VALLEY HOSP

PHYSICAL ASSESSMENT - SHIFT _____

NEURO

LOC	ORIENTATION	SPEECH
❏ ALERT	❏ X3 ❏ FOR AGE	❏ APPROPRIATE
❏ SEDATED	❏ PERSON	❏ APHASIA
❏ LETHARGIC	❏ PLACE	❏ SLURRED
❏ UNRESPONSIVE	❏ TIME	❏ RAMBLING

SENSATION	FONTANELS	
❏ INTACT	❏ FLAT	❏ NA
❏ NUMBNESS	❏ SUNKEN	
❏ TINGLING	❏ BULGING	

CARDIOVASCULAR

RHYTHM	PULSE	EDEMA	CAP. REFILL
❏ REGULAR	❏ STRONG	❏ ABSENT	❏ < 3 SEC.
❏ IRREGULAR	❏ WEAK	❏ _____	❏ > 3 SEC.
❏ MURMUR	❏		

MONITOR RHYTHM

RESPIRATORY

EFFORT		BREATH LU LL SOUNDS RU RL
❏ NORMAL	❏ DYSPNEA	❏❏ CLEAR ❏❏
❏ LABORED	❏ COUGH	❏❏ CRACKLES ❏❏
❏ NASAL FLARING	❏ SPUTUM	❏❏ RHONCHI ❏❏
❏ RETRACTIONS	❏ CRYING	❏❏ WHEEZING ❏❏
❏ IRREGULAR		❏❏ DIMINISHED ❏❏
		❏❏ ABSENT ❏❏

GASTROINTESTINAL

ABDOMEN

❏ FLAT	❏ FIRM	❏ NAUSEA
❏ ROUNDED	❏ TENDER	❏ VOMITING
❏ DISTENDED	❏ NON-TENDER	
❏ SOFT		
❏ GIRTH_____ CM		

BOWEL SOUNDS	STOOL	
❏ ACTIVE	❏ REGULAR	LAST BM
❏ ABSENT	❏ CONSTIPATED	
❏ HYPER	❏ DIARRHEA	_____
❏ HYPO	❏ INCONTINENT	

SUCTION

❏ INTERMITTANT	❏ CONSTANT	❏ CLAMPED
❏ FEEDING TUBE		❏ PATENT
❏ NG		❏ PLACEMENT ✔

DRNG COLOR:

GU

URINE		❏ CATHETER
❏ CLEAR, YELLOW / AMBER ❏ QS		❏ PAIN
❏ OTHER _____	❏ FREQUENT	
	❏ RETENTION	❏ INCONTINENT

MUSCULOSKELETAL

MOBILITY	MUSCLE TONE	ROM
❏ NORMAL	❏ GOOD	❏ FULL
❏ ASSIST X _____	❏ OTHER	❏ LIMITED
❏ AMBULATORY		
❏ BED REST		
❏ OTHER	❏ P.T. CONSULT	

SKIN

CONDITION	TURGOR	MUCOUS MEM
❏ WARM, DRY INTACT	❏ ADEQUATE	❏ MOIST
❏ BREAKDOWN	❏ DECREASED	❏ DRY

COLOR ❏ NORMAL
❏ PALE ❏ CYANOTIC ❏ FLUSHED ❏ _____

WOUND/INCISION/ DRESSING

LOCATION/CONDITION/DRAINAGE	HEALING NO S/S INFECTION
_____	❏
_____	❏
_____	❏

TUBES/DRAINS

LOCATION/CONDITION/DRAINAGE	GRAVITY	SUCTION
_____	❏	❏
_____	❏	❏
_____	❏	❏

IV'S

IV SITE / CONDITION	PATENT, NO REDNESS OR SWELLING	PUMP
_____	❏	❏
_____	❏	❏
_____	❏	❏

NURSING ASSESSMENT   PATIENT NAME

PAIN

❏ ABSENT	PAIN SCALE _____
❏ PRESENT	LOCATION _____
❏ CONTROLLED	

PSYCHOSOCIAL

EYE CONTACT ❏ YES ❏ NO

❏ APPROPRIATE	❏ RESTLESS	❏ COMBATIVE
❏ FLAT AFFECT	❏ AGITATED	❏ BELLIGERENT
❏ UNCOOPERATIVE	❏ CRYING	❏ ODOR
❏ ANXIOUS	❏ SUBSTANCE USE	

DISCHARGE

DISCHARGE PLAN

❏ NA	❏ ONGOING	❏ COMPLETED
❏ D.P. CONSULT	❏ O.T CONSULT	❏ H.H. CONSULT

EQUIPMENT

❏ BED ALARM	❏ CARDIAC MONITOR
❏ CPM	❏ FEEDING PUMP
❏ IV PUMP X_____	❏ K - PAD
❏ OXIMETER	❏ PCA PUMP
❏ PASSPORT	❏ POLAR ICE
❏ SUCTION	❏ TELEMETRY
❏ _____	❏ _____
❏ _____	❏ _____

SIGN

SIGNATURE X_____ TIME_____

REASSESSED BY X_____ TIME_____

OBSERVATION / INTERVENTION / EVALUATION

(TIME & INITIAL ENTRIES)

PHYSICAL ASSESSMENT - SHIFT _____

NEURO

LOC	ORIENTATION	SPEECH
❏ ALERT	❏ X3 ❏ FOR AGE	❏ APPROPRIATE
❏ SEDATED	❏ PERSON	❏ APHASIA
❏ LETHARGIC	❏ PLACE	❏ SLURRED
❏ UNRESPONSIVE	❏ TIME	❏ RAMBLING

SENSATION	FONTANELS	
❏ INTACT	❏ FLAT	❏ NA
❏ NUMBNESS	❏ SUNKEN	
❏ TINGLING	❏ BULGING	

CARDIOVASCULAR

RHYTHM	PULSE	EDEMA	CAP. REFILL
❏ REGULAR	❏ STRONG	❏ ABSENT	❏ < 3 SEC.
❏ IRREGULAR	❏ WEAK	❏ _____	❏ > 3 SEC.
❏ MURMUR	❏		

MONITOR RHYTHM

RESPIRATORY

EFFORT		BREATH LU LL SOUNDS RU RL
❏ NORMAL	❏ DYSPNEA	❏❏ CLEAR ❏❏
❏ LABORED	❏ COUGH	❏❏ CRACKLES ❏❏
❏ NASAL FLARING	❏ SPUTUM	❏❏ RHONCHI ❏❏
❏ RETRACTIONS	❏ CRYING	❏❏ WHEEZING ❏❏
❏ IRREGULAR		❏❏ DIMINISHED ❏❏
		❏❏ ABSENT ❏❏

GASTROINTESTINAL

ABDOMEN

❏ FLAT	❏ FIRM	❏ NAUSEA
❏ ROUNDED	❏ TENDER	❏ VOMITING
❏ DISTENDED	❏ NON-TENDER	
❏ SOFT		
❏ GIRTH_____ CM		

BOWEL SOUNDS	STOOL	
❏ ACTIVE	❏ REGULAR	LAST BM
❏ ABSENT	❏ CONSTIPATED	
❏ HYPER	❏ DIARRHEA	_____
❏ HYPO	❏ INCONTINENT	

SUCTION

❏ INTERMITTANT	❏ CONSTANT	❏ CLAMPED
❏ FEEDING TUBE		❏ PATENT
❏ NG		❏ PLACEMENT

DRNG COLOR:

GU

URINE		❏ CATHETER
❏ CLEAR, YELLOW / AMBER ❏ QS		❏ PAIN
❏ OTHER _____	❏ FREQUENT	
	❏ RETENTION	❏ INCONTINENT

MUSCULOSKELETAL

MOBILITY	MUSCLE TONE	ROM
❏ NORMAL	❏ GOOD	❏ FULL
❏ ASSIST X _____	❏ OTHER	❏ LIMITED
❏ AMBULATORY		
❏ BED REST		
❏ OTHER	❏ P.T. CONSULT	

SKIN

CONDITION	TURGOR	MUCOUS MEM
❏ WARM, DRY INTACT	❏ ADEQUATE	❏ MOIST
❏ BREAKDOWN	❏ DECREASED	❏ DRY

COLOR ❏ NORMAL
❏ PALE ❏ CYANOTIC ❏ FLUSHED ❏ _____

WOUND/INCISION/ DRESSING

LOCATION/CONDITION/DRAINAGE	HEALING NO S/S INFECTION
_____	❏
_____	❏
_____	❏

TUBES/DRAINS

LOCATION/CONDITION/DRAINAGE	GRAVITY	SUCTION
_____	❏	❏
_____	❏	❏
_____	❏	❏

IV'S

IV SITE / CONDITION	PATENT, NO REDNESS OR SWELLING	PUMP
_____	❏	❏
_____	❏	❏
_____	❏	❏

FIGURE 16–2 A portion of a nursing assessment checklist.

- Directions for using the medication, including frequency
- Historical information about prescriptions, pharmacies used, refills authorized

Inpatient Facilities

If you work in an inpatient facility, you will be responsible for administering the patient's medications. An inpatient medication record not only contains a list of medications ordered, but also tracks medication administration and usage. The record is frequently called the MAR, or medication administration record. The MAR includes the following:

- Drug name
- Dosage
- Route of administration
- Frequency
- Scheduled times of administration
- Charting of medication administration
- Signatures of nurses administering medications

The MAR includes **scheduled medications**—medications that are to be given on a regularly scheduled basis—as well as stat and PRN medicines.

Stat is an abbreviation for *immediately,* or *now.* Stat medications are often handwritten on the medication record. After giving the medication, you would record it on the MAR. Because this is an unusual event, you will also need to make a narrative note that describes the events leading up to the stat order, the time of administration, and the patient's response to the medication.

PRN is an abbreviation for the Latin term *pro re nata,* or *as needed.* Typical PRN medications include medicines for pain, fever, mild discomfort, nausea, and constipation. You administer a prescribed PRN medicine when you assess that the patient needs it or when the patient requests it.

You will often need to record additional information on the MAR, as in the following circumstances:

- *Injections.* If you administer an injection, you must chart the site of administration. Your documentation prevents the patient from receiving repeated injections in the same location.
- *Assessment required prior to administration.* To ensure that it is safe to administer some medications, you may need to make an assessment. For example, digoxin should be held (not given) if the heart rate is below 60 per minute, or per institutional protocol. Therefore, you will need to chart the heart rate on the medication form at the time you administer the drug. Blood pressure medications, insulin, anticoagulants, and pain medications also require assessments

before administration. The assessment data are recorded directly on the MAR.

- *Drug allergies.* Drug allergies are always noted on the MAR. If the patient has an allergic reaction to a medicine, be sure to document this response on the medication sheet and make note of this change in the nurses' notes.
- *PRN medication.* Chart the time of administration of the PRN medication on the MAR. Make a narrative note that briefly describes your assessment findings, your time of administration, and the patient's response to the medication. For example, your patient is having pain and has an order for morphine sulfate 1–2 mg IV push q1hr PRN for moderate to severe pain. In your note, you would make an entry such as the following when charting administration of the medicine:

  9/8/06 1940 Morphine sulfate 1 mg IV Push given for back pain rated as 9 on a scale of 1–10.

  9/8/06 2000 Pt. states back pain is now 7 on a scale of 1–10. Additional 1 mg morphine sulfate given IV Push.

  Many PRN orders provide a range of medication to be given based on your assessment of the patient. In the previous example, the range was 1 to 2 mg of morphine sulfate. When a choice is available, clearly state the amount of medication given. Initially your patient received only 1 mg of a possible 2 mg dose of morphine. The range provides an opportunity for you to administer an additional 1 mg of morphine to treat the pain if it continues.

- *Patient refusal.* If the patient refuses a medication, note the refusal on the MAR. Agency policy will dictate how this is recorded. Often you draw a circle around the scheduled time of administration. Also document the patient's actions or reason for refusal in the nurse's notes.
- *Omitted medications or delayed administration.* It may be necessary to withhold a medication, for example, if the patient is undergoing tests and is to take nothing by mouth (NPO). Some institutions provide a boxed section at the bottom of the MAR with a letter or number to indicate why the medication was withheld or given at a different time. Circle the scheduled time, and fill in the symbol. You will also document the omission or delay in the nurses' notes.

Progress Notes

Progress notes are used to document nursing interventions and the patient's response to them. Frequently progress notes are written on lined paper. Narrative, SOAP, PIE, or FOCUS charting may be used in the progress notes. Be sure to date and time all your entries.

Kardex or Patient Care Summary

As discussed in Chapter 5, the Kardex, or patient care summary, is a special form that briefly summarizes the patient's plan of care. Often the form is a folding card. Information on the Kardex usually includes the following:

- Demographic data (e.g., age, sex, emergency contact information, name of admitting physician)
- Medical diagnoses as well as a list of diagnostic testing, surgeries, or procedures performed during admission
- Medication or other allergies
- Diet and activity orders
- Safety precautions
- Intravenous therapy orders
- Ordered treatments, such as wound care, physical therapy, or respiratory treatments
- Ordered laboratory and diagnostic tests
- A summary of medications ordered
- Special instructions, such as preferred intensity of care or isolation orders

Each client has a separate Kardex form; however, all Kardex forms are usually kept together in a portable file in a central location in the nurses' station to allow all team members access to clients' summary information. For example, suppose your patient asks a nursing assistant for something to drink. He can review the Kardex to check for fluid or dietary restrictions and provide the patient with an appropriate drink without having to find you or search the chart. In most facilities, the clerk updates these forms as new orders are received. These forms may also be computer generated. The Kardex is not a part of the permanent chart. For an example of a Kardex,

 Go to Chapter 5, **Tables, Boxes, Figures: ESG Figure 5–1,** on the Electronic Study Guide.

Integrated Plans of Care (IPOCs)

Integrated plans of care (IPOCs) are a combined charting and care plan form. Each maps out, day by day, the patient outcomes, interventions, and treatments for a specific diagnosis or condition from admission to discharge. Lab work, diagnostic testing, medications, and therapies are all included in the pathway as well as standardized interventions listed in the plan. For examples of IPOCs,

 Go to Chapter 5, **Tables, Boxes, Figures: ESG Figure 5–2,** and Chapter 16, **Supplemental Materials,** on the Electronic Study Guide.

Administrators applaud IPOCs because they help predict length of stay, monitor costs of care, and assist with staffing. They also offer other advantages: They eliminate duplicate charting, increase team effort, and enhance the nurse's teaching about what the patient can expect during the hospital stay.

Multiple diagnoses in a patient, however, challenge the format of IPOCs. For example, an IPOC may be instituted for a patient who has undergone a radical mastectomy (removal of the breast and surrounding lymph nodes). However, if the patient has severe arthritis, she may not be able to follow the planned postoperative physical therapy. To adapt the IPOC to this patient's needs, you would need to document her special issues in the space provided for narrative comments. Special considerations that may require adaptation of an IPOC include developmental delay (as with our patient Steven Stellanski), more than one medical diagnosis, mental health concerns, and social issues, such as homelessness. If you find that you are adapting the IPOC frequently for a patient who does not "fit," this may signal a need for the agency to develop a new IPOC.

Discharge Summary

A discharge summary is the last entry in the chart. It is completed when the patient is discharged from or transferred within the facility. It may be a multidisciplinary document or each discipline may write a separate summary. The forms are different in each institution; however, in general, discharge summaries contain the following data:

- Time of departure
- Method of transportation
- Condition of client at discharge (vital signs and assessment data)
- Name and relationship of person(s) accompanying patient at discharge
- Teaching conducted or reinforced
- List of medications sent home with patient
- Handouts or informational matter sent home with patient
- Discharge instructions (including medications, dressings, diet, or activity)
- Follow-up appointments or referrals given

It is important to clearly document the patient's condition on discharge. Many patients require follow-up care. The discharge summary serves as baseline data for the healthcare professionals who will follow up on the patient after discharge. For an example of a discharge summary,

 Go to Chapter 5, **Discharge Planning Form,** in Volume 2.

BOX 16-1   Events Requiring an Occurrence Report

- Patient fall or other injury
- Medication error
- Needlestick injury
- Loss of patient belongings
- Injury of visitor
- Unsafe staffing situation
- Lack of availability of essential patient care supplies
- Inadequate response to emergency situation

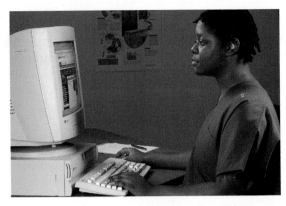

FIGURE 16–3   Many healthcare institutions are adopting computerized patient records.

Occurrence Reports

An **occurrence report,** or *incident report,* is a formal record of an unusual occurrence or accident. This is an agency report and is not part of the patient's chart. Examples of events requiring an occurrence report include falls, loss of patient belongings, or administration of the wrong medicine (Box 16–1). Occurrence forms are used to track problems and identify areas for quality improvement.

When completing an occurrence form, be sure to clearly identify the patient, date, time, and location. Briefly describe the incident in objective terms. Quote the patient or persons involved if possible. Avoid drawing conclusions or placing blame. Identify any witnesses to the event or any equipment involved.

Although you would document a patient's fall, medication error, or similar occurrences in the nurses' notes, you would not make reference to the occurrence report itself. Remember that the nurses' notes reflect the patient's response to the plan of care. In contrast, the occurrence report is an agency report aimed at solving agency problems or improving care. Chapter 45 provides additional information on occurrence reports.

Computerized Charting

Many healthcare institutions are adopting computerized patient record systems (Figure 16–3). Facilities vary in how extensively they use computers; some institutions use them only for limited charting, such as medication administration, whereas others use computers for all aspects of care, including care planning (see Chapter 5).

The following are some helpful hints for charting on a computer:

- Do not leave patient data displayed on a computer screen where others may view it. This is a breach of patient confidentiality.
- Follow your institution's protocol for correcting errors. Entries are part of the patient's permanent record and cannot be deleted. Follow protocol for correcting an erroneous entry.
- Never leave a computer terminal unattended after you have logged on. To do so allows others access to confidential data or may lead to other staff charting under your name.
- Never give your personal password or computer signature to anyone. You are responsible for the data recorded under your password. If someone has entered data under your password, you will be considered the source.

Whether stationed in the patient room or nurses' station, mobile, or hand-held, computers promote efficient use of time and interdisciplinary collaboration. For instance, pharmacy and radiology services can access patient data such as lab results and body weight. They can use this information to calculate drug dosages or to plan procedures. Computerized records also serve as an excellent resource. For example, the computer program may remind you of side effects to monitor for when administering medications. Perhaps the most obvious benefits of computerized charting are improved legibility, decreased paper waste, and decreased need for storage space. For further discussion of computerized charting, see Chapter 39.

KnowledgeCheck 16–3

- Identify at least five types of charting forms.
- What should you document after administering a PRN medication?
- What is the purpose of an occurrence report?
- Identify the following abbreviations (see Volume 2):

abd	OOB
BRP	pc
DM	PRN
fx	STD
NKDA	tid
q	

 Go to Chapter 16, **Knowledge Check Response Sheet and Answers,** on the Electronic Study Guide.

What Is Unique About Documentation in Home Health Care?

Although you will perform many of the same assessments and interventions in home care that you do in other areas of health care, the documentation is unique. Health Care Financing Administration (HCFA) guidelines govern home health care documentation. Among the requirements for care are (1) certification of homebound status, (2) a plan of care, and (3) ongoing assessment of the need for skilled care.

The most commonly used home health documentation form is known as OASIS—the Outcome and Assessment Information Set. You will need to write a progress note at each visit. Include the following in your note:

- Your assessment highlighting changes in the client's condition
- Interventions performed (wound care, teaching, and so on)
- The client's response to interventions
- Any interaction or teaching that you conducted with caregivers
- Any interaction with the patient's physician

For an example of the OASIS form,

 Go to Chapter 16, **Supplemental Materials: OASIS,** on the Electronic Study Guide.

Many home health nurses use laptop computers to record their notes. The computer is brought directly into the home to allow data retrieval as well as entry of notes. The computer also allows the nurse to order supplies needed for home care and to coordinate scheduling of follow-up visits.

In home care, a monthly summary describing the patient's status and ongoing needs is required. The patient's physician signs this form, which is submitted for reimbursement. Chapter 44 provides further information about home care.

 CriticalThinking 16–2

Why do you think it is essential to document homebound status and the ongoing need for skilled care?

What Is Unique About Documentation in Long-Term Care?

Documentation requirements for long-term care depend on the level of care the client requires. All clients in long-term care facilities must have a comprehensive assessment at admission. Federal law requires that a resident be evaluated using the Minimum Data Set for Resident Assessment and Care Screening (MDS) within 14 days of admission. The MDS must be updated every 3 months and with any significant change in client condition. For an example of an MDS form,

 Go to Chapter 16, **Supplemental Materials: Minimum Data Set,** on the Electronic Study Guide.

Legal requirements to protect older adults mandate that you report changes in a client's condition to the primary care provider as well as the client's family. Document your reports in narrative notes. If you are caring for a client receiving Medicare-reimbursed services, such as IV therapy, wound care, or rehabilitation services, documentation is required with each shift. In addition, a summary written by an LVN/LPN or RN must be recorded weekly. The weekly summary must include the following:

- A summary of the client's condition
- An evaluation of the client's ability to perform ADLs
- The client's level of orientation and mood
- Hydration and nutrition status
- Response to medications
- Any treatments provided
- Safety measures (e.g., bed rails, bed alarm, wander guard)

Long-term care facilities also provide intermediate-care services for clients who need assistance with medications, nutrition, and ADLs. These clients require a nursing care summary every 2 weeks.

KnowledgeCheck 16–4

How do home care and long-term care documentation differ from hospital-based documentation?

 Go to Chapter 16, **Knowledge Check Response Sheet and Answers,** on the Electronic Study Guide.

 CriticalThinking 16–3

Why do long-term care clients require less frequent charting than clients in acute care settings?

ORAL REPORTING

You will make oral reports to inform other caregivers of the patient's condition. You may communicate to another nurse, to a physician, to another hospital department, or to the patient's family. In giving an oral report, you deliver a message immediately and receive immediate feedback. Questions may be raised and answered immediately. To be efficient, restrict your oral reports to patient-focused discussion and limit extraneous details and social conversation.

How Do I Give Change-of-Shift Report?

The purpose of **change-of-shift report** is to alert the next caregiver about the client's status or recent

changes in the client's condition and to discuss planned activities, tests, procedures, or concerns that require follow-up.

Change-of-shift reports are usually given orally. Some institutions use written reports, but they offer no opportunity to interact and ask questions. As a student nurse, you will receive report from either the outgoing nurse or from the nurse assigned to the client during the shift you will be working. The staff nurse has entrusted you with the care of the client. Report any changes to the registered nurse assigned to the client during your shift, and always give report before leaving the unit.

Change-of-shift report may be given at the bedside or in a conference room. Bedside report, sometimes known as "walking rounds," allows you to observe important aspects of care, such as patient appearance, IV pumps, and wounds. With bedside report, the outgoing nurse can introduce you to the patient, and you can begin your assessment. If the patient is alert, give him the opportunity to participate in the report and ask questions. Although this type of report is time consuming, it encourages continuity of care.

Oral report may also be given in a conference room. This report may involve only the outgoing and oncoming nurse or may include the entire oncoming shift. When given in a conference room, oral report does not let you directly observe the patient, but it is less time consuming and still allows interaction between nurses.

Taped report is a convenient way to transmit information. The outgoing nurse tape-records report on the clients under her care. This method can be time consuming, especially if you must listen to the entire unit report before hearing about your own assigned patients. It also does not allow you to ask questions about the client. If you have questions, you will need to find the appropriate nurse when report is completed. Unfortunately, taped report is often used to allow the outgoing staff to leave promptly, and it may be impossible for you to speak directly with the previously assigned nurse. You will need to review the written notes from the previous shift if you are unable to speak with the nurse directly.

For key points to include in shift reports,

 Go to Chapter 16, **Technique 16–1: Giving Oral Reports,** in Volume 2.

Currie (2002) suggests that to improve the quality of change-of-shift reports, nurses should follow guidelines outlined by the acronym CUBAN:

Confidential. When giving report, always make sure you are in a private location so that confidentiality is maintained. Avoid giving report where others may overhear.

Uninterrupted. Uninterrupted report is focused and less time consuming. Distractions, such as the telephone, inquiring relatives, doctors, nurses, and other staff reduce the attention span of delivering and listening nurse.

Brief. Keep report concise and centered on the patient(s). Avoid extraneous comments.

Accurate. Include all of the pertinent and important information. Have the Kardex or flowsheet in front of you to make sure that the information you provide is current.

Named nurse. It is best to receive report from the nurse who has delivered care directly to the patient. Receiving report from anyone but the assigned nurse raises the risk of inaccuracy or omission of vital data. When the assigned nurse is not available, review the nurse's notes from the previous shift after receiving report.

KnowledgeCheck 16–5

- What data should be included in a change-of-shift report?
- What are the types of change-of-shift report?

Go to Chapter 16, **Knowledge Check Response Sheet and Answers,** on the Electronic Study Guide.

What Are Transfer Reports?

Transfer reports are given when a patient is transferred from unit to unit or facility to facility. For information to include in an oral transfer report,

 Go to Chapter 16, **Technique 16–1: Giving Oral Reports,** in Volume 2.

If the patient is being transported to another unit in the same facility, you will need to transport the chart with the patient. For transfers to another facility, you will send copies of chart entries with the patient or fax them to the facility prior to transfer. Your facility will have a policy on what is to be copied and how material should be transmitted.

How Do I Receive and Document Telephone Orders and Verbal Orders?

You will need to communicate with the patient's primary care provider about changes in the client's condition. Frequently, the care provider will give orders over the telephone. **Telephone orders** offer more room for error because of differences in pronunciation, dialect, or accent; background noise; and unfamiliar terminology. Once you receive the order, you must transcribe it into the patient's chart. Faxes and e-mail have reduced the need for oral orders; however, telephone orders will probably always be necessary.

For guidelines for use with telephone orders,

Go to Chapter 16, **Technique 16–2: Receiving Telephone and Verbal Orders,** in Volume 2.

The following is an example of a telephone order:

12/17/06 0815 Morphine 2 mg IVP x1 for pain now
TO: Dr. Kent/ S. Hogan R.N.

Verbal orders are spoken orders given to you in person. Often these are given in an emergency situation. Never use verbal orders as a routine method of communicating orders. Follow the same guidelines as for telephone orders. The verbal order consists of date, time, text of order, and "VO" for verbal order, followed by the provider's name and your name.

The following is an example of a verbal order:

03/11/06 1600 Morphine 2 mg IVP x1 for pain now
VO: Dr. Davidson/ P. Smith R.N.

To reduce errors in verbal and telephone orders, the JCAHO Patient Safety Goals for 2003 recommend reading back the complete order to the prescriber for verification.

KnowledgeCheck 16–6

- What important factors should you document when receiving a telephone order?
- What is the purpose of a verbal order? When should it be used?

Go to Chapter 16, **Knowledge Check Response Sheet and Answers,** on the Electronic Study Guide.

Practical Knowledge
knowing how

To document care effectively, you need to be familiar with the forms and requirements of your institution. Chart routine nursing actions, such as maintaining hygiene, on the designated flowsheets, and chart your assessments, interventions, and patient responses to care in the format approved by your facility. It is important to chart accurately, completely, and consistently so that the patient's progress can be tracked and appropriate care given.

GUIDELINES FOR DOCUMENTING CARE

Begin your charting at the beginning of your shift. Document the condition of your patient when you first observed him. Was he awake? Was he in bed? Did he have any complaints? What did you *do*? As your shift progressed, you performed your assessment and nursing interventions. What were your findings? Did any abnormalities exist? Finally, what was the patient's response to your interventions? Did any changes from the initial assessment occur?

Document accurately, and use nonjudgmental language. Avoid labeling patients. For example, if a patient refuses an ordered medicine, simply chart, "Patient refuses medication." If the patient offers an explanation for his refusal, you may quote the patient in your notes. Do not chart judgments, such as "Patient belligerent and obnoxious and refuses ordered medicine."

Know the requirements of reimbursement. Home care, hospitals, and long-term care facilities have specific guidelines for the frequency of charting and the type of data that must be recorded. Clinic and office settings also have requirements that must be met so that services can be reimbursed. Familiarize yourself with these requirements each time you work in a new setting.

Provide details about the patient's condition. When possible, give examples. For instance, if you were to chart, "Patient requires the assistance of two personnel to transfer to chair," anyone reading the chart has a clear idea of the patient's abilities. Including such details as this allows oncoming staff members to obtain adequate help and alerts other team members, such as discharge planners, about the patient's needs.

Remember that the patient's record is permanent and that information contained in the chart is confidential. As a student, you are granted access to patients' charts for educational purposes. You are expected to keep the information private and confidential. In most cases, you will be asked to use only the patient's initials on school projects. The Department of Health and Human Services (DHHS) issued updated regulations to protect health information in April 2003. As part of the reform of the Health Insurance Portability and Accountablity Act (HIPAA), the new rules affect access, storage, transfer, and discussion of patient information. Patient files should be kept in designated areas to which only healthcare providers have access. In addition, you must not provide written or verbal patient information to anyone outside the care of the patient, unless the patient has consented to allow access.

You should document as soon as possible after you make an observation or provide care. The longer you wait, the less you will recollect. If you leave your charting until the end of the shift, you may forget important details. Flowsheets, bedside progress notes, and bedside computers facilitate prompt charting. Discipline yourself to document promptly, but never chart ahead; to do so risks inaccuracy and jeopardizes the record's credibility.

Chart chronologically to demonstrate the changing status of the patient. If you forget to make an important entry while charting, you will need to make

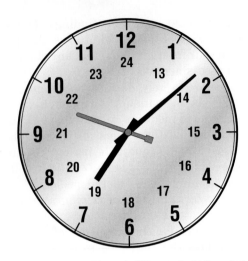

FIGURE 16–4 **Many healthcare facilities use the 24-hour clock.**

an addition to the narrative notes. This is known as a **late entry.** Generally a late entry is added to the first available line. Record the time and date you are charting, but in the body of the entry, clearly designate that this is a late entry. For example:

> Late entry 11/12/04 1300 Pt vomited 100 mL of bloody fluid at 0930 11/12/06. ——— J. Long, RN

If you know legal action is pending, do not place a late entry in the chart without notifying the nurse manager or risk management.

Date and time all of your notes. To avoid confusion between A.M. and P.M., many institutions use a 24-hour clock or military time (Figure 16–4). The day begins at 0001, which is equivalent to 12:01 A.M., and ends at 2400 (12 midnight). Most people have little difficulty with early morning hours. For example, 8:15 A.M. would be written 0815 in military time. However, after 12 noon, the changes are more noticeable. For instance, 1:00 P.M. is written as 1300. Simply add 12 to the P.M. time (e.g., 7:30 P.M. + 12 = 1930 in military time).

For complete charting guidelines,

 Go to Chapter 16, **Technique 16–3: Guidelines for Documentation,** in Volume 2.

KnowledgeCheck 16–7
- What aspects of care should be documented?
- When should care be documented?

 Go to Chapter 16, **Knowledge Check Response Sheet and Answers,** on the Electronic Study Guide.

CriticalThinking 16–4
You are caring for two clients on a medical-surgical unit. One of your clients is short of breath and complaining of chest pain. Your other client is recovering from abdominal surgery.

He is alert, stable, and free from pain at this time. After stabilizing your first client, you realize you are 45 minutes late administering a medication to the abdominal surgery patient. You are not sure how to proceed.

- What theoretical knowledge do you need?
- You give the medicine as soon as you can (50 minutes late). How and where should you chart the medication administration?
- If you had been aware that you were going to be late with the medication, what might you have done to be sure it was given on time?

Can I Delegate Charting?

In some facilities, each member of the team is responsible for documenting her part in the care of the patient. Nursing assistants or other unlicensed assistive personnel (UAPs) often chart ADLs, activity, and intake and output on graphic records. You are responsible for documenting the care you provided. Never chart the actions of others as though you had performed them. If an action is crucial to a chain of events, you may document that action if you observed it. For example, imagine that your patient fell while attempting to get out of bed. If you observed the fall, document what you observed. If the patient fell in the presence of the UAP, document the information given to you by the UAP and your assessment of the circumstances:

> 04/12/06   1110 Informed by UAP Smith that Pt. fell while getting OOB to go to the BR. Pt. seen and examined. No open areas, bruising, or pain. Pt. states, "I just slipped. It's nothing." Pt. instructed on call bell use. ——————— R. Smoot, RN

How Do I Question a Physician's Order?

If you feel uncertain about an order, you must question it. As a student, you will first want to discuss your concerns with your clinical instructor. Remember, your goal is to provide safe care. If you have concerns, act on them.

As a registered nurse, you will follow your institution's policy for clarifying orders. If an order is illegible or incomplete, contact the provider directly to seek clarification. If you believe an order is inappropriate or unsafe, you are legally and ethically required to question the order. Generally you should contact the provider who wrote the order. If the provider leaves the order as is and you still don't feel comfortable with it, you may refuse to carry it out. Inform your chain of command of your refusal. Usually this is the charge nurse. The charge nurse may then contact the nurse manager or nursing supervisor. The nature of the order will determine how this situation is handled.

As a new nurse, you may feel uncomfortable about questioning an order. Even experienced nurses sometimes feel uncomfortable undertaking this challenge. If you are uncertain how to proceed, you can discuss your concerns with your colleagues, the charge nurse,

or the supervisor before contacting the provider. Your efforts to clarify orders help to protect your patient. If you do refuse an order, you must document your refusal and the actions you took to clarify the order.

KnowledgeCheck 16–8

- Can charting be delegated?
- You are a student nurse on a medical-surgical unit. You review your patient's chart and notice that the physician has written orders that do not appear to be appropriate for your patient. How would you handle this situation?

 Go to Chapter 16, **Knowledge Check Response Sheet and Answers,** on the Electronic Study Guide.

 Suggested Readings: Go to Chapter 16, **Reading More About Documenting and Reporting,** on the Electronic Study Guide.

 Bibliography: Go to Volume 2, Bibliography.

| toward evidence-based practice |

Wise, L., Mersch, J., Racioppi, J., Crosier, J. & Thompson, C. (2000). Evaluating the reliability and utility of cumulative intake and output. *Journal of Nursing Care Quality, 14*(3), 37–42.

This quality improvement study examined the accuracy of intake and output (I&O) recording for estimating fluid balance. Three nurse managers examined the I&O records of 73 patients for a 48-hour period. I&O recordings were correlated with daily weight measures for the same patients. Recorded I&O measures were found to poorly correlate with weights. I&O records seriously underestimated fluid balance. For example, although a patient's record

indicated that the patient had a negative fluid balance (more output than input), the patient's weight was up by 3 pounds.

---

1. What kinds of things might have caused the nurses to record inaccurate I&Os?

2. What consequences might result from inaccurate recordings of intake and output?

 Go to Chapter 16, **Toward Evidence-Based Practice Suggested Responses,** on the Electronic Study Guide.

17 CHAPTER

Measuring
Vital Signs

Learning Outcomes

After completing this chapter, you should be able to:

* State at least one nursing diagnosis that might be used to describe a problem for each of the four vital signs: temperature, pulse, respirations, and blood pressure.
* Describe the process of thermoregulation in the body.
* Describe the process for taking oral, rectal, axillary, and tympanic membrane temperatures.
* Convert between the Fahrenheit and centigrade temperature scales.
* For different patient situations, choose the best way to take the temperature, including site and equipment.
* State the normal oral temperature range for adults.
* Explain the physiological mechanisms of fever.
* Describe at least four nursing interventions for the patient with a fever.
* Describe at least six nursing interventions for the patient with temperature alterations.
* Describe a method for obtaining a peripheral pulse and for an apical pulse.
* Given a client's age and pulse rate, rhythm, quality, and equality, differentiate between normal findings and those that should be referred to the primary healthcare provider.
* Explain how respirations are regulated in the body.
* Given a client's age and respiratory rate, depth, and rhythm; chest movement; and associated clinical signs, differentiate between normal findings and those that should be referred to the primary healthcare provider.
* Define *arterial oxygen saturation, hypoxia, hyperventilation,* and *hypoventilation.*
* Discuss at least five nursing interventions for the client with impaired respiratory status.
* Describe the physiology of blood pressure, including references to systolic, diastolic, pulse pressure, and mean arterial pressure.
* State the normal blood pressure range for the average adult.
* Explain why it is important to interpret a client's blood pressure pattern rather than relying on a single reading.
* Describe the process of obtaining a brachial blood pressure reading.
* Discuss the importance of cuff size when obtaining a blood pressure reading.
* Define *hypotension, hypertension, essential hypertension,* and *secondary hypertension.*
* Identify at least three nursing interventions for the client with hypertension.

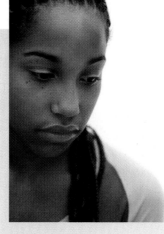

Your Patients

Your instructor has scheduled a clinical day at a local community health fair. Students from your program will be available to answer health-related questions, administer flu vaccines, check blood sugar levels, and take vital signs—temperature, pulse, respiratory rate, and blood pressure. You have been asked to check vital signs.

The first person you encounter is Rosemary, a young mother who arrives at the booth with Jason, her 2-year-old son. She tells you he has been eating poorly and is very irritable. You note that the child's skin is warm and dry, and he is flushed. The mother explains that she does not have a thermometer, and she would like you to take her son's temperature. Jason's axillary temperature is 101.8°F (38.8°C).

Now it is time to think like a nurse! What may be the meaning of this temperature reading? What, if any, additional data should you collect? How will you explain your findings to Rosemary? What action would you advise Rosemary to take? You may not yet have all the theoretical knowledge you need to answer these questions, but try to do so anyway, based on your present knowledge base and your life experiences.

The next person to arrive at the booth is Ms Sharma, an active 80-year-old woman who works part time in a local literacy program and walks 3 miles, four times per week. Ms Sharma notes that she has "lost a little pep. I don't feel sick, but I'm tired lately." Her pulse is difficult to feel. The rhythm is irregular, and the strength of the pulse is uneven—some beats are strong, while others are weak.

What might this finding mean? What questions do you have for Ms Sharma? What, if any, additional data should you collect? How will you explain your findings to Ms Sharma? What action would you advise her to take?

Mr. Jackson stops by to have his vital signs checked. As he sits down next to you, you notice he is short of breath. His respiratory rate is 28, and he appears to be struggling to breathe.

What do you think this respiratory rate means? What should be your next action? What would you say to Mr. Jackson?

The next client to arrive is Lucas. Lucas is a 35-year-old accountant who works for a firm in a nearby office building. Lucas tells you he has been under a lot of stress and is worried about his blood pressure. You measure his blood pressure as 150/98.

Is this an acceptable blood pressure? What does this reading mean? What should you discuss with Lucas? What advice should you offer?

You will gain the theoretical knowledge you need to answer the preceding questions as you work through this chapter and learn more about vital signs.

WHAT ARE VITAL SIGNS?

The term **vital signs (VS)** suggests assessment of vital or critical physiological functions. Variations in temperature, pulse, respirations, or blood pressure are indicators of a person's state of health and function of the body systems. Therefore, these four important measurements are among the most frequent assessments you will make as a nurse (Boxer & Kluge, 2000). Because of the importance of each of the vital signs, you must be very accurate in your measurements and recordings. A fifth vital sign, a measure of *pain,* has recently been proposed. See Chapter 30.

Do not become complacent when a client's vital signs are within normal limits. Although stable vital signs *indicate* physiological well-being, they do not *guarantee* it. Vital signs alone are limited in detecting some important physiological changes; for example, vital signs may sometimes remain stable in the presence of moderately large blood loss. Vital signs must be evaluated in the context of your overall assessment of the client.

Some experts recommend that *pulse oximetry* be added to the four traditional measures of physiological status when accurate assessment and monitoring are essential. Pulse oximetry is a technique for assessing oxygenation and is discussed later in the chapter. Also, although it does not fit with the traditional concept,

TABLE 17-1 Vital Signs: Average/Normal Findings for Adults

Core Temperature	
Average normal range	
Oral	96.2–100.4°F (35.7–38°C)
Rectal	97.2–101.4°F (36.2–38.6°C)
"Ideal" average	
Oral and tympanic	98.6°F (36.7–37°C)
Rectal	99.5°F (37.5°C)
Axillary	97.7°F (36.5°C)
Pulse	
Normal range	60–100 bpm
Average	80 bpm
Respirations	
Normal range	12–20 per min
Blood Pressure	
Normal range	100–120 systolic and 60–80 diastolic
Prehypertensive range	120–130 systolic and 80–89 diastolic
Average	Until recently, 120/80 was considered an "average" BP. However, recent guidelines (Joint National Committee on Prevention, Detection, Evaluation, and Treatment of High Blood Pressure, 2003) suggest that the number should be considerably lower, perhaps 110/70, the middle of the "normal" range.

some researchers suggest that *smoking status* be considered a vital sign during the initial patient encounter ("Vital Signs," 1999).

When Should I Measure a Patient's Vital Signs?

In the community health fair scenario, clients asked you to take their vital signs. However, in many clinical settings you and other care providers will determine how often to measure and record the vital signs. In general, the frequency depends on the patient's condition and the events taking place. The following are common occasions for assessing vital signs:

- On admission to the hospital
- At a visit to the healthcare provider's office or clinic

- Before, during, and after surgery or special procedures
- To monitor the effects of certain medications or activities
- Whenever the patient's condition changes

Although there has been little research on the optimal frequency for assessing vital signs, agency policies usually require that nurses monitor and record vital signs on a regular basis. The frequency varies by setting and situation. Below are commonly used frequencies:

- In the hospital: once every 4 to 8 hours
- In the home health setting: at each visit
- In the clinic: at each visit
- In skilled nursing facilities, also known as convalescent hospitals: weekly to monthly

When a client's VS vary from normal, you should assess and document them more frequently, perhaps every 5 to 15 minutes. As a beginning practitioner, you should validate your clinical assessments with a more experienced nurse.

In hospital settings, it is up to the nurse to decide whether VS need to be monitored more frequently than the primary care provider has ordered. Initially, you will measure VS to establish the patient's baseline. A baseline is important because (1) a change in VS may be caused by a disease state, the effect of therapies, or merely by changes in activity and environment; and (2) there are normal variations in VS among individuals. Table 17–1 shows average or normal findings for adults, but it is important to remember that each person has his or her own baseline for "normal." If a patient's VS vary from established norms, compare the finding to that person's baseline to determine the degree and severity of the variation.

How Do I Record Vital Signs?

Most agencies have special flowsheets for recording vital signs. For examples, see Figure 3–4 and forms in Chapter 16 of Volume 2. If the vital signs are not within normal limits, you will also document them in the nurses' notes, along with any associated symptoms (e.g., cyanosis [blue-grey skin] with abnormal respirations). Document any interventions as well (e.g., elevating the head of the bed when the patient has shortness of breath). The following sections will explain the meaning of each of the vital signs and how to assess them.

BODY TEMPERATURE

Body temperature is the degree of heat maintained by the body. It is the difference between heat produced by the body and heat lost to the environment.

Theoretical Knowledge
knowing why

To assess and support regulation of body temperature, you will need to know the normal temperature range, how heat is produced by and lost from the body, and factors that influence body temperature.

What Is a Normal Temperature?

No single number can be considered "normal," because body temperature fluctuates with age, exercise, and environmental conditions. However, the body functions optimally within a narrow temperature range. The adult's internal temperature, called the body's **core temperature,** normally ranges from 96.2 to 100.4°F (36.2 to 38°C), although a range of 98 to 98.6°F (36.7 to 37°C) is considered "average" for a healthy adult. Core body temperature is typically 1 to 2°F (0.6 to 1.2°C) higher than **surface temperature.** Rectal and tympanic membrane measurements reflect core temperatures; oral and axillary measurements reflect surface temperatures. Table 17–1 in this chapter identifies normal adult temperatures. For age-related variations for all vital signs, including temperature,

 Go to Chapter 17, **Tables, Boxes, Figures: ESG Table 17–1,** on the Electronic Study Guide.

Temporary, slight variations of temperature above or below normal usually are not significant. Greater variations indicate a disturbance of function in some system or region of the body (Figure 17–1). The degree of temperature elevation does not always indicate the seriousness of the underlying disease or condition. For example, some acute, even fatal, infections may cause only a mild temperature elevation. However, a continuously elevated temperature, even if slight, is always cause for concern and indicates a need for further evaluation.

How Does the Body Regulate Temperature?

The process of temperature regulation is called **thermoregulation.** To keep the body temperature constant, the body must balance heat production and heat loss. This balance is controlled by the hypothalamus, located between the cerebral hemispheres of the brain. Similar to a thermostat, the hypothalamus recognizes even small changes in body temperature that are sent to it by sensory receptors in the skin.

• *Decreasing the body temperature.* When heat sensors in the hypothalamus are stimulated, they send

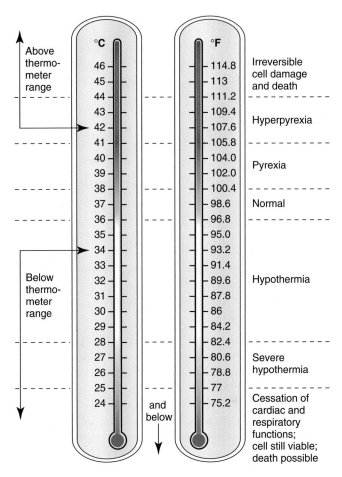

FIGURE 17–1 Ranges of normal and altered body temperatures.

out impulses to reduce the body temperature. This activates compensatory mechanisms, such as peripheral vasodilation, sweating, and inhibition of heat production. Vasodilation diverts core-warmed blood to the body surface, where heat can be transferred to the surrounding environment.

• *Increasing the body temperature.* When the sensors in the hypothalamus detect cold, they send out impulses to increase heat production and reduce heat loss. To produce heat, the body responds with shivering and the release of epinephrine, which increases metabolism. To reduce heat loss, the blood vessels constrict. Vasoconstriction conserves heat by shunting blood away from the periphery (where heat is lost) to the core of the body, where the blood is warmed. **Piloerection** (hairs standing on end) also occurs, but it is not an important heat-conserving mechanism in humans.

• *Behavioral control of temperature.* In addition, temperature is under our behavioral control. When people feel cool, they can turn up the furnace, put on more clothing, or move to a warmer place. When they feel too warm, they can turn on an air conditioner, remove clothing, or take a cool shower.

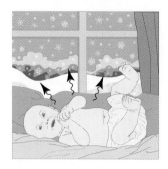
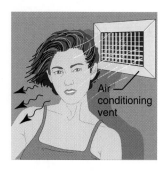
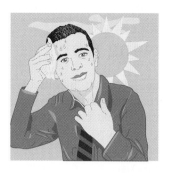
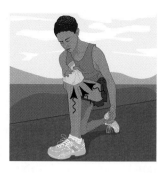

FIGURE 17–2 Mechanisms of heat exchange with the environment: Radiation, convection, evaporation, and conduction.

How Is Heat Produced in the Body?

The body produces heat through the interaction of three factors: metabolism, the movement of skeletal muscles, and nonshivering thermogenesis.

1. *Metabolism* is the sum of all physical and chemical processes and changes that take place in the body. Metabolism uses energy and generates heat. The **basal metabolic rate (BMR)** is the amount of energy required to maintain the body at rest. Body size, lean muscle mass, and numerous hormones influence BMR. For example, *hyperthyroidism* (an increase in the thyroid hormone thyroxine) increases the BMR. Clients with hyperthyroidism often complain of feeling warm even when they are in a cool environment. By contrast, when the thyroxine level is low (*hypothyroidism*), less heat is produced. Clients who are in a hypothyroid state frequently complain of feeling cold. Epinephrine and norepinephrine, produced from stimulation of the sympathetic nervous system, also increase BMR and heat production.
2. *Skeletal muscles* are used in all movement of the body. Muscles need fuel to function. The breakdown (*catabolism*) of fats and carbohydrates in the muscle produces energy and heat. It requires very little muscle activity to sit and read this text. However, if you were to go to a local track for a run, you would use more skeletal muscles. After your run, your body temperature would be higher, perhaps as high as 101 to 104°F (38.3 to 40°C). In contrast, if you were to go outside without a coat when the temperature was 35°F (1.6°C), you would begin to feel cold. Your hypothalamus would sense a drop in body temperature, and shivering would begin in the skeletal muscles. This mechanism is so efficient that body heat production can rise to about four times the normal rate in just a few minutes.
3. *Nonshivering thermogenesis* is the metabolism of brown fat to produce heat. It is used by infants because they cannot produce heat through shivering, as do adults and children. This mechanism disappears in the first few months following birth.

How Is Heat Exchanged Between the Body and the Environment?

Heat moves from an area of higher to an area of lower temperature; that is, cool air and objects "pick up" heat from warmer ones. The mechanisms that effect the exchange of heat between the body and the environment are radiation, convection, evaporation, and conduction. (Figure 17–2).

Radiation is the loss of heat through electromagnetic waves emitting from surfaces that are warmer than the surrounding air. If the uncovered skin is warmer than the air, the body loses heat through the skin. This is why a cool room warms by radiation when it is filled with many people. In contrast, a person can acquire heat by turning on a heat lamp or sunbathing. Radiation accounts for almost 50% of body heat loss.

Convection is the transfer of heat through currents of air or water. Nurses use this principle to intentionally effect changes in a patient's body temperature. Immersion in a warm bath may raise body temperature for a hypothermic client. In contrast, the currents of cool air produced by a fan can help reduce a fever. Together, the processes of conduction and convection account for approximately 15 to 20% of all heat loss to the environment.

Evaporation occurs when water is converted to vapor and lost from the skin (as perspiration) or the mucous membranes (through the breath). Evaporation causes cooling. Water loss by evaporation is called **insensible loss.** Evaporation is affected by the relative humidity of the environment. If the air already contains much moisture (**humidity**), then less moisture evaporates from the skin and less cooling occurs.

Conduction is the process whereby heat is transferred from a warm to a cool surface by direct contact. Suppose that a patient's temperature was 98.6°F (37°C) while he is fully dressed in the exam room. If he were dressed in a thin hospital gown and lying on a cool metal x-ray table, his temperature would drop, possibly by a full degree in the first hour.

What Factors Influence Body Temperature?

The following are some examples of factors involved in the delicate balance of body temperature:

- *Developmental level.* Infants and older adults are most susceptible to the effects of environmental temperature extremes. Infants lose approximately 30% of their body heat through the head, which is proportionally larger than their body compared to adults. This places them at increased risk for decreased body temperature. Body temperature begins to stabilize during childhood and remains relatively stable until older adulthood. Older adults have difficulty maintaining body heat because of slower metabolism, decreased vasomotor control, and loss of subcutaneous tissue. It is common for older adults to have temperatures as low as 95°F (35°C) during the morning. For a comparison of normal vital signs for various ages,

 Go to Chapter 17, **Tables, Boxes, Figures: ESG Table 17–1,** on the Electronic Study Guide.

- *Environmental temperature.* The environment strongly influences body temperature. For example, warm room temperatures or hot baths can increase body temperature. Very high external temperatures can produce very high internal temperatures, causing heat stroke. In contrast, cold environments can lower body temperatures and, in severe cases, lead to hypothermia.

- *Hormones.* A woman's body temperature varies (as much as 1°F, or 0.6°C) with her menstrual cycle. Body temperature is lower when progesterone levels are low and increases as progesterone levels increase. Hormone fluctuations during menopause, when menses stop, often cause temperature fluctuations commonly known as *hot flashes,* which can produce episodes of intense body heat and sweating.

- *Exercise.* Because it increases metabolism, hard work or strenuous exercise can increase body core temperature to 101 to 104°F (38.3 to 40°C).

- *Emotions and stress.* Emotional stress, excitement, anxiety, and nervousness stimulate the sympathetic

---

| toward evidence-based practice |

Electronic thermometers, including the tympanic membrane infrared thermometer, have almost completely replaced mercury-and-glass thermometers in many healthcare settings. They save nursing time and are thought to be safer to use. Questions remain about their accuracy, though.

Kocoglu, H., Goksu, S., Isik, M., Akturk, Z., & Bayazit, Y. A. (2002). Infrared tympanic thermometer can accurately measure the body temperature in children in an emergency room setting. *International Journal of Pediatric Otorhinolaryngology, 65*(1), 39–43.

In this study, researchers randomly selected pediatric patients admitted to the emergency department. They found no statistically significant difference in temperatures obtained using the infrared tympanic thermometer and oral and rectal temperatures obtained using a glass thermometer.

Modell, J. G., Katholi, C. R., Kumaramangalam, S. M., Hudson, E. C., & Graham, D. (1998). Unreliability of the infrared tympanic thermometer in clinical practice: A comparative study with oral mercury and oral electronic thermometers. *Southern Medical Journal, 91*(7), 737–738.

Researchers in this study used a convenience sample of 137 adult inpatients and compared readings from an infrared tympanic thermometer, an electronic oral

thermometer, and a mercury-glass thermometer. When using the tympanic thermometer and comparing clients' right and left ears, researchers found significantly large variations in temperature between the ears. They concluded that infrared tympanic thermometers should not be used for routine temperature assessment.

Jensen, B. N., Jensen, F. S., Madsen, S. N., & Lossl, K. (2000). Accuracy of digital tympanic, oral, axillary, and rectal thermometers compared with standard rectal mercury thermometers. *European Journal of Surgery, 166*(11), 848–851.

This study included 200 patients. Researchers compared electronic tympanic, oral, axillary, and rectal measurements with those taken with a mercury-glass rectal thermometer. They concluded that when the mercury-glass rectal readings were used as the standard, the electronic rectal temperatures were the most accurate. They do not recommend electronic tympanic, oral, or axillary measurements.

---

1. Imagine you are in charge of an adult clinic. Based on the preceding studies, would you change from glass to electronic thermometers in your agency?

2. What assumption must you make in order to use these studies to answer your question?

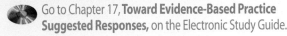 Go to Chapter 17, **Toward Evidence-Based Practice Suggested Responses,** on the Electronic Study Guide.

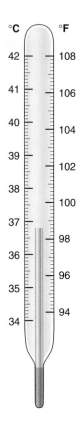

FIGURE 17–3 Glass thermometers are available with degree markings in Fahrenheit or centigrade. (left), Centigrade readings. (right), Fahrenheit readings. Note: Thermometers read only one scale. For demonstration purposes this figure includes both scales.

nervous system, causing production of epinephrine and norepinephrine. These biochemical agents trigger an increase in the metabolic rate, which in turn increases body temperature.

- *Circadian rhythm.* **Circadian rhythm** is a cyclical repetition of certain physiological processes (e.g., changes in temperature and blood pressure) that occurs every 24 hours. Temperature fluctuates 1 to 2°F (0.6 to 1.2°C) over the course of 24 hours. It is usually lowest in the early morning hours and highest in late afternoon or early evening.

 CriticalThinking 17–1

- You notice the following temperature readings in your client's chart:

    4:00 A.M.—97.4°F
    8:00 A.M.—97.9°F
    12:00 noon—98.4°F
    4:00 P.M.—99.6°F
    8:00 P.M.—100.9°F

    You are working the night shift. When you assess the client's temperature at midnight, it is 101.2°F. What do you notice about the pattern of the temperature readings?
- What is important in this scenario?
- As a nursing student, what should you do?

 KnowledgeCheck 17–1

- Which age groups are most susceptible to thermoregulation problems, and why?
- List five factors that affect body temperature.
- What are the compensatory mechanisms for decreasing body temperature?
- What are the compensatory mechanisms for increasing body temperature?

Go to Chapter 17, **Knowledge Check Response Sheet and Answers,** on the Electronic Study Guide.

Practical Knowledge
knowing how

Now that you understand the physiology of temperature regulation, you are ready to gain the practical knowledge of how to assess and support a patient's body temperature. To see the sequence of steps you will take when measuring a patient's temperature,

VOL 2   Go to Chapter 17, **Procedure 17–1: Assessing Body Temperature,** in Volume 2.

The accompanying Critical Aspects box for Procedures 17–1 through 17–6 summarizes that procedure.

| Assessment |

On a daily basis we commonly assess temperature by touch. For example, when you remove a blanket from a warming unit, you can feel that it is warm; however, it is difficult to pinpoint the exact temperature of the blanket. The same is true of body temperature. Although some research has shown that people can use simple touch to detect fever, they cannot differentiate *degrees* of fever. Because vital signs are used as indicators of a client's health status, it is essential to get an accurate measure.

Temperature Measurement Scales: Fahrenheit and Centigrade

Two scales are used for recording temperature: Fahrenheit and centigrade (or Celsius), a metric scale. Most people in the United States are familiar with the Fahrenheit scale; however, some healthcare agencies use centigrade. Electronic and tympanic membrane thermometers can usually measure temperature in either scale; all you need to do is to flip a switch. Glass thermometers read only one scale (Figure 17–3), so you may need to convert a reading from one scale to the other. For example, you may have obtained a centigrade reading for a child and wish to explain its significance to the mother, who is familiar only with Fahrenheit.

For steps to follow in *all* procedures, refer to the inside back cover of Volume 2.

critical aspects of procedures 17–1 through 17–6

Procedure 17–1: Assessing Body Temperature

- Select the appropriate site and thermometer type.

- "Zero" or shake down the thermometer as needed.

- Insert the thermometer in its sheath, or use a thermometer designated only for the patient.

- Insert the thermometer in the chosen site.

- Leave a glass thermometer in the site for the recommended time (oral, 3 to 5 minutes; rectal, 2 minutes; axillary, 6 to 8 minutes).

- Leave an electronic thermometer in place until it beeps.

- Read the temperature. Hold a glass thermometer at eye level to read.

- Shake down a glass thermometer, and clean or store it.

- For an oral temperature, obtain a reading 15 to 30 minutes after the patient consumes hot or cold food or fluids or smokes.

- Hold a rectal thermometer securely in place, and never leave it unattended.

Procedure 17–2: Assessing Peripheral Pulses

- Make sure the client is resting while you assess a peripheral pulse.

- Select and palpate the appropriate site.

- Count for 30 seconds if the pulse is regular; for 60 seconds if it is irregular.

- Note pulse rate, rhythm, and quality.

- Compare pulses bilaterally.

- Palpate the carotid pulse on only one side at a time.

Procedure 17–3: Assessing Apical Pulse

- Palpate the 5th intercostal space at the midclavicular line for stethoscope placement.

- Count for 60 seconds.

- Note pulse rate, rhythm, and quality and the S_1 and S_2 heart sounds.

Procedure 17–4: Assessing for an Apical-Radial Pulse Deficit

- Palpate the 5th intercostal space at the midclavicular line for stethoscope placement.

- Palpate the radial pulse.

- When possible, have two nurses carry out the procedure. (This is ideal; can be done by one person skilled in the procedure.)

- Count for 60 seconds.

- Compare the pulse rates at both sites.

Procedure 17–5: Assessing Respirations

- Count unobtrusively (e.g., while palpating radial pulse).

- Count for 30 seconds if respirations regular; for 60 seconds if they are irregular.

- Observe the rate, rhythm, and depth of respirations.

Procedure 17–6: Measuring Blood Pressure

- If possible, place the patient in a sitting position, with the feet on the floor and the legs uncrossed.

- Measure BP after the patient has been inactive for 5 minutes.

- Support the patient's arm at the level of the heart.

- Use a cuff of the appropriate size.

- Position the cuff correctly, and wrap it snugly.

- Inflate the cuff while palpating the radial artery. Inflate to 30 mm Hg above the point at which you can no longer feel the radial artery.

- Place the stethoscope on the brachial artery and release pressure at 2 to 3 mm Hg per second.

- Read the mercury manometer at eye level.

- Record systolic/diastolic pressures (first and last sounds heard—e.g., 110/80).

- Wait at least 2 minutes before remeasuring.

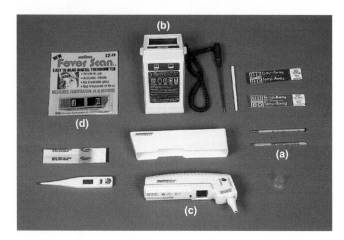

FIGURE 17–4 Types of thermometers. *A*, Glass thermometers. *B*, Electronic thermometer. *C*, Tympanic membrane thermometer (infrared). *D*, Tape or other chemical/paper thermometers.

You will probably have access to a conversion chart but you may sometimes need to convert mathematically. To convert between Fahrenheit and centigrade readings,

 VOL 2 Go to Chapter 17, **Conversion Table,** in Volume 2.

To convert from Fahrenheit to centigrade, subtract 32 from the Fahrenheit temperature and multiply by 5/9. For example:

A client has a temperature of 102°F. What is his temperature as measured in centigrade?

$$(102 - 32) \times 5/9 = 39°C$$

To convert a centigrade reading to Fahrenheit, multiply the centigrade temperature by 9/5, and add 32. As a cross-check we can verify the preceding example:

Client temperature = 39°C
$$(39 \times 9/5) + 32 = 102°F$$

What Equipment Do I Need?

Nurses measure temperature with various kinds of thermometers. Each type has advantages and disadvantages, so you will need to think critically about the type of thermometer best suited for each patient situation.

Glass Thermometers

The thermometer that has traditionally been used is a glass, mercury-filled tube marked in degrees Fahrenheit or centigrade that is read visually (Figure 17–4*A*). However, because of the dangers of exposure to mercury (e.g., when thermometers break), the U.S. Environmental Protection Agency (EPA) and the American Hospital Association advise against use of equipment containing mercury (USEPA, 2002). In recent years, electronic digital thermometers have replaced glass thermometers in many agencies. Glass thermometers

containing other liquids, such as alcohol or gallium-indium-tin (galinstan) are available.

Advantages

- Flexibility of use: can be used for measuring oral, rectal, or axillary temperature.
- Inexpensive initial cost.
- Accuracy, as indicated by several studies.
- Easily disinfected.

Disadvantages

- Fragile, so there is constant cost of replacement.
- Slow: it takes 3 to 6 minutes to obtain an accurate reading.
- Difficult for some people to read accurately.

Electronic Thermometers

An electronic thermometer is a rechargeable unit consisting of an electronic probe attached to a portable unit by a thin wire (Figure 17–4*B*). Disposable plastic sheaths are used to cover the probe. To prevent transmission of infection, the nurse discards the sheath after each use. Units are color-coded red and blue to prevent oral temperatures from being taken with rectal thermometers and vice versa.

Advantages

- Flexibility of use: can be used for measuring oral, rectal, or axillary temperature.
- Ease of use.
- Provide rapid measurement: it takes 15 to 45 seconds to measure the temperature. A beep sounds when the peak temperature is reached.

Disadvantages

- Expensive.
- Require frequent calibration.
- Conflicting data regarding their accuracy.
- Need to be kept charged.

Electronic Infrared Tympanic Membrane Thermometers

The electronic infrared tympanic membrane thermometer is a rechargeable unit that contains an infrared sensor at the tip of an ear probe (Figure 17–4*C*). The sensor measures heat radiating from the tympanic membrane.

Advantages

- Ease of use.
- Provide rapid measurement: it takes 2 to 5 seconds to measure the temperature. A beep sounds when the peak temperature is reached.
- May be the most cost-effective method because of their rapid reading capabilities and labor savings.

Disadvantages

- Expensive.
- Less accurate than electronic or glass thermometers, as some studies indicate.
- Require frequent calibration.
- Batteries require recharging.

Disposable Chemical Thermometers

The disposable chemical thermometer is a thin plastic strip, patch, or tape containing a matrix of chemicals that change color at designated body temperatures (Figure 17–4*D*). Clients use chemical thermometers at home. Nurses use them infrequently. If a chemical thermometer indicates above or below normal temperature, you should use a glass or electronic thermometer to validate the reading.

Advantage

- Ease of use; requires no special training.

Disadvantage

- Less accurate than glass or electronic thermometers.

What Sites Should I Use?

For accurate assessment, you must place the thermometer in contact with body tissues that are amply supplied with blood vessels. The usual sites are the mouth (in the right or left posterior sublingual pocket), rectum, axillae, and tympanic membrane.

 VOL 2 Go to Chapter 17, **Procedure 17–1: Assessing Body Temperature,** in Volume 2.

The temperature reading varies depending on the site used. From lowest to highest readings, the sites are as follows: axillary, oral, rectal, and tympanic membrane. There is approximately 1°F (0.6°C) difference between each site and the next higher one. To obtain a comparative oral temperature:

To an axillary reading, add 0.9°F (0.5°C)
To a rectal reading, subtract 0.9°F (0.5°C)
To a tympanic membrane reading, subtract 1.1 to 1.5°F (0.7 to 0.9°C)

For example, an axillary temperature of 98.1°F is comparable to an oral reading of 99.0°F, a rectal reading of 99.9°F, and a tympanic membrane reading of 100.1 to 100.5°F (Erickson & Yount, 1991). Each site has advantages and disadvantages, so you must choose the safest and most accurate site for each client.

Oral Site

The oral temperature is a simple, convenient, and comfortable method for most adults.

Disadvantages

- Eating and drinking affect the accuracy of the reading.
- The client must keep her mouth closed for several minutes.
- There is a risk of exposure to body fluids.
- It is slow. Some experts say it takes up to 7 minutes to ensure correct reading, depending on the type of thermometer.
- This site is contraindicated for clients who cannot cooperate with the instructions or who might be injured (e.g., infants and small children; patients who have had oral surgery, breathe through the mouth, have chills, or are confused or unconscious).

Rectal Site

The rectal temperature most accurately represents the core (internal) body temperature. Temperature is usually measured rectally in clients who may be unable to follow directions for oral temperature monitoring or in situations where an accurate temperature is crucial. However, because of the risk for injury to rectal mucosa, it is not recommended as the first choice of site.

Disadvantages

- Most clients find this method objectionable or embarrassing.
- It requires special positioning of the client.
- It does not reflect changes in core temperature as rapidly as the oral method.
- There is a risk of exposure to body fluids.
- There is risk for injury to the patient, especially infants.
- Presence of stool may cause inaccurate reading.

Contraindication

- Clients who may be injured by the method (e.g., clients who have a rectal disease, severe diarrhea, or rectal surgery; newborns, whose rectal mucosa is fragile).
- Because it can slow the heart rate by stimulating the vagus nerve, this method is sometimes contraindicated for clients with cardiac surgery and some heart conditions.

Axillary Site

The axillary temperature is safe and easy to measure. It can be used with newborns, children, and uncooperative or unconscious clients. It is recommended over rectal temperatures for routine measurements ("Vital Signs," 1999).

Disadvantages

- It is considered the least accurate of the sites.
- The thermometer must be left in place for a long time.
- Diaphoresis (sweating) can affect the reading.

Tympanic Membrane Site

Tympanic membrane temperatures are readily measured with the use of a special thermometer. This method is often used in settings where temperatures must be obtained quickly (2 to 5 seconds) or for patients who are unable to comply with the requirements for other temperature measures. For example, pediatric clinics often use this method because young children may not be able to comply with instructions (e.g., "Keep your mouth closed").

Disadvantages

- It requires a special instrument, an expensive initial purchase.
- Hearing aids must be removed.
- Presence of cerumen (earwax) may affect accuracy of reading.
- Questions about accuracy remain; using the "ear tug" technique is said to improve accuracy of the readings.

Contraindication

- Clients who have had ear surgery.

 CriticalThinking 17–2

- Convert the following temperatures, and analyze the readings. What might they mean?
  a. 38.5°C _____ °F
  b. 96.5°F _____ °C
  c. 37.0°C _____ °F
- Rank the expected early evening temperatures of the following individuals from lowest to highest.
  a. a 22-year-old college athlete
  b. a 5-year-old kindergartener
  c. an 88-year-old nursing home resident

Assessing Temperature in the Home

When teaching clients how to check their temperature at home, teach the same procedures that you have learned. This usually means teaching:

- How to use a glass or disposable chemical thermometer
- How to disinfect and store the thermometer
- How to maintain safety, such as not using the same glass thermometer for both oral and rectal temperatures and not using an oral thermometer to take rectal temperatures

For other home care adaptations,

 Go to Chapter 17, **Procedure 17–1: Assessing Body Temperature,** in Volume 2.

What Is Fever?

Fever—or **pyrexia**—is an abnormally high body temperature (>100.4°F, or 38°C). **Hyperpyrexia** is fever above 105.8°F (41.0°C). Fever occurs in response to **pyrogens** (fever-producing substances). When bacteria or other foreign substances invade the body, they stimulate **phagocytes** (specialized white blood cells), which ingest the invaders and secrete pyrogens (e.g., interleukin-1). Pyrogens induce secretion of substances (called *prostaglandins*) that reset the hypothalamic thermostat at a higher temperature. The body's heat-regulating mechanisms (vasoconstriction, increased metabolism, and shivering) then act to bring the core temperature up to this new setting. When the stressor is removed, the thermostat resets at normal. Fever occurs in three phases:

- *The initial phase (febrile episode or onset)*—the period when body temperature is rising but has not yet reached the new set point. The onset of fever may be sudden or gradual, depending on the condition causing it. The person usually feels chilly and generally uncomfortable and may shiver.
- *The second phase (course)*—the period when body temperature reaches its maximum (set point) and remains fairly constant at the new higher level. The person feels warm and dry during this phase, which may last from a few days to a few weeks.
- *The third phase (defervescence or crisis)*—the period when the temperature returns to normal. The person feels warm and appears flushed in response to vasodilation. Diaphoresis occurs, which assists with heat loss by evaporation. This phase is commonly referred to as the fever's "breaking."

There are four types of fever:

1. **Intermittent fever**—temperature alternates regularly between periods of fever and periods of normal or below-normal temperature.
2. **Remittent fever**—wide fluctuations in temperature (>3.6°F, or 2°C), all above normal, during a 24-hour period.
3. **Constant (sustained) fever**—temperature may fluctuate slightly but is always above normal.
4. **Relapsing fever**—short periods of fever alternating with periods of normal temperatures, each lasting 1 to 2 days.

At some time in your life, you most likely have taken Tylenol (acetaminophen) or aspirin for a fever. Can you think of a reason why this may or may not be a good idea? Why should you think carefully before administering antipyretic (fever-reducing) medications to a client?

The answer is that fever, up to a point, is beneficial. High temperatures (up to 102.2°F, or 39°C) enhance the immune response because they:

- Kill or inhibit the growth of many microorganisms.
- Enhance phagocytosis.

- Cause the breakdown of lysosomes and self-destruction of virally infected cells.
- Cause the release of interferon, a substance that protects cells from viral infection.

This does not mean that you should *never* administer, or take, antipyretic medications. They may be needed to keep the temperature from becoming dangerously high. Very high temperatures, 106°F (41°C) or greater, can damage cells throughout the body, especially in the brain, causing agitation, confusion, stupor or coma. Vascular collapse may follow, producing cerebral edema, shock, and death. Death usually results if body temperature becomes higher than 109 to 112°F (43 to 44°C) (McCance & Huether, 1998).

| Nursing Diagnosis |

Fever may be a medical diagnosis, a nursing diagnosis, or the symptom of other problems. The following nursing diagnoses may be used when the fever is considered to be a *client problem* and not just a symptom of an illness or other problem (for example, fever may be a symptom of problems such as Deficient Fluid Volume, or dehydration).

- Hyperthermia is diagnosed when a person's body temperature is above normal and the person complains of fatigue, feels warm, is flushed, and has an increased heart rate.
- Ineffective Thermoregulation applies to a person whose temperature fluctuates above and below the normal range.
- Risk for Imbalanced Body Temperature should be used when the temperature is normal but the client is at risk for failure to maintain body temperature within normal range (e.g., newborns and the frail elderly).

| Planning Outcomes/Evaluation |

Associated NOC standardized outcomes include the following:

- For the actual nursing diagnoses Hyperthermia and Ineffective Thermoregulation: Thermoregulation, Thermoregulation: Newborn, and Vital Signs
- For the potential problem Risk for Imbalanced Body Temperature: Adherence Behavior, Compliance Behavior, Risk Control, and Risk Detection

 Go to Chapter 17, **Standardized Language,** in Volume 2.

Individualized goals/outcome statements you might write for a client include the following:

- Oral temperature < 99°F (37.2°C).
- No clinical signs of fever present (e.g., no chills or flushing).
- Pulse and respiratory rates within normal range.

Use the goals set in the planning outcomes phase to evaluate clients' responses to nursing and medical interventions.

| Planning Interventions/Implementation |

Although overall care of the patient depends on the disease causing the fever and on specific orders from the physician, there are nursing interventions and activities that address fever, regardless of its cause. *NIC standardized interventions* for Hyperthermia include Fever Treatment, Malignant Hyperthermia Precautions, Temperature Regulation, Temperature Regulation: Intraoperative, and Vital Signs Monitoring.

 Go to Chapter 17, **Standardized Language,** in Volume 2.

Specific nursing activities for clients with fever and/or nursing diagnoses of Hyperthermia or Ineffective Thermoregulation include the following:

- *Provide focused assessments:*

  Help determine the cause of the fever. For example, you may collect specimens from various body sites for culture.

  Monitor the temperature and other VS at least every 2 hours, and more often if temperature is rising rapidly or if clinical symptoms are changing. Recall that the increased metabolism accompanying a fever also increases the pulse and respirations. There is conflicting research regarding the accuracy and sensitivity of electronic thermometers, especially the infrared tympanic thermometer; therefore, when you suspect fever, it would be wise to take a rectal reading (or oral reading, if the rectal site is contraindicated) with a glass thermometer for comparison.

  Observe for the clinical signs that accompany a fever. Symptoms vary, depending on the phase of the fever. The characteristic symptoms include flushed face; dry, hot skin; eyes that appear bright and somewhat apprehensive; rapid, shallow respirations; increased heart rate; unusual thirst; loss of appetite; headache; and complaints of nausea. If the fever is extreme, urine may be concentrated and decreased in volume. Seizures, confusion, or delirium can also be associated with very high fevers.

- *Provide collaborative care to treat the underlying cause of the fever.* For example, you may administer antibiotics that a physician prescribes to treat a bacterial infection.

- *Provide oral or intravenous fluids* to replace fluids lost through diaphoresis. They help prevent dehydration or **hypovolemia** (fluid deficiency) secondary to the fever.

- *Use nonpharmacological measures to reduce fever.* The following measures are likely to produce shivering,

which produces heat; therefore, they can actually raise instead of lower the patient's temperature. When using these measures, be careful not to cause your patient to shiver.

Cooling blankets that circulate water and decrease fever by conduction

Alcohol or tepid baths

Cloth-covered ice packs or cool washcloths to the groin, neck, or axillae

Circulating fan in the patient's room

Instructing the client to use minimal bed covers

- *Provide nutritional support.* Food is essential to meet the increased energy needs created by the high metabolic rate accompanying fever. However, lack of appetite often accompanies fever, so food must be made appealing to the patient.

- *Provide special mouth care.* Lubricate lips with petroleum jelly (e.g., Vaseline). Lips may become dry and cracked, the tongue may be swollen, and sores may be present.

- *Keep clothing and bed linens dry* to promote comfort and help prevent chilling. Recall that diaphoresis occurs during defervescence.

- *Provide emergency treatment,* if necessary. Heat stroke is an emergency because death can occur rapidly. Cooling blankets or cool water baths can be used successfully if the surface temperature is not lowered too quickly. Rapid lowering of the surface temperature causes vasoconstriction, which prevents core cooling.

What Is Hypothermia?

Hypothermia exists when the core temperature drops below normal (<96.8°F, or 36°C). It may be associated with extended exposure to cold, as during surgery, extreme weather conditions, immersion in cold water, or lack of shelter and clothing. As the body temperature drops, metabolic processes slow. Prolonged exposure to the cold is not correctable by shivering and may prove fatal (see Figure 17–1). **Severe hypothermia** occurs when body temperature drops below 82.4°F (28°C). Although survival has been noted at a core temperature of 60.8°F (16°C), death usually results when body temperature falls below 70 to 75°F (21 to 24°C). Hypothermia is sometimes deliberately induced to decrease the need for oxygen in body tissues (e.g., during cardiac or neurological surgery).

| Nursing Diagnosis |

The following nursing diagnoses may apply to the patient with hypothermia:

- Hypothermia is diagnosed when a person's body temperature is below normal range.

- Ineffective Thermoregulation applies to a person whose temperature fluctuates above and below the normal range. As you can see, Ineffective Thermoregulation can be used in both hypothermia and fever.

- Risk for Imbalanced Body Temperature should be used when the temperature is normal but the client is at risk for failure to maintain body temperature within normal range (e.g., newborns and the frail elderly). As you can see, this diagnosis can also apply to both hypothermia and fever.

| Planning Outcomes/Evaluation |

NOC standardized outcomes include the following:

- For the actual nursing diagnoses of Hypothermia and ineffective Thermoregulation, use Thermoregulation, Thermoregulation: Neonate, and Vital Signs

- For the potential nursing diagnosis Risk for Imbalanced Body Temperature, use Adherence Behavior, Compliance Behavior, Risk Control, and Risk Detection

 Go to Chapter 17, **Standardized Language,** in Volume 2.

Individualized goals/outcome statements you might write for a client with Hypothermia are as follows:

- Oral temperature >98.6°F (37°C).

- No clinical signs of Hypothermia present (e.g., no disorientation, no decrease in urine output).

- Pulse and respiratory rates within normal range.

Use the goals set in the planning outcomes stage to evaluate client responses to interventions.

| Planning Interventions/Implementation |

NIC standardized interventions recommended for Hypothermia include Hypothermia Treatment, Temperature Regulation, Temperature Regulation: Intraoperative, and Vital Signs Monitoring.

 Go to Chapter 17, **Standardized Language,** in Volume 2.

Specific nursing activities include the following:

- *Provide warm, dry clothing and warm drinks.* For mild cases of Hypothermia, this may be enough to restore normal temperature.

- *Use warmed intravenous fluids, heating pads or heating blankets, and/or warm baths,* in addition, for patients with a temperature below 86°F (30°C).

- *Rewarm a patient who is severely hypothermic gradually* to prevent complications, such as shock or dysrhythmias (abnormal heartbeats) and to ensure core, as well as surface, warming.

Focused assessments include the following:

- *Monitor the temperature and other VS frequently.* Hypothermia causes vasoconstriction, coagulation

in the microcirculation and tissue **ischemia** (lack of oxygen). In the heart, this can lead to dysrhythmias.

- *Observe for the following symptoms of hypothermia:*
  Body temperature below 96.8°F (36°C)
  Decreased or irregular pulse, respirations, and blood pressure
  A subjective feeling of being cold
  Severe shivering (only initially)
  Pale, cool, shiny skin
  Decreased urine output
  Disorientation and/or drowsiness

 CriticalThinking 17–3

Recall the clients you encountered at the community health fair. Two-year-old Jason's axillary temperature was 101.8°F (38.8°C); his skin was warm, dry, and flushed. His mother told you that he had been eating poorly and was very irritable.

- What changes in behavior alert you to know that something is wrong?
- Do you have enough theoretical knowledge or patient information to know what is going on?
- What, if any, additional information about the patient situation do you need?

PULSE

The **pulse** is the rhythmic expansion of an artery produced when a bolus of blood is forced into it by contraction of the heart.

Theoretical Knowledge
knowing why

To assess and support regulation of a client's pulse, you will need to know the normal pulse range, how the pulse is produced and regulated, and factors that influence pulse rate.

What Is a Normal Pulse Rate?

Pulse rate is measured in beats per minute (bpm). The normal range for healthy young and middle-aged adults is 60 to 100 bpm, with an average rate of 70 to 80 bpm. Table 17–1 identifies average pulse rates for adults. For average pulse rates for other age groups,

 Go to Chapter 17, **Tables, Boxes, Figures: ESG Table 17–1,** on the Electronic Study Guide.

When the heart rate is of concern, you will most likely use a cardiac monitor to determine not only the rate, but also the rhythm and pattern of the pulse. An important reason to assess the pulse is to identify when more advanced monitoring is required.

How Does the Body Produce and Regulate the Pulse?

The pulse wave begins when the left heart ventricle contracts and ends when it relaxes. Each contraction forces blood into the already filled aorta, increasing pressure within the arterial system. The intermittent pressure and expansion of the arteries causes the blood to move along in a wavelike motion toward the capillaries. You can palpate a light tap at the peak of the wave, when the artery expands. The trough of a pulse wave occurs when the artery contracts to push the blood along its way. The peak of the wave corresponds to **systole,** or the contraction of the heart; the trough corresponds to **diastole,** or the resting phase of the heart.

Stroke volume is the quantity of blood forced out by each contraction of the left ventricle. You will not usually know your patient's actual stroke volume, though it averages 70 mL in most healthy adults. If stroke volume decreases (as in a large blood loss, or *hemorrhage*), the body tries to maintain the same cardiac output by increasing the pulse rate. The **cardiac output** is the total quantity of blood pumped per minute. It is expressed in liters per minute and calculated as follows:

Cardiac output = stroke volume × pulse (heart) rate

For a person with a pulse of 80 bpm and an average stroke volume (70 mL), the cardiac output would be about 5600 mL (or 5.6 liters) per minute.

The pulse rate is regulated by the autonomic nervous system. Sympathetic stimulation increases the heart rate (and thus the cardiac output); parasympathetic stimulation decreases it. We'll discuss this in more detail in Chapter 35.

What Factors Influence the Pulse Rate?

In a healthy adult, the pulse rate is the same as the heart rate. Therefore, taking the pulse is a quick and simple way to assess the condition of the heart, blood vessels, and circulation. The pulse changes in response to changes in the volume of blood pumped through the heart, variations in heart rate, changes in the elasticity of the arterial walls, or any condition that interferes with the functioning of the heart. Because the heart and blood vessels are regulated by the nervous system, conditions that interfere with normal functioning of the nervous system also affect the pulse. Other factors that may cause variations in pulse rate, rhythm, or quality include the following:

- *Age.* Newborns have a rapid pulse rate. The rate stabilizes in childhood and gradually slows through old age.

 Go to Chapter 17, **Tables, Boxes, Figures: ESG Table 17–1,** on the Electronic Study Guide.

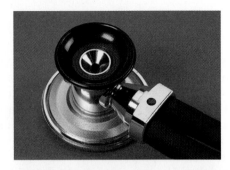

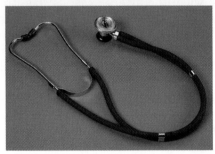

FIGURE 17–5 A stethoscope. Top, Use the bell when listening for low-frequency sounds, such as certain heart sounds. Bottom, Use the diaphragm when listening for high-frequency sounds, such as the blood pressure and lungs.

- *Sex.* Adult females have a slightly more rapid pulse rate than do adult males.
- *Exercise.* Increased muscle activity normally increases the pulse rate. After exercise, a well-conditioned heart returns to normal more quickly than a nonconditioned heart. Also, people who exercise regularly and are well conditioned have lower heart rates, both before and during exercise, than those who do not.
- *Food.* Ingestion of food causes a slight increase in pulse rate for several hours.
- *Stress.* Stress triggers the fight-or-flight sympathetic nervous system response, which increases both pulse rate and strength of the heart contractions (stroke volume).
- *Fever.* The pulse rate tends to increase about 10 bpm for each degree of temperature elevation. The reasons are that (1) the metabolic rate increases and (2) the body attempts to compensate for the decrease in blood pressure produced by the peripheral vasodilation that occurs with fever.
- *Disease.* For example, heart disease, hyperthyroidism, respiratory diseases and infections are generally associated with increased pulse rates. Hypothyroidism is associated with decreased pulse rates.
- *Blood loss.* Small blood losses are generally well tolerated and produce only temporary increases in pulse rates. Theoretically, a large blood loss stimulates the sympathetic nervous system, bringing about an increase in pulse rate to compensate for the decreased blood volume. However, some studies suggest that VS are limited in their ability to detect large blood losses; stable pulse and blood pressure do not, by themselves, guarantee that there has been no blood loss.

- *Position changes.* Standing and sitting positions generally cause a temporary increase in pulse rate and decrease in blood pressure as a result of blood pooling in the veins of the feet and legs. This decreases blood return to the heart, decreasing blood pressure and subsequently increasing heart rate.
- *Medications.* Stimulant drugs (e.g., epinephrine) increase pulse rate. Cardiotonics (e.g., digitalis) and opioids (e.g., narcotic analgesics) or sedative drugs decrease pulse rate.

Practical Knowledge
knowing how

Now that you understand some of the processes and factors that produce and affect the pulse, you are ready to gain the practical knowledge of how to assess and support this aspect of physical functioning.

| Assessment |

You will assess the pulse by **palpation** (feeling) or **auscultation** (listening with a stethoscope). To palpate the pulse, select the pulse site and lightly compress the client's artery against the underlying bone with the index and middle finger of one of your hands. When a client's pulse is difficult to palpate, you may need to use a Doppler device, which has an ultrasound transducer that transmits the pulse sounds to an audio unit. For the sequence of steps in assessing a client's peripheral pulse,

 Go to Chapter 17, **Procedure 17–2: Assessing Peripheral Pulses,** in Volume 2.

The Critical Aspects box summarizes the steps.

What Equipment Do I Need?

To count the pulse, you will need a watch with a second hand or digital display. To auscultate the pulse, you will need a stethoscope. A **stethoscope** consists of a sound-transmitting device (bell and diaphragm) that is attached to earpieces by rubber tubing and hollow metal tubes (Figure 17–5). The stethoscope does not magnify sounds, but rather blocks out noise so that you can hear blood pressure and other faint sounds. With the earpieces in place, you can use the bell to hear low-frequency sounds (e.g., certain heart sounds). Use the diaphragm to assess high-frequency sounds (e.g., lung sounds). Using the bell will enable

you to hear blood pressure sounds more accurately, especially at diastolic pressures (Perloff, as cited in AHA, 2002, p.1). However, most people use the diaphragm because it is easily placed and because some stethoscopes do not have a bell.

What Sites Should I Use?

Nurses assess the pulse at the apex of the heart (**apical pulse**) or at a place where an artery can be pressed by the fingers against a bone (**peripheral pulses**). Peripheral sites are shown in Figure 17–6 and include the radial, brachial, dorsalis pedis, posterior tibial, carotid, femoral, popliteal, and temporal arteries.

The choice of pulse sites depends on the reason for assessing the pulse and/or the accessibility of a site. To measure a peripheral pulse, you would, for example, use the:

- *Radial artery* for routine assessment of vital signs. This is the most commonly used site because it is easily found and readily accessible.
- *Brachial artery* when performing cardiopulmonary resuscitation (CPR) of infants.
- *Carotid artery* when performing CPR of adults and for assessing circulation to the brain.
- *Femoral artery* for infants and children, to determine circulation to the legs, and in cases of cardiac arrest.
- *Dorsalis pedis* (also called *pedal pulse*) and *posterior tibial arteries* for assessing peripheral circulation.
- *Popliteal artery* for assessing circulation to the lower leg.

 CriticalThinking 17–4
- If you obtain a very slow radial pulse, how might you check to be sure your count is accurate?
- What kind of nursing knowledge does this require (i.e., theoretical, practical, self, or ethical knowledge)?

When Should I Take an Apical Pulse?

The apical pulse is the most accurate of the pulses. In a healthy person, the apical and peripheral pulses should be about the same. However, in some cardiovascular diseases, they can differ. If the heartbeat is weak, for example, some beats may be too weak to be felt in a peripheral site. In this case, you would obtain a lower count for the radial pulse than for the apical pulse. The apical pulse would accurately reflect the heartbeat. Use the apical site when:

- The radial pulse is weak or irregular.
- The rate is less than 60 bpm or higher than 100 bpm.
- The patient is taking cardiac medications (e.g., digitalis).

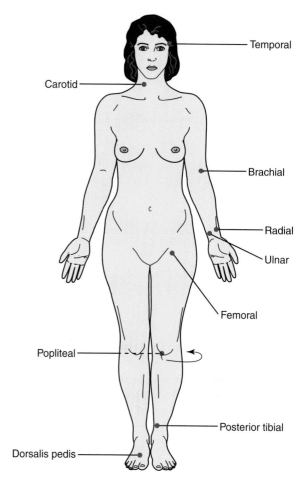

FIGURE 17–6 Sites commonly used for assessing a pulse.

- Assessing infants and children up to age 3 (because peripheral pulses may be difficult to palpate).

To assess the apical pulse, auscultate and count the number of heartbeats at the apex of the heart. For an adult, this site is on the anterior chest at 3 inches (8 cm) or less to the left of the sternum, at the 4th, 5th, or 6th intercostal space at the midclavicular line. For children, the location is different, depending on age (Figure 17–7). You will hear two sounds, "lub" and "dub," as the heart valves close. Count each pair of sounds ("lub-dub") as one heartbeat. For step-by-step instructions,

 Go to Chapter 17, **Procedure 17–3: Assessing the Apical Pulse,** in Volume 2.

See also the Critical Aspects box for a summary.

When Should I Take an Apical-Radial Pulse?

You will sometimes need to obtain a radial and apical pulse at the same time to assess for heart function or the presence of heart irregularities. A difference between the two counts (**pulse deficit**) indicates that not all apex beats are being transmitted or felt at the

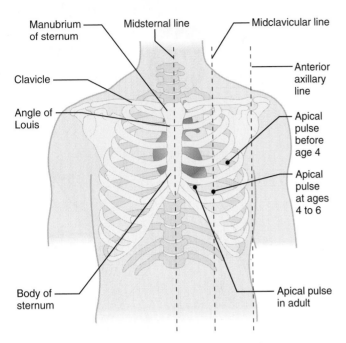

Manubrium of sternum
Midsternal line
Midclavicular line
Clavicle
Anterior axillary line
Angle of Louis
Apical pulse before age 4
Apical pulse at ages 4 to 6
Body of sternum
Apical pulse in adult

FIGURE 17–7 Location of apical pulse for adults and children.

radial artery. As you are listening at the apical site, you will hear a beat without feeling a pulse at the radial artery. You should report pulse deficits promptly to the primary care provider.

 Go to Chapter 17, **Procedure 17-4: Assessing for an Apical-Radial Pulse Deficit,** in Volume 2.

Also see the Critical Aspects box.

KnowledgeCheck 17–2

For each of the following, would you expect the pulse rate to be greater or less than the normal adult rate of 80 bpm?

- A healthy, professional tennis player
- A newborn infant
- An adolescent who has just finished running track
- A client who has just undergone a painful procedure
- A client with a fever
- An accident victim who is hemorrhaging
- A 90-year-old male

 Go to Chapter 17, **Knowledge Check Response Sheet and Answers,** on the Electronic Study Guide.

What Data Should I Collect?

Consider the following data, which a nurse has documented for several patients:

Patient A: Radial pulse 80 bpm, strong, regular, and equal bilaterally (the same in both arms).
Patient B: Pedal pulse 96 bpm, regular, moderate volume, but stronger in the left ankle.
Patient C: Brachial pulse 86 bpm, slightly irregular; skips about every fifth beat; weak but stronger in left arm.

Patient D: Apical pulse 60 bpm, slightly irregular; heart sounds clearly auscultated.
Patient E: Radial pulse 92 bpm, irregular—beats in triplets—weak, equal bilaterally.

What types of information has the nurse gathered about these patients' pulses? (At least three different characteristics of the pulse are represented in the nurse's charting; look for patterns.)

Did you see that for each patient the nurse recorded the rate, rhythm (or pattern), and quality (or volume) of the pulse? If so, well done. Notice also that the nurse compared each patient's left side to the right side.

Rate

To assess the pulse **rate,** count the number of beats per minute while palpating or auscultating. Begin the count with one, rather than zero (Hwu, Coates, & Lin, 2000). You can determine the rate of a regular heart rhythm by counting the pulse for 15 seconds and multiplying by 4. If the pulse is irregular or slow, count for a full minute. Rates below 60 bpm are known as **bradycardia** (*brady* = slow, *cardia* = heart). Rates in excess of 100 bpm are known as **tachycardia** (*tachy* = rapid, *cardia* = heart).

Rhythm

The intervals between heartbeats establish a pulse pattern known as the **rhythm.** Normally, the heart beats at regular intervals, much like a metronome. When the intervals between beats vary enough to be noticeable, the rhythm is abnormal (**dysrhythmia.** Abnormal rhythms may be single beats that occur too early or too late, or a group of irregular beats that form a pattern. When you are assessing an irregular pulse, it is important to determine whether the beat is *regularly irregular* (an irregular rhythm that forms a pattern) or *irregularly irregular* (an unpredictable rhythm). To make this distinction, you must count the rate for a full minute. An irregular heart rhythm can be very serious and may require additional assessment by **electrocardiogram (ECG),** a procedure that traces the electrical pattern of the heart.

Quality

The **quality** of the pulse is assessed by determining the pulse volume and bilateral (both sides) equality of pulses. **Pulse volume** refers to the amount of force produced by the blood pulsing through the arteries. Normally, the pulse volume for each beat is the same. The following terminology refers to pulse volume; numbers are assigned on a scale of 0 to 3.

0—Absent: pulse cannot be felt.
1—Weak or thready: pulse is barely felt and can be easily obliterated by pressing with the fingers.

2—Normal quality: easily palpated, not weak or bounding.

3—Bounding or full: easily felt with little pressure; not easily obliterated.

Bilateral equality is useful in determining whether the blood flow to a body part is adequate. Assess bilateral equality by comparing the pulses on both sides of the body for equal volume. For example, if you are concerned about the circulation to the left hand, assess both the right and left radial arteries to determine whether the volume is the same. If the pulses feel the same, they are said to be *equal bilaterally*. If one pulse is stronger than the other, then the pulses are *unequal bilaterally*. You would record, "Radial pulses unequal bilaterally; weaker in left arm." You may also comment on equality by using a pulse volume scale. For example, you might record, "Radial pulses unequal bilaterally; Right +2, Left +1."

If a peripheral pulse is absent or weak, the reason may be that the circulation is compromised in that extremity. If this is the case, then pallor or cyanosis may be present. **Pallor** refers to the paleness of skin when compared to another part of the body. **Cyanosis** is a bluish or grayish discoloration of the skin due to excessive carbon dioxide and deficient oxygen in the blood. For example, when circulation to the lower extremities is compromised, the feet often appear pale in comparison to the trunk or arms, the dorsalis pedis and/or posterior tibial pulses may be weak or absent, and the feet may feel cool to the touch.

Nursing Diagnosis

An abnormal pulse may present as weak, thready, bounding, dysrhythmic, or absent. Pulse changes are symptoms, not problems. Therefore, nursing diagnoses are useful for describing the condition that is *causing* the pulse changes. Note that by itself, a change in pulse (e.g., a dysrhythmia) is not adequate to support the following diagnoses. Other symptoms must also be present.

- Ineffective Tissue Perfusion (Peripheral) can be used when a pulse is absent or weak and cool, pale skin is present.
- Risk for Impaired Skin Integrity and Risk for Impaired Tissue Integrity may be used as secondary diagnoses when Ineffective Tissue Perfusion is present. If tissue is not adequately perfused, tissue ischemia and necrosis (death of tissue) may occur.
- Deficient Fluid Volume may cause the pulse to be weak and thready.
- Excess Fluid Volume may cause the pulse to be bounding and full.
- Decreased Cardiac Output may cause tachycardia, bradycardia, or changes in pulse volume.

Planning Outcomes/Evaluation

NOC standardized outcomes include the following:

- Vital Signs Status is the only outcome that directly pertains to assessing the pulse.
- Other outcomes depend upon the nursing diagnosis causing the pulse changes. For example, Ineffective Peripheral Tissue Perfusion can be monitored with the NOC label of Circulation Status.

Some *individualized goal/outcome statements* you might write for pulse status follow:

- Apical pulse will be 60 to 80 bpm when at rest.
- Pedal pulses will be 80 to 100 bpm, 2 (on a scale of 0–3), and equal bilaterally.

Planning Interventions/Implementation

NIC standardized interventions include the following:

- Dysrhythmia Management, which applies to monitoring an abnormal pulse
- Vital Signs Monitoring, which may be used for general evaluation of clients who do not have an identified problem with the pulse

 Go to Chapter 17, **Standardized Language,** in Volume 2.

Specific nursing activities and focused assessments for a patient with a dysrhythmia depend on the cause of the dysrhythmia and on specific orders from the physician. For example, a client with a pulse rate of 50 bpm is usually considered to have bradycardia. However, such a slow resting heart rate would be perfectly normal for a well-trained athlete. Some dysrhythmias are *benign;* that is, they are not dangerous to the client, and they require no interventions. Nursing strategies that address dysrhythmias, regardless of cause, include the following:

- *Focused assessments:*

    Closely monitor the patient's vital signs. A reduced heart rate may alter blood pressure and tissue perfusion. The extent of intervention depends on the effect of the dysrhythmia on the client's other vital signs.

    Monitor the patient's activity tolerance. Degree of activity, orientation, and level of fatigue while the dysrhythmia is present are indicators of the patient's ability to tolerate the dysrhythmia.

    Collect and assess laboratory data as ordered. Cardiac function depends on normal electrolyte balance, particularly potassium, calcium, and magnesium levels. If a client is receiving medications that affect cardiac rhythm, serum levels of these medications must be checked periodically.

- *Help determine the cause of the dysrhythmia.* Determine when the client experiences the dysrhythmia. Are there precipitating or alleviating factors?
- *Administer antidysrhythmic medications (if ordered)* at regular intervals to control the heart rhythm.
- *Provide emotional support.* The client experiencing a dysrhythmia may be frightened by the experience. Explain all procedures to the client, and maintain a calm presence. Family members may also be frightened. Be sure to include them in your explanations and teaching.

CriticalThinking 17–5

- Which of the following findings should be referred to the primary healthcare provider so that an ECG can be ordered? Why?

    Patient A, who has a radial pulse of 100 bpm, regular, and equal bilaterally

    Patient B, who has a regular apical pulse of 100 bpm

    Patient C, who has a very irregular apical pulse of 78 bpm

- Recall the clients you encountered at the community health fair. Ms Sharma is an active 80-year-old woman who works part time and exercises four times per week. She is complaining of feeling tired. You find that her pulse is irregular and uneven.

    What other patient data do you need to know? How would you go about getting this additional information?

    What actions should you consider taking while meeting with Ms Sharma?

    What theoretical knowledge (rationale) supports your beliefs and actions?

RESPIRATION

Respiration is the exchange of oxygen and carbon dioxide in the body. The process of respiration consists of two separate functions: mechanical and chemical. The mechanical aspects of respirations involve the active movement of air into and out of the respiratory system. This is known as **pulmonary ventilation** or, more commonly, breathing. The chemical aspects of respiration include the exchange of oxygen and carbon dioxide between the alveoli and the pulmonary blood supply **(external respiration),** the transport of these gases throughout the body **(gas transport),** and the exchange of these gases between the capillaries and body tissue cells **(internal respiration).** This chapter will focus on the mechanical aspects of respiration. Chapter 35 will explore gas exchange and transport throughout the body.

Theoretical Knowledge
knowing why

To assess and support clients' respirations, you will need to know the normal range of respiratory rates, how respiration is regulated, the mechanics of breathing, and factors that affect respiration.

What Is a Normal Respiratory Rate?

Like temperature and pulse, respiratory rate normally varies with age, exertion, emotions, and other factors discussed shortly. Normal adult respirations are identified in Table 17–1 on page 306. For normal respiratory rates at other developmental stages,

 Go to Chapter 17, **Tables, Boxes, Figures: ESG Table 17–1,** on the Electronic Study Guide.

How Does the Body Regulate Respiration?

Special respiratory centers in the medulla oblongata and pons of the brain, along with nerve fibers of the autonomic nervous system, regulate breathing in response to minute changes in the concentrations of oxygen (O_2) and carbon dioxide (CO_2) in the arterial blood. The primary stimulus for breathing is the level of CO_2 tension in the blood. **Central chemoreceptors,** located in the respiratory centers, are sensitive to CO_2 and hydrogen ion (pH) concentrations. Minor increases in either stimulate respirations. When the partial pressure of oxygen in arterial blood (PaO_2) falls below 100 mm Hg (normal), **peripheral chemoreceptors** in the carotid and aortic bodies stimulate respirations.

Normally breathing is an involuntary action that requires little effort. However, it is possible to exert conscious control over respiration through breath holding. For example, a young child who holds his breath during a temper tantrum is exerting conscious control over breathing. Swimming also involves conscious control of breathing. A swimmer can resume respiration through conscious control, or, if the swimmer collapses, the autonomic nervous system would resume breathing automatically.

Mechanics of Breathing

Pulmonary ventilation depends on changes in the capacity of the chest cavity (Figure 17–8). In response to impulses sent from the respiratory center along the phrenic nerve, the thoracic muscles and the diaphragm contract. The ribs move upward from midline 1/2 to 1 inch (1.2 to 2.5 cm), the diaphragm moves downward and out about 0.4 inch (1 cm), and the abdominal organs move downward and forward, expanding the thorax in all directions. As expansion causes airway

pressure to decrease below atmospheric pressure, air moves into the lungs. This stage of respiration (drawing air into the lungs) is termed **inspiration.**

When the diaphragm and thoracic muscles relax, the chest cavity decreases in size, and the lungs recoil, forcing air from the lungs until the pressure within the lungs again reaches atmospheric pressure. This stage, which involves the expelling of air from the lungs, is called **expiration.** Expiration is passive and normally takes 2 to 3 seconds, compared to 1 to 1.5 seconds for inspiration. During normal breathing, you can observe the chest wall and the abdomen gently rising and falling.

KnowledgeCheck 17–3

- What two gases are exchanged through respiration?
- Which respiratory process involves the movement of air into and out of the lungs?
- What is external respiration?
- What is the primary stimulus for breathing?
- What mechanical forces allow the lungs to expand?

 Go to Chapter 17, **Knowledge Check Response Sheet and Answers,** on the Electronic Study Guide.

What Factors Influence Respiration?

To interpret the meaning of your clients' respiratory data, you need to be aware of some factors that influence breathing.

- *Age.* A newborn's respiratory rate ranges from 40 to 90 breaths per minute. As a child ages, the rate gradually decreases until it reaches the normal adult rate of 12 to 20 breaths per minute. The respiratory rate decreases slightly in older adults.

 Go to Chapter 17, **Tables, Boxes, Figures: ESG Table 17–1,** on the Electronic Study Guide.

- *Exercise.* Muscular activity causes a temporary increase in respiratory rate and depth so as to increase oxygen availability to the tissue and to rid the body of excess carbon dioxide.
- *Pain.* Acute pain causes an increase in respiratory rate but a decrease in depth.
- *Stress.* Psychological stress, such as anxiety or fear, may markedly influence respiration. The most common change is an increase in rate.
- *Smoking.* Chronic smoking increases resting respiratory rate as a result of changes in airway compliance (elasticity).
- *Fever.* When heart rate increases because of fever, respiratory rate also increases. For every 1°F (0.6°C) the temperature rises, the respiratory rate may increase up to 4 breaths per minute.
- *Pulse rate.* If a client's pulse rate increases, the respiratory rate usually also shows an increase. The usual ratio of respiratory rate to pulse rate is approximately

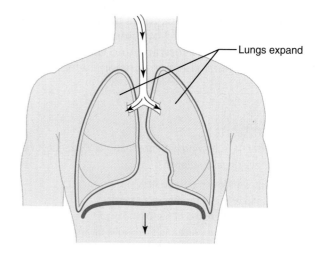

(a) During inspiration (diaphragm contracting)

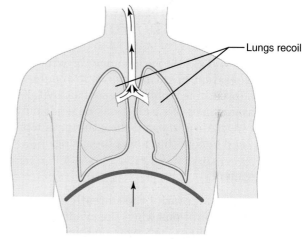

(b) During expiration (diaphragm relaxing)

FIGURE 17–8 Changes in thoracic cavity during inspiration and expiration. A, During inspiration. B, During expiration.

1:4. Thus, a client with a respiratory rate of 16 would be expected to have a pulse rate of at least 64.

- *Hemoglobin.* Respiratory rate and depth increase as a result of anemia (reduced hemoglobin), sickle cell anemia (abnormally shaped red blood cells), and high altitudes. To maintain adequate oxygenation to the tissue in spite of a decreased amount of hemoglobin or an abnormality in hemoglobin, the rate and depth of respirations, as well as the heart rate, may be increased. High altitudes inhibit the binding of oxygen to hemoglobin and trigger similar compensation efforts.
- *Disease.* The rate of breathing may be increased or decreased by various diseases. For example, brain stem injuries and increased intracranial pressure may interfere with the respiratory center, inhibiting respirations or altering respiratory rhythm.
- *Medications.* Central nervous system depressants, such as morphine or general anesthetics, cause slower, deeper respirations. Caffeine and atropine can cause shallow, fast breathing.

• *Position.* Respiratory depth is maximized by standing up and is hampered by lying flat. Slumping (sitting with shoulders forward, and the back curved in a "C") prevents chest expansion, which impedes breathing.

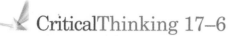 CriticalThinking 17–6

Consider the following patient situations. What effect would they have on respirations?

• A client with four fractured ribs.
• A woman who is 9 months pregnant.
• A young child excited at her birthday party.
• An adult who has consumed alcoholic beverages.

Practical Knowledge
knowing how

Although you will assess the adequacy of external and internal respiration in various ways, it is pulmonary ventilation (breathing) that you assess as a vital sign. Accurate assessment of respirations depends on your ability to recognize normal breathing, abnormal breathing, and factors that affect breathing.

| Assessment |

Because people can control their breathing rate, it is best to count respirations when the client is unaware of what you are doing. One way to do this is to palpate and count the radial pulse, and then count the respirations before removing your fingers from the client's wrist. For the sequence of steps,

 Go to Chapter 17, **Procedure 17-5: Assessing Respirations,** in Volume 2.

The Critical Aspects box summarizes the procedure.

What Equipment Do I Need?

The only equipment you need for measuring respiratory rate is a watch with a second hand or digital display. You will need a stethoscope if you decide to auscultate respirations. Many electronic thermometers have counter displays and signals that indicate 15-, 30-, and 60-second time intervals for counting respirations.

What Data Should I Collect?

In addition to measuring the rate of respirations, you will also observe several other indicators of overall respiratory function, including depth, rhythm, effort,

and others. For additional information on respiratory assessment,

 Go to Chapter 19, **Procedure 19-12: Assessing the Chest and Lungs,** in Volume 2.

See also Chapter 19 in this volume.

Rate

The number of times a person breathes (or completes a cycle of inhalation and exhalation) within a full minute is the **respiratory rate.** You can easily count and observe respirations by:

• Placing your hand on the client's chest (palpation) or observing (inspection) the number of times the client's chest or abdomen rises (inspiration) and falls (expiration).
• Placing your stethoscope on the client's chest (auscultation) and counting the number of inhalation and exhalation cycles.

Whether auscultating the rate or measuring by palpation or observation, you should count for a full minute to ensure accuracy ("Vital Signs," 1999). If respirations vary from normal, you should count for a full minute by auscultation.

A person can tolerate **apnea,** cessation of breathing, for only a few minutes. If apnea continues for more than 4 to 6 minutes, brain damage and even death can occur. An abnormally slow respiratory rate is called **bradypnea. Tachypnea** (also called *polypnea*) is abnormally fast breathing. **Eupnea** is the term used for people who have respirations that fall within normal parameters (Table 17–2). The respiratory rate is an important measure of the client's general condition, but rate alone is not a good indicator of the adequacy of respiration. You must also assess other characteristics of the respirations.

Depth

Tidal volume is the amount of air taken in on inspiration—about 300 to 500 mL for a healthy adult. Specialized equipment is required to measure tidal volume. However, you can estimate the adequacy of tidal volume by observing the depth of a client's respirations. This is a subjective evaluation of how much or how little the chest or abdomen rises during breathing. Respiratory depth is described as *deep* (taking in a very large volume of air and fully expanding one's chest or abdomen), *shallow* (when the chest barely rises and is difficult to observe), or *normal* (falling between shallow and deep).

Rhythm

Rhythm is assessed simply as *normal* or *abnormal.* Generally, the period between each respiratory cycle is the same, and there is a regular breathing pattern (see

TABLE 17-2	Respiratory Rates and Rhythms	

Type	Description	Illustration
Eupnea	Normal respirations, with equal rate and depth, 12–20 breaths per minute	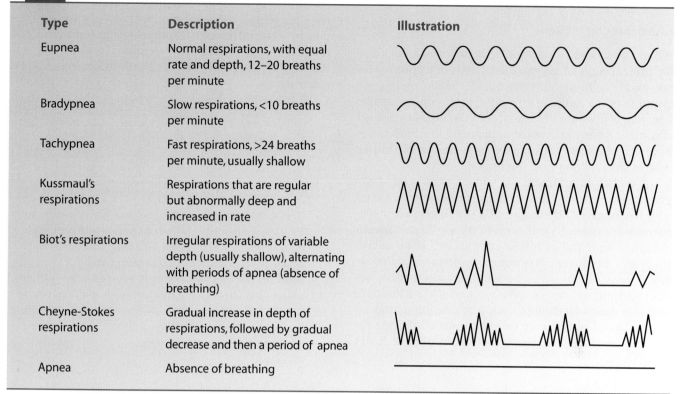
Bradypnea	Slow respirations, <10 breaths per minute	
Tachypnea	Fast respirations, >24 breaths per minute, usually shallow	
Kussmaul's respirations	Respirations that are regular but abnormally deep and increased in rate	
Biot's respirations	Irregular respirations of variable depth (usually shallow), alternating with periods of apnea (absence of breathing)	
Cheyne-Stokes respirations	Gradual increase in depth of respirations, followed by gradual decrease and then a period of apnea	
Apnea	Absence of breathing	

Table 17–2). Infant breathing rhythms are more likely to be irregular than adult rhythms. An abnormal breathing pattern may be an indicator of other health care problems and deserves further assessment. Two abnormal breathing patterns, Cheyne-Stokes and Biot's breathing, are discussed in Chapter 35.

Effort

Respiratory effort refers to the degree of work required to breathe. Normal breathing should be effortless. When diseases such as asthma or pneumonia are present, the person must work harder to breathe. Increased effort with breathing is called **dyspnea** or labored breathing. It is uncomfortable for the client and frequently produces fatigue and fear. **Orthopnea** is the inability to breathe when the person is in a horizontal position. As discussed in Chapter 35, you will observe this in some clients with respiratory or cardiac conditions.

Breath Sounds

You will use a stethoscope to listen for breath sounds. Normal respirations are quiet. Abnormal sounds include the following.

- **Wheezes** are high-pitched, continuous musical sounds, usually heard on expiration. Wheezes are caused by narrowing of the airways.

- **Rhonchi** are low-pitched, continuous sounds caused by secretions in the large airways. They often clear with coughing.

- **Crackles** are discontinuous sounds usually heard on inspiration, but they may be heard throughout the respiratory cycle. They may be high-pitched, popping sounds or low-pitched, bubbling sounds.

- **Stridor** is a piercing, high-pitched sound that is primarily heard during inspiration in infants who are experiencing respiratory distress.

- **Stertor** refers to labored breathing that produces a snoring sound.

See Chapter 19 for further discussion of abnormal breath sounds. To listen to the sounds,

 Go to **Sound File, Breath Sounds,** on the Electronic Study Guide.

Chest and Abdomen Movement

The chest or abdomen normally rises with inspiration and falls with expiration in a gentle and rhythmic pattern. When a person is having difficulty moving air into or out of the lungs, respiratory patterns change. **Intercostal retraction** refers to the visible sinking of tissues around and between the ribs that occurs when the person needs to make additional effort to breathe. **Substernal retraction** exists when tissues

are drawn in beneath the sternum (breastbone), and **suprasternal retraction** exists when tissues are drawn in above the clavicle (shoulder girdle).

Associated Clinical Signs

When you assess respiration, it is important to assess for clinical signs of oxygenation. Signs of **hypoxia** (inadequate cellular oxygenation) include pallor or cyanosis of the nails, lips, or skin; restlessness; apprehension; confusion; dizziness; fatigue; decreased level of consciousness; tachycardia; tachypnea; and changes in blood pressure. Chronic hypoxia causes **clubbing** (loss of the nail angle) of the fingers.

A **cough** is a forceful or violent expulsion of air during expiration. Coughs may be *constant* (occurring frequently and consistently) or *intermittent* (occurring occasionally). If secretions are expectorated (coughed up), the cough is *productive*. If no secretions are produced, the cough is *nonproductive* or *dry*. A *hacking cough* is a series of dry coughs that occur together, whereas a *whooping cough* is a sudden, periodic cough that ends with a whooping sound on inspiration. Coughs may be symptoms of allergic reactions, lung disease, respiratory infection, or heart conditions.

KnowledgeCheck 17–4

- How can you estimate a client's tidal volume?
- What is the range of normal for an adult's respiratory rate?
- Besides the rate, what other characteristics of a client's respirations should you observe?
- What are some common clinical signs associated with poor oxygenation?

Go to Chapter 17, **Knowledge Check Response Sheet and Answers,** on the Electronic Study Guide.

Arterial Oxygen Saturation

The rate, quality, and depth of the respirations are indicators of the general health of the respiratory system. However, they do not measure the amounts of oxygen and carbon dioxide present in the blood—information that is essential for evaluating the effectiveness of respiratory effort. Two methods exist to measure O_2 and CO_2 blood levels. One method is invasive; the other is not.

Arterial Blood Gas Sampling

Arterial blood gas (ABG) sampling directly measures the partial pressures of oxygen and carbon dioxide and blood pH, in other words, the gases in the arterial blood. This method requires the puncture of an artery followed by laboratory testing of the sample. It provides comprehensive data, but it is invasive, time-consuming, and relatively expensive.

Pulse Oximetry

A noninvasive method of monitoring respiratory status involves the use of a **pulse oximeter,** a device that measures **oxygen saturation** (amount of oxygen in arterial blood). A photosensor placed on the client's finger or earlobe calculates a pulse saturation (SpO_2) that is a good estimate of arterial oxygen saturation.

For the procedure for performing pulse oximetry,

 Go to Chapter 35, **Procedure 35–2: Pulse Oximetry Monitoring,** in Volume 2.

 ## CriticalThinking 17–7

- Mrs. Dowell has smoked two packs of cigarettes per day for 45 years. She has recently been diagnosed with pneumonia—an infection of the lungs. What vital sign assessments would be important for Mrs. Dowell, and why?
- Recall the clients you encountered in the community health fair scenario. Mr. Jackson is short of breath and struggling to breathe. His respiratory rate is 28. What else do you need to know about the patient situation? What is important and what is not important in this scenario? What is probably least important?

What Are Some Alterations in Respiration?

As noted earlier, *hypoxia* refers to inadequate cellular oxygenation. It results from decreased oxygen intake, decreased ability of tissues to remove oxygen from blood, impaired ventilation or perfusion, impaired gas exchange between the blood and alveoli, or inadequate levels of hemoglobin.

Hyperventilation occurs when rapid and deep breathing result in excess loss of CO_2 (*hypocapnia*). Causes of hyperventilation include anxiety, infection, shock, hypoxia, drugs (aspirin, amphetamines), diabetes mellitus, or acid-base imbalance. A client who is hyperventilating may complain of feeling lightheaded and tingly.

Hypoventilation occurs when the rate and depth of respirations are decreased and CO_2 is retained or alveolar ventilation is compromised. Hypoventilation may be related to chronic obstructive pulmonary disease (COPD), general anesthesia, or other conditions that result in decreased respirations.

This chapter discusses only assessment of respirations. For nursing diagnoses, outcomes, and interventions for respiratory problems, see Chapter 35.

BLOOD PRESSURE

Blood pressure (BP), an important indicator of overall cardiovascular health, is the pressure of the blood as it is forced against arterial walls during cardiac contraction. **Systolic pressure** is the peak

TABLE 17-3 Classification of Adult Blood Pressure*

Category	Systolic (mm Hg)		Diastolic (mm Hg)	Follow-Up
Normal	<120	and	<80	Encourage lifestyle modification if there are risk factors. Recheck in 1–2 years or sooner if there are risk factors.
Prehypertension	120–139	or	80–89	Encourage lifestyle changes; recheck in 1 year or sooner if indicated. Antihypertensive are pre-scribed only with compelling indications, such as renal disease.
Stage I hypertension	140–159	or	90–99	Encourage lifestyle modification. Follow up with primary care provider in 1–2 months. (Most patients will be started on thiazide-type diuretics.)
Stage II hypertension	≥160	or	≥100	Encourage lifestyle modification. Refer for care within 1 week, or immediately if warranted. (Most patients will be given a two-drug combi-nation therapy, for example, thiazide-type di-uretics with ACE inhibitors.)

*For adults age 18 and older, based on the average of two or more readings taken at each of two or more visits after an initial screening.

Source: Data from the Joint National Committee on Prevention, Detection, Evaluation, and Treatment of High Blood Pressure. (2003). *JNC Express 7: The seventh report of the Joint National Committee on Prevention, Detection, Evaluation, and Treatment of High Blood Pressure.* Bethesda, MD: National Institutes of Health. Retrieved May 22, 2003, from http://www.nhlbi.nih.gov/guidelines/hypertension/index/htm

pressure exerted against arterial walls as the ventri-cles contract and eject blood. **Diastolic pressure** is the minimum pressure exerted against arterial walls, between cardiac contractions when the heart is at rest.

Blood pressure is measured in millimeters of mer-cury (mm Hg) and is recorded as systolic pressure over diastolic pressure (e.g., 120/80 mm Hg). The pulse that can be palpated to determine heart rate is due to the difference between the systolic and diastolic pressures. This difference is known as the **pulse pres-sure.** The pulse pressure for a BP of 120/80 mm Hg is 40 mm Hg. The difference between systolic and dia-stolic pressure is an indication of the volume output of the left ventricle. Generally, the pulse pressure should be no greater than one-third of the systolic pressure, as in the example of a BP of 120/80, with a pulse pres-sure of 40 (1/3 × 120 = 40).

KnowledgeCheck 17–5

- For a client whose BP is 150/80, what is the pulse pressure?
- Is that normal? If so, explain. If not, what should the pulse pressure be?

 Go to Chapter 17, **Knowledge Check Response Sheet and Answers,** on the Electronic Study Guide.

Theoretical Knowledge
knowing why

To assess and support clients' blood pressure, you will need to know what constitutes a normal reading for a client, how the body regulates blood pressure, and what factors affect the blood pressure.

What Is a Normal Blood Pressure Reading?

There is some controversy about what constitutes a normal blood pressure reading. According to the American Heart Association (Perloff et al. (1993), as cited in AHA, 2002), a blood pressure of less than 120 to 129 systolic and less than 80 to 84 diastolic is con-sidered "optimal" for adults (Table 17–3). Up to 130 systolic and 85 diastolic is considered "normal" for adults. More recently, the National High Blood Pres-sure Education Program, an expert panel, has classi-fied "normal" as systolic BP below 120 and diastolic BP below 80 (Joint National Committee on Preven-tion, Detection, Evaluation, and Treatment of High Blood Pressure, 2003).

How Does the Body Regulate Blood Pressure?

Blood pressure regulation is a highly complex process that is influenced by three factors: cardiac function, peripheral vascular resistance, and blood volume. The body constantly regulates and adjusts arterial pressure to supply blood to body tissues via perfusion of the capillary beds. For in-depth discussion, see Chapter 35.

Cardiac Function

Recall that *cardiac output* is the volume of blood pumped by the heart per minute and reflects the functioning of the heart. An increase in cardiac output causes an increase in BP; a decrease in cardiac output causes a decrease in BP (if all other factors remain the same). A change in either stroke volume or heart rate alters cardiac output.

Conditions that *increase* cardiac output by increasing stroke volume include:

- Increased blood volume (as occurs during pregnancy, for example).
- More forceful contraction of the ventricles (as occurs during exercise, for example).

Conditions that *decrease* cardiac output by decreasing stroke volume include:

- Dehydration.
- Active bleeding.
- Damage to the heart (as seen after myocardial infarction, or heart attack).
- A very rapid heart rate. Up to a point, an increase in heart rate increases cardiac output. However, a very rapid heart rate limits the time allotted for the ventricles to fill, resulting in decreased stroke volume and decreased cardiac output.

Peripheral Resistance

Peripheral resistance refers to *arterial* and *capillary* resistance to blood flow as a result of friction between blood and the vessel walls. An increase in peripheral resistance creates a temporary increase in BP. The amount of friction or resistance depends on blood **viscosity** (thickness) and arterial size and **compliance** (elasticity). The walls of the veins are thin and very distensible, so they have little influence on peripheral resistance and BP.

- *Blood viscosity.* Blood viscosity influences the ease with which blood flows through the vessels. Viscosity is determined by the percentage of red blood cells in plasma, or **hematocrit.** Any disorder that increases hematocrit (e.g., dehydration) increases blood viscosity and, therefore, BP. Similarly, a low hematocrit, as seen in anemia, lowers viscosity and may reduce BP.

- *Arterial size and compliance.* The smaller the radius of a blood vessel, the more resistance it offers to blood flow. Constricted arteries prevent the free flow of blood and, subsequently, increase BP. Dilated arteries allow unrestricted flow of blood, thereby reducing blood pressure. The sympathetic nervous system controls vasoconstriction and vasodilation. Arteries with good elasticity can distend and recoil easily and adequately. When age- or disease-related changes in arterial structure cause a loss of elasticity, peripheral resistance and possible BP increase. **Arteriosclerosis** (hardening of the arteries) is a common contributor to increased BP in middle-aged and older adults.

Blood Volume

The normal volume of blood in the body is about 5000 mL. A significant volume decrease, as occurs with hemorrhage or other fluid losses, reduces vascular volume, and BP falls. When vascular volume is increased above the norm, as occurs with renal (kidney) failure, BP increases.

What Factors Influence Blood Pressure?

Blood pressure normally changes from minute to minute with changes in activity or even changes in body position. Therefore, you must establish BP *patterns* rather than relying on individual BP readings when determining whether a client's BP is normal or abnormal. This is even more important for older adults because their BP tends to fluctuate more. The following are some factors that affect the BP.

- *Age.* An average newborn has a BP of about 40 systolic. It increases gradually throughout childhood. A child or adolescent's BP depends on body size; therefore, a smaller child or adolescent has a lower blood pressure than a larger child does. Both systolic and diastolic BP continue to increase with age as a result of decreased arterial compliance. Blood pressures over 140/90 mm Hg are considered hypertensive and require further evaluation. A BP of more than 120 systolic or 80 diastolic is considered prehypertensive.

 Go to Chapter 17, **Tables, Boxes, Figures: ESG Table 17-1,** on the Electronic Study Guide.

- *Sex.* The average BP for men is slightly higher than that for women of comparable age, although the difference is not considered significant. Following menopause, a woman's BP tends to increase, probably due to a decrease in estrogen.

- *Family history.* A family history of hypertension markedly increases the likelihood of an individual's developing hypertension.

- *Lifestyle.* Factors such as increased sodium consumption, smoking, and consumption of three or more alcoholic drinks per day have been shown to elevate BP.

Caffeine may raise BP for a short while after ingestion, but it has no long-term effect on the BP.

- *Exercise.* Participation in a consistent exercise program over time has been shown to reduce BP in many individuals. However, muscular exertion temporarily increases BP as a result of increased heart rate and cardiac output. You should, therefore, wait about 30 minutes before you assess BP for someone who has been physically active.

- *Body position.* BP is higher when a person is standing than when sitting or lying down. Readings are higher if taken with the client's arm above heart level or if the arm is unsupported at the client's side. Seated readings are higher if the client's feet are dangling rather than resting on the floor.

- *Stress.* Fear, worry, excitement, and other stressors cause BP to rise sharply because of sympathetic nervous system stimulation (fight-or-flight response). One example of this is "white-coat hypertension." This occurs when a patient's BP is elevated in the physician's office or clinic—a situation in which he is likely to experience stress—but not at other times.

- *Pain.* Pain often causes the BP to increase. However, severe pain can significantly decrease BP.

- *Race.* African Americans have a higher rate of hypertension than do European Americans, and they have a higher incidence of complications and hypertension-related deaths (McCance & Heuther, 1998).

- *Obesity.* As a rule, obesity increases the BP. This increase is related to the additional vascular supply required to perfuse the large body size and the resultant increase in peripheral resistance.

- *Diurnal variations.* Generally, BP varies according to the person's daily schedules and routines.

- *Medications.* Many medications alter BP. This effect may be intended, as with antihypertensive medications, or unintended, such as the drop in BP that often results when a client receives pain medication. Many over-the-counter preparations, herbal products, and illicit drugs can effect BP.

- *Diseases.* Diseases that affect the circulatory system or any of the major organs of the body (e.g., the kidneys) may affect BP.

CriticalThinking 17–8

- Evaluate the following blood pressures. Are they high, low, or normal?

    116/90

    80/50

    184/102

    140/90

    40/0

- What theoretical knowledge did you use in evaluating the blood pressures?

Practical Knowledge
knowing how

Now that you understand how blood pressure is maintained and regulated, you are ready to gain the practical knowledge of how to assess and support this aspect of physical functioning.

|Assessment|

Blood pressure may be assessed directly or indirectly. As a rule, you will measure BP via the *indirect,* or *noninvasive, method.* This is an accurate estimate of arterial BP that can be performed in any clinical or community setting. In the *direct method,* a catheter is threaded into an artery under sterile conditions and attached to tubing that is connected to an electronic monitoring system. The pressure is constantly displayed as a waveform on the monitor screen. Although this method of measuring BP is very accurate, its use is confined to critical care areas and surgery because of the risk of sudden arterial blood loss.

 VOL 2   Go to Chapter 17, **Procedure 17–6: Measuring Blood Pressure,** in Volume 2.

See also the Critical Aspects box for a summary of the procedure.

What Equipment Do I Need?

You will need a stethoscope, a blood pressure cuff and sphygmomanometer, or an electronic blood pressure monitor to assess blood pressure. A common stethoscope is generally sufficient to hear most clients' blood pressures. When blood pressure is weak, ultrasonic stethoscopes are useful for magnifying sound waves occurring during systole.

A **sphygmomanometer** (Figure 17–9) consists of a vinyl or cloth cuff, a pressure bulb with a regulating valve, and a manometer. Blood pressure cuffs contain an inflatable rubber bladder. The cuff is attached to a gauge or manometer and a valved pressure bulb that inflates the bladder (Figure 17–10). Cuffs can be placed on either the upper arm or midthigh and are supplied in various sizes.

Sphygmomanometers are either aneroid or mercury. **Aneroid** manometers have dials that register BP by pointers attached to a spring (Figure 17–9). **Mercury** manometers measure BP using a calibrated upright tube containing mercury (Figure 17–9). As the bladder of the cuff is inflated, the pressure pushes the column of mercury up the tube. The column of mercury falls as the cuff is deflated. Mercury manometers are not as popular as aneroid manometers because they pose a health hazard if the mercury tube is broken. They are, however, easier to maintain and more

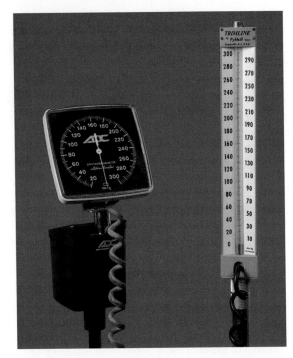

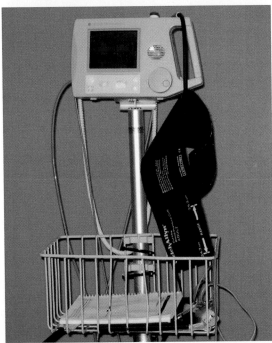

FIGURE 17–9 Types of manometers: top left, aneroid; top right, mercury; bottom, electronic.

accurate than aneroid manometers, which require frequent calibration. Since 1998, the American Hospital Association and the Environmental Protection Agency have recommended that the health care industry eliminate mercury-containing waste by the year 2005 (USEPA, 2002). This would include phasing out mercury manometers.

Electronic blood pressure monitors use either microphones to sense sounds or sensors that detect pressure waves as blood flows through arteries (Figure 17–9). They can be set to monitor and record BP at timed intervals and do not require the use of a stethoscope. They measure systolic, diastolic, and mean arterial pressures. Electronic monitors are useful when you must monitor BP frequently (e.g., during surgery or when a client is critically ill). They are, however, less accurate than auscultated blood pressures, so you should auscultate a baseline BP prior to initiating automatic monitoring.

Many clients use a version of the electronic BP monitor in their homes. These devices can be purchased in grocery stores and pharmacies. They are useful for screening, but clients should seek follow-up care when readings are not within their normal range. The Home Care box on page 332 identifies teaching topics for clients using electronic BP monitors.

What Cuff Size Should I Use?

As shown in Figure 17–11, the *width* of the bladder of a properly fitting cuff will cover approximately two-thirds of the *length* of the upper arm (or other extremity) for an adult, and the entire upper arm for a child (National Institutes of Health, 1996). Alternatively, you can check that (1) the *cuff width* is 20% greater than the diameter of the midpoint of the limb or (2) the *length* of the bladder encircles 80 to 100% of the arm in adults (Joint National Committee, 1997; Perloff et al., 1993).

Using a cuff or bladder of the incorrect size can result in a measurement error of as much as 30 mm Hg. If the cuff is too narrow, you will obtain an erroneously high reading; if it is too wide, the reading will be too low. Although cuffs are manufactured in various sizes, in practice, you will probably have access to only two or three different adult sizes (small adult, adult, large adult, and thigh). If you must use a cuff of the improper

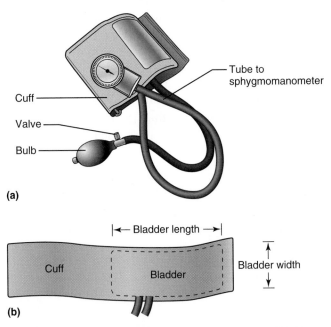

FIGURE 17–10 A blood pressure cuff showing placement of bladder within the cuff.

size, it is better to use one that is too large than one that is too small—be sure to document the cuff size along with the BP reading. Refer to Figure 17–11 and Table 17–4 for information about cuff sizes in centimeters.

Which Site Should I Use?

You will usually use the *brachial artery* for assessing BP. The condition of the client's arm and other factors can interfere with accurate BP measurement, however. Avoid assessing blood pressure in an arm that has an intravenous access device, renal dialysis fistula, or skin graft; that is paralyzed, diseased, or has extensive trauma; that has a cast or dressings; or from an arm on the same side of breast or shoulder surgery. In these and similar instances, you can use the popliteal artery.

 Go to Chapter 17, **Procedure 17-6: Measuring Blood Pressure,** in Volume 2.

Systolic pressure may be 20 to 30 mm Hg higher in the lower extremities than in the arms, but diastolic pressures are similar.

Auscultating Blood Pressure

Blood pressure can be measured indirectly by auscultation or palpation. The preferred, and most commonly used, method is auscultation; however, palpation is useful in certain situations. When auscultating BP, place your stethoscope over an artery, inflate the cuff, and listen for sounds as you deflate the cuff.

As you *inflate* the cuff, the artery is occluded as the pressure of the cuff exceeds the pressure in the artery. At that point, blood flow through the artery is halted, and no sound can be heard. As you *deflate* the cuff, blood begins to flow rapidly through the partially open artery, producing turbulence that you will hear through the stethoscope as a tapping sound.

- *The first sound* you hear is measured on the manometer and recorded as the systolic pressure.
- *The disappearance of sound* defines the diastolic BP. When the artery is no longer compressed, blood flows freely, and no sound is heard.

The sounds you listen for when you assess BP are called **Korotkoff sounds.** These sounds, described by Russian neurologist Nicolai Korotkoff in 1906, are used to describe the sounds of blood pulsating through arteries (Figure 17–12).

1st sound—As you deflate the BP cuff, you will initially hear a sound that occurs during systole. It is a tapping sound that corresponds to the pulse (systolic BP).

2nd sound—Occurs as you further deflate the cuff. It is a soft, swishing sound caused by blood turbulence.

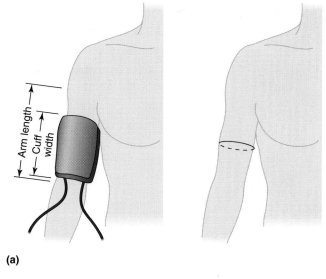

(a)

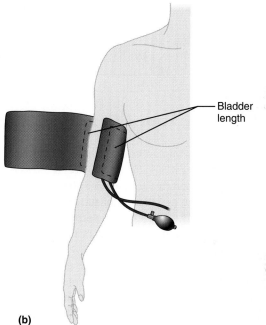

Bladder length

(b)

FIGURE 17–11 Determining correct BP cuff size. *A,* The cuff width should be two-thirds of the length of the upper arm or 20% wider than diameter of the upper arm. *B,* The length of the bladder should encircle 80% of the upper arm.

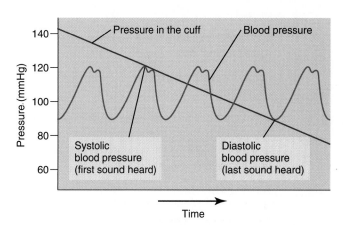

FIGURE 17–12 Relationship of blood pressure to changes in cuff pressure and the first and fifth Korotkoff sounds (BP 120/80).

TABLE 17-4 Blood Pressure Cuffs: Acceptable Bladder Sizes

Cuff Type	Arm Circumference at Midpoint (cm)*	Bladder Width (cm)	Bladder Length (cm)
Newborn	<6	3	6
Infant	6–15	5	15
Child	16–21	8	21
Small adult	22–26	10	24
Adult	27–34	13	30
Large adult	35–44	16	38
Adult thigh	45–52	20	42

*Arm circumference is half the distance from the acromion to the olecranon process. If correct size not available, use next larger (rather than smaller) size.

Used with permission. Sperloff, D., et al. (1993). *Recommendation: Human blood pressure determination by sphygmomanometer.* Copyright © 2002 American Heart Association.

Teaching Your Client Self-Monitoring of Blood Pressure

There are two common, acceptable BP devices available for self-monitoring (finger monitors are inaccurate). One is a portable home device. The client simply pushes a button, and the cuff inflates and deflates automatically. The device has an electronic digital readout, so it does not require use of a stethoscope. Because of the sensitivity of these devices, arm movement or improper cuff placement can cause inaccurate readings. Also, these devices must be recalibrated at least every 6 months. Some grocery stores, fitness clubs, and other public places have stationary automatic BP devices for public use. The person places his arm in the cuff, which fits over his clothing. The machine gives a visual display of the BP reading. The accuracy of these machines varies, however.

Benefits of Self-Monitoring

- May detect high BP in those who have not previously had a problem (screening).

- Allows for observation of the BP *pattern* in those with high normal BP.

- Distinguishes "white-coat hypertension" from actual hypertension (the BP of persons with hypertension tends to be higher when measured in the clinic or office than when measured at home).

- For clients with hypertension, self-monitoring increases participation in treatment and may improve compliance with treatment.

Disadvantages of Self-Monitoring

- Possible incorrect use of the BP device.

- Needless alarm over one elevated reading.

- Clients with hypertension may make adjustments to their medications based on the BP readings without consulting their care provider.

Nursing Implications

- Teach proper use of the self-measurement devices.

- Periodically evaluate client's technique.

- Teach the meaning of BP readings and the need to look for patterns, not just a single reading.

- Explain the need for frequent calibration of the home-monitoring device.

- Have the client bring the home-monitoring device to clinical visits so that readings can be compared with simultaneously recorded auscultatory readings.

- Teach the client to have abnormally high or low readings (on more than one occasion) rechecked by a healthcare provider. Home readings of 135/85 or higher should be considered elevated.

- Advise the client to keep a written record of BP readings, including the date and time for each, and bring it to each clinic or office visit.

3rd sound—Begins midway through the BP and is a sharp, rhythmic tapping sound.

4th sound—Like the third sound, but softer and fading.

5th sound—Silence; it corresponds with diastole (diastolic BP).

You will not always be able to identify each of the five sounds. In some clients the sounds are distinct, but in others you will note little difference between beginning and ending sounds. To hear these sounds,

 Go to **Sound File, Blood Pressure Sounds,** on the Electronic Study Guide.

Palpating Blood Pressure

When the BP is difficult to hear (e.g., when there are cardiac conditions, shock, or other conditions that compromise circulation) you can use palpation alone. You can usually palpate only the systolic BP, because diastolic pressure is difficult to feel. Apply the cuff, and feel for the radial or brachial pulse. Begin to inflate the cuff. When you can no longer feel the pulse, inflate the cuff about 30 mm Hg more. As you release the valve and slowly deflate the cuff, note the reading on the manometer at which you once again feel the pulse. Record the palpated blood pressure according to the way it was assessed (e.g., "Palpated, low Fowler's, left arm 86/——").

Using Palpation with Auscultation

You will use palpation with auscultation for calculating the proper cuff inflation pressure before auscultating the BP and for detecting an auscultatory gap, to be discussed shortly.

Calculating Proper Inflation Pressure

The first time you measure a client's BP, you do not know what the systolic BP will be. Should you pump the cuff to 200 mm Hg, just to be sure you don't miss the first sound? The answer is NO. If you overinflate the cuff, the patient will feel discomfort. However, if you underinflate it (e.g., stop inflating at 110 mm Hg), you may miss the first sound and obtain an incorrect reading.

There is a method that allows you to estimate the systolic BP to ensure that you inflate the cuff to the proper level to obtain an accurate reading. Inflate the cuff rapidly to 70 mm Hg, and then palpate the radial pulse while you increase more slowly, in 10 mm Hg increments. Note the pressure at which the pulse disappears and reappears with deflation. When taking the actual measurement, inflate the cuff to a pressure that is 20 to 30 mm Hg above the palpated level.

Recognizing an Auscultatory Gap

If the client has hypertension, as you auscultate the BP during deflation of the cuff you may note the loss of sounds for as much as 30 mm Hg followed by the return

of sound. This loss and later return of sound is referred to as an **auscultatory gap.** Palpating first and then auscultating (as described in the preceding paragraph) ensures that you will not miss the isolated first sound. You should record the range of pressures in which the gap occurs (e.g., BP LA sitting, 170/90 with an auscultatory gap from 170 to 140). It is important to recognize an auscultatory gap because it can result in a serious misreading of the systolic BP. For tips that will help ensure the validity of your BP measurements,

 Go to Chapter 17, **Technique 17-1: Taking an Accurate Blood Pressure,** in Volume 2.

KnowledgeCheck 17–6

- Which of the Korotkoff sounds would you record as the systolic pressure?
- Which of the Korotkoff sounds would you record as the diastolic pressure?
- A nurse is auscultating a BP. He hears the first sound at 170 mm Hg. The sound disappears immediately. At 150 mm Hg, the sound appears again and continues until there is silence at 80 mm Hg. The pressures were taken in the client's right arm while the client was lying down.

  How should the nurse record these pressures?
  How do you explain what happened?

 Go to Chapter 17, **Knowledge Check Response Sheet and Answers,** on the Electronic Study Guide.

What Is Hypotension?

Hypotension is diagnosed when systolic blood pressure is less than 100 mm Hg. A low blood pressure is usually not considered a problem. However, further evaluation is always called for if:

- The client is also experiencing dizziness, fatigue, concentration problems, activity intolerance, or shortness of breath.
- The low blood pressure is of sudden onset.

Hemorrhage and heart failure are two causes of hypotension. Inappropriately low BP (hypovolemic shock) is a medical emergency. For more information on hypovolemic shock, consult a medical-surgical nursing text.

Orthostatic or **postural hypotension** occurs when a person's BP drops suddenly on moving from a lying position to a sitting or standing position. The *JNC 7 Express* report (Joint National Committee, 2003) defines it as a decrease of 10 mm Hg in standing blood pressure when associated with dizziness and/or fainting. Postural hypotension results from peripheral vasodilation without a compensatory increase in cardiac output. It is most likely to occur in older adults, pregnant women, clients on prolonged bed rest, and clients with decreased blood volume (e.g., from dehydration or recent blood loss).

Nursing Diagnosis

Hypotension is a medical diagnosis or, more commonly, a symptom rather than a nursing diagnosis. However, it may be the etiology of nursing diagnoses—for example, Risk for Falls related to orthostatic hypotension.

Planning Outcomes/Evaluation

The *NOC outcomes and goals* you use will depend on the nursing diagnosis (the problem caused by the hypotension). For Risk for Falls, you might use NOC's Falls Occurrence. You might write *an individualized goal* such as, "Patient will have no falls while walking."

Planning Interventions/Implementation

NIC standardized interventions will be determined by the nursing diagnosis you use. In the case of Risk for Falls related to orthostatic hypotension, you might use the following: Fall Prevention, Self-Care Assistance: Transfer, and Surveillance: Safety.

 Go to Chapter 17, **Standardized Language,** in Volume 2.

Specific nursing activities, regardless of the nursing diagnosis used, must address the etiology: the orthostatic hypotension. When you detect orthostatic hypotension:

1. Help the client lie down, and then notify the physician or nurse in charge.
2. Then obtain *orthostatic vital signs*—that is, take the pulse and BP with the client supine, sitting, and standing. Take each reading 1 to 3 minutes after the client changes position.
3. When documenting orthostatic vital signs, record the client's position in addition to the pulse and BP measurements (e.g., supine P = 80, BP = 150/90; sitting P = 84, BP = 140/84; standing P = 90, BP = 104/60).

What Is Hypertension?

A transient elevation in BP is a normal response to physiological or psychological stress (e.g., after eating, after exercise). **Prehypertension** is a BP reading of 120 to 130 systolic or 80 to 89 diastolic, obtained with two readings taken 6 minutes apart, with the patient sitting (Joint National Committee, 2003). **Hypertension** is a persistently higher than normal BP. It is diagnosed when BP is above 140 mm Hg systolic or above 90 mm Hg diastolic on two or more separate occasions. Hypertension is a major cause of illness and death in the United States. Hypertension increases the stress on the heart and blood vessels, and if untreated, it may lead to heart attack, heart failure, peripheral vascular disease, kidney damage, or stroke. The severity of the disorder is directly related to the degree of elevation; however, the latest guidelines (Joint National Committee, 2003)

recommend that even prehypertension be treated by lifestyle modifications to prevent coronary artery disease. The diagnosis of hypertension is often delayed because symptoms are mild or absent. Those who experience symptoms may complain of early morning suboccipital headaches, fatigue, and visual changes.

Primary, or *essential, hypertension* is diagnosed when there is no known cause for the BP elevation. Essential hypertension accounts for at least 90% of all cases of hypertension. Although no single cause is identified, family history, age, race, obesity, diet, heavy alcohol consumption, smoking history, high cholesterol levels, and stress all contribute to the development of essential hypertension. Physiologically, hypertension is related to thickening of the arterial walls and decreased elasticity of the arteries.

Secondary hypertension occurs when there is a clearly identified cause for the persistent rise in BP. A variety of renal and endocrine disorders may lead to secondary hypertension. Treatment is directed at eliminating the underlying cause.

Nursing Diagnosis

Hypertension is a medical, rather than nursing, diagnosis. However, there are nursing diagnoses associated with it. For a full discussion of nursing care for clients having hypertension, consult a medical-surgical nursing text.

- Risk for Decreased Cardiac Output occurs as a response to hypertension (i.e., hypertension is the etiology of this nursing diagnosis). As blood pressure rises, peripheral resistance increases. Over time the heart is unable to compensate, and cardiac output declines.
- Some nursing diagnoses may be the contributing factors for hypertension, for example:

  Imbalanced Nutrition: More than Body Requirements may be used if obesity (>20% above ideal body weight) is a factor in a patient's hypertension

  Imbalanced Nutrition: More than Body Requirements (for salt) could be used for a client whose high dietary sodium intake is contributing to hypertension.

  Excess Fluid Volume may also occur as a result of high salt intake.

- Hypertension may be a defining characteristic (symptom) of some nursing diagnoses, for example: Anxiety and Pain may cause an increase in BP.
- Hypertension may create the need for a diagnosis of Deficient Knowledge related to the need to make lifestyle changes.

Planning Outcomes/Evaluation

The NOC standardized outcome for assessing the blood pressure is Vital Signs Status. If it becomes necessary

to monitor cardiac output, you could use the labels of Cardiac Pump Effectiveness and Circulation Status.

Individualized goals/outcome statements will depend on the nursing diagnosis. For example, for Decreased Cardiac Output, goals might be, "BP will be at least 110/80," and "Extremities will be warm to the touch with quick capillary refill." If the nursing diagnosis were Imbalanced Nutrition: More Than Body Requirements, the desired outcomes would address the target weight for the client and the ideal number of calories to be consumed.

 VOL 2 Go to Chapter 17, **Standardized Language,** in Volume 2.

| Planning Interventions/Implementation |

NIC standardized interventions include the following:

Vital Signs Monitoring applies to monitoring an abnormal blood pressure.
Hemodynamic Regulation would be used to evaluate Decreased Cardiac Output.

Specific nursing activities for the patient with hypertension depends on whether hypertension is primary or secondary and on specific orders from the physician. Nursing activities and focused assessments that address hypertension, regardless of its cause, include the following:

- *Perform focused assessments:*
  Monitor all vital signs. An elevated blood pressure may affect the client's other vital signs. Watch for increases in pulse and respiratory rate.
  Monitor the patient's activity tolerance. The patient's degree of involvement in care, orientation, and level of fatigue while experiencing hypertension are all important indicators of decreased cardiac output.
  Accurately measure intake and output. If intake is appreciably more than output, the increased blood volume will cause the BP to rise further. Pay attention to free fluids as well as fluid in food sources. Also monitor for edema, which is an indicator of fluid retention.
  Weigh the client regularly. Weight loss of as little as 10 lb (4.5 kg) lowers BP in many overweight persons with hypertension. Weight gain may signal poor compliance with the treatment plan and/or indicate fluid retention.
  Collect and assess laboratory data as ordered. Blood urea nitrogen (BUN), creatinine, electrolytes, hemoglobin, hematocrit, and lipid levels must all be assessed on a regular basis.
- *Administer antihypertensive medications (if ordered)* at regular intervals to control blood pressure.
- *For self-monitoring of BP,* see the Home Care box on page 332.

- *For client teaching regarding hypertension,* see the Self Care box on page 336.

KnowledgeCheck 17–7

- Which of the following patients has hypertension? One with a BP of:

  150/80 on two separate occasions
  180/100 on one occasion
  138/88 on two occasions

- Which of the following client(s) has/have *primary* hypertension?

  Client A, who is obese and has a high sodium intake
  Client B, who is in renal failure
  Client C, who has hypertension induced by pregnancy
  Client D, who has a family history of hypertension

 Go to Chapter 17, **Knowledge Check Response Sheet and Answers,** on the Electronic Study Guide.

CriticalThinking 17–9

Recall the clients you encountered at the community health fair. Lucas is 35 years old. He has been under a lot of stress. His blood pressure is 150/98.

- To evaluate his BP, what else do you need to know about Mr. Lucas's situation (the context)?
- What possible actions should you consider while meeting with Lucas?
- What is the theoretical knowledge (rationale) to support your decisions?

PUTTING IT ALL TOGETHER

In the hospital setting, you will usually take a complete set of vital signs on patients at regular intervals. In ambulatory care settings, the VS you measure may vary according to the client's chief complaint. Regardless of setting, you will need to use clinical judgment about which VS to measure and how often to measure them.

Evaluating Vital Signs

You should evaluate the client's VS on the basis of known norms as well as the particular client's trends. Suppose your client's BP has consistently been 150 to 160/90 over the last 3 days. This morning his BP is 108/60. Although this BP is theoretically normal, it is significantly different from the client's norm. Therefore, you must evaluate the cause of the change. Has there been a change in the other VS? Has there been a change in the client's medications or condition? How does the client feel? Has his activity level been altered by the change in BP? This change may be positive or negative. You must put all the VS and other clinical signs together to determine your course of action.

A high fever can cause BP to drop precipitously, for instance. Suppose this client's temperature is

Teaching Your Client About Hypertension

Teach the client and family about lifestyle changes for preventing and managing hypertension.

- Limit salt intake (no more than 2.4 g sodium or 6 g sodium chloride per day).

- Consume a diet high in potassium (e.g., fresh fruits and vegetables, such as bananas, potatoes, yogurt, and acorn squash).

- Consume a diet high in calcium (e.g., milk and milk products, sardines, molasses, tofu).

- Limit alcohol intake (no more than the equivalent of 2 oz 100-proof whiskey per day—less for women).

- Lose weight if overweight.

- For overall cardiovascular health, reduce saturated fat and cholesterol intake.

- Eliminate smoking.

- Engage in aerobic exercise (30–45 minutes, several days a week).

- Try to reduce stress and stressful situations.

- Teach the client that even one lifestyle change has effects similar to treatment with a single antihypertensive drug. More than one change has an even more positive effect on the BP.

Teach the need for follow-up assessments.

- If BP is "normal," recheck at each healthcare encounter or at least every 2 years.

- If BP is above 120 mm Hg systolic or above 80 mm Hg diastolic, review lifestyle modifications and consult primary health provider within 1 to 2 months.

- If BP is above 140 mm Hg systolic or above 90 mm Hg diastolic, review lifestyle modifications and schedule follow-up with a healthcare provider within 1 to 2 months.

- If BP is 160 mm Hg systolic or higher, or 100 mm Hg diastolic or higher, consult the primary care provider within 1 week, or immediately if the clinical situation warrants.

- When readings are obtained by self-monitoring, reduce all numbers in the three preceding items by 5 mm Hg (e.g., a BP above 115 mm Hg systolic or above 75 mm Hg diastolic would merit lifestyle modifications and consultation with the primary health provider).

103.5°F (39.7°C). In that case, in addition to his drop in BP, you should also anticipate a rise in pulse and respiratory rate. So what should you do? Your action depends on the client's condition and the context. What else is going on in the situation? If the client has orders for medication for the fever, you would administer the medication and evaluate the VS again at frequent intervals. If the VS do not improve, you would then notify the primary care provider.

Now change the context slightly. Add to your preceding data that the client has undergone a surgical procedure and is not taking any antibiotics. Now what should you do? If your answer is to notify the primary care provider, you are correct. Always evaluate the vital signs as a unit. A sudden change in the client's condition requires you to thoroughly assess the client and report your findings to the physician or primary care provider.

A change in a client's vital signs may also be a positive sign. For instance, if the client has been in severe pain for 3 days and has finally obtained pain relief, a decrease in BP probably indicates that the current medication regimen has provided better control of the pain. You would still need to monitor the VS at more frequent intervals, however, to ensure that the BP does not continue to fall.

Delegating Vital Signs

In many healthcare settings, several providers interact with the clients. Vital signs may be obtained by nursing assistants or other unlicensed personnel. However, if you are working in a team nursing model as the registered nurse (RN), you are responsible for reviewing and interpreting the findings of all unlicensed assistive personnel (UAP). This includes evaluating the technique of UAPs and the accuracy of their measurements. The registered professional nurse *never* relinquishes the responsibility for interpretation of vital signs, vital sign trends, and decisions based on abnormal vital sign findings. As a student nurse, you are responsible for functioning within your scope of knowledge. If you are unsure how to interpret the meaning of VS you have obtained or that have been supplied to you by a UAP, you must discuss the findings with your instructor and/or the RN assigned to care for your client. Even though you are participating in the client's care, the RN maintains responsibility for client oversight.

 Go to Chapter 17, **Resources for Caregivers and Health Professionals,** on the Electronic Study Guide.

 Suggested Readings: Go to Chapter 17, **Reading More About Vital Signs,** on the Electronic Study Guide.

 Bibliography: Go to Volume 2, Bibliography.

Communicating
& the Therapeutic Relationship

Learning Outcomes

After completing this chapter, you should be able to:

* Define communication.

* Identify the three basic levels of communication.

* Discuss the elements of the communication process.

* List the characteristics of verbal and nonverbal communication.

* Analyze factors that influence the communication process.

* Explain how relationships and roles influence communication.

* Describe the role of communication in each of the four phases of the therapeutic relationship.

* Compare and contrast techniques that enhance communication to those that hinder communication.

* Write a nursing care plan for a client experiencing impaired communication.

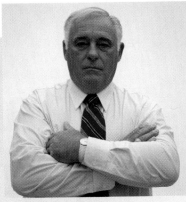

MEET Your Patient

You have been assigned to care for John Barker, a 56-year-old man admitted to the hospital with bleeding in the lower gastrointestinal tract. When you approach Mr. Barker to introduce yourself, you find him in his room with his wife at the bedside. They are holding hands, and clearly both have been crying. You begin by saying, "Good afternoon, Mr. Barker, I am a nursing student from the nearby university. I've been assigned to care for you tomorrow." Mr. Barker swallows hard and says, "I don't think you'll be able to do anything for me!" His wife says, "Don't take it personally. It's not a good time right now. Please just leave us alone."

You leave the room unsure how to respond. When you go to the unit station to review the chart, the charge nurse says, "Oh my! You've been assigned to him? I hope you've got a lot of experience." As you review the chart, you realize that Mr. Barker was just informed that he has metastatic colon cancer and probably has only a few months to live.

Theoretical Knowledge
knowing why

As a nurse, you may encounter situations similar to the one involving Mr. Barker. To respond effectively, you need therapeutic communication skills. As you read this chapter, you will gain theoretical and practical knowledge to help you to deal with this and similar situations.

WHAT IS COMMUNICATION?

Communication is a dynamic, reciprocal process of sending and receiving messages. The messages may be verbal, nonverbal, or both, and they may involve two or more people. As such, communication forms the basis for sharing meaning and building effective working relationships among individuals, families, and the healthcare team.

Communication is more than the act of talking and listening (Box 18–1). It is a basic function of human life. From the first cry of a newborn to the whisper of a patient who is dying, the primary purpose of communication is to share information and obtain a response. People use communication to meet their physical, psychosocial, emotional, and spiritual needs.

Communication Occurs on Three Levels

When we think about communication, we usually imagine a dialogue between two individuals. But communication actually occurs on any of three levels. The ability to use all levels of communication improves your effectiveness as a full-spectrum nurse.

Intrapersonal communication is conscious internal dialogue, sometimes known as *self-talk*. Constructive affirmations, or positive self-talk (e.g., "This will work!"), promote success in a task. In contrast, negative self-talk (e.g., "I can't do this") may adversely affect the person's ability to complete a task. Nurses often engage in intrapersonal communication. For example, if you enter a room and notice that your patient is pale, diaphoretic, and moaning, you may ask yourself, "What's happened? This client appears to be in a lot of pain."

Interpersonal communication is communication between two or more people. Face-to-face conversation between two people is the most frequent form of

---

BOX 18–1 **What Is Communication?**

Communication is ....

- Sharing or transmitting thoughts or feelings

- A way to meet physical, psychosocial, emotional, and spiritual needs

- A process—the act of sending, receiving, interpreting, and reacting to a message

- Content—the actual subject matter, words, gestures, and substance of the message

interpersonal communication. Nurses use interpersonal communication to gather information during assessment, to teach about health issues, to explain care, and to provide comfort and support. In addition to communicating directly with clients, nurses communicate with other nurses and healthcare team members to provide a comprehensive plan of care for the client. Because professional nurses are accountable for appropriate delegation of activities, they must also communicate effectively with the members of the nursing team.

Group communication is interaction that occurs among several people. *Small-group communication* occurs when you engage in an exchange of ideas with two or more individuals at the same time. Examples of small-group communication include staff meetings, committee meetings, educational groups, and self-help groups. Working with groups requires effective communication skills and a basic understanding of group processes. These processes will be discussed later in the chapter.

Public speaking is a unique form of group communication. Generally, the speaker addresses a dozen to hundreds of people, and varying degrees of interaction occur. Speakers may deliver a speech, talk directly with a small group of audience members, or have open discussion with the group. Nurses often engage in public speaking to educate groups of people about health issues, to lobby for legislation related to health promotion, and to address professional groups at conferences and conventions.

KnowledgeCheck 18–1
- What is the purpose of communication?
- Describe the three levels of communication.
- What level of communication was used in the "Meet Your Patient" scenario?

 Go to Chapter 18, **Knowledge Check Response Sheet and Answers,** on the Electronic Study Guide.

 ## CriticalThinking 18–1
Evaluate your own skills with the three levels of communication.

Communication Involves Both Content and Process

Communication has two major components: content and process. This distinction may seem obvious, but understanding the content and process of your communication helps you communicate more effectively.

The Content of Communication

The **content** of communication describes the actual subject matter, words, gestures, and substance of the

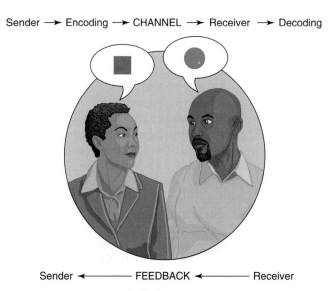

Sender → Encoding → CHANNEL → Receiver → Decoding

Sender ← FEEDBACK ← Receiver

FIGURE 18–1 Communication: A sender encodes and transmits a message to a receiver, who decodes it and transmits feedback.

message. It is the message that everyone may hear or see. For example, suppose your client said, "I slept through lunch." This statement is open to interpretation. We cannot tell—without also observing him, knowing his history, and so on—whether he thinks this is a good thing because he wanted or needed rest, or a bad thing because he is so exhausted, or a complaint about the staff for not waking him for lunch, or an apology and request for a late lunch. As you can see, the message is just a part of communication. You must also consider the process.

The Communication Process

Process refers to the act of sending, receiving, interpreting, and reacting to a message. The communication process has five elements: sender, message, receiver, feedback, and channel. Figure 18–1 illustrates the relationship among these elements.

The **sender** initiates the conversation to deliver a message (content) to another individual. The sender, sometimes called the *source* or the *encoder,* uses verbal and nonverbal methods to transmit the message. **Encoding** refers to the process of selecting the words, gestures, tone of voice, signs, and symbols used to transmit the message. For example, consider the case of Mr. Barker. As a beginning nursing student, you might feel anxious about being assigned to provide care to Mr. Barker. How could you communicate your concerns to your instructor? You might directly state, "It makes me nervous to be assigned to him," or you might avoid eye contact with your instructor and tell her, "I'm going to need some help today." Both styles communicate your anxiety, but they are encoded differently. Encoding is not always consciously intentional,

but it is affected by the nature of the message, the relationship between the sender and receiver, and the mood of the sender.

The **message** is the verbal and/or nonverbal information that the sender communicates. It might be a conversation, a speech, a gesture, a letter, and so forth. Effective messages are complete, clear, concise, organized, timely, and expressed in a manner that the receiver can understand. The message must be appropriate for the situation and for the developmental level of the person receiving the message. For instance, to family members awaiting the results of a life-saving procedure, seeing the patient's nurse walk toward them smiling broadly may give them an immediate nonverbal message about the outcome of the procedure.

The **channel** is the medium used to send the message. Face-to-face communication is a commonly used channel. Nurses frequently use touch as a nonverbal way to communicate caring and concern. Other channels include written pamphlets, audiovisual aids, recordings, and telephone messages. The type of message, the purpose, and the size of audience influence the choice of what channel is best suited for the communication. For example, in the case of Mr. Barker, by touching his hand while you remain silent, you would send a clear message of caring during this troubled time.

The **receiver** is the observer, listener, and interpreter of the message. Interpretation, also called **decoding,** refers to relating the message to one's past experiences to determine the sender's meaning. The receiver uses visual, auditory, and tactile senses to decode the message. If the decoded meaning matches the intended meaning, then the message was effective. However, messages are sometimes misinterpreted, especially when the receiver is not physically or emotionally ready to receive the message. For example, if you approached your instructor to discuss your concerns about Mr. Barker when she was assisting with an emergency on the unit, she might be unable to receive your message.

Once the receiver has received and interpreted the message, he may be stimulated to respond by providing feedback to the sender. **Feedback** validates that the receiver received the message and understood it as the sender intended. Feedback may be verbal, nonverbal, or both. Verifying the message avoids confusion.

KnowledgeCheck 18–2

Using the "Meet Your Patient" scenario, identify at least one sender, one message, one receiver, and one channel, and one example of feedback.

 Go to Chapter 18, **Knowledge Check Response Sheet and Answers,** on the Electronic Study Guide.

Communication Can Be Verbal or Nonverbal

People send and receive messages both verbally and nonverbally. The two forms of communication occur spontaneously and simultaneously in interpersonal and group interactions.

Verbal Communication

Verbal communication is the use of spoken and written words to send a message. It is influenced by such factors as educational background, culture, language, age, and past experiences. Verbal communication is generally a conscious act in which the sender is able to select the most effective words to communicate a message. When delivering a verbal message, keep the following factors in mind.

Vocabulary

Healthcare workers have a large vocabulary of technical terms. However, laypersons are often unfamiliar with the language of health care and find its use intimidating or frightening. Consider the following example:

> "You are scheduled for surgery tomorrow. You need to be NPO after 2400. I'll be in to prep the op site at about 8. You'll need to void before your premed. After that we'll move you to a litter and transfer you to the holding area."

Do you think most clients would understand this message? Do you understand all the words? Clients are often confused by medical terms and technical jargon, but for various reasons (e.g., being embarrassed at not knowing), they often hesitate to ask questions to clarify what was said. It is your responsibility to deliver messages that the client can understand; therefore, use medical terms only when you are certain the listener understands them. When encoding a message, consider the receiver's age, knowledge, education, and any cultural differences. (These factors are discussed shortly.) Encourage feedback to ensure that the recipient understood the message as you intended.

Denotative and Connotative Meaning

Denotation is the literal (dictionary) meaning of a word. In contrast, **connotation** is the implied or emotional meaning of the word. Consider the following examples:

> A mother says to her infant, "Don't cry, baby."

> A 40-year-old man says to his nurse, "Would you rub my back, baby?"

> A 10-year-old boy says to another boy, "You're a baby!"

The denotative meaning of *baby* is a very young child who is not yet able to walk. However, the connotative meaning is different in each example. In the first example, the connotative meaning is the same as the denotative meaning. In the second example, the nurse might understandably feel offended; and in the last example, the 10-year-old boy undoubtedly meant *baby* as an insult. As these examples illustrate, words are often value-laden or biased. The situation, qualities of the participants, and the words they choose all affect interpretation. Use terms that provide clear, objective data and are not open for misinterpretation.

 CriticalThinking 18–2

Think of two other examples in which the connotative meaning may be different from the denotative meaning.

Pacing

The pace and rhythm of the delivery can alter the receiver's interpretation of the message. A rapid pace, which does not allow the receiver to track what the speaker is saying, is frustrating and can cause the receiver to lose interest. The pace must be slow enough for the receiver to interpret one thought before the sender moves on to the next thought. By pausing at intervals, the speaker also gives the listener time to interpret the words and respond.

However, the pace must be fast enough to maintain the listener's interest. What happens when a professor talks very slowly during a lecture? Do you find your mind wandering: "I need to take the dog to the vet. . . . What shall we have for dinner? . . ."

Intonation

Intonation reflects the feeling behind the words. We get a sense of a person's "tone of voice" by noting the pitch (high or low), cadence (rising and falling of the pitch), and volume (soft or loud). These variables help a speaker convey confidence, enthusiasm, sadness, fear, anger, anxiety, or boredom. For example, experiment with the variety of ways you might state, "Your tests results are in."

Pitch, cadence, and volume can either reinforce or contradict the message. When spoken at a moderate pitch and volume, with a falling cadence, the words, "I understand that I am to report at noon" can be a simple confirmation that the person has received the message. When spoken quietly, hesitantly, and with a rising cadence, it can convey the message that the person actually does not understand at all. Monitor your intonation and that of your clients as you communicate.

People tend to lose interest when someone speaks in a monotone (does not vary the pitch, cadence, and volume). Before presenting lengthy information, whether as individualized teaching or an address to a group, experiment with these variables to ensure that you maintain the listener's engagement with your topic.

Clarity and Brevity

Clarity in communication requires that you select words that convey the intended meaning and that you make sure your spoken words and the nonverbal message are congruent. You can achieve brevity by using the fewest words possible. A conversation that is clear and brief holds the interest of all parties and effectively conveys the message.

Timing and Relevance

Timing is crucial to the communication process. Before starting a conversation, assess your client. A person who is distracted by pain, hunger, or other physiological needs will not receive the message as you intended it. Similarly, a client attempting to cope with stressors, such as limited finances, an upcoming surgery, or a terminal diagnosis, may be unable to listen effectively.

The presence of others is another consideration in timing. For example, asking a client about a personal issue in a public corridor may inhibit his response. You will receive a different response if you ask the same question in a more private setting. In contrast, if you are instructing a client about a recommended diet, be sure that the person who is responsible for shopping and cooking is also present. If your client does neither in his household, he may pay little attention to your instruction.

Timing also involves relevance and response time. Communication is effective when both parties value the interaction and find the discussion relevant. For example, to teach your client about his medicines, choose a time when he is alert, pain-free, and not distracted, and begin by reminding him of the purpose of the discussion: "I'm going to teach you how to take this medication so that it effectively controls your pain." The interaction must also allow time for response. Incessant questions or one-sided conversations inhibit interaction. The conversation must also be relevant.

Credibility

Clients judge the credibility of the message on the credibility of the sender. A pattern of honest and timely response to patient concerns fosters credibility. As a nurse, you will be called on to provide information on a wide variety of topics. Provide information only if you are certain of the facts. A response such as, "I don't know, but I'll find out and let you know" is far more credible than an incorrect answer or guess.

Never lie to the patient; lying destroys trust. Lying can take many forms. If you tell the patient you

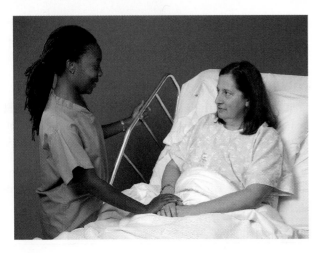

FIGURE 18–2 The nurse's facial expression is appropriate if the nurse and patient are discussing an improvement in the patient's condition or other optimistic news. However, this expression is inappropriate if the patient is conveying discomfort or worry.

will be right back with pain medication but do not return until she reminds you an hour later, she may doubt your credibility. If a patient care situation makes you uncomfortable it is best to acknowledge your discomfort rather than risk loss of credibility. For example, you may feel uncomfortable talking to Mr. Barker ("Meet Your Patient") about his recent diagnosis. You may be tempted to say, "Maybe the test results are wrong," or "The timeline is just a guess. I bet you can beat this." This approach avoids uncomfortable discussion and may make the patient feel better temporarily. However, a more honest approach would be to tell Mr. Barker that you would like him to meet with a counselor or hospital chaplain.

To be credible, your nonverbal communication must match your spoken words. This cannot be overemphasized. For example, if your client asks you if his wound is "ugly," he will pay attention to your facial expressions as well as your spoken response. If you respond that "The wound looks good," but you frown, the client will most likely believe that you are not being completely honest. This may jeopardize future interactions.

Humor

Humor and laughing can have a positive influence on attitude and healing. Laughter can create physiological changes that contribute to well-being and provide an emotional release in a tense situation. However, use humor cautiously. Humor is highly subjective and depends on cultural norms. Never direct humor at the client, disease process, or treatment team. Misused humor can have a negative effect on self-esteem, self-confidence, or the client's confidence in the treatment team. Consider the different affects the following uses of humor might have. Imagine that your patient has

had vomiting and diarrhea for the last 8 hours. When you enter the room you jokingly say, "Oh my! You look like you had too much to drink last night." Although the intent was to lighten the mood, this statement may offend your patient. In contrast, imagine that you notice that an older patient thoroughly enjoys visits from his young grandchildren. You might consider sharing with him an amusing story about your own children.

Nonverbal Communication

Nonverbal communication (or body language) is the exchange of messages without the use of words. Verbal communication is a highly conscious activity in which we choose words to communicate. However, nonverbal communication occurs on a more unconscious level. Because nonverbal language communicates how someone is feeling, it more accurately conveys the true meaning of a message. It may thereby reinforce or contradict the spoken message. For example, in the "Meet Your Patient" scenario Mr. Barker uses few words. However, he is tearful and distressed. His body language gives you valuable insight into how he is adjusting to the news of his cancer.

Facial Expression

Expressions of the face and especially the eyes are some of the most demonstrative forms of nonverbal communication. Facial expressions communicate joy, anger, sadness, concern, or fear. Raised eyebrows, staring, squinting, or darting eyes all convey meaning.

Smiling is one expression that is understood universally. In contrast, the interpretation of many other facial expressions is culturally dependent. For example, downcast eyes may indicate sadness, poor self-esteem, a desire to avoid the conversation, respect, powerlessness, or submissive behavior. In Western cultures, eye contact usually indicates an interest in the conversation and a willingness to communicate; however, in Eastern cultures, the amount of eye contact considered acceptable varies. Chapter 13 discusses cultural variations.

A mismatch between your verbal message and facial expression may cause the client to doubt your credibility (Figure 18–2). For example, suppose that a patient states, "I just had my pain pill. How come my pain is still so bad?" You answer, "The medication should take effect within a few more minutes. If it doesn't, call me." Imagine the different effect this reply would have if you were smiling, frowning, raising one eyebrow, or evading the client's eyes.

Posture and Gait

Body position, gait, and posture offer clues to a person's attitudes, emotions, physical well-being, and self-concept. When you see someone with an erect posture, head held high, and a quick gait, what do you

think? In Western culture, these are nonverbal indicators of health and a sense of self-assuredness. In contrast, a slow, shuffling gait may signify someone who is ill, is depressed, or has poor self-esteem.

Personal Appearance

Clothing and personal appearance can provide clues to a person's feelings, socioeconomic status, culture, and religion. A person who is ill, tired, or depressed may not have the energy to invest in hygiene and grooming. Lack of attention to personal appearance is especially significant in an individual who typically engages in meticulous grooming. As with all nonverbal data, you need to investigate the meaning of personal appearance to avoid drawing erroneous conclusions.

Dress and adornments are powerful cultural clues. Does the patient dress in a style that differs from local custom? Are pieces of jewelry or religious medallions visible? These are clues to the patient's values, as well as the patient's socioeconomic status. Pay attention to these clues, but do not make assumptions from them. A person who wears an elaborate religious medal may like the ornamentation but not espouse the beliefs that are attached to the symbol.

Gestures

Hand and body gestures emphasize and clarify the spoken word. They are good indicators of the feeling tone behind the conversation. Imagine that your client says, "I'm OK." What might it mean if he accompanies his statement with a broad grin and raised arms? What might it mean if, instead, he lowers his head to his hands?

Gestures vary widely among individuals and cultures, so use them with caution. For example, consider the gesture of a "V" made with the second and third fingers of the hand. To some people, this is a peace sign; to others, it is a victory sign; and still others may attach no meaning to it at all. Gestures can help you communicate with individuals with impaired verbal communication. Be careful, however, that you and the patient agree on the meaning of the gestures.

Touch

Touch can convey affection, caring, concern, and encouragement. Avoid using touch when dealing with someone who is angry or mentally disturbed, because the touch may be misinterpreted (e.g., as a sign of aggression or sexual attraction). Although touch can be highly effective, use it with conscious awareness of the situation, environment, and receptivity of the patient. For examples of therapeutic nonverbal behaviors and how patients may interpret them,

 Go to **Technique 18-1: Enhancing Communication Through Nonverbal Behaviors,** in Volume 2.

 KnowledgeCheck 18–3

- Identify the components of verbal and nonverbal communication.
- What action should you take when there is a discrepancy between the client's spoken word and nonverbal body language?

 Go to Chapter 18, **Knowledge Check Response Sheet and Answers,** on the Electronic Study Guide.

CriticalThinking 18–3

- Observe an interaction between family members or your fellow students. Look for congruence between verbal and nonverbal communication. Strategize what you would say to validate the intended meaning when the two modes of communication are not in agreement.
- Recall the brief interaction with the charge nurse in the "Meet Your Patient" scenario. What might you say or do in response?

WHAT FACTORS AFFECT COMMUNICATION?

The following is a discussion of the major factors that affect communication.

Environment

Communication is most successful in a favorable environment. A favorable environment is quiet, private, free of noxious smells, and at a comfortable temperature. As a beginning student, you are aware of the noises and distractions in the clinical setting. However, experienced nurses become accustomed to such distractions. Be sensitive to how the environment is affecting your client. Background noise is distracting, impedes hearing, and can create confusion. Lack of privacy hinders information sharing. Being around others in pain or distress creates anxiety and fear.

Think creatively to secure the most comfortable environment possible for communicating with patients and families. Hospital chapels, foyers, and activity rooms may be ideal locations for conversation. To discuss private matters, consider talking with the patient in a conference room rather than a shared room.

Developmental Variations

Physical and cognitive development, language skills, level of education, and maturity influence the communication process. Thus, you will need to modify your communication strategies to fit your client's developmental level. For detailed information on expectations for each developmental stage,

 Go to **Chapter 9** on the Electronic Study Guide.

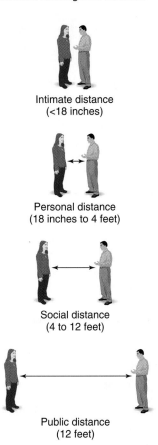

Intimate distance
(<18 inches)

Personal distance
(18 inches to 4 feet)

Social distance
(4 to 12 feet)

Public distance
(12 feet)

FIGURE 18–3 The distance that individuals engaged in communication maintain between one another is influenced by the relationship of the individuals, the nature of the conversation, the setting, and cultural influences.

Infants and young toddlers with limited language skills communicate nonverbally. Your response may combine verbal and nonverbal communication. For example, if a hospitalized 1-year-old cries out for his mother, you might cuddle the child with his favorite toy and explain that "Mama will be back very soon." Older toddlers and preschoolers have more verbal ability. Although they may prefer to have a parent present, they are likely to talk with you and answer questions. School-age children are usually quite comfortable interacting verbally. Pay attention to their vocabulary as they speak, and be sure to match it to the extent possible, using words and phrasing the child will understand. By the time children reach adolescence, most can process abstract concepts. As a result, they are usually able to understand disease processes, treatments, and other health issues. Bear in mind that children with chronic health problems that have required frequent interventions are often more knowledgeable than would be expected for their age.

Older adults may be affected by sensory alterations, such as hearing loss or vision changes, or any of a variety of healthcare problems that affect cognition. Communication strategies for these situations are discussed in the "Planning Interventions/Implementation" section of the chapter.

Gender

Males and females communicate differently and may interpret the same communication differently. Deborah Tannen, a linguist from George Washington University and author of *You Just Don't Understand: Women and Men in Conversation* (1990), states that women communicate to form connections and establish relationships. In contrast, male communication styles focus on maintaining independence and favorable positions in a hierarchy. In essence, women want to "be connected," whereas men want to "be one up."

The roots of these communication patterns are early socialization differences. Traditionally boys are socialized to participate in hierarchical team sports. Through this play, they learn how to compete, strategize, and win or lose. In contrast, young girls are more likely to engage in one-on-one or fantasy play that requires cooperation and focuses on fairness and negotiation. This early socialization is carried over into communication patterns. Men are more likely to be comfortable in situations that result in a win or loss, whereas women are more likely to attempt to reach consensus.

Gender differences in communication are important to nurses for a number of reasons. Male and female patients may communicate their needs very differently. Similarly, the gender of the nurse may affect the response to the patient's requests. For example, a female patient might state, "I feel so lousy today." A female nurse may interpret this as a desire to talk. In contrast, a male nurse may discuss pain control.

Personal Space

People vary in the amount of physical space they are comfortable with when communicating. The distance that individuals engaged in communication maintain between one another is influenced by the relationship of the individuals, the nature of the conversation, the setting, and cultural influences (Figure 18–3). (See Chapter 13 for cultural preferences for personal space.) Hall (1969, p. 45) describes four distinct distances influencing communication: intimate distance, personal distance, social distance, and public distance.

Intimate distance is the area immediately surrounding people that they define as their "private space." It is the distance people prefer to maintain between themselves and others during interactions. In Western cultures, intimate distance is within 18 inches of the other person. Within this distance, people can sense each other's smell and body heat and usually can hear each other speaking at a low volume. It is also at this distance that body contact occurs. As a nurse, you invade a client's intimate distance to perform assessments and procedures. You even breach a client's intimate distance when touching a hand or shoulder to

offer support. It is important to recognize that this may make some clients uncomfortable. Before providing nursing interventions in the client's intimate distance, discuss what you are about to do. It is best to ask the client's permission, even for gentle touch, if you are in the slightest doubt about his receptivity.

Personal distance is from 18 inches to 4 feet. Your interactions with clients and healthcare team members will commonly occur in this range. This distance facilitates sharing of feelings or personal thoughts and is appropriate to maintain when communicating caring or concern.

Social distance is a distance of 4 to 12 feet. It is used in more formal interaction or when communicating with a group of individuals at the same time. The volume of the spoken words may be loud enough for others to overhear. At this distance, individuals are not within range to be physically touched. Personal feelings and thoughts are shared less often at this distance. If you maintain a social distance from your clients, expect that the clients may be less willing to share personal thoughts. For example, if you stand by a client's door and ask how she is feeling, you will likely receive a more impersonal response than if you were to ask the same question at her bedside.

Public distance is considered to be beyond 12 feet. This distance requires loud and clear enunciation for communication. Public speakers and large educational groups use this form of personal space. This distance is characterized by a lack of individuality and a greater focus on the group or community.

Territoriality

Territoriality refers to the space and things that an individual identifies as belonging to him. Territories may be bounded and visible to others or may be defined by the individual in a way not noticeable to others. In a hospital setting, many clients consider everything within the curtain boundary to be their territory. Clients may be offended if you invade, rearrange, or interfere with this territory by moving furniture, discarding objects, or borrowing items from the client's room, even if they are institutional property. Be aware of this and request permission to rearrange your client's personal territory. Also recognize that hospitalized clients are not in their "home" territory and are therefore likely to be less at ease during interactions.

Sociocultural Factors

Culture and socioeconomic status strongly influence communication. Facial expressions, nonverbal communication, and even the selection of who to interact with are affected. For example, in some cultures it would be unacceptable for a male nurse to address and provide care to a female patient.

Social status also plays a role in communication. Have you ever been present while a physician explained a treatment plan to a patient? Often the patient asks no questions or nods approval, yet barrages you with questions when the physician leaves. One reason for this behavior is that many clients perceive less social distance between themselves and the nurse. Consequently they are more likely to ask you questions or to discuss concerns with you. Social distance can also play a role in how health professionals view clients. For example, you may see impoverished clients being treated with less respect than wealthy members of the community, although this is certainly not ideal.

Roles and Relationships

The roles of the sender and receiver and the relationship between them affects communication. Relationships affect the choice of vocabulary, tone of voice, use of gestures, and distance associated with the communication. Think of the way you interact with your instructor. Compare your approach with the way you interact with your classmates. What are the differences?

Many patients have preconceived notions about nursing. Some may view you as an authority figure. Others may perceive nursing as a lowly occupation and limit conversation with you to matters of comfort and hygiene. Still other clients become confused by the fact that many healthcare workers, such as medical assistants and nursing aides, call themselves nurses in spite of the fact that they cannot legally use the title. This makes it unclear whom the patient should speak with about concerns. If you are working with UAPs or other team members, be sure to clarify their roles with the patient.

As a member of the healthcare team, you will also need to communicate effectively with physicians and health professionals from other disciplines. Each of you shares the common goal of providing optimal patient care. This goal should guide the manner in which you communicate, whether at the bedside, at the nurse's station, in care conferences, or via the chart.

KnowledgeCheck 18–4

- What are the major factors that affect communication?
- In what distance(s) do most nurse-client interactions occur?

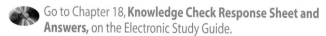 Go to Chapter 18, **Knowledge Check Response Sheet and Answers,** on the Electronic Study Guide.

WHAT IS THE ROLE OF COMMUNICATION IN THERAPEUTIC RELATIONSHIPS?

The **therapeutic relationship** focuses on improving the health of the client, whether an individual or community. The client gains information and knowledge

and works through issues, concerns, and problems related to health status, treatments, and nursing care. **Therapeutic communication** promotes this helping relationship. It is client-centered communication directed at achieving client goals. It is used to establish the therapeutic relationship, provide and obtain healthcare information, and express interest and concern for the client and family.

Communication Is Essential to All Phases of the Therapeutic Relationship

The therapeutic relationship consists of four phases. As you read about each phase, notice the fundamental role of client-focused communication.

The **pre-interaction phase** occurs before you meet the client. In this phase you will gather information about the client. As a student, you initiate this phase as you prepare for clinical days. The client also experiences a pre-interaction phase, which begins when she identifies the need for health care. This can be an anxious time for the client. In this phase, the nurse and client do not have direct communication.

The **orientation phase** begins when you meet the client. The goal in this phase is to establish rapport and trust. This phase begins with introductions, followed by an initial exchange of information. Information may include the client's purpose for the visit or chief concerns. Ideally there is time to exchange pleasantries and begin to develop a level of comfort. In some clinical situations, such as during an emergency, this phase is extremely brief. This phase ends when the relationship has been defined. During this phase, verbal and nonverbal communication occurs. All of the factors that affect communication (discussed above) influence the interaction.

The bulk of therapeutic communication occurs in the **working phase,** the active part of the relationship. During this phase, caring is communicated, thoughts and feelings are expressed, mutual respect is maintained, and honest verbal and nonverbal expression occurs. Key communication goals are to assist the client to clarify feelings and concerns. A professional relationship is courteous, trustworthy, and confidential, and accomplished by active listening and other techniques of therapeutic communication presented later in this chapter.

The **termination phase** is the conclusion of the relationship, whether at the end of the nurse's shift or on the client's discharge from the unit, facility, or service. Reviewing and summarizing help to bring the relationship to a comfortable conclusion. If communication has been effective, the termination phase prepares the nurse and client for future interactions. Unsuccessful communication may affect the client's health outcomes or understanding of his disease process, as well as affect the nurse's job satisfaction.

CriticalThinking 18–4
Recall the scenario of Mr. Barker ("Meet Your Patient").
- What phase of the therapeutic relationship is illustrated in the scenario?
- How might the interaction between you and Mr. Barker change if it occurred in a different phase of the therapeutic relationship?
- What could you have done differently?

Therapeutic Communication Has Five Key Characteristics

The therapeutic relationship requires conscious use of your knowledge and skills to effect change in the client. This is often called the *therapeutic use of self.* Five qualities characterize communication in the therapeutic relationship: empathy, respect, genuineness, concreteness, and confrontation.

Empathy

Empathy is the desire to understand and be sensitive to the feelings, beliefs, and situation of another person. To empathize with a client, you must look beyond outward appearance or behavior. Empathy is more than sharing of information. Instead, it involves putting yourself, mentally and emotionally, in the client's place so that you acknowledge the uniqueness of the client. Empathy requires you to be willing to adapt your style, tone, vocabulary, and behavior to create the best approach for each client situation.

Respect

In the therapeutic relationship, you communicate respect by valuing the client and being flexible to meet the needs of your client. As a nurse, you must be willing to adjust to your client rather than expecting the client to adjust to you, the healthcare environment, or hospital routines. Most healthcare experiences strip the client of power—clothes are removed, roles are discontinued, clients are separated from loved ones and familiar surroundings, and schedules are altered. When a relationship is grounded in respect, both parties maintain power and self-esteem. You show your respect for clients in the way you address them, the words and intonation you choose, and in your acknowledgment of their strengths and needs. Making even minor adjustments, such as putting off breakfast for an hour to allow the client to sleep, communicates that you respect the client's wishes.

Genuineness

When interviewing clients, we expect them to respond truthfully. After all, many healthcare decisions are

based on the client's responses. Similarly, clients have a right to expect truthful responses from healthcare providers as well. Genuineness is the ability to respond honestly. If you are unable to answer a client's question, do not offer guesses. Be honest. Tell the client you need assistance before you can answer the question. Genuineness also involves willingness to self-evaluate. How well did I communicate? Did I handle that situation appropriately? How could I improve my communication?

Concreteness and Confrontation

In a therapeutic relationship, you must offer understandable responses to a client's questions or concerns. To do so requires you to express in concrete terms what you mean. The message must be constructed and delivered in a manner that is suitable for the client. Communication is a reciprocal process. If your client is unable to express his thoughts clearly, you must be willing to confront her to request clarification. Similarly, you must be willing to be confronted if you are unclear.

Therapeutic communication requires practice. A strategy commonly used to improve communication skills is called *process recording*. In process recording, two people converse while a third transcribes the conversation. Afterward, the participants analyze the interaction. A tape recorder can facilitate process recording. It effectively captures the words and intonation of the conversation, but it must be supplemented by notes on nonverbal communication. Videotaping allows participants to examine both verbal and nonverbal communication. As you examine an interaction, look for the five qualities just discussed. Box 18–2 identifies skills associated with these qualities. Later, the chapter presents specific strategies for enhancing communication, as well as barriers to therapeutic communication. Look for these techniques and barriers in any conversation you analyze.

Communication Is Also Important in Group Helping Relationships

One-on-one communication has been the focus of most of our previous discussion. However, nurses frequently communicate with groups. Group communication occurs when you interact with a family, a community, or a committee. Groups can enhance problem solving and creativity, generate understanding and support, enhance morale, and provide affiliation.

Task groups are developed to address a task or need. Members are chosen based on ability to complete the task. **Short-term groups** dissolve once the task is completed. Short-term groups might include a task force to address holiday scheduling or a panel to critique response to a disaster drill. Because the time together is limited, the focus of communication is on

---

> ## BOX 18–2 Skills Needed in a Therapeutic Relationship
>
> The ability to:
>
> - Appreciate experiences and beliefs that differ from your own
> - Recognize and interpret verbal and nonverbal messages
> - Guide the interaction to accomplish goals
> - Determine *whether* communication is taking place
> - Speak when appropriate and remain silent when appropriate
> - Adapt to the pace, tone, and vocabulary of the client
> - Evaluate your own participation in an interaction

---

the task at hand. Often time to develop rapport or relationships is limited. Direct verbal communication with congruent nonverbal communication allows the group to function most effectively.

Ongoing groups address issues that are recurrent. Committees are a form of a task group. Common ongoing committees in healthcare organizations include quality assurance, infection control, and discharge planning. A committee has a chairperson that may be elected from within or appointed. Members have designated roles within the groups (e.g., recorder, time keeper). The size of the group strongly affects communication. In small groups, all members have an opportunity to communicate their opinions. In larger groups, patterns of communication form; some members voice their opinion regularly, whereas others are often silent. When not all members speak, it is essential to examine nonverbal behavior to determine whether the nonspeaking members are in agreement.

Self-help groups are voluntary organizations composed of individuals with a common need. Members who have met the goals of the group often run meetings. Alcoholics Anonymous is the most widely recognized self-help group. Other well-known self-help groups include Weight Watchers, Narcotics Anonymous, and Reach for Recovery (for women with breast cancer). Nurses may be members, facilitators, or consultants for self-help groups. Members are encouraged to share experiences and seek help from other members of the group. The facilitator may serve as a leader of the group or may coordinate room arrangements and schedules but acts as a member during sessions. The facilitator is usually chosen by the members. Consultants may be health professionals or experts in the field who offer advice or education to the group.

Characteristics of a Successful Group

A successful group has:

- A clearly defined purpose
- A set of guidelines apparent to all members under which the group functions
- A sense of shared responsibility
- Shared leadership
- Mutual trust
- Comfort among members
- A climate that is cohesive but does not stifle individuality
- Members who are willing to share feelings, concerns, or beliefs
- Flexibility to change what is not working

Several channels are available to self-help groups. They may have face-to-face meetings, participate in Internet chat groups, or communicate via newsletters. Communication of shared interests is the link that holds these groups together.

Therapy groups are formed to help individual members cope with issues, improve relationships, or address stress. They may be ongoing or have a designated length of operation. Community, public health, and psychiatric nurses sometimes facilitate therapy groups. Group facilitators arrange the time and place of the group and often introduce topics for discussion. Many groups are organized around themes, such as coping with divorce, loss of a spouse, or motherhood. These groups are also called self-awareness or growth groups.

Work-related social support groups help members of a profession cope with the stress associated with their work. The helping professions can be quite emotionally draining. These social support groups provide an opportunity to share concerns and offer mutual support through formal meetings with a facilitator or informal drop-in events.

The formation of a group does not guarantee its success. To be successful, a group must have characteristics that allow the group to function and achieve its goals. Box 18–3 describes characteristics of a successful group.

KnowledgeCheck 18–5

- Identify and describe the phases of the therapeutic relationship.
- What are the five characteristics of therapeutic communication?
- Describe the difference between a task group and a self-help group.

- Compare and contrast the role of a therapy group with a work-related support group.

 Go to Chapter 18, **Knowledge Check Response Sheet and Answers,** on the Electronic Study Guide.

 CriticalThinking 18–5

Review the local newspaper, phone book, hospital bulletin board, and school directory. Identify at least three group helping experiences available. How might you learn more about these organizations? How would you determine whether they are resources that you might make available to your patients?

Practical Knowledge
knowing how

Therapeutic communication is used throughout the nursing process. In the next few sections we will explore communication problems as well as therapeutic interventions.

Assessment

Assessment is essential to effective communication. Your assessment should look for factors that alter a client's ability to receive, process, or transmit information, such as the following:

- *Language barrier.* Clients with limited knowledge of the dominant language often find it difficult to communicate their needs or respond to communication from healthcare providers. Imagine how difficult it would be if you became seriously ill while traveling in a country where you were unable to speak or read the language. How would you communicate that you were nauseated or in pain; how would you tell them when the symptom started or what makes it worse?

- *Cognitive skills.* Difficulty understanding or engaging in communication may signal cognitive impairment. Developmental delays and physiological conditions involving the central nervous system affect language skills. Gather data about the client's abilities. Does the client have problems with short-term memory, long-term memory, or both? Does the client function at, below, or above expectations for her age?

- *Sensory perceptual alterations.* Assess for hearing deficits, use of hearing aids, or visual problems. Aphasia is a problem that may develop after cerebrovascular accident (stroke) or neurological disease. **Receptive aphasia** is the inability to receive or interpret verbal or nonverbal messages. **Expressive aphasia** is the inability to express verbal or nonverbal messages. It is important to distinguish the type of aphasia your client is experiencing. The type dictates the solutions that are effective.

• *Physiological barriers.* Difficulty speaking may be due to respiratory problems, such as dyspnea or the use of artificial airways, or oral problems, such as loose-fitting dentures or cleft palate.

| Nursing Diagnosis |

Several NANDA diagnoses directly pertain to communication. Note that communication problems may involve the inability to receive, interpret, or express spoken, written, and nonverbal messages.

• Readiness for Enhanced Communication is appropriate when the client expresses willingness to enhance communication.

• Impaired Verbal Communication is an appropriate diagnosis if the client has (1) expressive aphasia or a physiological problem (e.g., dyspnea, stuttering, or laryngeal cancer) that impairs the ability to speak; or (2) receptive aphasia or sensory deficits (e.g., vision or hearing loss) that impair the ability to receive messages.

• Impaired Communication is the preferred nursing diagnosis if the client is unfamiliar with the dominant language or has some other difficulty receiving and sending messages. Note that this is not a NANDA label.

Etiologies of Communication Diagnoses

Other nursing diagnoses may be the cause of communication problems. For example, clients with Acute or Chronic Confusion often have difficulty expressing or receiving verbal and nonverbal messages. Confusion may be related to physical health problems or mental health problems or be a side effect of medications or sleep deprivation. Mental health problems can also lead to communication difficulties. For example, Anxiety impairs the ability to deliver and receive messages, and Chronic or Situational Low Self-Esteem often results in limited interaction with others. Your assessment data will help you determine whether communication impairment is the primary problem or whether it is a result of other health problems.

Communication as Etiology of Other Nursing Diagnoses

Impaired Verbal Communication may be the etiology of other nursing diagnoses, for example:

• Anxiety related to inability to communicate needs

• Social Isolation related to difficulty maintaining relationships secondary to Impaired Verbal Communication

• Impaired Social Interaction related to inability to carry on conversation

• Chronic Low Self-Esteem related to fear of conversing with others secondary to stuttering

| Planning Outcomes/Evaluation |

For *NOC standardized outcomes* associated with Impaired Verbal Communication,

 Go to Chapter 18, **Standardized Language,** in Volume 2.

With selected indicators, you can use these to write goals for clients' communication problems.

Individualized client outcomes and goals depend on the nursing diagnosis you identify. For example, for Impaired Verbal Communication, you might write the following desired outcomes. The client:

• Uses alternative methods of communication (e.g., writing, picture board, gestures) effectively (specify time frame).

• Demonstrates minimal frustration with communication difficulties (specify time frame).

• Communicates effectively using a translator or interpreter.

• Interprets messages accurately, as evidenced by appropriate verbal or nonverbal feedback.

| Planning Interventions/Implementation |

For *NIC standardized interventions* and selected nursing activities for Impaired Verbal Communication,

 Go to Chapter 18, **Standardized Language,** in Volume 2.

Specific nursing activities for communication problems depend on the etiology of the problem and on the goals selected.

Enhancing Therapeutic Communication

The following are activities you can implement immediately to improve your communication with patients and others.

Active Listening

At first glance, the term *active listening* appears to be an oxymoron. People often think of listening as a passive activity. If you have ever been in a one-sided conversation, you are very aware that listening can be passive. In contrast, an active listener focuses on the sender's message with all senses.

An active listener gives undivided attention and allows the sender the opportunity to complete comments without interruption. Active listening requires paying attention to verbal and nonverbal communication and looking for congruence. If a message is

BOX 18-4

Characteristics of an Assertive Nurse

- Maintains eye contact, as culturally appropriate
- Speaks clearly and firmly
- Projects a clear tone of voice
- Is self-confident
- Maintains professional composure
- Communicates in a positive manner
- Refrains from sarcasm
- Provides congruence between verbal and nonverbal messages
- Guides the direction of the discussion

unclear, seek clarification through use of probing questions or reflective comments, such as, "Tell me more," or "When you say . . . what do you mean?"

As a nurse, you can demonstrate active listening by facing your client, making eye contact, and focusing the conversation on issues of importance to the client. If you must take notes during the conversation, record only key words to stimulate your memory at another time, because taking copious notes distracts you from active listening. Active listening behaviors signal a willingness to listen, convey caring, and provide a comfortable environment for the client to share his concerns.

Establishing Trust

Mutual trust is an essential component of therapeutic communication because it facilitates disclosure and honesty. As you and the client establish trust, the client can more easily relay information and share feelings. To establish trust, always greet the client by name, listen actively, respond honestly to the client's concerns, and provide care competently and consistently.

Being Assertive

There are many communication styles. In fact, it may be best to think of these styles as a continuum from passive, through assertive, to aggressive. A passive approach avoids conflict and allows others to take the lead. "Whatever you want. I don't want you to change anything for me," is an example of a passive approach. In contrast, an aggressive approach forces others to lose. The goal is to win and be in control. "My way is the correct way. You don't know what you're talking about," typifies an aggressive approach.

Assertiveness is the ability to express your beliefs or feelings without infringing on another's rights. Assertive communication conveys respect for others,

encourages honest feedback, and aims to establish balance and fairness without blame. Assertive communication techniques include the following:

- *Make "I" statements.* "I think this approach might be the best, but I'd like to hear your thoughts." This approach focuses on the issue, not the participants.
- *State facts, avoid judgments.* "The patient is in pain and needs medication," instead of, "Why haven't you given the patient his medications yet?"
- *Don't invite negative responses.* "I would really appreciate it if you could help me weigh Mr. Max on the bed scale," rather than, "Can you help me weigh him?"
- *Use assertive body language.* Face the client, stay calm, make eye contact, and speak clearly.

An assertive individual is one who is confident and comfortable and remains in charge of where the conversation is going. Assertive communication enables you to deal directly with stressful interpersonal communication. An assertive nurse also serves as a role model for the client. The therapeutic relationship is a safe place for clients to practice being assertive and receive feedback about their communication. See Box 18–4 for characteristics of an assertive nurse.

Restating, Clarifying, and Validating Messages

Restating means using your own words to summarize the message you received from the client. This demonstrates concern and active listening. Below is an example:

Client: I'm so worried about this diabetes. I have young kids. I want to see them grow up. Every diabetic I've known has died young.

Nurse: Diabetes is a serious disease. I understand why you would worry about its effects on you. However, we want to focus on becoming well controlled so that you can avoid complications.

Clarify messages to ensure that you have accurately interpreted the information. For instance, you might state, "I'm not sure what you mean when you say you're so worried about your diabetes." Or, "When you say you're worried, what do you mean?"

To validate the message, ask the client whether you are making a correct interpretation: "When you say you're worried about your diabetes, do you mean you are afraid you will die soon?" These techniques help to identify client concerns and focus communication. They are especially helpful if the client is unclear or vague with his message.

Interpreting Body Language and Sharing Observations

Be attentive to what the patient says and how she says it. Note the tone of voice, rate of speech, distance,

eye movement, facial expressions, and gestures. Look for congruence between the spoken message and the nonverbal message. If there is a disparity, share your observations with the patient. You can share your observations by describing the patient's body language or tone or voice. For example, you might state, "I know you said you feel well, but your voice and hands are trembling. How can I help you?" Or more simply, "You're frowning. Has something upset you?"

Exploring Issues

Ask open-ended questions to obtain a clear understanding of an issue and follow your client's thoughts (see Chapter 3). Probing comments such as "Tell me more" encourage your client to share information.

Using Silence

Learn to be comfortable with silence. When you remain silent but attentive, clients are unlikely to interpret your silence as a gap in rapport. Silence demonstrates acceptance and allows clients to compose their thoughts and provide further information. It is especially effective if your client is emotionally upset.

Summarizing the Conversation

At the end of the conversation, summarize what you have heard. For example, you might say, "Today we talked about diet, exercise, and medications for high blood pressure. Your job is to review the handouts and start taking your medication every morning. I will see you in 2 weeks when you return for your follow-up visit." Summarizing demonstrates active listening and allows the client to clarify any misunderstandings.

Barriers to Therapeutic Communication

As you learn to communicate therapeutically, you may find yourself thinking, doing, or saying things that seem to close down your conversation. If so, acknowledge your error and return to therapeutic patterns. The following sections describe the most common barriers to therapeutic communication.

Asking Too Many Questions

Asking questions at the appropriate time is important. However, asking too many questions, especially closed questions (requiring only a yes or no answer) can make clients feel they are being interrogated. Excessive questioning may suggest lack of respect or sensitivity to the client's issues, as in the following dialogue:

Patient:	I feel lousy today.
Nurse:	Didn't you sleep well?
Patient:	No, hardly at all.
Nurse:	Did you take anything to help you sleep?
Patient:	No.
Nurse:	Don't you think you should have taken something?
Patient:	I guess.
Nurse:	Why didn't you tell the night nurse you needed something?
Patient:	I don't know.

As you can see, this approach controls the range and nature of responses that the client provides. In contrast, open-ended questions stimulate conversation and exploration. Contrast the preceding conversation with the conversation below.

Patient:	I feel lousy today.
Nurse:	Lousy? Tell me more.
Patient:	Well, my back and neck hurts, and I hardly slept at all. I thought it would go away, but I just lay in bed last night worrying.
Nurse:	What kind of things are you worrying about?
Patient:	I'm worried about . . .

In the second conversation, the nurse asked open-ended questions. These prompts encouraged the patient to discuss his concerns.

Asking Why

In many health situations, we want to learn why a patient acted or responded as he did. However, asking why suggests criticism to some people. If you ask, "Why did you stop taking your medication?" the patient may become defensive and halt further communication. A more subtle approach is usually more comfortable for the patient. You might ask, "What concerns do you have about your medicines?" or "Tell me more about your experience with the medicines." Both of these approaches will help you gather more information about the client's concerns, without suggesting criticism.

Review the first dialogue in the previous section, "Asking Too Many Questions," for another example of the effect of "why" questions. How do you think this patient felt?

Changing the Subject Inappropriately

Abruptly changing the topic of discussion makes you appear uninterested. This often occurs when the nurse is intent on one issue and the client is focused on another. For example, imagine that you want to tell the patient about a change in the scheduling for a diagnostic test before you forget. As you enter the room, your patient says, "I am having a lot of pain in my

knee today." This situation requires you to address the patient's concern first and postpone discussing the schedule change until the patient can be receptive to the information.

In an ongoing dialogue, changing the subject can stop the flow of conversation cold. Both patients and nurses sometime use this tactic to avoid discussing sensitive topics. The following is an example:

Nurse:	This must be a tough time for you. Your wife is very sick. How are you handling this?
Patient's husband:	Yes, it's tough, but I went out to a movie last night. Have you seen that new Spielberg movie? It's all about . . .

Your relationship with the patient's husband and the facts of the patient situation would determine whether you would redirect this conversation back to the original subject or allow him to wander. You may choose to give the husband more time to be comfortable with you prior to approaching this topic again.

Failing to Listen

Failure to listen to your client will result in missed messages or misinterpretation. Consider this example:

Patient:	I guess I'm going to surgery tomorrow.
Nurse:	(Checking the IV fluids and hanging a medication) Uh-huh.
Patient:	The surgeon says I'll be in intensive care for a few days.
Nurse:	(Looking at the drainage in the urine collection bag) OK. Your urine looks good.
Patient:	I guess this is pretty risky surgery.
Nurse:	(Recording on the flowsheet) Yep.

How do you think the patient must feel in this situation? The patient is clearly expressing concern about his upcoming surgery. However, the nurse is busy with a variety of tasks and is not paying attention to the conversation. Undoubtedly the patient will continue to feel anxiety. In fact, his unsuccessful attempts to communicate may even increase his anxiety. If the nurse were listening, this would be an excellent opportunity to discuss the patient's concerns, provide preoperative teaching, and help the patient ease his anxiety.

Failing to Probe

The quality of your care is affected by the interchange between you and your client. A thorough assessment requires you to explore issues in detail. Failing to probe results in incomplete assessment. Review the following conversation.

Patient:	I'm having a lot of discomfort in my back.
Nurse:	How much does it hurt?
Patient:	Quite a bit. I had trouble sleeping last night.
Nurse:	I'll get you something for pain.

Compare this conversation with the next example, in which the nurse gathers additional data.

Patient:	I'm having a lot of discomfort in my back.
Nurse:	Tell me about the discomfort.
Patient:	It hurts a lot. I had trouble sleeping last night.
Nurse:	When did you first notice this pain?
Patient:	It started in the middle of the night.
Nurse:	What does it feel like?
Patient:	I feel sore. I'd like to turn over to my side, but I can't because of this heavy cast.
Nurse:	Let me help you turn. (Assists patient to turn and uses pillows to hold the patient on her side)
Patient:	Oh, that feels better!
Nurse:	How is the discomfort now?
Patient:	It's pretty much gone.
Nurse:	I'm glad you're feeling better. Would you like something for pain as well?
Patient:	I think I'm OK now.

In the second example, the nurse followed her original question with additional probing questions. A few additional questions helped clarify what the patient needed and led to immediate comfort.

Expressing Approval or Disapproval

We offer our friends and family members approval when they do something well or disapproval for doing something wrong. But you should exercise caution when providing approval or disapproval in the nurse-client relationship. Even approval can inhibit further sharing—it puts you in the position of being the judge of what is "right." This often prompts the patient to continue to seek approval. He thinks, "I'd better be careful; she may not approve of the next thing I was going to tell her. She expects me to be

this way." Consider instead offering recommendations and allowing the client to choose. Read the following exchange.

Patient: I've decided I'm going to have the surgery.

Nurse: That's great. I think you made the right choice.

Compare this conversation with the following example.

Patient: I've decided I'm going to have the surgery.

Nurse: Tell me about your decision.

Patient: Well, my shoulder has been bothering me for several months now. I know I said I wanted to put off surgery, but I think I'll have a faster recovery if I just get the surgery done now.

Nurse: So your choices are to do a trial of physical therapy and anti-inflammatory medicines, to try a steroid injection, or to have surgery.

Patient: Right. But there's a good chance I'll still need surgery even if I try the therapy or medicines. The only thing that will actually fix the problem is surgery. The others don't guarantee improvement.

Can you see how different the conversation becomes if the nurse does not express approval? By allowing the patient to discuss the choices, the nurse has empowered the patient to make his own healthcare decisions.

Offering Advice

Offering an opinion is rarely helpful. Avoid statements such as, "If I were you . . ." or, "You should . . ." These statements impose your opinion on your clients. In effect, your statements function as approval if they agree with the client's thoughts or disapproval if they do not. As with other forms of approval or disapproval, conversation halts. If the client asks, "What should I do?" help her clarify her options, and provide her with information about the choices. Telling the client what you think negates the client's opportunity to participate as a mutual partner in the decision-making process.

Providing False Reassurance

Providing reassurance helps to ease concern, offers comfort, and communicates empathy. Thus, it is an appropriate and therapeutic action—if the reassurance is warranted. For example, consider the client who presents to the emergency department (ED) for treatment of an acute episode of asthma. Because anxiety exacerbates asthma, reassuring the client that he will be cared for promptly and effectively is certainly therapeutic. In contrast, false reassurance is a barrier to therapeutic communication. When patients or family members ask for information or tell you that they are worried, it is easy to reassure them that everything will be okay. However, such responses are uninformed, inaccurate, and may feel dismissive—even condescending—to the receiver. Examine the following scenario:

You are a nurse working at the triage station in the local ED. Your role is to evaluate the condition and prioritize the care of all clients presenting for treatment. An ambulance arrives with a man complaining of severe chest pain. He is ashen and short of breath. He tells you his pain is "crushing." Suspecting a heart attack, you immediately move him to the critical care bay of the ED and request urgent evaluation. Several minutes later his wife arrives by private car and approaches the triage station. She anxiously asks, "How is my husband?" How would you respond?

It may be tempting to offer a response such as, "Don't worry, everything will be all right." But do you really know that will be the case? A better approach is to provide accurate information: "I had him immediately taken in for treatment. I'll get you in to see him as soon as I can. Please have a seat, and I'll check on him." This comment is accurate, calming, and avoids misstatements.

Stereotyping

As discussed in Chapter 13, racial, cultural, religious, age-related, or gender stereotypes distort assessment and prevent you from recognizing the uniqueness of the patient. Examples of statements reflecting a stereotype include, "He's old, he won't remember anything you tell him," or "Men are always the biggest crybabies about pain." Such comments may shut down communication and escalate tension. Avoid their use with patients and colleagues.

Stereotypes may be blatant or subtle. Blatant examples, such as those above, are easily recognized and may create an intense reaction. Subtle stereotypes, however, may be equally disruptive to care. Subtle stereotypes common in healthcare include the following:

• Believing a patient will be calm and know what to expect because he has had previous hospitalizations for the same diagnosis or has had previous surgeries or other procedures

- Assuming that patients will understand their health care because of their educational level or work experience, for example, expecting that a physician who has suffered a heart attack needs no explanation of her care
- Expecting all patients with the same surgery or diagnosis to experience similar responses

Using Patronizing Language

Patronizing language communicates superiority or disapproval. Statements such as, "You know better than that," are patronizing and offensive to the client.

Condescending approaches, such as, "You should have used the call button before you got up. You're lucky you didn't hurt yourself," do not communicate respect for the client.

Patronizing language may seem innocent. Have you heard staff call patients "Sweetie," "Dearie," or "Mama"? Although the intent is to be endearing, many patients are offended. When you first meet your client, use a formal title—Mr., Ms, and so on. In the orientation phase of the relationship, ask your patient how he would prefer to be addressed. If the patient is unable to respond, ask family members how to address the patient.

| toward evidence-based practice |

A group of Finnish researchers are conducting a series of studies on nurse-patient communication. Three of their recent studies are described below. Review the studies, and answer the questions below.

Poskiparta, M., Liimatainen, L., Kettunen, T., & Karhila, P. (2001). From nurse-centered health counseling to empowermental health counseling. *Patient Education Counseling, 45*(1), 69–79.

In this study, the researchers videotaped, transcribed verbatim, and analyzed 38 health counseling sessions. These counseling sessions began with checkup questions about the patients' conditions and continued with factual questions about their illnesses and healthcare measures. During nurse-centered discussions, the nurses' advice did not correspond to the patients' need for information. During health counseling sessions, the nurses made use of the patients' knowledge of their circumstances and supported their ability to reflect on their health behavior. Strategies for questioning and advising clients were found to be crucial for empowerment and enhancing the impact of health counseling.

Kettunen, T., Poskiparta, M., & Gerlander, M. (2002). Nurse-patient power relationship: Preliminary evidence of patients' power messages. *Patient Education Counseling, 47*(2), 101–113.

This research examined the nurse-patient power relationship from the patient's perspective through analysis of 38 health counseling sessions that the researchers videotaped, transcribed verbatim, and analyzed. The purpose of this research was to describe in detail how patients exercised control during hospital counseling. Nurses' power is associated with their healthcare knowledge.

However, patients construct their power and influence the flow of interaction by directing the counseling with questions, interruptions, and extensive disclosure.

Karhila, P., Kettunen, T., Poskiparta, M., & Liimatainen, L. (2003). Negotiation in type 2 diabetes counseling: From problem recognition to mutual acceptance during lifestyle counseling. *Qualitative Health Research, 13*(9), 1205–1224.

Researchers analyzed strategies used by nurses in 73 videotaped diabetes counseling sessions. Negotiation was found to be a frequently used tool. Negotiation consists of recognizing the problems in the patients' health behavior, offering proposals as solutions to the problems, and reaching an agreement on them.

Make a list of the results and findings of the three studies. This will help you to answer the critical-thinking questions that follow.

---

1. Suppose you are an inservice educator in a hospital. Which study supports your idea to develop a program to train nurses to improve their listening skills? Explain your reasoning.

2. Study 2 indicates that nurses' power comes from their healthcare knowledge. What does the study say about patients' power? What could nurses do to make patients' power resemble nurses' power more closely?

3. Look at study 3. Write a short scenario to illustrate how a nurse might negotiate with a patient.

 Go to Chapter 18, **Towards Evidence-Based Practice Suggested Responses,** on the Electronic Study Guide.

KnowledgeCheck 18–6

Identify at least five barriers to communication.

 Go to Chapter 18, **Knowledge Check Response Sheet and Answers,** on the Electronic Study Guide.

Using a Translator

Many health facilities have in-house translation services available for communication with non-English-speaking patients. Translators may also be available through telephone contact. Avoid using relatives as translators unless there are no other options. It is often culturally unacceptable to have family members ask personal questions. As a result, translations may be altered or questions remain unasked. See Chapter 13 for additional information on the use of translators. For a list of useful Spanish terms,

 Go to Chapter 18, **Technique 18–2: Some Useful Spanish Words and Phrases,** in Volume 2.

Enhancing Communication with Clients Who Have Impaired Hearing or Speech

For guidelines to help you communicate with clients who have hearing or speech deficits,

 Go to Chapter 18, **Technique 18–3: Communicating with Clients Who Have Sensory Deficits,** in Volume 2.

Enhancing Communication with Clients with Impaired Cognition or Reduced Level of Consciousness

Communicating with cognitively impaired clients can be difficult, time-consuming, and frustrating for even the most experienced healthcare provider. Make every effort to communicate regardless of whether or not the client can understand you. For guidelines to help you communicate with clients with impaired cognition or consciousness,

 Go to Chapter 18, **Technique 18–4: Communicating with Clients Who Have Impaired Cognition or Consciousness,** in Volume 2.

 Go to Chapter 18, **Resources for Caregivers and Health Professionals,** on the Electronic Study Guide.

 Suggested Readings: Go to Chapter 18, **Reading More About Communicating & the Therapeutic Relationship,** on the Electronic Study Guide.

 Bibliography: Go to Volume 2, Bibliography.

CHAPTER 19

Health Assessment: Performing a Physical Examination

Learning Outcomes

After completing this chapter, you should be able to:

✳ Identify the purposes and components of a physical examination.

✳ Discuss the differences among a comprehensive, focused, and ongoing physical examination.

✳ Describe how to prepare for a physical examination.

✳ Demonstrate the skills used in physical examination.

✳ Explain adaptations that may be required when you examine clients of various ages.

✳ Identify the components of the general survey.

✳ Conduct a full physical examination of a client.

✳ Discuss the expected findings of a physical examination.

✳ Document the findings of a physical examination.

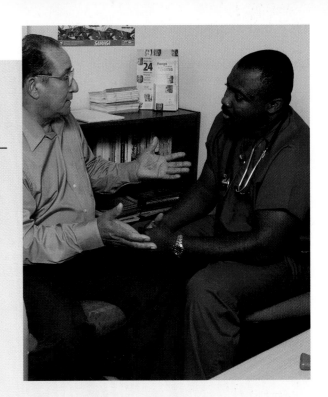

MEET Your Patients

Joseph Garcia is scheduled for a comprehensive physical exam at the family health center at 2:00 P.M. today. As you may recall, he has previously been seen and evaluated by Jordan Miller, FNP. Mr. Garcia has medical diagnoses of hypertension, degenerative joint disease, obesity, and tobacco abuse. During his earlier visit, Jordan instructed Mr. Garcia in a low-salt, low-fat diet and advised him to lose weight and quit smoking. Jordan also ordered lab work. You will find the results of Mr. Garcia's lab work in the figure on page 358.

At today's visit, Jordan will perform a comprehensive physical examination of Mr. Garcia and review his lab work. Later in the day, Flordelisa Garcia will also have a comprehensive exam.

Theoretical Knowledge
knowing why

Health assessment is a comprehensive assessment of the physical, mental, spiritual, socioeconomic, and cultural status of an individual, group, or community. A complete health assessment includes both a nursing history and a physical examination. Nursing assessments focus on the client's functional abilities and physical responses to illness and other stressors. In contrast, a medical assessment focuses on disease and pathology. As a nurse practitioner, Jordan Miller combines the nursing and medical approach.

PHYSICAL EXAMINATION

We usually think of **physical examination,** or **physical assessment,** as the techniques we use to gather objective data about the body. However, you will also ask questions to obtain subjective data about each body system or area. This may be done in a separate nursing interview or as you perform the physical examination.

What Are the Purposes of a Physical Examination?

A physical examination is performed for any of several reasons:

- *To obtain baseline data about a patient.* Data about the patient's physical status and functional abilities serve as a basis for comparison as the patient's health status changes.

- *To identify nursing diagnoses, collaborative problems, and wellness diagnoses.* Problem statements serve as the basis for the care plan and help you to address the patient's nursing care needs.

- *To monitor the status of a previously identified problem.* For example, Mr. Garcia has already begun treatment for hypertension. Today's examination will further investigate his hypertension and will be correlated with the lab results.

- *To screen for health problems.* Regular checkups identify health problems at early stages. Examples include annual breast examinations for women and testicular examinations for men. Mr. Garcia's PSA test was done to screen for prostate cancer.

The type of physical examination you perform will depend on the client's health status, the nature of the client encounter, and the setting. For example, at an outpatient appointment for an annual physical, on a client's admission to an inpatient setting, or at the initial home health visit, you would perform a **comprehensive physical assessment,** which includes an interview and a complete head-to-toe examination of every body system. Data from a

Laboratory Data for Joseph Garcia

Name: Joseph Garcia	**DOB:** 7/12/50	
Acct#: K00205412	Family Medicine Center, J. Miller	

Test	Result	Reference Range*
CBC/Differential		
WBC	$5.6 \times 10^3/mm^3$	$5–10 \times 10^3/mm^3$
Hemoglobin	14.8 g/dL	M: 14–18 g/dL
		F: 12–16 g/dL
Hematocrit	45.1%	M: 42–52%
		F: 37–47%
RBC count	5.1 million/mm^3	M: 4.7–5.14 million/mm^3
		F: 4.2–4.87 million/mm^3
MCV	84 mm^3	85–95 mm^3
MCH	29 pg	28–32 pg
MCHC	34%	33–35%
Neutrophils	57%	59%
Lymphocytes	30%	34%
Monocytes	5%	4%
Eosinophils	2.5%	2.7%
Basophils	0.7%	0.5%
Platelet count	197,000/mm^3	150,000–400,000/mm^3

Test	Result	Reference Range
Lipid Panel[†]		
Total cholesterol	201 mg/dL	< 160 mg/dL: optimal
		160–200 mg/dL: borderline high
		> 200 mg/dL: high
Triglycerides	196 mg/dL	< 150 mg/dL: normal
		150–199 mg/dL: borderline
		200–499 mgdL: high
		> 500 mg/dL: very high
LDL	140 mg/dL	< 100 mg/dL: optimal
		< 130 mg/dL: near optimal
		130–159 mg/dL: borderline high
		> 160 mg/dL: high
HDL	34 mg/dL	< 40 mg/dL: low

[†] To interpret lipid panel results, follow the most recent guidelines of the National Cholesterol Education Program (NCEP) Expert Panel on Detection, Evaluation, and Blood Cholesterol in Adults available at www.nhlbi.nih.gov/chd. The reference range figures in this table will undoubtedly be revised (and lowered) by NCEP in the near future.

Also, the norms for an individual patient's lipid panel depend on the calculation of risk factors. Joe is hypertensive, is obese, and has an elevated blood sugar. His norms reflect high risk for coronary heart disease; they would be about <160 for total cholesterol, <100 for triglycerides, <100 for LDL, and >45 for HDL.

Test	Result	Reference Range
Comprehensive Metabolic Panel		
Sodium	138 mEq/L	135–145 mEq/L
Potassium	4.3 mEq/L	3.5–5.0 mEq/L
Chloride	101 mEq/L	97–107 mEq/L
Carbon dioxide	27 mEq/L	23–29 mEq/L
BUN	16 mg/dL	10–31 mg/dL
Creatinine	0.8 mg/dL	M: 0.6–1.2 mg/dL
		F: 0.5–1.1 mg/dL
Glucose	156 mg/dL	75–110 mg/dL
Albumin	4.0 g/dL	19–60 years: 3.2-4.8 g/dL
Total protein	7.2 g/dL	6.8–8.0 g/dL
ALT (alanine aminotransferase, also called SGPT)	18 units/L	M: 10–40 units/L
		F: 7–35 units/L
ALP (alkaline phosphatase)	43 units/L	M: 35–142 units/L
		F: 25–125 units/L
AST (aspartate aminotranspeptidase, also called SGOT)	26 units/L	M: 19–48 units/L
		F: 9–36 units/L
Bilirubin, total	0.7 mg/dL	0.3–1.2 mg/dL
Calcium	8.5 mg/dL	8.2–10.2 mg/dL

Test	Result	Reference Range
Urinalysis		
Appearance	Clear	Clear
Color	Amber	Light yellow to amber
Odor	Aromatic	None–aromatic
pH	6.0	5.0–9.0
Specific gravity	1.012	1.001–1.035
Leukocyte esterase	Negative	Negative
Nitrites	Negative	Negative
Ketones	Negative	Negative
Protein	5 mg/dL	< 20 mg/dL
Crystals	None	In acid urine: uric acid, calcium oxalate, amorphous urates In alkaline urine: triple phosphate, calcium phosphate, ammonium biurate, calcium carbonate, amorphous phosphates
Casts	None	None, except rare hyaline
Glucose	Negative	Negative
WBC	1/hpf	< 5/hpf
RBC	1/hpf	< 5/hpf
PSA (prostate-specific antigen)	2.8 ng/mL	< 4 ng/mL
Fecal occult blood screen		

Sample #1 — negative
Sample #2 — negative
Sample #3 — negative

*For most studies, each laboratory establishes its own reference range.

Source: Van Leeuwen, A.M., Kranpitz, T.R., & Smith, L. (2006). *Davis's comprehensive handbook of laboratory and diagnostic tests with nursing implications,* 2e. Philadelphia: F.A. Davis Company.

comprehensive physical assessment provides guidance for planning care and determines the need for further assessment.

In an urgent situation, your assessment will be rapid and focused on the presenting problem. A **focused physical assessment** is performed to obtain data about an actual, potential, or possible problem that has been identified. It focuses on a particular topic, body part, or functional ability rather than on overall health status, and it adds to the database created by the comprehensive assessment. The following are examples of focused physical assessment:

- An abdominal exam for a client who is having abdominal pain
- Listening to the breath sounds of a client who has a cough

Ongoing assessment is performed as needed, after the initial database is completed, and, ideally, at every interaction with the patient. For example, on a medical-surgical unit, each nurse who provides care to a client conducts a brief ongoing assessment to update the client's status. Ongoing assessment data reflect the dynamic state of the client and are used in evaluating client outcomes. For more detail on the types of assessment, see Chapter 3.

How Do I Prepare to Perform a Physical Examination?

You should develop a systematic approach to physical examination and follow the same order each time you perform an exam. This will help you recall the steps and include all important data. You may use a **head-to-toe approach,** starting at the head and neck, progressing down the body, and examining the feet last. Or you could use a **body systems approach,** examining each system in a predetermined order (e.g., musculoskeletal, cardiovascular, neurological). Before beginning the physical examination, prepare yourself, the environment, and the client.

Prepare Yourself

Preparing for a physical examination requires theoretical knowledge of anatomy and physiology, examination equipment and techniques, therapeutic communication, and documentation. Self-knowledge is also important. How comfortable are you when performing an examination? What skills do you need to review or practice? Will you need assistance to perform some aspects of the exam? Will you need help charting your findings? Honestly evaluate your strengths and areas that need improvement. Assessment findings are the basis of many healthcare decisions, so be sure to seek help from your instructor, an experienced nurse, fellow students, or other healthcare providers as needed.

Before approaching the patient, familiarize yourself with the patient situation. What are the patient's main health concerns? What is the purpose of your exam? For instance, if you are doing a focused assessment of a client's wound, you will need to learn about the wound being examined. Is there a dressing over the wound? What supplies will you need to remove and replace the dressing? Has the patient required pain medication prior to past exams? Reviewing previous findings helps you to formulate any questions you might want to ask the patient.

Finally, unless this is an initial assessment, review the nursing plan of care and keep it in mind as you examine the patient. Your assessment data may lead to modification or updating of the care plan.

Prepare the Environment

Physical examination requires you to observe and touch the client's body, so privacy is essential. You will need a room with curtains or a door to shield the client from view. For additional privacy, drape your client and uncover only the area you are examining. For convenience you may use bed linens and/or a gown to drape. Disposable paper drapes are also available.

Because you will need to hear the patient and listen to a variety of sounds during the exam, turn off the television and radio. You will need good lighting for observing subtle changes in skin and body contours. Adjust the temperature of the room according to patient comfort.

Determine the instruments and equipment you will need. Take everything you need so that you will not have to leave the client to obtain supplies.

Prepare the Client

In most clinical settings, you must conduct examinations often to evaluate a client's changing status, and timing will be dictated by the client's condition rather than by convenience. However, timing is important. When possible, select a time when the client is relaxed and receptive to the examination.

Help the client to relax by taking the time to develop rapport. Introduce yourself, ask the client how he wishes to be addressed, and explain what you will be doing. Have the client void before the examination; this promotes relaxation and also makes it easier to palpate the abdomen. Always alert the client before touching him. For example, before you start to palpate the neck for lymph nodes, say, "I'm going to feel your neck now." Proper positioning during the exam also promotes comfort (see the following section).

Consider cultural differences. For example, some clients may wish to have a family member present; some may require a same-sex examiner. If the client's language is different from yours, arrange to have an interpreter present.

KnowledgeCheck 19–1

- What are the purposes of physical examination?
- Describe how you would prepare for a physical exam.

 Go to Chapter 19, **Knowledge Check Response Sheet and Answers,** on the Electronic Study Guide.

CriticalThinking 19–1

- Joe and Flordelisa Garcia (see "Meet Your Patients") are being examined at an outpatient clinic. Discuss the differences between their planned experience and a focused physical exam of a hospital inpatient.
- Identify a plan to practice and improve your assessment skills.

How Do I Position the Client for a Physical Examination?

The client will need to assume a variety of positions during a comprehensive physical examination. To begin the examination, seat the client on the side of the bed or examination table. Face the client, and establish eye contact. This helps to build rapport and put the client at ease. If your client is unable to sit, lay him flat on his back with the head of the bed elevated. An upright position allows the client to fully expand his lungs and is useful for assessing vital signs, the head and neck, the heart and lungs, the back, and the upper extremities. Table 19–1 illustrates and discusses the major positions you will need to use.

As you place your client in positions that allow you to best observe the body system you are examining, be alert to special needs that call for you to modify the position. For example, a patient with a cervical spine problem would need a neck roll when lying supine.

KnowledgeCheck 19–2

Identify the best position for examining the lungs, heart, pulses, and abdomen.

 Go to Chapter 19, **Knowledge Check Response Sheet and Answers,** on the Electronic Study Guide.

What Skills Do I Need to Perform a Physical Examination?

The skills used in physical examination include inspection, palpation, percussion, auscultation, and sometimes olfaction. You will use these skills in that order except when performing an abdominal assessment, in which case you will perform auscultation before percussion and palpation to avoid disturbing the abdominal sounds.

Inspection

Inspection is the use of sight to gather data. You begin to use inspection the moment you meet the client and continue as you observe the person's gait, personal hygiene, affect, and behavior during the general survey. You will also use inspection as you evaluate each body system. Adequate lighting and proper positioning aid inspection. The otoscope, ophthalmoscope, and penlight also enhance your inspection abilities.

Palpation

Palpation is the use of touch to gather data. Use palpation to assess temperature, skin texture, moisture, anatomical landmarks, and such abnormalities as edema, masses, or areas of tenderness. Following is a list of the most common palpation techniques, using different parts of the hand.

- *Fingertips:* use for fine tactile discrimination, including assessment of skin texture, swelling, and specific locations of pulsations and masses.
- *Dorsum of hand:* use for temperature determination.
- *Palmar surface of hand:* use for locating general area of pulsations.
- *Grasping with fingers and thumb:* use to detect the position, shape, and consistency of a mass.

Again, advise the client that you are about to touch him, and use a gentle approach. Be certain your hands are warm. Begin with light pressure to detect surface characteristics. Then move to deep palpation to assess the underlying structures. Examine last any areas of discomfort.

Percussion

Percussion is tapping your fingers on the skin using short strokes to assess underlying structures. Tapping produces vibrations. The resulting sound allows you to determine location, size, and density of underlying structures. Percussion is especially useful when assessing the abdomen and lungs. Percussion may be direct or indirect. For **direct percussion,** tap lightly with the pads of the fingers directly on the skin. **Indirect percussion** is used more frequently and requires two hands (Figure 19–1). Percussion takes practice. For the best results keep your fingernails short. A quiet environment allows you to perceive the

TABLE **19-1** Positioning the Client

Name	Description	Comments
Sitting 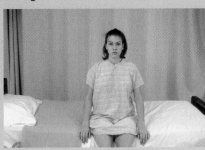	Sitting upright at side of bed or exam table	Use to assess vital signs, head and neck, chest, cardiovascular system, and breasts. If your client is weak, he may need assistance to maintain this position.
Supine (including Fowler's and semi-Fowler's positions) 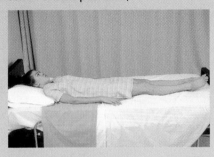	Lying flat on the back with arms and legs fully extended	Use to assess the abdomen, breasts, extremities, and pulses. If your client becomes short of breath, raise the head of the bed (HOB). In **Fowler's** position, the head is elevated 60°. In **semi-Fowler's** position, the head is elevated only 30–45°.
Dorsal recumbent 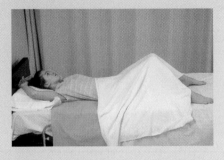	Supine with knees flexed	Use for abdominal assessment if your client has abdominal or pelvic pain. Flexing the knees promotes relaxation of the abdominal muscles.
Lithotomy 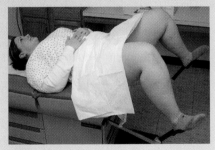	Dorsal recumbent position at end of table with feet in stirrups, legs flexed, and widely open	Use for a female pelvic exam; provides maximum exposure of genitals. Older patients may need support to assume and maintain this position. The patient's legs are exposed here to illustrate position. To see a privacy drape see Procedure 22-4 in Volume 2.
Sims' 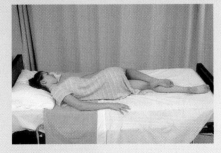	Flexion of the hip and knees in a side-lying position	Use to examine the rectal area. Use for a female pelvic exam if the patient is unable to assume the lithotomy position. Do *not* use if the client has had total hip replacement.

➤

TABLE 19-1 Positioning the Client *(continued)*

Name	Description	Comments
Prone 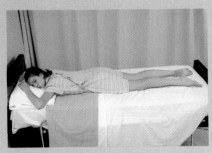	Lying on stomach (A small pillow under the abdomen makes this position more comfortable.)	Use to examine the musculoskeletal system, especially hip extension; may also be used to examine the back and buttocks. May be difficult to assume by clients with respiratory problems.
Lateral recumbent 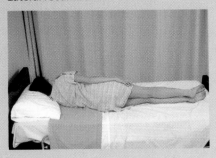	Lying on the side in a straight line	Left lateral recumbent is used to evaluate heart murmur or during a thorough cardiovascular assessment. This position brings the heart closer to the chest wall. If the client cannot assume this position, listen to the heart with the client seated and bending forward.
Knee-chest 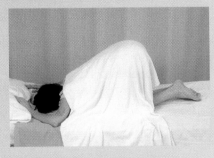	On hands and knees with head down and buttocks elevated	Provides good visualization for examining the rectal area. However, it is not used often because it is embarrassing and uncomfortable for the client.
Standing 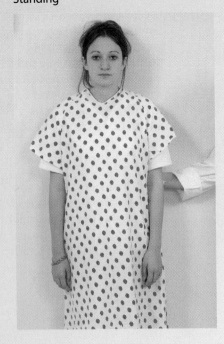	Upright posture with both feet flat on the ground	Use to examine the musculoskeletal and neurological systems and to assess gait and cerebellar function. Clients who are weak or who have poor balance may not be able to assume this position.

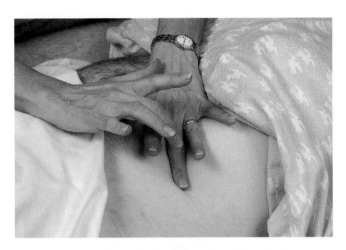

FIGURE 19–1 When performing indirect percussion, strike your stationary finger like a hammer to produce the best sound.

subtle differences in percussion notes. To learn terminology for the notes you may hear when assessing your clients,

 Go to Chapter 19, **Technique 19–1: Performing Percussion,** in Volume 2.

 Go to **Sound Files** on the Electronic Study Guide.

Auscultation

Auscultation is the use of hearing to gather data. **Direct auscultation** is listening without using an instrument. If you have heard wheezing or chest congestion without the use of a stethoscope, you have already performed direct auscultation. **Indirect auscultation** is listening with the help of a stethoscope. The stethoscope has two end pieces, the diaphragm and the bell.

- *Use the diaphragm* to listen to high-pitched sounds that normally occur in the heart, lungs, and abdomen. Press the diaphragm hard enough to produce an obvious ring on the patient's skin.

- *Use the bell* to hear low-pitched sounds, such as extra heart sounds (murmurs) or turbulent blood flow, known as bruits. Always apply the bell lightly with just enough pressure to produce an air seal with its full rim.

To improve your skill in indirect auscultation,

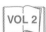 Go to Chapter 19, **Technique 19–2: Performing Auscultation,** in Volume 2.

Olfaction

Olfaction is the use of the sense of smell to gather data. Some clinicians may not consider this a formal assessment skill; however, you will certainly use this skill in the clinical setting. Olfaction adds information to the

data you collect through inspection, palpation, percussion, and auscultation. Consider these examples:

- If a client is slurring his words, you will want to look for data that reveal the cause of the problem. Slurred speech might be caused by a stroke or by sedative medications. However, if the client smells of alcohol you would first investigate recent alcohol use as a probable cause for the slurred words.

- If an older client smells of urine, you would want to assess for problems with leakage of urine or inability to perform self-care.

- If the client's breath has a "fruity" or "acetone" odor, you would suspect ketoacidosis (which may accompany diabetes). You would know to assess the urine for ketones and contact the primary care provider if necessary. You would also ask the client about dietary patterns, because a high-protein, high-fat, low-carbohydrate diet can cause a buildup of ketones in the blood.

KnowledgeCheck 19–3

- Identify five physical assessment skills.
- In what order are these skills performed?

 Go to Chapter 19, **Knowledge Check Response Sheet and Answers,** on the Electronic Study Guide.

CriticalThinking 19–2

 Think about olfaction as an assessment technique. Give two or three additional examples of data you might collect through the use of smell.

How Do I Modify Assessment for Different Age Groups?

The basic techniques of physical assessment remain the same for all age groups. However, your approach will vary according to the developmental stage of your patient. The most common modifications are discussed below.

Infants

Infants usually feel most secure if a parent holds them during the examination, either against the chest or, for older infants who can sit without support, on the parent's lap. Otherwise, position an infant on a padded examination table. If there are siderails, raise them to prevent falling. Do not leave the infant's side or turn your back on the infant. Use the assessment as an opportunity to teach the parent normal growth and development.

Toddlers

Toddlers can be challenging to examine. They are interested in exploring the environment, but they also like to

stay close by a parent, often in the parent's lap. Because they may be fearful of invasive procedures, such as examination of the oral cavity or inner ear, perform these procedures last. Most toddlers enjoy making choices, so use this characteristic to promote the toddler's cooperation. For example, you might provide a choice by saying, "Would you like to sit on the exam table or in your mother's lap?" or "Should I listen to your chest first, or should we see how much you weigh?" Allow the child to show you his developmental skills. If he needs assistance to remove clothing, have the parent help, and observe how the parent and child interact. Always praise the toddler for his abilities and cooperation. This sets the stage for positive feelings about health care.

Preschoolers

Preschool children are developing initiative and, as a result, usually cooperate with an examination. However, children of this age have fantasies and fears that may arise during the examination. For example, they may object to a noninvasive procedure because they believe it will cause pain or injury, or they may refuse to step on the scale because to them it resembles a monster. In such cases, it may be helpful to demonstrate the procedure on a doll or have the parent step on the scale prior to approaching the child.

As appropriate, allow the preschool child to sit in the parent's lap if she wishes. By age 5, most children will be comfortable enough to lie on the examination table if the parent is present. Let the child help with the exam. For example, have her hold equipment or remember her height and weight. Give reassurance as you go through the examination: for example, "Your lungs sound very healthy." Always compliment the child on her cooperation.

School-Age Children

The school-age child has a rapidly expanding vocabulary and usually seeks approval of parents, teachers, and healthcare providers. Develop rapport by asking the child about his favorite school or play activities. Allow the child to undress himself and get up and down from the exam table. Demonstrate your equipment before you use it. The school-age child will be interested in how his body works, so use this opportunity for teaching.

Adolescents

The adolescent is self-conscious and introspective and should be examined without parents or siblings present. Adolescents often worry about the "normalcy" of their changing bodies and appreciate attempts to respect their privacy. Be certain to discuss the normal physiological changes that accompany puberty (see Chapter 9). Adolescent behavior may be strongly influenced by peer values, so emphasize lifestyle habits that promote wellness, including a healthful diet, adequate rest and exercise, and avoidance of smoking, alcohol, and other drugs. Because suicide is the third leading cause of death in adolescents, you should also use this opportunity to screen for depression and suicide risk.

Young and Middle Adults

Most young and middle adults are able to cooperate during a physical examination and do not require a modified approach. Modifications may be required if the client has acute or chronic illness.

Older Adults

Older adults are adjusting to changes in physical abilities and health. As part of a comprehensive exam, assess the client's support system and ability to perform activities of daily living. Observe your client's energy level during the physical examination and provide rest periods if needed. If the client tires easily, arrange the exam sequence to limit position changes. Also be aware that stiff muscles and arthritic joints may make it impossible for the client to assume certain positions. Older adults may have impaired vision or hearing, so you may need to adapt your techniques to compensate for this. Obtain feedback to be sure the patient is seeing and hearing you adequately.

KnowledgeCheck 19–4

What exam modifications, based on developmental stage, should you consider for the following clients ("Meet Your Patients"):

- Joe Garcia?
- Joe's 3-year-old granddaughter, Bettina?
- Joe's elderly mother, Katherine?

 Go to Chapter 19, **Knowledge Check Response Sheet and Answers,** on the Electronic Study Guide.

Practical Knowledge
knowing how

The remainder of the chapter will discuss each of the components of a comprehensive physical examination. For a step-by-step approach to perform each assessment,

 Go to Chapter 19, **Procedures,** in Volume 2.

The Critical Aspects box on pages 393–396 summarizes the entire comprehensive physical assessment, including a summary of the general survey.

As you perform your physical assessments, you may wish to refer to laboratory tests associated with

each of the systems you are assessing. For a list of laboratory tests,

 Go to Chapter 19, **Supplemental Materials: Laboratory and Diagnostic Tests by System,** on the Electronic Study Guide.

THE GENERAL SURVEY

The general survey is your overall impression of the client. It begins at first contact with the client and continues as you gather data throughout the exam. When you discover a deviation from normal in the general survey, you will explore it further during focused assessment of that body system. For example, if on meeting the patient you notice a drooping eyelid (ptosis) on one side of her face, you will keep that in mind as you perform the neurological assessment (ptosis may be caused by a stroke or neurological injury). For a step-by-step approach,

 Go to Chapter 19, **Procedure 19–1: Performing the General Survey,** in Volume 2.

The following are aspects of the general survey.

Appearance and Behavior

Observe the client's general characteristics. Does he look his age? Are his speech and behavior appropriate for his developmental stage? Does he make eye contact with you? Be sure to consider cultural background, because this may influence your findings and interpretation. Look for any signs of distress, either physical or emotional. What is his mood? Observe the condition of your client's face: Are his facial features symmetrical? Note also the visible skin; for example, excessive wrinkling of the skin from sun exposure, tobacco use, or illness may make the client appear older than his stated age.

Body Type and Posture

Next, observe your client's body size, build, and gait. As you introduce yourself and greet him, assess his muscle strength, mobility, and skin temperature and texture. Are his body movements smooth and coordinated? Does he use a cane or other assistive device? If your client is bedridden, observe his ability to move from side to side and change positions. Posture is also a clue about overall health status. A slumped position may indicate fatigue, depression, or pain. An unsteady gait may be associated with joint, muscle, or neurological disorders. Focused assessments in the remainder of the exam will help to reveal the exact meaning of such cues.

Speech

As you talk with the client and ask health-related questions, look for clues offered by his speech.

- Inappropriate or illogical responses may be associated with psychiatric disorders.
- Difficulty speaking or changes in voice quality may indicate a neurological problem.
- Rapid speech may be a sign of anxiety, hyperactivity, or use of stimulants.
- Slow speech may be due to depression, sedation from medications, or neurological disorders.
- Vocabulary and sentence structure provide information about the client's educational level and comfort with the language.
- A foreign accent with hesitancy and/or sparse verbalization may signal a language barrier and a need for an interpreter.

Dress, Grooming, and Hygiene

A client's ability to dress and groom is affected by physical and emotional well-being. An unkempt appearance may reflect chronic pain, fatigue, depression, or low self-esteem. Poor hygiene may indicate a self-care deficit or lack of easily accessible bathroom facilities.

Mental State

Mental state includes level of consciousness and capacity to interact. Notice whether your client seems awake, alert, and oriented to time, place, person, and self. If the client has an altered mental status, ask a family member about the onset of the change. Keep in mind that many medications, especially in older adults, may contribute to a change in mental status.

- Bizarre responses may signal a psychiatric problem.
- Lethargy may be due to medications, depression, or a neurological, thyroid, liver, kidney, or cardiovascular disorder.
- Confusion and irritability may indicate hypoxia or medication side effects.
- Inability to provide a health history or to recall information may indicate a neurological disorder.

Vital Signs

You should assess vital signs as a part of the general survey and with each subsequent assessment. Analyze for trends. See Chapter 17 for a complete discussion of vital signs.

Height and Weight

Height and weight provide valuable information about your client's growth and development, nutritional status, overall general health, and required

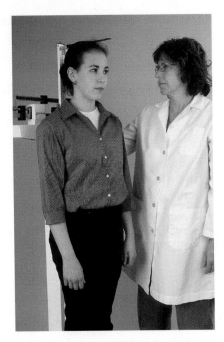

FIGURE 19–2 For adults, measure height with the client's back to the platform scale.

dosages for medication. For adults who can stand, measure height and weight using a platform scale with a sliding ruler (Figure 19–2). When possible, the client should wear minimal clothing (gown) and no shoes. If the client cannot stand, use a bed scale. To measure an infant's length, use a stationary measure. Because children have frequent changes in growth, their measurements are documented on growth charts for easy monitoring. For growth charts for males and females from birth to 20 years of age,

 Go to Chapter 19, **Supplemental Materials: Growth Charts,** on the Electronic Study Guide.

Body mass index (BMI) evaluates the relationship between height and weight. You can calculate the BMI for adults using a BMI calculator or table. For a BMI table,

 Go to Chapter 19, **Procedure 19–1: Performing the General Survey,** in Volume 2.

Because the proportion of fat to muscle affects BMI calculation, the BMI is not useful for athletes (who have a larger proportion of muscle), for pregnant and lactating women (who have a larger blood and tissue volume), for growing children, or for frail and sedentary older adults.

Once you have completed your general survey of the client, you can begin to focus on each body system. Whether you are doing a complete or focused physical assessment, remember that all body systems are interrelated. A problem in one system may affect or be affected by other systems.

THE INTEGUMENTARY SYSTEM

The integumentary system consists of the skin, hair, and nails. In a comprehensive exam, you assess this system by cursory exam and then in greater detail as you move through the exam. This allows the client to remain draped as long as possible.

The Skin

To perform a skin assessment, observe skin color, lesions, and other characteristics. As you observe the skin, also notice unusual odors. An unpleasant body odor may be a sign of poor hygiene, the presence of a wound, or underlying disease. Excessive sweating may be related to activity (for example, if the client has just completed exercise), thyroid problems, or overactive sweat glands. An odor of urine or stool may indicate a nursing diagnosis of Self-Care Deficit or Bowel or Urinary Incontinence.

For step-by-step instructions on performing a skin assessment,

 Go to Chapter 19, **Procedure 19–2: Assessing the Skin,** in Volume 2.

For a summary, refer to the Critical Aspects box on pages 393 to 396 of this volume.

Skin Color

Skin color varies according to age, culture, and ethnicity, but each person's skin color is fairly uniform. Exposed areas, such as the hands, face, and neck, are usually darker than unexposed areas, whereas the palms, soles, and nail beds are lighter than the rest of the skin. In people with dark skin, the lips are also usually lighter than surrounding skin. Variations in skin color commonly seen in neonates and infants include the following:

- **Mongolian spots** are blue-black areas seen on the lower back and buttocks of African American, Native American, and Asian babies. They are due to pigmented cells in the deeper areas of skin and fade as the child matures.
- **Capillary hemangiomas,** sometimes known as "stork bites," are small, irregular pink-red areas that are often seen around the face and neck in newborns. They typically disappear in infancy.

Table 19–2 discusses the significance of other skin color variations that may be seen in clients of any age.

Skin Characteristics

In addition to color, the temperature, texture, and turgor of the skin offer clues to the client's health status.

TABLE 19-2 Common Skin Color Variations

Color Variation	Description	Significance
Pallor	In light-skinned clients: extreme paleness; skin appears white; loss of pink or yellow tones In dark-skinned clients: a loss of red tones	May be related to poor circulation or a low hemoglobin level (anemia). Best sites to assess for pallor include the oral mucous membranes, conjunctiva, nail beds, palms, and soles of feet.
Cyanosis	A blue-gray coloration of the skin, often described as ashen	If seen in the lips, mucous membranes, and facial features, it is known as *central cyanosis* and is associated with hypoxia. May also be seen in the extremities, especially hands and feet, after exposure to extreme cold.
Jaundice	A yellow-orange cast to the skin	Often associated with liver disorders. Best sites to assess for jaundice include the sclera, mucous membranes, hard palate of the mouth, palms, and soles.
Flushing	A widespread, diffuse area of redness	Generalized redness of the face and body may occur as a result of fever, excessive room temperature, sunburn, polycythemia (an abnormal increase in red blood cells), or vigorous exercise.
Erythema	A reddened area	Associated with rashes, skin infections, and prolonged pressure on the skin.
Ecchymosis	Bruised (blue-green-yellow) area	May be seen anywhere on the body. The color will vary based on the age of the injury. May indicate physical abuse.
Petechiae	Tiny, pinpoint red or reddish-purple spots	Visible in the skin due to extravasation (leakage from vessels) of blood into the skin. May be associated with a variety of disorders and medications.

Although it is not technically a skin characteristic, you should also check for edema while you are assessing the skin.

Skin Temperature

Use the dorsum of the hand or fingers to assess skin temperature. Compare the temperature of the hands with that of the feet, and compare the right side of the body with the left. The skin should feel warm, but keep in mind that the temperature should be consistent with the room temperature and the patient's activity level.

If the patient's skin feels excessively warm, validate your data: Check her temperature to determine whether she has a fever. Hyperthyroidism stimulates the metabolism and may also cause an elevation in skin temperature. Excessive coolness may be due to poor peripheral circulation, shock, exposure to cold, or hypothyroidism.

Be sure to check the temperature of the skin over any area of erythema. Erythema accompanied by warmth may indicate infection or inflammatory changes.

Skin Moisture

Normally the skin is warm and dry. Excessive moisture may result from hyperthermia, thyroid hyperactivity, anxiety, or hyperhidrosis (excessive sweating). Oily skin is often seen with acne. Dry skin may result from dehydration, chronic renal failure, hypothyroidism, excessive exposure, or overzealous hygiene.

TABLE 19-3 Assessing Pitting Edema

Scale	Description
Trace	A minimal depression is noted with pressure.
+1	Creates a depression of about 2 mm. No visible distortion and rapid return of skin to position.
+2	Creates a depression up to 4 mm in depth that disappears in about 10–15 seconds.
+3	Creates a depression of approximately 6 mm in depth that lasts about 1–2 minutes. The area appears swollen.
+4	Creates a depression up to 8 mm in depth that persists for about 2–3 minutes. Area is grossly edematous.

Skin Texture

Normal skin is smooth and soft. The following factors affect skin texture:

- *Exposure.* Exposed areas tend to be drier and coarser in texture, as do the elbows and knees.
- *Age.* The skin of infants and young children is very smooth because of lack of exposure to the environment.
- *Hyperthyroidism and other endocrine disorders* may cause the skin to become coarse, thick, and dry.
- *Impaired circulation.* Peripheral arterial insufficiency is associated with smooth, thin, shiny skin with little to no hair. In contrast, venous insufficiency leads to thick, rough skin that is often hyperpigmented.

Skin Turgor

Turgor refers to the elasticity of the skin, which provides data about hydration status. To assess turgor, lift ("pinch up") a fold of skin (e.g., over the clavicle) and allow it to return to its normal position. Normally, skin returns immediately to original position. Skin that takes 3 seconds or longer to return to original position (**tenting**) may be a sign of dehydration. Elasticity decreases with age, so tenting may also be seen with normal aging. With edema or scleroderma, the skin turgor is increased, and the tension does not allow the skin to be pinched up.

Edema

Edema, or an excessive amount of fluid in the tissues, is an abnormal finding. It is common in clients with congestive heart failure, kidney disease, peripheral vascular disease, or low albumin levels. A client with edema may tell you his skin feels "tight" or say, "My shoes don't fit any more." Swollen tissue may feel tender to touch. Table 19–3 presents a grading system for edema.

Skin Lesions

Any **lesion,** variation in pigment, or break in continuous tissue requires assessment. Lesions considered to be normal variations include *milia,* white raised areas on the nose, chin, and forehead of newborns. These lesions, which resemble "white heads," are due to retention of sebum in the maturing sebaceous glands and disappear in infancy. Other normal variations are **nevi** (moles), freckles, birthmarks, **skin tags** (tiny tags or buds of skin usually around skin creases) in middle and older adults, and **striae** (silver-to-pink stretch marks) in pregnant women, women who have had children, and anyone who has experienced significant weight fluctuations. These are not harmful.

Abnormal lesions are classified as primary or secondary. **Primary skin lesions** develop as a result of disease or irritation. The pustules of acne are an example. **Secondary skin lesions** develop from primary lesions as a result of continued illness, exposure, injury, or infection, such as the crusts that form from ruptured pustules. The table at the end of Procedure 19–2 should also help you to categorize lesions. When you observe a lesion, evaluate it for size, shape, pattern, color, distribution, texture, surface relationship, exudate, tenderness, pain, or itching.

 VOL 2   Go to Chapter 19, **Procedure 19–2: Assessing the Skin,** in Volume 2.

Also see the Abnormal Atlas at the end of chapter 19 in Volume 2 to view abnormal lesions associated with particular conditions, such as cellulitis and scabies.

Evaluate all skin lesions for the possibility of malignancy. Ask the client whether he has any newly developed moles or skin lesions or whether there has been any change in the appearance of existing lesions. You can remember the warning signs of malignant lesions by thinking of the letters ABCDE:

A—is for asymmetry.
B—is for border irregularity.
C—is for color variation.
D—is for diameter greater than 0.5 cm.
E—is for elevation above the skin surface.

KnowledgeCheck 19–5

- What aspects of the skin should you assess?
- What assessments should you perform if you find a lesion?
- What warning signs lead you to suspect a malignant lesion?

 Go to Chapter 19, **Knowledge Check Response Sheet and Answers,** on the Electronic Study Guide.

The Hair

When assessing the hair, inspect and palpate for color, texture and distribution, as well as the condition of the scalp. The hair should be clean and free of debris. A client who does not properly groom her hair may need help with ADLs or may be neglecting herself.

- *Color.* There is a wide range of naturally occurring hair color. Age-related graying of the hair varies among individuals according to their genetic background. White hair accompanied by very pale skin is seen in a condition known as **albinism,** or lack of pigment.
- *Texture.* Hair texture varies normally from fine to coarse. However, hair that is exceptionally dry and coarse hair may be a sign of hypothyroidism; very fine, silky hair may indicate hyperthyroidism.
- *Distribution.* Generally the hair is evenly distributed on the scalp, and fine body hair is present over the body. Men often have more hair on the face, chest, and back. Alterations in hair distribution may be signs of disease.

  Alopecia (hair loss) along the temples and in the center of the scalp is considered a normal balding pattern in men and is largely genetically based. Diffuse alopecia can be caused chemotherapy for the treatment of cancer, by nutritional deficiencies, or by endocrine disorders.

  Patchy hair loss may be due to fungal infections of the scalp, hair pulling, constant wearing of caps, or *alopecia areata,* a benign autoimmune disorder.

  Hirsutism (excess facial or trunk hair) may be due to endocrine disorders or steroids.
- *Scalp.* Normally the scalp is smooth, firm, symmetrical, nontender, and without lesions. Common deviations include an asymmetrical or bumpy scalp due to trauma or lesions, and scaly flakes or patches due to fungal infection (e.g., dandruff), dermatitis, or psoriasis. Tenderness may indicate a localized infection or trauma. In newborns, *cradle cap*—scaly white patches over the scalp due to secretion of sebum—is common. It can be removed with washing and gentle scrubbing.

In addition, the hair should be free of debris and **pediculosis** (head lice infestation). Head lice are tiny, very mobile, and difficult to see. You may find it easier to see the eggs, or **nits,** that are deposited on the hair shaft close to the scalp.

 Go to Chapter 19, **Procedure 19–3: Assessing the Hair,** in Volume 2.

See also the Critical Aspects box, on pages 393 to 396 of this volume, for a step-by-step description of assessing the hair.

The Nails

Healthy nail beds are level, firm, and similar to the color of the skin. The nail is smooth and uniform in texture with a 160° nail plate angle. Examine nails on both hands and feet. However, you may defer examination of the toenails until you are assessing the peripheral circulation. Variations in color, shape, or texture may indicate health problems.

For a step-by-step description of nail assessment, see the Critical Aspects box on pages 393 to 396, and

 Go to Chapter 19, **Procedure 19–4: Assessing the Nails,** in Volume 2.

For illustrations of nail variations, go to the Abnormal Atlas at the end of chapter 19 in Volume 2.

Nail Color

Pale or cyanotic nail beds are seen in clients with circulatory or respiratory disorders that result in anemia or hypoxia. Other color abnormalities that you may encounter include the following:

- *Half-and-half nails,* in which a distal band of reddish-pink covers 20 to 60% of the nail. These occur in clients with low albumin levels or renal disease.
- *Mee's lines,* which are transverse white lines in the nail bed. They are seen in clients who have experienced severe illnesses.
- *Splinter hemorrhages,* which are small hemorrhages under the nail bed. They are associated with bacterial endocarditis or trauma.
- *Black nails,* due to blood under the nail, are seen after local trauma.
- *White spots* may indicate zinc deficiency.

Nail Shape

A change in nail shape may indicate underlying disease. Figure 19–3 illustrates the typical nail plate angle of 160°. Clubbing, in which the nail plate angle is 180° or more, is associated with long-term hypoxic states, such as occurs with chronic lung disease. Spoon-shaped nails may result from iron deficiency.

Nail Texture

Nails are normally smooth in texture. You may see the following indications of problems:

- Thickened nails may result from poor circulation.
- A thick nail with yellowing is an indication of fungal infection known as *onychomycosis.*

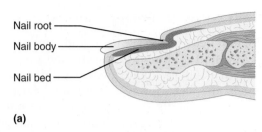

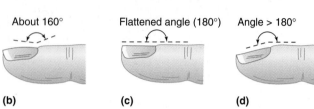

FIGURE 19–3 Nails. *A,* Parts of the nail. *B,* The normal nail plate angle is 160°. *C,* A nail plate angle of 180° or more is known as clubbing. *D,* Late clubbing from long term hypoxia.

- Brittle nails are seen with hyperthyroidism, malnutrition, calcium and iron deficiency, and repeated use of harsh nail products.
- Soft, boggy nails are seen with poor oxygenation.

The tissue surrounding the nail should be smooth epidermis. Chronic nail-picking results in callus formation around the nail. Occasionally the surrounding skin becomes inflamed. This condition, known as *paronychia,* is painful and may require drainage if infection is present.

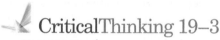 CriticalThinking 19–3

You are caring for a woman who has no hair on her head. How might you determine the cause of her hair loss? What other assessments should you perform?

THE HEAD

Assessment of the head is often referred to by the acronym HEENT: head, eyes, ears, nose, and throat. You will use all the assessment techniques—inspection, palpation, percussion, and auscultation—in the HEENT exam.

The Skull and Face

Taking individual variation into account, the skull should be rounded and the face symmetrical in appearance and movement. Inspect head size; if it seems unusual, measure it.

- A large head in an adolescent or adult may be associated with **acromegaly,** a disorder associated with excess growth hormone.
- **Microcephaly,** an abnormally small head size, is seen in clients with certain types of mental retardation.

- In infants, abnormal shape or flattening of the skull may result from trauma during a vaginal birth or placing the baby in the same position for several hours every day.
- In infants and children, a head that is growing disproportionately faster than the body may be a sign of **hydrocephalus** (an accumulation of excessive cerebrospinal fluid).
- Asymmetry may be the result of trauma, surgery, neuromuscular disorder, paralysis, or congenital deformity.
- Facial appearance that is inconsistent with gender, age, or racial/ethnic group may indicate an inherited or chronic disorder, such as Graves' disease, hypothyroidism with myxedema, or Cushing's syndrome.

The skull should be smooth to palpation, with no unusual contours or bulges. Jaw motion should be symmetrical with no pain, clicking, or crepitus (cracking). Contour abnormalities, bulging, or tenderness result from trauma, congenital anomalies, or surgery. Irregular jaw movement or cracking of the jaw may indicate **TMJ** (temporomandibular joint) **syndrome.** The Critical Aspects box on pages 393 to 396 summarizes the assessment of the face. For the entire procedure, and an Abnormal Atlas of facial abnormalities,

 Go to Chapter 19, **Procedure 19–5: Assessing the Head and Face,** in Volume 2.

The Eyes

In examining the eyes, you will inspect and palpate the external eye structures, assess vision, and examine the internal eye structures. Have the patient assume a sitting position for the exam. The Critical Aspects box on pages 393 to 396 summarizes the eye exam. For step-by-step instructions.

 Go to Chapter 19, **Procedure 19–6: Assessing the Eyes,** in Volume 2.

For convenience, you may wish to perform some cranial nerve testing along with the eye exam (e.g., corneal reflex, pupillary reaction, accommodation, and extraocular movements). For instructions on performing a cranial nerve examination,

 Go to Chapter 19, **Procedure 19–16: Assessing the Sensory-Neurological System,** in Volume 2.

External Structures

To review the structure of the external eye, see Figure 19–4. Normal eyelid margins are moist and pink with short lashes that are evenly spaced and curl outward.

The lower eyelid margin appears at the bottom edge of the iris, and the upper eyelid covers half the upper iris. The conjunctiva is smooth, glistening, and peach in color, with minimal blood vessels present. There should be no pallor, dryness, or edema. The following are common abnormal findings of the eyelids:

- Crusting, scales, or swelling of the lid is associated with infection of the eyelids or eyelashes.
- A **pterygium** is a growth or thickening of conjunctiva from the inner canthus toward the iris.
- **Ectropion,** an everted eyelid, is commonly seen in older adults secondary to loss of skin tone. It can lead to excessive dryness of the eyes.
- **Entropion,** an inverted eyelid, can lead to corneal damage.
- **Ptosis,** or drooping of the lid, may be seen in clients who have experienced a stroke (cerebrovascular accident, or CVA) or Bell's palsy (paralysis of the facial nerve). To see ptosis and other abnormalities,

 Go to Chapter 19, **Procedure 19–5: Assessing the Head and Face,** and the **Abnormal Atlas,** in Volume 2.

The **sclera** should be smooth, glistening, and blue-white in color with tiny vessels visible. Dark-skinned patients may have a yellowish cast to the peripheral sclera or small brown spots more centrally. Numerous disorders may affect the sclera and conjunctiva, including infection, allergies, injuries, and liver disorders. For example, yellow (**icteric**) sclera may be seen with an elevated bilirubin. Blood visible in the sclera is known as a **subconjunctival hemorrhage** and may be related to trauma or hypertension.

The lens and the **cornea,** or outermost layer of the eyeball, are transparent, smooth, and moist. A white ring encircling the outer rim of the cornea is known as **arcus senilis** and is a normal variant in older adults. Lens opacities, known as **cataracts,** are frequently seen in older adults and may impair vision. Roughness or irregularity of the cornea is seen with trauma or a corneal abrasion.

The **pupils** should be uniform in color, equal in size, and round. They should **accommodate** equally; that is, the pupils constrict and the eyes converge (cross) as a person attempts to focus on an object moving toward him. This is typically charted as PERRLA: pupils equal, round, reactive to light and accommodation. The following are common pupil abnormalities:

- Sluggish accommodation may be caused by anticholinergic drugs or advanced age.
- Failure of one or both pupils to accommodate may reflect a cranial nerve III problem or **exophthalmos** (associated with hyperthyroidism).

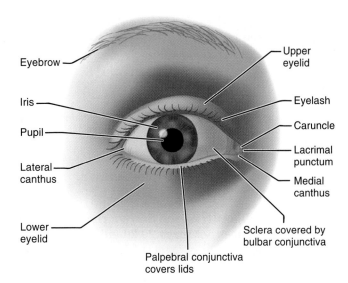

FIGURE 19–4   The external eye and eyelid.

- Cloudy pupils, a sign of cataracts, are commonly seen in older adults.
- **Mydriasis** (enlarged pupils) may be seen with glaucoma, an increase in intraocular pressure.
- Many medications affect pupil size. Medications called *mydriatics* are used to dilate the pupil to allow better visualization of the internal eye during examination. **Miosis** (constricted pupils) often results from medications to treat glaucoma.
- **Anisocoria** (unequal pupils) may be seen with central nervous system disorders such as stroke, head trauma, or cranial nerve injuries.

Visual Acuity

Visual acuity is a measure of the eye's ability to detect the details of an image. When testing visual acuity, you will assess distant, near, peripheral, and color vision. Nurses usually perform screening tests of visual acuity. Other testing is performed by nurses in advanced or specialty practice or by an optometrist or ophthalmologist as needed.

Distance Vision

Use the Snellen chart from a distance of 20 feet to assess distance vision. Assess each eye separately, and then reassess both eyes simultaneously. Normal vision is a measure of 20/20 in the right eye, left eye, and both eyes without hesitation. If a patient hesitates, document "with hesitation." If the person misses one or two items in a line, document the number missed.

Myopia, or diminished distant vision, is associated with a smaller fraction. For example, 20/100 vision implies that to see lines of print that a person with normal vision can read at 100 feet, the client has

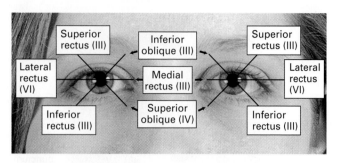

FIGURE 19–5 Cranial nerves and the extraocular muscles.

to stand just 20 feet from the Snellen chart. A child's distance vision does not reach 20/20 until around 6 or 7 years of age.

Near Vision

Test near vision by having the client read newsprint from a distance of 35.5 cm (14 in.). A client with normal near vision will be able to read the newsprint without hesitation with either eye and both eyes. With **hyperopia,** or diminished near vision, the client must hold the paper more than 35.5 cm (14 in.) away. As we age, the lens of the eye naturally loses some ability to accommodate to near objects. In a client over 45 years of age, diminished near vision is known as **presbyopia.**

Color Vision

Color vision is the ability to detect color. **Color blindness** may be genetically inherited (usually seen in males), or it may result from macular degeneration or other diseases that affect the cones of the eye. Use the color bars at the base of the Snellen chart to test color vision. *Ishihara cards,* specialized cards that enable thorough testing for color blindness, contain embedded figures within a field of color. An individual with normal color vision will be able to successfully identify the figures in the cards or the bars on the base of the Snellen chart, whereas a person who is color blind will not.

Visual Field

Visual field is the area observable with the eye. It is related to peripheral vision and extraocular muscle (EOM) function. **Peripheral vision** describes the boundaries of the visual field while the eye is in a fixed position. The common phrase, "I see you out of the corner of my eye," refers to peripheral vision.

The EOMs control the movement of the eye and eyelids and allow you to track movement. Three cranial nerves (CN) innervate the EOM. They are CN III (oculomotor), CN IV (trochlear), and CN VI (abducens). CN III also works together with CN II (optic)

to control the pupillary reaction to light. Figure 19–5 illustrates the eye positions affected by the EOM and the corresponding cranial nerves.

Visual field abnormalities may be caused by problems with the cranial nerves III, IV, and VI or with the retina. Poorly controlled diabetes, cataracts, macular degeneration, and advanced glaucoma are disorders that limit the visual field.

Internal Structures

To visualize the internal structures of the eye, use an ophthalmoscope in a darkened room. Examine the optic disc, physiological cup, retinal vessels, retinal background, and macula. This is an advanced assessment technique; however, advanced practice nurses and registered nurses on specialty units do perform it with training. Advanced practice nurses use this technique to gain information about certain diseases that affect the eye, such as hypertension and diabetes.

KnowledgeCheck 19–6

- What are the major components of an eye assessment?
- Identify the cranial nerves involved with eye movement and function.

 Go to Chapter 19, **Knowledge Check Response Sheet and Answers,** on the Electronic Study Guide.

The Ears and Hearing

The ear is involved in hearing and equilibrium. The **external ear** collects and conveys sound waves to the middle ear. It protects the middle ear from environmental factors such as humidity and temperature and prevents entry of foreign matter. The **middle ear** contains the tympanic membrane and cavity, the eustachian tube, and the **ossicles** (the small bones of the middle ear: the malleus, incus, and stapes). The middle ear conducts sound waves to the inner ear. The **inner ear** is responsible for hearing and equilibrium. Figure 19–6 illustrates the structures of the ear.

You will use an otoscope and tuning fork to examine the ears. For procedure steps and guidelines for using the otoscope and tuning fork,

VOL 2 Go to Chapter 19, **Procedure 19–7: Assessing the Ears and Hearing,** in Volume 2.

See also the Critical Aspects box on pages 393 to 396.

As with the eyes, registered nurses are usually responsible for screening and making referrals. However, in some settings nurses perform advanced assessments.

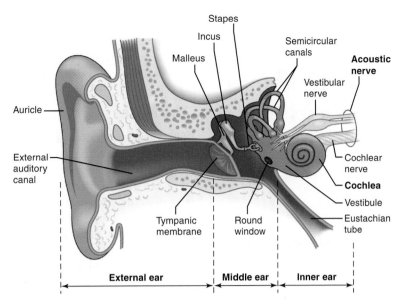

FIGURE 19–6 Cross-section of the ear.

Examining the External and Middle Ear

On inspection, the ears should be of equal size and similar appearance. Normally the pinna is level with the corner of the eye and within a 10° angle of vertical position (Figure 19–7). Altered placement of the ear may be a sign of hearing deficit or genetic disorders, including Down syndrome. There should be no lesions or drainage. Bloody drainage may result from trauma. Purulent drainage may be seen with infection.

On palpation, the external structures of the ear are smooth, nontender, pliable, and without nodules. A painful auricle or tragus may be associated with **otitis externa** (an outer ear infection), whereas tenderness behind the ear is seen with **otitis media** (a middle ear infection).

As you begin the otoscopic examination, you may notice that the external auditory canal contains **cerumen** (wax), which protects the middle ear from excessive drying. However, it should not completely obstruct the ear canal. Cerumen may be black, dark red, gray, or brown in color and waxy, flaky, soft, or hard, with no odor; all are normal variations. The auditory canal walls are smooth and free of redness or drainage. Be careful as you manipulate the otoscope, because the inner two-thirds of the canal is tender to the touch.

Normally the **tympanic membrane (TM)** is pearly gray, shiny, and translucent. The structures of the middle ear should be visible through the membrane. Changes in its appearance arise from abnormalities such as otitis media (which causes a red, bulging TM) and the presence of pressure equalization tubes in young clients with chronic ear infections.

Assessing Hearing

To assess hearing, you will need a quiet room and a tuning fork. Gross hearing ability includes the ability to hear both high- and low-pitched tones. A client who hears low tones will be able to hear and repeat words whispered from 1 to 2 feet behind him. The client can

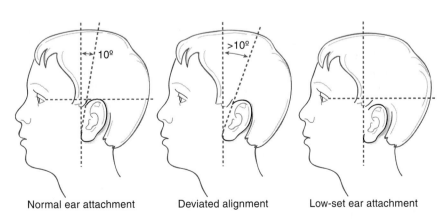

Normal ear attachment   Deviated alignment   Low-set ear attachment

FIGURE 19–7 Normally the pinna is level with the corner of the eye and within a 10° angle of vertical position.

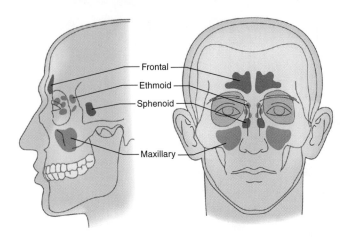

FIGURE 19–8 Paranasal sinuses: frontal, ethmoid, sphenoid, and maxillary.

hear high tones if he is able to hear a watch ticking at 5 inches (12 to 13 cm) from each ear.

The Weber and Rinne Tests

Hearing involves transmission of sound vibrations and generation of nerve impulses along CN VIII. The **Weber test** assesses both aspects. When you place a vibrating tuning fork on the center of the client's head, he should be able to sense the vibration equally in both ears. Record a positive Weber test if the vibration is louder in one ear.

If the Weber test is positive, you will need to perform the Rinne test to assess the type of hearing problem. The **Rinne test** also uses a tuning fork to compare air conduction (AC) and bone conduction (BC). Normally AC is twice as long as BC. For step-by-step instructions for performing the Weber and the Rinne tests,

 Go to Chapter 19, **Procedure 19-7: Assessing the Ears and Hearing,** in Volume 2.

The Romberg Test

Vestibular cells in the ear are responsible for maintaining equilibrium. To assess equilibrium, perform the Romberg test. Have the client stand with feet together and eyes closed. The client should be able to maintain balance with minimal swaying. Swaying and moving (positive Romberg) may indicate a vestibular disorder.

KnowledgeCheck 19–7

Your client has a negative Weber test. What further testing is required?

 Go to Chapter 19, **Knowledge Check Response Sheet and Answers,** on the Electronic Study Guide.

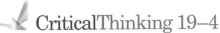 CriticalThinking 19–4

What type of symptoms would you expect a client to be experiencing if he had a positive Romberg test?

The Nose

The nose and sinuses (Figure 19–8) are part of the respiratory system and are the organs of smell. Vaporized molecules sniffed into the upper nasal cavities trigger receptors that generate impulses along the olfactory nerve (CN I) that travel to olfactory centers in the temporal lobes. The sense of smell diminishes in older adults because of a gradual decrease in and atrophy of the olfactory nerve fibers.

The external nose should be smooth, nontender, and symmetrical, with a midline septum. The client should be able to breathe freely through both sides of the nose. Normally the mucous membrane inside the nose is pink and moist and without lesions. To assess the nose and sinuses, you will need a penlight and nasal speculum or an otoscope with broad-tipped speculum. See the Critical Aspects box on pages 393 to 396 of this volume and

 Go to Chapter 19, **Procedure 19-8: Assessing the Nose and Sinuses,** in Volume 2.

The Mouth and Oropharynx

The structures of the mouth include the lips, tongue, teeth, **gingiva** (gums), uvula, hard and soft palate, and salivary glands and ducts (Figure 19–9). On external inspection, the mouth and lips should be

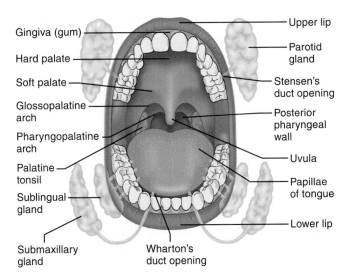

FIGURE 19–9 Structures of the mouth.

symmetrical and without lesions, swelling or drooping. For instructions on examining the mouth and oropharynx,

 Go to Chapter 19, **Procedure 19–9: Assessing the Mouth and Oropharynx,** in Volume 2.

The Critical Aspects box on pages 393 to 396 summarizes the procedure.

The Lips, Buccal Mucosa, and Gingiva

The lips, **buccal mucosa** (mucous membrane of the cheeks), and gums should be smooth, moist, and pink in color. Increased pigmentation (e.g., bluish or dark patches) occurs in dark-skinned clients. No lesions should be present. The following are abnormal findings:

- Paleness may indicate anemia or inadequate oxygenation.
- **Canker sores** are painful vesicles that erupt with allergies and stress.
- **Gingivitis** is a sign of periodontal disease. You will see red, swollen, or spongy, bleeding gingiva and receding gum lines. The gums may be tender.
- **Parotitis** is an inflammation of the parotid salivary gland.
- **Stomatitis** is inflammation of the oral mucosa.
- **Leukoplakia** (thick, elevated white patches) that do not scrape off may be precancerous lesions; white, curdy patches that scrape off and bleed indicate **thrush** (a fungal infection).
- Redness or abrasions of the gingiva may be caused by poorly fitted dentures.
- **Aphthous ulcers** are small, painful vesicles with a reddened periphery and a white or pale yellow base. They are believed to be caused by viral infection, stress, or trauma.

Be sure to ask your client about use of tobacco, either smoked or chewed. Both forms of tobacco are associated with increased risk for oral cancer.

The Teeth

The upper teeth rest on top of lower teeth, with the upper incisors slightly overriding lower ones. A healthy adult should have 28 teeth, or 32 if the wisdom teeth are present. The teeth should be fixed to the gum and without obvious debris or darkening that may indicate caries. Tooth decay and periodontal (gum) disease are common. Both arise from poor oral hygiene. As you examine the mouth and teeth, talk to the patient about his oral care. Recommend tooth brushing after each meal, daily flossing, and dental

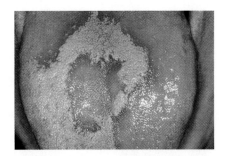

FIGURE 19–10   A geographic tongue is a common normal variant.

checkups every 6 months. See Chapter 22 for a more complete discussion of oral hygiene and prevention of periodontal disease.

The Tongue

When inspecting the mouth, carefully examine all aspects of the tongue: dorsal, ventral, and lateral. The **tongue** should be moist, symmetrical, slightly rough, smooth, pink, and freely movable. A fissured, or geographic, tongue is a common normal variation (Figure 19–10). The following are abnormal findings:

- Deviation from the midline, which may be caused by damage to the hypoglossal nerve (CN XII)
- Limited mobility of the tongue
- **Glossitis** (inflammation of the tongue)
- A dry, furry tongue, which is associated with dehydration
- A black, "hairy" tongue, which is associated with fungal infections
- Absence of papillae, reddened mucosa, and ulcerations, which may indicate allergy, inflammation, or infection
- Swelling, nodules, or ulcers
- A smooth, red tongue, which may occur in clients who have a deficiency of iron, vitamin B_{12}, or vitamin B_3

The Hard and Soft Palates and Oropharynx

The hard palate, soft palate, and oropharynx should be pink, moist, and intact. No lesions, swelling, erythema, or discharge should be present. If the tonsils are present, they should be symmetrical, small in size, and free of exudate in a healthy person. The uvula is midline and should rise on **phonation** (vocalization).

THE NECK

The neck has components of the musculoskeletal, neurological, vascular, respiratory, endocrine, and lymphatic systems. The sternocleidomastoid and trapezius muscles form the landmarks of the neck, known as the

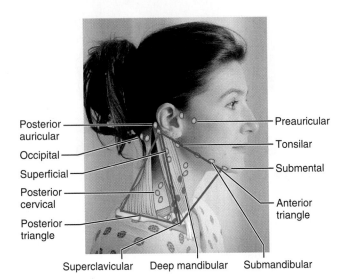

FIGURE 19–11 The anterior and posterior triangles of the neck and the cervical lymph nodes.

anterior and posterior triangles (Figure 19–11). The symmetrical neck muscles center and coordinate movement of the head. Asymmetrical head position may result from damage to the muscles, swelling, or masses. Painful or erratic movement may be due to a benign condition, such as muscle spasm, or to significant problems, including meningitis, neurological injuries, or chronic arthritis.

The trachea, thyroid gland, anterior cervical nodes, and carotid arteries are positioned in the anterior triangle; the posterior cervical nodes are in the posterior triangle. You will palpate the tracheal rings and the cricoid and thyroid cartilage in the midline of the anterior neck (Figure 19–12).

For instructions in assessing the neck,

 Go to Chapter 19, **Procedure 19-10: Assessing the Neck,** in Volume 2.

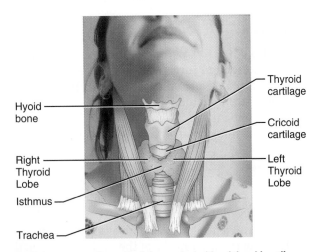

FIGURE 19–12 The tracheal rings and cricoid and thyroid cartilage are palpable in the midline of the anterior neck.

See also the Critical Aspects box on pages 393 to 396 of this volume.

The Thyroid Gland

Normally the thyroid is smooth, firm, and nontender. It is often nonpalpable. Thyroid abnormalities are common. An enlarged thyroid may be associated with either hypothyroidism or hyperthyroidism. Thyroid tenderness usually results from inflammation. Thyroid masses may be malignant but are usually benign. If the thyroid is palpable, you will need to auscultate it for bruits.

The Cervical Lymph Nodes

The cervical lymph nodes occur in three chains (Figure 19–11). The anterior chain is in the anterior triangle, the posterior chain in the posterior triangle. There is a deep cervical chain under the sternocleidomastoid muscle. The lymph nodes are generally not palpable, although occasionally nodes can be felt, especially in young children. Normal nodes are small in size (less than 1 cm) mobile, soft, and nontender. You should describe enlarged nodes (greater than 1 cm in diameter) according to their location, size, shape, consistency, mobility, and tenderness.

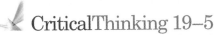

CriticalThinking 19–5

A client complains of sore throat, fever, chills, and runny nose. What assessments should you perform?

THE BREASTS AND AXILLAE

The breasts (Figure 19–13) consist of glandular, adipose, and connective tissue; smooth muscle; and nerves. The functions of the female breast are sexual stimulation and nourishing offspring. Breast size and shape varies among women, and commonly one breast is slightly larger than the other. At puberty, the ovaries produce estrogen and progesterone, which stimulate the breasts to develop. The menstrual cycle, pregnancy, and breastfeeding all stimulate breast tissue. Although breasts are thought of as female organs, men also have breasts. However, because of limited estrogen and progesterone levels, male breasts develop only minimally.

Breast tissue and lymph drainage for the breast extend up into the axilla. The majority of breast tumors are found in the tail of Spence or in the axilla. A breast exam therefore always includes an exam of the axillae. Many women have breast reconstruction, either after breast removal due to cancer or for cosmetic reasons. These women should not omit breast examination, and it is performed in exactly the same way as for natural breasts.

Currently there is some controversy about whether or not we should continue to encourage breast self-examination (BSE). Some studies indicate that it does

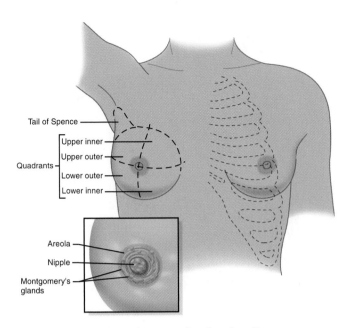

FIGURE 19–13   **Breast tissue extends up into the axilla.**

not reduce death rates from breast cancer, but others found increased rates of cancer discovery and earlier detection in groups who perform BSE (Green & Taplin, 2003; Hackshaw & Paul, 2003; Kösters & Gøtzsche, 2003; Thomas et al., 2002; Weiss, 2003). So until there is more evidence, it seems reasonable to continue to encourage BSE. See Chapter 9 for a discussion of breast self-exam as an important health promotion activity. Chapter 41 includes a thorough discussion of teaching your client how to perform a breast self-exam. For a step-by-step guide to examining the breasts and axillae,

VOL 2 Go to Chapter 19, **Procedure 19–11: Assessing the Breasts and Axillae,** in Volume 2.

The Critical Aspects box on pages 393 to 396 of this volume summarizes the procedure. You should perform

this procedure for the woman if she cannot do it herself and demonstrate the procedure as part of client teaching for self-care.

 CriticalThinking 19–6

What strategies might encourage more women to regularly perform breast self examination?

THE CHEST AND LUNGS

The chest, or thorax, is the bony cage that protects the heart, lungs, and great vessels. The ribs, sternum, and vertebrae form the chest. Be systematic in your assessment: always assess the areas of the chest and lungs in the same order.

Chest Landmarks

Before beginning the thoracic exam, review the following important landmarks that will help you visualize the underlying structures and perform an accurate assessment.

- Identify positions vertically on the anterior chest in relation to the ribs. For example, the space between the 5th and 6th ribs is known as the 5th intercostal space (5th ICS). You can easily palpate the ribs and count the spaces if you remember that the 1st rib is tucked up next to the clavicle (Figure 19–14A).

- On the posterior chest, identify positions vertically in relation to the vertebra (Figure 19–15B). The prominent vertebra at the base of the neck is the 7th cervical vertebra (C7). The next one down is T1 (1st thoracic). Counting down to about T9 should be adequate.

- Use a series of imaginary vertical lines to further aid in identifying locations. Figure 19–14B illustrates the location of these lines. Use them with the rib spaces to describe locations on the anterior chest.

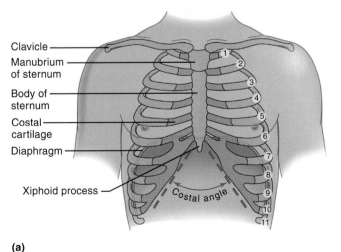

(a)

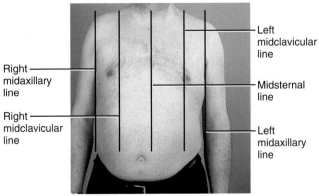

(b)

FIGURE 19–14   *A*, The anterior thoracic cage and the bony landmarks. *B*, A series of imaginary vertical lines is used to describe locations on the chest.

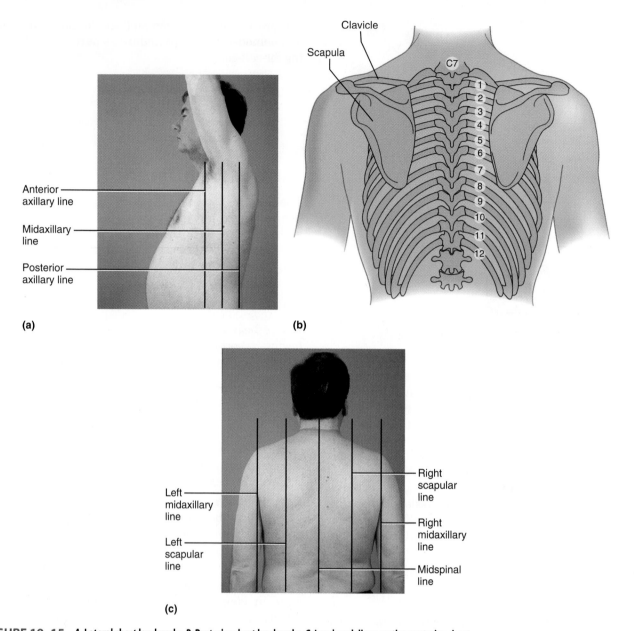

(a)

Anterior axillary line
Midaxillary line
Posterior axillary line

(b)

Clavicle
Scapula
C7
1
2
3
4
5
6
7
8
9
10
11
12

(c)

Left midaxillary line
Left scapular line
Right scapular line
Right midaxillary line
Midspinal line

FIGURE 19–15   *A,* Lateral chest landmarks. *B,* Posterior chest landmarks. *C,* Landmark lines on the posterior chest.

For instance, the apex of the heart is usually located in the 5th intercostal space at left midclavicular line (5th ICS MCL).

- Use imaginary lines on the lateral and posterior chest as well (see Figure 19–15). Notice that the anterior axillary line can be used to locate sounds on both the anterior and lateral chest.

Chest Shape and Size

The normal adult chest is symmetrical and rises and falls with respirations. The chest diameter expands up to 3 inches (7.6 cm) with deep inspiration. The anteroposterior diameter of the chest is twice the size of the lateral diameter. The slope of the ribs is less than 90°. In young children, the chest is apple-shaped. Musculoskeletal changes associated with aging result

in a gradual increase in the anteroposterior diameter. This change is also seen, regardless of age, in clients who have chronic obstructive pulmonary disease (COPD), a disorder associated with long-term smoking. Figure 19–16 illustrates the normal chest ratio and the barrel chest appearance that develops with COPD, in which the anteroposterior and lateral diameters may be equal.

Spinal alterations, such as *kyphosis* (excessive curvature of the thoracic spine) and *scoliosis* (lateral curvature of the spine) alter the shape of the thoracic cage. Osteoporosis, a common disorder associated with aging, is associated with increased porosity of the vertebrae. As a result, vertebrae may compress or collapse, shortening the length of the spine and pushing the ribs forward and downward.

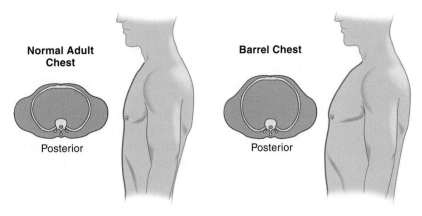

FIGURE 19-16 The normal anteroposterior to lateral ratio is 1:2. The lateral aspect of the chest increases dramatically with COPD, leading to a barrel chest appearance.

Breath Sounds

Listen to breath sounds in a quiet room by auscultating one full respiratory cycle at each site. Directly apply the stethoscope to the client's skin. Compare breath sounds bilaterally. Three types of breath sounds are heard (Figure 19–17):

- **Bronchial breath sounds** are loud, high-pitched, tubular sounds; expiration is of longer duration than inspiration. Air moving through the trachea produces these sounds, which you will hear best over the trachea on the anterior chest and below the nape of the neck on the posterior chest.

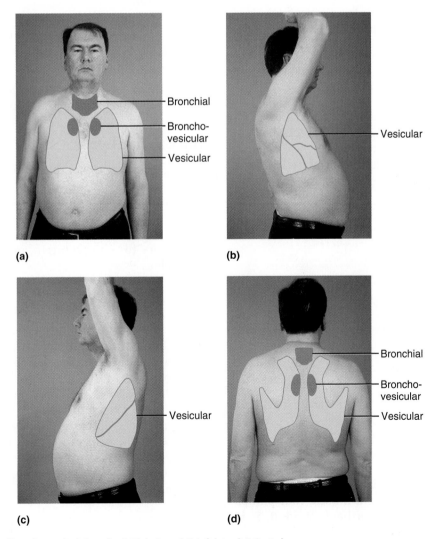

FIGURE 19-17 Normal breath sounds. *A,* Anterior. *B,* Right lateral. *C,* Left lateral. *D,* Posterior.

- **Bronchovesicular breath sounds** are medium-pitched with an equal inspiratory and expiratory phase. Air moving through the large airways of the bronchi produces these sounds, which are best heard over the 1st and 2nd ICS adjacent to the sternum on the anterior chest and between the scapula on the posterior chest.

- **Vesicular breath sounds** are soft, low-pitched, breezy sounds with a lengthy inspiratory phase and a short expiratory phase. Air moving through the smaller airways produces these sounds, which are best heard over the lung fields.

Breath sounds that differ from those above are abnormal. **Diminished breath sounds** are heard with poor inspiratory effort, in the very muscular or obese, or with restricted airflow. **Misplaced breath sounds** (e.g., bronchial breath sounds heard over the lung fields) indicate constriction of flow. **Adventitious breath sounds** are sounds heard over normal breath sounds. If an abnormal sound is heard, have the client cough and listen again.

Other abnormal findings include bronchophony, whispered pectoriloquy, and egophony. These are abnormal voice sounds that result from consolidation of lung tissue. To find a discussion of these,

 Go to Chapter 19, **Supplemental Materials,** on the Electronic Study Guide. Also go to **Sound Files,** to listen to normal and adventitious breath sounds.

For more information about the respiratory system, see Chapter 35. The Critical Aspects box on pages 393 to 396 of this chapter summarizes respiratory assessment. For a table describing abnormal lung sounds and the procedure for performing a respiratory assessment,

 Go to Chapter 19, **Procedure 19–12: Assessing the Chest and Lungs,** in Volume 2.

KnowledgeCheck 19–8

- List and describe the location of the horizontal and vertical landmarks of the anterior chest.
- List and describe the location of the horizontal and vertical landmarks of the posterior chest.
- List and describe the location of the vertical landmarks of the lateral chest.

 Go to Chapter 19, **Knowledge Check Response Sheet and Answers,** on the Electronic Study Guide.

THE CARDIOVASCULAR SYSTEM

The cardiovascular system consists of the heart and the blood vessels. The heart is a muscle that pumps blood throughout the body. In a healthy adult, it is about the size of a clenched fist. The blood vessels, which make up the vascular system, have two main networks: the pulmonary circulation and the systemic circulation. See Chapter 35 for illustrations of the anatomy of the cardiovascular system.

Oxygen-depleted blood circulates from the heart into the lungs, where it is oxygenated, then back to the heart. This system is known as the **pulmonary circulation.** From the heart the blood enters the **systemic circulation.** The left ventricle is the largest chamber of the heart. It pumps blood into the systemic circulation via the arterial system. The arteries subdivide many times, becoming smaller and smaller until they separate, in the tissues and organs, into capillaries. It is at the capillary level that oxygen is delivered to the tissues. The venous system collects the oxygen-depleted blood and returns it to the right atrium of the heart to begin the circuit again. **Coronary circulation,** which circulates blood through the heart itself, is a part of the systemic circulation. For further discussion on pulmonary circulation and oxygenation, see Chapter 35. For instructions in assessing the heart and vascular system,

 Go to Chapter 19, **Procedure 19–13: Assessing the Heart and Vascular System,** in Volume 2.

The Critical Aspects box on pages 393 to 396 of this volume summarizes the procedure.

The Cardiac Cycle

During a cardiac cycle, the atria and ventricles alternately contract and relax to fill and empty; while the atria are contracting (emptying), the ventricles are relaxing (filling), and vice versa. **Systole** refers to the contraction, or emptying, of the ventricles. **Diastole** refers to the relaxation, or filling, phase of the ventricles.

Cardiac Landmarks

The heart sits at an angle on the left side of the chest in the 3rd, 4th, and 5th intercostal spaces. You will be able to hear heart sounds from any location on the anterior chest wall. However, the four sites located over the heart valves are the preferred listening areas. Table 19–4 and Figure 19–18 illustrate these locations. Be systematic. Always listen in the same order to all the areas in Figure 19–18. To help minimize your client's anxiety, explain that it always takes time to examine the heart and circulatory system.

TABLE 19-4 Locations for Assessing the Heart

Title	Structure Assessed	Location
Base right	Aortic valve	2nd ICS right sternal border
Base left	Pulmonic valve	2nd ICS left sternal border
Left lateral sternal border	Tricuspid valve	4th ICS left sternal border
Apex	Mitral valve	5th ICS MCL

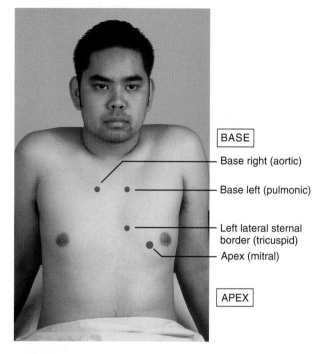

BASE

— Base right (aortic)

— Base left (pulmonic)

— Left lateral sternal border (tricuspid)

— Apex (mitral)

APEX

FIGURE 19–18 Cardiac auscultation sites.

To facilitate auscultation of specific heart sounds, perform the cardiac assessment with the client in three positions: sitting, supine, and left lateral recumbent. Clients with chronic heart or lung problems may have little cardiac reserve, so minimize position changes to conserve your client's energy.

Inspection and Palpation of the Heart

Begin your assessment of the heart with the client sitting. Observe the **precordium,** the area of the chest over the heart, for visible pulsations. A small pulsation at the 5th ICS midclavicular line, also known as the **point of maximal impulse (PMI),** is normal. Other visible pulsations on the precordium, known as **heaves** or **lifts,** are associated with an enlarged ventricle.

Also palpate for vibrations. A **thrill** is a vibration or pulsation palpated in any area except the PMI. A thrill is associated with abnormal blood flow and usually has an accompanying **murmur** (additional heart sound).

Heart Sounds

You will auscultate to establish cardiac rate and rhythm and to identify normal and abnormal heart sounds. A quiet room is essential. To thoroughly assess heart sounds, auscultate in an orderly fashion. Start at the aortic area, and move gradually through each landmark. The following is a mnemonic you may use to recall the order of the heart sound landmarks:

Aunt   Aortic
Polly   Pulmonic
Takes   Tricuspid
Meds   Mitral

$S_1, S_2, S_3,$ and S_4 Heart Sounds

Listen carefully at each site to each component of the heart sounds. Listen first with the diaphragm of your stethoscope. Then retrace your steps with the bell.

- *The first heart sound (S_1, or lub)* results from the closure of the valves between the atria and ventricles. It may be heard in all locations on the chest but will be loudest over the mitral and tricuspid areas. S_1 marks the beginning of systole. S_1 ("lub") is a dull, low-pitched sound.

- *The second heart sound (S_2, or dub)* corresponds to closure of the semilunar valves (between the ventricles and the great arteries exiting the heart). S_2 marks the beginning of diastole. "Dub" is higher in pitch and shorter than the S_1 "lub." You can hear the S_2 in all locations, but it is loudest at the aortic and pulmonic areas.

  Normally, the mitral and tricuspid valves and the aortic and pulmonic valves close within a fraction of a second from each other. This near simultaneous closure results in a singular S_1 and S_2 sound. However, a split sound may occur, at either S_1 or S_2, if there is a delay in closure of one of the valves.

- *A third heart sound (S_3),* immediately heard after S_2, has a gallop cadence that follows the rhythm of the word *KenTUcky.* It is normal in young children and adolescents when they are sitting or lying, but it disappears when they stand or sit up. An S_3 is also a normal variant in the third trimester of pregnancy. In

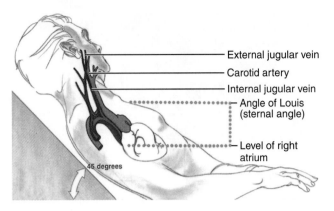

External jugular vein
Carotid artery
Internal jugular vein
Angle of Louis (sternal angle)
Level of right atrium
45 degrees

FIGURE 19–19 **The central vessels.**

adults, an S_3 that does not disappear with position change is abnormal and represents heart failure or volume overload.

- *A fourth heart sound (S_4),* heard immediately before S_1, has a rhythm that follows the word *FLOrida.* An S_4 is normal in trained athletes and some older clients. It may also be heard in adults with coronary artery disease, hypertension, and pulmonic stenosis. Both S_3 and S_4 are best heard at the apical site, with the client lying on his left side, and using the bell of the stethoscope. To listen to heart sounds,

 Go to **Sound Files** on the Electronic Study Guide.

Murmurs

Murmurs are additional sounds produced by turbulent flow through the heart. Identifying and classifying a murmur are advanced skills that require practice. To learn more about assessing murmurs,

 Go to Chapter 19, **Procedure 19-13: Assessing the Heart and Vascular System,** in Volume 2.

 Also go to Chapter 19, **Supplemental Materials: Heart Murmurs,** on the Electronic Study Guide.

 CriticalThinking 19–7

What findings would you anticipate when assessing Mr. Garcia's ("Meet Your Patients") thorax?

The Vascular System

The vascular system consists of a network of arteries and veins that transport oxygen, carbon dioxide, and nutrients to the cells of the body. Arteries carry blood away from the heart: The pulmonary arteries carry oxygen-depleted blood from the right ventricle to the lungs, whereas the systemic arteries carry oxygenated blood from the left ventricle to the body periphery. Veins carry blood toward the heart: The pulmonary

veins transport oxygenated blood from the lungs to the left atrium, whereas the systemic veins return oxygen-depleted blood from the periphery to the right atrium of the heart.

The Central Vessels

The carotid arteries and internal jugular veins run alongside the sternocleidomastoid muscle on both sides of the neck (Figure 19–19). These central vessels provide circulation to the brain.

The Carotid Arteries

Because the carotid arteries are large and close to the heart, you can easily feel a pulse over the carotid artery even when it is difficult to palpate a peripheral pulse. Never palpate both carotid arteries at the same time, because bilateral pressure may impair cerebral blood flow. Avoid massaging the carotid artery as you palpate, because increased pressure on the carotids will lead to a drop in the pulse rate.

Turbulent blood flow through the carotid artery produces a whooshing sound known as a **bruit,** which you can auscultate using a stethoscope. Bruits are common among older adults. The following conditions cause turbulence: **carotid stenosis** (narrowing from plaque), increased cardiac output secondary to fluid overload, use of stimulants, or hyperthyroidism. If you hear a bruit, lightly palpate the neck for thrills (pulsations or vibrations), which further confirm turbulent flow.

The Jugular Veins

The jugular veins return blood from the brain to the superior vena cava. The external jugular veins are superficial; the internal jugular veins are deep. Normally the jugular veins are flat when the client is in an upright position and distend when the client lies flat. Jugular venous distention (JVD) is seen when the right side of the heart is congested due to inadequate pump function. The best position for assessment of JVD is semi-Fowler's (30 to 45° angle). Normally the neck veins are flat at this angle.

The Peripheral Vessels

There are over 60,000 miles of arteries, arterioles, capillaries, venules, and veins in the peripheral system. The peripheral vessels supply blood to all the body cells. The **arteries** are a high-pressure system with several palpable pulse sites. The **veins** are a low-pressure system with valves that return blood to the heart via the continuing pressure from the arterial system and pumping action of the adjacent muscles.

Assess the peripheral vascular system by:

1. Measuring the blood pressure (see Chapter 17). Usually you will measure the blood pressure at the start of the exam as part of the general survey.
2. Palpating the peripheral pulses (see Chapter 17). In a healthy individual, pulses will be regular, strong, and equal bilaterally. Weak, absent, or asymmetrical pulses may indicate partial or complete occlusion of the artery. Other signs of arterial occlusion include pain, pallor, cool temperature, paresthesia, or paralysis.
3. Inspecting and performing tests for adequate perfusion.

The data you obtain when inspecting and palpating the integumentary system provides some information about peripheral tissue perfusion. Recall that when an area is not adequately oxygenated, the skin may be pale, cyanotic, cool, and shiny; hair growth may be sparse, and there may be clubbing of the nails. Recall that inadequate oxygenation may be a result of chronic pulmonary problems; however, it can also result from impaired central or peripheral circulation.

Also assess the venous system. Inspect the veins for signs of distention. Superficial spiderlike veins, especially on the lower extremities, may occur with normal aging. Ropelike distended veins, or **varicosities,** may be painful. If a client has varicosities, assess for valve competence with the **manual compression test** discussed in Volume 2.

KnowledgeCheck 19–9

- Identify the precautions to take when evaluating the carotid arteries.

 Go to Chapter 19, **Knowledge Check Response Sheet and Answers,** on the Electronic Study Guide.

THE ABDOMEN

The method most commonly used to identify the location of assessment findings is the four-quadrant method, which divides the abdomen into four sections by "drawing" a line vertically from the xiphoid process to the symphysis pubis and a horizontal line at the level of the umbilicus (Figure 19–20). For the rarely used nine-region method,

 Go to Chapter 19, **Tables, Boxes, Figures: ESG Table 19–2,** on the Electronic Study Guide.

Examination of the abdomen differs in sequence from all other body systems. Percussion and palpation stimulate the bowel and may alter bowel sounds. Therefore, you should inspect and auscultate before performing percussion and palpation. To promote

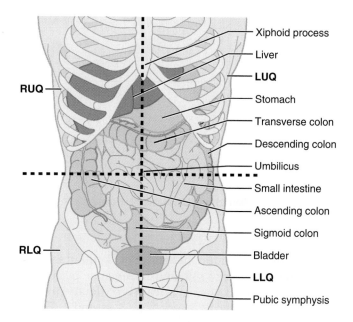

FIGURE 19–20 **The four abdominal quadrants.**

comfort, have the client empty his bladder prior to your examination. Have the client assume a supine position with flexed knees. This relaxes the abdominal muscles and is usually the most comfortable position. If the client has a painful area, examine that area last to minimize discomfort during the rest of the exam.

- *Inspection.* The skin over the abdomen is usually more pale than other parts of the body. Fine veins, silver-white striae, and surgical scars are normal variations. The abdomen should be symmetrical with a rounded contour and sunken umbilicus. See Figure 19–21 for normal variations in abdominal shape. You may be able to see peristalsis and aortic pulsations on a very thin client, but in most clients usually you will see no movement. In clients with abdominal distention, the skin will appear taut. Distention may be normal, as with pregnancy, or it may be due to gas or fluid retention or to bowel obstruction.

- *Auscultation.* Proceed in an organized manner, listening in several areas in all four quadrants. Use the same pattern for every examination so that it becomes a habit.

1. *Auscultate bowel sounds.* Bowel sounds are high-pitched, irregular gurgles or clicks lasting one to several seconds and occurring every 5 to 15 seconds (or 5 to 30 times per minute) in the average adult. If the client has a nasogastric (NG) tube that is attached to suction, discontinue the suction or clamp off the tube while listening for bowel sounds. Otherwise you may mistake the sound of suction in the stomach for bowel sounds. Bowel sounds may be **absent**

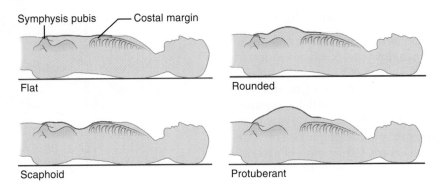

FIGURE 19–21   Normal variations in abdominal contour.

(none heard after listening for 5 minutes), **hypoactive** (very soft and infrequent, perhaps 1 per minute), or **hyperactive** (loud rushing sounds occurring every 2 or 3 seconds). Bowel sounds may be absent or hypoactive after abdominal surgery or with bowel obstruction, infection, or innervation problems. Bowel sounds may be hyperactive with diarrhea, early bowel obstruction, or gastroenteritis (infection of the gastrointestinal tract). To listen to bowel sounds,

 Go to **Sound Files** on the Electronic Study Guide.

2. *Auscultate the major arteries.* Major arterial vessels lie in the abdomen below the intestines. Listen over the aorta and the renal, iliac, and femoral arteries for the presence of bruits.

- *Percussion.* Use indirect percussion to assess for fluid, air, organs, or masses. Normally there is generalized tympany over the bowels (due to the presence of gas) and the abdomen is nontender, soft, and without masses. You will hear dullness when percussing organs, masses, or fluids. Some practitioners include percussion of the kidney with the abdominal examination.

- *Palpation.* Begin with *light palpation* to put the patient at ease. Palpate for tenderness and guarding in all four quadrants. Use *deep palpation* to assess organs and for masses and tenderness. The liver border should be smooth and without masses, and the spleen is not normally palpable. Palpation of the liver and spleen is an advanced technique not usually performed by staff nurses, except perhaps in some specialty areas.

The Critical Aspects box on pages 393 to 396 summarizes abdominal assessment; for the complete procedure,

 Go to Chapter 19, **Procedure 19–14: Assessing the Abdomen,** in Volume 2.

KnowledgeCheck 19–10

- What strategies can you use to make the client more comfortable during an abdominal assessment?
- Identify the sequence of assessment for the abdominal exam.

 Go to Chapter 19, **Knowledge Check Response Sheet and Answers,** on the Electronic Study Guide.

THE MUSCULOSKELETAL SYSTEM

The musculoskeletal system consists of bones, muscles, and joints. Bone is complex living tissue that responds to nutrition, stress, and illness. The bones include *long bones,* such as the humerus and tibia; *flat bones,* such as the sternum and ribs; and *irregular bones,* such as the vertebrae and pelvis. Tendons, ligaments, and cartilage serve as connecting structures. **Bursae,** small disc-shaped, fluid-filled sacs, act as cushions to reduce friction. The musculoskeletal system provides shape and support to the body, allows movement, protects internal organs, produces red blood cells in the bone marrow, and stores calcium and phosphorous.

Assessment of the musculoskeletal system includes evaluation of the client's posture, gait, bone structure, muscle function, and joint mobility. To assess this system, you will need a tape measure to measure limb lengths and circumference and a goniometer (Figure 19–22) to measure joint range of motion.

Assessment of the musculoskeletal system is summarized in the Critical Aspects box on pages 393 to 396 of this volume. For step-by-step instructions,

 Go to Chapter 19, **Procedure 19–15: Assessing the Musculoskeletal System,** in Volume 2.

Body Shape and Symmetry

To assess bone structure, examine body shape and symmetry. Normally the difference in length between the right and left arm and the right and left leg is less

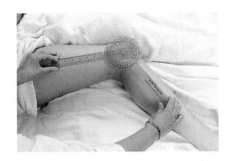

FIGURE 19–22 Use a goniometer to measure joint range of motion.

than 1 cm. A greater difference may alter gait and posture or trigger pain.

Major deformities in bone structure affect posture and gait. The client should be able to stand upright with the neck and head midline. There are four normal curvatures of the spine. The cervical and lumbar are concave, and the thoracic and sacral are convex. Commonly seen abnormalities include **kyphosis** (accentuated thoracic curve), **scoliosis** (lateral "S" deviation of the spine), and **lordosis** (accentuated lumbar curve).

Balance, Coordination, and Movement

Walking is a complex task involving balance, coordination, and movement. Pay attention to the *base of support* and *stride* as the client walks. The average base of support (distance between the feet) in adults is 5 to 10 cm (2 to 4 in.). Stride length (distance between each step) is 30 to 35 cm (12 to 14 in.). A wide base of support or shortened stride may indicate a balance problem. If the client has an altered gait, try to identify the specific portion of the gait that is abnormal. Abnormal gait may be caused by muscle hypertonicity (e.g., from stroke or brain tumor), lumbar disc problems, muscle atrophy, nerve damage, Parkinson's disease, cerebral palsy, multiple sclerosis, or spinal tumors. For additional information on gait, see Chapter 31.

To assess *balance and movement,* have the client perform tandem walking (heel-to-toe), heel-and-toe walking, deep knee bends, and hopping in place. The Romberg test is also used to assess balance; in a comprehensive exam, you would have already performed this test as part of the ear exam.

Two simple measures for assessing *coordination* are finger-thumb opposition and running the heel of one foot down the shin of the other. When performing these activities, the patient's movements should be smooth and controlled.

As you perform each assessment, pay attention to the client's stability and level of comfort. Do not attempt movements that may produce pain or cause the

client to fall. For example, recall that Mr. Garcia ("Meet Your Patients") has bilateral knee pain. Before asking him to perform deep knee bends or hop in place, you will want to assess his pain and its triggers.

Joint Mobility and Muscle Function

Healthy joints are smooth, nontender, warm to touch, and of similar color to the surrounding tissue. Any joint deformity requires investigation. Color changes in a joint indicate inflammation or infection. If you see erythema or swelling, investigate further by feeling for warmth. Determine any effect the deformity has on function.

Joints should move freely and without pain or **crepitus** (clicking or grating at a joint). To assess function, test range of motion (ROM) and muscle strength. **Active ROM** requires the client to move the joint through its full ROM. **Passive ROM** is used when the client is unable to exercise each joint independently. Instead, you support the body and move each joint through its ROM. **Muscle strength** is assessed in conjunction with movement by asking the patient to perform ROM while you apply resistance to the part being moved. Muscle strength should be strong (5 on a scale of 0 to 5) and equal bilaterally. For more information about the musculoskeletal system, see Chapter 31.

 CriticalThinking 19–8

As you may recall, Mr. Garcia ("Meet Your Patients") is obese and has been having pain in both of his knees.

- What history questions would you ask him to assess his knee pain?
- What would you do to examine his knees?

THE NEUROLOGICAL SYSTEM

The neurological system controls or affects the function of all body systems and allows interaction with the external world. Its work is carried out through the transmission of chemical and electrical signals between the body and the brain. The basic functions of the nervous system are cognition, emotion, memory, sensation and perception, and regulation of homeostasis. When interpreting a neurological exam, consider the developmental changes described in Box 19–1.

A comprehensive neurological assessment takes hours to complete and is usually reserved for clients with symptoms of neurological problems. As a staff nurse in general practice, you will usually perform only portions of a neurological exam. In the next few sections we will look at the components of a focused neurological exam.

The Neurological System over the Life Span

- *Infants.* Reflexes present at birth include rooting, sucking, palmar grasp, tonic neck reflex (fencing), and Moro. (Go to Chapter 9 to review these reflexes). These reflexes disappear during infancy. With neurological injury, as may occur with stroke or trauma, these reflexes may return, indicating severe neurological problems.

- *Young children.* Because language skills and motor development are age-dependent, the Denver Developmental Screening Test II (DDST) is used as a neurological screen for young children. The DDST examines motor, language, and coordination skills. Chapter 9 provides additional information on the DDST. Once a child has reached toddlerhood, you can usually perform a comprehensive neurological exam with age-appropriate modifications; for example, when testing for smell use materials that a young child knows, such as peanut butter or apples.

- *Older adults.* Throughout life, neurons are lost. With advanced age, changes commonly observed are slowing of reaction time, a decreased ability for rapid problem solving, and slower voluntary movement. However, intelligence, memory, and discrimination do not change with normal aging. Neurological deficits in older adults are usually the result of adverse effects of medications or medication interactions, nutritional deficits, dehydration, cardiovascular changes that alter cerebral blood flow, diabetes, degenerative neurological changes (e.g., Parkinson's disease or Alzheimer's dementia), alcohol or drug use, depression, or abuse.

For a summary see the Critical Aspects box on pages 393 to 396 of this volume. For the complete procedure,

 Go to Chapter 19, **Procedure 19–16: Assessing the Sensory: Neurological System,** in Volume 2.

Cerebral Function

Cerebral function refers to the client's intellectual and behavioral functioning. It includes level of consciousness, mental status and cognitive function, and communication.

Level of Consciousness

Level of consciousness (LOC) includes arousal and orientation. Arousal may range from alert to deeply comatose. Arousal is classified based on the type of stimuli (auditory, tactile, or painful) required to produce a response from the client. An alert client responds to *auditory stimuli* (e.g., verbal communication or noise). Remember, however, that if your client does not speak your language he may not respond to questions or commands.

If the client does not respond to auditory stimuli, try *tactile stimuli.* Begin with gentle touch. Many clients who have hearing deficits lip-read to compensate. If you catch the client's attention by touching her hand, she may be able to respond to the combined auditory and visual stimuli. If the client does not respond to gentle touch, shake her shoulder.

If still no response is obtained, turn to *painful stimuli.* Painful stimuli include squeezing the trapezius muscle, rubbing on the sternum, putting pressure on the mandible, or putting pressure over the moon of a nail. Clients who respond to painful stimuli withdraw when pressure is applied.

Document LOC by describing the client's response or grading the response based on the Glasgow Coma Scale (Table 19–5). Often you will read descriptions of a client's behavior. Box 19–2 identifies commonly used terms to describe LOC. Although these terms are widely used, a thorough description is preferable. Look at the following two chart entries:

Pt lethargic.

Pt responds to repeated tactile and verbal stimulation. Quickly drifts off to sleep if stimulation is discontinued.

As you can see, the second charting entry provides significantly more information than the first.

Orientation refers to the client's awareness of time, place, and person. **Time orientation** includes awareness of the year, date, and time of day. Older adults who become disoriented to time usually think it is an earlier date. If a client offers a bizarre time or futuristic date, consider psychiatric concerns as the cause of disorientation. Hospitalized patients easily become disoriented to time: They are subjected to lights and noise around the clock; are roused in the middle of night for medications or time-sensitive treatments; and are given anesthesia and pain medications that alter their sense of awareness.

Orientation to place involves awareness of surroundings. The patient should know that he is, for example, in the hospital and not in church. Patients who have been moved (e.g., from the emergency department to a ward bed) may not recall their room number but are easily reoriented.

Orientation to person involves recognition of familiar persons and self-identity. The client should be able to state her name or identify people in photographs at the bedside. Because a client may meet many health professionals during a hospitalization, she may not be able to recall your name unless you have had repeated encounters with her.

TABLE 19-5	Glasgow Coma Scale	
Observation	**Response**	**Score**
Eye response	Opens spontaneously	4
	Opens to verbal commands	3
	Opens to pain	2
	No response	1
Motor response	Reacts to verbal commands	6
	Reacts to localized pain	5
	Flexes and withdraws (general body response)	4
	Assumes flexor posture (decorticate posturing—arms flexed to chest, hands clenched and internally rotated); indicates problem is at or above the brainstem	3
	Assumes extensor posture (decerebrate posturing—arms extended, hands clenched and hyperpronated); indicates problem at the brainstem level	2
	No response	1
Verbal response	Oriented and converses	5
	Disoriented but converses	4
	Uses inappropriate words	3
	Makes incomprehensible sounds	2
	No response	1

BOX 19-2 Terms Commonly Used to Describe Level of Consciousness

- *Alert:* Follows commands in a timely fashion.
- *Lethargic:* Appears drowsy, easily drifts off to sleep.
- *Stuporous:* Requires vigorous stimulation before responding.
- *Comatose:* Does not respond to verbal or painful stimuli.

Mental Status and Cognitive Function

Mental status and cognitive function include behavior, appearance, response to stimuli, speech, memory, communication, and judgment. By this point in the exam, you would have already interviewed the client, so you would have a good deal of information about his mental status and cognitive function. You would have already assessed posture, gait, motor movements, dress, and hygiene through the general survey and the musculoskeletal exam; and you would be aware of the client's mood based on his tone of voice, actions, and statements.

Many clinicians choose to screen for mental status and cognitive function by working questions into the interaction with the client as they assess other body systems. The advantage of this type of informal assessment is increased comfort for the client. If you choose this method, observe for clarity of thought, appropriate content, concentration, memory, and ability to perform abstract reasoning. Normal findings include the ability to:

- Express and explain realistic thoughts with clear speech
- Follow multistep directions
- Listen
- Answer questions
- Recall significant past events

Formal screening of mental and cognitive status allows you to perform serial assessment of the client. Several screening tools are used.

 Go to Chapter 19, **Procedure 19-16: Assessing the Sensory-Neurological System,** in Volume 2.

Cranial Nerve Function

Cranial nerve assessment is a key component of the neurological exam. The cranial nerves control a variety of sensory and motor functions, as you will see in Table 19–6. Also see Figure 19–23.

Reflex Function

Reflexes are automatic responses that do not require conscious thought from the brain. A reflex produces a rapid, involuntary response that occurs at the level of the spinal cord (Figure 19–24). Because the brain is not involved, response is instantaneous. Intact sensory and motor systems are required for a normal reflex response. The simplest reflex, a **deep tendon reflex (DTR),** involves communication across a single synapse between one sensory neuron and a motor neuron. To test DTRs, you will use a rubber percussion hammer to tap a slightly stretched muscle. A

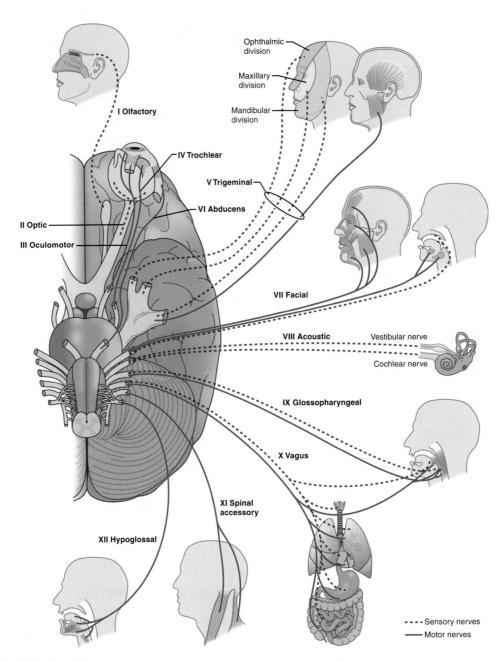

FIGURE 19–23   Origin of cranial nerves.

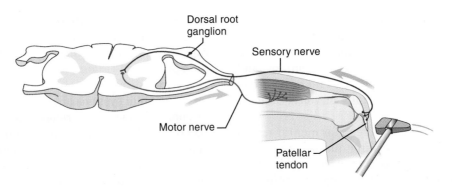

FIGURE 19–24   Reflex arc.

TABLE 19-6 Cranial Nerves

Cranial Nerve #	Name	Type of Nerve	Function of Nerve
I	Olfactory	Sensory	Smell
II	Optic	Sensory	Visual acuity, visual fields, and ocular fundi
III	Oculomotor	Motor	EOM, pupil size
IV	Trochlear	Motor	EOM
V	Trigeminal: 3 branches	Sensory and motor	Corneal reflex, facial sensation, and jaw movement
VI	Abducens	Motor	EOM
VII	Facial	Motor and sensory	Facial movement
VIII	Auditory	Sensory	Hearing and equilibrium
IX	Glossopharyngeal	Motor and sensory	Swallowing, gag response, tongue movement, taste
X	Vagus	Motor and sensory	Sensation of pharynx and larynx; motor activity of swallowing and vocal cords
XI	Spinal accessory	Motor	Head movement and shoulder elevation
XII	Hypoglossal	Motor	Tongue movement

normal response is muscle contraction. Responses are graded on the following scale:

   0   No response detected
   +1 Diminished response
   +2 Response normal
   +3 Response somewhat stronger than normal
   +4 Response hyperactive with **clonus** (involuntary contractions that continue after the first contraction is elicited by the hammer)

You can elicit **superficial reflexes** by swiftly stroking a body part. Use the base of the reflex hammer or a tongue blade. Avoid pressure. Superficial reflexes are graded as positive or negative. For a description of methods to test the most common reflexes,

 Go to Chapter 19, **Procedure 19–16: Assessing the Sensory-Neurological System,** in Volume 2.

Sensory Function

Tests of sensory function include light touch, light pain, temperature, vibration, position sense, **stereognosis** (the ability to recognize the form of solid objects by touch), **graphesthesia** (the ability to recognize outlines, numbers, or symbols written on the skin), two-

point discrimination, point localization, and extinction. For specific techniques for these assessments,

 Go to Chapter 19, **Procedure 19–16 : Assessing the Sensory-Neurological System,** in Volume 2.

To assess sensory function, ask the client to keep his eyes closed as you apply various stimuli. Ask him to indicate when he feels a sensation. Vary your location and approach so that you test sensation, not pattern recognition. If you notice an area of altered sensation, systematically assess the area to define the border of the change.

Usually you will limit your testing to the upper and lower extremities and the trunk. If the client has known or suspected deficits, you should test at numerous other sites.

Motor and Cerebellar Function

The neurological system coordinates the function of the skeleton and muscles. Motor pathways transmit information between the brain and muscles and the muscles control movement of the skeleton. The cerebellum helps coordinate muscle movement, regulate muscle tone, and maintain posture and equilibrium. The cerebellum is also largely responsible for **proprioception,** or body

positioning. Disorders of motor and cerebellar function result in pain or problems with movement, gait, or posture. Thus, when you assess the musculoskeletal system, you also assess the motor functions of the neurological system.

KnowledgeCheck 19–11

• Identify and describe the components assessed in the neurological exam.
• What approach to assessment should you take if:

   Your client has no neurological problems but you are performing a comprehensive exam?

   Your client is hospitalized for a documented cerebrovascular accident?

   Your client has been admitted with an acute head injury and the extent of neurological injury is unknown?

 Go to Chapter 19, **Knowledge Check Response Sheet and Answers,** on the Electronic Study Guide.

THE GENITOURINARY SYSTEM

In most practice settings, nurses assess only the patient's external genitalia and inguinal lymph nodes. Nurse practitioners and physicians perform comprehensive examinations of the female and male reproductive and urinary systems. However, even as a novice nurse you may be called upon to assist with exams or just to be present to provide emotional support to the client.

Because a genitourinary (GU) assessment focuses on sexual and reproductive function, it is embarrassing for many people. As a result, the assessment requires a competent, straightforward approach. Your comfort with these topics will help the client to feel more comfortable.

The Male Genitourinary System

The male genitourinary system includes the reproductive system and the urinary system. A complete examination includes assessment of the external genitalia, evaluation for hernias, and a rectal exam for prostate screening. The penis and scrotum are examined by inspection and palpation. You will assess some of the urinary system organs when examining the back (kidneys, ureters) and the abdomen (bladder); the prostate gland is palpated during the exam of the rectum and anus (discussed later in this chapter). For steps to follow in examining the male genitourinary system,

 Go to Chapter 19, **Procedure 19–17: Assessing the Male Genitourinary System,** in Volume 2.

Also see the Critical Aspects box on pages 393 to 396 of this volume.

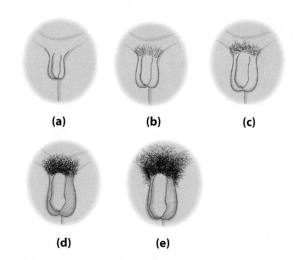

FIGURE 19–25 **The stages of male sexual development: A, Stage I: Preadolescent; B, Stage II; C, Stage III; D, Stage IV; E, Stage V: Adult.** *Source:* Tanner, J.M. (1962). *Growth at adolescence* (2nd ed.). Oxford: Blackwell Scientific Publications.

The appearance of the external genitalia depends on the client's developmental stage. Figure 19–25 illustrates the stages of male reproductive development.

Historically, the United States has had a high rate of **circumcision** (excision of the foreskin of the penis). Circumcision was routinely performed at birth, based on the belief that it had long-term health benefits. Over time, studies have not shown this to be true, and circumcision is no longer recommended as a routine practice. However, circumcision is tied to some religious and cultural beliefs (e.g., among Jews and Muslims), so it is still common.

A **hernia** is a protrusion of the intestine (or other organ). In men, this is most likely to be a protrusion of the intestine through the inguinal wall. A hernia may be a small protrusion or it may cause pain and distention as a loop of bowel extends into the scrotum.

During your examination, be sure to reinforce the importance of testicular self-examination (TSE), an important health promotion measure. See Chapter 41 for full discussion of TSE.

KnowledgeCheck 19–12

• What assessment techniques are used when examining the male genitourinary system?
• How and where would you examine for an inguinal hernia?

 Go to Chapter 19, **Knowledge Check Response Sheet and Answers,** on the Electronic Study Guide.

The Female Genitourinary System

Advance practice nurses and physicians perform comprehensive examinations of the female reproductive system, as do nurses working in specialty settings, such as maternity nursing. As a nurse, you may be called upon to assist with a comprehensive examination. Therefore, we include discussion of a complete pelvic examination in this chapter.

For a discussion of inspection of external female genitalia and palpation of inguinal lymph nodes,

 Go to Chapter 19, **Procedure 19–18: Assessing the Female Genitourinary System,** in Volume 2.

The Critical Aspects box on page 393 to 396 of this volume summarizes the procedure.

External Examination

For adolescents and young women who are not sexually active, an external GU examination includes the following:

- Inspect the amount and distribution of pubic hair and correlate with stages of sexual maturation.
- Inspect the skin of the pubic area for evidence of swelling, lesions, or pubic lice.
- Inspect the external genitalia: labia, clitoris, urethral orifice, and vaginal orifice. Look for lesions, inflammation, swelling, or discharge.
- Palpate the inguinal lymph nodes.

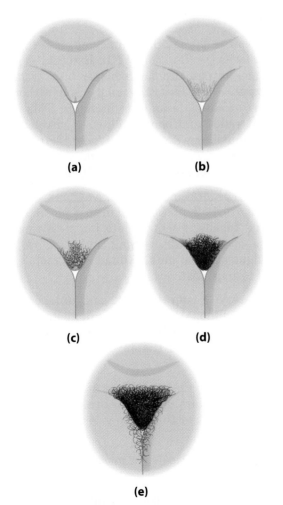

(a)   (b)

(c)   (d)

(e)

FIGURE 19–26   The stages of female sexual development: A, Stage I: Preadolescent; B, Stage II; C, Stage III; D, Stage IV; E, Stage V: Adult. *Source:* Tanner, J. M. (1962). *Growth at adolescence* (2nd ed.). Oxford: Blackwell Scientific Publications.

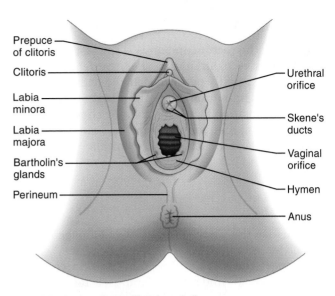

FIGURE 19–27   External female genitalia.

The appearance of the external genitalia depends on the developmental stage of the client. Figure 19–26 illustrates the changes that occur with maturation.

Internal Examination

Women who are sexually active, who have abnormal findings on external examination, who have abdominal, pelvic, or genitourinary complaints, or who are on hormone therapy require an internal genital examination. This includes the following:

- Palpation of Bartholin's glands and Skene's ducts (Figure 19–27)
- Assessment of vaginal muscle tone and pelvic musculature
- Speculum examination

Sexually active women should have a Papanicolaou test (Pap smear) annually to screen for cervical and uterine cancer. Additional cultures or screens may be done if there is unusual discharge or risk of sexually transmitted infection. A **speculum examination** is performed to collect specimens and assess the cervix. You will need to gather equipment, prepare the patient, assist the client and examiner during the procedure, assist the client after the procedure, and document your findings.

For a description of these responsibilities and a step-by-step guide to external genital examination,

 Go to Chapter 19, **Procedure 19–18: Assessing the Female Genitourinary System,** in Volume 2.

KnowledgeCheck 19–13

What are the responsibilities of the nurse during an internal exam of the female genitourinary system?

 Go to Chapter 19, **Knowledge Check Response Sheet and Answers,** on the Electronic Study Guide.

The Anus, Rectum, and Prostate

Examining the rectum and anus is the last aspect of a comprehensive examination. For the female client, this exam is usually performed at the end of a bimanual pelvic examination while the client is still in the lithotomy position. Usually a male client assumes Sims' position, and you perform the exam after completing your examination of the genitals.

 Go to Chapter 19, **Procedure 19-19: Assessing the Anus and Rectum,** in Volume 2.

See also the Critical Aspects box on pages 393 to 396 of this volume.

Inspect the anus and rectum for skin condition and hemorrhoids and palpate for muscle tone, masses, and tenderness. Skin irritation and erythema are common in clients who have diarrhea and infants and toddlers who wear diapers. **Hemorrhoids** (dilated, usually painful, anal vessels) may be seen in clients with a history of constipation. Many women develop hemorrhoids with pregnancy and childbirth.

A comprehensive examination for a man should include a digital rectal examination to assess for prostate enlargement. An enlarged prostate may indicate benign enlargement of the prostate, which is common in men over age 50; or it may indicate prostatitis. A hard nodule or multiple nodules may indicate prostate cancer.

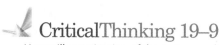 CriticalThinking 19–9

How will examination of the rectum and anus differ for Joe and Flordelisa Garcia ("Meet Your Patients")?

DOCUMENTING PHYSICAL ASSESSMENT FINDINGS

Jordan Miller has completed his physical assessment of Joe Garcia ("Meet Your Patients"). Below is his charting entry. Recall that Jordan is an advanced practice nurse and has performed a comprehensive physical assessment. Therefore, this examination and charting entry are more extensive than what would be expected of a staff nurse. All of the abbreviations have been used in the chapter. See if you can recall their meaning as you read through the charting.

General Survey: 56 y.o. obese ♂ presents to the clinic for a physical exam in no apparent distress. Pt appears stated age, is well dressed and groomed, AA&O x 3, speech clear, response and affect appropriate. MAE well, gait steady and balanced. Smells of cigarettes.

Height	5′ 10″
Weight	229 lb
BP	166/100
Pulse	88
RR	22
Temp	98.5°F oral
BMI	33

Integumentary: Skin even in color, warm & dry, good turgor, no suspicious lesions. Well healed scar in R inguinal area. Hair clean, coarse, evenly distributed. Some graying. Nails pink, brisk capillary refill, no clubbing.

Head & Neck: Normocephalic, erect, midline. Scalp mobile, no lesions, tenderness, or masses. Facial features symmetrical. Thyroid and cervical lymph nodes not palpable.

Eyes: Snellen = right eye 20/100, left eye 20/100, both eyes 20/100. Color vision intact. Difficulty noted with near vision. Visual fields normal by confrontation. Extraocular movements intact. PERRLA at 3 mm by direct and consensual. Eyes clear and bright, + blink, no lid lag or abnormalities. Anterior chamber clear. Cornea & iris intact. Sclera white, conjunctiva clear. Lacrimal glands and ducts nontender. + red reflex bilateral, discs flat c̄ sharp margins, vessels intact, retina & macula even in color.

Ears, Nose & Throat: Skin intact, no masses, lesions, or discharge. Position WNL. External ears nontender to palpation. + whisper test. Weber—no lateralization. External canals clear without redness, swelling, lesions, or discharge. TMs intacts, light reflex and bony landmarks visible; frontal and maxillary sinuses nontender. Nares patent, able to distinguish familiar odors, mucosa pink, no discharge, septum intact with no deviation.

Mouth: Lips, oral mucosa, gingivae pink with no lesions. All teeth present and in good repair. Pharynx pink, tonsils absent, palate intact. Symmetrical rise of the uvula, + gag and swallow reflex. Tongue smooth, pink, symmetrical, mobile, without lesions, taste intact.

Respiratory: Respirations 22 and unlabored. Trachea midline, AP < transverse diameter. Chest expansion symmetrical. No tenderness, scars, masses, or lesions. Diaphragmatic excursion 5 cm. Lungs CTA.

Cardiovascular: PMI @ MCL at 5th ICS, P 85, regular, no murmurs, gallops, or thrills present; pulses +2, no bruits or thrills, no varicosities; JVP 2 cm at 45°.

Breasts: Symmetrical. No masses, lymphadenopathy, or discharge.

Abdomen: Abdomen soft, rounded, no masses or pulsations. Surgical scar R inguinal area. + BS, + tympany throughout.

Musculoskeletal: Normal spinal curvature. Joints and muscles symmetrical, no deformity. + Bilateral knee pain R > L; Full ROM in upper and lower extremities, +5 muscle strength, some crepitus R knee.

Neurological: AA&O x 3, CN I–XII intact. Gait steady and coordinated; negative Romberg; unable to do deep knee bends due to pain. Point-point localization, superficial and deep sensation intact, +2 DTRs.

GU: Circumcised male; penis nontender, no masses, urethral meatus midline, no discharge; testicles descended bilaterally, nontender, inguinal and femoral canals free of masses, prostate small, smooth, mobile, nontender. Rectal wall smooth, no masses, stool hemoccult negative.

Comprehensive Physical Examination: Summary

 VOL 2 For steps to follow in *all* procedures, refer to the inside back cover of Volume 2.

Note: Throughout the assessment compare findings on both sides of the body.

Procedure 19–1: The General Survey

- Observe the patient's apparent age, gender, race, facial expression, body size and type, posture, movements, speech, grooming, dress, hygiene, mental state, and affect.
- Identify any signs of distress.
- Measure vital signs.
- Measure height and weight, and calculate BMI.
- Consider the client's cultural/ethnic background, gender, and developmental stage.
- Review history data that may influence general survey findings, including usual state of health, current health problem, allergies, and unexplained changes in weight.
- Note verbal and nonverbal responses throughout exam.

Procedure 19–2: Assessing the Skin

- Techniques: inspection, palpation, and olfaction.
- Assess both exposed and unexposed areas.
- Inspect skin color; note any unusual odors.
- Inspect and palpate any lesions. Describe their size, shape, color, distribution, texture, surface relationship, and exudate. Note the presence of tenderness or pain.
- Evaluate the lesions for the possibility of malignancy, remembering the mnemonic ABCDE.
- Palpate skin for temperature with the dorsal aspect of your hand.
- Palpate skin for turgor by gently pulling up skin, noting its return when you release it.
- Palpate skin for texture, moisture, and hydration.
- In interpreting data, consider the client's cultural/ethnic background, gender, and developmental stage.

- Review history that may influence skin findings, including usual state of health, current health problem, allergies, and occupation.

Procedure 19–3: Assessing the Hair

- Techniques: inspection and palpation.
- Assess both scalp hair and body hair.
- Consider the client's cultural/ethnic background, gender, and developmental stage.
- Inspect hair for color, quantity, distribution, condition of scalp, and presence of lesions or pediculosis.
- Palpate the texture of the hair.
- Palpate the scalp for mobility and tenderness.

Procedure 19–4: Assessing the Nails

- Techniques: inspection and palpation.
- Inspect the nails for color, condition, and shape.
- Palpate the texture of the nails.
- Assess capillary refill by pressing on the nails and releasing.
- Assess factors that may alter nail assessment findings (e.g., a cold environment may cause peripheral cyanosis).
- Examine nails on both hands and feet. However, you may defer examination of the toenails until the assessment of peripheral circulation.

Procedure 19–5: Assessing the Head and Face

- Techniques: inspection, palpation, auscultation.
- Inspect the head for size, shape, symmetry, and position.
- Inspect the face for expression and symmetry.

critical aspects of procedures 19–1 through 19–19

Comprehensive Physical Examination: Summary *(continued)*

- Palpate the head for masses, tenderness, and scalp mobility.

- Palpate the face for symmetry, tenderness, muscle tone, and TMJ function.

Procedure 19–6: Assessing the Eyes

- Techniques: inspection and palpation.

- Assess distance vision using a Snellen chart.

- Test near vision by measuring the client's ability to read newsprint at a distance of 14 inches (35.5 cm).

- Test color vision by using color plates or the color bars on the Snellen chart.

- Assess peripheral vision by determining when an object comes into sight.

- Assess EOMs by examining the corneal light reflex, assessing the ability to move through the six cardinal gaze positions, and performing with the cover/uncover test.

- Inspect the external eye structures.

- Test the corneal reflex with a cotton wisp.

- Check pupillary reaction for direct and consensual response.

- Assess accommodation by having the patient focus on an approaching object.

- Palpate the external eye structures.

Procedure 19–7: Assessing the Ears and Hearing

- Techniques: inspectation and palpation.

- Inspect the external ear for placement, size, shape, symmetry, and the condition of the skin.

- Palpate the external structures of the ear for the condition of the skin and for tenderness.

- Inspect the tympanic membrane and bony landmarks.

- Assess gross hearing with the whisper and watch-tick tests.

- Perform the Weber test to assess hearing loss.

- Perform the Rinne test to identify whether hearing loss is conductive or sensorineural.

- Perform the Romberg test to assess balance.

Procedure 19–8: Assessing the Nose and the Sinuses

- Techniques: inspection and palpation.

- Insert the speculum about 1 cm, and then open it as much as possible.

- Inspect the external and internal structures of the nose.

- Transilluminate and palpate the sinuses.

- Palpate the external structures of the nose.

Procedure 19–9: Assessing the Mouth and Oropharynx

- Techniques: inspection and palpation.

- Inspect the lips, oral mucosa, gums, teeth, and bite.

- Inspect the hard/soft palate, tonsils, and uvula.

- Inspect the tongue and frenulum; inspect under the tongue.

- Palpate the lips and tongue for tenderness and muscle tone.

- Test the gag reflex by touching the back of the soft palate with a tongue blade.

Procedure 19–10: Assessing the Neck

- Techniques: inspection and palpation (auscultation as needed).

- Inspect the neck. Note symmetry, range of motion (ROM), and the condition of the skin.

- Palpate the cervical lymph nodes. Note the size, shape, symmetry, consistency, mobility, tenderness, and temperature of any palpable nodes.

- Palpate the thyroid. If it is enlarged or if there is a mass, follow up with auscultation of the gland.

Procedure 19–11: Assessing the Breasts and Axillae

- Techniques: inspection and palpation.

- Inspect the breasts and axillae for skin condition, size, shape, symmetry, and color.

- If you notice an open lesion or nipple discharge, wear procedure gloves to palpate the breasts.

- Inspect the nipples for discharge. Culture any discharge, if present.

- Palpate the breasts using the vertical strip method, pie wedge method, or concentric circles method.

- Palpate the nipples, areolae, and lymph nodes.

Procedure 19–12: Assessing the Chest and Lungs

- Techniques: inspection, palpation, percussion, auscultation.

Comprehensive Physical Examination: Summary *(continued)*

- Assess respirations by counting the respiratory rate and observing the rhythm, depth, and symmetry of chest movement.

- Inspect the chest for anteroposterior (AP): lateral ratio, costal angle, spinal deformity, respiratory effort, and skin condition.

- Palpate the trachea.

- Palpate the chest for tenderness, masses, or crepitus.

- Palpate chest excursion.

- Palpate the chest for tactile fremitus.

- Percuss the chest.

- Percuss diaphragmatic excursion.

- Auscultate the chest.

Procedure 19–13: Assessing the Heart and Vascular System

- Techniques: inspection, palpation, auscultation.

- If possible, work from your patient's right side.

- Inspect the neck for pulsations.

- Measure jugular venous pressure (JVP).

- Inspect the precordium for pulsations.

- Palpate the carotid arteries.

- Palpate the precordium for pulsations, lifts, heaves, or thrills.

- Auscultate the carotid arteries with the bell of the stethoscope.

- Auscultate the jugular veins with the bell of the stethoscope.

- Auscultate the precordium at the apex, left lower sternal border, base left, and base right. Use the bell and then the diaphragm of the stethoscope.

- Palpate the peripheral pulses. Any abnormalities require further evaluation.

Procedure 19–14: Assessing the Abdomen

- Techniques: inspection, auscultation, percussion, palpation (in that order).

- Have the client void prior to the exam.

- Position the client supine with the knees slightly flexed.

- Inspect the abdomen.

- Auscultate the abdomen for bowel sounds and bruits.

- Use indirect percussion to assess at multiple sites in all four quadrants.

- Using your fist or blunt percussion, percuss the costovertebral angle bilaterally to assess for kidney tenderness.

- Lightly palpate throughout the abdomen by pressing down 1 to 2 cm in a rotating motion. Identify surface characteristics, tenderness, muscle resistance, and turgor.

- Use deep palpation to palpate organs and masses.

Procedure 19–15: Assessing the Musculoskeletal System

- Techniques: inspection, palpation.

- Assess posture, body alignment, and symmetry.

- Assess the spinal curvature.

- Examine the gait by assessing the base of support (distance between the feet), stride length (distance between each step), and phases of the gait.

- Assess balance through tandem walking, heel-and-toe walking, deep knee bends, hopping, and the Romberg test.

- Assess coordination by testing finger-thumb opposition, rhythmic movements of lower and upper extremities, and rapid alternating movements.

- Test the accuracy of movements by having the client touch his finger to his nose with his eyes closed.

- Measure limb length and circumference. Compare limbs on both sides of the body.

- Inspect muscle symmetry.

- Perform ROM at all joints.

- Assess muscle strength by having the client perform ROM against resistance.

Procedure 19–16: Assessing the Sensory-Neurological System

- Assess behavior.

- Determine level of arousal.

- Determine level of orientation.

- Assess memory.

- Assess mathematical and calculation skills.

- Assess general knowledge.

➤

critical aspects of procedures 19–1 through 19–19

Comprehensive Physical Examination: Summary *(continued)*

- Evaluate thought processes.
- Assess abstract thinking.
- Assess judgment.
- Assess communication ability.
- Test cranial nerves.
- Test superficial sensations.
- Test deep sensations.
- Test discriminatory sensations.
- Test deep tendon reflexes.
- Test superficial reflexes.

Procedure 19–17: Assessing the Male Genitourinary System

- Techniques: inspection and palpation.
- Inspect the external genitalia, including the pattern of hair distribution.
- Palpate for lumps, masses, hernias, and enlarged lymph nodes.

Procedure 19–18: Assessing the Female Genitourinary System

- Techniques: inspection and palpation.
- Inspect the external genitalia.
- Palpate lymph nodes and possible hernia sites.

Procedure 19–19: Assessing the Anus and Rectum

- Inspect the external anal area, sphincter tone, and stool for occult blood.
- Palpate the anus and rectum for muscle tone and masses.
- For females, assessment of the anus and rectum is usually performed at the end of the internal pelvic exam; for males, it is done after the genitourinary exam.

 Go to Chapter 19, **Resources for Caregivers and Health Professionals,** on the Electronic Study Guide.

 Bibliography: Go to Volume 2, Bibliography.

Promoting Asepsis
& Preventing Infection

Learning Outcomes

After completing this chapter, you should be able to:

* Discuss the six links in the chain of infection.

* Describe the stages of a typical infectious process.

* Summarize the roles of the various barriers involved in the body's primary defenses.

* Describe four processes involved in secondary defense.

* Compare and contrast humoral and cell-mediated immunity.

* Identify activities that promote immune function.

* Discuss the factors that place an individual at increased risk for infection.

* Identify standard precautions to prevent transmission of infection through blood and body fluids.

* Describe additional precautions that must be taken when there is concern about contact, droplet, or airborne disease transmission.

* Compare and contrast methods of preventing infection by breaking the chain of infection.

* Implement measures to prevent nosocomial infections.

* Use medical asepsis when providing care to clients.

* Implement sterile technique in selected patient care activities.

Your Nursing Role Model

Stephanie Sergi is the 7-year-old daughter of Jason Sergi. Jason works as a nurse on a busy labor and delivery unit in a major medical center. One night at the dinner table, Stephanie asks, "Daddy, what was the most important thing you did at work today?" Jason has shared many stories about his work with his family. He takes a few minutes to consider his reply. Finally Jason answers, "I washed my hands—a lot."

Jason tells his daughter that he also assisted in the birth of five infants, resuscitated one of the infants who was initially struggling for breath, and identified several problems that prevented complications or even death of mothers in labor. "Daddy, I don't understand why you think washing your hands was so important," Stephanie protested. "Look at all the *really* important things you did today!"

As you read this chapter, think back to Jason's discussion with his daughter. Perhaps you will someday say the same thing to your child or anyone who asks about your day.

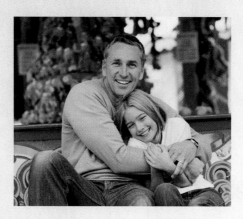

Theoretical Knowledge
knowing why

Nosocomial infections (infections acquired in a healthcare facility) are one of the top 20 health problems in the United States and are a concern of healthcare providers worldwide. They cost over $4.5 billion each year and are a leading cause of death (Adams & Corrigan, 2003). It may surprise you that people can acquire infections in a healthcare facility; this is where people go to be healed, not harmed. But this is also where people cluster together for care and where they come into contact with other patients, healthcare equipment, and health workers. Many of those clients are ill and therefore either (1) a source of infectious organisms or (2) especially susceptible to infectious organisms. In fact, most infection among patients is spread through the hands of healthcare providers! In this chapter you will learn how infections occur. You'll also learn how to promote **asepsis,** a term that means absence of contamination by disease-causing microorganisms. Asepsis is essential to prevent nosocomial infections, reduce the transmission of infection, and protect your patients and yourself from infections.

HOW DOES INFECTION OCCUR?

Imagine that your clinical instructor alerts you to an outbreak of infectious disease in the hospital where you have your assignment. The hospital census is currently over 200 patients, and so far 14 have become infected, and one has died. Have you ever wondered how infections are spread and why they seem to affect some people more than others?

Infections Develop in Response to a Chain of Factors

The process by which infections spread is commonly referred to as the **chain of infection.** It is made up of six links, all of which must be present for the infection to be transmitted from one individual to another (Figure 20–1). Here we describe each of the six links. Later in the chapter we will discuss how to interrupt the chain to limit the spread of infection.

Infectious Agent

Some microorganisms live on or in the human body without causing harm. For instance, the *Staphylococcus* bacteria growing on human skin usually cause no

harm. Other microorganisms are beneficial or even essential for human health and well-being. Such organisms are referred to as **normal flora.** For example, normal flora in the intestine aid in digestion and synthesize vitamin K, and release vitamin B_{12}, thiamine, and riboflavin when they die. In addition, they limit the growth of harmful bacteria by competing with them for available nutrients.

In contrast, some microorganisms are **pathogens,** that is, organisms capable of causing disease. In fact, the precise definition of the term **infection** is successful invasion of the body by a pathogen (Bauman, 2004). The largest groups of pathogenic microorganisms are bacteria, viruses, and fungi (which include yeasts and molds). Less common pathogens are protozoa, such as amoebae, helminths (commonly called worms), and prions, which are infectious protein particles that cause neurological disease. In addition, normal flora may become pathogenic if disease or injury permit them to enter body regions they do not normally inhabit. For instance, rupture of the bowel through trauma or disease allows intestinal microbes to enter the abdominal cavity or bloodstream, where they cause infection.

Research continues to lead to the discovery of new pathogens. Disease outbreaks, such as the 2003 outbreak of severe acute respiratory syndrome (SARS), often lead to intensive study. Currently researchers are also investigating the role of viruses in the development of cancer; virally induced cancers include Hodgkin's disease, Kaposi's sarcoma, cervical cancer, and others. Other research is investigating the role that certain species of bacteria play in producing heart disease (Fouad, Mamer, Sauriol, Khayyal, Lesimple, & Ruhenstroth-Bauer, 2004). Another area of intensive study is the ability of microorganisms to mutate to develop resistance to antimicrobial drugs. Antibiotic resistance is one of the most significant challenges of treating patients with severe infectious diseases today.

Reservoir

A **reservoir** is a source of infection: a place where pathogens survive and multiply. Animals, insects, and humans are living reservoirs of infection. Soil, water, food, and environmental surfaces can be nonliving reservoirs.

To support microbial growth, a reservoir needs to maintain a hospitable environmental temperature. Environments that are either too hot or too cold for a particular species will slow its growth or even kill the entire population. In part, the microbes that are pathogenic to humans are so because they thrive at about the same temperature as the human body. Thus, a fever in response to infection can inhibit and even kill invading pathogens.

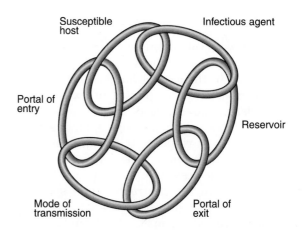

FIGURE 20–1 All six links in the chain of infection must be present for infection to be transmitted from one individual to another.

To thrive in the human body, microbes also must be able to use the body's precise balance of moisture, nutrients, electrolytes, and pH to support their own reproduction. Microbes that aren't pathogenic to humans require environments that are more wet or dry than the body or have a higher or lower concentration of salts, sugars, pH, and so on. That's why, for example, the bacteria that thrive in the Great Salt Lake would not cause infection in your body.

As noted earlier, food may serve as a nonliving reservoir. Bacteria can rapidly multiply in food left at room temperature. To prevent the growth of pathogens, many foods are cooked at high temperatures and stored in a cool environment. Alternatively, many foods are deliberately prepared with a concentration of solutes that inhibits the growth of pathogenic microbes. This concept underlies the salting of meats and the production of fruit jellies, jams, and preserves. Other nonliving reservoirs of infection include contaminated water, stagnant ponds, garbage, soiled diapers, discarded wound dressings, and raw sewage.

In healthcare facilities, many surfaces act as reservoirs. Microorganisms have mass, and they eventually fall to the floor or onto bedside tables, chairs, or equipment. Other surfaces, such as sinks, toilets, bed rails, and bed linens may also become reservoirs because of their proximity to patients, family members, and healthcare providers harboring pathogens.

Some people are capable of defending themselves from active disease but harbor the pathogenic organism within their body. These individuals, called **carriers,** have no symptoms of disease, yet they can pass the disease to others.

KnowledgeCheck 20–1

- What is a pathogen?
- What is the role of normal flora?
- Identify at least five reservoirs of infection.

 Go to Chapter 20, **Knowledge Check Response Sheet and Answers,** on the Electronic Study Guide.

Portal of Exit

A contained reservoir is only a potential source of infection. For infection to spread, a pathogen must exit the reservoir. In the case of human or animal reservoirs, the most frequent **portal of exit** is through body fluids, including blood, mucus, saliva, breast milk, urine, feces, vomitus, semen, or other secretions. The body's natural response to foreign materials, including pathogens, is to try to expel them. If you have a pathogen in the respiratory system, you cough and sneeze. If it is in the gastrointestinal system, you vomit or experience intense intestinal cramping and diarrhea. Microbes responsible for sexually transmitted infections can exit via semen, vaginal secretions, or blood that is present during sex.

Cuts, bites, and abrasions also provide an exit for body fluid. Blood and pus seeping from a wound help transport pathogens away from the patient's broken skin but become a portal via which infection may be transmitted to others. In nosocomial infections, puncture sites, drainage tubes, feeding tubes, and intravenous lines commonly serve as routes for pathogens to exit the body.

Mode of Transmission

Contact, either direct or indirect, is the most frequent **mode of transmission** of infection. *Direct contact* between two people usually involves touching, kissing, or sexual intercourse. Animals commonly transmit infection via scratching and biting as well. *Indirect contact* involves contact with a **fomite,** a contaminated object that transfers a pathogen. For example, suppose that while you are charting you begin to sneeze or cough. If you cover your nose and mouth with your hand and then resume charting, you may transmit pathogens to the pen, paper, and chart. Shoes, eyeglasses, stethoscopes, and other items we wear also commonly serve as fomites, as do contaminated needles.

Droplet transmission occurs when the pathogen travels in water droplets expelled when an infected person exhales, coughs, sneezes, or talks. It may also occur during suctioning and providing oral care. The usual method of transmission is for the droplet to be inhaled or enter the eye of a susceptible person. Although droplets can travel only a few feet from the infectious person, within that distance they may readily contaminate fomites that then transmit the organism by contact.

Airborne transmission occurs with much smaller organisms that can float considerable distances on air currents. Airborne pathogens can travel through heating and air conditioning systems to infect large numbers of people. Sweeping a floor or shaking out contaminated bed linens can stir up airborne microorganisms and launch them on air currents. The agents of measles and tuberculosis, as well as many fungal infections, are commonly transmitted in this manner.

A **vector** is an organism that carries a pathogen to a susceptible host, either by biting or by carrying the pathogen on its body. A common vector for diseases, including malaria, yellow fever, and the West Nile virus, is the mosquito. Ticks carry several diseases, as do fleas, mites, and other insects.

Modern air travel allows spread of pathogens in many ways. Infected travelers serve as reservoirs for pathogens. The close quarters and recirculated air system in modern planes provide an ideal environment for the transmission of airborne pathogens and both direct and indirect contact contamination between passengers. Air travel also enables a person to infect multiple individuals headed for diverse locations, often even before the reservoir shows symptoms of the disease. The 2003 SARS outbreak is an excellent example of flight travel as a means of transmission: a Chinese physician unknowingly infected at least a dozen guests at a hotel in Hong Kong where he was staying, and the guests then flew to Vietnam, Singapore, and Canada, prompting outbreaks in those countries.

Portal of Entry

Pathogens can enter the body through various **portals of entry.** Normal body openings, such as the conjunctiva of the eye, the nares (nostrils), mouth, urethra, vagina, and anus are potential portals of entry, as are abnormal openings, such as cuts and scrapes. Vectors such as mosquitos create abnormal portals of entry when they bite through the skin. In healthcare settings, common portals of entry include wounds, surgical sites, and insertion sites for tubes or needles.

Susceptible Host

A **susceptible host** is a person with inadequate defenses against the invading pathogen. Once a pathogen gains entry into a host, three factors determine whether the person develops infection:

1. The virulence of the organism (its power to cause disease)
2. The number of organisms transmitted (the greater the number, the more likely they are to cause disease)
3. The ability of the host's defenses to prevent infection

KnowledgeCheck 20–2

- Identify the six links in the chain of infection.
- What kinds of microbes favor the human body as a reservoir of infection?

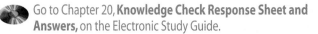 Go to Chapter 20, **Knowledge Check Response Sheet and Answers,** on the Electronic Study Guide.

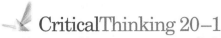 CriticalThinking 20–1

You are working as a nurse on a medical-surgical unit. What roles might you play in the chain of infection?

Infections Can Be Classified by Location and Duration

Some infections cause harm in a limited region of the body, such as the upper respiratory tract, the urethra, or a single bone or joint. Such infections are said to be **local.** In contrast, **systemic** infections occur when pathogens invade the blood or lymph and spread throughout the body. **Bacteremia** is the clinical presence of bacteria in the blood, whereas **septicemia** is symptomatic systemic infection spread via the blood.

In addition, it is helpful for healthcare providers to distinguish between primary and secondary infections. A **primary infection** is the first infection that occurs in a patient. Following a primary infection, especially in immunocompromised patients, may be one or more **secondary infections.** For example, a frail client infected with pneumonia develops herpes zoster (shingles, a viral infection related to past infection with varicella) related to the stress of illness.

Healthcare providers also need to determine the source of pathogens in a patient infected while he is in the facility. In **exogenous nosocomial infections,** the pathogen is acquired from the healthcare environment. In **endogenous nosocomial infections,** the pathogen arises from the patient's normal flora, and some form of treatment (e.g., chemotherapy or antibiotics) causes the normally harmless microbe to multiply and cause infection. For example, candidal vaginitis (yeast infection) may develop in a client receiving antibiotics after abdominal surgery.

Infections that have a rapid onset but last only a short time, such as a head cold, are said to be *acute.* In contrast, *chronic* infections develop slowly and last for weeks, months, or even years. Some chronic infections, such as relapsing fever, recur after periods of remission. *Latent* infections cause no symptoms for long periods of time, even decades. Human immunodeficiency virus (HIV) is an example. It typically causes an initial, brief illness that is then followed by about 6 years of latency before the patient begins to experience symptoms of AIDS.

Infections Follow Predictable Stages

Many infections follow a fairly predictable course of events, although the precise duration and intensity of symptoms in each stage vary from one individual to another:

• **Incubation** is the stage between successful invasion of the pathogen into the body and the first appearance of symptoms. In this stage, the person does not suspect that he or she has been infected but may be capable of infecting others. This stage may last only 1 day, as with the influenza virus, or as long as several months or even years.

• The **prodromal stage** is characterized by the first appearance of vague symptoms. For example, a person infected with a cold virus may experience a mild throat irritation. Not all infections have a prodromal stage.

• **Illness** is the stage marked by the appearance of the signs and symptoms characteristic of the disease. If the patient's immune defenses and medical treatments (if any) are ineffective, this stage can end in the death of the patient.

• **Decline** is the stage during which the patient's immune defenses, along with any medical therapies, successfully reduce the number of pathogenic microbes. Thus, all signs and symptoms of the infection begin to fade.

• **Convalescence** is characterized by tissue repair and a return to health as the remaining number of microorganisms approaches zero. Convalescence may require only a day or two or, for severe infections, as long as a year or more.

WHAT ARE THE BODY'S DEFENSES AGAINST INFECTION?

The human body has three "lines of defense" against infectious disease. First, certain anatomical features limit the entry of pathogens. Second, protective biochemical processes fight pathogens that do enter. Third, the presence of pathogens activates immune responses against specific, recognized invaders.

The first two lines of defense are nonspecific; that is, they have no means of adapting their response to each specific invader. Instead, they act in precisely the same way against any and all intruders, from a simple cold virus to deadly fungal spores.

Primary Defenses

The "soldiers" in the first line of defense are the structural barriers of the human body. These **primary defenses** prevent organisms from entering the body.

• *Skin.* The surface of intact, healthy skin is tough and resilient and prevents entry of many pathogens.

• *The respiratory tree.* The nares, trachea, and bronchi are covered with mucous membranes that trap pathogens, which are then expelled. The nose contains hairs that filter the upper airway, and the nasal passages, sinuses, trachea, and larger bronchi are lined with cilia, tiny hairlike cells that sweep microorganisms upward from the lower airways. Coughing and sneezing forcefully expel organisms from the respiratory tract.

- *Eyes.* The lacrimal glands produce tears that contain lysozyme, an antimicrobial enzyme. Thus, tears help the body wash infective organisms from the eyes.
- *The mouth.* The mouth normally has a large number of pathogenic microorganisms, but saliva, like tears, contains lysozyme and helps continually wash microbes from the teeth and gums. The rich blood supply of the mouth swiftly transports defensive blood cells (discussed later in this section) that keep the microorganisms in check. In addition, normal flora of the mouth compete for nutrition with invading organisms, thereby limiting the number of pathogens.
- *The gastrointestinal tract.* Many pathogens that reach the stomach are destroyed in its acidic environment. Those that successfully enter the small intestine face the antimicrobial action of bile. Simple peristalsis, as well as diarrhea and vomiting, are other first-line defense mechanisms for pathogens that invade the gastrointestinal tract.
- *The genitourinary tract.* Like the respiratory tree, the genitourinary tract is protected with mucous membranes. The epithelial cells lining the urethra and anus secrete mucus, which adheres to pathogens to promote their excretion through urine and stool. Urine itself is highly acidic and contains lysozyme. Mucous membranes lining the vagina also inhibit establishment of pathogens. In addition, the high acidity and normal flora of the vagina hold pathogens in check.

Secondary Defenses

Pathogens that dodge the primary defenses and gain entry into the body begin to release wastes and secretions and to cause the breakdown of cells and tissues. The presence of such chemicals activates a set of **secondary defenses.**

- *Phagocytosis*—the process by which white blood cells (WBCs) called *phagocytes* engulf and destroy pathogens directly. Phagocytic white blood cells include neutrophils, monocytes, and eosinophils. Monocytes also have the ability to differentiate into macrophages that specialize in cleaning up sites of injury or infection by phagocytizing pathogens, used WBCs, and cellular debris. Eosinophils are occasionally phagocytic; however, they are responsible mainly for binding to helminths and releasing harmful toxins onto their surface.
- *The complement cascade*—a process by which a set of blood proteins called **complement** triggers the release of chemicals that attack the cell membranes of pathogens, causing them to rupture. Complement also signals white blood cells called basophils to release a chemical called histamine, which prompts inflammation.

- *Inflammation*—a process that begins when histamine and other chemicals are released either directly from damaged cells, or from basophils in response to the activation of complement. Histamine and other inflammatory chemicals cause dilation and increased permeability of blood vessels, increasing the flow of phagocytes, antimicrobial chemicals, oxygen, and nutrients to the damaged area.
- *Fever*—a rise in core body temperature that increases metabolism, inhibits multiplication of pathogens, and triggers specific immune responses (discussed shortly). Believing that low-grade fevers are a necessary natural defense mechanism, many clinicians do not treat a fever lower than 102°F (38.9°C).

The classic signs and symptoms of inflammation are localized heat and erythema (redness), which develop as blood flow is increased. In addition, fluid leaking from the more permeable blood vessels accumulates in the surrounding tissue, causing edema, which in turn prompts pain as pressure is exerted on nerve endings (Bauman, 2004).

Table 20–1 summarizes the types of white blood cells and their roles in defending against infection.

Tertiary Defenses

Why is it that people who recover from an infectious disease like measles or chickenpox never get the disease again, even if they are repeatedly exposed to the virus? The answer lies in **specific immunity:** the process by which the body's immune cells "learn" to recognize and destroy pathogens that they have encountered before.

The cells involved in specific immunity are white blood cells called **lymphocytes,** which are produced from stem cells in the red bone marrow. Lymphocytes that grow to maturity in the bone marrow are designated *B lymphocytes,* or *B cells,* whereas those that mature in the thymus are designated *T lymphocytes,* or *T cells.* After they have matured, most B cells and T cells travel to the lymph nodes, spleen, and other sites of lymphatic tissue. Some circulate in blood and lymph. From all of these locations, lymphocytes seek out foreign cells and other matter to target for destruction. Lymphocytes recognize foreign substances by the molecules that they present on their surfaces. These molecules that trigger a specific immune response are called **antigens.**

B cells are involved in the humoral immune response. T cells are responsible for cell-mediated immunity. These two types of specific immunity are discussed next.

Humoral Immunity

The humoral immune response acts directly against antigens. In response to the presence of antigens,

TABLE 20-1 Types and Functions of White Blood Cells

Type	Function
Granular	
Basophils: 0.5–1% of total WBCs	Release histamine and heparin granules as part of the inflammatory response
Eosinophils: 1–3% of total WBCs	Destroy helminths; mediate allergic reactions; have limited role in phagocytosis
Neutrophils: 55–70% of total WBCs	Phagocytize pathogens
Agranular	
Lymphocytes: 20–35% of total WBCs	T cells—responsible for cell-mediated immunity; recognize, attack, and destroy antigens B cells—responsible for humoral immunity; produce immunoglobulins to attack and destroy antigens
Monocytes: 3–8% of total WBCs	Able to phagocytize directly as well as to differentiate into macrophages, which help clean up damaged or injured tissue

macrophages and a class of T cells called *helper T cells* stimulate B cells to become plasma cells and produce **antibodies,** also called **immunoglobulins (Ig).** Antibodies are proteins with a base region and two arms (somewhat like the letter Y). They bind to target antigens and destroy them by any of the following methods (Figure 20–2):

- *Phagocytosis.* Antibodies do not phagocytize directly, but instead signal leukocytes (macrophages and neutrophils) to phagocytize the pathogens to which the antibodies are bound.

- *Neutralization.* By binding to a pathogen's attachment sites, antibodies disable the pathogens' machinery for adhering to and invading body cells; thus, although they are not destroyed, the pathogens are effectively neutralized.

- *Agglutination.* Antibodies have two attachment sites, and therefore each antibody can attach to two pathogenic cells in a population. This quality causes the cells to clump together (agglutinate), reducing the cells' activity and increasing the likelihood that the group will be detected by leukocytes and phagocytized.

- *Activation of complement and inflammation.* Antibodies trigger the complement cascade and stimulate the release of inflammatory chemicals to destroy the antigen.

Immunoglobulins are antibodies secreted by B lymphocytes. Five classes of immunoglobulins (Ig) are formed.

- *IgM.* IgM is produced when an antigen is encountered for the first time. This is a large molecule and cannot pass through the placenta to protect a fetus.

- *IgG.* IgG is the most common immunoglobulin in the body. Once the body recognizes the antigen and

produces IgG, special B memory cells are formed that remember the antigen and rapidly produce IgG in response to subsequent infection. However, it takes at least 10 days for IgG to be produced in response to an initial infection. Eventually the IgG

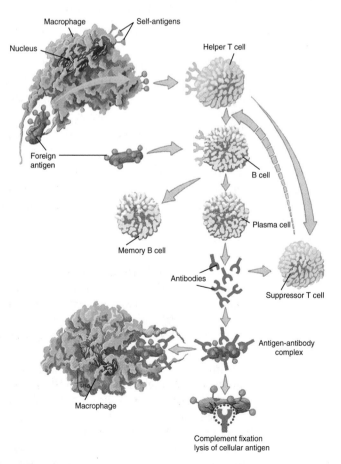

FIGURE 20–2 **The humoral immune response produces antibodies to destroy antigens.**

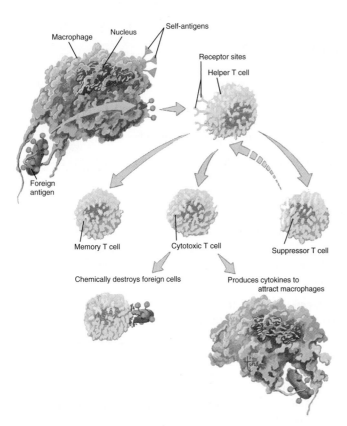

FIGURE 20–3 **The cell-mediated immune response causes white blood cells to attack antigens.**

response fades. The length of time the body remembers how to produce IgG for a specific pathogen depends on the characteristics of the pathogen, the strength of the initial response, and the health of the person.

IgG is small enough to pass through the placenta. If the mother has developed IgG through previous exposure, IgG will pass through the placenta and provide protection from the pathogen. Infants are born with **passive immunity** from their mother's IgG. Additional IgG is passed to the child through breast feeding. Passive immunity can also be given to individuals by administering immune globulins (an injectable medication). Passive immunity is maintained only as long as the IgG molecule exists.

- *IgE.* IgE is the immunoglobulin primarily responsible for the allergic response. The body identifies an allergen as a potential pathogen and begins efforts to destroy or excrete the allergen. Subsequent exposure to the allergen results in a more severe response. Individuals vary in their response to allergens, but a typical allergic response includes some or all of the following symptoms: increased production of mucus, itching (this is actually a defense designed to stimulate the person to rub off the allergen), hives, rashes, eczema, sneezing (to clear the upper airway), wheezing (caused by constriction of the airways in an effort to prevent further penetration of the allergen into

the lungs), and in the most severe responses, a life-threatening anaphylactic shock.

- *IgA.* The mucous membranes secrete IgA around the body openings. They provide additional protection for these vulnerable portals of entry.
- *IgD.* These antibodies form on the surface of B cells and trap the potential pathogen to prevent it from replicating and causing disease.

Cell-Mediated Immunity

Whereas the humoral immune response acts directly against antigenic cells, the cell-mediated immune response acts to destroy body cells that have become infected, in most cases by viruses. T cells are responsible for the cell-mediated immune response. Four types of T cells play a role (Figure 20–3):

- *Cytotoxic (killer) T cells* directly attack and kill body cells infected with pathogens.
- *Helper T cells* help regulate the action of B cells in humoral immune responses, and of cytotoxic T cells in cell-mediated responses.
- *Memory T cells.* The first time an antigen invades the body, T cells form that respond to that specific antigen. With subsequent infections, the memory T cells are able to increase the speed and amount of the T cell response.
- *Suppressor T cells* are thought to stop the immune response when the infection has been contained (also see Figure 20–2).

KnowledgeCheck 20–3

- Identify and describe the purpose of the body's three major lines of defense against infection.
- Mr. Jefferson has an acute infection. If lab work reveals that IgM, but not IgG, is present in his blood, what can you conclude about this infection?

 Go to Chapter 20, **Knowledge Check Response Sheet and Answers,** on the Electronic Study Guide.

HOW CAN THE HOST DEFENSES BE SUPPORTED?

Efforts to promote wellness help break the chain of infection by strengthening an individual's defenses against invading pathogens. Lifestyle factors essential for promoting host defenses are healthful nutrition, adequate hygiene, rest and exercise, stress reduction, and immunizations.

Nutrition

Adequate nutrition, including protein, vitamins, minerals, and water, is essential for combating infection. An acute infection depletes the body's nutritional

stores. Nutrients are required to replace these lost stores, to maintain production of white blood cells, and to repair damaged tissues. Fever and increased mucus secretions, which are common defenses against infection, increase water losses. Additional water is needed to supplement this lost fluid and to support the increased metabolic rate. Chapter 26 will further discuss the importance of adequate nutrition.

Hygiene

Hygiene is a crucial aspect of maintaining skin integrity. Intact skin is one of the best defenses against infection. Frequent hand washing, as well as regular showering or bathing, decreases the bacterial count on the skin. However, overzealous cleanliness diminishes the skin's natural oils and may lead to cracking of the skin. Chapter 22 focuses on the importance of hygiene for health.

Rest and Exercise

Both rest and exercise are necessary to rejuvenate the body. Adequate rest and sleep renew the body and mind and conserve strength. Sleep needs vary among individuals. There is really no "correct" amount or pattern of sleep. However, sleep of 7 to 8 hours per night is considered fully restorative. Research demonstrates that exercise is just as important. Too little activity causes circulation to slow and the lungs to supply less oxygen. Excessive exercise leads to fatigue. Chapters 31 and 33 provide in-depth discussion on rest, sleep, activity, and exercise.

Stress Reduction

Stress, whether physical or mental, decreases the body's immune defenses. Numerous studies demonstrate a correlation between increased stress and increased disease (Clark, 2003; Franco, de Barros, Nogueira-Martins, & Michel, 2003; Cousins, 1979). Laughing, in contrast, increases oxygenation, promotes body movement, and increases immune responses. See Chapter 25 for further detail on the effects of stress.

Immunizations

Immunization via vaccination can protect against several infectious diseases. Immunizations expose the body to weakened or killed pathogens, stimulating an immune response. At a later date, if the body encounters the pathogen, immune cells are available to ward off an infection. Unfortunately, some pathogens, like the virus that causes the common cold, mutate too rapidly for an immunization to be developed. Chapter 41 discusses recommended immunizations throughout the life span and their role in health promotion.

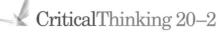 CriticalThinking 20–2
Consider your current lifestyle. How would you evaluate your ability to support your body's defenses?

WHAT FACTORS INCREASE THE RISK FOR INFECTION?

Anything that weakens the defenses makes a person more susceptible to infection. In addition, any factors that increase the person's exposure to pathogens, such as working at a day care center or being a nurse, increase the risk for infection. Some of the most common factors are discussed below.

- *Developmental stage.* Young children are vulnerable because their immune systems are immature and have had limited exposure to pathogens. Children frequently have an increased number of infections when they start interacting with people outside their family (e.g., when they begin child care or start school). This is a natural process known as acquiring **active immunity.** Also, older adults are more susceptible hosts because their immune response declines with aging. Skin, a primary defense, becomes less elastic and more prone to breakdown with aging. Elders also tend to be less active, and their nutrition may be inadequate.

- *Breaks in the first line of defense.* A break in the skin, whether caused by a surgical procedure, skin breakdown, or insertion of an intravenous device, creates a portal of entry for infectious microorganisms.

- *Illness or injury.* Recuperation from infection or injury limits the physical resources available to combat a new pathogen.

- *Smoking.* Smoking is a major risk factor for pulmonary infections. Smoking interferes with normal respiratory functioning, including the ability to move the chest, cough, sneeze, or have full air exchange. Chemicals in tobacco paralyze cilia; thus, secretions pool in the lower airways, creating a hospitable environment for bacterial growth. Although smokers are most profoundly affected by these changes, people exposed chronically to secondhand smoke, (e.g., bartenders, children of smokers) are also affected by these changes and are at increased risk for infection.

- *Substance abuse.* Alcohol curbs hunger because it contains many calories. As a result, many chronic alcohol users do not consume an adequate diet. Alcohol is also directly toxic to the liver and to the cells lining the intestinal mucosa. Smoked substances, such as marijuana and cocaine, affect respiratory cilia in a manner similar to tobacco. Any substances that affect orientation and energy level will negatively alter food intake, activity, rest, and hygiene—factors that support host defenses. Injecting substances leads to breaks in skin integrity, increasing the risk of infection.

- *Multiple sexual partners.* The number of sexual partners is directly related to the risk of sexually transmitted infections and cervical cancer.
- *Environmental factors.* Increased exposure to pathogens in one's work situation (e.g., kindergarten teacher, healthcare worker), living situation (e.g., nursing home, parents with young children who are in preschool), and other environmental factors increase one's risk for infection.
- *Chronic disease.* Many chronic diseases diminish the body's ability to fend off infection. Diseases that impair peripheral circulation, such as uncontrolled hypertension (high blood pressure) and diabetes mellitus, make the patient prone to infection in the extremities. Poor circulation prevents antibodies and T cells from reaching the pathogens and damages tissue, making it easier for pathogens to enter. Leukemia, a form of cancer, increases the production of abnormal white blood cells, but these cells are ineffective in fighting infection. Because HIV infects T cells, a patient with AIDS has a reduced ability to fight off secondary infections.
- *Medications.* Some medications are given for the purpose of reducing the immune response, for example, to patients receiving organ or tissue transplants. For most patients, however, decreased immunity is a side effect of treatment. Even common medications, such as nonsteroidal anti-inflammatory agents (e.g., ibuprofen, aspirin) decrease the immune response. As a side effect, some medications, such as chemotherapeutic agents, decrease the production of white blood cells or cause the cells produced to be abnormal. Even antibiotics can increase the risk for infection. For example, an antibiotic given for a respiratory infection may cause a vaginal yeast infection because it destroys colonies of normal flora, allowing the harmful microbes to thrive. Such infections are called **superinfections** (opportunistic growth of harmful transient pathogens that are normally kept in check), and some can be extremely challenging to treat.
- *Nursing and medical procedures.* Several procedures are associated with an increased risk of infection. For example, urinary catheterization may damage the fragile urethral mucosa, provide a direct pathway for pathogens into the bladder, and prevent the normal flushing of the urethra. Also an IV line inserted to infuse an antibiotic may serve as a portal of entry for pathogens to enter a patient's body.

KnowledgeCheck 20–4

- What factors increase a client's risk for infection?
- What activities decrease the likelihood of infection?

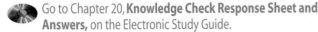 Go to Chapter 20, **Knowledge Check Response Sheet and Answers,** on the Electronic Study Guide.

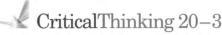 CriticalThinking 20–3

Recall the scenario of Jason Sergi, the labor and delivery nurse, and his daughter. Why did Jason say that hand washing was the most important thing he did at work that day? Explain your answer by referring to all of the links in the chain of infection.

Practical Knowledge
knowing how

As a nurse you will have direct contact with patients who are infected with a variety of pathogens or who are at increased risk for infection. The remainder of this chapter provides practical information for preventing infection in your clients and for caring for clients with infection.

| Assessment |

Some elements of the nursing history and physical assessment focus specifically on the risk factors and symptoms of infection.

Nursing History

To elicit information related to infection, ask the client about the following:

- Any exposure to pathogens in the environment, including at work, recent travel, contact with people who are ill, and unprotected sexual behavior
- Any unusual foods or products ingested
- Past and present disease or injury history
- Medications, over-the-counter preparations, herbal products, alcohol intake, and any substances currently in use
- Current level of stress
- Immunization history
- Symptoms of illness

Physical Assessment

Observe the patient's general appearance: Does he seem tired or fatigued? Is he diaphoretic? Is he wrapped in blankets or complaining of feeling chilled? Does the patient appear well nourished? Are the mucous membranes dry? Does the patient have good skin turgor?

Physical assessment includes a thorough examination of the skin. Look for signs of local infection evidenced by pain, redness, swelling, and warmth. Note the presence or absence of any rashes, along with any breaks or reddened areas of the skin. Patients with poor peripheral circulation often have skin discoloration, rather than signs of inflammation, when experiencing

an infection. Swollen lymph nodes indicate the possible presence of an infection in the area that drains into the nodes. An elevated temperature and pulse rate are classic signs of an infection.

It is important to remember that the presence of one infection does not eliminate the risk for an additional infection. For example, a patient being treated with intravenous medications for a wound infection is at risk for infection at the intravenous site, as well as for a super-infection or an infection related to insufficient immunizations. The accompanying Diagnostic Testing box lists common tests used to evaluate evidence or risk of infection. The specific test(s) should be evaluated based on the patient's condition, age, and coexisting conditions.

Nursing Diagnosis

Virtually any patient in a healthcare setting is at Risk for Infection due to exposure to pathogens in the environment. Use this diagnosis only for patients who are at higher risk than usual (e.g., those with poor nutritional status) and who need nursing interventions to help prevent infection. Do not use it for the generic assessments you do routinely for all patients (e.g., assessing temperature, routine examination of surgical incision). Examples of appropriate use of this diagnosis include the following:

- Risk for Infection r/t altered immune response secondary to corticosteroid therapy
- Risk for Infection r/t impaired skin integrity and poor nutritional status

Patients with actual infection will be managed collaboratively with the healthcare team.

Infection may be a medical diagnosis or the etiology of other nursing diagnoses, such as Fatigue, Risk for Imbalanced Body Temperature, or Pain. Patients with infection may experience other nursing care problems due to their infected status. For example:

- Social Isolation r/t communicable disease (e.g., tuberculosis [TB])
- Diversional Activity Deficit r/t inability to leave room secondary to protective isolation

Other diagnostic statements may apply, depending upon the patient's condition, treatment ordered, and the patient's response to illness.

For a care plan and care map for Risk for Infection,

 Go to Chapter 20, **Care Plan,** on the Electronic Study Guide.

Planning Outcomes/Evaluation

Associated NOC standardized outcomes for Risk for Infection include:

- Community Risk Control: Communicable Disease
- Immune Status

---

diagnostic testing

Common Tests for Evaluating the Presence of or Risk for Infection

Test	Description
White blood cell (WBC) count with differential	A breakdown of the types of WBCs; normal WBC count is 5,000–10,000/cu mm
Blood cultures	A sample of blood placed on culture media and evaluated for growth of pathogens
Disease titers	Blood tests for specific disease immunity (e.g., to rubella)
Panels to evaluate specific disease exposure	Blood tests to evaluate exposure to specific diseases (e.g., HIV, hepatitis)
Immunoglobulin (IgG, IgM) levels	Blood tests to evaluate humoral immunity status
C-reactive protein (CRP)	A blood test to measure inflammatory change or bacterial infection
Agglutinins, warm or cold	Used to diagnose atypical infections by detecting antigens in the blood
Erythrocyte (red blood cell) sedimentation rate (ESR or sed rate)	A measure of inflammatory changes

- Immunization Behavior
- Knowledge: Infection Control
- Nutritional Status
- Risk Control: Sexually Transmitted Diseases (STD)

Individualized goals/outcomes statements depend on the specific nursing diagnosis and etiology. For example, for an undernourished woman, if the nursing diagnosis is Risk for Infection related to intravenous puncture site and potential for invasive procedure due to active labor, an appropriate goal would be:

Patient will show no signs of localized infection at the infusion site, as evidenced by the absence of

swelling, redness, excessive warmth, pain, or drainage.

You will evaluate the nursing care plan by examining the extent to which such goals have been met.

| Planning Interventions/Implementation |

When caring for a client at risk for infection, nursing activities are aimed at breaking the chain of infection at every possible link. Some of the most common reasons clients are diagnosed with Risk for Infection are exposure to pathogens, bypass of their normal defense mechanisms, increased physiological stress, or inadequate immune response. Direct nursing care toward these concerns, and provide the following global interventions:

- Reduce exposure to pathogens through the use of aseptic technique (discussed shortly).
- Maintain skin integrity and natural defenses against infection.
- Reduce stress.
- Promote immune function through collaborative care.

NIC standardized interventions for Risk for Infection include:

- Communicable Disease Management
- Immunization/Vaccination Management
- Infection Protection
- Nutrition Management
- Skin Surveillance
- Vital Signs Monitoring
- Wound Care

Specific nursing activities will be based on the unique situation of the client, as described in the etiology of the diagnostic statement. For example:

- For clients who have had surgery and general anesthesia or who are at risk for pneumonia, promote coughing and deep breathing on a regular basis.
- For clients who are at risk for disease based on age, debilitated state, community living arrangement, or employment in healthcare facilities, facilitate participation in vaccination programs, which can help them acquire immunity from some communicable diseases.
- Community health nurses can limit disease transmission through surveillance of the community, tracking of disease patterns, and initiation of prompt treatment.
- For clients with breaks in the skin or incision sites, provide regular assessment for infection status.
- For all clients at risk for infection, provide care that is based on principles of medical asepsis.

Medical Asepsis

Medical asepsis refers to a state of cleanliness that decreases the potential for the spread of infections. You probably already practice aseptic technique in other settings without realizing it. For example, when preparing dinner, before chopping food on a cutting board, you make sure the cutting board is clean and that the utensils you use have been washed. After using it, you wash the board with hot, soapy water. You also wash your hands before and after handling raw foods. These are all examples of medical asepsis.

Maintaining a Clean Environment

The goal of medical asepsis is to keep all public and patient care areas within the facility clean and free from dust, debris, and contamination. Any spilled liquids, dirty surfaces, or potentially contaminated areas should be cleaned immediately. In your home you use hot water and general cleaning supplies. However, healthcare facilities use special techniques and cleaning solutions formulated to inhibit microbial growth. Reusable equipment and supplies that have been or are suspected of being contaminated are disinfected or sterilized according to agency policy. **Disinfection** removes pathogens by physical or chemical means, including steam, gas, chemicals, and ultraviolet light. Disinfection reduces microbial populations, but it does not guarantee that all pathogens are eliminated, because certain viruses and other pathogenic microbes can remain (Bauman, 2004). In contrast, **sterilization** is the elimination of all microorganisms (except prions) in or on an object. Thus, it is used when absolute purity of an object or surface is critical, such as in situations requiring surgical asepsis, discussed shortly.

To promote medical asepsis in healthcare settings, keep the patient care area as clean and free of clutter as possible. Do not stock rooms with unnecessary supplies. Consider supplies that are brought into a patient room contaminated. Do not return them to the linen or supply cart; instead, handle them according to agency policy. Also consider contaminated any items brought from the patient's home, gifts from visitors, and so forth. The Home Care box discusses the differences encountered when providing care in the home.

Maintaining Clean Hands

The most important aspect of medical asepsis is hand cleanliness. Clean hands will markedly decrease the transmission of infection. Although you may feel you already know how to wash your hands, remember that in healthcare settings you are coming in contact with pathogens that are potentially dangerous to you and your patients.

In October 2002 a federal task force on hand hygiene made the following recommendations for hand

Infection Control

- Clients and caregivers in their own home are usually at less risk for infection than they are in the hospital. The client and caregiver share the same potential pathogens and antibodies, and there is limited exposure to others with illness.

- Teach clients and family members the importance of hand washing and keeping the environment clean to create an optimal environment for care.

- Procedures performed using sterile technique in the hospital (e.g., urinary catheterization) are often performed by clean procedure in the home because of the decreased risk of infection.

- Healthcare workers in the home are a potential source of pathogens and should use caution to avoid infecting the client.

- If the client or family member is capable and willing to perform the required treatment, provide the necessary teaching; the client will have less exposure to pathogens than he would if a healthcare provider came to the home to provide care.

- Assess for subtle signs of infection: temperature increase, fatigue, lymph gland enlargement, delayed healing of wounds, fever, chills, or drainage.

- Instruct clients and family members in the signs and symptoms of infection and how and when to contact their primary care provider to report these findings.

- To disinfect the home environment, teach caregivers to create a dilute bleach solution. Mix 1 part regular-strength bleach to 50 parts water. The mixture may be stored for a month in an opaque container. Instruct caregivers NEVER to mix the solution with other household cleaners.

- For additional information on home care practices, see Chapter 43.

---

cleanliness. Healthcare workers must clean their hands with either an alcohol-based solution or wash with soap and water:

- When arriving on a patient care unit.
- When leaving the patient care unit.
- Before and after using the restroom.
- Before and after any contact with a patient or articles in the patient's vicinity.
- Before putting on gloves.
- After removing gloves.
- Before and after touching any area on the face.
- Before and after eating.
- After touching anything that might be contaminated.
- Whenever the hands are visibly dirty.

If there is a potential for contact with bacterial spores, the hands must be washed with soap and water; alcohol-based solutions are ineffective against spores (Boyce, Pittet, Healthcare Infection Control Practices Advisory Committee, & Hand Hygiene Task Force, 2002).

Hand washing involves five key factors: time, water, soap, friction, and drying (Figure 20–4).

1. *Time.* In a nonsurgical setting, wash the hands for at least 15 seconds. In a surgical setting, wash the hands for 2 to 6 minutes, depending on the soap used.
2. *Water.* Use warm water to wet the hands prior to applying soap and to completely rinse off the soap. Using hot water will increase the potential for skin breakdown.
3. *Soap.* Use agency-approved soap.

4. *Friction.* Rub all surfaces of the hands and wrists, including the backs of the hands and between the fingers. Clean areas underneath jewelry. Clean underneath the fingernails if they are visibly dirty or possibly contaminated, using an orangewood stick.
5. *Drying.* Use single-use towels or hand dryers to remove all moisture after washing the hands.

For further instructions on hand washing for medical asepsis,

Go to Chapter 20, **Procedure 20–1: Hand Washing,** in Volume 2.

The Critical Aspects box on page 410 highlights the essential components of this procedure.

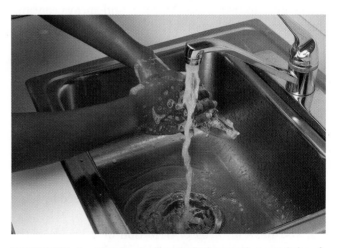

FIGURE 20–4   Clean hands will markedly decrease the transmission of infection.

Hand Washing

Hand Washing Steps:

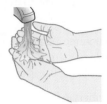

1. Wet hands.

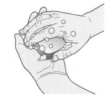

2. Soap (at least 15 seconds).

3. Scrub backs of hands, wrists, between fingers, under fingernails.

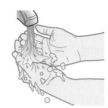

4. Rinse.

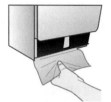

5. Towel-dry.

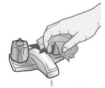

6. Turn off taps with towel.

If using alcohol-based handrubs:

1. Use alcohol-based handrubs when hands are not soiled.

2. Cover all surfaces of fingers and hands.

3. Rub until dry.

When you have no access to hand-washing supplies, you can use solutions, rubs, and sprays containing at least 60% alcohol to decontaminate your hands. Follow the manufacturer's recommendations for the use of the product. Rub the liquid on all areas of the hands until it dries. Table 20–2 identifies the effectiveness of components of hand-hygiene antiseptic agents.

To promote clean hands, follow these guidelines:

• Keep fingernails short. Do not wear artificial nails or nail extenders for patient care. If you do wear fingernail polish, be sure it is not chipped.

• Apply non-petroleum-based hand lotion at least twice a day to decrease the irritation caused by hand cleansing.

• If you have an area of irritation or a break in the skin, wear gloves or apply an occlusive dressing during patient contact.

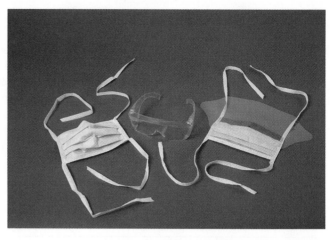

FIGURE 20–5 Several types of face masks and eye shields are available.

In addition to maintaining a clean environment and hand washing, you should follow other precautions to protect yourself and your patients. CDC guidelines provide for two tiers of protection. *Tier One* includes recommendations that pertain to all patients. These recommendations are known as standard or universal precautions. *Tier Two* outlines precautions to be taken based on the mode of transmission of the infection (Garner & Hospital Infection Control Practices Advisory Committee (HICPAC), 1996, updated 1997).

The United States Occupational Safety and Health Administration (OSHA) requires employers to provide personal protective equipment for healthcare workers (e.g., gloves, gowns, face masks, and eye protection). This equipment is to be used in standard precautions as well as Tier Two precautions. Figure 20–5 provides examples of face masks and eye protection equipment. For instructions in how to don and remove these items,

VOL 2 Go to Chapter 20, **Procedure 20–2: Donning and Removing Personal Protective Equipment (PPE),** in Volume 2.

The Critical Aspects box for Procedures 20–2 through 20–6, on page 414, highlights the main points.

CDC Tier One: Standard Precautions

Standard precautions (also called *universal precautions*) apply to all clients and should be used whenever there is a possibility of coming in contact with blood, body fluids (except sweat), excretions and secretions, mucous membranes, and breaks in the skin. These precautions are designed to protect you from exposure to potential pathogens, to decrease the likelihood that you will transmit pathogens among patients, and to protect the patient from microorganisms that you may carry. Box 20–1 provides a detailed description of the precautions you should take with all patients.

Antimicrobial Spectrum and Characteristics of Hand-Hygiene Antiseptic Agents

TABLE 20-2

Group	Gram-Positive Bacteria	Gram-Negative Bacteria	Mycobacteria	Fungi	Viruses	Speed of Action	Comments
Alcohols	+++	+++	+++	+++	+++	Fast	Optimum concentration 60–95%: no persistent activity
Chlorhexidine (2% and 4% aqueous)	+++	++	+	+	+++	Intermediate	Persistent activity: rare allergic reactions
Iodine compounds	+++	+++	+++	++	+++	Intermediate	Causes skin burns: usually too irritating for hand hygiene
Iodophors	+++	+++	+	++	++	Intermediate	Less irritating than iodine: acceptance varies
Phenol derivatives	+++	+	+	+	+	Intermediate	Activity neutralized by nonionic surfactants
Triclosan	+++	++	+	—	+++	Intermediate	Acceptability on hands varies
Quatemary ammonium compounds	+	++	—	—	+	Slow	Used only in combination with alcohols: ecological concerns

Note: +++ = excellent: ++ = good, but does not include the entire bacterial spectrum; + = fair; — = no activity or not sufficient. Hexachlorophene is not included because it is no longer an accepted ingredient of hand disinfectants.

Source: Boyce, J. M., Pittet, D. & Healthcare Infection Control Practices Advisory Committee & the HICPAC/SHEA/APIC/IDSA Hand Hygiene Task Force. (2002). Guideline for Hand Hygiene in health care settings. Available at http://www.cdc.gov/mmwr/preview/mmwrhtml/rr5116a2.htm

Following Standard Precautions

BOX 20-1

- Immediately wash your hands with soap and water after contact with blood, body fluids (except sweat), excretions and secretions, mucous membranes, any break in the skin, or contaminated objects, REGARDLESS of whether you have been wearing gloves.

- Wear clean gloves whenever there is potential for contact with blood, body fluids, secretions, excretions, nonintact skin, or contaminated materials.

- Remove gloves immediately after use. Avoid touching clean items, environmental surfaces, or another patient.

- Change gloves between tasks or procedures on the same patient if you have made contact with material that may contain a high concentration of microorganisms.

- Wash your hands with soap and water after removing gloves, between patient contacts, and between procedures on the same patient to prevent cross-contamination of different body sites.

- Wear a mask and eye protection or a face shield to protect mucous membranes of the eyes, nose, and mouth during patient care activities that are likely to generate splashes or sprays of blood, body fluids, secretions, and excretions.

- Wear a clean, nonsterile gown to protect skin and prevent soiling of clothing whenever there is a risk of spray or splash onto clothing. Promptly remove the gown

once it is soiled. Avoid contaminating clothing when removing the gown. Wash hands after removing the gown.

- Clean reusable equipment that is soiled with blood or body fluids according to agency policy.

- Do not reuse equipment for the care of another patient until it has been cleaned and reprocessed appropriately.

- Dispose of single-use equipment that is soiled with blood or body fluids in appropriate biohazard containers.

- Carefully handle contaminated linens to prevent skin and mucous membrane exposures, contamination of clothing, and transfer of microorganisms to other patients or the environment.

- Never recap used needles, or otherwise manipulate them using both hands, or use any other technique that involves directing the point of a needle toward any part of the body; rather, use either a one-handed "scoop" technique or a mechanical device designed for holding the needle sheath.

- Use puncture-resistant containers for disposal of "sharps"—scalpels, needles, and so on.

- Use mouthpieces, resuscitation bags, or other ventilation devices as an alternative to mouth-to-mouth resuscitation methods in situations when the need for resuscitation is predictable.

KnowledgeCheck 20–5

Under what circumstances are standard precautions used?

 Go to Chapter 20, **Knowledge Check Response Sheet and Answers,** on the Electronic Study Guide.

CDC Tier Two: Transmission-Based Precautions

Recall from the discussion on the chain of infection that pathogens may be transmitted by contact, droplet, or air. Each mode of transmission requires a different approach to prevent infection. For a summary of precautions to take for each mode of transmission,

 Go to Chapter 20, **Technique 20-2: Following Transmission-Based Precautions,** in Volume 2.

Contact Precautions

Contact precautions are used when direct contact with the organism can lead to spread of the pathogen. This is the most common form of transmission. Draining wounds, dressings, patient supplies, and secretions are sources of infection. Indirect contact, or contact with fomites, can also transmit pathogens that spread by this method.

Contact precautions include the following:

- Follow all standard precautions.
- Place the patient in a private room or in a room with a patient with an active infection caused by the same organism and no other infections.
- Wear a clean gown and gloves when you anticipate any contact with the patient or with any contaminated items in the room.
- Either dispose of all items entering the room within the room, or disinfect them per institution policy prior to removing them from the room.
- Double bag all linen and trash, and clearly mark them contaminated.
- Follow any additional precautions specific to the microorganism.

Droplet Precautions

Droplet precautions are used when the pathogen can be spread via moist droplets (e.g., sneezing, coughing, talking). Droplets can spread infection by direct contact with mucous membranes or through indirect contact, for example, touching a bedside table that was contaminated with moist droplets and then rubbing your eyes.

Droplet precautions include the following:

- Follow all standard precautions.
- Follow all contact precautions.
- Wear a mask and eye protection when working within 3 feet of the patient.

Airborne Precautions

Airborne precautions are used to control the spread of infections that are transmitted on air currents. Airborne infections include tuberculosis, varicella (chickenpox), severe acute respiratory syndrome (SARS), and rubeola (measles). Pathogens that are spread by this method are very small and can be easily transmitted through ventilating systems as well as by any activities that stir the air, such as fanning sheets, shaking out towels, or sweeping the floor.

Airborne precautions include the following:

- Follow all standard precautions.
- Follow all contact precautions.
- Place the patient in a private room or in a room with a patient with an active infection caused by the same organism and no other infections. Make sure that the room has negative air pressure and that the air is discharged through a filtration system.
- Wear a clean gown and gloves when you anticipate any contact with the patient or with any items in the room.
- Wear a special mask (N95 respirator) if the patient is suspected of having pulmonary tuberculosis.
- If the patient is known to have or is suspected of having measles (rubeola) or varicella (chickenpox), only immune caregivers should provide care. Immune caregivers do not need to wear masks.

Protective Isolation

Patients at high risk for infection are placed in a special form of isolation called **protective** (or **reverse**) **isolation.** The goal of protective isolation is to protect an unusually vulnerable patient from organisms brought in by healthcare workers and visitors. This type of isolation may be used for clients with low WBC counts, clients undergoing chemotherapy, or clients with large open wounds or weak immune systems. Some units, such as neonatal intensive care units, burn units, and labor and delivery suites, may follow some aspects of protective isolation all the time. Protective isolation includes the following:

- Follow all standard precautions.
- Healthcare workers caring for patients in protective isolation should not also be providing care for other patients with active infections.
- When patients in protective isolation need to leave the room, they should wear a mask and have minimal contact with others.
- All persons entering the patient's room should wear a mask and wash their hands thoroughly with soap and water.
- After hand washing, caregivers and visitors should put on a clean or sterile gown over clothing and take

care to keep the outside of the gown from any contact with surfaces outside the room.

- Once the gown is placed, don gloves.
- If the mask or gown becomes wet while you provide care, change it.
- On exiting the room, remove the mask, gloves, and gown. Do not use them again.

Go to Chapter 20, **Technique 20–3: Maintaining Protective Isolation,** in Volume 2.

Control of Potentially Contaminated Equipment and Supplies

Whenever possible, use disposable equipment in an isolation room. Nondisposable equipment and supplies require special handling.

- *Protective isolation.* If a client is in protective isolation, be sure that equipment has been disinfected *before* it is taken into the room. Take linen and dishes directly to the protective isolation room, and hand them to someone wearing the required protective garb.
- *Transmission-based isolation.* If the client is in transmission-based isolation, disinfect the equipment *on removal* from the room. When removing linen or nondisposable dishes from a room with contact, droplet, or airborne isolation, place them in special isolation bags. This process requires two healthcare workers. The worker inside the room wears protective garb and handles only contaminated items. The second worker stands at the door and holds the isolation bag open. The first worker places items inside the bag without touching the outside of the bag. If the bag contains linens, the isolation bag is closed and placed in a laundry hamper.

Place contaminated disposable equipment and materials containing body fluids in special isolation bags. Securely close the isolation trash bag, and place it in a special isolation trash container. Special disposal methods are used to prevent these objects from going into a landfill, where they could become a reservoir of infection. Because this trash is much more expensive to process, take care to put *only* contaminated materials in the contaminated trash.

Always place disposable needles, syringes, and other sharp items, such as broken glass, in special disposable sharps containers immediately after their use. Never recap a contaminated needle. Refer to Chapter 21 for further information on preventing needlestick injuries.

Laboratory specimens contain blood and body fluids and are always considered contaminated. Label the specimen container in a clean area prior to taking it to the patient. Have the specimen collected by a healthcare worker wearing appropriate protective clothing. Once the specimen is collected, place it in a special transport bag. Do not allow the outside of the bag to touch any contaminated item, including your gloves.

Supporting the Psychological Needs of Patients in Isolation

It is important to remember that isolation precautions are designed to prevent the spread of disease. It is the disease that is being isolated, *not* the person who has the disease. Patients who are in isolation continue to have a need for human contact. In fact, isolation may actually produce anxiety and increase the desire for human contact. When caring for a client in isolation, search for ways to maintain contact with the patient. Possible solutions include the following:

- When wearing the required protective equipment, touch the patient.
- Organize the time you spend in the patient's room to include time for discussion about how the client is coping with isolation.
- If the patient is in droplet isolation, remember that the danger area is 3 feet from the patient. You can go to the door of the room and speak to the patient without a mask.

Surgical Asepsis

Sterile means without life. If an object is sterile, it contains no life and therefore no infectious organisms. The exception is *prions,* the protein particles that cause severe neurological degeneration in animals and humans. Researchers have not yet determined what types of antimicrobial techniques are successful in destroying prions. Inanimate objects, such as surgical equipment, gauze dressings, or wound irrigation fluid may be sterile. However, humans will always have pathogens in and on their bodies.

Surgical asepsis requires creation of a sterile environment and use of sterile equipment. It differs from medical asepsis in that it is more complex and it is not required for use with all patients. Sterilization can be accomplished through the use of special gases or high heat. Surgical equipment and implanted devices are examples of materials that must be sterilized.

To create a sterile area, housekeeping personnel perform extensive cleaning using special solutions and procedures. All health personnel working in the area must wear appropriate surgical attire and perform a surgical hand scrub. A **surgical scrub** is a modification of the hand-washing procedure described earlier. It involves an extended scrub of the hands using brush, nail cleaner, and a bactericidal scrubbing agent. For the steps involved,

Go to Chapter 20, **Procedure 20–3: Surgical Hand Washing,** in Volume 2.

For steps to follow in *all* procedures, refer to the inside back cover of Volume 2.

critical aspects of procedure 20–2 through 20–6

Procedure 20–2: Donning and Removing Personal Protective Equipment

- Prior to exposure, don appropriate personal protective equipment according to standard precautions or transmission guidelines.

- Avoid contaminating self or others when removing equipment.

- Remove the most soiled item first.

Procedure 20–3: Surgical Hand Washing

- Apply surgical shoe covers, cap, and face mask before the scrub.

- Use warm water.

- Perform an initial hand wash, and lather up to 2 inches above your elbows.

- Clean under your nails.

- Wet the scrub brush, and apply a generous amount of antimicrobial soap.

- Using a circular motion, scrub all surfaces of nails, hands, and forearms at least 10 times.

- Rinse hands and arms by keeping your fingertips higher than your elbow.

- Grasp a sterile towel, and back away from the sterile field.

- Thoroughly dry your hands before donning sterile gloves.

Procedure 20–4: Donning Sterile Gown and Gloves (Closed Method)

- Grasp the gown at the neckline, and slide your arms into the sleeves without extending your hands through the cuffs.

- Have a co-worker pull the shoulders of the gown up and tie the neck tie.

- Don gloves using the closed method by keeping your hands covered at all times, first with the gown cuffs, and then with the sterile gloves.

- Secure the waist tie on your gown by handing it to a co-worker.

- Keep your hands within your field of vision at all times.

Procedure 20–5: Applying Sterile Gloves (Open Method)

- Place the glove package on a clean, dry surface.

- Open the inner package so that the cuffs are closest to you.

- Apply the glove of your dominant hand first by touching only the inside of the glove (the folded-over cuff) with your nondominant hand.

- Apply the second glove by touching only the outer part of the glove with your already-gloved hand.

Procedure 20–6: Preparing and Maintaining a Sterile Field

- Check to ensure that all supplies are ready for the procedure.

- Clear the area for the sterile field.

- Position the patient appropriately for the procedure.

- Establish the sterile field with a sterile drape or sterile package wrapper.

- Add items to the sterile field by gently dropping them onto the sterile field.

- Pour sterile solutions into a sterile bowl or receptacle without touching the bowl or splashing onto the sterile field.

- Don sterile gloves, and perform the procedure.

See also the Critical Aspects box for Procedures 20–2 through 20–6.

Surgical Attire

Burn units, labor and birth units, and some surgical wards, intensive care units, nurseries, and oncology wards require special surgical attire for patient caregiving. In each of these units, nurses care for clients who are at increased risk for infection or are undergoing an invasive procedure that places them at in-

creased risk. The goal on all of these units is to protect the patient from infection transmitted by healthcare workers.

All personnel on these units don surgical attire, or scrub suits, when they arrive on the unit. These scrub suits should *not* be worn outside the unit. If you must transport a patient to another area or leave the unit to gather supplies, wear a covering over the scrub suit. Remove the covering on your return to the unit. Additional precautions include a disposable hat to cover the hair, shoe coverings, and face masks.

Personnel engaged in surgery or invasive procedures must dress in *sterile* surgical attire. As a beginning student, you will soon find yourself in such a situation. Initially your role will be limited to observation, but you will need to be prepared for these experiences.

First you will change into a scrub suit, apply shoe coverings, and put on a disposable hat. Wash your hands, and apply a face mask. If there is potential for spray of fluids, wear a face mask with eye shield. Be sure to adjust the mask so that it is comfortable to breathe through. Once you have adjusted the mask, perform the surgical scrub.

If a surgical gown is required, don it after the hand scrub. Put on the gown by opening it without touching the outside. Carefully slip your arms into the gown. Avoid pushing your hands through the openings. A co-worker will assist you with tying the back of the gown.

If you are applying full surgical attire, you will need to apply gloves using a closed method. In the closed method, gloves are applied after the gown is donned. The gloves are applied so that the cuffs extend over the cuffs of the gown sleeves. Once you don sterile gloves, you may touch only sterile items. For step-by-step instructions on how to apply surgical garb,

 Go to Chapter 20, **Procedure 20–4: Donning Sterile Gloves and Gown (Closed Method),** in Volume 2.

See also the Critical Aspects box for Procedures 20–2 through 20–6.

Sterile gloves are often applied for procedures that do not require full surgical attire. The glove packaging must be opened slowly. Avoid fanning the wrapping or touching the gloves. With the fingers of your nondominant hand, pick up the glove to be applied to your dominant hand by touching only the inside cuff of the glove. Slip the hand being gloved into the glove. Figure 20–6 illustrates how to apply the first glove.

A general rule to consider when applying the second glove is to touch glove to glove, and skin to skin. The already-gloved hand may touch any of the sterile surfaces of the second glove. The second hand may touch only the inside of the glove—the portion that will have contact with the skin. Figure 20–7 illustrates the hand positions used to apply the second glove. Although this process sounds very awkward, you will develop comfort with practice. For detailed instructions,

 Go to Chapter 20, **Procedure 20–5: Applying Sterile Gloves (Open Method),** in Volume 2.

See also the Critical Aspects box for Procedures 20–2 through 20–6.

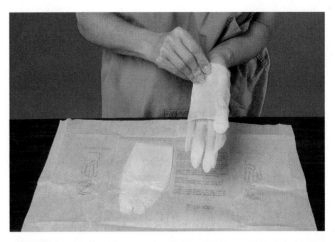

FIGURE 20–6 When applying the first glove, touch only the inside cuff of the glove.

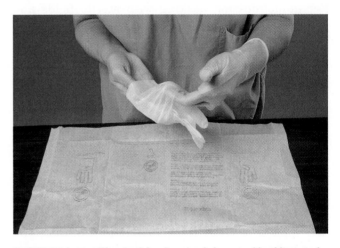

FIGURE 20–7 When applying the second glove, consider this general rule: glove to glove, skin to skin.

Sterile Technique

Healthcare providers use sterile technique to perform a variety of procedures that do not require full surgical attire. You will use sterile technique (in addition to general principles of asepsis) when administering an injection, starting an IV line, or performing a sterile dressing change. Prior to performing a sterile procedure, gather as much information as possible about the procedure. Determine what supplies you will need and whether you will need assistance. If the patient is unable to maintain a position required for the procedure, you will need a helper to hold the patient during the procedure.

Wash your hands before getting materials from the sterile supply area, and then gather the required supplies and equipment. Check the expiration date on each package. Check the package to make sure it is

intact. If it has paper or cloth wrapping, be sure there are no indications that it has ever been wet.

Donning sterile attire and working with sterile equipment require special attention. In a sterile field, only the horizontal plane is considered sterile. Consider nonsterile any material that drapes over the horizontal plane. A 1-inch margin around the field is also considered unsterile because it is in contact with contaminated surfaces. Do not allow persons without sterile garb within 1 foot of the sterile field. Handle sterile equipment only if you are wearing sterile gloves. If you are wearing sterile attire, you are considered sterile only in the front of your body from shoulders to waist. Never turn your back to a sterile field, because your back is considered unsterile and will contaminate the field if it makes contact. Finally, never assume an item is sterile. If there is any doubt about its sterility, consider it contaminated. For guidelines for working with sterile fields and equipment,

 Go to Chapter 20, **Technique 20–4: Using Sterile Technique,** in Volume 2.

Sterile Fields

When performing a sterile dressing change, you will use both medical and surgical asepsis. Use medical aseptic technique to remove the old dressing. The old dressing is considered contaminated, and you must observe standard precautions. Take care to avoid touching the contaminated dressing against the sterile supplies, bedding, or surrounding skin. Once you have removed the old dressing, discard the nonsterile gloves, and wash your hands. Now you are ready to set up the sterile field and begin the procedure.

 Go to Chapter 20, **Procedure 20–6: Preparing and Maintaining a Sterile Field,** in Volume 2.

See also the Critical Aspects box for Procedures 20–2 through 20–6. See Chapter 34 for more information about sterile dressing changes.

Some supplies come in special packaging with a wrapping that can form the sterile field. You must open these packages in a way that does not contaminate the field. Other packages are opened by pulling apart two flaps of the package. The outside of these packages is considered clean, and the inside is sterile.

Be cautious when adding supplies to the sterile field. If they are light and small, gently add them to the sterile field by separating the package flaps and popping them onto the field. If the object is large, such as an irrigation bowl, slowly unwrap the packaging and, touching only the outside wrapper, place the bowl

on the field. If any object falls only partly on the field, it is no longer sterile. For detailed instructions on how to add supplies to a sterile field,

 Go to Chapter 20, **Procedure 20–6: Preparing and Maintaining a Sterile Field,** in Volume 2.

Add sterile liquids to a sterile field by gently pouring them into a container on the field. As an alternative, you may use a sterile drape that contains an impermeable membrane between its layers. This membrane serves as a barrier to moisture and prevents wicking. With this type of drape, you may pour sterile liquid directly on gauze pads on the field. Pour only an amount of liquid that is sufficient to make the gauze pads damp. Excess fluid may run off the field, causing the field to become contaminated. For step-by-step instruction in how to add sterile solutions to a sterile field,

 Go to Chapter 20, **Procedure 20–6: Preparing and Maintaining a Sterile Field,** in Volume 2.

INFECTION CONTROL FOR HEALTHCARE WORKERS

It is critical that you learn how to protect yourself from infections. You want not only to avoid personal illness, but also to avoid becoming a reservoir for infection. Nurses and other patient care workers are at great risk of acquiring infections because they come in contact with a large number and variety of pathogens. Skin contact, mucous membrane contact, and puncture wounds often serve as portals of entry.

Unlicensed assistive personnel, ancillary personnel, and housekeeping and maintenance workers are often present on nursing units. Visitors, volunteers, and family are also on the unit. It is essential that you protect them from potential hazardous exposure as well as protect yourself and patients from possible problems brought into the unit. As a nurse you need to monitor other healthcare workers, patients, and visitors for possible breaks in infection control.

What Should I Do If I Am Exposed to Bloodborne Pathogens?

Exposure to blood, body secretions, or body tissues containing blood or secretions requires immediate action. The first step is to minimize the exposure. If the fluid is on your skin, on mucous membranes, or in the eyes, wash the area thoroughly with running water. If the contaminated fluid is on intact skin, use soap and water or an alcohol rub.

Contact the infection control or employee health nurse as soon after the exposure as possible, and complete an injury report. If an exposure occurs while you are a student, you must also contact your clinical instructor. Anyone exposed to bloodborne pathogens should have baseline lab work conducted to check for hepatitis and HIV. If the patient source is known, the infection control nurse will arrange to have the patient tested. Subsequent testing and possible prophylactic treatment are based on the type of exposure and what is known about the source and the injured person. To limit risks from the exposure, the infection control team will provide counseling and recommendations as soon as possible after the event. Chapter 21 presents information on preventing needle stick injuries.

What Role Does the Infection Control Nurse Play?

The task of the infection control nurse is to minimize the number of infections in the healthcare facility. Because it is not possible to provide absolute protection all the time, the nurse must balance the risks for infection with the costs of protective measures and the benefits of various strategies. Infection control nurses must keep current with information concerning pathogens, antibiotic resistance, and infection control. The nurse also functions as an epidemiologist, tracking down the source of nosocomial infections and strengthening measures to prevent their recurrence. Finally, all members of the infection control team enforce compliance with federal, state, and local regulations related to infection control.

How Can I Minimize the Effects of Bioterrorism and Infectious Outbreaks?

In 2001 anthrax spores were sent through the United States mail. This incident brought new attention to the possibility of biological agents being used as weapons, especially by terrorists. In addition, new infectious organisms are continually emerging, including numerous drug-resistant bacterial strains, the Ebola virus, the West Nile virus, the SARS virus, and the prions involved in Creutzfeldt-Jakob disease (the human form of mad cow disease).

A key factor in minimizing infectious outbreaks is recognizing unusual disease patterns. Special pattern identification programs are being included in some computerized patient record systems to detect these outbreaks. The use of these systems supplements, but does not replace, clinical observation skills. Nurses need to assess not only the individual patient's condition, but also clusters of symptoms. Hospital, emergency department, and clinic nurses are in key positions to recognize outbreaks because they see patients from multiple primary care providers. Nurses must keep the following questions in mind:

- Am I seeing an unexpected number of infectious diseases, or diseases possibly caused by infectious organisms?
- Am I seeing similar cases that are not responding to medical treatment?
- Are healthcare workers who come in contact with infectious patients becoming ill?

After identifying a suspicious pattern, you should notify the institution's infection control nurse or safety officer as soon as possible. Appropriate cultures will be needed, and the federal and state health departments should be notified. If the infectious organism is unknown, samples must be preserved for future analysis. Patients with similar symptoms should be cared for by a minimum number of healthcare personnel, and those personnel must use appropriate precautions. If the etiology and transmission route of the causative organism are unknown, standard, contact, and airborne precautions should be implemented.

| toward evidence-based practice |

Lawson, C., Juliano, L., & Ratliff, C. R. (2003). Does sterile or nonsterile technique make a difference in wounds healing by secondary intention? *Ostomy & Wound Management, 49*(4), 56–60.

Using a nonexperimental longitudinal design, surgical nurses at a university medical center implemented a study to evaluate the cost and outcomes of wound care performed with clean technique as opposed to sterile technique. All wounds evaluated were healing by secondary intention (left open, not sutured closed) and required three dressing changes per day. For the first 3 months of the study, traditional (sterile) wound care was given. Nine of 1,070 (0.84%) admissions to the surgical units had a surgical site infection. During the second 3-month cycle,

clean technique was utilized for wound care. Eight of 963 (0.83%) of surgical site infections were documented. An average of $380 per patient was saved with the use of clean dressings versus sterile.

---

1. What potential explanations might account for these findings?

2. Suppose you were a nurse manager. On the basis of this study, would you change your policies and discontinue sterile dressing changes on the unit? Why or why not?

 Go to Chapter 20, **Toward Evidence-Based Practice Suggested Responses,** on the Electronic Study Guide.

 Go to Chapter 20, **Resources for Caregivers and Health Professionals,** on the Electronic Study Guide.

 Suggested Readings: Go to Chapter 20, **Reading More About Promoting Asepsis and Preventing Infection,** on the Electronic Study Guide.

 Bibliography: Go to Volume 2, Bibliography.

Promoting Safety

Learning Outcomes

After completing this chapter, you should be able to:

✳ List the three leading causes of accidental death in the United States.

✳ Identify factors that create safety risks.

✳ Identify at least five safety hazards in the home environment and interventions to prevent injury from them.

✳ Discuss the steps to follow when you suspect that a client has ingested a poisonous substance.

✳ Describe the Heimlich maneuver, and identify instances when it is appropriate to use it.

✳ Describe the four main physical hazards that are found in the community and interventions to prevent injury from them.

✳ Describe and give examples of hazards that we encounter in the healthcare agency.

✳ Identify four interventions to prevent falls in the healthcare agency.

✳ Discuss when it is appropriate to use siderails in the healthcare agency.

✳ Properly apply restraints and discuss measures to prevent injury in clients who are restrained.

✳ Discuss at least one instrument that is used to assess the client who is at risk for falls.

✳ Formulate a nursing diagnosis in relation to preventing injury in the environment.

✳ Write an individualized goal for clients with a nursing diagnosis of Risk for Falls.

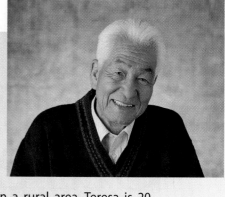

MEET Your Patients

1. You have been assigned to care for Alvin Lin, a 79-year-old man who was just transferred from a long-term care facility to your medical unit. His admitting diagnosis is dehydration and pneumonia. The report you received stated that he had rested well during the night and was alert and oriented. When you enter his room, he is confused and does not know where he is. He is becoming combative and is trying to get out of bed. How should you respond to the situation?

2. Suppose you are a nurse making a home visit to Teresa, who lives in a rural area. Teresa is 20 years old and has a 2-year-old daughter. She is also responsible for caring for her 78-year-old grandmother, who is recovering from a hip fracture. Teresa states that it is getting more difficult to keep up with her toddler, who is "into everything," and to care for the needs of her grandmother. Her grandmother has a fear of falling and is very reluctant to do anything for herself.

Safety is a basic human need, second only to survival needs such as oxygen, nutrition, and fluids. As a nurse, you will be fundamentally concerned with the safety of patients in the healthcare setting, in the home, and in the community. You must also be concerned with your own safety and the safety of other care providers in your place of work. Many accidental injuries can be prevented by being aware of hazards and taking reasonable precautions. This chapter will increase your ability to recognize safety hazards and to plan interventions that promote safety for clients of all ages in a variety of settings, such as the two in "Meet Your Patients." To simplify organization, nursing interventions to promote safety are included with the discussion of each of the safety hazards in the "Theoretical Knowledge" section.

Theoretical Knowledge
knowing why

According to the National Safety Council, 98,000 deaths occurred from unintentional injury in the United States in 2001—up 2% from the year before. A fatal injury occurs every 5 minutes; a disabling injury, nearly every second (2001b, p. 4). Accidents or unintentional injuries are the fifth leading cause of deaths in the United States (National Safety Council, 2001a). Motor vehicle accidents continue to be the number-one cause, followed by poisonings and falls (National Safety Council, 2001a). Table 21–1 lists the leading causes of accidental death in the United States.

Environment includes the physical and psychosocial factors that contribute to each person's life and well-being. It can be further defined as any setting in which the nurse and client interact. **Environmental hazards** are situations or conditions in which something in the environment can cause human illness or injury (World Health Organization [WHO], 1997). This section (1) discusses specific developmental and individual safety risks factors and (2) describes hazards in three environments: the home, the community, and the healthcare agency.

TABLE 21-1 Leading Causes of Unintentional Deaths in the United States in 2001	
Cause	**Total Annual Deaths**
Motor vehicles	42,900
Poisoning	14,500
Falls	14,200
Suffocation by inhalation or ingestion	4,200
Fires, flames, and smoke	3,900

Source: National Safety Council. (2001). *National Vital Statistics Report, 2001.* Retrieved February 15, 2003, from www.nsc.org/index.htm

WHAT FACTORS AFFECT SAFETY?

To assess and plan for client safety, you will need theoretical knowledge about developmental stages and individual factors that affect clients' ability to avoid accidental injury.

Developmental Factors

The type and incidence of accidents vary among age groups. You will find interventions for all age groups integrated into the topics of home, community, and healthcare agency throughout the rest of this chapter. For supplemental discussion of safety needs during different developmental stages,

 Go to **Chapter 9** on the Electronic Study Guide.

- *Infant/toddler.* Motor vehicle accidents are the leading cause of death during the first 3 years of life (Polan & Taylor, 2003), followed by burns. Sudden infant death syndrome (SIDS), choking, drowning, and ingesting poisons are other critical safety concerns. Infants and toddlers are completely dependent on others for their care. Their locomotion and manipulative skills advance before they have the judgment necessary to recognize dangers such as falling. In addition, infants and toddlers explore the environment by putting objects in their mouth, so the incidence of lead poisoning is highest between 6 months and 3 years of age. As mobility continues to improve, toddlers gain more freedom, and their curiosity leads them to explore cupboards, stairs, open windows, swimming pools, and other hazards.

- *Preschooler.* After age 3, children are less prone to falls because their gross and fine motor skills, coordination, and balance have improved. However, the extension of play to the outside environment (playgrounds, pools, front yards, and so on) creates additional safety concerns. Although this age group is more aware of dangers and limitations (e.g., "Mommy says don't touch the stove!"), adult supervision continues to be essential (Polan & Taylor, 2003).

- *School-age child.* Children in this age group have developed more refined muscle coordination and control, and their decision-making skills have improved (Wong, Perry, & Hockenberry, 2002). However, because school-age children become more involved in activities outside the home, bone and muscle injuries are common. Injuries are often related to sports or bicycle riding. "[M]ost children at this stage are ready to attempt any new skill with or without practice or training. . . . [T]hey are much less fearful than they were during earlier years" (Polan & Taylor, 2003, p. 162). Being in the wider school and neighborhood environment also puts this group at greater risk for injury from strangers (e.g., abduction).

- *Adolescent.* Peak physical, sensory, and psychomotor functions give teenagers a feeling of strength and confidence, yet they lack the judgment of adults. This combination, along with feelings of indestructibility, makes them more likely to participate in risk-taking behavior and makes them particularly prone to injury. The leading cause of death in this age group is motor vehicle accidents, followed by homicide. Both of these are associated with alcohol and drug use (Polan & Taylor, 2003). Sports and recreational injuries, including diving and drowning incidents, are also common, especially when drinking and drug use are involved.

- *Adult.* Motor vehicle accidents continue to contribute to death and injury in this age group (Polan & Taylor, 2003). Workplace injury may also be a significant concern. Other injuries to adults are related to lifestyle (e.g., excessive alcohol use), stress, and decline in strength and stamina. Work and family responsibilities often leave little time for regular physical activity, increasing the risk of musculoskeletal injury in the so-called weekend athlete.

- *Older adult.* Although many older adults have intact senses that enable them to continue to enjoy life as they age, physiological changes do occur. These changes may include loss of muscle strength and joint mobility, slowing of reflexes, decreased ability to respond to multiple stimuli, and sensory losses, particularly hearing and vision. These changes increase the older adult's risk for falls, burns, car accidents, and other injury (Kennedy-Malone, Fletcher, & Plank, 2004; Tyson, 1999).

Individual Risk Factors

In addition to developmental stage, individual factors also influence a person's risk for unintentional injury. These include lifestyle, cognitive awareness, sensoriperceptual status, ability to communicate, mobility status, physical and emotional health, and awareness of safety measures. Table 21–2 summarizes individual risk factors.

KnowledgeCheck 21–1

- What are some important developmental considerations when providing a safe environment for a preschool child?
- What is the main cause of injuries during the adolescent period?
- What are some ways that the aging process makes the older adult more prone to injury?
- Based on your theoretical knowledge and the scant patient data you have, why do you think Teresa's toddler ("Meet Your Patients") is at risk for accidents? What about Teresa's grandmother?

 Go to Chapter 21, **Knowledge Check Response Sheet and Answers,** on the Electronic Study Guide.

TABLE 21-2   Individual Risk Factors for Injury

Risk Factors	Behavior Manifestation
Lifestyle	Smoking, alcohol abuse, risk-taking behaviors
Cognitive awareness	Impaired thought processes due to confusion and stress, loss of short-term memory
Sensory and perceptual status	Loss of senses (e.g., vision, hearing, pain), which provide first line of defense
Impaired communication	Language barriers and hearing and speech impairment related to disease processes
Impaired mobility	Impaired strength with accompanying problems in mobility, balance, and endurance
Physical and emotional well-being	Reduced physical stamina and depression, with feelings of loss of control and helplessness
Safety awareness	Reduced cognitive awareness (e.g., of older adult) and immature development of the child

BOX 21-1   Poisonous Agents Most Commonly Ingested by Children

- Household cleansers
- Medicines and vitamins, including cough and cold preparations, pain medications, antidepressants, anti-convulsants, and iron tablets, which to children may look like M&M candies
- Indoor house plants, including poinsettia, diffenbachia, philodendron, and many others
- Cosmetics
- Pesticides
- Kerosene, gasoline, furniture polish, lighter fluid, and other chemicals

Source: Data from the National Ag Safety Database (NASD). (2002). Protect your children from poisons at home. Retrieved November 13, 2003, from *http://www.cdc.gov/ nasd/documents/d001501-d001600/d001584/ d001584.html*

WHAT SAFETY HAZARDS ARE IN THE HOME?

What safety issues in the home environment would you need to assess with regard to Teresa's toddler and grandmother? The following discussion provides an overview of conditions within the home that increase the risk for injury and death. It should help you to answer the question about Teresa's family and home.

Except for motor vehicle accidents, most fatal accidents occur in the home. The leading causes of death in the home are poisonings, falls, fires and burns, and suffocation by ingested object (National Safety Council, 2001b). For a checklist to assess home safety hazards,

 Go to Chapter 21, **Assessment Guidelines and Tools, Home Safety Checklist,** in Volume 2.

Poisoning

Poison ingestion is one of the major causes of death in children younger than 5 years. Poisoning resulted in 14,500 accidental deaths in all age groups in 2001

(National Safety Council, 2001a). In many more instances, the person does not die but becomes ill or suffers other effects. Most poisoning of young children occurs because of improper storage of household chemicals, medicines and vitamins, and cosmetics, but even house plants can cause poisonings (National Ag Safety Database [NASD], 2003). See Box 21–1 for a list of poisons most commonly ingested by children.

Lead poisoning has been a problem in the United States since the 1900s, when white lead was added to paints and tetraethyl lead was added to gasoline. The use of lead in paint has been banned since 1978, but lead-based paint can still be found in older homes, and some soil (which young children often put in their mouths) contains high lead content.

Older children and adolescents may attempt suicide by overdosing with medicines or be poisoned accidentally when experimenting with drugs. In adults, most poisonings occur as a result of illegal drug use or misuse or abuse of prescription drugs, especially tranquilizers and antidepressants.

Interventions: Preventing and Treating Poisoning

It is important for all homes to be equipped to handle an emergency when a poisonous substance is involved. Teach parents to keep the telephone number for the nearest poison control center easily accessible. If there are no young children in the home, advise families with older adults to prevent accidental overdose of prescribed medications by using a medication

organizer that may be filled once a week by the patient or family member (Figure 21–1). See the Home Care box for prevention of and first aid for poisoning.

Treatment choice depends on the poison ingested. Medical treatments for poisoning include gastric lavage, dialysis, administration of activated charcoal orally or by gastric tube, administration of antidotes, and forced diuresis. For most poisonings, the most effective intervention is professional administration of activated charcoal orally or via gastric tube. However, charcoal is not effective for ethanol, alkali, iron, boric acid, lithium, methanol, or cyanide. For a list of medical treatments for commonly ingested poisons,

 Go to Chapter 21, **Tables, Boxes, Figures: ESG Table 21–1,** on the Electronic Study Guide.

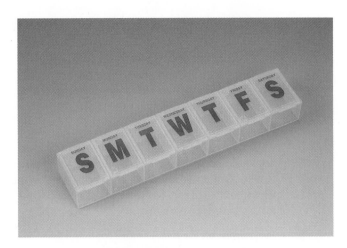

FIGURE 21–1   Medication organizer.

Preventing and Treating Poisoning in the Home

home care

Prevention

Young children will eat and drink almost anything. Most victims of accidental poisoning are children under the age of 5. Tips to prevent poisoning include the following:

- Never leave a child unattended near household cleaners or medicines, even for a moment. If you must answer the phone or doorbell, take the child with you. Children act fast; it takes only a moment for them to swallow something.

- Do not store medicines or household chemicals on kitchen counters or bathroom surfaces. Instead, store them on high shelves or in locked cabinets and drawers.

- Store all household chemicals away from food.

- Keep medicines and household chemicals in their original containers. Leave the original labels on. Especially do not store chemicals in containers that normally hold food.

- Use child-resistant packaging for medicines and household chemicals. Close the container securely after each use. However, do not assume that your child is safe around substances in child-resistant containers; research has shown that many toddlers and preschoolers can open them.

- Avoid taking medicines in front of children. Children tend to imitate grown-ups.

- Never call medicines or vitamins "candy." Instead, use the correct name ("cough medicine," and so on).

- Throw away all old medications by flushing them down the toilet, and rinse the container before discarding it. Do not throw away medicines in a wastebasket, where children can find them.

- A wide variety of plants can cause illness and even death in young children. Before purchasing a house plant, verify that it is nontoxic. Find out whether any plants growing in your yard are poisonous, and, if so, remove them. Teach children that they must never eat berries, wild mushrooms, or other edible-looking plants in yards, fields, and forests.

- Lead-based paint can still be found in older homes, and some soil (which young children often put in their mouths) contains a high lead content. Warn parents to keep children from chewing on window sills, and so on, and to carefully clean up flakes of paint. Advocate for clients who need to have lead-based paint replaced in their homes.

Signs of Poisoning

You should also be able to recognize the tell-tale signs of poisoning:

- Unusual stains or odors on clothes or skin

- Unusual odor on breath

- Burns around the mouth

- Drowsiness, stomach pain, vomiting, breathing problems, sweating, drooling, irritability, signs of fear, or other sudden changes in behavior

- Drugs or chemical containers that are open and/or out of place

First Aid

If you suspect that your child has ingested a poisonous substance, speed is crucial. Be sure to keep all emergency numbers near the phone. Include your physician's number and the number of the nearest poison control center (PCC). The universal number in the United States is (800) 222-1222.

➤

Preventing and Treating Poisoning in the Home *(continued)*

They will connect you to a local PCC. Also keep your name, address, and phone number accessible in case someone else needs to call. Take these self-help actions for the following situations:

- *For poisons in the eye.* Flood the eye with lukewarm water poured from a cup 2 to 3 inches from the eye. Continue flooding the eye for 15 minutes. Tell the child to blink as often as possible during flooding, but do not allow the child to rub the eye. Have someone call the PCC as soon as possible.

- *For poisons on the skin.* Remove contaminated clothing as quickly as possible. Flood the area with lukewarm water for 10 minutes. Then gently wash the area with soap and water, and rinse. Have someone call the PCC as soon as possible. Later, destroy contaminated clothing.

- *For inhaled poisons.* Protect yourself from exposure to the fumes by taking several deep breaths of fresh air and then holding your breath. If possible, hold a wet cloth over your nose and mouth. Then immediately get the child to fresh air. Loosen the child's clothing. If the child is not breathing, tell someone to call 911, and start artificial respiration. Continue until breathing resumes or help arrives. Even if the child seems OK, call the PCC immediately.

- *For swallowed poisons.* Examine the child's mouth, and remove all tablets, powder, or other material. Look for burns, swelling, and so on, and rinse and wipe the

mouth with a cloth. If the child is awake and able to swallow, and you suspect that the poison is corrosive (e.g., a household chemical), give one-half glassful of water immediately. Then call the PCC. The American Academy of Pediatrics does not advise giving children syrup of ipecac. Give it only if advised to do by the PCC or a qualified medical professional. Call 911 if a child is having convulsions, stops breathing, or loses consciousness. If the child is not breathing, start artificial respiration and continue it until breathing resumes or help arrives.

In all cases of suspected poisoning, if you are unsure of what to do, contact your local poison control center, physician, or emergency personnel (911) immediately.

Sources: American Academy of Pediatrics. (2003). *Q and A: Poison treatment in the home.* Retrieved January 10, 2004, from http://www.aap.org/advocacy/releases/novpoisonqanda.htm; National Ag Safety Database (NASD). (2003). Symptoms and First Aid for Poisonings. Retrieved January 10, 2004, from http://www.cdc.gov/nasd/docs/d00801-d00900/d000817.html; National Ag Safety Database (NASD). (2003). Protect Your Children from Poisons at Home. Retrieved January 10, 2004, from http://www.cdc.gov/nasd/docs/d001501-d001600/d001584/d001584.html; Personal communication with National Poison Control Center. They can be contacted at (800) 222-1222 or at their web site, www.aapcc.org (retrieved January 4, 2004).

Although the American Academy of Pediatrics (2003) no longer recommends inducing emesis (e.g., with syrup of ipecac), some practitioners may still do so. As of the time this text was prepared, the National Poison Control Center did not support the routine stocking of ipecac in all households with young children. They state that it should be given only on specific recommendation from a poison center or qualified medical personnel (Manoguerra, Cobaugh, & Members of the Guidelines for the Management of Poisonings Consensus Panel, 2004).

Carbon Monoxide Poisoning

Carbon monoxide (CO) is a colorless, tasteless, odorless, toxic gas. Exposure can cause headaches, weakness, nausea, and vomiting; prolonged exposure leads to unconsciousness, brain damage, and death. CO poisoning is the means of more than 1700 suicides and also causes over 500 unintentional deaths every year in the United States (Parmet, 2002). It accounts for a majority of deaths at the scene of fires.

The burning of fuel, such as wood, oil, gasoline, natural gas, kerosene, and coal produces carbon monoxide.

Dangerous levels of CO can build up because of a faulty furnace, and CO can build up quickly in an unventilated garage when a car is running. Other consumer products involved in CO-related deaths include lawn mowers, charcoal grills, gas water heaters, camp stoves or lanterns, and gas ranges or ovens. Many unintentional deaths occur during cold weather among older adults and the poor who seek nonconventional heat sources (e.g., gas ranges and ovens) to stay warm.

Interventions: Preventing and Treating Carbon Monoxide Poisoning

If carbon monoxide (CO) intoxication is suspected, the person should be treated with 100% humidified oxygen. A simple blood test may be done to confirm CO levels in the blood. Interventions to prevent CO poisoning include teaching clients the following (Children's Environmental Health Network, 1999):

- Buy, install, and maintain a home CO detector.

- Never use a gas oven or range to heat a house.

- Ensure that gas or wood-burning appliances are adequately vented to the outside.

- Never operate gasoline-powered engines, such as automobiles or lawn mowers, in confined spaces, such as garages or basements.
- Never burn charcoal inside a home, cabin, recreational vehicle, or tent.
- Do not use kerosene heaters indoors.
- Repair rust holes or defects in vehicles that could allow exhaust fumes to enter the passenger compartment.

Scalds and Burns

Scald injuries (e.g., from hot water or grease) are the single most common cause of burns in children under the age of 3. Warming food or formula in the microwave may cause the food to become hotter than intended, leading to burns in infants. Sunburn can be a source of first- or second-degree burn, and burns may occur from contact with metal surfaces and vinyl seats when cars are parked in the sun. Scalding burns (especially on both feet or both hands) and cigarette burns in children and vulnerable older adults should always prompt you to assess for abuse. The risk of contact burns in all age groups is greater in the presence of such heating devices as kerosene heaters and wood-burning stoves. People may use these as alternative heat sources when they cannot afford the cost of natural gas, heating fuel, or other traditional furnace fuels. Chemical agents, such as acid, alkali, or other organic compounds, can also cause localized burns (Wong, Perry, & Hockenberry, 2002).

| Interventions: Preventing Burns and Scalds |

Teach the client the following important safety tips for preventing burns and scalds in the home:

- Turn pot handles toward the back of the stove so that children cannot tip them over.
- Place guardrails in front of radiators and fireplaces.
- Avoid warming infant formula and food in the microwave. You will find that many parents ignore this advice, so also tell them to always check the temperature of formula and food carefully before giving it to the child.
- Remove lids or other coverings from microwaved food carefully.
- Never wear loose-fitting clothing when cooking.
- Stress the danger of open flames; do not use candles near curtains or other flammable materials.
- Always check bath water temperature for children and older adults, and set water heater temperature low enough to prevent scalds.
- Wear protective clothing and sunscreen when outside.

Fires

Home fires are a major cause of death and injury, and seniors (age 65 years and over) and children under the age of 5 have the greatest risk of fire death (National Fire Protection Association, 2001). Cooking fires are the number-one cause of home fires and home fire injuries. However, most *fatal* home fires occur while people are asleep, and most fire-related deaths occur from smoke inhalation. Smoking (e.g., cigarettes) is the leading cause of fatal home fires, but during the winter months, heating equipment is equally responsible. Other causes include unsupervised children playing with matches, the improper use of candles, and faulty wiring.

| Interventions: Preventing Injury from Fires in the Home |

Teach families measures to prevent fires and measures to take should a fire occur. Refer to the Home Care box on page 426.

Falls

Falls are the third leading cause of unintentional death. Over half of all falls occur in the home, and about 80% involve people age 65 years and older (*Accident Facts,* 1998). Falls are the leading cause of injury-related deaths in that group (National Center for Injury Prevention and Control, 2000). Environmental factors that contribute to falls include slippery floors and bathtubs, lack of grab bars, low toilet seats, and high beds. Health issues that increase the risk for falls include poor vision, hypotension (low blood pressure), a history of falls, dizziness, pain, and alcohol use (Tyson, 1999).

| Interventions: Preventing Falls in the Home |

Teach clients, especially older adults, the following measures to increase the safety of their home environment:

- Ensure that shoes fit properly, and wear slippers with nonskid soles.
- Avoid loose, trailing clothes.
- Clean eyeglasses frequently.
- Make sure rooms are adequately lighted, and use dim light at night.
- Use shower chairs and raised toilet seats; use a bath or shower mat.
- Keep clutter out of the walkways.
- Wipe up all foods and fluids from the floor immediately.
- Remove all scatter or throw rugs (or at least be sure they have nonskid padding under them).

Preventing Injury from Fires in the Home

- Do not smoke, especially in bed.
- Have working smoke alarms (Figure 21–2); change batteries every 6 months or more frequently.

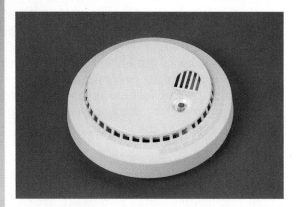

FIGURE 21–2 Smoke alarm.

- Develop and practice a home fire escape plan.
- If fire occurs, crawl or stay low to the floor to avoid the smoke as much as possible.
- Keep a rope or other type of ladder for escape from rooms above ground level.
- Have a fire extinguisher in the home, and know where it is located and how to use it; check it regularly and replace it when it becomes outdated.
- Never pour water on a grease fire.
- Never discharge a fire extinguisher onto a pan fire.

- If there is an oven fire, turn off the heat and keep the door closed.
- If there is a microwave fire, keep the door closed, and unplug the microwave.
- When decorating Christmas trees, always use fire-safe tree lights.
- Always unplug Christmas tree lights before leaving home.
- Never leave burning candles unattended.
- With charcoal grills, only use charcoal starter fluids designed for barbecue grills.
- With gas grills, be sure that the hose connection is tight, and check hoses for leaks.
- Store flammable materials (e.g., oil-soaked rags) in appropriate containers.

Promoting Electrical Safety in the Home

- Make sure electrical outlets have covers.
- Routinely inspect electrical appliances for damaged cords.
- Make sure electrical cords do not hang off of tables and countertops.
- Do not place electrical cords under carpets.
- Replace frayed electrical cords.

- Install handrails and slip-resistant floor coverings on staircases.
- Check tips of canes, walkers, and crutches for the presence of intact nonskid covers.
- Apply an ice-melt product, salt, or sand to icy sidewalks, steps, and porches.
- Be sure that children wear helmets and other appropriate protective gear for bicycling, skateboarding, and other active sports.

Firearm Injuries

Gun ownership is a sensitive issue. Some people keep guns in the home for protection and/or recreation (e.g., hunting, target shooting). However, guns are one source of unintentional injury and death. Gun safety is especially important when there are children in the home. Young children may encounter a loaded gun with tragic results, and household access to firearms has been implicated as a risk factor for youth suicides and

domestic homicides (Grossman, Cummings, Koepsell, Marshall, D'Ambrosio, Thompson, et al., 2000).

| Interventions: Promoting Firearm Safety |

The frequency and severity of unintentional firearm injuries involving children make education an essential intervention. The American Academy of Pediatrics and other groups have mounted efforts to educate parents about firearm safety. Even if parents avoid having guns in their own home, it is possible that children will encounter them in other places. Some important actions include the following:

- Provide information to parents so that they will be able to make smart choices related to gun safety.
- Teach children safe behavior around firearms.
- Teach children what to do if they see a gun (e.g., at a friend's house or in school): (1) stop, (2) don't touch it, (3) leave the area, (4) tell an adult (Kakkuri, 2000).
- Participate in gun safety courses.

- Store firearms unloaded and in a secure container when not in use.
- Store ammunition in a different location from the firearm.

Suffocation and Asphyxiation

Suffocation may be caused by drowning, choking on a foreign object, or inhaling gas or smoke. Suffocation causes the most home fatalities to children up to 4 years of age (National Safety Council, 2001c). Food items, including hot dogs, raw vegetables, popcorn, hard candies, nuts, and grapes, are responsible for most nonfatal choking incidents. Nonfood items, such as latex balloons and plastic bags, cause the majority of suffocation deaths in young children. Suffocation of infants is often related to bed or crib hazards, such as excess bedding or pillows, or toys hung from long ribbons inside the infant's crib. Infants can become entangled in cords from venetian blinds or in the ribbon or string used to hang a pacifier around an infant's neck.

Children up to age 4 are especially at risk for accidental drowning and should never be left unattended in or near a bathtub, hot tub, swimming pool, or other source of water. Even wading pools, toilets, and mop buckets hold enough water to drown an infant.

Interventions: Preventing Suffocation and Asphyxiation

To prevent suffocation or choking in an infant or child, instruct parents and caregivers to do the following:

- Inspect toys for small, removable parts.
- Do not attach pacifiers, rattles, or other infant toys to ribbons or strings.
- Do not use sweatshirts or jackets with necktie strings.
- Position mobiles well above the crib, out of the infant's reach.
- Store plastic bags away from young children in a secure place.
- Ensure that the crib is designed to meet federal regulations: Crib slats must be less than $2\frac{3}{8}$ inches (6 cm) apart, and the mattress must fit snugly.
- When feeding children meat, cheese, or other firm foods, cut the food into very tiny pieces.
- Do not give a young child hard candy, chewing gum, nuts, popcorn, grapes, or marshmallows.
- Keep venetian blind cords out of the child's reach.
- Supervise children's balloon play, and dispose of burst balloons promptly.
- Supervise activity when the child is near any source of water, including buckets.
- Do not allow children to run around a pool or to dive in shallow areas.

- If you have a pool, be sure it has a barrier (e.g., tall fence) to prevent children from gaining access.
- Insist that children use personal flotation devices (e.g., lifejackets, not float toys). (This is controversial. Some authorities regard flotation devices as toys that provide false security; others say anything that reduces a child's fear of the water is positive, because it is the fear reaction that leads to drowning.)
- Recognize and teach the universal sign for choking: grasping the neck between the thumb and index finger or clutching the neck with both hands.
- Teach adults the Heimlich maneuver for choking, realizing that this is a psychomotor skill that is best taught using supervised practice with a mannequin.

 CriticalThinking 21–1
- What are some initial questions you might ask Teresa regarding the home environment?
- What are some basic interventions that could be suggested to Teresa to help *child-proof* her home? To answer this question, you will need to recall information about:

    Safety hazards that we encounter in the home
    Developmental and lifestyle factors that affect safety
    Specific nursing activities that can be used to prevent accidents or injuries related to the environmental hazards (e.g., firearms)

Heimlich Maneuver

The **Heimlich maneuver** is an emergency procedure for removing a foreign object lodged in the airway. It lifts the diaphragm and forces enough air from the lungs to create an artificial cough. The cough should move and expel the obstruction from the airway. If you suspect airway obstruction in an adult, determine whether the victim is able to speak or cough (ask, "Are you choking?"). If the person cannot speak or indicates that he is choking, perform the Heimlich maneuver. Note that the management of choking for the adult differs from that of a child, and the American Heart Association does not recommend using the Heimlich maneuver for infants under 1 year of age.

 Go to Chapter 21, **Technique 21–1: Performing the Heimlich Maneuver on an Infant or Child** and **Technique 21–2: Performing the Heimlich Maneuver on an Adult,** in Volume 2.

KnowledgeCheck 21–2
- What are the most common poisonous agents ingested by children?
- Name one source of CO poisoning.
- Identify four safety measures that decrease the risk of burns in the child.

- What are some specific activities that reduce the possibility of fires in the home?
- What should parents teach their children to do if they encounter a firearm?
- What specific safety measures would you discuss with a mother to prevent choking in her 9-month-old child?

  Go to Chapter 21, **Knowledge Check Response Sheet and Answers,** on the Electronic Study Guide.

CriticalThinking 21–2

You are having dinner in a restaurant and notice that the guest at the table beside you seems to be choking.

- What is the universal sign for choking?
- What is the first action you should take?

Take-Home Toxins

Take-home toxins are hazardous substances transported from the workplace to the home. The National Institute for Occupational Safety and Health (NIOSH) reports that pathogenic microorganisms, asbestos, lead, mercury, arsenic, pesticides, caustic farm products, and dozens of other agents cause significant morbidity and mortality in workers' homes (NIOSH, 2003). These toxins are most likely transported to workers' homes on the workers themselves, on their clothing, or on objects brought from the workplace. In the home, contamination occurs via any of three sources (Worthington, 2001):

1. Direct skin-to-skin contact, or direct contact with contaminated clothing
2. Arthropod vectors, such as ticks that are responsible for Lyme disease
3. Transmission on dust particles that are inhaled (e.g., anthrax spores, arsenic in mine and smelter dust)

Most preventive measures apply to the workplace. However, you can teach clients who are at risk to remove work clothing and to shower, preferably in an open-air shower, before leaving work (NIOSH, 2003). If facilities for showering are not available, patient advocacy may be appropriate (see Chapter 44). Before entering their homes, exposed workers who have not showered should remove their clothing. Then they should shower immediately. When handling contaminated clothes or objects, they should wear gloves to reduce the risk of skin transmission. Laundering may not be effective in removing certain toxins in clothes.

WHAT SAFETY HAZARDS ARE IN THE COMMUNITY?

Hazardous agents in the community are a major contributor to illness, disability, and death worldwide. This section discusses four major topics of concern: motor vehicle accidents, pathogens, pollution, and electrical storms.

Motor Vehicle Accidents

Motor vehicle accidents (MVAs) are the leading cause of accidental death in American adults and children over 1 year of age (National Center for Injury Prevention and Control, 2003; National Safety Council, 2001b). Failure to use seat belts and proper child car seats continues to be the major contributing factor. Severe injuries and death also occur from air bag deployment when young children are improperly placed in the front passenger seat. Many of the fatal MVAs during adolescence involve abuse of alcohol or other substances.

Interventions: Preventing Motor Vehicle Accidents

Anticipatory guidance and educational programs are important measures for improving motor vehicle safety for all age groups. Teach families to observe the following measures:

- Be cautious when walking or bicycling on the roadway, and observe the laws.
- Do not drink and drive; have a designated driver.
- Observe the speed limits.
- Always wear seat belts while driving, and periodically check belts to ensure safe operation.
- Make certain children are properly buckled in age-appropriate safety seats in the back seat of the car. Use rear-facing seats for infants (Figure 21–3) and forward-facing seats for toddlers. For children ages 4 to 8 years, booster seats are safer than a seat belt alone. If in doubt about the appropriateness or use, ask the local police department to check the installation of your child safety seat.

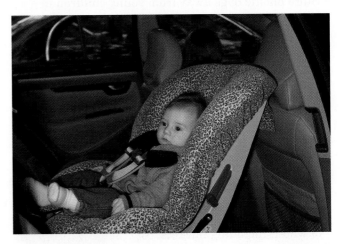

FIGURE 21–3 Infant car seat with infant in rear-facing position in the middle of the back seat.

- Do not allow children under age 12 to ride in the front seat. Riding in the back seat is associated with at least a 30% reduction in the risk of fatal injury, and up to 46% in cars with airbags (National Center for Disease Prevention and Control, 2003). Some experts recommend that anyone weighing under 110 lb, regardless of age, ride in the back seat.

For in-depth information about child safety seats,

Go to the **American Academy of Pediatrics web site at http://www.aap.org/family/cps.htm**

You may also wish to become politically active on the issue of motor vehicle safety. For instance, you might petition your city council for a stop sign at a particularly dangerous intersection or a reduced speed limit on a highway in your area. Or you might lobby for the enactment of graduated licensing laws in your state to more closely regulate teenage driving or for stronger seat belt laws nationwide.

KnowledgeCheck 21–3

Which of the preceding safety measures apply most directly to Teresa's toddler ("Meet Your Patients")?

Go to Chapter 21, **Knowledge Check Response Sheet and Answers,** on the Electronic Study Guide.

Pathogens

A **pathogen** is any microorganism capable of causing an illness. Pathogens can enter the body through several sources in the environment: food, mosquitoes and other insects, rodents and other animals, and unclean water.

Food-Borne Pathogens

Food poisoning is a nonspecific term that describes illness caused by ingesting bacteria and other microorganisms, or their toxins, in food. Improper food storage and preparation are a major cause of food poisoning (Krieger & Higgins, 2002). Poisonous chemicals in the environment, such as mercury, arsenic, zinc, and potassium chlorate, may also contaminate foods.

| Interventions: Preventing Food Poisoning |

Education is an important component of preventing food poisoning. This includes teaching clients to refrigerate perishable foods, wash foods before preparing them, use clean surfaces and utensils for food preparation, cook foods at a temperature high enough and a period of time long enough to destroy microbes, and promptly refrigerate leftovers. See the Home Care box on page 430 on food safety for other measures.

Vector-Borne Pathogens

Vectors are organisms that transmit pathogenic bacteria, viruses, and protozoa from one host to another. They include mosquitoes and other insects, rodents, birds, and other animals.

Almost everyone has been bitten by mosquitoes. The severity of the reaction depends on the person's degree of allergy to the mosquito's saliva. In addition to the discomfort caused by mosquito bites, infected mosquitoes can transmit diseases such as West Nile virus and malaria. They can also transmit parasites to domestic animals (e.g., dog heartworm, equine encephalitis). Other insects, such as roaches, fleas, ticks, sand flies, and lice, can also transmit serious diseases.

Rodents and other animals can also act as vectors. For example, rabies can be spread through the bite of a rabid animal, and some fungal diseases can spread via the inhalation of bird droppings. Structural defects in roofs and walls permit entry of birds, rodents, and other small animals, and dead spaces in walls permit their circulation among apartments in multi-unit dwellings (Krieger & Higgins, 2002).

| Interventions: Fighting Vectors |

Mosquito control is the responsibility of both the individual and governmental agencies. Strategies include spraying programs and digging ditches to promote drainage from stagnant areas. All pesticides, whether used by an agency or the consumer, should have the name and amount of active ingredient on the label. No pesticide is 100% safe, so people must use them cautiously. Teach clients the following strategies for fighting mosquitoes (U.S. Environmental Protection Agency, 1998):

- Empty standing water in old tires, buckets, toys, or other outdoor containers.
- Change water in bird baths, fountains, and wading pools at least once a week.
- Keep rain gutters unclogged.
- Keep swimming pools treated with the proper chemicals.
- Use mosquito repellents when necessary, and follow label directions carefully.
- Make sure window and door screens do not have holes in them.
- Replace outdoor lights with yellow "bug" lights.
- Use head nets, long sleeves, and long pants if you go into areas with high mosquito populations (e.g., salt marshes, deep woods).
- Use "bug zappers" or citronella candles for evening outdoor activities.
- Contact your local health department if you have questions about mosquitoes or about a spraying program.

Food Safety

Cleaning

- Wash hands before and after handling food or eating.

- Never use a cutting board, knife, or other object that was used to prepare meat, poultry, or fish for any other purpose until it has been thoroughly washed in hot, soapy water.

Cooking

- Eat only meats that are fully cooked. Use a thermometer to check internal food temperature:

  Leftovers and casseroles, 165°F
  Beef, lamb, and veal 145°F
  Pork and ground beef, 160°F
  Whole poultry and thighs, 180°F
  Poultry breasts, 170°F
  Ground chicken or ground beef, 165°F
  Stuffed fish, 165°F
  Roast meats at an oven temperature of 300°F or above
  Hold hot food above 140°F and for no more than 2 hours

- Do not eat raw or partially cooked eggs.

Storing

- Cover and date food.

- Store vegetables and fruit separately from uncooked meats.

- Do not store food in decorative containers unless they are labeled safe for food. Some crystal and pottery, for example, have high lead content.

- Store cleaning supplies away from food.

Refrigerating

- Refrigerate foods promptly after meals.

- Do not buy partially thawed items. Be sure they are frozen solid.

- Use a cooler to transport foods when the temperature is above 80°F.

- Store deli meat for only 1 or 2 days.

- Use thermometers in the refrigerator and freezer.

  Keep freezer temperature at 0°F or below.
  Keep refrigerator temperature at 40°F or below.

- Thaw foods in the refrigerator or under cold running water. Use the microwave to thaw foods only if you are going to continue cooking them at that time.

- Chill cooked foods rapidly in a shallow (2-inch-deep) container.

- Pack lunches in insulated containers. You can refrigerate or freeze sandwiches before packing, to keep them cold.

Other

- Never eat any food that has an odor or that might be spoiled.

- Be aware that imported folk remedies, such as *greta* (which is used by some Hispanic patients for colic), may be contaminated with lead.

- Observe sanitation reports for selecting eating establishments in the community.

Source: U.S. Food and Drug Administration, Center for Food Safety and Applied Nutrition. Last updated 3/17/04. Consumer advice on food safety, nutrition, and cosmetics. Retrieved July 11, 2004, from http://www.fda.gov

---

To control rodents, raccoons, and other small animals, remove as many food and water sources as possible. Advise clients to:

- Cover food and clean up immediately after meals.
- Keep garbage in closed containers that cannot be overturned.
- Repair holes and cracks in the exterior structure of the home, as well as in walls, closets, attic, around sinks and cabinets, and so on.
- Use commercial traps or hire professional exterminators.
- Participate in neighborhood cleanup projects.
- Caution clients that rat and mice poisons and baits can be fatal and should not be used in areas accessible to children and pets.

Water-Borne Pathogens

Sanitation refers to measures to promote and establish favorable health conditions, especially those related to the community's water supply. People who live in substandard housing may not have safe drinking water, hot water for washing, or adequate methods of waste disposal. People in rural areas often depend on private wells, which may not be adequately maintained and tested for pathogens. These are primarily community health problems (see Chapter 42).

Pollution

Pollution is any harmful chemical or waste material discharged into the air, water, or soil. Examples of pollutants are gaseous fumes, asbestos, carbon monoxide,

and cigarette smoke. Hospitals in the United States produce 6600 tons of waste daily, partly because of the increased use of disposable items (Hospitals for a Healthy Environment, 2002).

- *Air* pollution occurs outdoors and indoors. Motor vehicle emissions are the primary cause of *outdoor air pollution* in the United States. Other toxic air pollutants include asbestos, toluene, and metals such as mercury, chromium, and lead compounds. *Indoor pollutants* include radon, carbon monoxide, and allergens from dust mites, cockroaches, mold, rodents, and pets. These allergens are an important health issue because people spend the majority of their time indoors. It is well documented that passive exposure to tobacco smoke is associated with respiratory disease (U.S. Department of Health and Human Services, 2000).

- *Water* contamination in lakes, rivers, and streams ultimately affects both the recreational and food production of these waters. Pollution occurs when inadequately treated or inappropriate quantities of human, industrial, or agricultural wastes are released into the water systems (U.S. Department of Health and Human Services, 2000). If the pollution is severe enough, the water may become unsafe for human consumption.

- *Noise.* Substantial exposure to noise has been associated with a range of adverse health effects, including hearing loss, stress, elevated blood pressure, and loss of sleep. Noise is pervasive in our society, for example, from road traffic, jet planes, garbage trucks, construction equipment, lawn mowers, and loud music. People who live or work near major roads, bus depots, airports, and trucking routes are at greater risk, as are those in certain work environments (e.g., railroad workers) (U.S. Department of Health and Human Services, 2000).

- *Soil* can become contaminated by improper waste disposal and excessive use of pesticides. Agricultural, industrial, and manufacturing processes create solid and toxic waste. Animal, radioactive, and medical wastes pose special problems. Household products such as paints, cleaners, oils, batteries, and pesticides contain corrosive or toxic ingredients that contaminate the environment when disposed of improperly (e.g., when they are put in the trash or poured down the drain, on the ground, or into storm sewers).

| Interventions to Reduce Pollution |

Teach families that proper disposal and recycling of solid wastes helps to prevent pollution. The following measures are appropriate:

- Contact the local refuse disposal company for instructions about proper disposal of hazardous wastes.

- Encourage the use of products that are nonhazardous or less hazardous, and use only the amount necessary for a project. Share leftover materials with neighbors.

- *Solid waste.* The EPA suggests the following:

    Reduce the amount of trash discarded (e.g., don't buy products that have unnecessary packaging).

    Reuse containers, bags, and products; sell or donate instead of throwing items out.

    Recycle. Use and buy recyclable and recycled products; compost yard trimmings.

    Respond by educating others, expressing preferences for less waste (e.g., to manufacturers, merchants).

For a more complete discussion of reducing solid waste,

 Go to Chapter 21, **Supplemental Materials: The Consumer's Handbook for Reducing Solid Waste,** on the Electronic Study Guide.

- *Air pollution.* Pay attention to air quality warnings, and restrict time spent in high-traffic areas. Participate in car pools or use public transportation whenever possible.

- *Noise pollution.* Take actions to help prevent irreversible hearing loss: (1) avoid exposure to continuous high noise levels and (2) wear protective devices (e.g., ear plugs) in environments with a high noise level.

Electrical Storms

According to the National Weather Service, deaths from lightning strikes lead all other categories of weather-related fatalities.

| Interventions: Preventing Injury from Electrical Storms |

Weather conditions play a major role in outdoor recreation programming. It is important for professionals, participants, and outdoor recreation providers to understand severe weather conditions, specifically thunderstorms and lightning, and the dangers associated with them. The following are guidelines for activities and evacuation procedures (Trapasso & Owens, 1996):

- Stay away from tall objects, particularly individual trees, in the open.

- Crouch or sit in the lowest spot possible.

- Seek shelter in large buildings.

- Stay away from open vehicles, including bicycles and motorcycles.

- Get out of the water or off small boats.

- Drop all metal objects, such as golf clubs and fishing gear.

BOX 21-2 JCAHO Patient Safety Goals for 2003

1. Improve the accuracy of patient identification, for example:
   - Use at least two identifiers when administering medications or blood products.

2. Improve effectiveness of communication among caregivers, for example:
   - Require a "read-back" to verify verbal or telephone orders.
   - Standardize abbreviations and acronyms used in the organization, and use only those on the list.
   - Clarify orders with the physician when a nonstandard abbreviation is used.

3. Improve the safety of using high-alert medications, for example,
   - Do not keep concentrated electrolytes (e.g., potassium chloride, or KCl) on patient care units.

4. Eliminate wrong-site, wrong-patient, and wrong-procedure surgery.
   - Use a preoperative verification process (e.g., a checklist) to be sure that all necessary records (e.g., x-ray studies) are available.
   - Involve the patient in marking the surgical incision site.

5. Improve the safety of using infusion pumps, for example, by having built-in protection to ensure that patients do not receive an unintended free-flowing solution.

6. Improve the effectiveness of clinical alarm systems, for example:
   - Conduct regular testing and maintenance of alarm systems.
   - Ensure that all staff know how to use all alarms in their practice area.

Source: Kirkpatrick, C. (2003, April 21). Safety first: The JCAHO introduces new patient safety goals. *NurseWeek,* 19–21.

KnowledgeCheck 21–4
- What are the major causes of MVAs?
- List at least three tips for preventing food poisoning.
- What other forms of pollution can invade a healthful environment?

 Go to Chapter 21, **Knowledge Check Response Sheet and Answers,** on the Electronic Study Guide.

 CriticalThinking 21–3

Identify an environmental problem in your neighborhood. What are some possible solutions?

WHAT SAFETY HAZARDS ARE IN THE HEALTHCARE FACILITY?

Several areas within healthcare facilities pose safety hazards for residents and workers. Box 21–2 lists the Joint Commission on Accreditation of Healthcare Organizations (JCAHO) National Patient Safety Goals for 2003, which should give you an idea of the types of accidents that occur in healthcare agencies.

Falls

Although anyone can fall, infants and older adults are especially at risk for injury from falls. Although most falls occur in the home, they are a major concern in healthcare facilities, as well. Falls are by far the most common incident reported in hospitals and long-term care facilities (Fortin, Yeaw, Campbell, & Jameson, 1998; Ray et al., 1997; Walker, 1998). Many patients have risk factors such as poor vision, cognitive impairment, difficulty with walking or balance, orthostatic hypotension, weakness or dizziness from disease or therapy, and drowsiness from medications. Most agencies have established procedures and safety features to prevent falls.

| Interventions: Preventing Falls |

Nursing interventions to prevent falls will, of course, depend on the risk factors that were identified at the initial assessment. For an example of a falls risk assessment,

 Go to Chapter 21, **Tables, Boxes, Figures: ESG Figure 21–1,** on the Electronic Study Guide.

For clients at risk for falls, repeat the falls assessment every 8 hours, and increase the frequency of rounds. For a care plan for Risk for Falls,

 Go to Chapter 21, **Care Plan: Risk for Falls,** on the Electronic Study Guide.

Also consider the following interventions:
- Perform falls risk assessments for all resident patients; identify medications that increase the risk of falling.
- Place the call light within reach. Have client demonstrate ability to call for the nurse.
- Orient the person to surroundings (e.g., bathroom, chairs; you may need to label items).
- Place disoriented patients in rooms near the nurse's station.

- Keep the bed in a lowered position, except when giving care, with wheels locked (Figure 21–4A).
- Make sure wheels of wheelchairs are locked, as appropriate, especially during transfer activities (Figure 21–4B).
- Offer to assist with toileting and transfer activities.
- Provide nonskid slippers (Figure 21–4C).
- Keep water, urinal, bedpan, and tissues within easy reach of client.
- Provide adequate lighting, and use floor-level lighting.
- Place holdbars and handrails in bathrooms and hallways.
- Determine the appropriate use of siderails based on the patient's cognitive and functional status.
- Provide a night light.
- Keep floors dry and free of clutter.
- Monitor the patient regularly.
- Educate the patient and family regarding fall prevention strategies.
- For patient at risk for falls, place a warning sticker on the chart or door.

Equipment-Related Accidents

Equipment-related accidents usually occur when equipment malfunctions or is used improperly, for example, when suction devices and infusion pumps are not working properly, oxygen cylinders are transported incorrectly or wheelchairs and beds are not locked during transfer activities.

Interventions: Preventing Equipment-Related Accidents

The following interventions help ensure safe use of equipment.

- Seek advice if you are unsure how to operate the equipment.
- Make sure medical equipment has been properly inspected.
- Be alert to signs that the equipment is not functioning properly.
- Make sure that rooms are not cluttered with equipment.
- Follow agency policies regarding equipment brought from the patient's home (e.g., hair dryers, electric shavers, radios); usually these should be inspected for proper grounding and safe cords.

Fires and Electrical Hazards

Because most institutions promote a smoke-free environment, fire in a healthcare agency is more often

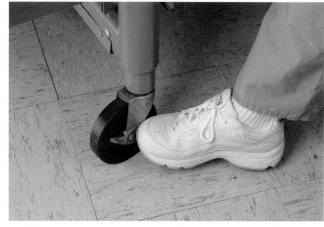

(a)

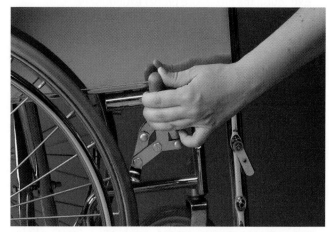

(b)

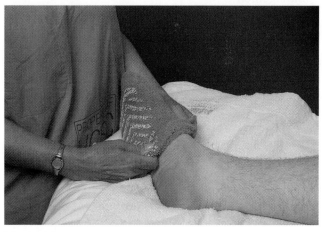

(c)

FIGURE 21–4 Preventing falls. *A,* Locking bed. *B,* Safety locks on wheelchairs. *C,* Applying nonskid slippers.

related to anesthesia or improperly grounded or malfunctioning electrical equipment. Nevertheless, patients and guests do break the rules and smoke, so smoking cannot be discounted as a hazard.

VOL 2 Go to Chapter 21, **Procedure 21–1: Using a Bed Monitoring Device,** in Volume 2.

BOX 21-3 Response to Fire in the Healthcare Facility

Rescue the patient	From immediate danger. Move client into corridor. Close doors to affected area.
Activate the alarm	Report fire as to location and kind, and identify yourself. Activate nearest alarm.
Confine the fire	Close all doors and windows. Turn off all oxygen valves after coordinating with the charge nurse.
Extinguish the fire	Use proper extinguisher. Stay between the fire and path to safety. Keep low.

| Interventions: Fires and Electrical Hazards |

All personnel must know the fire escape route and follow hospital policy regarding fires (Box 21–3). Most healthcare agencies have policies for preventing electrical hazards. The following activities promote safety in the healthcare agency:

- Prior to use, have all electrically powered equipment and accessory equipment evaluated by facilities management.
- Participation in education and training programs for electrical safety are mandatory for all employees as established by JCAHO standards.
- If an electrical safety hazard is suspected, clearly label the malfunctioning equipment and send it for inspection.
- Use three-pronged electrical plugs whenever possible.
- Observe for breaks or frays in electrical cords.

Restraints

The Health Care Financing Administration (HCFA) defines a **restraint** as "any device that restricts a patient's voluntary movement or access to his body and that can't easily be removed by the patient" (HCFA, 2000). The most obvious form of restraint is the use of physical force by another person. A restraint may also be (1) a mechanical device (e.g., a siderail), material, or equipment attached or adjacent to the patient's body; or (2) a chemical restraint (i.e., medications such as sedatives and psychotropic agents) given to control disruptive behavior. HCFA requires that restraints be medically ordered and that you try all less restrictive interventions before using them.

Restraints have traditionally been used as a safety measure to reduce the chance for patient and staff injury; however, research indicates that restraints are themselves a safety hazard, increasing the risk of injury. A restrained person has a natural tendency to struggle and try to remove the restraint and, as a result, can become entangled, suffer nerve damage, circulatory impairment, and even suffocation. Restraint-imposed immobility can cause pressure ulcers, contractures, and other hazards of immobility. Emotionally, the person may suffer anger, fear, humiliation, and diminished self-esteem.

Siderails

Siderails are often used to promote a safe environment or as an aid to independence. It is important to note that, based on the HCFA standards, siderails can be viewed as a restraint. A full-length side rail is a restraint when it is used to prevent the patient from getting out of bed regardless of whether he is able to do so safely (Tyson, 1999). A half- or quarter-length upper siderail can be an aid to independence if it is used by the patient for the purpose of getting into and out of bed. Similarly, split rails are not considered restraints if a client requests them in order to feel more secure (Talerico & Capezuti, 2001).

Remember that older or cognitively impaired adults may regard siderails as a barrier rather than as a reminder that they need assistance. Several studies have shown that siderails may lead to serious falls and injuries. These findings have led healthcare providers to reevaluate the use of restraints and to recommend that siderails not be used routinely (Capezuti, Talerico, Sturmpf, & Evans, 1998; Brusch & Capezuti, 2001).

Ambularm and Bed Alarms

The Ambularm is one device that is used as an alternative for restraints with clients who climb out of bed and are in danger of falling. The Ambularm is worn on the leg and signals when the leg is in a dependent position, such as over the siderail or on the floor. Another type of alarm is an integral bed alarm, which beeps if the patient's weight is off the mattress for more than a few seconds.

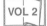

The Critical Aspects box for Procedures 21–1 and 21–2 summarizes the key points.

| Interventions: Using Restraints Safely |

In 2001 the Joint Commission on Accreditation of Healthcare Organizations (JCAHO) put into effect pa-

For steps to follow in *all* procedures, refer to the inside back cover of Volume 2.

critical aspects of procedures 21–1 and 21–2

Procedure 21–1: Using a Bed-Monitoring Device

- Explain to the patient and family that the device alerts the staff when the patient tries to get out of the chair or bed.

- Apply or place the device; connect the control unit to the sensor pad.

- Connect the control unit to the nurse call system, if possible.

- Explain that the patient will need to call for assistance when she wants to get up.

- Disconnect or turn off the alarm prior to assisting the patient out of the bed or chair.

- Reactivate the alarm after assisting the patient back to the bed or chair.

Procedure 21–2: Using Restraints

- Follow agency policy and state laws for using restraints.

- Medicare standards allow for restraints only if the patient (1) is a danger to self or others, or (2) must be immobilized temporarily so that a procedure may be performed.

- Obtain a medical order for the restraint; in an emergency, apply restraints, and obtain a medical order within 24 hours. The order must be renewed every 24 hours. Guidelines are more restrictive when drugs are used for behavior management.

- Obtain patient and family consent when feasible; explain the need for the restraints.

- Pad bony prominences (e.g., wrists, ankles) as needed before applying the restraint.

- Tie and knot the restraints so that they can be released quickly in an emergency.

- Never tie restraints to a siderail.

- Adjust restraints to maintain good body alignment, comfort, and safety.

- Be sure that restraints do not impair blood circulation to any body area.

- At least every 2 hours:

  Release restraints and provide skin care, passive and active range of motion, ambulation, toileting, hydration, and nutrition. Document. Assess circulation, skin integrity, and need for continuing restraint. Document.

- Check the restraints every 30 minutes.

---

tient safety standards for maintaining and improving patient safety in healthcare settings (Abrahamsen, 2001). The JCAHO guidelines also aim to reduce the use of restraints. To comply with the standards and to provide the safest possible care environment, healthcare facilities are encouraged to:

- Promote among all direct-care staff a commitment to reduce the use of restraints and seclusion.

- Educate caregivers before they take part in any restraint-related activity.

- Document restraint episodes specifically, in detail.

- Maintain one-on-one viewing of patients in restraint and seclusion.

- Include staff members when deciding whether to explore new technology that's considered a safe alternative to traditional restraint devices.

- Budget for an adequate number of qualified staff to attend to patients.

Alternatives to using restraints for confused clients include the following:

- Orient clients and families to their surroundings; reorient as often as necessary. This helps to relieve anxiety and prevent wandering.

- Use one-to-one supervision as needed; encourage family members and friends to stay or to hire sitters for clients who need supervision.

- Use Ambularms and integrated bed alarm systems.

- Provide pain relief and other comfort measures to decrease agitation.

- Discontinue treatments that cause discomfort or agitation as soon as possible. For example, some patients become agitated and pull at or try to escape sensations from indwelling catheters, intravenous catheters, and nasogastric tubes. Provide oral feeding and hydration as soon as possible, and assist with toileting routines.

- Provide music therapy; this is calming to many patients.

- Use therapeutic touch and relaxation techniques, such as massage (see Chapter 40).

- Place near the nursing station clients with cognitive deficits or who need supervision for other reasons; check on them frequently.

- Keep the environment and the caregivers as consistent as possible.

- Provide diversional activities.

TABLE 21-3 Potential Health Effects of Mercury		
Primary Route	**Potential Health Effects**	
Acute Effects		
Inhalation	Respiratory damage, wakefulness, muscle weakness, anorexia, headache, ringing in the ears, chest pain, inflammation of the mouth, and pneumonitis	
Eye	Irritation and corrosion	
Skin	Irritation and allergic dermatitis	
Ingestion	Intestinal obstruction	
Chronic Effects		
Primarily central nervous system	Numbness or tingling of the hands, lips, and feet; behavior and personality changes	

- Use low beds for clients who are likely to fall or wander.

- Use wedge cushions and body props for patients sitting in chairs to help them maintain good posture in the chair; these help keep them from slumping and falling out of the chair.

- Keep doors to the unit locked if this is feasible and acceptable; in long-term care facilities, also lock outside doors. Have a staff member at main entrances and exits.

Use restraints only as a last resort. They make care more time-consuming and do not reduce falls. If you must use them, follow organization policies and the following guidelines:

- Obtain a physician's order for physical restraints.

- In an emergency you may apply restraints for behavior management, but a physician or advanced practice nurse must evaluate the patient within 1 hour. Orders must be renewed daily, and cannot be "prn" (as needed) orders.

- If you must restrain a patient, release restraints periodically and check circulation. You must document continual visual and audio monitoring of the patient's status.

For directions and further explanation of how to care for patients in restraints,

 Go to Chapter 21, **Procedure 21–2: Using Restraints,** in Volume 2.

See also the Critical Aspects box for Procedures 21–1 and 21–2.

KnowledgeCheck 21–5

- What is a typical cause of fire in healthcare facilities?
- What measures should you take, and in what order, if a fire occurs in the hospital?
- List three measures for preventing patient falls in the hospital.

 Go to Chapter 21, **Knowledge Check Response Sheet and Answers,** on the Electronic Study Guide.

Mercury Poisoning

Mercury exists as a heavy, odorless, silver-white liquid metal. Highly toxic in both acute and chronic exposure, mercury is commonly found in high school and university laboratories, healthcare facilities, and old industrial sites. Products containing mercury include thermometers, thermostats, batteries, fluorescent light bulbs, blood pressure devices, and electrical equipment and switches (Zeitz, Orr, & Kaye, 2002). Mercury can be inhaled, ingested, or absorbed through the skin. It accumulates in muscle tissue and can cause renal and neurological disorders, especially in fetuses and neonates. Because of mercury's shiny color and ability to form beads or balls, it is appealing to curious children. See Table 21–3 for potential health effects.

| Interventions: Preventing Mercury Poisoning |

As a nurse, one way you can help prevent mercury poisoning is to take an active role in eliminating mercury-containing items from your workplace. Since 1998, the American Hospital Association (AHA) and the Environmental Protection Agency (EPA) have recommended that the healthcare industry eliminate mercury-containing waste by the year 2005 (USEPA, 2002). This includes phasing out mercury thermometers and blood pressure manometers. Some hospitals conduct thermometer exchanges, providing free or low-cost nonmercury thermometers to anyone who brings in a mercury thermometer.

If a mercury spill is not properly cleaned, the mercury can remain in the cracks and crevices for long periods of time and cause continuous exposure to mercury vapors. In most cases, you will not encounter mercury exposure in acute care and ambulatory agencies. However, if you need to, you can clean small mercury spills by wearing disposable gloves, using a paper towel, and washing your hands well after removing the spill (Wong & Hockenberry-Eaton, 2001). Place the item causing the spill, the gloves, and the paper towel in a plastic bag, and discard them. Ventilate the area well for several days. Larger spills usually must be cleaned by a pollution control agency and can be very costly (Zeitz, Orr & Kaye, 2002). It is especially difficult to remove mercury spills from carpets, and they usually have to be disposed of as hazardous waste.

Hazards to Healthcare Workers

Nursing is an active profession, and workplace injuries are all too common. Common accidents include back injuries, needlestick injuries, and radiation injury. Workplace violence also occurs. Nurses sometimes hesitate to report that they have been injured because they fear they will be denied opportunities for promotion and fear other repercussions. However, OSHA requires that employers show employees how to report a workplace injury and prohibits discrimination against employees who make such reports (de Castro, 2003). You should always report an injury. By reporting your injury, you help (1) pinpoint trends and areas of need in safety, and (2) ensure that you will receive necessary treatment and follow-up.

Back Injury

Nursing has one of the highest rates of back injuries in all professions. In 2000, the incidence rate for back injuries involving days lost from work was 90.1 per 10,000 full-time workers in hospitals—more than for construction workers (American Nurses Association, 2005; Bureau of Labor Statistics, 2000b). The American Nurses Association (ANA) reports that 52 percent of nurses complain of chronic back pain. This is not surprising, as many nursing tasks require bending and twisting of the torso, activities that can cause injury when the nurse does not use correct body mechanics. Among the most stressful activities are transferring patients (e.g., from toilet to chair), weighing patients, lifting a patient in bed, repositioning patients in beds or chairs, and changing bed linens (Owen & Garg, 1990). In a recent position paper, the ANA (2005) recommends that nurses use assistive equipment and devices for such patient-handling activities in order to prevent injury to themselves and patients. The ANA states that "manual" patient handling should be used only in exceptional situations when it cannot be avoided. For those situations, you can reduce your risk to some degree by using appropriate body mechanics. Refer to Chapter 31 for information about body mechanics and lifting patients. For information about ANA's campaign to prevent musculoskeletal injuries,

 Go to **http://www.nursingworld.org/handlewithcare/**

Needlestick Injury

Healthcare workers, mostly nurses and housekeeping staff, suffer up to 1 million injuries per year from needles and other "sharps," putting them at risk for infectious diseases such as hepatitis B and AIDS. Since 1992 the Occupational Safety and Health Administration (OSHA) has required employers to provide "engineering controls," such as safer medical devices and needleless systems. A federal Needlestick Safety and Prevention Act became law in 2000. It is enforced by new OSHA standards, which also require employers to maintain a log of sharps injuries and to involve nonmanagerial employees in selecting safer needle devices. Although OSHA has fined hospitals for noncompliance, many employers still have not complied completely with the regulations (American Nurses Association [ANA], 2003; Wilburn, 2003). For suggestions to prevent needlestick injuries,

 Go to Chapter 21, **Technique 21–3: Preventing Needlestick Injury,** in Volume 2.

For more discussion on how to handle needles safely,

Go to Chapter 23, **Procedure 23–10: Recapping Needles Using One-Handed Technique,** in Volume 2.

Radiation Injury

Radiation is the process of emitting radiant energy in the form of waves or particles. Ionizing radiation is used in computerized tomography in diagnostic radiology, linear accelerators in radiotherapy, and positron emission tomography in nuclear medicine. Patients are deliberately exposed to radiation during diagnostic tests and certain medical treatments. Healthcare workers who care for these patients are unavoidably exposed to small doses of radiation.

Take precautions to avoid excessive radiation exposure for the patient and yourself during x-ray procedures. Follow the principles of time, distance, and shielding when caring for a patient who is being treated with an internal radioactive implant:

- Organize nursing care to limit the amount of time with the patient.
- Perform near the patient only the nursing care that is absolutely necessary.
- Wear protective shielding (e.g., a lead apron), if available, and wear a film badge if you deliver care that exposes you to radiation regularly. The film badge will indicate any radiation exposure (Lewis, Heitkemper, & Dirksen, 2005).

Violence

Hospital security may not be sufficient to protect you from injury if violence breaks out among patients, visitors, and/or staff. This is especially true in the emergency department (ED), which has 24-hour accessibility and may sometimes be cramped and chaotic. Gang activity, which is widespread in U.S. cities, is a potential source of violence. As gangs spread, so does the

likelihood that gang members will be treated in the ED or admitted to the hospital. When a gang member's reputation is threatened or when disrespect is shown, the tendency is to retaliate—sometimes even weeks later—in an effort to restore reputation and respect (Grossman, 2003). Although gangs are a significant risk in the ED, other patients and family members may also become violent, especially when they are intoxicated. For guidelines for coping with the presence of gang members in the hospital,

 Go to Chapter 21, **Tables, Boxes, Figures: ESG Box 21-1,** on the Electronic Study Guide.

KnowledgeCheck 21–6

- What measures can healthcare workers use to reduce exposure to radiation?
- What safety measures help reduce equipment-related injuries in the healthcare facility?
- As a nurse, what can you do to help prevent injuring your back?

 Go to Chapter 21, **Knowledge Check Response Sheet and Answers,** on the Electronic Study Guide.

Practical Knowledge
knowing how

This section focuses on assessing for safety risks and using standardized nursing language for nursing diagnoses, patient outcomes, and interventions. Specific nursing interventions were discussed with their related safety hazards in the "Theoretical Knowledge" section.

| Assessment |

It is important to assess the client's immediate environment, developmental stage, and individual risk factors. For example, assess all inpatients for falls risk on admission to the healthcare setting. Several useful tools have been developed for assessing safety risks.

Morse Fall Scale

The Morse Fall Scale uses the following questions to assess a person's risk for falls:

1. Does the patient have a history of falling?
2. Does the person have more than one medical diagnosis?
3. Does the person use ambulatory aids, such as crutches or a walker?
4. Does the person have an IV line or a heparin lock?

5. Is the person's gait normal or stooped or otherwise impaired?
6. What is the person's mental status (e.g., disoriented, forgetful)?

These six variables are quick and easy to score, tally, and record on the patient's chart. The risk of falling varies greatly with different patient populations, different times of day, and different stages of the patient's illness. Age alone is not a predictor of falls, but the items scored by the scale are more common in older adults (Morse, 2001). Ideally, the Morse Fall Scale should be calibrated for each particular unit so that fall prevention strategies are targeted to those most at risk and so that proper cut-off scores may be established. Institutions implementing the Morse Scale should train personnel in the proper use of the scale (Morse, 1997).

 Go to Chapter 21, **Tables, Boxes, Figures: ESG Figure 21–1,** on the Electronic Study Guide.

Home Safety Assessment

As you know, many accidents occur in the home (e.g., fire, poisoning). Everyone should take a few minutes to check for environmental safety hazards.

- A **home safety checklist** is a convenient way for clients to identify potential hazards.

 Go to Chapter 21, **Assessment Guidelines and Tools, Home Safety Checklist,** in Volume 2.

- **Safety assessment scale (SAS).** The home safety assessment scale (SAS) is an objective way to evaluate the dangers incurred by people with memory and cognitive deficits who live alone at home. The short version of the SAS will enable you to assess the individual's risk status (a client who receives 15 or more out of a possible 47 points should have an in-depth evaluation). In addition to assessing the person's risk injury, this scale evaluates whether the cognitively impaired person is capable of cooking, taking medications independently, shopping, and performing other activities of daily living by asking questions such as the following:

  Does the person live alone?
  What, if any, are the person's health problems?
  What is the risk for fire and burns (e.g., does the person smoke; is the stove gas or electric; does the person forget to turn it off)?
  Is the person capable of cooking, taking medications independently, shopping, and performing other activities of daily living?
  Can the person recognize food that is fresh and that which is spoiled?

Does the person get lost in familiar places? Can he find his way home?

For the complete short form of the SAS,

 Go to Chapter 21, **Tables, Boxes, Figures: ESG Figure 21–2,** on the Electronic Study Guide.

KnowledgeCheck 21–7

- Which assessment tool would you use for a slightly confused home care client to assess her ability to safely live alone and perform activities of daily living?
- List the six risk factors that are assessed on the Morse Fall Scale.

 Go to Chapter 21, **Knowledge Check Response Sheet and Answers,** on the Electronic Study Guide.

| Nursing Diagnosis |

Consider the following nursing diagnoses. How would your interventions differ for the two diagnoses?

Risk for Falls related to poor vision secondary to cataracts

Risk for Falls related to muscle weakness, joint instability, and poor sense of balance

The nursing diagnoses listed above illustrate that problem etiologies are important because they affect your choice of interventions. Etiologies may include environmental hazards as well as the developmental and individual risk factors discussed in the preceding sections. Keep in mind that you must state *specific* etiologies for each individual—not just general ones, such as "environmental hazards." For example:

Correct: Risk for Falls related to cluttered home environment and joint instability

Incorrect: Risk for Falls related to environmental and physical factors

For NANDA labels that are useful in describing safety problems,

 Go to Chapter 21, **Standardized Language, NANDA Diagnoses and NOC Outcomes for Safety Problems,** in Volume 2.

Use the diagnosis Risk for Injury only when the risk cannot be described by one of the more specific nursing diagnoses.

| Planning Outcomes/Evaluation |

The *NOC standardized outcomes* you use will depend on the nursing diagnosis. For some examples,

 Go to Chapter 21, **Standardized Language, NANDA Diagnoses and NOC Outcomes for Safety Problems,** in Volume 2.

Individualized goals/outcome statements you might write for a client's safety diagnoses include the following:

- The child will be free of injury.
- Environmental hazards will be identified and eliminated.
- Will experience no physical injury due to environmental hazards.
- Falls will not occur.
- Family members will describe their planned escape routes in case of fire.
- Will not experience latex allergy response.

| Planning Interventions/Implementation |

NIC standardized interventions will be determined by the nursing diagnosis you use. To see examples of the approximately 50 interventions in the NIC domain (category) of Safety, as well as some interventions from other NIC domains that are applicable to safety needs,

 Go to Chapter 21, **Standardized Language, Examples of NIC Interventions Related to Safety,** in Volume 2.

Nursing Activities Related to Safety

Specific nursing activities are designed to monitor and manipulate the physical environment to promote safety in all types of settings and circumstances. Specific nursing interventions aimed at preventing accidents in the home, the community, and the healthcare setting were discussed in detail in the "Theoretical Knowledge" section. General activities include the following:

- Ongoing assessment of the safety needs of patients, based on their level of physical and cognitive function and past history of behavior
- Ongoing assessment of safety hazards in the environment (i.e., physical, biological, and chemical)
- Removing hazards from the environment, when possible
- Providing clients with emergency phone numbers
- Modifying the environment to minimize hazards and risk
- Teaching clients about specific safety measures
- If an accident or injury occurs in the healthcare setting, you should file an incident report according to agency policy. See Chapter 16 for more information on this topic.

Which Safety Interventions Can I Delegate?

As nurse manager on a clinical unit or as a primary care nurse, you may need to delegate safety promotion

interventions to unlicensed assistive personnel (UAP). Which safety interventions would you delegate?

For all delegation decisions, refer to the discussion and guidelines in Chapter 7. One safety activity you might delegate is applying restraints. As in all delegation, you must first be sure that the UAP is competent to perform the skill. You may delegate the application of the restraints; however, you may *not* delegate the assessment of the patient's status nor the evaluation of the patient's response to the restraints.

You may assign the UAP to (1) remove and reapply restraints to provide skin care and allow for supervised movement, and (2) assess for skin excoriation under or around restraint location and report it to you.

You should be sure that assistive personnel are aware of and follow all safety measures and institutional procedures. For example, you can expect the UAPs to remove clutter and spills in patient rooms, to provide patients with nonskid slippers, and to lock beds and wheelchairs.

| toward evidenced-based practice |

Whitman, G., Davidson, L., Sereika, S. & Rudy, E. (2001). Staffing and pattern of mechanical restraint use across a multiple hospital system. *Nursing Research 50*(6), 356–362.

This study was conducted to determine the rates, frequencies, duration, and timing of restraint use in a multiple hospital system. It was also conducted to determine the relationship between restraint use and staffing. The research revealed that more restraints were applied on night shifts than on day or evening shifts. Most were applied at midnight. There was a weak positive relationship between staffing and restraint use.

Karlsson, S., Bucht, G., Rasmussen, B., & Sandman, P. (2000). Restraint use in elder care: Decision making among registered nurses. *Journal of Clinical Nursing 9*(6), 842–850.

This study aimed to identify reasons for using physical restraint in nursing practice. It also attempted to explore the relationship between nurses' attitudes and decisions regarding use of physical restraints. The results showed that although nurses strive to act in the client's best interests, this ambition is affected by a variety of variables,

especially in relation to the working conditions and the nurses' willingness to take the risk when not restraining the client.

To enhance client safety in healthcare settings, initiatives have been established to limit the use of mechanical restraints. The use of physical restraints in acute care settings continues to cause concern because restraints can negatively impact patient safety. There are additional concerns that restraint use will increase as staffing levels or skill mix changes.

---

1. Imagine that you are in charge of a unit in an acute care facility. Based on the preceding studies, how would you defend the use of restraints on a fall-prone client with dementia who refused to be restrained? **Dementia** is a broad impairment of intellectual (cognitive) function that usually is progressive and that interferes with normal social and occupational activities.

2. What assumptions must you make to use these studies to answer this question?

 Go to Chapter 21, **Toward Evidence-Based Practice Suggested Responses,** on the Electronic Study Guide.

 Go to Chapter 21, **Resources for Caregivers and Health Professionals,** on the Electronic Study Guide.

 Suggested Readings: Go to Chapter 21, **Reading More About Promoting Safety,** on the Electronic Study Guide.

 Bibliography: Go to Volume 2, Bibliography.

Facilitating Hygiene

Learning Outcomes

After completing this chapter, you should be able to:

❋ Explain how personal hygiene relates to health and well-being.

❋ Identify factors influencing personal hygiene practices.

❋ Discuss delegation of hygiene activities to unlicensed assistive personnel (UAP).

❋ Discuss the nurse's role in determining a client's self-care ability.

❋ Identify nursing diagnoses related to self-care ability and hygiene practices.

❋ Describe normal and abnormal assessment findings of the skin, feet, nails, mouth, hair, eyes, ears, and nose.

❋ State the importance and purpose of bathing.

❋ Describe the following types of baths: complete, help, partial, towel, bag, shower tub, and therapeutic.

❋ Apply the nursing process to common hygiene-related problems of the skin, feet, nails, mouth, hair, eyes, ears, and nose.

❋ Demonstrate nursing skills to promote patient hygiene, such as bathing, foot care, and bed making.

❋ Demonstrate care of the eyes, ears, and teeth, including glasses, contacts, hearing aids, and dentures.

❋ Discuss the relationship between a patient's overall well-being and the immediate environment.

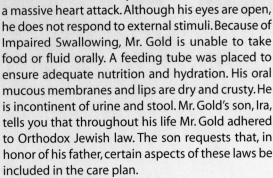

MEET

Your Patients

Your instructor has assigned you to assist the following patients with their hygiene. You must assess the needs of each person, gather information on their bathing habits and preferences, plan nursing measures necessary to meet individual needs, and together with a UAP (unlicensed assistive personnel), provide care.

The first person on your assignment is Mrs. Williams, a 76-year-old Indian American woman who was admitted yesterday after suffering a stroke that paralyzed her right side. Since the stroke, she has been unable to speak clearly and becomes frustrated as she attempts to communicate her needs. Her daughter says Mrs. Williams is a proud, independent, and tidy woman who has been living alone since her husband's death last year. She has been driving her car, cleaning the house, doing her grocery shopping, and maintaining the yard and garden. She wears eyeglasses for reading and driving and has a hearing aid, although she rarely uses it.

The second person on your assignment is Mr. Gold, a 68-year-old Orthodox Jewish man admitted last week after he experienced a massive heart attack. Although his eyes are open, he does not respond to external stimuli. Because of Impaired Swallowing, Mr. Gold is unable to take food or fluid orally. A feeding tube was placed to ensure adequate nutrition and hydration. His oral mucous membranes and lips are dry and crusty. He is incontinent of urine and stool. Mr. Gold's son, Ira, tells you that throughout his life Mr. Gold adhered to Orthodox Jewish law. The son requests that, in honor of his father, certain aspects of these laws be included in the care plan.

What immediate concerns come to your mind about each of these patients? How will you ensure that their hygiene needs are met? Are there any safety issues? Which parts of their hygiene care can you delegate, if any?

Theoretical Knowledge
knowing why

This chapter will provide the theoretical knowledge you need to answer the preceding questions, as well as others that will arise as you care for patients.

HYGIENE AND SELF-CARE

Hygiene describes activities involved in maintaining personal cleanliness and grooming. Personal hygiene contributes to our physical and psychological well-being. **Activities of daily living (ADLs),** such as taking a bath or shower, washing our hair, or brushing and flossing our teeth promote comfort, improve self-image, and decrease infection and disease. Healthy people maintain their own personal hygiene, but some patients need assistance because of illness or injury. As a nurse, you are responsible for providing the necessary assistance and, at the same time, promoting as much self-care as possible. Self-care in ADLs promotes increased activity, independence, and self-esteem.

What Factors Influence Hygiene Practices?

Every patient is unique, so as you would expect, personal hygiene practices vary greatly. The following are a few of the factors that influence a person's hygiene practices.

- *Personal preferences.* Some people prefer a shower, others a bath. One person may shower in the morning, whereas another bathes in the evening to relax before going to sleep. Choice of soaps, deodorants, shampoos, and moisturizers varies from person to person, as well. Respect and accommodate each person's preferences whenever possible. This will reflect your caring and promote maximum participation and independence.

- *Culture and religion or spirituality.* Our cultural and family values and beliefs about hygiene form the foundation for our beliefs as adults. Of course, you will respect and accommodate such differences to the extent possible. Generally, people in North America consider daily bathing, use of deodorant, and brushing of the teeth necessary to eliminate body odors. However, people from some cultures may not be as sensitive about body odor and may

bathe less frequently, finding a weekly bath sufficient. Some religious or spiritual beliefs also influence hygiene practices. For example, some religions consider a menstruating woman unclean and require a ritual cleansing bath 7 days after the menstrual bleeding stops. As another example, Orthodox Judaism prohibits providing personal care by a member of the opposite sex.

- *Economic status or living environment.* Inadequate bathing facilities or lack of money for hygiene supplies can influence how frequently a person bathes. For example, homeless individuals or migrant workers, although they may value cleanliness and grooming, might not have access to running water or soap with which to bathe. People living in poverty must focus on meeting basic needs for food and shelter before they can spend money and energy on hygiene. For some patients you may need to be a patient advocate and initiate contact with appropriate community social service agencies.

- *Developmental level.* Parents and other caregivers perform hygiene care for infants and young children. Older children learn practices that become habits, such as brushing and flossing the teeth. As older children begin to perform their own hygiene independently, they are influenced by the media and societal norms. As a result, they pick and choose hygiene practices that seem important to them. For example, preteens may avoid water and bathe only under parental duress, but teenagers, who are typically very self-conscious, may begin to take several showers a day. Many teenagers have oily skin and can tolerate frequent bathing, but as we age, the oil-producing sebaceous glands become less active. For mature adults, frequent bathing and the use of deodorant soap further dries the skin. Older adults may find it necessary to bathe only every 2 or 3 days, use less soap, and increase the use of skin moisturizers.

- *Knowledge level.* Not everyone has the knowledge necessary to make appropriate decisions. For example, some people who are careful to brush their teeth daily may not know the importance of flossing. Or, some women may not be aware of the importance of cleansing the perineum from front to back after using the toilet. Patient teaching is an important part of your hygiene care because most people will, eventually, be responsible for their own personal hygiene.

How Does Health Status Affect Self-Care Ability?

Both physiological and emotional factors can interfere with a person's ability or willingness to perform hygiene measures.

- *Pain* severely limits the person's ability and motivation to perform hygiene and grooming. The pain itself, limited mobility caused by the pain, and drowsiness from analgesics used to manage the pain may all contribute to a self-care deficit.

- *Limited mobility* (e.g., from injury, weakness, surgery, prescribed bedrest, or pain) decreases the ability to perform hygiene activities. For example, a patient may be unable to bend over to wash her lower legs and feet, cut her toenails, or even raise her arms to wash and dry her hair. A patient who is weak or "lightheaded" may be afraid of falling and be reluctant to move about. Such a person needs help, especially getting into the bathtub or shower. Obstacles such as intravenous lines, oxygen tubing, nasogastric tubes, indwelling urinary catheters, or casts may also interfere with the patient's ability to perform self-care.

- *Sensory deficits* diminish a person's ability to perform hygiene measures safely and independently. Safety is a priority for patients with sensory deficits. Consider these examples:

   A patient with macular degeneration (a visual deficit) is admitted to the hospital. Because he is unfamiliar with the new surroundings, he is unable to gather necessary supplies for grooming. You would need to provide direction, assistance, and understanding.

   A patient with a hearing loss is taking an anticoagulant (a medication to delay blood clotting). You may need to provide explicit written instructions about the importance of using an electric razor rather than his preferred double-edged razor.

- *Cognitive impairment,* such as is found in patients with dementia, delirium, psychoses, stroke, Alzheimer's disease, or traumatic brain injury, may make it impossible for the person to initiate his own grooming. The patient may be unable to determine the need for hygiene, much less know how to accomplish related tasks. For example, a patient with advanced Alzheimer's disease may actually forget how to care for himself and will need step-by-step direction. Because the person may also have difficulty interpreting stimuli in the environment, he may be fearful and resistant to hygiene measures performed by the nurse. Such cognitive deficits may require new or modified hygiene plans.

- *Emotional disturbances* may diminish a person's ability to perform hygiene measures. Patients experiencing altered reality states, such as psychoses, delusions, or hallucinations, may dress inappropriately and have poor hygiene practices. Some are unable to make decisions about "what to do next" when bathing, dressing, and so on. Many people with depression neglect their grooming and hygiene because of a profound lack of energy or motivation.

KnowledgeCheck 22–1

- What are the benefits of personal hygiene?
- Why should you respect and accommodate your patients' hygiene preferences?
- Identify two economic or living environment factors that may influence how frequently a person bathes.
- Identify one example of a cognitive impairment that may make independent initiation of grooming impossible.
- Why may people experiencing depression neglect their grooming and hygiene?

 Go to Chapter 22, **Knowledge Check Response Sheet and Answers,** on the Electronic Study Guide.

 CriticalThinking 22–1

Think about your patients, Mrs. Williams and Mr. Gold ("Meet Your Patients"). After reviewing each of the factors presented determine the following for each patient.

- Which factor(s) will have the most influence on the hygiene practices of this patient?
- Why do you think so?
- How will this factor impact the individual plan of care?

Practical Knowledge
knowing how

Although cleanliness can contribute to well-being, comfort and health, it can also be stressful. As you have learned, bathing tends to create a high level of discomfort in people with dementia (Dunn, Thiru-Chelvam, & Beck, 2002). In another study involving patients in an intensive care unit, an "adverse event" occurred in 48% of the hygiene interventions performed. Adverse events included decreased oxygenation or ventilation, hypertension, hypotension, intracranial hypertension, and even one cardiorespiratory arrest (Robles et al., 2002). This does not imply that you should avoid hygiene care for such patients, but that you may need to modify it and evaluate patient responses constantly as you work. You might provide care in small segments, allowing the patient to rest after brushing his teeth, for example.

| Assessment |

Even when a patient needs assistance with hygiene measures, the overall goal is to promote eventual self-care. Of course, critically ill patients need rest, so you will not push them to perform at their highest level of function. Even if the patient is able to perform self-care, you might allow him to rest while you perform part of the care, for example washing his feet and legs. As a professional nurse, in consultation with the patient you must assess his willingness and ability to perform ADLs, determine the type of help needed, and encourage him to strive for optimal functioning. Plan hygiene care around the patient's needs, not facility routines or staff convenience. For guidelines for assessing hygiene needs,

 Go to Chapter 22, **Assessment Guidelines and Tools, Assessment Guidelines: Hygiene,** in Volume 2.

Assessing Self-Care Abilities

Begin your assessment of self-care ability by conducting an initial interview with the patient and/or family.

- *Obtain a health history.* Identify underlying illness, injury, or disease which might contribute to a self-care deficit or affect the person's ability to tolerate hygiene procedures.

- *Assess the patient's cognitive ability and physical functioning* by determining overall grooming and cleanliness, level of consciousness, short- and long-term memory, ability to follow instructions, range of motion and mobility, level of knowledge, and energy level.

- *Identify other factors (e.g., cultural, religious)* that may influence the patient's hygiene practices and preferences.

- *Assess for sensory disturbances* (auditory, visual, tactile, or olfactory) that interfere with self-care ability. For example, a person who has decreased tactile sensation (sense of touch) may be at risk for burns because he is not able to determine the temperature of the bath water.

- *Determine preferences and practices.* Identify the patient's previous hygiene measures, normal routines, preferences, need for assistive devices, or any other existing problem areas.

Assess your patient's functional status regularly to identify the need for care plan modifications. Focus your assessments on the patient's *ability* to perform self-care hygiene measures and the need for assistance, not necessarily on the *quality* of these measures. To assess a patient's self-care abilities, you can use a standardized functional status rating scale such as the basic 0–4 scale in Box 22–1.

 CriticalThinking 22–2

Answer the following questions for Mrs. Williams (from the "Meet Your Patients" scenario).

- What factor(s) may interfere with Mrs. Williams's self-care ability?
- How can you ensure maximum independence with hygiene for her?
- How might you encourage her to strive toward optimal functioning?

| Nursing Diagnosis |

When a person is unable to perform one or more activities of daily living, a self-care deficit exists. NANDA International (2005) Self-Care Deficit diagnoses related to hygiene are (1) Bathing/hygiene, (2) Dressing/grooming, (3) Toileting, and (4) Feeding. Each is described below, except for Feeding Self-Care Deficit, which will be included in Chapter 26.

Nursing Diagnoses Related to Self-Care

Bathing/Hygiene Self-Care Deficit is a state in which the individual experiences an impaired ability to perform or complete bathing and hygiene activities independently.
  Defining Characteristics. Inability to wash body or body parts, obtain or get to water source, regulate temperature or flow of bathwater, get bath supplies, dry body, get in and out of the bathroom.

Dressing/Grooming Self-Care Deficit is a state in which the individual experiences an impaired ability to perform or complete dressing and grooming activities independently.
  Defining Characteristics. Impaired ability to put on or take off necessary items of clothing, fasten clothing, obtain or replace articles of clothing. Inability to put clothing on upper body or lower body, choose clothing, use assistive devices, use zippers, remove clothes, put on socks, put on shoes, maintain appearance at satisfactory level, pick up clothes.

Toileting Self-Care Deficit is a state in which the individual experiences an impaired ability to perform or complete toileting activities independently.
  Defining Characteristics. Inability to get to toilet or commode, sit on or rise from toilet or commode, manipulate clothing for toileting, carry out proper toileting hygiene, flush toilet or commode.

Total Self-Care Deficit occurs when a patient has all of these Self-Care Deficits, plus a Feeding Self-Care Deficit.

  The following are common etiologies for the Self-Care Deficit diagnoses:

Decreased or lack of motivation
Pain and/or discomfort
Anxiety
Weakness and/or fatigue
Activity intolerance (e.g., as in emphysema, pneumonia)
Decreased strength and/or endurance (e.g., as in heart failure)
Neuromuscular impairment (e.g., secondary to spinal cord injury)
Musculoskeletal impairment (e.g., secondary to arthritis, multiple sclerosis)

BOX 22-1 Classification of Self-Care Abilities

Completely independent	0
Requires use of equipment or device	1
Requires help from another person for assistance, supervision, or teaching	2
Requires help from another person and equipment or device	3
Totally dependent; does not participate in activity	4

Source: NANDA International. (2005). Nursing diagnoses: Definitions and classification, 2005–2006. Philadelphia: Author, pp. 119.

Impaired mobility status (e.g., secondary to casts, traction, prescribed bedrest)
Impaired transfer ability
Perceptual or cognitive impairment (e.g., blindness, Alzheimer's disease)
Environmental barriers (e.g., doorway too narrow to accommodate walker)

  When writing these diagnoses, you should classify the patient's functional level as 0 to 4, as in Box 22–1. The following are examples of diagnostic statements you might write for a client with Self-Care Deficit:

• Bathing/Hygiene Self-Care Deficit (2) related to severe knee pain secondary to degenerative joint disease
• Toileting Self-Care Deficit (4) related to inability to walk to the bathroom secondary to muscle weakness

✗ CriticalThinking 22–3

• Which of the preceding NANDA self-care diagnoses apply to Mrs. Williams and Mr. Gold ("Meet Your Patients")?
• Explain the reasoning for your choices.
• For each patient, what are the related factors for their Self-Care Deficit?
• Using the diagnostic label, Total Self-Care Deficit, write a diagnostic statement for Mrs. Williams and Mr. Gold.

| Planning Outcomes/Evaluation (Self-Care) |

For a sample care plan,

Go to Chapter 22, **Nursing Care Plan: Bathing/Hygiene Self-Care Deficit,** on the Electronic Study Guide.

  The NOC standardized outcome Self-Care: Activities of Daily Living (ADL) is appropriate for all of the

Self-Care Deficit diagnoses. For outcomes for specific diagnoses,

VOL 2 Go to Chapter 22, **Standardized Language, Selected Standardized Outcomes and Interventions for Self-Care Deficit Diagnoses,** in Volume 2.

Individualized goals/outcome statements you might write for Self-Care Deficit include the following examples:

• Verbalizes satisfaction with body cleanliness and oral hygiene after A.M. care.

• Accepts assistance with ADLs or total care, if needed.

• By October 4, will comb hair unassisted.

• By October 4, will complete bath independently, except for back and feet, after nurse provides equipment and assists patient to the bathroom.

You will use the outcomes developed in the planning outcomes phase of the nursing process as the criteria for evaluating patient responses to self-care interventions.

Planning Interventions/Implementation (Self-Care)

For *NIC standardized interventions* for Self-Care Deficit diagnoses,

VOL 2 Go to Chapter 22, **Standardized Language, Selected Standardized Outcomes and Interventions for Self-Care Deficit Diagnoses,** in Volume 2.

Individualized interventions depend on the level (0–4) of the client's Self-Care Deficit, as well as the etiology of the problem. The following are some examples:

• Demonstrate the use of assistive devices (e.g., to help patient grasp and pull on socks).

• Use Velcro fasteners instead of buttons and zippers.

• Allow sufficient time for all ADLs to prevent fatigue and frustration.

• Offer pain medication prior to ADLs.

You will find a thorough discussion of specific hygiene-care activities (e.g., care of the skin, oral hygiene) in the remainder of this chapter.

Types of Scheduled Hygiene Care

The following types of scheduled hygiene care are provided in most inpatient facilities (e.g., hospitals and long-term care settings). Although they are scheduled routinely, you should individualize them to meet patient needs and preferences as much as possible. Always promote self-care to the extent possible.

Early morning care is provided soon after the patient awakens. It includes preparing the patient for

breakfast or other activities, such as diagnostic tests. You will, as needed, assist with toileting, washing the face and hands, giving mouth care, and providing comfort measures.

A.M. (morning) care is hygiene care that occurs after breakfast. Depending on the patient's self-care ability, you will assist with toileting, bathing, oral hygiene, skin care, hair care (including shaving if needed), dressing, and positioning or helping the patient transfer to a chair. You will also change or straighten bed linens, according to agency policy, and tidy the room.

P.M. (afternoon) care consists of preparing patients to receive visitors or afternoon rest. You may assist nonambulatory patients with toileting, hand washing, and oral care; straighten bed linens; reposition the patient; and offer other comfort measures (e.g., pain medications).

H.S. (hour of sleep) care is given before the patient goes to sleep. In addition to the care given in the afternoon, you should offer a back massage to help relax the patient (see Chapter 33). Also place within easy reach the call light, water glass, urinal, or anything else the patient may need during the night. Turn off lights and TV, and close the door before leaving the room (according to patient needs and preferences).

Delegating Hygiene Care to Unlicensed Assistive Personnel

In many institutions, unlicensed assistive personnel (UAP) perform most of the hygiene care. As you have learned, hygiene care can be stressful. Therefore, you will need to carefully assess patients to ensure that it is safe to delegate their care to a UAP. If the patient is very ill or the UAP inexperienced, you will need to assist or perform the care yourself. Read "What Should I Know about Delegation and Supervision?" in Chapter 7 for a review of making delegation decisions.

Prior to assigning a UAP to assist with a bath, shower, or toileting, instruct the UAP about the following:

• Patient's limitations and restrictions, and the amount of assistance necessary

• Use of any assistive devices (e.g., cane, walker, or gait belt)

• Specific safety precautions to follow (e.g., use of gait belt or shower chair)

• Any obstacles present, such as drainage tubes, catheters, IV tubing, or bandages, and how to maintain them during bathing or toileting

• Observations to make during the procedure (e.g., skin condition; the presence of any lesions; areas of special concern over bony prominences and under abdominal folds and breasts; presence, appearance, and amount of urine or stool, or the need to collect a specimen). Explain why the observations are important.

Remember, as the professional nurse, you are responsible for making assessments and determining the meaning of the data reported to you by the UAP. Assisting with or supervising care (especially a bath) is an excellent opportunity for you to assess the patient's level of consciousness, short- and long-term memory, ability to follow instructions, range of motion, skin condition, activity tolerance, and overall self-care ability.

 CriticalThinking 22–4

Think of Mrs. Williams ("Meet Your Patients"). You have delegated her bathing and oral hygiene to a UAP.

- What information do you need to share with the UAP about this patient's needs, limitations, or preferences?
- What, if any, specific observations will you ask the UAP to make for Mrs. Williams?
- What, if any, specific observations will *you* need to make for Mrs. Williams?
- What action will you take if you determine that the patient's needs and preferences were not met by the UAP?

CARE OF THE SKIN

The preceding sections introduced you to the broad topic of hygiene and activities of daily living. The rest of the chapter will deal with specific topics, such as care of the skin.

Theoretical Knowledge
knowing why

To assist patients with skin care, you must have theoretical knowledge about personal hygiene measures and the structure and function of the **integument** (skin).

Anatomy and Physiology of the Skin

The **integumentary system** consists of the skin, the subcutaneous layer directly under the skin, the hair, nails, and the sweat and sebaceous glands. The skin covers the internal structures of the body and protects them from the environment. It has two distinct layers, the epidermis and the dermis (see Figure 34–1, in Chapter 34).

The **epidermis** (the thicker, outer layer) consists of stratified squamous epithelial tissue composed of keratinized (dead) cells, which are fused to make the skin waterproof. The epidermis continually sheds **(desquamates)** and is completely replaced every 3 to 4 weeks. The epidermis contains **melanin,** a pigment that provides protection against the ultraviolet rays of

the sun and that, together with circulating blood, gives skin its color. The **dermis** (the thinner, second layer) contains blood and lymphatic vessels, nerves, bases of hair follicles, and sebaceous and sweat glands.

Functions of the Skin

The skin has five main functions: protection, sensation, regulation, secretion/excretion, and formation of vitamin D.

1. *Protection.* Intact skin is the body's first line of defense against bacteria and other microorganisms that can enter the body and cause infection. It also provides protection from thermal, chemical, and mechanical injury to underlying tissues. **Sebaceous glands** secrete an oily substance called *sebum,* which helps to waterproof and lubricate the skin and decrease bacterial growth.
2. *Sensation.* The skin contains sensory organs or receptors for heat, cold, pressure, touch, and pain.
3. *Regulation.* The skin helps maintain fluid and electrolyte balance by preventing the escape of excess water and electrolytes from the body. It helps to regulate body temperature through the processes of dilating and constricting blood vessels and activating or inactivating sweat glands. **Sweat glands,** concentrated in the axillae and external genitalia, excrete water in the form of perspiration; evaporation produces a cooling effect on the skin.
4. *Secretion/excretion.* The sweat glands secrete fatty acids and proteins and excrete nitrogenous wastes (*urea*), sodium chloride, and water in perspiration.
5. *Vitamin D formation.* The skin contains a form of cholesterol that on exposure to ultraviolet light from the sun is changed to vitamin D. This is why vitamin D is sometimes referred to as the "sunshine vitamin."

See Chapter 34 for more information about the structure and functions of the skin.

Factors Affecting the Skin

In addition to a person's hygiene practices, health status and developmental stage also affect skin condition.

Health Status

Anything that interferes with the hydration, circulation, and nutrition of the skin creates a risk to skin integrity. Which of the following factors do you think would be present for Mr. Gold ("Meet Your Patients")?

- *Dampness* of the skin is caused by excessive perspiration (e.g., in fever and certain illnesses) and incontinence of urine or bowel. The skin breaks

down more easily when it is damp, especially in the skinfolds.

- *Dehydration* is caused by fluid loss (e.g., from vomiting, diarrhea, or fever) and by insufficient fluid intake. This causes the skin to become dry and to crack easily.

- *Insufficient circulation* may be caused by immobility, vascular disease, and overall inadequate nutritional status. This predisposes the patient to local tissue death and ulceration when skin cells do not receive enough oxygen.

- *Nutritional status* is also a factor. People who are very thin or very obese are more likely to experience skin irritation and injury.

- *Skin diseases,* such as impetigo (bacterial infection of the skin), and *systemic diseases,* such as measles and chickenpox, cause lesions that create discomfort and require special hygiene care.

- *Jaundice,* yellow discoloration caused by accumulation of bile pigments in the skin, is a symptom of certain diseases. Jaundice causes the skin to be itchy and dry.

Developmental Stage

Infants have fragile, easily injured skin that is at increased risk for infection. As a child matures, the skin becomes more resistant to injury and infection, but children need adults to provide or supervise the cleanliness of their skin. In adolescence, the sebaceous glands enlarge, and secretions increase. The skin becomes oily and susceptible to acne.

The effects of aging on the skin are numerous and visible. With age, the skin and subcutaneous tissues become thinner and more fragile. As collagen and elastin fibers in the dermis deteriorate, the skin becomes wrinkled. Sebaceous and sweat gland activity decreases, causing the skin to become dry, scaly, and itchy. Temperature regulation in hot weather becomes more difficult. At the same time, vascularity of the skin decreases, causing coolness and pallor. As the number and activity of hair follicles and pigment cells (melanocytes) decrease, hair becomes thin, turns gray or white, and grows more slowly; skin may become unevenly pigmented. Nails thicken, and the growth rate diminishes; nails become softer and tear easily. These changes increase the risk for skin problems.

KnowledgeCheck 22–2
- What are five functions of the skin?
- How does the skin help regulate body temperature?
- What changes take place in the skin as a person ages?

 Go to Chapter 22, **Knowledge Check Response Sheet and Answers,** on the Electronic Study Guide.

Practical Knowledge
knowing how

| Assessment (Skin) |

Assisting a patient with a bath provides an excellent opportunity to assess the patient's skin. Although you can instruct a UAP to report her observations of the patient's skin, you are ultimately responsible for making the assessments. For a thorough discussion of skin assessment, including how to describe and document your observations, see Chapter 19. However, you should routinely make the following assessments as you provide skin care interventions.

Subjective Data

Patients may be sensitive about skin problems or poor hygiene practices, so as you direct your questions to the patient, do so in a nonjudgmental, respectful manner. Ask about the patient's:

- Usual bathing and skin care practices and preferences
- Past and current skin problems, including their effect on the patient's life
- Prescription and over-the-counter (OTC) or herbal remedies used to treat any skin problems
- Allergic skin reactions to food, medications, plants, skin care products, or other substances
- History of diseases or other factors that are known to cause skin problems; for example, decreased mobility, decreased circulation, incontinence, inadequate nutrition, or deficient knowledge

Objective Data

Inspect each area of the skin in an orderly, head-to-toe manner, noting overall cleanliness, condition, color, texture, turgor, hydration, and temperature. Also look for rashes, lumps, lesions, and cracking. Look for drainage from wounds or around tubes. Protect the patient's privacy by closing the curtain and exposing only the area being bathed or examined. Be mindful of the room temperature, and try to reduce drafts to avoid chilling the patient. Observe for four significant color changes:

1. **Pallor** in a light-skinned person may appear as pale skin without underlying pink tones. However, in a dark-skinned person, you will need to observe for an ashen gray or yellow color.
2. **Erythema** is redness of the skin. It is related to vasodilation and inflammation. It is difficult to see in dark-skinned people, so you may discover it by palpating the skin for areas of increased warmth.
3. **Jaundice,** a yellow discoloration of the skin, occurs in a person with impaired liver function. It is best seen in the sclera of the eye.

4. **Cyanosis,** a bluish coloring of the skin, is caused by decreased peripheral circulation or decreased oxygenation of the blood. It may be related to cardiac, pulmonary, or peripheral vascular problems (e.g., arteriosclerosis). In dark-skinned patients, you can best see cyanosis by examining the conjunctivae, tongue, buccal mucosa, and palms and soles for a dull dark color.

KnowledgeCheck 22–3

- True or False: The professional nurse is responsible for making assessments.
- True or False: Assisting with the bath is an excellent time to assess the patient.
- To inspect for pallor in a dark-skinned person, which areas would you assess for an ashen gray or yellow color?
- What is the term that means "a bluish discoloration of the skin"?
- Name two causes of erythema.
- Where can you best see jaundice?

 Go to Chapter 22, **Knowledge Check Response Sheet and Answers,** on the Electronic Study Guide.

| Nursing Diagnosis (Skin) |

You should be familiar with the following common skin problems:

- **Pruritus** (itching), which may lead to scratching and breaks in the skin.
- **Dry skin,** which tends to crack.
- **Maceration** is softening of the skin from prolonged moisture (e.g., urinary incontinence). It makes the epidermis more susceptible to injury.
- **Excoriation** is a loss of the superficial layers of the skin caused by the digestive enzymes in feces.
- **Abrasion,** a rubbing away of the epidermal layer of the skin, especially over bony areas or prominences, is often caused by friction or shearing forces that occur when a patient moves or is moved in bed.
- **Pressure ulcers** (decubitus ulcers) are lesions caused by tissue compression and inadequate perfusion. See Chapter 34.
- **Acne** is an inflammation of the sebaceous glands that is common among adolescents and young adults.

Impaired Skin Integrity as Problem

When you wish to focus on prevention or treatment of the *skin condition,* use the following NANDA (2005) diagnostic labels.

- **Risk for Impaired Skin Integrity.** *Definition:* At risk for skin being adversely altered.
  Risk factors: NANDA lists about 20 specific risk factors (e.g., radiation, obesity). It may be easier for you to remember the general conditions that affect the skin: dampness, dehydration, insufficient circulation,

nutritional status (thin or obese), skin diseases, systemic diseases, and jaundice.

- **Impaired Skin Integrity.** *Definition:* Altered epidermis or dermis (NANDA, 2005).
  Defining characteristics: Invasion of body structures, destruction of skin layers (dermis), disruption of skin surface (epidermis).

Examples of diagnostic statements for skin problems include the following:

Risk for Impaired Skin Integrity related to immobility secondary to casts and traction
Risk for Impaired Skin Integrity related to dehydration and malnutrition
Impaired Skin Integrity related to decreased peripheral circulation secondary to arteriosclerosis
Impaired Skin Integrity related to skin fragility secondary to severe peripheral edema

Impaired Skin Integrity as Etiology

Impaired Skin Integrity may be associated with the development of other nursing diagnoses. Certain skin problems place the patient at risk for infection by causing cracks or breaks in the skin. Others may contribute to discomfort and low self-esteem. The following are examples:

Risk for Infection related to skin lacerations and abrasions
Situational Low Self-Esteem related to appearance and self-consciousness about skin lesions secondary to severe eczema

CriticalThinking 22–5

- Why are Mrs. Williams and Mr. Gold ("Meet Your Patients") at risk for Impaired Skin Integrity?
- What are the specific kinds of skin integrity problems that pose an increased risk to both patients?

| Planning Outcomes/Evaluation (Skin) |

For *NOC standardized outcomes* for problems of the skin, feet, nails, mouth, teeth, hair, eyes, ears, and nose,

 Go to Chapter 22, **Standardized Language, Selected Standardized Outcomes and Interventions for Hygiene Problems,** in Volume 2.

Individualized goals/outcome statements you might write for a patient with skin problems include the following:

- Skin will remain intact and free of secretions.
- Skin will remain free of lesions.
- Will follow regimen to improve skin dryness.

| Plan

For *NIC* s
and skin

Go t
Out
Volu

Individua
paired Sk
which are

Rationa

As the fa
mix with
odor resu
ria from
odor. The
of bathing
the skin,
lates dept
It can als
relationsh
hance wel
have alrea
make a va

Choosin
to Meet

The type
judgment
and endu
know, fun
pendent t
baths are
"Help" ba
the nurse
difficult to
correspon
Box 22–1.
you may s
will clean
comfort, s
ing section

Bed Bath

A **bed ba**
but who a
by placing
basin of w
other bath
metics if
device wit

---

critical aspects of procedures 22–1 through 22–14

Hygiene Procedures *(continued)*

Procedure 22–10: Providing Beard and Mustache Care

- Assess the skin for redness, dry areas, or lesions.
- Trim the beard and mustache to the desired length with a comb and a scissors or beard trimmer.
- Shampoo the beard and mustache.
- Apply conditioner, if desired.
- Towel-dry the beard and mustache, and comb and style as desired.

Procedure 22–11: Shaving a Patient

- Wear procedure gloves.
- Assess the skin for redness or dry areas.
- To soften the beard and moisten the skin:
  - Apply a warm, damp towel to the face.
  - Apply shaving cream or soap.
- To prevent skin irritation:
  - Hold the skin taut, and shave the face and neck.
  - If using a safety razor, hold the blade at a 45-degree angle to the skin.
- Apply after-shave product, if desired.

Procedure 22–12: Removing and Caring for Contact Lenses

- Instill 1 to 2 drops of wetting solution.
- Gently remove contact lenses; use your finger pads, not your fingernails.

- Clean and store contact lenses in sterile solution.
- Mark the containers "L" and "R" to identify the correct eye.

Procedure 22–13: Making an Unoccupied Bed

- Remove soiled linens without cross-contaminating other items in the room.
- Remake the bed with clean linens.
- Do not "shake" or "fan" linens.
- Work efficiently and safely.
- Ensure that there are no wrinkles in the bottom sheet or drawsheet.

Procedure 22–14: Making an Occupied Bed

- Maintain patient safety during the procedure.
- Position the patient laterally near far siderail, and roll soiled linens under him.
- Place clean linens on the side nearest you, and then tuck under the soiled linens.
- Roll the patient over the "hump," and position him on his other side, near you. Raise the near siderail.
- Move to the other side of bed; pull soiled and clean linens through, and complete the linen change as in Procedure 22–13.
- Place the bed in a low position, raise the siderails, and fasten the call light to the pillow.

CriticalThinking 22–7

- Which of your patients ("Meet Your Patients") will require nurse-assisted perineal care? Explain your reasoning.
- Which patient, if you are a woman, is most likely to be embarrassed by perineal care? Explain your reasoning.
- If you need more theoretical knowledge to answer these questions, what is it? Where could you find the information?

Towel Bath

A **towel bath** is a modification of the bed bath, in which you place a large towel and a bath blanket in a plastic bag, saturate them with a commercially prepared mixture of moisturizer, disinfectant, non-rinse cleaning agent, and water; warm them in a microwave, and use them to bathe the patient. Because the solution dries rapidly, there is no need to towel-

dry the patient. Some agencies prefer towel baths because they take less time than a traditional bed bath and because patients find them satisfactory. This is a preferred method for patients who have mild to moderate Impaired Skin Integrity or Activity Intolerance and for patients with dementia (e.g., Alzheimer's disease).

 Go to Chapter 22, **Procedure 22-2: Bathing: Providing a Towel Bath,** in Volume 2.

Bag or Packaged Bath

A **bag bath** is a modification of the towel bath, in which you use 8 to 10 washcloths instead of a towel and bath blanket. Each part of the patient's body is cleansed with a fresh cloth. A **packaged bath** simply refers to a set of commercially prepared and packaged,

home care

Showers and Baths

- Assess the patient's self-care abilities: sensorimotor, musculoskeletal, and cognitive function; activity tolerance; level of knowledge.

- Advise parents never to leave a child alone in the tub or shower and to have a way to unlock the bathroom door from outside the room.

- For patients who have impaired mobility or activity intolerance:

    Advise use of a shower chair (see below) in the shower or tub.

    Encourage patients and families to install hand bars on the sides of the bathtub and on the wall next to the tub.

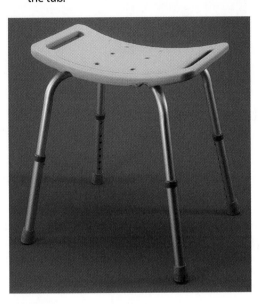

Shower chair

- Advise patients not to lock the bathroom door while bathing so that help can be summoned if needed (e.g., if they become faint).

- Ensure that there is a nonskid surface or mat in the shower or tub. Handrails and grab bars also help prevent falls.

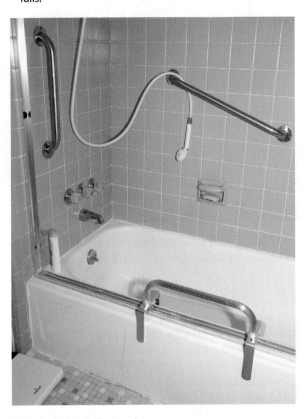

Bathtub with handrail and grab bars

premoistened, disposable washcloths that are used in the same way as a bag bath.

 Go to Chapter 22, **Procedure 22–3: Bathing: Providing a Packaged or Bag Bath,** in Volume 2.

CriticalThinking 22–6

Suppose you have been providing towel baths to a patient who has mild dementia. One day a visiting family member says, "My father tells me that he has not had a bath all week. What's going on here?" What would you do? How could you help to prevent this misunderstanding in the future?

Shower

Most ambulatory patients prefer a shower. It is a time-saver and refreshing as well as cleansing. In a hospital or long-term care facility, some clients can manage a shower mostly on their own. Even so, you will still

need to be sure that the shower or tub is clean and safe. Most hospitals and long-term care facilities have grab bars and handrails in the bathrooms, but these may need to be installed in the home. You may also need to prepare the client's bathing supplies, assist her to the shower, and help with areas of her body that she cannot reach. For complete information, refer to the accompanying Home Care box. Also,

 Go to Chapter 22, **Technique 22–1: Assisting with a Shower or Tub Bath,** in Volume 2.

Tub Bath

If a client is ambulatory but requires much assistance with bathing (for example, because of pain and stiffness in the hands and arms) you may prefer a tub bath. It will be easier for you to wash and rinse the patient, and you will not get as wet as when you help with a shower. Immersion in the water also helps to soak areas that

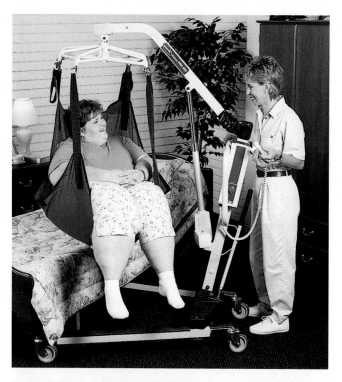
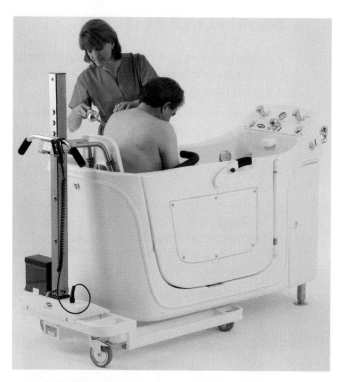

FIGURE 22–1 *A,* A hydraulic lift allows you to transport a patient to a bath or shower. *B,* A tub with a side-opening door enables patients to safely and easily enter the tub. *Source:* Courtesy of Carroll Health Care, London, Ontario, Canada.

are crusty, scaly, or soiled and is relaxing to stiff, sore muscles and joints. Overall, tub baths are thought to be of greater benefit than a sponge or bed bath. Your responsibilities for a tub bath are similar to those of a shower if the patient is ambulatory, and similar to a help bath if the patient requires a great deal of support.

The tub should have handrails and a nonskid surface to prevent falls (see the Home Care box on page 453). Some patients need assistance getting into and out of a tub. To assist, have the patient grasp the handrails near the tub, and steady her as she places first one foot, then the other, in the tub. Or, you can place a chair beside the tub and help the patient place her feet in the tub; then she can reach for the handrail on the opposite side of the tub, stand up, and ease down into the tub. Some patients kneel or squat first and then sit in the tub. For completely dependent patients, there are specially designed tubs that reduce the effort necessary to lift patients into and out of the tub. You can also use a hydraulic lift and a regular tub (Figure 22–1). For more information about tub baths,

 Go to Chapter 22, **Technique 22–1: Assisting with a Shower or Tub Bath,** in Volume 2.

Therapeutic Bath

The physician may prescribe **therapeutic baths** for some patients. The order will include specific instructions for the type of bath and solution to be used, area of the body to be treated, and water temperature. Oatmeal or coal tar baths are examples of therapeutic baths used to treat specific skin conditions, such as chickenpox lesions or psoriasis. It is your responsibility to add the medically ordered substance, ensure appropriate temperature, assist the patient into the tub, and clean the tub at the end of the bath. A warm sitz bath is another type of therapeutic bath; it helps to cleanse the perineum and soothe inflammation of perineal, vaginal, or rectal tissues.

Bathing Patients with Dementia

Bathing should be a pleasant time, not a stressful one. However, this is not true for all patients, especially those with dementia. One study found that more than 90% of people with dementia became agitated when told it was time to bathe (Kovach & Meyer-Arnold, 1996). They commonly yell, scream, pinch, or hit their caregivers (Rasin & Barrick, 2004). The reason behind the patients' agitation, it has been found, is that they experience pain, cold, fear, and loss of control. When the nurse meets these needs, the aggressive behavior declines significantly. Simply by changing the water temperature or taking special care when washing arthritic joints, you may make the patient more comfortable and less agitated.

Nurses and UAPs sometimes focus, mistakenly, on the need to give a daily tub bath or shower instead of individualizing the procedure to meet patient

needs. Caregivers can significantly reduce aggressive behaviors by giving a towel bath instead (Rasin & Barrick, 2004). Despite the common myths about bathing, keep in mind that:

- It does not take a lot of water (e.g., a shower) to get a person clean.
- The bath does not have to be performed at the same time every day, nor in the way "we have always done it here."
- You can educate families that a shower or tub bath are not the only ways to get clean.
- The patient will not be at more risk for skin problems or infections if a towel bath is used.
- It is not necessary to bathe a person who is resisting. You can adapt the approach, method, and time.
- Patients who are forced to bathe do not "just forget about it"; many stay upset and agitated for hours.

For more discussion of bathing myths and for instructions about providing a towel bath for a person with dementia,

 Go to **www.bathingwithoutabattle.unc.edu/main_page.html**

Back Massage

Regardless of the type of bath used, when possible end the bath with a back massage to provide relaxation and stimulate circulation. As with all procedures, be sure there are no contraindications to massage (e.g., fractured ribs, burns, recent heart surgery).

 | VOL 2 | Go to Chapter 33, **Procedure 33–1: Giving a Back Massage,** in Volume 2.

KnowledgeCheck 22–5

- A nurse has given a bath in which he washed a bedridden patient's entire body without assistance from the patient. What is the term for this bath?
- What are the advantages of a towel or bag bath?
- For which type of bath will you most likely have a medical order?

 Go to Chapter 22, **Knowledge Check Response Sheet and Answers,** on the Electronic Study Guide.

 CriticalThinking 22–8

- Which type of bath would be most appropriate for each of your patients ("Meet Your Patients")?
- Provide rationale for your choices.

CARE OF THE FEET

Foot care is a necessary part of hygiene and essential at any age for tissue health, proper posture, and ambulation.

Theoretical Knowledge
knowing why

When providing foot care, you will need theoretical knowledge about the structure of the feet, life span variations, and common foot problems. The feet provide support for the weight of the entire body and absorb a significant amount of shock during walking. Their musculoskeletal structure is complex, consisting of 26 bones and many muscles, tendons, and ligaments. The feet can be affected by congenital malformations, injuries, improper footwear, and medical conditions. For example, a person with diabetes mellitus or peripheral neuropathy (nerve damage) may experience decreased sensation and delayed healing of open areas on the feet, and people with arthritis experience pain and decreased mobility.

Developmental Variations

The feet are fully grown at about age 20 and, if healthy, change little throughout life. However, risk factors do increase with aging. Because of diseases such as arteriosclerosis and peripheral vascular insufficiency, older adults often have decreased circulation to the lower extremities. This decreased circulation increases their risk for foot ulcers and infection. The incidence of diabetes is high among older adults, creating further risk for infection secondary to delayed healing. Additionally, the skin becomes dry with aging, predisposing the person to cracking of the skin.

Common Foot Problems and Nursing Implications

Over 43 million people in the United States have foot abnormalities (e.g., pain, deformity, and disability). Many of these problems are the result of improperly fitting shoes (American Academy of Orthopedic Surgeons, 2001).

- **Corns.** A corn is a cone-shaped thickening of the epidermis caused by continuous pressure (e.g., from improperly fitting shoes) over bony prominences, such as the toe joints. Corns are often painful.
- **Calluses.** Calluses are usually found over bony prominences in the weight-bearing part of the foot: the heels, soles, or plantar surfaces of the feet. They are similar to corns but cover a wider area and are not painful.
- **Tinea pedis.** Athlete's foot, a fungal infection of the skin, is aggravated by moisture accumulation in unventilated shoes. Symptoms include itching and burning skin with blisters, scaling, and cracking,

especially between the toes. Athlete's foot may be contracted by walking barefoot in public showers.

- **Ingrown toenail.** Improperly trimming the toenails and wearing poorly fitting shoes may cause an ingrown toenail, in which the toenail grows inward into the soft tissues around it. The tissue at the nail border becomes swollen, inflamed, and painful; the nail may need to be surgically removed.
- **Foot odor.** Microorganism growth on the feet interacts with perspiration to produce foot odor. The warm, moist environment created by shoes encourages both perspiration and bacterial growth.
- **Plantar wart.** A painful growth caused by a virus. It may occur on any part of the sole of the foot.
- **Pressure ulcers.** A lesion caused by unrelieved pressure that impairs the circulation; this usually occurs over a bony prominence. Pressure ulcers are not limited to the foot; in bedridden patients, the back of the heels, the ankles, and the great toes are common locations.

Practical Knowledge
knowing how

The nursing focus for foot care is on prevention and early identification of problems.

| Assessment (Feet) |

Careful assessment of the feet allows for early detection of common foot problems. For a thorough discussion of foot assessment, see Chapter 19. This chapter describes routine observations that you can make when giving foot care.

You will need information about the patient's normal foot care routine, the type of footwear he usually wears, any foot problems or treatments for them, and any diseases (e.g., diabetes mellitus and peripheral vascular disease) that create risks for foot problems.

As you observe the feet, compare findings for both feet. Assess cleanliness, odor, and skin integrity. Inspect for redness, drainage, and swelling. Palpate for edema, and check for cracks or signs of fungal infection between the toes. The color and temperature of the feet provide data about circulation and oxygenation. For example, cold, dusky feet may indicate impaired circulation or tissue perfusion secondary to peripheral vascular disease. Check capillary refill. For specific questions to ask,

 Go to Chapter 22, **Assessment Guidelines and Tools, Assessment Guidelines: Hygiene,** in Volume 2.

| Nursing Diagnosis (Feet) |

The following are examples of nursing diagnoses related to the feet:

- Impaired Skin (or Tissue) Integrity (feet) related to mechanical pressure from wearing shoes that do not fit properly
- Risk for Impaired Skin Integrity (feet) related to (1) decreased sensation secondary to diabetes mellitus and (2) decreased circulation to the feet secondary to arteriosclerosis
- Impaired Walking related to foot pain secondary to arthritis
- Risk for Injury (to feet) related to deficient knowledge of foot hygiene

 Go to Chapter 22, **Standardized Language, Selected NOC Outcomes and NIC Interventions for Hygiene Problems,** in Volume 2.

| Planning Outcomes/Evaluation (Feet) |

For associated *NOC standardized outcomes* for patients with common foot problems,

 Go to Chapter 22, **Standardized Language, Selected NOC Outcomes and NIC Interventions for Hygiene Problems,** in Volume 2.

Individualized goals/outcome statements you might write for a patient with foot problems include the following:

- Demonstrates proper cleansing, rinsing, and drying of the feet.
- Avoids trimming calluses.
- Wears shoes that fit properly.
- Inspects feet regularly.

| Planning Interventions/Implementation (Feet) |

For *NIC standardized interventions* related to care of the feet,

Go to Chapter 22, **Standardized Language, Selected NOC Outcomes and NIC Interventions for Hygiene Problems,** in Volume 2.

Individualized nursing activities related to care of the feet are those that prevent infection, odor, and trauma to the soft tissues of the feet. While performing foot care, teach the patient about self-care measures for care of the feet (see the accompanying

Teaching Your Client About Foot Care

Use the time during foot care to teach your client the following self-care activities. These measures are good advice for most people, but they are especially important for people who have diabetes or poor peripheral circulation.

Daily Foot Inspection

- Inspect the feet daily, using a mirror to view all surfaces. Check between the toes for cracks or redness. Look for calluses or dry areas. If you cannot check your own feet, have someone else do it.

- Report any signs of foot problems to the physician.

- If you have diabetes, have your feet checked regularly by a professional.

- Seek professional help for foot problems, such as poor circulation, corns, and ingrown toenails, and for trimming very thick nails—especially if you have diabetes.

Hygiene for Feet and Nails

- Wash, rinse, and dry the feet well.

- Avoid soaking the feet (if you are diabetic, or if there is decreased circulation to the feet).

- Apply a water-soluble lotion to feet, but do not use lotion between the toes, because it may cause maceration.

- Use an antifungal powder, if necessary, for athlete's foot.

- Do not cut or file callused areas.

- Cut and file toenails straight across. Do not use a razor blade on the nails or feet.

Shoes and Stockings

- Wear cotton or wool socks, which absorb perspiration.

- Wear well-fitted, sturdy shoes with nonskid soles and arch support. Natural materials, such as canvas and leather, are best because they allow air to circulate and perspiration to evaporate. Shoes should allow $^1/_2$ to $^3/_4$ inch of toe room.

- Avoid open-toed shoes, sandals, high heels, and thongs. They do not protect the feet.

- Before putting on shoes, check for foreign objects; check that the inside of the shoe is smooth.

Protecting the Feet

- Avoid measures that impair circulation to the feet, such as wearing tight garters or knee stockings, or crossing the legs.

- Do not go barefoot, even when getting out of bed at night. Wear slippers.

- Do not put tape or over-the-counter corn medicines or pads or other medications (e.g., hydrogen perioxide) on the feet.

- Do not smoke. This further decreases circulation to the feet.

Self-Care box). To learn how to administer foot care,

 Go to Chapter 22, **Procedure 22–5: Providing Foot Care,** in Volume 2.

Also see the Critical Aspects box for Procedures 22–1 through 22–14.

Diabetic Foot Care

Because of impaired circulation and increased risk for infection, people who have diabetes are at high risk for problems with their feet. If they have neuropathy, they may not experience pain with a foot injury, so treatment may be delayed. If untreated, a seemingly minor foot lesion can progress to gangrene and require amputation. The instructions in the Self-Care box, "Teaching Your Client About Foot Care," are especially important for people with diabetes (as well as for those with impaired peripheral circulation).

KnowledgeCheck 22–6

- What are some causes of ingrown toenails?
- What is the cause of foot odor?
- Why should you *not* apply lotion between the toes?

 Go to Chapter 22, **Knowledge Check Response Sheet and Answers,** on the Electronic Study Guide.

CARE OF THE NAILS

Composed of epithelial tissue, the nails are part of the integumentary system. Healthy nailbeds are usually clean, pink, smooth, convex, and evenly curved. Present at birth, the nails change very little throughout life; however, as one ages, nails thicken, become ridged, and may yellow or become concave in shape. Other changes are caused by certain pathological conditions. For example, inadequate diet or metabolic changes can cause the nails to become brittle. Also, patients with diabetes mellitus are much more prone to infection and must be vigilant about toenail care.

Teaching Your Client About Nail Care

- Inspect the nails daily.
- Trim nails with a nail clipper. (People with diabetes or circulatory problems should file only, because cutting poses a risk for injury to the tissues.)
- File the nails straight across, rounding the corners slightly to prevent scratching. Do not cut deeply into the lateral corners, because this may cause ingrown nails.
- Remove hangnails by carefully cutting them off.
- Clean under the nails with an orangewood stick or other blunt instrument.
- Push back the cuticles gently.
- Use a moisturizing lotion to soften cuticles.
- Avoid biting nails.
- Consult a podiatrist for ingrown toenails or other nail problems.
- Recommend to patients with diabetes, circulatory insufficiency, or nail problems that they seek nail care from a podiatrist.

| Assessment (Nails) |

Unclean or rough fingernails may scratch or abrade the skin and pose a risk for infection secondary to impaired skin integrity. Other nail changes may reflect an underlying disease process. When assessing the nails, you should obtain *subjective data* about the patient's usual nail care practices, any history of nail problems, and their treatments. To obtain *objective data,* inspect the nails for shape, contour, and cleanliness. Look for redness or swelling of the skin around the nails, and observe whether they are neatly manicured and trimmed appropriately, straight across.

For more information about physical assessment of the nails, see Chapter 19, and

 Go to Chapter 22, **Assessment Guidelines and Tools, Assessment Guidelines: Hygiene,** in Volume 2.

| Nursing Diagnosis (Nails) |

There are no NANDA labels to describe nail problems. However, the following are some examples of nursing diagnoses related to nail care:

- Risk for Impaired Tissue Integrity related to ingrown nails secondary to trimming too close to the cuticle

- Risk for Infection related to loss of skin integrity secondary to hangnails, cracked cuticles, or trauma from using sharp scissors or nail clippers

 Go to Chapter 22, **Standardized Language, Selected NOC Outcomes and NIC Interventions for Hygiene Problems,** in Volume 2.

| Planning Outcomes/Evaluation (Nails) |

Associated NOC standardized outcomes are determined by the nursing diagnosis. For some examples,

 Go to Chapter 22, **Standardized Language, Selected NOC Outcomes and NIC Interventions for Hygiene Problems,** in Volume 2.

Individualized goals/outcome statements you might write for a patient with problems related to the care of the nails may include the following:

- Demonstrates proper care of the nails.
- Trims fingernails with supervision.
- Seeks care of a **podiatrist** (physician who specializes in foot care) for toenail care.

| Planning Interventions/Implementation (Nails) |

For *NIC standardized interventions* related to care of the nails,

 Go to Chapter 22, **Standardized Language, Selected NOC Outcomes and NIC Interventions,** in Volume 2.

Individualized nursing activities related to proper care of the nails include the following:

- Teaching for self-care (see the Self-Care box, "Teaching Your Client About Nail Care")
- Providing nail care for dependent patients (the procedure for care of the fingernails is the same as for care of the toenails).

 Go to Chapter 22, **Procedure 22–5: Providing Foot Care,** in Volume 2.

KnowledgeCheck 22–7

- True or False: Healthy nails are usually clean, smooth, and convexly curved.
- List at least three nail changes that occur with aging.
- List at least four things you should teach clients about self-care of their nails.

 Go to Chapter 22, **Knowledge Check Response Sheet and Answers,** on the Electronic Study Guide.

ORAL HYGIENE

To maintain the integrity of the mucous membranes, teeth, and gums, and to prevent tooth loss and gum disease, it is important to have (1) routine dental checkups, (2) adequate nutrition, and (3) daily mouth care or oral hygiene. Mouth care removes food particles and secretions. In addition, a clean mouth helps to promote a better appetite.

Theoretical Knowledge
knowing why

Digestion of food begins in the mouth (oral cavity). The tongue and teeth begin digestion by breaking up food and mixing it with the saliva. Saliva, produced by three pairs of salivary glands in the mouth, also acts as a mechanical cleaner of the mouth. The structures of the mouth pertinent to oral hygiene include the tongue, **gingiva** (gums), and teeth.

Developmental Variations

The first set of teeth (the **deciduous teeth**) erupts between 6 months and 2 years of age. By age 2, a child usually has 20 teeth (Figure 22–2). Between ages 6 and 12 years, the deciduous teeth loosen, fall out, and are eventually replaced with 32 permanent teeth (Figure 22–3). **Wisdom teeth** are the very back molars on either side of each jawbone. Some people have no room for the four wisdom teeth to erupt, so they may need to be extracted to prevent damage to other teeth.

With aging, tooth surface is abraded, and the gums may begin to recede, resulting in bone and tooth loss and necessitating the use of dentures or false teeth. Poorly fitted or loose dentures can lead to chewing difficulties and even nutritional deficiencies. Other changes that may occur with aging are a brownish pigmentation of the gums and dryness of the oral mucosa, which is caused by decreased saliva production.

Risk Factors for Oral Problems

Oral health is influenced by heredity, nutrition, and oral hygiene. Therefore, any condition that prevents good oral hygiene can lead to oral problems. Such risk factors include the following:

- *History of periodontal disease.*
- *Lack of money or insurance for dental care.*
- *Pregnancy.* Increased estrogen during pregnancy increases the vascularity of the gingiva. The gums may bleed easily and become puffy and tender. The condition disappears after birth, but good hygiene is needed meanwhile to prevent infection.

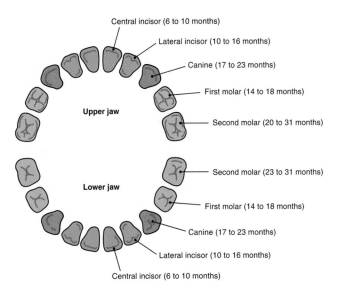

FIGURE 22–2   The 20 deciduous teeth typically erupt by age 2. *Source: Courtesy of P. Dillon (2003), Nursing Health Assessment. Philadelphia: F. A. Davis.*

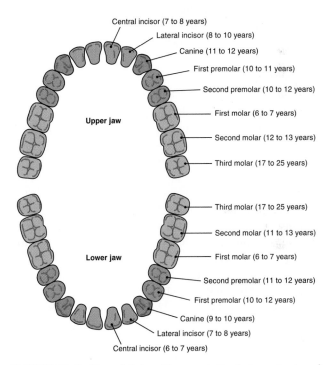

FIGURE 22–3   Most adults have 32 permanent teeth. *Source: Courtesy of P. Dillon (2003), Nursing Health Assessment. Philadelphia: F. A. Davis.*

- *Poor nutrition or eating habits.* Adequate intake of calcium, phosphorus, and vitamin D is essential for healthy teeth and gums. Excessive intake of refined sugars leads to dental decay. One example of this is **baby-bottle tooth decay,** which occurs when parents put an infant or toddler to bed with a bottle of milk or fruit juice. Carbohydrates in the fluid cause demineralization of the tooth enamel, leading to major decay of the upper and lower teeth.
- *Some medications and medical treatments.* The anticonvulsant phenytoin (Dilantin), causes gingival **hyperplasia** (excessive growth of cells). Other

medications cause dryness of the mouth. These include diuretics, laxatives (used excessively), medications used to treat cancer, and tranquilizers such as chlorpromazine (Thorazine) and diazepam (Valium). Medical treatments affecting the oral cavity include the following:

Jaw surgery, which requires scrupulous oral hygiene to prevent infection

Radiation treatments of the head and neck. These can permanently damage the salivary glands, resulting in dryness of the mouth. Radiation can also damage teeth and jaw structure.

Oxygen therapy, which dries the oral mucosa, especially if the client must breathe through the mouth.

Presence of nasogastric tubes, especially if the person breathes through his mouth.

• *Any situation that causes dry mouth predisposes to cracking* of the mucosa:

Heavy cigarette smoking

Excessive alcohol use

Inadequate fluid intake or dehydration (e.g., being NPO)

Mouth breathing

• *Compromised self-care abilities* may be caused by:

Decreased level of consciousness (e.g., a person who is comatose or heavily sedated). Such patients are, in addition, likely to breathe through the mouth, causing dryness of the mucous membranes.

Serious illness or injury, weakness, activity intolerance, or paralysis.

Cognitive impairment, as seen in patients with developmental delay, dementia, and certain mental illnesses.

Depression.

Lack of knowledge or motivation to perform self-care (e.g., lack of daily brushing and flossing).

KnowledgeCheck 22–8

• How do the teeth aid in digesting food?
• How many deciduous teeth does a child usually have?
• List at least three factors that cause dry mouth.
• List at least two medications or medical treatments that can cause oral problems.
• Name four situations that can compromise self-care ability for oral hygiene.

 Go to Chapter 22, **Knowledge Check Response Sheet and Answers,** on the Electronic Study Guide.

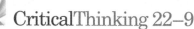 CriticalThinking 22–9

• For which of your patients, Mrs. Williams or Mr. Gold, does the scenario provide *actual data* to indicate that the patient is at risk for oral problems? What is the data?

• Why is the patient's nursing diagnosis Risk for Impaired Oral Mucous Membrane instead of Impaired Oral Mucous Membrane?

Common Problems of the Mouth

Dental caries (cavities) and periodontal disease are the two most frequent problems affecting the teeth. They are discussed here along with other common mouth problems:

• **Halitosis,** or bad breath, results from poor oral hygiene, eating certain foods (e.g., garlic, onions), tobacco use, dental caries, infections, or even a systemic disease such as uncontrolled diabetes or liver disease.

• **Dental caries,** or cavities, are caused primarily by a failure to remove **plaque,** an invisible, destructive bacterial film that builds up on the teeth. Plaque buildup eventually leads to destruction of the tooth enamel. Factors that contribute to the formation of cavities include excessive intake of refined sugars, a lack of brushing and flossing, and infrequent visits to the dentist.

• **Gingivitis** is inflammation of the gum tissue surrounding the teeth. If untreated, it may progress to periodontal disease.

• **Periodontal disease (pyorrhea)** is the major cause of tooth loss in adults 35 years and older. It is an inflammation characterized by bleeding and receding gums and destruction of the surrounding bone structure. The patient experiences halitosis and complains of a bad taste in the mouth. When pyorrhea is advanced, the gums become infected, and the teeth loosen and may fall out or need to be removed.

Tooth loss is the result of untreated plaque, which builds up with dead bacteria and forms hard deposits at the gum lines **(tartar).** The tartar causes deterioration of the supporting structures that hold the teeth in the gums and also attacks the bone tissue, causing the teeth to become loose.

• **Stomatitis,** an inflammation of the oral mucosa, has numerous causes, including bacteria, mechanical trauma, irritants, nutritional deficiencies, and systemic infection. Symptoms may include pain, halitosis, and increased salivation.

• **Glossitis,** an inflammation of the tongue, is caused by deficiencies of vitamin B_{12}, folic acid, and iron.

• **Cheilosis** is a cracking and/or ulceration of the lips, in the form of reddened fissures at the angles of the mouth. It is usually caused by vitamin B-complex deficiencies.

• **Oral malignancies** must be detected as early as possible. The patient should be taught to see a dentist

immediately if any of the following are present in the mouth: lumps, ulcers, white or red patches, bleeding, pain, persistent sores, or numbness.

KnowledgeCheck 22–9

* Define and identify several causes of halitosis.
* What are the two most common problems affecting the teeth?
* What is the end result of severe periodontal disease?

 Go to Chapter 22, **Knowledge Check Response Sheet and Answers,** on the Electronic Study Guide.

Practical Knowledge
knowing how

| Assessment (Oral Cavity) |

You might begin your subjective assessment by asking the client about his usual hygiene practices. You should also interview the patient or examine his records for the risk factors for oral problems discussed on page 459–460 (i.e., history of oral problems, nutritional status, access to dental care, medications such as anticonvulsants or diuretics, radiation therapy, oxygen therapy, NPO status, dehydration, and nasogastric tubes). Ask about smoking and alcohol use.

As part of your objective assessment during hygiene care, inspect the lips, oral mucosa, gums, and tongue. Mucosa and gums should be pink and moist without lesions or bleeding. Look for loose, missing, or decaying teeth, and note any unusual odors or halitosis.

To learn more about physical assessment of the oral cavity, refer to Chapter 19. Also,

 Go to Chapter 22, **Assessment Guides and Tools, Assessment Guidelines: Hygiene,** in Volume 2.

| Nursing Diagnosis (Oral Cavity) |

In addition to Self-Care Deficit, discussed in the first part of the chapter, the following are examples of nursing diagnoses that may be useful in describing problems of the mouth:

* Risk for Infection related to mouth lesions
* Impaired Dentition (caries) related to inability to afford dental care
* Impaired Oral Mucous Membrane related to inability to manage mouth care secondary to impaired mobility
* Deficient Knowledge related to lack of interest in learning about oral hygiene

Oral and dental problems can be the etiology of other nursing diagnoses, for example:

* Imbalanced Nutrition related to lack of teeth for mastication
* Pain related to mouth lesions

 Go to Chapter 22, **Standardized Language, Selected NOC Outcomes and NIC Interventions for Hygiene Problems,** in Volume 2.

| Planning Outcomes/Evaluation (Oral Cavity) |

For *NOC standardized outcomes* for Impaired Oral Mucous Membrane, Risk for Impaired Oral Mucous Membrane, and Impaired Dentition,

 Go to **Chapter 22, Standardized Language, Selected NOC Outcomes and NIC Interventions for Hygiene Problems,** in Volume 2.

Individualized goals/outcome statements you might write for mouth problems include the following:

* Oral mucous membranes will remain pink, moist, and intact.
* Brushes teeth after each meal.
* Flosses daily.
* Demonstrates correct technique for brushing and flossing.
* Makes preventive dental visits every 6 months.

| Planning Interventions/Implementation (Oral Cavity) |

For some patients, you may need only to provide the necessary supplies for mouth care. For others, you will need to assist or even completely provide care as often as necessary to keep the mouth clean and moist. Mouthwash is not a substitute for a thorough cleaning of the teeth and mouth.

For *NIC standardized interventions* you might use for potential and actual Impaired Oral Mucous Membranes and Impaired Dentition,

 Go to Chapter 22, **Standardized Language, Selected NOC Outcomes and NIC Interventions for Hygiene Problems,** in Volume 2.

Individualized nursing activities related to oral hygiene include (1) teaching for self-care (see the Self-Care box, "Teaching Your Client about Oral Hygiene") and (2) assisting with and providing oral hygiene for dependent patients.

Teaching Your Client About Oral Hygiene

Measures to promote oral health and prevent periodontal disease and caries include the following:

Preventing Caries and Periodontal Disease

- Eliminate sweet snacks between meals (ice cream, soft drinks, candy, gum, jams and jellies).

- Include in the diet cleansing, fibrous foods, such as raw fruits and vegetables.

- Include an adequate intake of calcium, phosphorus, and vitamins A, C, and D.

- Have regular dental checkups every 6 months.

- Brush teeth with a soft brush and toothpaste after each meal and at bedtime (some dentists say twice a day). Bacteria do the most damage to the teeth in the first 24 hours after eating.

- Floss between the teeth daily to remove food debris.

- Use a fluoride toothpaste, or make your own cleanser by combining one part baking soda with two parts salt.

- Follow the dentist's recommendations for topical applications of fluoride.

Brushing and Flossing

- Make sure the brush is small enough to reach all teeth. If it is too firm, it can injure enamel and gum tissue.

- Electric toothbrushes are effective; however, you should consult your dentist about using waterspray units, because they can force debris into pockets of the gums.

- Brush at a 45-degree angle, from the gum to the tooth crown, using small circular or vibrating motions.

- When flossing, (1) wrap one end of the floss around each of your middle fingers. (2) Hold about 1 to 2 inches of floss tightly between the fingers. (3) Insert

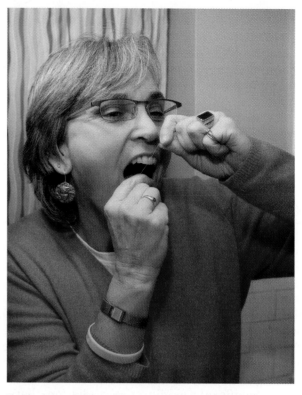

Flossing between the teeth is an essential part of oral hygiene.

floss between the teeth by gently moving it back and forth; do not force it. (4) Floss adjacent sides of both teeth to the gum tissue, but not into the gum, because you may injure the tissue. (5) Use a fresh section of floss when it becomes soiled or frayed. (6) Rinse your mouth well when you are finished.

Oral Hygiene for Children

- Begin oral hygiene when the first tooth erupts. Use a washcloth, cotton ball, or gauze pad moistened with water.

- Do not put the child to bed with a bottle.

Oral Care for Unconscious Patients

Oral care for unconscious patients is particularly important because they often breathe through the mouth. If the patient is receiving oxygen per cannula or has a nasogastric or feeding tube inserted, the mucous membranes dry out even more. When providing oral care for an unconscious person, place him on his side, and use a minimal amount of solution to prevent aspiration. An unconscious patient often responds to oral stimulation by biting down, so use a padded tongue blade instead of your fingers to hold the mouth open.

Follow agency practices for the type and frequency of special mouth care. Some patients may need it every

hour or two. You may use commercially packaged applicators or foam swabs to clean the mouth. However, lemon-glycerine swabs are not recommended for long-term use because they are drying to the mucosa and may causes changes in tooth enamel. You should not use hydrogen peroxide because it is irritating to oral mucosa and may alter the balance of normal flora of the mouth. To learn more about how to provide oral care for unconscious patients,

 Go to Chapter 22, **Procedure 22–6: Brushing and Flossing the Teeth; Procedure 22–7: Providing Denture Care;** and **Procedure 22–8: Providing Oral Hygiene for an Unconscious Patient,** in Volume 2.

(continued)

- Begin brushing the child's teeth with a soft toothbrush when she is about 18 months old. Start first using water only. Later, switch to a fluoride-containing toothpaste.

- Follow your dentist's instructions for giving a fluoride supplement.

- Schedule a visit to the dentist when all 20 deciduous teeth have erupted.

- See your dentist if you notice any problems such as chipping, redness or swelling, caries, or misalignment.

- For school-age children, parents may need to supervise mouth care to be sure it is done adequately.

Care of Dentures

- If you have dentures or other removable prostheses ("bridges"), wear them. If you do not, the gums are likely to shrink, and you will have further gum loss.

- Clean dentures and bridges at least once a day, preferably after each meal.

- Remove dentures from the mouth to clean them.

- Use regular toothpaste or special denture-cleaning compounds.

- Do not use hot water on dentures; it may damage them.

- If the dentures have metal parts, do not soak them overnight in cleaning solutions.

- Store dentures in a denture cup, in water, to prevent drying. Do not wrap them in tissues because they may accidentally be thrown away.

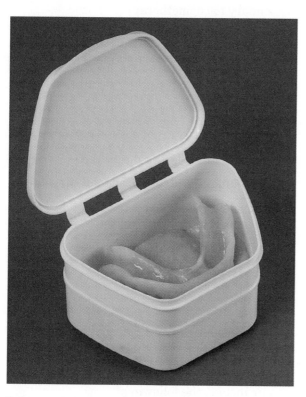

Patients may have an upper, lower, or partial denture.

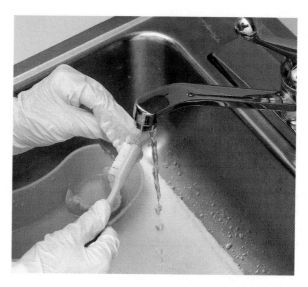

Dentures must be cleaned thoroughly as a part of daily oral hygiene.

See also the Critical Aspects box for Procedures 22–1 through 22–14.

Denture Care

A patient may have a complete set of removable dentures or just an upper or lower plate. Another type of appliance is a **bridge** or partial plate, which consists of one or more artificial teeth. A bridge may be permanently fastened to other teeth, or it may be removable. Artificial teeth are fitted to the individual and should not be used by anyone else. If the person leaves the prosthesis out of his mouth for long periods, the shape of the gums will change, and it will no longer fit properly. The nurse's role is to assure cleanliness by teaching for self-care (see the Self-Care box, "Teaching Your Client About Oral Hygiene") or providing denture care for dependent patients.

 Go to Chapter 22, **Procedure 22–7: Providing Denture Care,** in Volume 2.

See also the Critical Aspects box for Procedures 22–1 through 22–14.

KnowledgeCheck 22–10

How would you position Mr. Gold ("Meet Your Patients") to perform his oral hygiene?

 Go to Chapter 22, **Knowledge Check Response Sheet and Answers,** on the Electronic Study Guide.

CARE OF THE HAIR

Hair is an accessory structure of the skin. The hair helps to maintain body temperature, serves as a receptor for tactile sensation, and influences a person's self-image. **Vellus hair** is the short, fine hair present over much of the body. **Terminal hair,** which is coarser, darker, and longer, is found on the scalp, eyebrows, axillae, perineum, and legs. Sebaceous glands found at the base of the hair follicle secrete sebum, or oil, to lubricate hair and scalp. The condition of the hair is a measure of a person's overall health. See Chapter 19 to read more information about changes in hair that occur through the life span and as a result of illness.

| Assessment (Hair) |

For the purposes of hygiene, you will need information about the patient's history of hair problems or current conditions needing treatment (e.g., pediculosis), diseases or therapy that affect the hair (e.g., chemotherapy), and factors influencing the patient's ability to manage her hair and scalp care (e.g., Impaired Mobility). Ask the patient about special products she uses and about her preference for styling of the hair. Inspect the condition and cleanliness of the hair, and inspect the scalp for dandruff, lesions, and so forth. For more complete information about assessing the hair, see Chapter 19. Also,

 Go to Chapter 22, **Assessment Guidelines and Tools, Assessment Guidelines: Hygiene,** in Volume 2.

| Nursing Diagnosis (Hair) |

Common problems associated with the hair and scalp include the following (also see Chapter 19):

- **Dandruff** is a condition in which there is excessive shedding of the epidermal layer of the scalp. Primary symptoms include itching and flaking of the scalp, which may be caused by fungal infection.
- **Pediculosis** is an infestation of head lice. Though frequently associated with poor hygiene practices, it knows no socioeconomic boundaries. Head lice spread through sharing of combs, brushes, hair ornaments, hats, and caps.
- **Alopecia,** or hair loss, can be very stressful and affect self-image. Abnormal hair loss, which may be gradual or sudden, can be caused by an autoimmune disorder, hormonal imbalance, thyroid disease, stress, fever, certain medications, or chemotherapy.

There are no NANDA labels that apply specifically to the hair. When the difficulty lies with self-care ability, you can of course use Dressing/Grooming Self-Care Deficit and Bathing/Hygiene Self-Care Deficit. Examples of other nursing diagnoses that may apply include the following:

- Risk for Impaired Skin Integrity related to secretions on the scalp
- Situational Low Self-Esteem related to inability to perform grooming tasks
- Situational Low Self-Esteem related to alopecia secondary to chemotherapy

KnowledgeCheck 22–11

- List at least four assessments you should make of a patient's hair.
- What is pediculosis?
- What is alopecia?

 Go to Chapter 22, **Knowledge Check Response Sheet and Answers,** on the Electronic Study Guide.

| Planning Outcomes/Evaluation (Hair) |

For *NOC standardized outcomes* for patients with problems related to care of the hair,

 Go to Chapter 22, **Standardized Language, Selected NOC Outcomes and NIC Interventions for Hygiene Problems,** in Volume 2.

As always, you will select outcomes based on the client's nursing diagnoses.

Individualized goals/outcome statements you might write for a patient with problems related to the hair include the following:

- Scalp and hair are clean.
- States preferences for hair styling.
- By 9/18, brushes own hair.
- Hair and scalp are free from infestation, infection, irritation, or dryness.
- Verbalizes improved comfort and self-esteem.

| Planning Interventions/Implementation (Hair) |

For *NIC standardized interventions* related to self-care of the hair,

 Go to Chapter 22, **Standardized Language, Selected NOC Outcomes and NIC Interventions for Hygiene Problems,** in Volume 2.

Individualized nursing activities related to the care of the hair include daily brushing and combing of the hair, shampooing, and, for men, shaving and beard care.

Hair Care

Hair should be brushed daily to remove tangles, massage the scalp, stimulate the circulation, and distribute oil down the hair shaft. Use a stiff-bristled brush, but be sure the bristles are not sharp enough to injure the patient's scalp. Likewise, a comb with broken or uneven teeth or one that is too fine can break or snarl the hair or scrape the scalp. Hair that is tightly curled or kinky is best combed with a wide-toothed comb or pick (Figure 22–4). Encourage patients to brush and comb their own hair, if they are able to do so. Encouraging a family member to assist with hair care will involve them in the patient's care and reduce feelings of helplessness. Do not cut a patient's hair unless he or she consents to the haircut.

Hair Care for African Americans

Hair care is equally important for all patients. However, because Caucasian, Hispanic, Asian, and Native American nurses may not know how to do it, they sometimes omit hair care for African American patients. The hair of African Americans varies in texture—it may be long or short, straight or kinky, thick or thin. Worn naturally, African American hair can easily become entangled or matted, and it is quite fragile and easily broken. The scalp also tends to be dry. The hair requires careful handling, especially if it has been chemically straightened, relaxed, or permed. Do not apply chemical relaxers to a patient's hair. Only a licensed beautician should do this.

Shampooing and grooming should, of course, be done according to the person's preference, but in general, you should comb and brush the hair daily and apply a light oil to the scalp (e.g., mineral oil or a light moisturizing cream). Ask a family member to bring from home the product that the patient prefers to use. If the person's hair is corn-rowed or braided, you can massage, oil, and shampoo it without unbraiding it simply by applying a stocking cap to the client's head prior to shampooing.

Shampooing the Hair

Shampooing cleans the hair and scalp. It is soothing and relaxing to many patients. Hair can be shampooed while the person is in the shower, standing or sitting over a sink, or in bed. Protect the patient's eyes with a dry washcloth, and make sure the water temperature is appropriate for the patient. Although not as effective as shampooing with water, a dry shampoo is an alter-

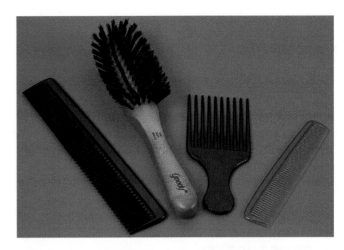

FIGURE 22–4 There are several types of combs for use with various hair types.

native for patients who may not be able to tolerate a standard shampoo procedure. For more information,

 Go to Chapter 22, **Procedure 22-9: Shampooing Hair for the Patient on Bedrest,** in Volume 2.

See also the Critical Aspects box for Procedures 22–1 through 22–14.

Beard and Mustache Care

Beards and mustaches tend to collect food particles. They should be washed daily during a bath or shower and combed and trimmed as necessary. Do not shave a patient's mustache or beard without permission to do so. For details of beard and mustache care,

 Go to Chapter 22, **Procedure 22-10: Providing Beard and Mustache Care,** in Volume 2.

See also the Critical Aspects box for Procedures 22–1 through 22–14.

Shaving

Shaving is an important part of grooming and helps patients feel better about their appearance. Most men shave their facial hair every day. Women may shave to remove axillary and leg hair. If the patient has a bleeding disorder or is taking anticoagulant medication, you should use an electric razor. For important points about shaving,

 Go to Chapter 22, **Procedure 22-11: Shaving a Patient,** in Volume 2.

See also the Critical Aspects box for Procedures 22–1 through 22–14.

Some dark-haired men (e.g., African Americans and Italian Americans) have tightly curled facial hair, which curls back into the skin when shaved. An immune reaction may occur, resulting in the formation of papules and pustules. In such cases, the man may wish to use a **depilatory** (hair-removing agent) instead of shaving. If you apply a depilatory, be sure to keep the chemical from contacting the patient's eyes, nose, mouth, and ears. Do not use a straight or safety razor to remove the depilatory, because it will irritate the skin. Some men with this condition prefer to grow a beard, especially when they are ill and unable to care for themselves.

CARE OF THE EYES

Generally you will not need to provide special hygiene care for the eyes. The eyelids and lashes keep dust and debris from entering the eyes, and tears continually cleanse and lubricate them. When necessary, you may gently cleanse the eyes, from the inner to the outer canthus, with a moistened washcloth (but with no soap). If there is drainage or crusting, use a different cloth for each eye to prevent cross-contamination.

| Assessment (Eyes) |

When performing hygiene care, inspect the eyes for redness, lesions, swelling, crusting, excessive tearing, or discharge. Also check the color of the conjunctivae. You should also ask the patient or check his records to see whether he wears glasses or contact lenses. If the patient wears glasses, ask when he uses them (e.g., for reading, for driving), and ask how well he sees without them. If the patient wears contact lenses, determine:

- The type of lens (hard, soft, long-wearing, disposable)
- How often he wears them (daily, occasionally) and for how long at a time
- Whether they are worn during sleep
- History of or current problems with lens usage (e.g., cleaning, removal)
- Usual practices for cleaning and storage
- History of or current problems with the eyes (e.g., redness, tearing, irritation, dryness, or "scratchy feeling")

This should be adequate data for hygiene care. However, it is not a complete eye assessment. For detailed information about assessing the eyes, see Chapter 19.

| Nursing Diagnosis (Eyes) |

Other than Bathing/Hygiene Self-Care Deficit, there is only one NANDA label specific to the eyes: Dis-

turbed Sensory Perception: Visual. This label is of limited use for hygiene care. Other diagnoses that might occur include:

- Risk for Infection related to improper hand washing and improper lens cleaning
- Risk for Injury (to eyes) related to wearing lenses longer than recommended

| Planning Outcomes/Evaluation (Eyes) |

The only *NOC standardized outcome* specific to the eyes is Sensory Function: Vision. Its use is limited with regard to hygiene care; instead, you would use it if the client has a diagnosis of Disturbed Sensory Perception: Visual. *Individualized goals* you might write for eye care include these examples:

- Demonstrates proper cleaning and storage of contact lenses
- Uses adequate light when reading to avoid eyestrain
- Eyes appear clean and without redness or drainage

| Planning Interventions/Implementation (Eyes) |

For *NIC standardized interventions* related to eye care,

Go to Chapter 22, **Standardized Language, Selected NOC Outcomes and NIC Interventions for Hygiene Problems,** in Volume 2.

Individualized nursing activities related to the care of the eyes include providing eye care to unconscious clients, caring for eyeglasses and contact lenses, and caring for artificial eyes.

Eye Care for the Unconscious Client

Having lost the blink (corneal) reflex, comatose or critically ill patients may need more frequent eye care (every 2 to 4 hours). You will need to keep their eyes lubricated with saline or artificial tears to protect them from corneal abrasions and drying. Instill eye ointment or drops in the lower lids as ordered (see Chapter 23). You may also need to use a protective eye shield to keep the patient's eyes closed.

Go to Chapter 23, **Procedure 23–2: Administering Ophthalmic Medications,** in Volume 2.

Caring for Eyeglasses and Contact Lenses

Eyeglasses need to be cleaned at least once a day. They are expensive, so take care to see that they are not lost or damaged. Using warm water and a soft cloth, clean gently to prevent scratching of the lens.

If possible, ask the patient whether the lenses require a special cleaning solution; some patients bring their own. Label each patient's glasses, and store them in a safe place within the patient's reach, preferably in a glasses case in the drawer of the bedside table.

Contact Lens Wearing Times

Contact lenses are an alternative to eyeglasses. They are discs made of hard or soft plastic and are worn on the cornea over the pupil. They float on the tears of the eye and stay in place because of surface tension. The cornea is nourished mainly by oxygen from the atmosphere and from tears, so in order to ensure an optimal supply of oxygen, contact lenses must be removed periodically. General rules for wearing times are as follows:

- Hard lenses should not be worn for more than 12 to 14 hours and should be removed before going to sleep.
- Extended-wear soft lenses can be worn for 1 to 30 days, depending on the brand. However, they should be removed and cleaned at least weekly.
- Other soft lenses, depending on the type, can be worn day and night for 7 days or during waking hours only for 14 days.
- Disposable lenses are replaced daily.

These are only general rules. Advise your patients to remove the lenses whenever there is pain, redness, mucus accumulation, blurred vision, or excessive tearing of the eyes.

Cleaning and Storing Contact Lenses

Contact lens users must be very careful to keep them free of microorganisms that could cause eye infections and to be careful to avoid eye irritation. Advise patients to:

- Always wash their hands before touching the eyes or the lenses.
- Be careful not to allow the lenses to come in contact with soaps, hair sprays, or cosmetics.
- Be aware of the risk for eye irritation when in the presence of smoke or chemical vapors.

People usually care for their own contact lenses. Cleaning and disinfecting procedures and solutions vary among manufacturers. Depending on the type of lens, saline solutions or special rinsing and soaking solutions may be used. There should be a special container for the lenses, with a cup labeled for the left and right lens. Usually the cups are marked "L" and "R" (Figure 22–5). Some lenses are stored in a solution; others are stored dry.

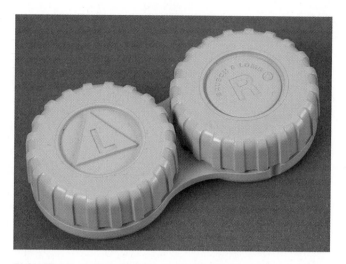

FIGURE 22–5 To avoid placing a contact lens in the wrong eye, lens cases are marked to ensure that the correct lens is stored in the appropriate cup.

If you need to remove a patient's lenses during an emergency, follow these guidelines:

- You may store the lenses in normal saline.
- Prior to inserting or removing contact lenses, wash your hands, and apply gloves.
- It is very difficult to remove a lens when wearing gloves, so you may need to take them off, but this is a last resort. For hard lenses, if you have a small suction cup available for this purpose, use that instead.
- Do not use your fingernails to remove a lens. You may scratch the eye or damage the lens.
- Handle and safeguard lenses as you would any other valuable patient property.

For more information about removal and care of contact lenses,

 Go to Chapter 22, **Procedure 22–12: Removing and Caring for Contact Lenses,** in Volume 2.

Also see the Critical Aspects box for Procedures 22–1 through 22–14.

Caring for Artificial Eyes

An artificial eye is made to look like a natural eye. It can be made of glass or plastic. Some artificial eyes are permanently implanted in the socket, but others must be removed daily for cleaning of the prosthesis and the eye socket. If the patient is not able to perform his own eye care, ask about and follow his usual routines, when possible.

To remove an artificial eye, wear procedure gloves. Using your dominant hand, raise the upper eyelid and depress the lower lid. Apply slight pressure below the

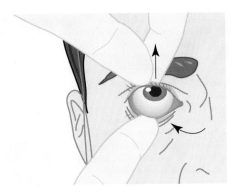

FIGURE 22–6 To remove a prosthetic eye, apply pressure just below the eye.

eye to release the suction holding it in place (Figure 22–6). Alternatively, you can use a small bulb syringe, place it directly on the eye, and squeeze to create suction and lift the eye from the socket. For guidelines to remove, clean, and replace an artificial eye,

 Go to Chapter 22, **Technique 22–2: Caring for Artificial Eyes,** in Volume 2.

KnowledgeCheck 22–12

- True or False: Eyes should be cleansed from the outer to the inner canthus.
- How can a contact lens wearer help prevent eye infections?
- After you have cleaned a prosthetic eye, should you dry it before reinserting it, or leave it wet? To answer this question,

 Go to Chapter 22, **Technique 22–2: Caring for Artificial Eyes,** in Volume 2.

 Go to Chapter 22, **Knowledge Check Response Sheet and Answers,** on the Electronic Study Guide.

CARE OF THE EARS

Healthy ears require minimal care. However, you will need to provide help for patients who have limited self-care abilities and teach others about self-care. For example, **cerumen** (wax) impaction is a common cause of hearing loss, especially in older adults. People sometimes conclude that hearing loss is a normal part of aging and fail to seek treatment. Encourage them to see their primary care provider whenever hearing loss occurs. Also teach patients to avoid using rigid objects, such as bobby pins or toothpicks to clean their ears. Such instruments can traumatize the ear canal and may rupture the **tympanic membrane** (eardrum). Likewise, never use cotton-tipped applicators; they will push the cerumen further into the ear, causing a blockage.

Providing Ear Care

For dependent patients, assess for drainage, excess cerumen, and hearing loss during the bath. Clean the auricle, and remove cerumen from the canal with the tip of the moistened washcloth. If cleansing with a washcloth is inadequate to remove excess cerumen buildup, obtain a physician's order for **cerumenolytic** drops and water irrigation. You can delegate ear cleaning and hearing aid care to the UAP if you are sure that the UAP knows how to perform these tasks. Describe what you want the UAP to observe and report to you. See Chapter 29 for information about ear irrigations.

Care of Hearing Aids

A hearing aid is a battery-powered device that amplifies sound. Three types of hearing aids are shown in Figure 22–7. In addition to these, some patients wear a hearing aid in the temple pieces of their eyeglasses.

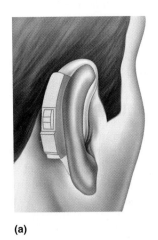
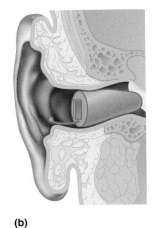
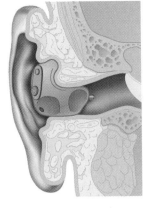

(a) (b) (c)

FIGURE 22–7 Hearing aids. *A,* The postaural (behind-the-ear) aid is the most widely used. A plastic tube connects it to an earmold. *B,* An in-the-canal aid is the least visible. *C,* The in-the-ear aid is made in one piece; all components are in the earmold.

People with severe hearing loss may wear a body hearing aid that clips onto the clothing or a harness-type carrier that connects by a cord to the earpiece.

Hearing aids are expensive, so handle and store them properly. They require regular cleaning and replacement of batteries. Even with good care, they usually need to be replaced every 5 to 10 years, and earmolds usually need adjustment more often than that. Never place a hearing aid in water. For guidelines to remove, clean, and replace a hearing aid,

 Go to Chapter 22, **Technique 22–3: Caring for Hearing Aids,** in Volume 2.

CARE OF THE NOSE

Usually no special care is required for the nose. Have the patient remove excess secretions by gently blowing into a tissue with both nostrils open. Holding one nostril shut can force secretions into the eustachian tubes. In debilitated or unconscious patients, dried secretions can interfere with respirations. Remove secretions by gently inserting a moistened cotton-tipped applicator into the nostrils. Occasionally you may need to instill saline into the nares and suction secretions to keep the airway patent. If the patient has a nasogastric (NG) tube, the constant pressure on the skin may cause breakdown. Provide special skin care at the point where the tube touches the nares.

THE CLIENT'S ENVIRONMENT

A comfortable environment contributes to the patient's well-being. It is your responsibility, as a nurse, to see that the bedside unit and surroundings are clean, safe, and comfortable. Each time you enter a patient's room, you should scan the environment to see whether you need to make adjustments to ensure patient safety and comfort:

- Is the room temperature comfortable?
- Are the siderails up, when indicated? Is the bed in low position?
- Are bed wheels locked?
- Are bed linens clean and free of wrinkles?
- Is the patient's call device within reach?
- Is the overbed table clean and uncluttered?
- Is there uncluttered walking space?
- Are there unpleasant odors?

Each time you leave the room, ask, "What else can I do for you?" This ensures that you have not overlooked anything.

In a hospital, standard bedside equipment usually includes a bed, bedside stand (end table), overbed table, and one or two chairs. The wall unit may consist of a call light, oxygen, suction and electrical outlets, and light fixtures and switches. The patient's personal items are usually kept in the bedside stand. Therefore, you should request permission from the patient before opening the stand. A wash basin, soap dish, bedpan, and urinal may also be kept in the lower cabinet of this stand. Keeping these items clean helps to prevent odor and possible infection.

Practical Knowledge
knowing how

Adequate ventilation, proper room temperature, low noise level, and neat, clean surroundings are important to ensure the patient's comfort.

Ventilation

In an inpatient facility or in the home, there may be odors associated with body secretions such as urine, feces, vomitus, or draining wounds. Odors can be offensive, and they often cause the patient embarrassment, so work quickly to free the environment of any sources of odors. Cleanliness is the best way to prevent odors. Other suggestions include the following:

- Provide good ventilation, if this is under your control. For example, open a window or use a fan.
- Empty urinals, bedpans, or emesis basins promptly.
- Dispose of soiled dressings or other malodorous items in appropriate containers, and immediately remove them from the room.
- Unless contraindicated by the patient's illness, you can use a room deodorizer to help eliminate odors.
- Most institutions ban smoking in patient rooms, in part because of the odor.

Room Temperature

Although preference may vary, a room temperature between 68 and 74°F (20 and 23°C) is usually comfortable for most patients. You may need to adjust the temperature to higher than normal for those who are very ill, very young, or very old. Provide blankets for warmth, as needed.

Noise

Persons who are ill are often sensitive to various environmental noises, such as an ice machine, suction equipment, paging systems, loud talking, and laughter. In addition, sleeping in a new and strange environment or in the presence of pain may be difficult and interrupted. Make it a priority to control noise in

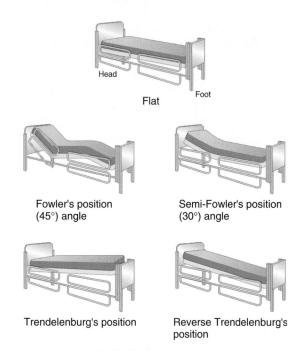

FIGURE 22–8 **Hospital beds adjust to several positions.**

the hospital setting. Keep unnecessary conversations to a minimum, and speak quietly.

Hospital Beds

Hospitalized patients spend a significant amount of time in bed. Hospital beds can be uncomfortable and may contribute to restlessness and poor sleep. Hospital beds are generally standard in size and higher and narrower than a home bed. This allows you to reach the patient more easily and safely.

Hospital beds are usually electronically controlled, so the patient can raise and lower the head and foot separately by the push of a button. You can also raise and lower the height of the bed electronically (see Figure 22–8 for bed positions). Patient safety is your priority, so although you may raise the entire bed to a working level that is comfortable for you, be sure to place the bed in the lowest position before leaving the bedside. Long-term care settings usually have low beds to make it easier for ambulatory patients to transfer into and out of bed. As a part of the admission procedure, you will teach patients how to use the bed controls.

 Go to Chapter 10, **Procedure 10–1: Admitting a Patient to a Nursing Unit,** in Volume 2.

Siderails may be used to provide assistance to patients moving into and out of bed or to prevent falls by patients with decreased consciousness. Siderails are considered a passive restraint and may pose risk to a patient with a cognitive impairment. See Chapter 21 for additional information about the safe use of siderails and other equipment.

Always be sure to lock the wheels on a hospital bed when it is stationary. For example, the bed could roll out from under an ambulatory patient who is moving from the bed to a chair. Ensure that the wheels are locked when you are helping the patient to a sitting position on the side of the bed or assisting with a transfer to a chair or stretcher.

Mattresses and Linens

Mattresses are usually firm and covered in a water-repellant material that resists staining and soiling and may be easily wiped down with a germicidal cleaner. A variety of special therapeutic mattresses are available to help reduce the effects of pressure over the bony prominences (e.g., sacrum, heels). See Chapter 34 for further discussion of special mattresses.

Using a mattress cover and/or pad promotes patient comfort and prevents soiling of the mattress. Sheets may be fitted or flat. Other linens include drawsheets, washable incontinent pads, pillow cases, blankets, bedspreads, and gowns.

Bed Making

Clean, wrinkle-free bed linens help to promote comfort and a sense of well-being. In contrast, wrinkled and soiled linen can contribute to skin breakdown and pressure areas. Linens are generally changed daily after the bath and when soiled. If the patients are up and about during the day, such as on a rehabilitation unit, beds are made daily, but bed linen may be changed weekly or only when soiled. If the patient is immobile or on bedrest, the bed is made while the patient occupies it. You or the UAP may make an unoccupied bed or an occupied bed. For more information about bed making,

 Go to Chapter 22, **Procedure 22–13: Making an Unoccupied Bed,** and **Procedure 22–14: Making an Occupied Bed,** in Volume 2.

Also see the Critical Aspects box for Procedures 22–1 through 22–14.

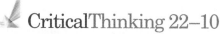 CriticalThinking 22–10
For which of your patients ("Meet Your Patients") will you most surely need to make an occupied bed? Why?

| toward evidence-based practice |

Shiomori, T., Miyamoto, H., Makishima, K., Yoshida, M., Fujiyoshi, T., Udaka, T., et al. (2002). Evaluation of bedmaking-related airborne and surface methicillin-resistant *Staphylococcus aureus* contamination. *Journal of Hospital Infection, 50*(1), 30–35.

Researchers used an air sampler to measure the number of airborne methicillin-resistant *Staphylococcus aureus* (*MRSA*) before, during, and after bed making. They took samples from surfaces such as tables, floors, and bedsheets. They found that the number of MRSA was significantly higher 15 minutes after bed making than during the period before bed making, suggesting that MRSA was recirculated in the air, especially after movement.

Warshaw, E., Nix, D., Kula, J., & Markon, C. E. (2002). Clinical and cost effectiveness of a cleanser protectant lotion for treatment of perineal skin breakdown in low-risk patients with incontinence. *Ostomy and Wound Management, 48*(6), 44–51.

Perineal dermatitis due to urinary and/or fecal incontinence is a common problem. Nineteen elderly patients (mean age 73.1 years) who were considered to be "at low risk" for perineal dermatitis participated in this study. Researchers compared the effectiveness of a one-step cleanser protectant lotion to their standard protocols for perineal care (which was a traditional bathing-plus-skin-barrier procedure). After 7 days, scores for erythema and pain were significantly lower for both methods. They calculated that the one-step product would cost $136 per patient per year less than their standard protocols, and would reduce caregiver time by an average of 23 seconds per episode of care.

1. What implications do the findings of the first study have for your nursing practice? That is, how might you change some of your activities, or what new ones might you add (assuming, of course, that the study methods were adequate and the results valid)?

2. You have decided, as a nurse manager, to switch to the one-step product for perineal care described in the second study. You wish to use this study to support the rationale for your decision. Which of the following is/are supported by this study? The one-step method will:
   a. Save the hospital money.
   b. Reduce the incidence of perineal dermatitis.
   c. Be more efficient in terms of caregiver time.

 Go to Chapter 22, **Toward Evidence-Based Practice Suggested Responses,** on the Electronic Study Guide.

 Go to Chapter 22, **Resources for Caregivers and Health Professionals,** on the Electronic Study Guide.

 Suggested Readings: Go to Chapter 22, **Reading More About Facilitating Hygiene,** on the Electronic Study Guide.

 Bibliography: Go to Volume 2, Bibliography.

23 CHAPTER

Administering Medications

Learning Outcomes

After completing this chapter, you should be able to:

* Name at least five sources of medication information.

* Discuss the agencies and legislation that help to ensure drug quality and safety.

* Discuss the routes by which medications are absorbed in the body, including each one's advantages and disadvantages.

* State the primary site of drug metabolism (biotransformation) in the body.

* Explain how drug excretion occurs at each of the following sites: kidneys, liver, gastrointestinal tract, lungs, and exocrine glands.

* Define *onset, peak,* and *duration of drug action; therapeutic level, peak level,* and *trough level*; and *biological half-life.*

* Compare and contrast primary effects, secondary effects, side effects, adverse reactions, toxic reactions, allergic reactions, anaphylactic reactions, and idiosyncratic reactions.

* Define *drug-drug interaction, antagonistic drug relationship, synergistic drug relationship, drug incompatibility, and medication contraindications.*

* Correctly calculate drug dosages, including (1) conversion among the metric, apothecary, and household measurement systems and (2) working with units and milliequivalents (mEq).

* Describe nursing assessment before, during, and following the administration of a drug.

* Plan care for clients with problems of Risk for Injury and Noncompliance related to medications.

* Administer medications using the "three checks" and "six rights."

* Demonstrate the correct procedure for administering medications by the oral, enteral, and parenteral routes.

* Demonstrate the location of the following intramuscular injection sites: ventrogluteal, deltoid, vastus lateralis, dorsogluteal, and rectus femoris.

* List five steps you can incorporate in your practice to ensure safe medication administration and prevent a medication error.

MEET Your Patients

You are scheduled to administer medications to five patients on the medical-surgical unit today. You will be administering medications unsupervised for the first time. Your clinical instructor will be available as a resource. Your patients are:

- Margaret Marks, an 82-year-old woman who has a fractured hip and experiences periods of confusion
- Cary Pearson, a 70-year-old man with feeding and swallowing difficulties who receives his medications through a gastrostomy tube
- Cyndi Early, a 32-year-old woman with diabetes who is scheduled for surgery at 10:00 A.M. today
- James Bigler, a 44-year-old man who has had a repair of a compound fracture of the right arm and is receiving intravenous fluids and medications
- Rebecca Jones, an 84-year-old woman with compression fractures of the vertebrae resulting from a fall at a nursing home.

You have reviewed your assignment but are unsure of where to begin. Should you visit your patients first and perform an assessment? Should you review the charts first? What should you do with the MARs (medication administration records)? There are so many questions running through your head, and you are a little nervous being on your own. Perhaps you could use the model of full-spectrum nursing (Chapter 2) to focus your thinking. In general, any time you give a medication, you will need to incorporate the following:

1. *Theoretical knowledge:* Find out about the actions and expected effects of the medications you are to give.
2. *Patient situation:* Assess the health status (e.g., disease process) of each patient as it relates to his medications.
3. *Critical thinking:* Why is the drug being given? Is there anything about the patient's physiology that may alter his responses to the drug? Do you need to modify the administration procedure in any way?
4. *Practical knowledge:* Be sure that you know the procedures for administering each medication safely.

By the time you complete this chapter, you will have the detailed information you need to make those kinds of judgments. And remember that while you are a student, your instructor and the staff nurses will be there for support.

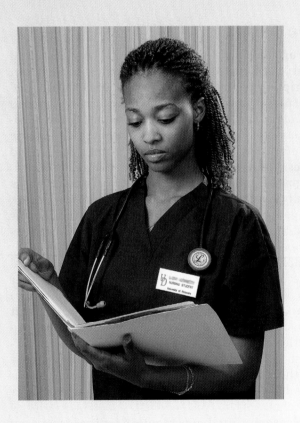

Theoretical Knowledge
knowing why

Pharmacology is the science of drug effects. It deals with all drugs used in society, legal and illegal, prescription and nonprescription, and street drugs. Because of their potential for harm as well as benefit, you should thoroughly understand all the medications you administer.

HOW ARE DRUGS NAMED AND CLASSIFIED?

A **drug** is a chemical that interacts with a living organism and alters its activity. In health care, drugs are used in diagnosing, treating, or preventing a disease or other medical condition. The term *drug* is used interchangeably with *medication,* although some people think of the term *drug* as meaning an illegal substance.

Drug Names

A drug may have multiple names. The **chemical name,** rarely used in nursing practice, is the exact description of the drug's chemical composition and molecular structure. For example, *2-(p-isobutylphenyl) propionic acid* is the chemical name of the anti-inflammatory drug ibuprofen. When the developing manufacturer is ready to market a drug, the United States Adopted Name Council (USAN Council) assigns the **generic (nonproprietary) name.** This is usually similar to the chemical name, but it is simpler. The generic name is also the **official name** that is listed in publications such as the *United States Pharmacopeia (USP)* and *National Formulary (NF)*. For example, *ibuprofen* is both a generic and an official name. When the drug is marketed, the manufacturer sells it under a **brand (trade** or **proprietary) name.** The brand name is easily recognized because it begins with a capital letter and sometimes has a registration mark ® at the upper right of the name. Different manufacturers of the same medication may give the medication different brand names. For example, Advil, Nuprin, and Motrin are all brand names for ibuprofen.

Prescription drugs require a written order from a healthcare provider (e.g., physician or nurse practitioner) who is licensed by the state to prescribe or dispense drugs. **Nonprescription,** or **over-the-counter (OTC),** drugs may be purchased without a prescription and are assumed to be safe if consumers follow the manufacturer's directions. Some drugs are nonprescription at low doses but require a prescription for the consumer to purchase in a higher dose. For example, naproxen sodium 200 mg is sold over the counter as Aleve, whereas naproxen 550 mg is sold as Naprosyn and requires a prescription.

Drug Classifications

Drugs are grouped according to their use (clinical indication), body system, and chemical or pharmacological traits. Drugs in a certain classification share similar actions; for example, the opioid analgesics meperidine HCl (Demerol) and morphine both decrease pain and have side effects of drowsiness, constipation, and nausea. You need only learn the common characteristics for each drug classification. Then, when you encounter a new drug, you will be able to associate it with its classification and make inferences about its basic characteristics. It is not realistic to know everything about every drug, so "looking it up" should become second nature. See Table 23–1 for a summary and examples of classifications.

A drug can be placed in more than one category in a classification system. Classified by usage, for example, ibuprofen (Motrin) can be an analgesic, anti-inflammatory, and an antipyretic agent. A drug can act on more than one body system, as well; in fact, most do. For example, meperidine HCl (Demerol) is used for its central nervous system effects, but it also decreases the activity of the intestinal system and other smooth muscles.

KnowledgeCheck 23–1

- Name three ways a drug may be classified.
- List at least four ways a drug could be named.

 Go to Chapter 23, **Knowledge Check Response Sheet and Answers,** on the Electronic Study Guide.

WHAT MECHANISMS PROMOTE DRUG QUALITY AND SAFETY?

In the United States until the 20th century, there were no mechanisms for publishing drug ingredients, no regulations to govern the contents of drugs, and no limitations about their sale. People could buy medicines containing potent and dangerous ingredients, such as opium, morphine, heroin, and alcohol. Besides the great deal of money that people wasted on ineffective drugs, drug addiction and deaths from drug overdose were common. Now, reliable sources of drug information, state and federal regulations and standards controlling drug administration, and a variety of systems for storing and distributing medications in healthcare agencies all work together to protect consumers.

Drug Listings and Directories

When in doubt, look it up! As a nurse, you are professionally, morally, legally, and personally responsible

TABLE 23-1 Drug Classification Systems

Classification	Explanation	Examples
Usage (why the drug is used)	This refers to the clinical indication for the medication or to the clinical effect it is intended to achieve.	• Analgesics—used to manage pain (e.g., by this system, Demerol would be an analgesic) • Anticoagulants—used to prevent the blood from clotting • Antineoplastics—used to destroy cancer cells • Laxatives—used to produce a bowel movement
Body systems (where the drug works)	This refers to the body system that the drug targets.	• Central nervous system drugs (e.g., by this system, Demerol would be a central nervous system drug) • Endocrine system drugs
Chemical or pharmacological class (what the drug is made of)	This refers to the drug's structure or composition.	• Opiates (e.g., by this system, Demerol would be an opiate) • Digitalis glycosides • Rauwolfia alkaloids • Corticosteroids • Barbiturates

for every dose of medication you administer. Always use current information when researching a medication. The following references have become the official standards for the healthcare industry:

• *United States Pharmacopoeia (USP).* This directory of drugs approved by the Food and Drug Administration (FDA) lists the physical and chemical composition for each drug. Any drug included in this book has met rigorous standards of quality, strength, and purity and is permitted to use the letters USP after the drug name.

• *National Formulary* (United States). This resource identifies the therapeutic value of drugs as well as their formulas and prescriptions.

• *British Pharmacopoeia.* This is the British version of the USP. Drugs listed in the *British Pharmacopoeia* are considered official and subject to legal control in Great Britain. It is also used in Canada.

• *Canadian Formulary.* This is a listing of all drugs and formulas used in Canada. Not all the drugs listed in this formulary are in the *British Pharmacopoeia.*

In addition to the pharmacopoeia and formularies, the following are reliable resources for medication information:

• *Nursing drug handbooks.* Several nursing drug handbooks are available from textbook and other publishers. They serve as a quick resource for information (e.g., dosage, side effects) and nursing interventions associated with a drug.

• *Physician's Desk Reference (PDR).* This book, financed by the pharmaceutical companies, lists several thousand drugs with complete drug information and is a standard resource for physicians and pharmacists. The information contained in the PDR is the same information found in drug package inserts. The PDR does not include nursing interventions but does contain information on dosing, routes of administration, and side effects.

• *Pharmacology texts.* A textbook provides more information about physiology and pathophysiology, and provides broader information, than the PDR or a handbook. It may or may not have detailed information about the specific drug you are giving, but it will include a thorough discussion of the drug's classification.

• *Pharmacist.* A clinical pharmacist can assist you with medication-related concerns (e.g., dosage calculations, compatibility, admixture administration, and adverse reactions).

• *Medication package inserts.* Most medications are packaged with an insert that provides information identical to that found in the PDR. Inserts also contain instructions that are specific for that particular drug.

• *Institutional medication policies and procedures.* Every institution has policies and procedures governing medication administration. You should know the policies and procedures for each institution in which you practice.

CriticalThinking 23–1

Mr. Pearson ("Meet Your Patient") has a medication, metoprolol (Lopressor), due at 0800. You are not familiar with this medication.

*   What do you need to know before giving the drug?
*   What resources might you use to learn about this medication?
*   Which is the generic and which is the brand name of this medication?
*   Select a nursing drug handbook and research this medication. What kinds of information are available to you in the book?
*   Now look up the drug in a pharmacology text. How is that information similar to and different from the information in the handbook?

Legal Considerations

In the United States and Canada, drug administration is controlled by federal, state or provincial, and local laws. Standards of nursing care, state nurse practice acts, and organizational policies and procedures define your role and responsibilities for administering medications. You must be familiar with them to know what you can and cannot do. In addition, you must recognize the limits of your own experience, skills, and knowledge.

The Food and Drug Administration (FDA) of the U.S. Department of Health and Human Services regulates the manufacturing, sale, and effectiveness of all medications. It also regulates, through controlled clinical trials, the testing of any medication that is to be marketed and sold in the United States. This process helps to ensure that ineffective or unsafe drugs are not marketed; if later found unsafe, they are subject to a recall. However, many medicinal products are *not* regulated by the FDA. For example, herbal remedies and some naturopathic supplements are considered "food products" and are not controlled. Yet they are advertised as having health benefits.

Nurse Practice Acts

In most states, a nurse (other than an advanced practice nurse) cannot prescribe or administer medications without a physician order. If you violate the state's nurse practice act by giving medications without an order, your state board of nursing could revoke your license to practice nursing.

CriticalThinking 23–2

Obtain a copy of your nurse practice act for the state in which you live. To find a copy,

Go to the **National Council of State Boards of Nursing web site** at **http://www.ncsbn.org/**

What does your state's nurse practice act tell you about administering medications?

U.S. Drug Legislation

Various state and federal agencies regulate the manufacturing and sale of medications. Table 23–2 presents the more important medication-related legislation enacted in the United States. Each state must conform to federal regulations concerning medications. The states may, in turn, institute additional controls. Finally, local governments may enact regulations for the use of alcohol and tobacco.

Canadian Drug Legislation

Drug regulation is carried out through the Health Protection branch of the Canadian government. Under this branch, the Drugs Directorate oversees the bureaus that deal with specific areas of regulation, such as prescription drugs, nonprescription drugs, biological agents, drug research, and control of drug quality. The Canadian Food and Drugs Act (1953) protects consumers from contaminated, adulterated, and unsafe drugs.

Regulation of Controlled Substances

Controlled substances are drugs considered to have either limited medical use or high potential for abuse or addiction. Under the Controlled Substance Act of the Comprehensive Drug Abuse Prevention Act of 1970, it is illegal to possess a controlled substance without a valid prescription. For a summary of categories of controlled substances,

Go to Chapter 23, **Tables, Boxes, Figures: ESG Table 23–1,** on the Electronic Study Guide.

Controlled substances must be stored, handled, disposed of, and administered according to regulations established by the U.S. Drug Enforcement Agency (DEA). Facilities using controlled substances must store them in locked drawers within a second locked area. (This process is known as **double locking.**) The facility must also keep a record of every dose administered. A count of all controlled substances is performed at specified times, usually at change of shift. To facilitate counting and tracking, drug manufacturers

TABLE 23–2 U.S. Legislation for Drug Quality and Safety

Date	United States Law	Provisions
1906	Pure Food and Drug Act	Established official standards for listing or labeling dangerous and addictive ingredients; set standards for proper labeling of medications.
1914	Harrison Narcotic Act	Regulated importation, manufacture, sale, and use of opium, cocaine, marijuana, and similar drugs likely to cause dependence.
1938	Food, Drug, and Cosmetic Act	Required that a drug be proven safe before it was marketed; provided for governmental approval of new drugs before marketing; defined labeling requirements.
1952	Durham-Humphrey Amendment	Specified which drugs need a prescription to be sold and which do not. Required that all prescription drugs be clearly marked with, "Caution: Federal Law prohibits dispensing without prescription." Established over-the-counter (OTC) as a separate group of drugs.
1962	Kefauver-Harris Amendment	Authorized FDA to establish official names for drugs; required proof of safety and efficacy before approval for use.
1970	Comprehensive Drug Abuse and Control Act	Classified drugs by abuse potential and medical usefulness; regulated manufacture, distribution, and sale of controlled substances; provided for treatment and rehabilitation for drug abuse and dependence.
1983	Orphan Drug Act	Provided tax credits to companies to develop drugs used to treat rare diseases.
1988	Food and Drug Administration Act	Established the FDA within the Department of Health and Human Services.

package many narcotics in sectioned containers, with each tablet separately and consecutively numbered (Figure 23–1).

The Canadian Narcotic Control Act (1961) regulates the manufacture, distribution, and sale of narcotics in Canada. Possession of narcotics for any reason other than those related to medical use is an offense subject to severe penalties.

CriticalThinking 23–3

Locate the controlled substance area on your nursing unit.

- Is there a double lock present?
- Who is responsible for "carrying" the narcotics keys?
- What is done if there is a discrepancy between a narcotic sign-out sheet and the actual number of narcotic doses present?

Systems for Storing and Distributing Medications

Most inpatient healthcare facilities have specific areas designed for preparation of medications. Usually this is a central room ("medication room") or mobile cart. Some nursing units keep drugs and supplies in a locked cabinet in or near patient rooms. Whatever the method, all drugs are secured in designated areas accessible only to nurses.

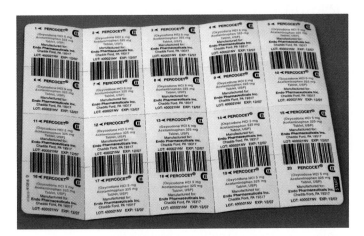

FIGURE 23–1   To facilitate counting, many narcotics are packaged in sectioned containers with each tablet numbered consecutively.

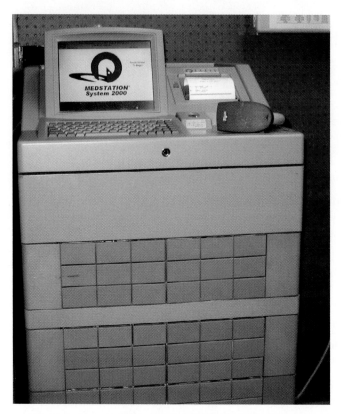

FIGURE 23–2   Medications may be kept in locked, mobile carts, with a drawer for each patient. Some carts are a part of an automated (computerized) dispensing system.

Stock Supply

Medications used most frequently may be kept in **stock supply** (bulk quantity), labeled, and in a central location. For example, Tylenol Elixir and cough syrups may be kept in large multidose bottles, from which you measure doses for more than one patient. Stock supplies require you to measure the dose each time a patient needs it, so the potential for measurement error is present each time a dose is poured. However, a bulk supply of medication is often extremely cost-effective.

Unit-Dose System

A locked, mobile cart is used, with drawers containing separate compartments for each patient's medications (Figure 23–2). Extra drawers contain supplies, such as medication cups, syringes, and alcohol swabs. The pharmacy staff refills the drawers each shift or every 24 hours. Limited amounts of **PRN** ("give according to patient need") medications and stock medications are also kept in the mobile cart.

A **unit dose** is the ordered amount of drug the patient receives at a single time (e.g., for an ordered 800 mg of ibuprofen [Motrin], to be given every 8 hours, the unit dose is 800 mg). Each unit dose (usually one tablet) is individually packaged and labeled with drug name, dose, and expiration date. The pharmacist checks each unit dose before sending the drug to the nursing unit, and you will recheck the drug and dose when preparing it for administration. The unit-dose system not only saves nursing time, but also is the safest method because of the double-check system.

Automated Dispensing System

An automated dispensing system is a computerized system similar to unit dosage (see Figure 23–2). The locked cart contains all the medications frequently used on a particular nursing unit, and the computer database contains records and counts of the medications, as well as the medication orders for each patient on the unit. Each nurse uses a password to access the machine and enters the data about the needed drug, after which the machine dispenses the medication. The machine tracks dispensed medications for billing and controlled-substances monitoring. The medications are usually packaged in unit doses, but some bulk medications may also be kept on the cart. This method allows for immediate administration of newly ordered medications, PRN medications, controlled substances, and emergency medications because the drugs are available on the unit, so that the nurse does not need to wait for the pharmacy to fill an order.

Self-Administration

At times, even in the hospital, patients may self-administer their medications. For example, sublingual nitroglycerine (used for chest pain) is frequently self-administered. The prescribed drugs are supplied in individual containers for the patient and stored at the bedside. Remind the patient to tell you when he takes the drug. This method promotes independence and allows you to evaluate prior to discharge the patient's ability to manage medications safely and accurately.

KnowledgeCheck 23–2

- What legislation defines controlled substances in both the United States and Canada?
- How is quality in medications managed?

 Go to Chapter 23, **Knowledge Check Response Sheet and Answers,** on the Electronic Study Guide.

WHAT IS PHARMACOKINETICS?

Pharmacokinetics refers to the absorption, distribution, metabolism, and excretion of a drug (Figure 23–3). These four processes determine the intensity and duration of a drug's actions. Each drug has unique pharmacokinetic characteristics.

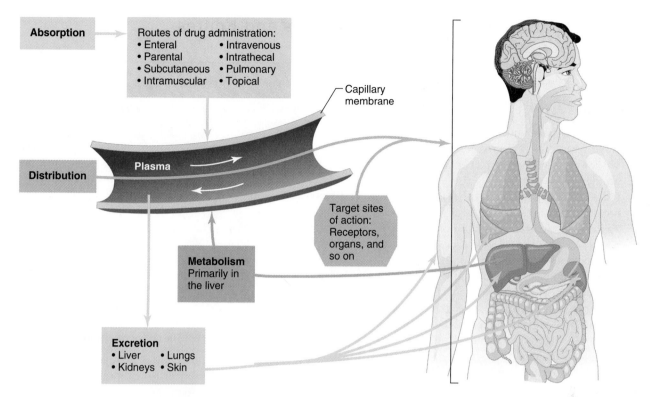

FIGURE 23–3 Pharmacokinetics is the study of drug absorption, distribution, metabolism, and excretion, which determine the intensity and duration of a drug's actions in the body.

What Factors Affect Drug Absorption?

Absorption refers to the movement of the drug from the site of administration into the bloodstream. The rate of absorption determines when a drug becomes available to exert its action; thus, absorption also influences metabolism and excretion. Absorption depends on the route of administration, form of the drug, drug solubility, effects of pH, blood flow to the area, and body surface area.

Route of Administration

Drugs are given for either local or systemic effect. The **local effects** of a drug occur at the site of application (e.g., certain topical applications of drugs to the skin), so no absorption occurs. When a medication is given for a **systemic effect,** the drug must be absorbed into the bloodstream before it can be distributed to a distant location. A drug may enter the circulation either by injection into a vein or by absorption from other areas into which it has been placed (e.g., muscle, mucous membranes, skin).

Drugs are designed for a specific route of administration: oral, sublingual, buccal, topical, enteral, and parenteral. Drugs are absorbed at different rates from each of these routes. The form (preparation) of a drug usually determines its route of administration. Medications are available in a variety of forms.

Table 23–3 summarizes the preparations and the advantages and disadvantages for the various routes of administration. The choice of route is crucial in determining the suitability of the drug for an individual patient. For example, if your patient is vomiting, an oral drug will not be absorbed in the stomach and will likely be expelled during vomiting. If the patient has diarrhea, the rapid motility of the gastrointestinal tract will decrease absorption. If your patient, Cary Pearson ("Meet Your Patient"), has an order for an oral medication, would you question it? Why or why not?

Solubility of the Drug

Solubility refers to ability of a medication to be transformed into a liquid form that can be absorbed into the bloodstream. **Enteric-coated** drugs cannot be decomposed by gastric secretions; the coating thus prevents the medication from being diluted before it reaches the intestines. The coating thereby provides delayed action of the medication. It also decreases irritating effects of the medication on the stomach. **Timed-release (sustained-release)** medications are formulated to dissolve slowly, releasing small amounts for absorption over several hours.

To be absorbed, oral preparations must be water soluble so that they can dissolve in the *aqueous* (watery) contents of the gastrointestinal (GI) tract. *Liquids* (e.g., suspensions or solutions) are absorbed

Text continues on page 483.

TABLE 23-3   Preparation Types and Advantages and Routes of Administration

Route: Oral   The drug is swallowed and absorbed from the stomach or small intestines.

Preparation Types

- **Capsule**—A gelatinous container that holds the liquid, powder, or oil form of the drug. When swallowed, the gelatin container dissolves in the gastric juices.
- **Pill**—This term is rarely used now. *Tablet* is the preferred term.
- **Tablet**—A powdered drug is compressed into a hard, compact form (e.g., round, oval) that is easy to swallow and then breaks up into a fine powder in the stomach. The tablet is the most common oral preparation. *Enteric-coated tablets* have an acid-insoluble coating to keep them from dissolving in the stomach; they disintegrate in the alkaline secretions of the small intestine.
- **Time-released tablet or capsule**—A tablet or capsule formulated so that it does not dissolve all at once, but gradually releases medication over a few hours.
- **Elixir**—A liquid containing water and about 25% alcohol that is sweetened with volatile oils (e.g., aromatic elixir); not as sticky or as sweet as syrups.
- **Extract**—A very concentrated form of a drug made from animals or vegetables; may be a syrupy liquid or a powder.
- **Fluid extract**—An alcohol-based solution of a drug from a vegetable source (e.g., belladonna); the most concentrated of the fluid preparations.
- **Spirits**—A concentrated alcohol-based solution of a volatile (easily evaporated) substance or oil (e.g., ammonia, peppermint oil, orange oil); it contains larger amounts of the substance than can be dissolved in water.
- **Syrup**—An aqueous solution of sugar, used to disguise unpleasant taste of drugs.
- **Tincture**—An alcohol or water-and-alcohol (with a high percentage of alcohol) solution made by extracting potent plants; may also be used externally (e.g., tincture of iodine).
- **Powder**—Finely ground drug(s), usually mixed with a liquid before ingesting; some are used internally, others externally. (Some are mixed with a diluent for parenteral injection.)
- **Solution**—Drug(s) dissolved in a liquid carrier. *Aqueous solutions* are medications dissolved in water. (May be used orally, externally, and parenterally.)
- **Suspension**—Drug(s) that are suspended (not completely dissolved) in a liquid. *Aqueous suspensions* are suspended in water. *Never* used for IV or intra-arterial routes.

Advantages

- Convenient
- Sterility is not needed for oral use
- Economical
- Noninvasive, low-risk procedure
- Easy to administer, good for self-administration
- Capsule can mask unpleasant taste of a drug

Disadvantages

- Unpleasant taste may cause noncompliance
- May irritate gastric mucosa
- Patient must be conscious
- Digestive juices may destroy drug
- Cannot use if patient has nausea and vomiting or decreased gastric motility
- Cannot use if patient has difficulty swallowing
- Potential for aspiration
- May be harmful to teeth
- Onset of action is slow

TABLE 23–3 *(continued)*

Route: Enteral   The drug is given directly into the stomach or intestine (e.g., through a nasogastric or gastrostomy tube).

Preparation Types	Advantages	Disadvantages
Same as for oral medications.	Can be used for patients with Impaired Swallowing as an alternative to parenteral administration	• Not all pills can be crushed; medications can clog the NG tube • NG tube itself presents some risk of aspiration

Route: Sublingual   (a variation of transmucosal administration)—Drug is held under the tongue and absorbed across the sublingual mucous membrane.

Preparation Types	Advantages	Disadvantages
• **Lipid-soluble lozenge (troche)**—A flat, round preparation that dissolves when held in the mouth. May act locally or be absorbed through mucosa for systemic effect. • **Tablet** (see oral route).	• Used for local or systemic effects • Convenient • Sterility not needed • Quick delivery to general circulation • Bypasses stomach and intestines; absorbed directly into bloodstream	• May inadvertently be swallowed in the saliva • Not useful for drugs with unpleasant taste • May irritate oral mucosa • Patient must be conscious • Useful only for highly lipid-soluble drugs • Patient must hold the drug in place until it is dissolved, which may take a few minutes • Limited period of effectiveness, requiring frequent redosing

Route: Buccal   Transmucosal administration: medication is held against mucous membrane of cheek until it dissolves.

Preparation Types	Advantages	Disadvantages
Lipid-soluble lozenge or tablet (see oral and sublingual routes).	Same as sublingual	Same as sublingual

Route: Topical (Skin)   Drug acts locally or is absorbed directly through skin (transdermal or percutaneous absorption).

Preparation Types	Advantages	Disadvantages
• **Aerosol** spray or foam—A liquid or foam that is sprayed by air pressure onto the skin. • **Cream**—A non-oily, semisolid substance applied to the skin. • **Gel** or **jelly**—A clear or translucent semisolid substance that liquefies when applied to the skin. • **Liniment**—An oily liquid to rub into the skin. • **Lotion**—An *emollient* (softening or soothing agent) for use on the skin; may be a clear solution, suspension, or emulsion. • **Ointment**—A semisolid, fatty (usually petroleum jelly– or lanolin-based) substance for skin or mucous membranes; usually not water soluble. • **Paste**—Similar to an ointment, but thicker and stiffer. • **Tincture** (see oral route). • **Transdermal patch**—Releases constant, controlled amounts of medication, for systemic effect.	• Continuous dosing • Sterility is not needed • For local or systemic effects • Long-acting systemic effect • Useful if patient is unable to take oral medications • Acceptable to most patients	• Effective only for lipid-soluble drugs and must be specially formulated • May cause local irritation, especially if the patient is allergic to latex or tape • Discarded patches may pose danger of poisoning • Leaves residue on skin • Accurate doses can be difficult to obtain when the drug is in a tube or jar

➤

Preparation Types and Advantages and Routes of Administration *(continued)*

TABLE 23-3

Route: Topical: Instillations The drug is placed into a body cavity (e.g., urinary bladder, rectum, vagina, ears, nose, eye).

Preparation Types	Advantages	Disadvantages
• **Solutions** (for nose, ears, and eyes; enemas per rectum)—Drug(s) dissolved in a liquid carrier. • **Suppositories** (for bladder, vagina, rectum)—Drug(s) mixed with a glycerin-gelatin or cocoa butter base and shaped for insertion into the body. It dissolves gradually at body temperature. • **Jellies, creams** (for vagina and rectum)—See skin route.	• Continuous dosing • Sterility is not needed • Useful if patient is unable to take oral medications • May be used for local or systemic effects	• May be embarrassing for patient • Drugs may be poorly absorbed from the rectum if stool is present or if patient defecates before suppository melts

---

Route: Topical: Inhalation A device (e.g., nebulizer, face mask) breaks the drug into finely dispersed particles, which are breathed into the respiratory passages. Some drugs are intended for local effects in the respiratory passages; others (e.g., anesthetic gases) are for systemic effects, especially in the brain.

Preparation Types	Advantages	Disadvantages
• **Aerosols**—Aerosols are liquids in very fine particles that can be inhaled into the lungs; they are sprayed under air pressure. • **Gases**—Gas is a basic form of matter (i.e., solid, liquid, and gas). A gas must be kept in a closed container; otherwise, the fast-moving molecules escape into the air. Examples are oxygen, nitrogen, carbon dioxide, and anesthetic gases.	• Quick and efficient local and systemic route through the lungs • May be given to unconscious patient • Allows continuous dosing, and dosage can be easily modified	• Requires special equipment • May irritate lung mucosa • Useful only for drugs that are gases at room temperature • May have unexpected systemic effect when only local effect is desired

---

Route: All Parenteral Routes

Preparation Types	Advantages	Disadvantages
Depends on Route	• Patient may be conscious or unconscious	• Requires sterile procedures • Poses risk for infection because skin is broken • Requires skill • May cause some pain • Produces anxiety • More expensive than oral administration

---

Route: Parenteral: Intravenous The drug is injected directly into the vein, either by bolus or slow infusion.

Preparation Types	Advantages	Disadvantages
Aqueous solutions—Drug(s) dissolved in water.	• Rapid effect because absorption is bypassed; therefore, good for emergency situations • Patient needs only one needlestick, even for multiple doses	• Poses risk of transient drug concentrations if drug is injected too rapidly • Limited to highly soluble medications • Poses risk for sepsis because pathogens may be introduced directly into bloodstream • Patient must have usable veins • Cost of supplies and medications

| TABLE | 23-3 | (continued) |

Route: Parenteral: Intramuscular The drug is injected into muscle mass.

Preparation Types	Advantages	Disadvantages
Primarily aqueous solutions (see intravenous route), although some preparations (e.g., penicillin) are suspensions	• Rapid absorption, except for oily preparations or suspensions • Allows use of drugs that are not stable in solution • Causes less pain (than do subcutaneous injections) from irritating drugs because they are deep in muscle • Allows administration of a larger volume than does subQ administration • Allows more rapid absorption than does subQ or oral administration	• May cause irritation and local reactions • Poses risk for tissue and nerve damage if site is improperly located • Cannot be used where tissue is damaged (e.g., bruised) or peripheral circulation is decreased

Route: Parenteral: Subcutaneous The drug is injected into the subcutaneous tissue under the skin.

Preparation Types	Advantages	Disadvantages
Primarily solutions—Drugs dissolved in a liquid carrier.	• Allows faster action than does oral administration • Allows better absorption of lipid-soluble drugs than does intramuscular administration	• Only very small amounts can be given • Absorption is relatively slow and often confined to the injected area

Route: Parenteral: Intradermal The drug is injected under the skin, into the dermis. Most commonly used for diagnostic testing or screening or for injecting local anesthetic.

Route: Parenteral

- **Intraspinal**—Injection of drug into spinal canal.
- **Intrathecal**—Injection of drug into the subarachnoid space around the spinal cord.
- **Epidural**—Injection of drug between the vertebral spines into the extradural space.

Most commonly used for regional anesthesia.
For advantages and disadvantages, see Chapter 37.

faster than tablets or capsules because the medications are already dissolved. To cross the lipid-rich cell membrane, drugs must also be at least somewhat lipid soluble. Lipid solubility depends partly on the drug's chemical structure and partly on the environment at the site of absorption. Lipid-soluble drugs can penetrate fat-containing cells, whereas water-soluble drugs, such as penicillin, cannot penetrate these areas. That is why a highly fat-soluble drug, such as nitrous oxide, can cross the blood-brain barrier and effect sedation.

Which of your patients ("Meet Your Patient") is almost certainly receiving a water-soluble medication?

Effects of pH and Ionization

The **pH** (relative acidity or alkalinity) of the local environment also affects the absorption of a drug. The acid content of the stomach aids in transporting the medication across the mucous membrane, so *acidic* medications, such as aspirin, are more readily absorbed in the stomach than *basic* (alkaline) medications, such as amphetamines, which are readily absorbed in the more alkaline small intestine. For best absorption, should Mr. Pearson's ("Meet Your Patient") medications be acidic or alkaline preparations?

In solution, some of a drug's molecules are in **ionized** (electrically charged) form, and others are **nonionized** (neutral or noncharged). The ionized molecules are lipid insoluble and, thus, cannot pass easily through the phospholipid layer of cell membranes. Drug molecules can be converted easily from one form to the other, depending primarily on the pH of the environment. For example, when aspirin is dissolved in the stomach acid, most of its molecules remain nonionized, so they easily pass through the membranes of the gastric mucosa and enter the bloodstream. If the person ingests an antacid before taking aspirin, however, it will likely reduce the effects of the aspirin.

Blood Flow to the Area

Medications are absorbed rapidly in areas where blood flow to the tissue is greatest (e.g., oral mucous membranes). Areas with poor vascular supply (e.g., the skin, scarred areas) experience delayed absorption. Consider the following examples:

1. Excessive exercise draws blood away from the stomach and intestines to the muscles. Which route would promote absorption for a person who has just exercised heavily: oral or intramuscular (IM)? Why?
2. A person in shock has poor peripheral circulation. Which route would promote faster absorption: intramuscular or intravenous (IV)? Why?

For question 1, the intramuscular route would be better because the medications are injected deep into the muscle, which has a rich blood supply; medications administered orally must first dissolve and be absorbed in the GI tract. For question 2, the IV route would be faster because (1) the drugs act faster, even in healthy people, because they are injected directly into the bloodstream and do not have to be absorbed into it, and (2) because intramuscular medications are usually given in muscles of the lower body, where the shock victim's circulation is poor.

KnowledgeCheck 23–3
- Define *absorption*.
- How are drugs absorbed?
- What factors affect absorption?

 Go to Chapter 23, **Knowledge Check Response Sheet and Answers,** on the Electronic Study Guide.

How Are Drugs Distributed Throughout the Body?

Distribution involves the transportation of a drug in body fluids (usually the bloodstream) to the various tissues and organs of the body. Because blood goes to all parts of the body, theoretically a drug can produce effects (intended or unintended) anywhere. The rate of distribution depends on the adequacy of local blood flow in the **target area** (the site where the drug effects occur), the permeability of capillaries to the drug's molecules, and the protein-binding capacity of the drug.

Local Blood Flow

The vascularity of the target site affects distribution. For example, it is difficult to deliver a systemic medication to the skin and toes, where the blood vessels are very small. Circulation in the tissues is affected by a variety of factors. Factors that cause vasodilation in an area (e.g., application of warmth to an injection site, fever, and rest) increase circulation to area tissues. Factors that cause vasoconstriction (e.g., shock and chilling of the body) decrease circulation to the target tissue.

Membrane Permeability

Drug molecules must leave the blood and cross capillary membranes to reach their sites of action. Some capillary membranes act as barriers. The capillary networks in some organs consist of tightly packed endothelial cells that prevent some drugs from crossing them. For example, the **blood-brain barrier** allows distribution into the brain and cerebrospinal fluid of only those drugs that are (1) lipid soluble (e.g., anesthetics and barbiturates) and (2) not tightly bound to plasma proteins. Many antibiotics are only water soluble and thus cannot be used to treat infections of the central nervous system. This barrier can be bypassed by injecting medications intrathecally (via the spinal canal) into the cerebrospinal fluid.

Protein-Binding Capacity

A drug's tendency to bind to plasma proteins in the blood also affects distribution. For a given amount of a drug, some molecules bind to plasma proteins, and the remainder will be "free." For example, nearly all acetaminophen (Tylenol) molecules are free in the bloodstream and are therefore pharmacologically active. By contrast, about 99% of the anticoagulant warfarin (Coumadin) is bound in the blood; its effects are produced by only the 1% of free warfarin molecules. Only free (unbound) drug molecules can produce pharmacological effects, because only free molecules can be metabolized or excreted. A drug's tendency to bind to plasma proteins depends mostly on its chemical structure. Some medical conditions also affect protein binding. For example, malnourishment and liver disease reduce the amount of protein (serum albumin) available for binding.

KnowledgeCheck 23–4
- Define distribution.
- What factors affect distribution of drugs in the body?

 Go to Chapter 23, **Knowledge Check Response Sheet and Answers,** on the Electronic Study Guide.

How Are Drugs Metabolized in the Body?

Metabolism (or **biotransformation**) is the chemical inactivation of a drug through its conversion into a more water-soluble compound or into metabolites that can be excreted from the body. Once a medication reaches its site of action, it is metabolized (changed into the inactive form) in preparation for excretion.

Metabolism takes place mainly in the liver, but medications also can be detoxified in the kidneys, blood plasma, intestinal mucosa, and lungs. If there is a decrease in liver function (e.g., due to liver disease or aging), the drug will be eliminated more slowly, and toxic levels may accumulate. Disease states also affect drug metabolism. For example, patients with diabetes do not metabolize sugar well, so they should not be given elixirs, which are high in sugar content.

Oral medications are absorbed from the gastrointestinal (GI) tract and circulate through the liver before they reach the systemic circulation. Many oral medications can be almost completely inactivated in this way. This inactivation is known as the **first-pass effect.** For this reason, oral medications are formulated with a higher concentration of the drug than are parenteral medications. Alternatively, some medications can be given parenterally, allowing the drug to be distributed directly to target sites before it passes through the liver. For example, nitroglycerine undergoes this first-pass effect when taken orally; therefore, it is given sublingually or intravenously so that it bypasses the stomach and liver and reaches therapeutic levels in the blood.

KnowledgeCheck 23–5

- Define metabolism.
- Where are drugs metabolized?
- What factors affect metabolism?

 Go to Chapter 23, **Knowledge Check Response Sheet and Answers,** on the Electronic Study Guide.

How Are Drugs Excreted from the Body?

A drug continues to act in the body until it is excreted. For **excretion** to occur, drug molecules must be removed from their sites of action and eliminated from the body. Drugs may be metabolized completely, partially, or not at all when they are excreted. The following are common organs of excretion.

- *Kidneys.* This is the primary site of excretion. Adequate fluid intake facilitates renal excretion. If your patient has decreased renal function (e.g., as indicated by an elevated creatinine level), you should monitor for medication toxicity; if signs of toxicity are present, obtain orders for adjusted dosing.

- *Liver and GI tract.* Some drugs broken down by the liver are excreted into the GI tract and eliminated in the feces. Others (e.g., fat-soluble agents) are reabsorbed by the bloodstream, distributed to the target site, and returned to the liver. This is called **enterohepatic recirculation.** The kidneys later excrete these compounds. Anything that increases peristalsis (e.g., diarrhea, laxatives, or enemas) accelerates drug excretion via feces. Inactivity, poor diet, and decreased peristalsis delay excretion, increasing the effects of a drug.

- *Lungs.* Most drugs removed by the lungs are not metabolized first. Gases and volatile liquids (e.g., general anesthetics) administered by inhalation usually are exhaled through the lungs. Other volatile substances, such as ethyl alcohol and paraldehyde, are highly soluble in blood and are excreted in limited amounts by the lungs. Exercising and deep breathing increase pulmonary blood flow and thereby promote excretion. By contrast, decreased cardiac output (as in shock) prolongs the period of time for drug elimination.

- *Exocrine glands.* Drug excretion through the **exocrine** (sweat and salivary) **glands** is limited. The elimination of metabolites in sweat is frequently responsible for such side effects as dermatitis. Drugs excreted in the saliva are usually swallowed and undergo the same fate as other orally administered agents.

 CriticalThinking 23–4

You are notified of a patient being transferred from ICU to your unit. The patient is 79-year-old Hattie Banks, admitted 2 days ago to ICU for digoxin toxicity.

- What theoretical knowledge do you have about the metabolism and excretion of digoxin (Lanoxin)?
- What assessments should you be sure to make for Ms Banks?

Concepts Relevant to Drug Effectiveness

In addition to the processes of absorption, distribution, metabolism, and excretion, you need to understand four other concepts related to a drug's effectiveness: (1) onset, peak, and duration of drug action; (2) therapeutic range; (3) bioavailability of the drug; and (4) concentration of the drug at target sites.

Onset, Peak, and Duration of Action

The **onset of action** is the time needed for drug concentration to reach a high enough blood level for its effects to appear. This is the **minimum effective concentration.** When the concentration of medication is highest in the blood, the medication has reached its **peak action.** The **duration of action** is

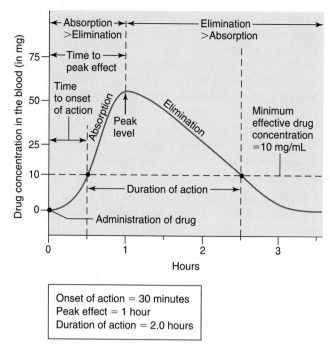

Onset of action = 30 minutes
Peak effect = 1 hour
Duration of action = 2.0 hours

FIGURE 23–4 Once the drug is administered and absorption begins, blood levels begin to rise. When the *minimum effective concentration* is reached, drug effects begin (*onset of action*). *Maximum effect* occurs at peak blood level.

that period of time in which the medication has a pharmacological effect (before it is metabolized and excreted) (Figure 23–4). If the serum level of a medication falls below the minimum effective concentration, then the drug is not effective during that time. If the drug level exceeds the peak level, toxicity occurs.

 CriticalThinking 23–5

Refer again to Table 23–3. James Bigler ("Meet Your Patient") is having right arm pain and needs relief quickly.

• Would you give him oral acetaminophen with codeine (Tylenol #3) or an IM injection of a similar-strength medication? Why?

• Do you have enough information to be 100% sure your choice of route will bring the quickest onset of action? Explain.

Therapeutic Range

When giving an ongoing medication (e.g., an antibiotic), the goal is to achieve a constant, therapeutic blood level. Because a fraction of the drug is constantly being excreted, repeated doses of the medication are given to achieve and maintain a constant therapeutic concentration. Even after absorption stops, distribution, metabolism, and excretion continue.

• **Therapeutic level** is the concentration of a drug in the blood serum that produces the desired effect without toxicity.

• **Therapeutic range** of a drug is a *range* of therapeutic concentrations. At *onset,* serum drug level is minimal.

• **Peak level** occurs when the drug is at its highest concentration (when the rate of absorption is equal to the rate of elimination). After that, metabolism and excretion begin to remove the drug from the tissues and blood.

• **Trough level** occurs when the drug is at its lowest concentration, right before the next dose is due.

A test called a *peak and trough level* helps to ensure the safety and effectiveness of certain drugs. The peak level must be measured when absorption is complete. This, of course, depends on all the factors that affect absorption. The trough level is usually measured about 30 minutes before the next dose of the drug is due. The drug's half-life and the time between doses affect the trough level. You will sometimes need to monitor serum drug levels so the primary care provider can adjust the dose and timing of a medication as needed. For a graphic illustration of peak, trough, and therapeutic levels,

Go to Chapter 23, **Tables, Boxes, Figures: ESG Figure 23–1,** on the Electronic Study Guide.

Biological Half-Life

A medication's **biological half-life** is the amount of time it takes for half of the drug to be eliminated. For example tramadol (Ultram), an analgesic, has a half-life of approximately 6 hours. This means if you take a 50 mg dose at 8:00 A.M., by 2:00 P.M. half of that dose (25 mg) will still be left in your body. In 12 hours, one-fourth of the initial dose (12.5 mg) will be left in your body. Because of their effect on metabolism and excretion, the following prolong half-life: liver and kidney disease, aging, absence of food, and slowed metabolic rate. Drug composition and distribution also affect half-life.

 CriticalThinking 23–6

Rebecca Jones ("Meet Your Patients") received Ultram 50 mg for pain at 8:00 A.M. Her order says she can have the drug every 6 hours. So at 2:00 P.M., you give her another 50 mg. Ultram is metabolized in the liver and excreted mainly in the urine.

• When this medication reaches onset of action, about how much Ultram does Ms Jones now have in her body?

• If the "normal" half-life of Ultram is 6 hours, you would expect Ms Jones to still have about 25 mg of her first dose left in her body at the time of the second dose. Given her age, though, do you think she probably has more or less than 25 mg left at 6 hours? Why?

TABLE 23-4 Drug Therapy Across the Life Span

Pharmacokinetic Process	Children	Older Adults
Absorption	• Exaggerated in infants as a result of lack of gastric acidity and shorter intestines. • More complete topical absorption resulting from a larger body surface and thinner epidermis. • Enteral route is unpredictable. • Decreased muscle tone makes absorption of parenteral drugs unpredictable. • Gastric pH is higher, so that medications absorbed in acid environments are absorbed much more slowly.	• Delayed but more complete. • Gastric pH is less acidic because of decreased acid production in the stomach. • Decreased gastric pH delays absorption of medications absorbed in acid environments. • Because of decreased intestinal motility, drugs remain in the system longer, allowing for more absorption.
Distribution	• Protein binding may be a problem. • Greater chance of toxicity because of low albumin levels. • Water content in the child's body is higher than in adults, so water-soluble drugs are less concentrated in the child and fat-soluble drugs are more highly concentrated.	• Low albumin level could create a problem with plasma protein binding. • Increased risk of toxicity due to multi-organ slowdown. • Altered because of less lean mass. • Less body water, greater body fat. • Dehydration, poor nutrition, and electrolyte imbalances decrease absorption.
Metabolism	• Metabolism may be altered because of immature liver. • Best to base dosage on body weight to avoid toxicity.	• Presence of diseases may decrease metabolism of the drug. • Changes due to age, higher blood concentration, and less excretion cause greater chances of toxicity. • Some drugs interfere with the liver's ability to metabolize another drug.
Excretion	• Delayed as result of immature kidneys. • Repeat dosing may cause problems.	• Decreased glomerular filtration rate inhibits excretion from the kidneys. • Diminished renal function inhibits excretion, thereby increasing the risk of toxicity.

Concentration of Active Drug at Target Sites

The effectiveness of a medication depends ultimately on its concentration at the intended site. For example, a medication such as nitrofurantoin (Macrodantin) may be ordered to treat a urinary tract infection. This drug is used because it is highly soluble in urine and therefore tends to accumulate and concentrate in the bladder and kidneys, where the infection exists.

What Factors Affect Pharmacokinetics?

A drug's pharmacokinetics and, therefore, its effectiveness and safety are affected by the following factors:

• *Age.* Infants and young children need smaller doses because of their smaller body mass and immature body systems. Older adults may have declining liver and kidney function and are therefore at higher risk for drug toxicity. Table 23–4 summarizes life span variations in pharmacokinetics.

• *Body mass (weight).* The average adult dose is based on the drug quantity that will produce a particular effect in 50% of people 18 to 65 years of age and weighing 150 lb. Obviously, a person who is much larger or smaller than this "average" requires an adjusted dose.

• *Sex.* Women are smaller than men and have different proportions of body fat and water, which affect drug absorption.

• *Pregnancy.* Most drugs are contraindicated during pregnancy because of their possible adverse effects

on the embryo or fetus. Drugs that are known to cause developmental defects are called **teratogenic** drugs. Examples are alcohol and the anticonvulsant phenytoin (Dilantin).

- *Environment.* For example, heat and cold affect peripheral circulation. A noisy environment may interfere with a person's response to antianxiety, sedative, or pain medications.
- *Timing of administration.* The presence or absence of food in the GI tract affects an oral drug's pharmacokinetics. Biorhythms and cycles (e.g., drug-metabolizing enzyme rhythms, blood pressure cycles) also influence drug action.
- *Fluids.* Insufficient fluid intake affects the absorption of solid dosage forms.
- *Pathological states.* Intense pain decreases the effect of opioids; diseases causing circulatory, hepatic, or renal dysfunction interfere with pharmacokinetic processes.
- *Genetic factors.* Abnormal susceptibility to certain chemicals is genetically determined. Enzyme deficiencies and altered metabolism change a patient's responses to a drug. For example, African Americans respond better to diuretics for blood pressure control than do other racial groups; and people of Asian descent metabolize some opioids at a slower rate. Use your critical thinking now. What important nursing intervention should you perform after you administer an opiate to an Asian patient?*
- *Psychological factors.* Some patients have the same response to a **placebo**—a pharmacologically inactive substance—as they do to the active drug. If a person has faith that a drug will help him, a *placebo effect* similar to the effect of an active drug may occur. Emotional states, such as anxiety, may cause resistance to tranquilizing drugs. Hostility toward or mistrust of medicine or health personnel can also interfere with a drug's effectiveness.

WHAT IS PHARMACODYNAMICS?

Pharmacodynamics is the study of *how* medications achieve their effects at various sites in the body—how specific drug molecules interact with target cells and how biological responses occur.

What Are Primary Effects?

Primary or **therapeutic effects** of medications are those effects which are predicted, intended, and desired. The primary effects, in short, are the reason the drug was prescribed. All other consequences are **secondary effects** (unintended, nontherapeutic). Both primary

and secondary effects are dose related, so increasing the dose increases the effects. Medications are given for the following effects:

- **Palliative effects** relieve the signs and symptoms of a disease but have no effect on the disease itself. For example, morphine sulfate may be given to a patient with cancer to manage pain, but it does not destroy cancer cells. The goal of palliative therapy is to make the patient as comfortable as possible when treatment options have been exhausted.
- **Supportive effects** support the integrity of body functions until other medications or treatments can become effective. For a patient with a bacterial infection, you may give acetaminophen (Tylenol) to control fever until blood levels of the prescribed antibiotic are effective in combating the infection causing the fever.
- **Substitutive effects** replace either body fluids or a chemical required by the body for improved functioning. You may, for example, administer insulin to a diabetic patient to replace the insulin no longer produced by the pancreas.
- **Chemotherapeutic effects** destroy disease-producing microorganisms or body cells. Two examples are (1) antibiotics, used to treat infections by killing or limiting the reproduction of certain bacteria; and (2) antineoplastic drugs, used to treat cancer by limiting cell reproduction and destroying malignant cells.
- **Restorative effects** return the body to or maintain the body at optimal levels of health. For example, vitamin and mineral supplements are administered to many patients recovering from surgery.

KnowledgeCheck 23–6

- Name and define the four pharmacokinetic processes.
- How does absorption differ in children and older adults?
- What factors affect excretion?
- You are to administer the following drugs to Cyndi Early ("Meet Your Patient"): (1) insulin for her diabetes, administered subcutaneously, and (2) morphine to relieve her pain, administered intravenously. For which primary effect is each of these drugs being given?

 Go to Chapter 23, **Knowledge Check Response Sheet and Answers,** on the Electronic Study Guide.

What Are Secondary Effects?

All medications can cause secondary effects (e.g., side effects, adverse reactions, allergic reactions), which can either be harmless or cause injury and which can sometimes be predicted.

Side Effects

Side effects are unintended, often predictable, physiological effects that are usually well tolerated by patients. They occur at the usual prescribed dose and may be

---

*How did you answer the question? If you said that you would need to observe closely for unexpected side effects, good thinking!

immediate (e.g., dizziness) or delayed (e.g., constipation). For hospitalized patients, you will most often see side effects caused by analgesics, antibiotics, antipsychotics, and sedatives. The most common side effects are nausea, vomiting, diarrhea, dizziness, drowsiness, dry mouth, abdominal distention or distress, and constipation.

If side effects are serious enough, the physician may discontinue the medication. For example, lanoxin (Digoxin), which is given to regulate and strengthen the heartbeat, can cause cardiac irregularities, a side effect that can be lethal. Persistent or troublesome side effects may require symptom management with laxatives, antidiarrheals, and antiemetics. For example, levofloxacin (Levaquin), an antibiotic, may cause diarrhea, which is treated with antidiarrheals (e.g., loperamide [Immodium]). Teach your patients what side effects to anticipate with medications and how to manage them.

Adverse Reactions

Adverse reactions are harmful, unintended, usually unpredicted reactions to a drug administered at the normal dosage. They are more severe than side effects and often require discontinuation of the drug.

- When adverse reactions are *dose related,* the undesired effects result from known pharmacological effects of the medication. For example, a diabetic patient treated with insulin may develop very low blood sugar if too much insulin is administered or he doesn't eat.

- Adverse reactions also occur because of *patient sensitivity,* meaning that the patient is unusually susceptible to the effects of the drug. Box 23–1 lists patients at high risk for adverse reactions.

The FDA defines **severe adverse reactions** as those that (1) are life-threatening, (2) require intervention to prevent permanent impairment or death, or (3) lead to congenital anomaly, disability, hospitalization, or death. You must document serious adverse reactions according to agency policy and report them to the FDA MedWatch program. To make a report, telephone (301)827-7240, or

Go to the **FDA Medwatch** web site at
http://www.fda.gov/medwatch/

Toxic Reactions

Toxic reactions are dangerous, damaging effects to an organ or tissue. They are more severe than adverse reactions, sometimes even causing permanent damage or death. It may help to think of toxicity as poisoning. Antidotes are available for some medications; for example, naloxone (Narcan) is given for opiate toxicity. Toxicity may be caused by any of the following:

- *Overdosing* (e.g., respiratory depression from excessive morphine or hypoglycemia from too much insulin)

> ## BOX 23–1 Risk Factors for Adverse Drug Reactions
>
> - Receiving treatment from two or more physicians at the same time
> - Concurrent illnesses (e.g., diabetes and renal failure)
> - A change in the ability to metabolize or excrete the drug
> - Taking multiple prescription drugs in addition to over-the-counter preparations
> - Taking a drug inconsistently
> - History of allergies
> - History of previous adverse drug reactions
> - Long-term use of a drug (may promote accumulation, leading to toxicity)
> - Very old or very young age
> - Obesity or extreme thinness
> - Impaired hepatic and renal function

- *Accumulation* of the drug in the tissues (related to long-term use or incomplete metabolism/excretion)
- *Abnormal sensitivity* to the drug

Toxic reactions are usually localized, reversible, and immediate. However:

- They can be localized to a particular tissue or organ, or they can affect several organ systems.
- They may be reversible (e.g., tinnitus caused by aspirin) or permanent (e.g., hearing loss caused by aminoglycoside antibiotics).
- They usually occur soon after administration; but, some require months or even years to develop (e.g., drug-induced cancers).

CriticalThinking 23–7

- You have just looked up a new antihypertensive drug, lisinopril (Zestril) and found the following side effects. What strategy could you use to help you remember all the side effects listed below?

  neutropenia, dizziness, headache, fatigue, depression, somnolence, paresthesia, hypotension, orthostasis, chest pain, nasal congestion, diarrhea, nausea, dyspepsia, impotence, rash, cough, muscle cramps, angioedema, lethargy, hypokalemia, decreased libido

- You have checked the medication record (MAR) for Margaret Marks ("Meet Your Patients") and prepared her next dose of antibiotic for intravenous administration. The MAR also indicates that she is receiving morphine for pain and that her last dose was given 1 hour ago. When you enter the room, you find her

TABLE 23–5   Medications Frequently Implicated in Allergic Reactions

Antibiotics	Cephalosporins Erythomycin Neomycin Penicillin Streptomycin Sulfonamides Tetracycline Vancomycin
Biological Agents	Antibiotics, antitoxins, corticotropin (ACTH), enzymes, gamma globulin, insulin, vaccines
Diagnostic Agents	Iodinated media contrasts, intravenous pyelogram (IVP) dye
Other Drugs	Acetaminophen (Tylenol), aspirin, benzocaine, dextran, histamines, iodines, iron, phenothiazines, quinidine, tranquilizers; anesthetic agents, such as tetracaine, phenylbutazone, procaine, lidocaine, cocaine

apparently sleeping. You are not able to awaken her to verify her identity. What do you suspect is happening, and how should you respond? (If you need information about antibiotics and morphine, look it up in an appropriate reference source.)

Allergic Reactions

In an **allergic reaction,** the immune system identifies a medication as a foreign substance that should be neutralized or destroyed. The patient experiences no problems with the first dose of the medication, but it acts as an antigen, activating the formation of antibodies against the drug. When the drug is again administered, the antigen-antibody binding prompts an allergic reaction.

Allergic reactions range from minor to serious; however, even a small amount of a medication has the potential to cause a severe reaction. Urticaria (hives), pruritus (itching), and rhinitis (inflammation of the nasal mucosa) usually occur within minutes to 2 weeks after exposure and are considered mild. Such reactions often disappear after the medication is discontinued and the blood level of the drug falls. Table 23–5 lists

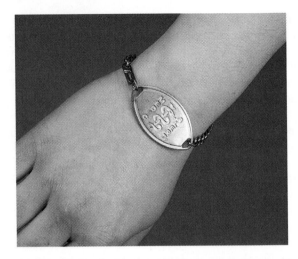

FIGURE 23–5   People with severe allergies to a medication should wear a MedicAlert bracelet.

medications most frequently implicated in allergic reactions.

An **anaphylactic reaction** is a life-threatening allergic reaction. It occurs immediately after administration, with sudden constriction of bronchioles, edema of larynx and pharynx, severe shortness of breath, wheezing, and severe hypotension (low blood pressure). Immediate treatment includes discontinuing the medication, giving epinephrine, IV fluids, steroids, and antihistamines. Respiratory support ranging from oxygen to intubation and ventilation may also be required. A patient who is allergic to one drug may also be allergic to other medications in the same class. For example, many patients who are allergic to penicillin are also allergic to cephalexin (Keflex), a synthetic penicillin.

Allergic reactions occur with 5 to 10% of all prescriptions, so always explore the patient's allergy history, use Allergy Alert bracelets and stickers, and document allergies in the patient's chart and care plan. People with severe allergic reactions should wear a MedicAlert bracelet (Figure 23–5).

 CriticalThinking 23–8

You are administering medications to your assigned patients ("Meet Your Patients"). What should you do in each of the following situations? Which patient should you attend to first? Explain your thinking.

- Mrs. Jones has ibuprofen (Motrin) ordered for her leg pain. She tells you she cannot take this medication because it makes her nauseated.
- Mr. Bigler had an open reduction internal fixation of his arm performed yesterday and is receiving an antibiotic, cefazolin (Ancef), 500 mg IV every 8 hours. He has already received three doses of this medication, and you initiated his 8:00 A.M. dose about 10 minutes ago. He tells you that he thinks his throat is closing shut.

Idiosyncratic Reactions

An **idiosyncratic** reaction is an unexpected, abnormal, or peculiar response to a medication. Idiosyncratic reactions may take the form of extreme sensitivity to a medication, lack of response, or a paradoxical (opposite of expected) response, such as agitation in response to a sedative. In children, for example, diphenhydramine (Benadryl) has been known to cause agitation or excitability instead of the expected drowsiness.

Cumulative Effect

Cumulative effect is the increased response to repeated doses of a drug when the rate of administration is greater than the rate of metabolism and excretion. This occurs when (1) the body cannot metabolize a dose of the medication before the next dose is given, (2) excretion is slowed but absorption is normal or rapid, or (3) absorption is slowed. Unless the dose is changed, the medication accumulates in the system until a toxic level is reached. Opiates and barbiturates are known for their cumulative effects.

KnowledgeCheck 23–7

- Differentiate between primary and secondary effects of medications.
- List one adverse reaction for each of the following systems: blood, gastrointestinal, central nervous system, cardiovascular, hepatic, renal.
- What are some of the symptoms you will see in an anaphylactic reaction?
- What type of patient is most likely to experience an allergic reaction?

 Go to Chapter 23, **Knowledge Check Response Sheet and Answers,** on the Electronic Study Guide.

How Do Medications Interact?

When one drug alters or modifies the action of another, a **drug interaction** occurs. In an **antagonistic drug relationship,** one drug interferes with the actions of another and decreases the resultant drug effect—that is, the combined effect is less than one drug given alone. In a **synergistic drug relationship,** there is an additive effect; that is, the effect of both drugs together is greater than the individual effects. **Drug incompatibilities** occur when multiple drugs are mixed together, causing a chemical deterioration of one or both the drugs. The result is an incompatible solution that should not be administered. You can usually recognize an incompatibility when the mixed solution takes on a change in appearance. However, you should always consult medication resources and compatibility charts *prior* to mixing medications. Then, after mixing, double-check the medication for changes in appearance.

As a nurse, you must be knowledgeable of drug interactions and monitor your patients for them. For a list of common drug-drug and drug-food interactions,

 Go to Chapter 23, **Tables, Boxes, Figures: ESG Table 23–2,** on the Electronic Study Guide.

The more drugs a patient takes, the higher the risk of a drug interaction. Other variables influence drug interactions: intestinal absorption, competition for protein binding, drug metabolism, renal excretion, and alteration of electrolyte imbalance.

Drugs may also interact with certain foods. For example,

- Fatty foods and foods low in fiber will delay stomach emptying and medication absorption by up to 2 hours.
- Acidic citrus fruits and juices enhance absorption of iron.
- Carbonated soft drinks can cause medications to dissolve faster, be neutralized, or experience a change in absorption rate in the stomach.
- When dairy products are taken with an antibiotic such as tetracycline, there is decreased absorption of the drug in the stomach.
- When foods containing tyramine (e.g. aged, dried, or fermented products) are ingested with MAO inhibitors, a hypertensive crisis may result.

For a list of several medications that should be taken with food and those that should be taken on an empty stomach,

 Go to Chapter 23, **Tables, Boxes, Figures: ESG Box 23–1,** on the Electronic Study Guide.

KnowledgeCheck 23–8

- What type of interaction occurs when one drug interferes with the action of another?
- What interactions occur when one drug has an additive effect on another drug?
- What is drug incompatibility?

 Go to Chapter 23, **Knowledge Check Response Sheet and Answers,** on the Electronic Study Guide.

What Should I Know About Drug Abuse or Misuse?

You should be able to differentiate between tolerance and dependence. **Tolerance** is a decreasing response to repeated doses of a medication. The person then requires more of the drug to achieve the desired effect. In contrast, a person's reliance on, or need for, a drug constitutes **drug dependence.** Dependence leads to compulsive patterns of drug use wherein the user's lifestyle centers on procuring and taking the drug.

Drug misuse is the nonspecific, indiscriminate, or improper use of drugs, including alcohol, over-the-counter (OTC), and prescription drugs. In performing self-care, people frequently misuse laxatives, aspirin, acetaminophen, ibuprofen, and cough and cold medications. Older adults are especially prone to misuse of laxatives.

Drug abuse is the inappropriate intake of a substance, continuously or periodically. For example, consuming alcohol at work is considered abuse, but consuming alcohol with dinner is not. Drug abuse may or may not lead to drug dependence. Alcohol, nicotine (tobacco), and opiates are the most frequently abused drugs. **Illicit drugs,** also known as street drugs, are drugs sold illegally. Many are prescription drugs (e.g., codeine) sought for their mood-altering effects.

HOW DO I MEASURE AND CALCULATE DOSAGE?

Medications are not always available in the exact dosage the patient needs. Therefore, you must be proficient in calculating drug dosages to be sure your patients receive the correct amount of medication.

Medication Measurement Systems

Medications are usually ordered and measured using the metric system; however, there are still a few medications that use the apothecary and household systems, so you need to learn how to work with all three systems. For a complete discussion of measurement systems and equivalents,

 Go to Chapter 23, **Measuring and Calculating Dosage,** in Volume 2.

- *Metric system.* The metric system is the preferred system. The metric system promotes accuracy by allowing for calculation of small drug dosages. A disadvantage of this system in the United States is its limited use among people outside the healthcare system.
- *Apothecary system.* The British apothecary system of measurement has been in use in the United States since Colonial times. Only a few medications (e.g., aspirin) are measured using this system because it is less convenient and less precise. Apothecary measurements are usually written using Roman numerals, but you may also see them in Arabic numerals. For example, *5 grains* might be written as *gr V* or *5 gr.*
- *Household system.* Because most people are familiar with the household system, it is easier to teach a patient about home medications using this system. However, nurses use it only occasionally because

dosages measured in this system are usually only approximate (e.g., teaspoons, ounces, cup).

Special Measurements: Units and Milliequivalents (mEq)

Insulin, a drug used by diabetics to assist in the control of blood sugar, is measured in **units,** with 100 international units (U100) being the standard strength preparation. In this strength, 1 mL of the fluid medication contains 100 units of insulin. Heparin, an anticoagulant, and penicillin are also ordered in units. Be aware that not all units are the same. For example, 1 mL of heparin does *not* contain 100 units of heparin. You must always read the container label to know the number of units per mL. The following is a medication order using units: "NPH insulin 14 units SubQ q A.M."

Milliequivalents (mEq) indicate the strength of the ion concentration in a drug. A milliequivalent is the number of grams of a solid contained in one mL of a solution. Electrolytes, such as potassium chloride (KCl), are measured in mEq. The following are medication orders using mEq:

KCl 20 mEq by mouth twice daily

D_5W 1000 mL with KCl 40 mEq q8hr

Note that units and mEq *cannot* be directly converted to the apothecary, metric, or household systems.

Calculating Dosages

You should be able to calculate accurately using several different methods and formulas. Inaccurate calculations result in incorrect dosages and could harm the patient. For expanded instructions on calculating dosages for adults and children,

 Go to Chapter 23, **Measuring and Calculating Dosage,** in Volume 2.

The Electronic Study Guide also contains several practice problems. To use them,

 Go to Chapter 23, **Practice Dosage Problems,** on the Electronic Study Guide.

WHAT MUST I KNOW ABOUT MEDICATION ORDERS?

Before administering any medication you must obtain a medication order from the care provider and verify that it is complete and correct. A complete medication order contains six essential elements:

- Patient's full name
- Date and time order was written
- Name of medication

- Dosage (including size, frequency, and number of doses)
- Route of administration
- Signature of prescriber

To verify a medication order, ask yourself the following questions:

Is the order legible enough for me to read?
Is the ordered dose within the normally prescribed dosage range?
Is the ordered route appropriate?
Is the drug appropriate for the patient? (For example, you would question an antihypertensive drug ordered to be given to a patient with hypotension.)
Is the patient allergic to the medication ordered?
Are the administration times appropriate? For example, is an antibiotic ordered for every 6 hours when the PDR indicates it should be taken every 24 hours?

A prescription and a physician order are similar, but the *prescription* is given to the pharmacy (often by the patient) to obtain medications for self-administration, whereas the *physician's order* is used in the hospital or ambulatory care setting. As shown in Figure 23–6, in addition to the components in an order, a prescription must contain the following:

- Address and license of person ordering
- Duration or dose quantity (e.g., the total number of tablets needed, often a 30-day supply, or "for 30 days")
- Number of refills

KnowledgeCheck 23–9

- What are the essential parts of a medication order?
- How does a medication order differ from a prescription?

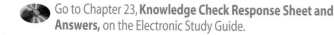 Go to Chapter 23, **Knowledge Check Response Sheet and Answers,** on the Electronic Study Guide.

What Abbreviations Are Used in Medication Orders?

For a list of abbreviations you may see used when ordering and documenting medications,

VOL 2 | Go to Chapter 23, **Medication-Related Abbreviations,** in Volume 2.

It is always safest to write words out in full when you deal with medications. Use abbreviations carefully, because some may be similar and confusing (Box 23–2). For example, qid (four times a day) and qd (daily) are easily confused if the handwriting is illegible. You should be familiar with institutional policies for use of abbreviations and know the acceptable abbreviations used by that facility.

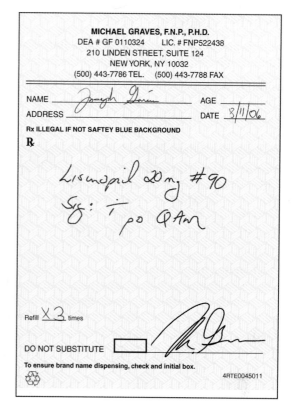

FIGURE 23–6 **Example of a prescription.**

BOX 23-2 **Easily Misunderstood Abbreviations**

Avoid using the following abbreviations because they are easily confused with other abbreviations.

CC*	po
d/c, D/C, DC*	IM
H.S.*	ID
qd*	U*
qid	IU*
qod*	MS*
os (O.S.)*	MSO$_4$*
od (O.D.)*	MgSO$_4$*
ou (O.U.)*	SC or SQ*
tid	cc*
bid	

*Indicates an abbreviation that has been disallowed by the Joint Commission on Accreditation of Healthcare Organizations (JCAHO).

Types of Medication Orders

Common types of medication orders are based on the duration, frequency, and/or urgency of the order.

- **Standard written orders** apply indefinitely until the prescriber writes an order to alter or discontinue the medication or indicates on the original order a specific stop date. For example, "Give Lasix 20 mg IV twice a day for 5 days."

- **Automatic stop dates** are protocols that hospitals use for discontinuing medications after a certain length of time. Most narcotic orders are in effect only for 7 days. If the medication is needed after the automatic stop date, the care provider must write another order.

- A **STAT order** means that a single dose of medication is to be given immediately and only once. The word *stat* or *now* should appear in the order, for example, "Give Lasix 20 mg IV STAT," or "Give Ativan 1 mg IV now."

- A **single order,** or *one-time order,* indicates that the medication is to be given only once at a specified time. Preoperative medications, given prior to surgery or diagnostic procedures or treatments, are single orders. For example:

    Versed 25 mg intramuscularly on call for OR [i.e., when the OR notifies you]

    Tetanus toxoid 0.5 mL intramuscularly before discharge

- **Standing orders.** When a unit frequently provides care to a standard population of patients—for example, coronary care patients or knee replacement patients—the physician may develop a set of *standing orders*. These are officially accepted sets of orders to be applied routinely by nurses for the care of patients under certain conditions or under certain circumstances. They establish guidelines for treating a particular disease or set of symptoms. For example:

    Coronary care or intensive care units (CCUs or ICUs) may have standing orders for the administration of nitroglycerine (NTG) or morphine for chest pain (e.g., "Give NTG 0.4 mg sublingually q3–5 min for chest pain, to a maximum of 3 doses in 15 min").

    Many postoperative patients receive a set number of doses of ketorolac (Toradol), an injectable analgesic medication. So, for all the postoperative patients on a unit, standing orders would include, "Toradol 30 mg IV q12hr × 2 days."

- **PRN orders.** The care provider may order a medication to be given whenever the patient requires (PRN). A PRN order requires the nurse to determine, in collaboration with the patient, when the medication is to be given. The order specifies (1) the condition for which the medication is to be given and (2) the minimum time intervals between doses. The medication cannot be given any more frequently than prescribed, even if symptoms persist. Pain medications, antiemetics (antinausea medications), and laxatives are usually given PRN. For example:

    Morphine 10 mg intramuscularly q3–4hr PRN incisional pain.

    Tylenol 650 mg po q4hr PRN for temp >101° F.

How Are Medication Orders Communicated?

Medication orders can be communicated in various ways. The nursing implications are slightly different for each.

- **Written orders** are those written (or preprinted) on a standard medication order form. Some agencies permit the physician to **fax orders** to the nurse and bring the original copy later. Although this step may save time, the risk of errors is greater because faxed copies may be illegible.

- **Verbal orders** are given orally rather than in writing, while the physician is present with the nurse. When you receive a verbal order, you, as the RN, will write the order and sign it with the physician's name followed by your name and credentials. You should then repeat the order to the physician to ensure accuracy. Avoid taking verbal orders and use them only in urgent situations, because they increase the risk for miscommunication and errors.

- **Telephone orders** are those that the physician gives you via a telephone. Usually this will be in response to a call you have placed to report a change in the patient's condition or the results of laboratory or other tests. The physician usually must cosign verbal and telephone orders within 24 hours.

What Steps Should I Take If I Think an Order Is Incorrect?

As a nurse, you are legally responsible for medications you administer. If you believe an order is incorrect, perform the following steps:

- Ask another nurse to check the order.
- Look up the medication in a reliable resource to verify spelling, usage, dosages, and routes.
- Contact the ordering physician for clarifications, concerns, or questions.
- Do not assume you are correctly interpreting the order if you have any question at all.

Use your knowledge, common sense, and intuition when administering medications. To avoid errors, you must know and understand the procedures at your facility, be familiar with the medications you give, and always check the orders. Each agency will have a policy

specifying the procedure for checking medication orders. For example, a unit clerk may copy the original order onto a medication administration record (MAR), but the nurse must check to be sure the transcription is correct.

 ## CriticalThinking 23–9

Find the errors in these medication orders. Look the medications up in a PDR or nursing drug handbook to check dosages, spelling, and so on

- Ancef 10 g q6hr IV
- Capatril 25 mg orally twice a day
- Digoxin 0.125 mg daily
- Lasix 400 mg by mouth
- NTG gr 1/150 PRN chest pain
- Tylenol orally PRN fever

Practical Knowledge
knowing how

Regardless of the type of medication or the route of administration, when administering a medication you should:

- Perform assessments relevant to the medication.
- Review the medication orders and the medication administration record (MAR); clarify any differences.
- Consult an appropriate reference source for medications unfamiliar to you.
- Explain to the patient the actions and the side effects of the medication.
- Administer the medication using the "six rights."
- Perform related interventions, for example:

    Explain the importance of drinking fluids, timing of medication in relation to food, and whether medication may be crushed.
    Assess vital signs.
    Assess for contraindications and adverse effects.

- Evaluate and record the patient's response to the medication.

The rest of the chapter will explain these activities to you. You should also

 Go to Chapter 23, **Medication Guidelines: Steps to Follow for All Medications (Regardless of Type or Route)**, in Volume 2.

 ## CriticalThinking 23–10

Mr. Pearson ("Meet Your Patients") refuses to take his 2:00 P.M. dose of antibiotic, stating that he had just taken it. What actions do you take to ensure sound decision making and maintain patient safety?

| Assessment |

During your initial patient assessment, you begin gathering data that you need to administer medications safely to the patient. The following are highlights of medication-related assessments to make.

Before administration, assess:

- Vital signs*
- Whether the patient's general condition is appropriate for the medication
- Your knowledge of the medication

During administration, assess the patient's:

- Perceptions
- Coordination
- Ability to self-administer the drug
- Swallowing (for oral medications)

Following administration, assess:

- Effectiveness of the drug
- For side effects
- For signs of toxicity

When taking a medication history, you should ask about the patient's history of illness, history of allergies, medications, attitudes toward medications, learning needs, and whether the patient (if a woman) is pregnant or breastfeeding. Also check relevant laboratory test results. For more discussion of the components to include in a medications history, and to print out a tool you can use for a full medications history and physical,

 Go to Chapter 23, **Supplemental Materials: Components of a Medication History,** on the Electronic Study Guide.

As with the nursing history, the physical examination allows you to identify potential problems and the need for adapting medication administration procedures. For example, you will assess relevant body systems to confirm the need for the drug and provide a baseline for evaluating the patient's responses to it. For oral medications, assess the patient's ability to swallow; for intramuscular medications, assess muscle mass. For more complete information about the physical examination related to medications,

 Go to Chapter 23, **Supplemental Materials: Physical Examination Related to Medications,** on the Electronic Study Guide.

---

*Except for certain medications, you will not need to take a new set of vital signs before administering; however, you should be aware of the patient's vital signs at the last assessment, as a reflection of his health status.

| Nursing Diagnosis |

The following are some examples of nursing diagnoses associated with patient medications:

- Deficient Knowledge related to lack of motivation to learn about medications
- Ineffective Management of Therapeutic Regimen related to confusion
- Risk for Aspiration related to Impaired Swallowing

For examples of other nursing diagnoses,

 Go to Chapter 23, **Standardized Language; Standardized Diagnoses, Outcomes, and Interventions Related to Medication Administration,** in Volume 2.

A few nursing diagnoses represent medication side effects; however, because a wide range of adverse effects is possible, no attempt was made to include them all. The following sections discuss Risk for Injury and Noncompliance.

Risk for Injury

Risk for Injury may be related to polypharmacy, misuse, overuse, or underuse of medications. Many people self-prescribe or rely on OTC medications for relief of symptoms such as insomnia, headaches, joint pains, and indigestion. They may continue taking them in combination with prescribed medications. This practice is **polypharmacy:** the ingestion of numerous medications in an attempt to treat many conditions simultaneously. Polypharmacy increases the potential for adverse reactions and dangerous drug and food interactions.

Older adults may be especially prone to polypharmacy. They typically take several medications prescribed for chronic diseases, and many experience symptoms related to the aging process (e.g., constipation) for which they self-medicate. The combination of polypharmacy with the increased sensitivity to medications and with declining cognitive and sensory function can be especially dangerous.

Some patients, especially older adults, misuse, overuse, underuse, and use drugs erratically. They may even use them when contraindicated (e.g., a patient with hypertension may self-prescribe a "diet pill" to lose weight, thus increasing his BP). When a person "feels better" after a few days of the medication, she may stop taking it or take it erratically as symptoms come and go. Such an inconsistent dosage schedule affects the body's ability to achieve a blood level high enough to treat the disease.

Noncompliance

Noncompliance (nonadherence) is failure to follow the treatment plan (e.g., not taking a prescribed medication, or skipping doses). You cannot assume that a noncompliant patient needs to be taught the importance of following the treatment plan. Prescription medications are expensive. Faced with choosing between food and pills, people on a limited budget often simply do not buy the more costly medications, or they may take only partial doses of maintenance medications (e.g., thyroid medications, oral hypoglycemics). Some patients, particularly older adults, may have visual and motor deficits that limit their ability to read labels and manipulate bottle caps, syringes, and so on. Other reasons for noncompliance include lack of symptoms, inability to tolerate side effects, forgetfulness, and impaired mental capacity. Always investigate the patient's reasons for nonadherence so that you can take appropriate actions.

KnowledgeCheck 23–10

- What are the risks involved for patients who engage in polypharmacy?
- List at least three reasons for noncompliance with a medication regimen.

 Go to Chapter 23, **Knowledge Check Response Sheet and Answers,** on the Electronic Study Guide.

| Planning Outcomes/Evaluation |

NOC standardized outcomes will depend on the specific nursing diagnoses you choose. For NOC outcomes for selected nursing diagnoses,

 Go to Chapter 23, **Standardized Language; Standardized Diagnoses, Outcomes, and Interventions Related to Medication Administration,** in Volume 2.

Individualized goals/outcome statements you might write for a client should be stated so that their achievement reflects resolution of the problem (NANDA label). The following are some examples:

- After explanation, and within 1 week, describes the expected actions and side effects of his medications.
- Self-administers his medications in the correct amounts and on the prescribed schedule.
- Describes possible interactions with other drugs; names the drugs to avoid taking with this medication.
- After demonstration and practice, and within 1 week, correctly draws up and self-administers insulin.
- Will consult primary care provider before adding any new OTC medications or herbal/other medications.

| Planning Interventions/Implementation |

NIC standardized interventions will depend on the patient's nursing diagnoses, especially on the etiologies.

 Go to Chapter 23, **Standardized Language; Standardized Diagnoses, Outcomes, and Interventions Related to Medication Administration,** in Volume 2.

Specific individualized nursing activities include preparing and administering medications. You will use specific, step-by-step procedures for these activities. However, only the general principles and the critical aspects of the procedures are presented in this volume. For specific procedures,

 Go to Chapter 23, **Procedures,** in Volume 2.

Nursing interventions also include activities to address specific nursing diagnoses and, for all patients, the following activities to ensure safe administration of medications.

ENSURING SAFE MEDICATION ADMINISTRATION

One study (*AJN* Reports, 2003) revealed that 19% of medication doses administered by nurses were incorrect. Errors included giving the dose at the wrong time, omitting doses, giving the wrong dose, and giving the dose without authorization. Seven percent of the errors were clinically significant. To help prevent errors, perform "three checks" and "six rights" when giving medications. Also,

 Go to Chapter 23, **Medication Guidelines: Steps to Follow for All Medications (Regardless of Type or Route),** in Volume 2.

Three Checks

Check each medication three times:

1. *BEFORE you pour, mix or draw up a medication,* check its label against the entry on the MAR. Be sure that the name, route, dose, and time match the MAR entry.
2. *AFTER you prepare the medication,* and before returning the container to the medication cart or discarding anything, check the label against the MAR entry again.
3. *AT THE BEDSIDE,* check the medication again before actually administering it.

Observing the "three checks" rule will help you to practice the "six rights."

Six Rights

Practicing the "**six rights**" will help to ensure accurate administration. This means that you will give the (1) right medication to the (2) right patient in the (3) right dose using the (4) right route at the (5) right time. You will also carry out (6) right documentation of the medication administration. Nurses regard these safeguards as the minimum requirements for safety and error prevention.

BOX 23-3 Medications with Similar-Sounding Names

Cefzil, Keflin	Keflex
glyburide	glipizide
Procardia	Procardia XL
Zantac	Xanax
Celebrex	Cerebrex, Celexa, Cerebyx
digoxin	digitoxin
quinine	quinidine
Keflex	Kantrex
Demerol	dicumerol
Percocet	Percodan
baclofen	Bactroban
Cytoxan	Ciloxan
ranitidine	amantadine
Zyrtec	Zantac
Lodine	iodine
Phenergan	Phenaphen
Zostrix	Zestril
Ophthalgan	Auralgan

1. **Right drug.** Obviously, you must always administer the correct medication. That is one reason for reading each label three times (see the "three checks"). The following are other ways to ensure that you give the correct drug:
   - Always check the order (especially after days off, after working a different shift, and after lunch) to see whether there have been changes in the medication dosage, route, and so forth.
   - Select the ordered medication from the *patient's* drug drawer (unless it is a stock drug). Do not substitute one medication for another.
   - Avoid selecting medications based on size and color, because many medications are the same size, shape, and color as others. Similarly, be alert for similar-looking labels and similarly spelled names. If you are accustomed to withdrawing Pitocin (given IV to stimulate uterine contractions) from a small vial with a green label, you might be surprised to find that the small, green-label vial in your hand is actually hydroxyzine (Vistaril), which would harm the patient if given IV.
   - Always repeat back verbal orders to be sure you have heard correctly. Spell the medication name. Medication names that sound the same can be very confusing and lead to administering the wrong drug. See Box 23–3 for examples.

- Review abbreviations that may be confusing, such as those listed in Box 23–2. Clarify dose form, especially with time-released drugs.

- If a label is hard to read or comes off the container, return the container to the pharmacy. Never give a medication from such a container.

- Do not transfer medications from one pharmacy container to another.

2. **Right dose.** The right dose is the dose prescribed for the particular patient. Be sure that the dose is within the recommended range for the patient's age and condition. Perform the "three checks" of the container against the MAR. If the pharmacist has sent a dose different from the one ordered, you may need to calculate how much of it to give. It is a good idea to have another nurse check your calculations.

How you prepare medications can affect the dose. When you must break a tablet, use a knife or a cutting device. If the tablet does not break evenly, you should discard it. Also, when crushing a tablet to mix with liquid or food, clean the crushing device completely before using it to remove any pieces of a previously crushed drug. Clean it after using it, as well.

3. **Right time.** Check the order against the time to give the drug, and document the exact time of administration on the MAR. Medications are administered at specific times to maintain constant therapeutic blood levels.

- Scheduled medications may be given within a "window" of one-half hour before and one-half hour after the scheduled time.

- "Right time" also includes timing of oral medications in relation to meals. Give drugs that are irritating to the stomach (e.g., potassium, aspirin) with food; give drugs that absorb better on an empty stomach (e.g., tetracycline) before meals.

- Determine whether your patient is scheduled for any diagnostic procedures, surgery, or blood tests that require him to remain NPO.

4. **Right route.** Recall that drug absorption is highly dependent on the route of administration. Perform the "three checks," and be sure that the drug is in the proper form for the route ordered. Many medications are available in multiple forms; others are made for one specific route. For example, cephalexin (Keflex), an antibiotic, comes in capsules, suspensions for oral use, and injectable forms for intramuscular and intravenous administration. By contrast, the antibiotic penicillin G procaine (Crystacillin) is prepared for intramuscular injection and is *not* to be given intravenously.

5. **Right patient.** Just before giving the medication, always double-check the patient's identification (ID) bracelet to ensure that you have the correct patient. The Joint Commission on Accreditation of Healthcare Organizations (JCAHO) national patient safety goals recommend using two methods of patient identification (JCAHO, 2003); so, also ask the patient to state his name. It is best to say, "Please tell me your name," because patients with hearing problems and confused patients may respond yes incorrectly when asked, for example, "Are you Mary Smith?" Never skip this step, even if you are familiar with the patient. If you are busy and distracted, it is possible to enter the wrong room. Also, patients, especially when they are confused or emotionally disturbed, may move about. You may enter room 214 with a medication for Mr. Jones but discover an entirely different person in Mr. Jones's bed!

Suppose you are taking an oral tablet to a patient's room. He is in the bathroom and says, "Just leave it; I'll take it when I come out." What would you do? If you leave the tablet, how would you know whether he really took it? And what might happen if another, confused, patient (or even a visiting child) wandered into the room and took the tablet?

6. **Right documentation.** Some nurses consider documentation the sixth right. After administering a medication, document it immediately on the patient's MAR, as in Figure 23–7. Be sure to document the following information:

- Name of medication given

- Dose of medication given

- Route of administration and injection site for parenteral medications

- Date and time administered

- Your name or initials as administering nurse

Most MARs are preprinted with the patient's name, name of the medication, dosage, and route administered (e.g., intramuscular, oral, or intravenous). If so, you need only to write the time you actually gave the medication, initial each medication, and sign the form one time. As for all charting, write legibly in ink.

If for some reason you do not administer an ordered medication, document that information on the MAR and write a nurse's note explaining the reason it was not given. Reasons may include patient refusal, NPO for surgery, tests, or procedures being performed. For example:

06/20/06 0800—Pt NPO for surgery this a.m. 0800 meds held as ordered ————— S. King, RN

When giving a PRN medication, in addition to recording on the MAR, you should write a nurse's note

HOSPITAL MEDICATION ADMINISTRATION RECORD

Codes For Injection Sites

A - Left Anterior Thigh
B - Left Deltoid
C - Left Gluteus Medius
D - Left Lateral Thigh
E - Left Ventral Gluteus
F - Left Lower Quadrant
G - Left Upper Quadrant

H - Right Anterior Thigh
I - Right Deltoid
J - Right Gluteus Medius
K - Right Lateral Thigh
L - Right Ventral Gluteus
M - Right Lower Quadrant
N - Right Upper Quadrant

Mary Smith 086432

age 46   *John Miller, M.D.*

ALLERGIES: *PCN, Sulfa*

DATE ORDERED	DATE REORD.	DRUG - DOSE - ROUTE - FREQUENCY	ADMIN. TIME	DATE 4.16.06	DATE 4.17.06	DATE 4.18.06
4.16.06		*Lanoxin 0.25mg po Q D*	*0900*	*09 JW*		
4.16.06		*Rocephin T̅ gm IV Q D*	*1200*	*1200 JW*		
4.16.06		*Zinacef T̅ gm IV Q 8 hr*	*0800*	*08 JW*		
			1600			
			2400			

SIGNATURE / SHIFT INDICATES			*7-3*	*JW*		
NURSE ADMINISTERING MEDICATIONS			*3-11*			
J Wilson, RN			*11-7*			

FIGURE 23–7   **After you administer a medication, document it as soon as possible on the MAR.**

documenting your assessment and the time the drug was given. Then, after allowing time for the medication to be absorbed and take effect, evaluate and document the patient's responses. For example:

0800—Pt c/o #6 (scale of 1–10) abd pain at incision site. Active bowel sounds auscultated. Resp 16, BP 130/84. Denies N/V. Morphine 10 mg given intramuscularly in right vastus lateralis (see MAR).
———————————————————— S. King, RN

0900—States pain relieved; "about 3" (scale of 1–10). Resp 14. BP 126/80. ———— S. King, RN

You are responsible for documenting the client's responses to all medications, including therapeutic effects, side effects, and unexpected or adverse reactions.

Other Rights

In addition to the "six rights" already discussed, patients also have the following rights:

• **Right reason.** This includes the right to *not* receive unnecessary medications. For example, a tranquilizer or sleeping pill should be given because the patient is very anxious or cannot sleep, not for the convenience of caregivers who are weary of his incessant demands.

• **Right to know.** This means that you tell the patient the name of the medication, why it is being given, its actions, and potential side effects.

• **Right to refuse.** The patient always has a right to refuse a medication regardless of her reasons and regardless of the consequences.

KnowledgeCheck 23–11

• What are the six rights?
• Give an example of each one.
• How many times, and when, should you check the medication against the MAR?

 Go to Chapter 23, **Knowledge Check Response Sheet and Answers,** on the Electronic Study Guide.

ADMINISTERING ORAL MEDICATIONS

The oral route is the one most commonly used for medications. Recall what you already know about oral medications: Where are they absorbed? What are their advantages and disadvantages? What assessments should you make? If you cannot answer these questions, review discussions of drug preparations and routes of administration, and review Table 23–3. To see the critical aspects of administering oral medications, see the Critical Aspects box on p. 522 for

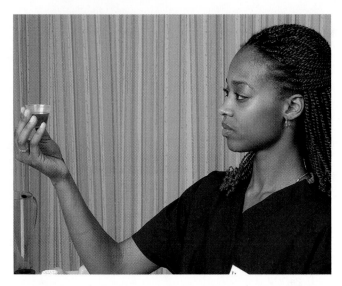

FIGURE 23–8 When pouring a liquid medication, measure the dose while holding the calibrated cup at eye level.

Procedures 23–1 through 23–16. To see procedural steps for administering oral medications,

Go to Chapter 23, **Procedure 23-1: Administering Oral Medications,** in Volume 2.

Pouring Liquid Medications

Liquid medications are frequently used for children and older adults. They usually come in multiple-dose bottles, so you will need to pour individual doses into a disposable, calibrated cup, as in Figure 23–8. When pouring, hold the bottle so the liquid does not run over the label, making it difficult to read.

- Measure the dosage with the calibrated cup at eye level.
- Read the dosage where the lowest part of the concaved surface (meniscus) of the fluid is on the line.
- When you are finished, wipe the rim of the bottle with a clean tissue or paper towel before replacing the cap.

If the patient has difficulty taking liquids from a cup, you can use a syringe without a needle to place the medication in his mouth. Place the patient in a side-lying or upright position to help prevent choking and aspiration. Place the syringe between the gum and cheek, and slowly push the plunger to administer the liquid slowly.

Buccal and Sublingual Medications

Buccal and sublingual medications, although placed in the mouth, are intended for absorption in the saliva rather than in the GI tract. Some medications and enzyme preparations are administered by this route and are rapidly absorbed, some within seconds. Buccal medications are held in the cheek; sublingual medications are held under the tongue.

Enteral (Nasogastric and Gastrostomy) Medications

For patients who cannot swallow or who have feeding tubes, you can give oral medications through nasogastric (NG), gastrostomy, or jejunal tubes. Observe the following precautions when administering enteral medications:

- Do not give hydrophilic medications, such as Metamucil, through feeding tubes because they attract water and will solidify in the tube.
- Some tablets should *not* be crushed, because crushing changes aspects of their action. Be sure to check that crushing is acceptable. Never crush an enteric-coated medication.
- Give medications separately, and flush with water between each. Some medications are less effective when given in combination with others.
- If the patient is receiving a continuous tube feeding, disconnect it before giving the medications; leave the tube clamped for a few minutes after administering the medication, according to agency protocol.
- If the enteral tube is connected to suction, you will usually discontinue the suction for 20 to 30 minutes after administration and keep the tube clamped, to allow time for the drug to be absorbed.
- Be sure to document on the intake and output record the amount of liquid medication and the water used for flushing.
- If the patient is on fluid restrictions, use the smallest amount of water possible to dissolve tablets and flush the tube.

For other procedures related to enteral tubes,

Go to Chapter 26, **Procedure 26-2: Inserting Nasogastric and Nasoenteric Tubes, Procedure 26-3: Administering Feedings Through Gastric and Enteric Tubes,** and **Procedure 26-4: Removing a Nasogastric or Nasoenteric Tube,** in Volume 2.

Special Situations

Some oral medications can discolor or damage the enamel of the teeth. Mix these drugs with a liquid, and have the patient drink it through a straw and drink water afterward. For medications (usually in liquid form) that have an objectionable taste, the following methods help to disguise the taste:

- Unless contraindicated, have the patient drink a liberal amount of flavored liquid (e.g., juice) or water to dilute the medication.

- Have the patient suck on ice chips for several minutes before taking the medication. Ice numbs the taste buds.
- Store the medication in the refrigerator. Especially if it is an oily liquid, its smell and taste will be less objectionable.
- Use a syringe to place the medication on the back of the patient's tongue. There are fewer taste buds there.
- Regardless of method, offer oral hygiene immediately after giving the medication.

Some patients have difficulty swallowing medications; they gag, or the pills become "stuck" in their throat. It may help to crush soluble tablets and place them in liquids or in a small amount of applesauce or pudding. Remember that some forms (e.g., time-released tablets) should *not* be crushed, so check your drug reference sources to be certain. Remember that you cannot give oral medications to patients who:

- Cannot swallow fluids. The risk for aspiration is too great.
- Have nausea or vomiting. The medication would be lost in the emesis.
- Are NPO.

In these situations you should obtain a medical order for an alternative route or, in the case of NPO, permission to give the medication with small sips of water.

KnowledgeCheck 23–12

- Describe two ways to ensure an accurate dosage when pouring liquid medications.
- What instructions should you give to a patient who is taking a sublingual medication?
- Explain the special steps required when administering enteral medications to a patient who is receiving continuous tube feedings.
- Describe three methods for disguising the taste of objectionable tasting drugs.
- For which patients are oral medications contraindicated?

 Go to Chapter 23, **Knowledge Check Response Sheet and Answers,** on the Electronic Study Guide.

Medicating Children

Young children present unique challenges because they cannot be motivated by logic. They cannot grasp the cause and effect of "Take this; it will make you feel better." If they do not like the taste, they will not swallow it. Another challenge is that before the age of 5 years, children may not be able to swallow tablets and capsules. For these reasons, most oral medications for children are prepared as sweetened liquids. For very young children and infants, you must take care to prevent choking and aspiration. Parents can often

self-care

Teaching Parents About Medicating Children

- If the child is old enough to understand, warn him when a medication has an objectionable taste (e.g., "John, this doesn't taste very good, but you can have a big drink of juice as soon as you swallow it."). You will lose his trust if you surprise him with a bad taste.

- Give the child a frozen fruit bar or frozen flavored ice pop just before the medication. This helps to numb the taste buds to weaken the taste of the medication.

- To mask bad-tasting medicines, you can crush tablets or empty the contents of a capsule and mix with soft foods, such as applesauce, hot cereal, or pudding. This is helpful for patients who might aspirate liquids, as well. (*Caution:* Check with a pharmacist or physician before crushing a tablet or emptying a capsule. Some medications should not be crushed.)

- Do not use essential foods in the child's diet (e.g., milk or orange juice) to mask the taste of medications. The child may later refuse a food that he associates with the medicine.

- Take care to prevent choking or aspiration. When giving liquids to infants and toddlers, hold the child in a sitting or semi-sitting position. Use a medicine dropper or syringe to place the medication between the gum and cheek. Apply gentle pressure; avoid giving too much medication too fast.

- Always praise the child after she swallows the medication.

suggest the best methods for getting their child to take medicines. For other parents, you may need to teach techniques for administering medications at home (see the accompanying Self-Care Box).

Medicating Older Adults

As you already know, because of physiological changes associated with aging, older adults usually require smaller dosages of drugs. In addition, their reactions to some medications are unpredictable. Therefore, you will need to observe carefully for both therapeutic and undesired effects. Other problems include the following:

- *Difficulty swallowing medications.* It may help to crush tablets or give drugs in liquid form. Gently massaging the area just below the chin may help to initiate swallowing. Consult a speech therapist for other suggestions.

- *Slow reflexes and reasoning ability.* You may need to allow more time to explain and administer medications to older adults. Some may not understand exactly what you want them to do.
- *Forgetting to take the medications.* Impaired memory is more common with age, so clients need simple plans that they can follow at home. A written schedule may help, especially if you schedule the drugs to be taken at mealtimes and at bedtime. Many people take their medication, only to forget shortly thereafter whether or not they did so. Advise the patient to use a divided pill container or a small glass filled with the medications for each dosage time during the day. If the A.M. container is empty, that means the person has taken the morning drugs.
- *Impaired visual acuity.* For patients who cannot see well, write out the home medication schedule in large letters, or ask family members to help.
- *Difficulty opening containers and administering medications.* Because of pain or stiffness in the hands and fingers, and also because of decreased visual acuity, older adults often find it difficult to open containers or to administer their own insulin injections, inhalers, eye medications, and so on. Help them find solutions or assistance from family and friends.
- *Lack of understanding of the need for the medication.* Some older adults accept unquestioningly everything a physician says, but they may not understand what each drug is for. For example, suppose a patient's tranquilizer is not effective. The physician prescribes a new one, but the patient does not understand that he should stop taking the old one; so for a period of time, he takes both medications. This type of situation can happen, too, when patients are being treated by more than one physician (e.g., a podiatrist and an internist may both prescribe a medication to treat toenail fungus).

  However, some patients do not see the need for the medication ("I don't feel any better when I take all this stuff"), so they simply do not take it. In the hospital, they may refuse to take medications, or they may put the tablets in their mouth but spit them out when you leave the room. You should stay with the patient until you see that he has swallowed the medications.

KnowledgeCheck 23–13

- What is the chief danger when administering oral medications to children?
- How can you help a person who has some difficulty swallowing oral medications?
- Keeping in mind that patients do have the right to refuse medications, how can you be sure that they are actually taking them and not spitting them out after you leave the room?

 Go to Chapter 23, **Knowledge Check Response Sheet and Answers,** on the Electronic Study Guide.

ADMINISTERING TOPICAL MEDICATIONS

Topical medications are applied directly to a body site or placed in body cavities by irrigation or instillation. They are usually used for their local effects (e.g., zinc oxide ointment to protect the skin against chafing and chapping associated with bowel and bladder incontinence), but some are absorbed through the skin and mucous membranes for their systemic effects (e.g., estrogen patches), depending on the drug preparation. Most require application to the skin two to three times per day for maximum effect.

Skin Applications: Lotions, Creams, and Ointments

To enhance absorption, cleanse the skin with soap and water and pat dry before applying lotions, creams, and ointments. If you warm the medication in your gloved hands, it will be more comfortable for the patient and make the preparation easier to apply. Use a sterile cotton swab, tongue blade, or gloved finger to apply corticosteroid creams and other topical medications so that your skin does not absorb them. For guidelines for applying skin medications, including powders and aerosols,

 Go to Chapter 23, **Technique 23–1: Applying Medications to the Skin,** in Volume 2.

Transdermal Medications

Designed to be absorbed through the skin, transdermal medications are prepared as patches that are made of a special membrane. Patches allow constant, controlled amounts of medications to be released over 24 hours or more, giving a prolonged systemic effect. Nitroglycerine (used to control angina or chest pain), scopolamine (used to treat motion sickness), nicotine (used to control smoking urges), and Fentanyl (used to treat chronic pain) are examples of drugs administered by patch. Most patches are made with the correct dose already applied; however, you must apply nitroglycerine (NTG) paste to NTG paper, wearing gloves to protect yourself from the medication.

  Also wear gloves when applying other transdermal patches (Figure 23–9). Avoid placing the patch on areas where there are skin lesions. When removing and discarding patches, be aware that they may still contain medication. Wear gloves, fold the medicated side to the inside, and dispose of the patches where they are not accessible to children or pets. For guidelines,

 Go to Chapter 23, **Technique 23–2: Applying Transdermal Medications,** in Volume 2.

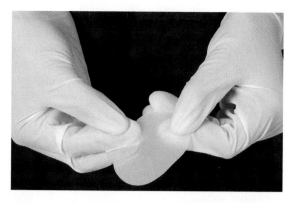

FIGURE 23–9 Patches allow constant, controlled amounts of medications to be released over an extended period, giving a prolonged systemic effect. Wear gloves when removing and applying patches.

Performing Irrigations and Instillations

Washing out a body cavity with a steady stream of fluid or water is called **irrigation.** Sterile water, saline, or antiseptic solutions are flushed into the eye, ear, throat, vagina, rectum, or urinary tract to wash out the cavity. **Instillation** is the insertion of medication into a body cavity (e.g., eye drops) so that the medication can be retained or absorbed through that body cavity. Some medications should remain in the body cavity for a period of time for maximum absorption and effect.

Irrigations and instillations are performed to remove discharge or foreign bodies (e.g., from the eye or ear), to apply heat and cold to an area, to apply medications such as antiseptics, and to prepare an area for surgery (e.g., an enema for cleansing the bowels). You will usually not use sterile technique unless there are breaks in the skin. Several types of syringes are used for irrigating and instilling medications and fluids. Each is calibrated to allow you to control the amount and speed of solution delivered into the cavity (Figure 23–10).

Ophthalmic Medications

Ophthalmic ointments or solutions are used for their local effects, for example, to treat eye irritations, infections, and glaucoma or to lubricate the eye. During an eye examination, eye medications may also be used to anesthetize the eye, dilate the pupil, or stain the cornea to identify abraded areas. Eye irrigation may be performed to remove foreign bodies, secretions, or harmful chemicals.

All ophthalmic medications are packaged in small bottles or tubes, which state, *"For ophthalmic use only."* Do not place any medication in the eye unless this statement appears on the container. The **cornea** (the transparent part of the sclera in front of the iris and pupil) is easily injured, so you should not place

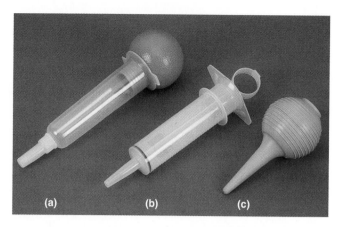

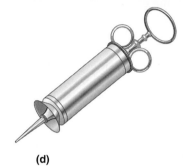

FIGURE 23–10 Syringes for administering enteral medications and performing irrigations and instillations. *A,* Asepto syringe: plastic syringe with a rubber bulb. *B,* Toomey (piston) syringe: calibrated plastic syringe with a tip that fits into the end of a tube (e.g., urinary catheter or enteral tube). This is used for deep wound irrigation, bladder irrigations, and administration of enteral medications. *C,* Rubber bulb syringe, for ear irrigations. *D,* Pomeroy syringe: metal syringe used to irrigate the ear for removal of wax by drainage.

medications directly onto the eyeball. Take care to not touch the tip of the dropper or tube to the eye or conjunctiva; doing so may lead to bacterial growth on the container.

See Chapter 29 for information about the structure and function of the eyes. The Critical Aspects box on p. 522 summarizes key points in performing ophthalmic instillations. For the step-by-step procedure,

VOL 2 Go to Chapter 23, **Procedure 23–2: Administering Ophthalmic Medications,** in Volume 2.

Otic Medications

Medications or solutions may be dropped into the ear to treat internal and external ear infections, to apply heat to the area, and to soften and remove earwax. Using sterile technique when administering otic medications will help prevent infection if the eardrum has been ruptured. Use solutions at room temperature, because a solution that is too hot or too cold may cause vertigo, nausea, and pain.

See Chapter 29 for information about the structure and function of the ear. The Critical Aspects box on p. 522 provides guidelines for performing otic instillations. For the complete procedure,

Go to Chapter 23, **Procedure 23-3: Administering Otic Medications,** in Volume 2.

Nasal Medications

Clients usually self-administer "nose drops" and sprays. The most frequently used nasal medications are used to shrink swollen mucous membranes and to loosen secretions and drainage for treatment of nasal cavity or sinus infections. Because many nasal medications are available without prescription, caution the patient regarding overuse. Long-term use of decongestants may cause a **rebound effect;** that is, they will be effective immediately after administration, but the nasal congestion will recur and even increase when the effects of the drug wear off. Frequent use of or swallowing excess decongestant can also cause systemic side effects, such as increased heart rate and increased blood pressure. These effects can be serious in children; saline drops are safer for them.

See Chapter 29 for information about the structure and function of the nose. The Critical Aspects box provides guidelines for performing nasal instillations. For the complete procedure,

Go to Chapter 23, **Procedure 23-4: Administering Nasal Medications,** in Volume 2.

Vaginal Medications

Vaginal medications come in various forms: foams, jellies, liquids (douches) creams, tablets, and suppositories. They may be used for contraception, to destroy bacteria in the vaginal area before gynecological surgery, to treat vaginal itching or infection, or to induce labor. Store suppositories in the refrigerator to keep them firm enough to insert. Insert them with a lubricated, gloved finger. After insertion, the body temperature causes the suppository to melt. Foams and jellies are inserted using an applicator or inserter. Apply a clean perineal pad if there is heavy drainage or if the woman is ambulatory (the medication may melt and drain from the vagina by gravity).

A **douche** is a vaginal irrigation using low pressure. Vaginal irrigations are used to administer antimicrobial solutions to prevent infection (e.g., before surgery), to remove irritating discharge, and to apply heat or cold (e.g., to reduce inflammation). In the acute care setting, you will usually use sterile supplies. However, this is not usually necessary when the irrigation is self-administered at home because people usually have some resistance to the microorganisms

in their daily environment. Teach women that douching is not necessary for ordinary female hygiene and that it may even be harmful because it disturbs the normal balance of microorganisms in the vagina.

The Critical Aspects box provides guidelines for administering vaginal medications. For the complete procedure,

Go to Chapter 23, **Procedure 23-5: Administering Vaginal Medications,** in Volume 2.

Rectal Medications

Rectal suppositories and liquid instillations (**enemas**) are used to encourage bowel movements or to treat systemic complaints. For example, antiemetic suppositories are often used to treat nausea. Absorption is slow and erratic because of rectal contents, local drug irritation, and uncertainty of drug retention in the rectum. Other disadvantages include embarrassment to the patient and possible rectal pain if the patient has hemorrhoids. However, the rectal route may provide for higher blood levels of the medication than does the oral route because the venous blood from the rectum does not pass through the liver before entering the general circulation (review the discussion of the first-pass effect, as needed). Also, rectal administration may be preferred when a drug has an unacceptable taste or odor or when it is not safe to use the oral route, as with a patient who is vomiting or unconscious. As a rule, rectal medications are contraindicated when there is active rectal bleeding.

The Critical Aspects box provides guidelines for administering a rectal suppository. For the complete procedure,

Go to Chapter 23, **Procedure 23-6: Inserting a Rectal Suppository,** and Chapter 28, **Procedure 28-3: Administering an Enema,** in Volume 2.

ADMINISTERING RESPIRATORY INHALATIONS

Nebulization is the production of a fine spray, fog, powder, or mist from a liquid drug. The patient inhales the medication mixture by breathing deeply through a mouthpiece attached to the nebulizer. The airways and alveoli are highly vascularized and therefore absorb inhaled medications rapidly.

Types of Nebulizers

The following are four types of devices for achieving nebulization:

- *Atomizers* disperse the medication in the form of large droplets.

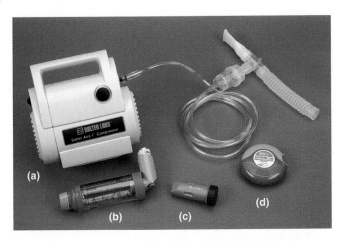

FIGURE 23–11 Inhalers. *A*, An ultrasonic nebulizer delivers medication and humidity as a fine mist. *B*, A metered dose inhaler delivers measured doses. This one has a spacer. *C*, A dry powder inhaler (Turbuhaler). *D*, A Diskhaler.

- *Aerosol sprayers* suspend the droplets of medication in a gas (e.g., oxygen).

- An *ultrasonic (hand-held) nebulizer* (Figure 23–11a) mixes a small volume of medication, usually less than 1 mL, with 3 mL of normal saline. The device forces air through the nebulizer and delivers medication and humidity as a fine mist. Because the particles are so small, the mist can be inhaled deep into the lungs.

- A *metered-dose inhaler (MDI)* (Figure 23–11b) is a type of nebulizer that delivers measured doses of a nebulized drug. A dry powder inhaler (DPI) is a type of MDI.

No matter which device is used, the smaller the droplets, the farther the medication can be inhaled into the respiratory tract.

Metered-Dose Inhalers

A *metered-dose inhaler (MDI)* is a pressurized container prefilled with several doses of a drug and a gas propellant. The patient inhales while pushing the canister's pump to release a measured dose of medication through a nosepiece or mouthpiece. Sometimes an extender (spacer) is attached to the mouthpiece (Figure 23–11b). The medication is pumped into the extender instead of directly into the patient's mouth. The patient inhales the drug from the chamber. Use of a spacer prevents coughing that may be triggered by the propellant.

A *dry powder inhaler (DPI)* does not have a propellant, but instead is activated by inhalation. Each powdered dose is in a blister pack that is activated according to the manufacturer's instructions. Once the dose is loaded, the patient simply takes a deep breath. Examples are Turbuhaler (Figure 23–11c), and Diskhaler (Figure 23–11d).

Patients frequently self-administer inhalations (most often bronchodilators or steroids) using an MDI. However, you may need to teach your patients how to use the device correctly (see the Self-Care box on page 506.).

The advantage of MDIs is that high doses of medication can be rapidly instilled in the lungs, producing local effects and avoiding systemic side effects. Disadvantages are the need for manual dexterity, which is often compromised in the older adult; skill in coordinating the inhaling of the medication and the pushing of the canister to administer the dose; and the ability to inhale and exhale deeply enough to allow penetration of the medication in the more distal bronchioles.

KnowledgeCheck 23–14

- Why should you use a cotton swab, tongue blade, or gloved finger to apply corticosteroid creams and other topical medications?
- Most of the following routes are used for both local and systemic effects. Which one is used *only* for medications intended for systemic absorption (that is, which one is *not* used to for local effects): lotions, creams, ointments, transdermal patches, or irrigations?
- When administering eye drops, how can you prevent injury to the cornea?
- When should you use sterile technique when performing otic instillations?
- What are two of the undesired effects of self-administered nasal decongestants?
- What possible harm can result from vaginal douching?
- When is rectal instillation of a drug preferred over oral administration?
- When, as a rule, are rectal medications contraindicated?
- Define *nebulization*.
- In terms of what the patient has to do to release a dose of the medication, what is the difference between a metered-dose inhaler and a dry powder inhaler?

 Go to Chapter 23, **Knowledge Check Response Sheet and Answers,** on the Electronic Study Guide.

ADMINISTERING PARENTERAL MEDICATIONS

Parenteral medications include those that are injected by the intradermal, subcutaneous, intramuscular, or intravenous routes. Parenteral injections are absorbed faster and more completely than drugs given by other routes; the results are more predictable; and the dosage can be measured more accurately. In addition, they can be used for patients who cannot take oral medications. However, injectable medications have some disadvantages:

1. They bypass the skin barrier, making infection more likely if aseptic technique is not used.

Teaching the Use of a Metered-Dose Inhaler (MDI)

Before teaching the steps of the procedure:

- Obtain the appropriate supplies for the procedure, including the inhaler and tissues.

- Explain to the patient when to use the inhaler and what side effects to anticipate.

- Demonstrate how the inhaler fits into the canister.

Then teach the following steps:

- Sit upright, preferably in a straight-backed chair.

- Remove the cap, and hold the canister upright in your dominant hand.

- Shake the canister several times to mix the medication in the canister.

- With a new inhaler, or when using an inhaler that you haven't used for a week or so, discharge the first two puffs into the air. Otherwise, you get a mouthful of the propellant instead of medication.

- Open your mouth, and hold the inhaler according to the care provider's or manufacturer's instructions. Either:

  Hold the mouthpiece 1 to 2 inches in front of your open mouth
  Or
  Place the mouthpiece over your tongue and into your mouth. Close your teeth and lips tightly around the mouthpiece. This is the method to use for all MDIs with a spacer or extender.

- Take a deep breath and breathe out until you can expel no more air from your lungs.

- Press the top of the canister firmly with your forefinger while inhaling deeply.

- Continue to inhale so the medication is drawn deep into your lungs. Then hold that breath as long as possible. Try to count to 10 seconds if possible.

- Exhale slowly through pursed lips to keep the small airways open during exhalation.

- Remove the inhaler from your mouth, and breathe normally.

- Wait at least 1 minute before giving the second puff, or 5 minutes before giving another inhaled medication, so the medication can enter the bloodstream and the canister can recharge.

- If you are using an inhaled steroid, rinse your mouth or gargle with water to prevent the steroid from being absorbed in the mouth.

- Clean the mouthpiece with a tissue, and replace the cap.

How to Tell When Your Inhaler Is Empty

- Each container is clearly marked with the number of sprays per container (30 to 100, usually); make a mark each time you use it.

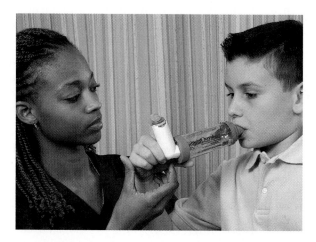

FIGURE 23–12   Using a metered dose inhaler with an extender.

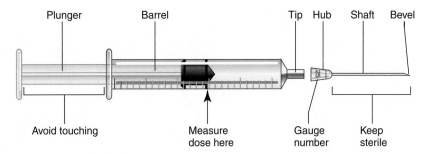

FIGURE 23–13   Parts of a needle and syringe.

2. Tissue damage may result if the pH, osmotic pressure, or solubility of the medication is not appropriate to the tissue where the medication is given. For example, medications intended for injection into muscle may damage subcutaneous tissue.

3. Preparation and administration must be performed accurately, because the onset of action is relatively rapid and the medications, once given, cannot be retrieved.

Preparing Injectable Medications

Injectable medications are those that are injected or infused into body tissues or into the bloodstream. When administering them, you must know about various kinds of needles and syringes. You will need to decide, based on each situation, what size and type of needle and syringe to use. For a summary of the sites and equipment used for parenteral injections,

 Go to Chapter 23, **Tables, Boxes, Figures: ESG Table 23–3,** on the Electronic Study Guide.

Needles

Needles are disposable, stainless steel sheaths that attach to a syringe. Figure 23–13 shows the parts of a needle. Needles are made in various lengths and gauges and with different bevel sizes.

• The **gauge** refers to the inside diameter of the needle lumen. The smaller the gauge, the larger the diameter (i.e., a 16-gauge needle has a larger diameter than a 20-gauge needle). Needle gauges are numbered 14 through 30. Choose the gauge based on the patient's size and skin condition, the viscosity of medication used, and the speed of administration desired. Smaller needles (26 to 30 gauge) cause less pain and trauma to the tissue, so they are especially useful for patients who must have frequent or long-term injections (e.g., for insulin and heparin). Larger needles (14 to 18 gauge) are used for blood and more viscous medications, such as penicillin, to mix intravenous (IV) medications, or for rapid infusion of IV medications.

• The **bevel** is the slanted tip with a narrow slit. The slant is designed to make an opening that will close

quickly to prevent leakage of medication, blood, and serum. A long bevel tip is sharper and narrower and therefore causes less discomfort during injection. Long bevels are usually used for subcutaneous (subQ) and intramuscular injections. Short bevels are used for intradermal or IV injections.

• The needle **length** (commonly $\frac{3}{8}$ to 3 inches) is the distance from the tip to the hub (bottom) of the needle. Use a longer needle for subQ and intramuscular injections, and a shorter one for intradermal and IV injections. Vary the length according to the thickness of the patient's muscle and adipose tissue. Although a $1\frac{1}{2}$ inch needle is common for intramuscular injections, you would use a shorter one for a child or a very thin person.

Filter needles and **filter straws** are used to trap rubber or glass fragments when drawing up a medication from a vial or an ampule. You must replace the filter needle with a regular needle before injecting the medication into the patient or into the IV solution.

 CriticalThinking 23–11
• You are to give repeated intramuscular injections to a client who is very thin (5 ft, 5 in. tall and weighing 96 lb) and has very little muscle mass. You are to give 1 mL of a thin, watery medication. You have these needle sizes available: 16 gauge, 20 gauge, 25 gauge. Which would you use, and why?
• For the same patient, you have needles available in 1 inch and $1\frac{1}{2}$ inch lengths. Which would you use, and why?

Syringes

A syringe consists of a barrel, plunger, and syringe tip (Figure 23–13). Because injections require strict sterile technique, you may touch the outside of the barrel and end of the plunger but not the inside of the barrel, hub, shaft of the plunger or needle.

Syringes are usually made of plastic and are disposable. Some have the needle attached; others do not. The syringe tip, either **Luer-Lok** (twist on) or **non-Luer-Lok** (slip on), fits into the needle hub (Figure 23–14). Syringes are made in various sizes, from 0.5 mL to 60 mL. The larger sizes are used for adding medications

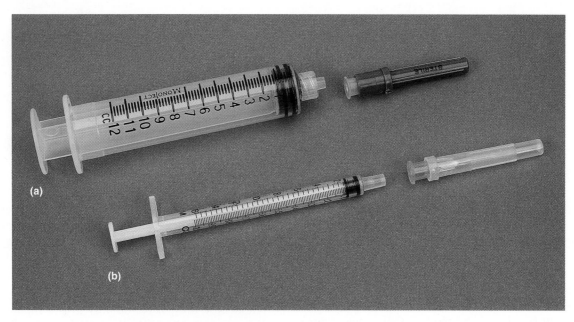

FIGURE 23–14   Syringe tips. *A*, Luer-Lok (twist-on) tip. *B*, Non-Luer-Lok (slip-on) tip.

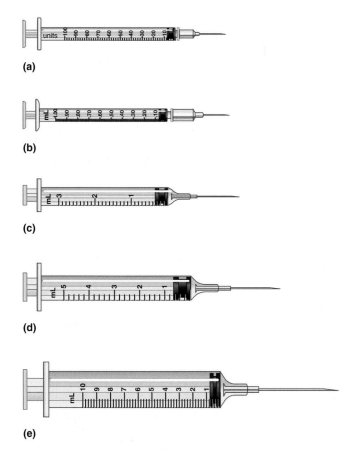

FIGURE 23–15   *A*, A 100-unit insulin syringe marked in units. *B*, A 1 mL tuberculin syringe marked in 0.01 (hundredths) and minims. *C*, A 3 mL standard syringe, marked in mL and 0.1 mL. *D*, A 5 mL standard syringe marked in mL and 0.2 mL. *E*, A 10 mL standard syringe marked in mL and 0.2 mL.

to IV solutions and for irrigating wounds. You will usually use a 2 mL or 3 mL syringe for intramuscular injections. Syringes larger than 5 mL are used for IV administration, instillations, and irrigations.

Five syringes are shown in Figure 23–15. **Standard syringes** are supplied in 3, 5, and 10 mL sizes. They are commonly supplied without needles or with 18-, 21-, 23-, or 25-gauge needles that are 0.5 to 3 inches long. They are calibrated and marked in 0.1 mL and 1 or 2 mL increments so that drugs can be measured accurately. **Tuberculin syringes** have a 1 mL capacity and are calibrated in 0.01 mL increments; they come with a small (usually 26- to 28-) gauge, short (0.5 to 0.625 inch) needle. Use tuberculin syringes to administer small, precise doses of medication (e.g., when medicating infants or children, for allergy tests, or when administering potentially dangerous medications, such as heparin). **Insulin syringes** are calibrated in units and are used to administer insulin. Insulin syringes are calibrated in 100 units per milliliter. They are made in 0.3, 0.5, or 1 mL sizes with very small-gauge needles (26 to 30 gauge).

Prefilled unit-dose systems (e.g., *Tubex* and *Carpuject*) are available for some medications. These are reusable syringe holders that house disposable, single-dose, prefilled medication cartridges (Figure 23–16). No medication preparation is necessary, but you must check each cartridge and dose carefully because all of the cartridges look alike. You simply insert the cartridge into the holder and lock it in place. After administering the medication, dispose of the cartridge; the holder is available for reuse. Currently, the use of Carpuject and Tubex prefilled systems is limited

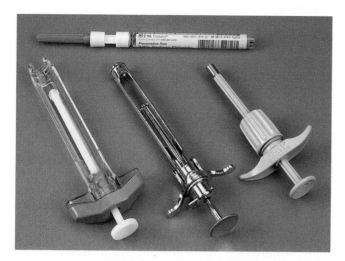

FIGURE 23–16 Prefilled unit-dose system: Prefilled sterile cartridge with needle and various holders.

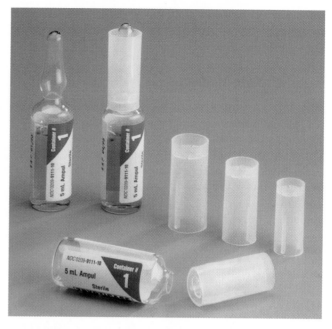

FIGURE 23–17 To prevent injury, break ampule necks with a special opener. *Source:* Courtesy of Medi-Dose®, Inc./EPS®, Inc.

to some office practices and to self-administration. They are no longer widely used in healthcare facilities because the manipulation required to remove the cartridge from the holder creates a needlestick risk for nurses.

 Go to Chapter 23, **Technique 23-2: Using Prefilled Unit-Dose Systems,** in Volume 2.

KnowledgeCheck 23–15

- What does the term *parenteral* mean?
- What are two disadvantages of the parenteral route?
- In order to maintain sterile technique, which part of a syringe must you *not* touch?
- You need to irrigate a wound. Which syringe size would you probably need: 0.5 mL, 3 mL, 5 mL, or 50 mL?
- Which syringe would you use for an intramuscular injection, as a rule: tuberculin syringe, 50 mL syringe, 5 mL syringe, or 3 mL syringe?

 Go to Chapter 23, **Knowledge Check Response Sheet and Answers,** on the Electronic Study Guide.

Drawing Up Medications from an Ampule

An **ampule** is a thin-walled, disposable glass container with a narrow neck that you must snap off to access the medication (Figure 23–17). To prevent injuries, use an ampule opener to snap the glass. Each ampule holds a single dose of a liquid medication, usually 1 mL to 10 mL, but some hold 50 mL. Because glass fragments may be introduced into the medication, most agencies require you to use a filter needle or filter straw to draw up the medication. See the Critical Aspects box. Also,

 Go to Chapter 23, **Procedure 23-7A: Preparing and Drawing Up Medications from Ampules,** in Volume 2.

Drawing Up Medications from a Vial

A **vial** is a single-dose or multidose plastic or glass container with a rubber stopper that seals the top. A plastic or metal cap covers the rubber stopper to protect it until it is used (Figure 23–18). Because the vial is a closed system, you must inject air into it to withdraw the solution. Otherwise, a vacuum is created in the vial that makes withdrawal difficult. See the Critical Aspects box. Also,

 Go to Chapter 23, **Procedure 23-7B: Preparing and Drawing Up Medications from Vials,** in Volume 2.

Nurses traditionally wipe the rubber stopper after removing the cap, even on a single-dose vial. However, there is little, if any, scientific justification for this practice. At least one study concluded that it is unnecessary as an infection control measure (Buckley, Dudley, &

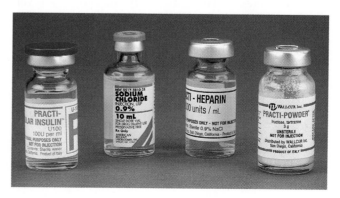

FIGURE 23–18 Medication vials.

Donowitz, 1994) and that using a filter needle prevents the aspiration of dust and rubber particles from the top of the vial.

Reconstituting Medications

Medications that are not stable in solution are dispensed as powders in vials. You must add a diluent or solvent to the powder to create a solution for injection. The diluent is usually sterile water or saline; however, each packaged vial includes the manufacturer's instructions for the amount and kind of solvent to add. For safety, use a plastic vial access cannula instead of a needle when possible. For guidelines,

 Go to Chapter 23, **Technique 23–3: Reconstituting Medications,** in Volume 2.

Mixing Medications in the Same Syringe

You can mix two medications in the same syringe (1) if they are compatible, (2) if the total dose is within accepted limits, and, obviously, (3) if they are both to be given by the same route. This technique allows for efficient use of supplies and allows the patient to receive fewer injections.

Medications are *compatible* if they can be mixed without affecting their constituents or actions. Package inserts and medication references usually include compatibility information. Always check the compatibility before mixing medications together. If the contents of the syringe become discolored, there are particles floating in the solution, or there is a change in consistency, do not administer the medications. When mixing medications in one syringe, you must follow these principles:

1. Maintain sterile technique.
2. Do not contaminate one container with medication from the other container. You must use a separate needle to withdraw from each vial (unless both are single-dose vials).
3. Ensure that the dosage of *each* medication is accurate. Calculate each dose before beginning, and draw the second drug up slowly and carefully. If you draw up too much of the second drug, you must discard the syringe and medication and begin again.
4. Ensure that the total, final, dosage is correct. Add the volumes calculated in step 3; when you have drawn up both medications, that total volume should be the amount you have in the syringe. Be sure at each measurement step either to expel or to account for air in the syringe.

See the Critical Aspects box for guidelines. For the complete steps,

 Go to Chapter 23, **Procedure 23–8: Mixing Medications in One Syringe,** in Volume 2.

Accounting for Needle "Dead Space"

Some nurses believe that a small amount of the patient's medication remains in the needle when an injection is given. Therefore, in the past, some recommended adding 0.2 mL of air to the syringe after measuring a medication for IM injection. Nurses are not in agreement about the need for adding air and, unfortunately, there is scant research to settle the question. Theoretically, on injection the air clears the needle of medication, ensuring that the patient receives the entire dose. However, because syringes are calibrated to account for medication left in the needle, and because the medication left in the needle after injection is the same amount as before the injection, many believe that air should not be added. We recommend that you add air only in the following situations:

1. *When the medication is irritating to subcutaneous tissues,* add 0.2 mL of air after measuring the proper dose. The air drives the medication deep into the muscle tissue; the air injected into the tissue creates an air lock above the medication, preventing it from tracking through subcutaneous tissue.
2. *When you change needles after drawing up the medication.* For example, when you draw up a dose using a filter needle, then replace it with a new needle, the new needle has air in it instead of medication. If you push the plunger until you see a drop of medication at the tip of the needle, you will see that you no longer have a complete dose in the syringe. Adding a 0.2 mL air lock will drive the entire dose into the patient's tissue.

 Go to Chapter 23, **Technique 23–4: Measuring Dosage When Changing Needles,** in Volume 2.

Preventing Needlestick Injuries

Healthcare workers suffer up to 1 million injuries per year from needles and other "sharps," putting them at risk for infectious diseases such as hepatitis B and AIDS (see Chapter 21). For this reason, special safety devices have been designed to reduce the risk of needlestick injuries. One such device is a special syringe with a guard that covers the needle immediately after it is withdrawn from the skin (Figure 23–19). You then dispose of both needle and sheath in a "sharps" container. The Centers for Disease Control and Prevention (CDC) and the Occupational Safety and Health Administration (OSHA) recommend the use of "needleless" systems. Most systems involve adapters that can be used with regular intravenous tubing and medication vials, permitting access through a valve system without a needle. Figure 23–20 is an example of needleless cannulae used to connect IV medication sets to a primary infusion. Figure 23–21 is a syringe with a needleless connection.

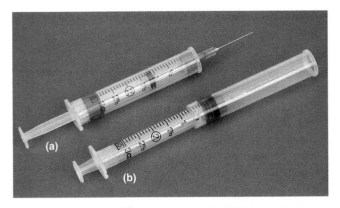

FIGURE 23–19 Special "safety" syringe. *A*, Needle guard position before injection. *B*, Needle guard position after injection.

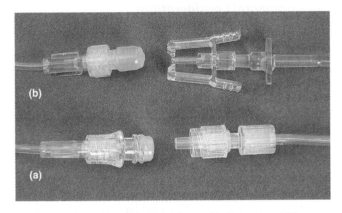

FIGURE 23–20 Needleless cannulae used to connect an additive to primary intravenous infusions. *A*, Threaded-lock cannula. *B*, Lever-lock cannula.

Always dispose of needles, glass, and other "sharps" in clearly marked, usually red, puncture-proof containers (Figure 23–22). Never force a needle into an already full container; you may be injured by sharps protruding from the top. Never put a needle or other sharp in a wastebasket, in your pocket, or at the patient's bedside.

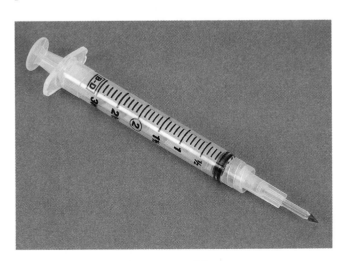

FIGURE 23–21 A syringe with a needleless connector.

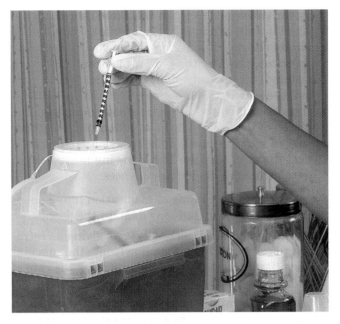

FIGURE 23–22 Always dispose of needles, glass, and other "sharps" in clearly marked, usually red, puncture-proof containers.

Recapping Contaminated Needles

You should never recap a contaminated needle (e.g., after giving an injection); place it uncapped, needle pointing downward, directly into a sharps container. However, you may occasionally find that you must recap a contaminated needle when there is "no feasible alternative" (U.S. Department of Labor, OSHA, 1999). For example, in some patient rooms the sharps container is not located near the bed. If there are several people (e.g., visitors) between you and the sharps container, you may need to recap the needle for their safety as well as for your own. In this case, use a *one-handed technique* for recapping the needle. For step-by-step instructions,

VOL 2 Go to Chapter 23, **Procedure 23-9: Recapping Needles Using One-Handed Technique,** in Volume 2.

You will find the critical elements of this procedure in the Critical Aspects box.

Recapping Sterile Needles

OSHA and the National Institute of Occupational Safety and Health (NIOSH) do not advise against recapping sterile needles (e.g., after drawing up a medication), except to recommend needleless systems and safety systems. We suggest that you not use the one-handed "scoop" technique to recap a sterile needle, because the risk of contaminating it is high. Consider one of the other methods described in Procedure 23–9.

Administering Parenteral Injections

Parenteral techniques are invasive. They carry the potential for tissue trauma and provide a portal of

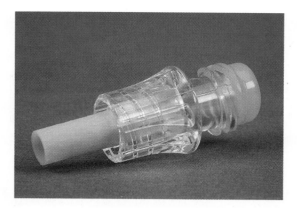

FIGURE 23–31   An intermittent injection port.

in water (D_5W) or normal saline. The drug is given over a period of time, usually 30 to 60 minutes, and at regular intervals (e.g., every 6 hours). The small bag of diluted medication (the "secondary" bag) is attached to the primary IV infusion line for administration. There are two types of setups for intermittent infusion using a primary IV line:

1. A **tandem setup** is connected to the primary IV line at the lower (secondary) port (Figure 23–32). The medication can be given intermittently or at the same time as the primary IV infusion—both bags can infuse at the same time.

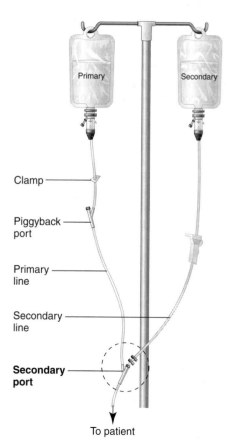

FIGURE 23–32   A tandem setup is attached to the primary (continuous infusion) IV line at the lower port, allowing for both intermittent and simultaneous infusion.

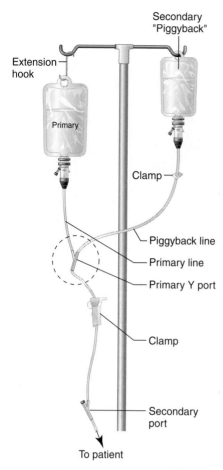

FIGURE 23–33   A piggyback setup is attached to the primary (continuous infusion) IV line at the upper port, allowing for intermittent infusion only.

2. With an **IV piggyback** setup the smaller (secondary) container is connected to the primary (continuous) infusion line at the upper (primary) port (Figure 23–33). This setup allows for intermittent use only.

Traditionally, the secondary tubing was attached to the primary set tubing by inserting a needle into the port and taping it in place. However, most agencies now use needleless systems (Figure 23–20), which use a threaded or lever-type lock to make the connection. In addition to helping prevent needlestick injuries, a needleless system prevents touch contamination at the IV connection site.

The Critical Aspects box provides guidelines for administering intermittent infusions. Also,

VOL 2 Go to Chapter 23, **Procedure 23–16: Administering Medications by Intermittent Infusion,** in Volume 2.

Volume-Control Infusion Sets

To effectively control the infusion of smaller amounts of solutions, particularly with pediatric patients, a volume-control infusion set (e.g., the Buretrol, Soluset, Volutrol, or Pediatrol) may be used (Figure 23–34). These are small fluid containers (100 to 150 mL) that

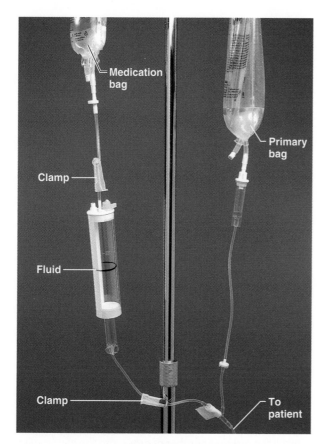

FIGURE 23–34 **A volume-control infusion set for intermittent infusion administration; used when the fluid volume is critical and must be carefully monitored.**

are attached directly below the primary fluid container. The medication and the desired amount of IV fluid are added to the volume-control container and administered through the primary line. This system decreases the risk of overhydration because the amount of fluid that can infuse into the client is limited to the amount that you place in the small container.

MEDICATION ERRORS

All medications are ordered, prepared, and administered with the best intentions. However, errors occur with surprising frequency. One observational study found that 19% of drug doses administered by nurses were erroneous. Of these, 43% were given at the wrong time; 30% were simply omitted or missed doses; 17% were the wrong dose, and 4% were an unauthorized drug (*AJN* Reports, 2003).

Why Do Errors Occur?

The following are a number of reasons why nurses make medication errors:

- Written order is not clear, is illegible, or is transcribed incorrectly.
- Telephone order is taken incorrectly.

- Wrong equipment is used to administer the drug.
- Equipment malfunctions or is not used properly.
- Medication is improperly handled or stored.
- Medication is given to a patient with contraindicating condition.
- Protocol is not understood or is violated.
- A drug is ordered for the wrong patient (written on the wrong patient's chart).
- The wrong dosage is ordered.
- The correct drug or dosage is ordered, but because of poor penmanship the wrong drug or dosage is administered.
- An error in calculating the dosage is made so the patient receives the wrong dose.
- A drug is given by the wrong route.
- The patient's identity is not checked, and the wrong patient receives the medication.
- The first person that administers the medication fails to record it immediately afterward. A second person checking the patient's chart thinks the drug has not been given so administers a dose. The patient receives a double dose.

How Can I Avoid Errors?

To prevent making a medication error, you should develop a set routine for administering medications. Practice this routine scrupulously when you are administering medications. Finally, learn from your mistakes and the mistakes of others. To administer medications safely, incorporate the following actions into your practice:

- Always practice the "three checks" and "six rights" of medication administration.
- Ask another nurse to check your calculations when you must calculate a dosage.
- Look at all medications closely for similar containers, colors, and shapes.
- Question orders of multiple tablets or vials as a single dose; most doses are one or two tablets or one single-dose vial.
- Beware of drugs with similar names (e.g., Keflex and Keflin).
- Check the decimal point! For example, Coumadin comes in both 1 mg and 10 mg sizes.
- Always write a zero before a decimal point (e.g., write "Lanoxin 0.125 mg," *not* "Lanoxin .125 mg"), and carefully read orders without a zero. It is easy to mistake .15 for 115 if the decimal point is written large or the 1 is written small.
- Question abrupt and excessive increases in dosage; most dosages increase gradually.

VOL 2 For steps to follow in *all* procedures, refer to the inside back cover of Volume 2. Also refer to Medication Guidelines: Steps to Follow for *All* Medications (Regardless of Type or Route), on page 450 of Chapter 23, Volume 2.

critical aspects of procedures 23–1 through 23–16

Procedure 23–1: Administering Oral Medications

- Observe the "three checks": before and after drawing up the medication, and at the bedside.

- Observe "six rights" of medication administration.

- *Tablets and capsules:* Pour the correct number into the medication cup.

- *Liquids:* Hold the plastic medication cup at eye level to measure the dose.

- Assist the patient to a high-Fowler's position, if possible.

- For enterically administered medications, check for correct placement of the nasogastric or gastric tube.

- Correctly administer the medication.

  Powder: Mix with liquid, and give it to the patient to drink.
  Lozenge: Instruct the patient not to chew or swallow it.
  Tablet or capsule: Place the tablet or medication cup in the patient's hand or mouth, and have the patient swallow with sips of liquid.
  Sublingual: Have the patient place the tablet under the tongue and hold it there until it is completely dissolved.
  Buccal: Have the patient place the tablet between the cheek and teeth hold it there until it is completely dissolved.

- Stay with patient until medications have been swallowed or dissolved.

Procedure 23–2: Administering Ophthalmic Medications

For Instillations

- Assist the patient to high-Fowler's position, with head slightly tilted back.

- If necessary, clean the edges of the eyelid from the inner to outer canthus.

- Apply the medication into the conjunctival sac.

- Do not apply the medication to the cornea.

- Do not let the dropper or tube touch the eye.

- For eye drops, press gently against the same side of the nose for 1 to 2 minutes to close the lacrimal ducts. For eye ointment, ask the patient to gently close the eyes for 2 to 3 minutes.

For Irrigations

- Assist the patient to low-Fowler's position.

- Check the pH in the conjunctival sac, if indicated.

- Use a Morgan lens or IV tubing to irrigate the eyes.

- For direct-flow irrigation, irrigate from the inner canthus to the outer canthus.

- Irrigate for 20 minutes or until desired pH is reached.

Procedure 23–3: Administering Otic Medications

- Warm the solution to be instilled.

- Assist the patient to a side-lying position, with the appropriate ear facing up.

- Straighten the ear canal. For an adult client, pull the pinna up and back; for a child 3 years or younger, down and back.

- Instill the ordered number of drops into the ear canal.

- Do not force the solution into the ear or occlude the ear canal with the dropper.

- Instruct the patient to remain on his side for 5 to 10 minutes.

Procedure 23–4: Administering Nasal Medications

- Determine head position: Consider the indication for the medication and the patient's ability to assume the position.

- Explain to the patient that the medication may cause some burning, tingling, or unusual taste.

- Position the patient with the head down and forward or supine with the head back.

- Have the patient blow his nose, occlude one nostril, and exhale.

- Administer the spray or drops while the patient is inhaling.

- Repeat for other nostril.

- If nose drops are used, ask the patient to stay in the same position for approximately 5 minutes.

Procedure 23–5: Administering Vaginal Medications

For Instillation

- Position the patient in a dorsal recumbent or Sims' position.

- Inspect and cleanse the vaginal area before administering the medication.

- Insert the suppository or applicator along the posterior vaginal wall about 8 cm (3 inches).

- Instruct the client to maintain the position for 5 to 15 minutes after the medication is inserted.

For Irrigation (Douche)

- Warm the irrigation solution to approximately 105°F (40.6°C).

- Hang the irrigation solution approximately 30 to 60 cm (1 to 2 ft) above the level of the patient's vagina.

- Position the patient in a dorsal recumbent position on a waterproof pad and bedpan.

- Insert the nozzle approximately 7 to 8 cm (3 inches) into the vagina, and start the flow of irrigation solution.

Procedure 23–6: Inserting a Rectal Suppository

- Before inserting the suppository, assess for contraindications, such as rectal surgery, rectal bleeding, or cardiac disease.

- Position the client in Sims' position (left lateral with the upper leg flexed).

- Lubricate the suppository.

- Never force the suppository during insertion.

- Insert the suppository past the internal sphincter about 10 cm (4 inches).

- Have the client stay on his side for 5 to 10 minutes and retain (not expel) the suppository for about 30 minutes.

Procedure 23–7: Preparing and Drawing Up Medications

- Maintain sterile technique.

- Recap the needle or injection cannula using a needle recapping device or the one-handed method (see Procedure 23–9).

- Change the needle, if indicated.

A. Ampules

- Tap the ampule to remove medication trapped in the top of the ampule.

- Use an ampule opener to break the ampule neck. If one is not available, wrap gauze around the neck of the ampule, and snap the ampule away from you.

- Use a filter needle or filter straw to withdraw the medication.

- Withdraw all of the medication from the ampule by inverting or tipping the ampule.

- Dispose of the top and bottom of ampule and filter needle in a sharps container.

B. Vials

- Thoroughly clean the rubber top of the vial with an alcohol prep pad (for a multiple-dose vial only).

- Draw air into the syringe equal to the amount of medication to be withdrawn.

- When inserting the needle through the rubber top of the vial, avoid coring by inserting the needle at a 45 to 60° angle, bevel up, or by using a filter needle.

- Keeping the needle above the fluid line, inject air into the vial before withdrawing the medication.

- Remove bubbles, hold the vial at eye level, and check that the dose is correct before removing the needle. (See Procedure 23–9).

Procedure 23–8: Mixing Medications in One Syringe

- Make sure the medications are compatible.

- Maintain the sterility of the needles and medication.

- Avoid contaminating a multidose vial with a second medication.

- Carefully expel air bubbles.

- When you withdraw the second medication, the medications are mixed as you pull back the plunger; therefore, you must withdraw the exact amount. If there is any excess, you must discard the contents of the syringe and start over.

- When opening ampules, protect yourself from injury.

- Use a filter needle or filter straw to withdraw medication from ampules; change to a needle of the proper length and gauge for administering the medication.

- When drawing up from a single-dose vial and ampule, draw up from the vial first.

- Do not use prefilled cartridges for intramuscular injections unless they have a safety device; transfer the medication to a syringe with a safety device before administering.

- Always recap a sterile needle using a needle capping device or the one-handed scoop method (see Procedure 23–9).

Procedure 23–9: Recapping Needles Using One-Handed Technique

Recapping Contaminated Needles

- Do not place your nondominant hand near the needle cap when recapping the needle or engaging the safety mechanism.

- If you are using a safety needle, engage the safety mechanism to cover the needle.

- If available, place the needle cap in a mechanical recapping device.

- If recapping devices are not available and you must recap the needle for your own and/or the patient's safety, use the one-handed scoop technique.

Recapping Sterile Needles

- Be sure to keep the needle and cap sterile.

- Do not place your nondominant hand near the needle cap when recapping the needle or engaging the safety mechanism.

- Use one of the following methods:

    Place the needle cap in a medication cup, and recap the needle.
    Place the cap on a clean surface so that the end of the needle cap protrudes over the edge of the counter or shelf, and scoop with the needle.
    Use a hard syringe cover: Insert the needle cap into the cover, and then insert the needle.
    Place the needle cap on a sterile surface, such as on open alcohol prep pad, and use the one-handed scoop technique (this is the least desirable method).

Procedure 23–10: Administering Intradermal Medications

- Maintain sterile technique and standard precautions.

- Use 1 mL syringe and a 25- to 28-gauge, $\frac{1}{4}$ to $\frac{5}{8}$ inch needle.

- Be aware that an intradermal dose is small, usually about 0.01 to 0.1 mL.

- Administer the injection on the ventral surface of the forearm, upper back, or upper chest.

- Hold the syringe parallel to the skin at a 5 to 15° angle, with the bevel up.

- Stretch the skin taut to insert the needle.

- Do not aspirate.

- Inject slowly, and create a wheal or bleb.

- Do not massage the site.

Procedure 23–11: Administering Subcutaneous Medications

- Maintain sterile technique and standard precautions.

- Use a 1 mL syringe and a 25- to 27-gauge needle that is less than 1 inch long (usually $\frac{3}{8}$ to $\frac{5}{8}$ inch).

- A subcutaneous dose must be no more than 1 mL.

- Injection sites: Use the outer aspect of the upper arms, abdomen, anterior aspects of the thighs, or the scapular area on the upper back.

- Pinch the skin to inject as a general rule.

- For an average-weight or thin client, inject at a 45° angle. For an obese client, inject at a 90° angle.

- Aspiration is optional, but do not aspirate when injecting heparin or insulin.

- Do not massage the site.

Procedure 23–12: Locating Intramuscular Injection Sites

- Always palpate the landmarks and the muscle mass to ensure correct placement.

- *Deltoid:* The injection site is an inverted triangle. The base is two to three fingerbreadths below the acromion process, and the tip is even with the top of the axilla.

- *Vastus lateralis:* Midlateral thigh: On adults, one handbreadth below the head of the trochanter and one handbreadth above the knee. The site is the middle third of this area. This is the preferred site for infants under 7 months.

- *Ventrogluteal:* On adults, a triangle formed between your fingers when you place your palm on the head of the trochanter, index finger on the anterior superior iliac spine, and middle finger on the iliac crest. This is the preferred site for adults and children over 7 months.

- *Dorsogluteal:* Locate the site by drawing an imaginary line between the head of the trochanter and the posterior superior iliac spine. At the middle of the line, go up approximately 1 inch. Use this site only if no others are accessible.

- *Rectus femoris:* Middle third of the anterior thigh. Use this site only if no others are accessible.

Procedure 23–13: Administering Intramuscular Injections

- Maintain sterile technique and standard precautions.

- Use a 1 to 3 mL syringe and a 21- to 25-gauge, 1 to $1\frac{1}{2}$ inch needle.

- The usual dose per injection is no more than 3 mL.

Procedure 23–13: (continued)

- Select an appropriate injection site, and identify the site using anatomical landmarks:

  Ventrogluteal site is preferred for IM injections. Deltoid site is acceptable for IM doses of 1 mL or less.

- Aspirate before injecting. If blood appears, remove the needle, discard it, and start over.

- Inject at a 90° angle.

- Z-track technique is recommended. Mnemonic:

Deliver	**D**isplace
All	**A**spirate
Injections	**I**nject (wait 10 seconds)
With	**W**ithdraw
Responsibility	**R**elease

Procedure 23–14: Adding Medications to Intravenous Fluids

- Check the compatibility of the intravenous solution and medication.

- Assess the patency of the intravenous site.

- Maintain the sterility of intravenous fluids and medication admixture.

- Affix the medication label to the bag, with the name and amount of medication, date and time administered, and your name or initials.

Procedure 23–15: Administering IV Push Medications

- Determine the type and amount of dilution needed for the medication.

- Determine the amount of time needed to administer the medication.

- Ensure the patency of the line prior to administration.

- Flush the line before and after administering the medication.

- Maintain sterility.

Procedure 23–16: Administering Medications by Intermittent Infusion

- Ensure the compatibility of the IV solution and medication, both the solution in the primary IV system and the diluent in the secondary system.

- Assess the IV site and the patency of the line.

- Calculate amount of medication to add to the solution.

- Use the correct amount and type of diluent solution.

- Use the correct rate of administration.

- Determine the correct primary line port in which to infuse the medication.

- Affix the correct label to the secondary bag, with start date and hour, discard date and hour, and your initials.

- When new or unfamiliar drugs are ordered, consult your resources for current information about the medication.

- Do not administer a drug ordered by a nickname or an unofficial abbreviation. Many providers refer to certain drugs by nickname (e.g., "MOM" for "milk of magnesia"); if you aren't familiar with the nickname used, then clarify the order so you select the correct medication.

- Do not attempt to decipher illegible handwriting. The chance of misinterpretation is great, so when in doubt, ask the prescriber to clarify.

- Be alert for patients with the same last names, and check arm bands carefully. It is common to have two patients with same or similar last names (e.g., Wilkinson, Wilson, Wilkerson). Special alerts on charts and MARs are helpful to prevent giving the medication to the wrong patient.

- Do not confuse measurements. It is easy to misread "mg" instead of "mL." There is a significant difference between 1 mg and 1 mL of intravenous morphine, for example.

- Double-check all orders transcribed to the MAR.
- Frequently review orders to make sure there have been no changes.

What Should I Do If I Commit a Medication Error?

Here are some steps to follow if you make a medication error.

- First check the patient. Take his vital signs, and perform assessments related to the medication that was given.

- If you are unfamiliar with the side effects of the medication, consult a drug reference source.

- Verify that you have made a medication error, and identify the type of error.

- Notify the nurse in charge for guidance if this is your first error.

- Notify the physician and follow her orders for intervention.

- Document on the chart that the medication was given, but do *not* indicate that the medication was given in error. This alerts anyone reviewing the chart that an error was made.
- Complete an incident report according to the facility's policies. Ask for assistance the first few times you complete this form so that the information you provide concerning the error is factual and accurate. Do *not* document in the patient's chart that an incident report was filed. This, again, alerts anyone reviewing the chart and makes the incident report available for legal review in the event of a lawsuit.
- Finally, when you have time to think carefully, critically review the error. Identify the influences that led to your making the error. Were you rushed? Did you check the order? Did you follow the six rights? Whatever the reason, use this situation as a learning experience to improve your practice.

| toward evidence-based practice |

You will encounter many nurses who have been in practice for years who flush indwelling catheters (known as heparin locks or saline locks) with 100 units of heparin. Only recently have studies indicated that saline works just as well at maintaining the patency of the catheter and preventing clotting.

Mudge, B., Forcier, D., and Slarrert, M. J. (1998). Patency of 24-gauge peripheral intermittent infusion devices: A comparison of heparin and saline flush solutions, *Pediatric Nursing 24*(2): 142–149.

This study used randomly selected pediatric patients with a 24-gauge peripheral intermittent device who were flushed with either heparin or saline. They found no statistical difference in the flush solutions but did find that frequency of use of the catheter improved patency.

American Society of Healthcare Pharmacists. (2003). ASHP therapeutic position statement on the institutional use of 0.9% sodium chloride injection to maintain patency of peripheral indwelling infusion devices. Retrieved June 23, 2003, from http://ww.ashp.org

This study resulted in a recommendation by the American Society of Healthcare Pharmacists that saline (sodium chloride 0.9%) should be used to flush peripheral indwelling devices. This group cites the risks related to heparin and the incompatibilities of medications being flushed though the lock with the heparin flush outweigh the risks for saline usage.

Le Duc, K. (1997). Efficacy of normal saline solution versus heparin solution for maintaining patency of peripheral intravenous catheters in children. *Journal of Emergency Nursing, 23*(4), 306–309.

This study was a prospective, randomized, double-blind controlled study using heparin and saline to flush peripheral indwelling infusion devices in children under the age of 12. The study yielded no significant differences between the two flushes for complications or diminished patency.

---

1. Based on the preceding three studies, would you choose to flush the indwelling catheter with heparin or saline?

2. What assumptions must you make to correlate these studies with your practice?

 Go to Chapter 23, **Toward Evidence–Based Practice Suggested Responses,** on the Electronic Study Guide.

 Go to Chapter 23, **Resources for Caregivers and Health Professionals,** on the Electronic Study Guide.

 Suggested Readings: Go to Chapter 23, **Reading More About Administering Medications,** on the Electronic Study Guide.

 Bibliography: Go to Volume 2, Bibliography.

Teaching Clients

Learning Outcomes

After completing this chapter, you should be able to:

✳ Discuss the role of teaching in professional nursing.

✳ Describe the processes of teaching and learning.

✳ Name, define, and give one example of each of Bloom's three domains of learning.

✳ Discuss how each of the following factors can affect learning: motivation, readiness, physical condition, emotions, timing, active involvement, feedback, repetition, environment, scheduling of the teaching session, amount and complexity of the content, communication, special needs (e.g., learning disability), developmental stage, culture, and literacy.

✳ List at least six barriers to teaching and learning.

✳ Describe some strategies for motivating learners.

✳ Develop strategies for working with clients with cultural or learning differences.

✳ Describe the content of a learning assessment.

✳ Discuss correct and incorrect uses of the nursing diagnosis Deficient Knowledge.

✳ Develop teaching plans for clients.

✳ List four methods for evaluating the outcomes of teaching and learning.

✳ Document teaching content, methods, and patient responses (learning).

Your Patient

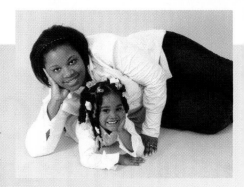

You are the student nurse assigned to Heather, a 20-year-old mother, and her 3-year-old toddler. They have come to a family practice clinic for a well-child checkup. You notice that the child speaks in one- or two-word phrases. The mother seems impatient with her and continually tells her to "stop using that baby talk." Your nursing instructor tells you that you need to assess for teaching needs and provide anticipatory guidance to the mother. How would you begin?

Heather says, "Gosh, I don't know what I'm doing wrong. All her little friends are bigger and talking more. She was even small when she was born, so I suppose it's my fault." How do you address Heather's learning needs without reinforcing her feeling that "it's my fault"?

Your assessment shows that the child is below the 5th percentile for height and weight. What teaching could you provide that might help address this problem?

Your anticipatory guidance should include information about safety measures for a 3-year-old, nutrition for toddlers, and expected growth and development. How can you evaluate whether or not the teaching has been effective and further promote Heather's retention of this new information?

By the time you finish working through this chapter, you should be able to answer these questions and provide teaching to meet the unique needs of other patients you encounter.

Theoretical Knowledge
knowing why

Much of your work as a nurse will involve client teaching. This has been true for well over 100 years—certainly since Florence Nightingale taught both nurses and patients about the importance of good nutrition, fresh air, exercise, and personal hygiene (Nightingale, 1860). Since that time, teaching has become progressively more important. The following are a few of the reasons why:

- *Patients participate in decisions.* No longer do patients wait passively for "the doctor's orders." Primary care providers have come to expect clients to take an active role in making decisions about their health; clients and families need information so that they make decisions that are *informed*. You can help clients get answers to their questions, find resources, recognize problems, and develop self-care behaviors.

- *Hospital stays are short.* With shorter hospital stays and more care being given in homes and the community, teaching takes on major importance. Patients are often sent home still needing medications, dressing changes, and even skilled procedures such as urinary catheterization. A major nursing

responsibility is to teach family members how to provide care and to teach patients to care for themselves as they are able.

- *Cost of health care is high.* Teaching can help to decrease the overall cost of health care. It does so by helping to increase patient compliance with medical and nursing regimens, which can shorten hospital stays and decrease frequency of medical treatments and admissions (Bastable, 2003).

As you may have guessed from the foregoing discussion, the basic purpose of teaching and learning is to provide information that will empower clients and families to (1) perform self-care and (2) make informed decisions about their healthcare options. Like other interventions, you can use teaching to promote wellness, prevent or limit illness, restore health, and facilitate coping with stress, illness, and loss.

WHO ARE THE LEARNERS?

As a nurse, you will teach clients, families, and others who care for the client. You may do informal one-to-one teaching as you care for a client. For example, as you give a medication, you will teach about its therapeutic and side effects. Or you may do more formal teaching to groups of people. For example, you might demonstrate a baby bath to several mothers of newborns.

Regardless of whether you work in a hospital, an ambulatory setting, home care, or in the community, you will teach clients about health promotion measures, about ways to prevent illness and accidents, and about measures for restoring health and adapting to changes in body function. As a community health nurse, you would be more likely to teach large groups of people; for example, you might teach safer sex to a class of college students or provide a class in CPR for a church group.

In the practice setting, you will be responsible for informal teaching of unlicensed assistive personnel, for example, when you observe an error in technique. Nurses in practice are also involved in clinical instruction of nursing students, new graduates, and new employees, as well as colleagues. Most of this teaching may be informal, but you may also present specific topics at unit meetings and conferences. For example, if there is a change in the agency's charting system, you might be asked to plan a class for teaching it to the nurses on your shift.

WHAT ARE MY TEACHING RESPONSIBILITIES?

Teaching is a major component of clinical practice skills and is an independent nursing function. In many states, the requirement to teach is included as a part of the Nurse Practice Act. According to the *American Nurses Association (ANA) Code of Ethics for Nurses* (2001), nurses are responsible for promoting and protecting health, safety, and rights of patients. Client teaching is essential in fulfilling that responsibility.

ANA standards of practice (2003), Standard 5B, states, "The nurse employs strategies to promote health and a safe environment." The following are the specific measurement criteria for that standard:

1. Provides health teaching that addresses such topics as healthy lifestyles, risk-reducing behaviors, developmental needs, activities of daily living, and preventive self-care.
2. Uses health promotion and health teaching methods appropriate to the patient's developmental level, learning needs, readiness, ability to learn, language preference, and culture.
3. Seeks opportunities for feedback and evaluation of the learning.

Joint Commission on Accreditation of Healthcare Organizations (JCAHO) standards require that educators in healthcare organizations consider the literacy, developmental and physical limitations, financial limitations, language barriers, culture, and religious practices of every client. Teaching must also include any person who will be responsible for the client's care (JCAHO, 2000).

The "Patient Care Partnership" (previously the "Patient's Bill of Rights") establishes the right of patients to receive complete and current information regarding diagnosis, treatment, and prognosis in ways they can understand, as well as the right to be informed of hospital policies and practices that relate to them (American Hospital Association, 2003).

The Pew Commission emphasizes that teaching for patients should focus on prevention rather than take a disease-oriented approach (Pew Health Professions Commission, 1998).

WHAT ARE SOME BASIC LEARNING CONCEPTS AND PRINCIPLES?

The educational process consists of both teaching and learning. **Teaching** is an interactive process that involves planning and implementing instructional activities to meet intended learner outcomes or providing activities that allow the learner to learn (Bastable, 2003). Teachers must have good communication skills to (1) adequately convey information, (2) assess verbal and nonverbal feedback, and (3) communicate effectively with individuals and groups of varying sizes. In patient education, nurses can use teaching, counseling, and behavioral modification together to achieve effective client learning.

Learning is a change in behavior, knowledge, skills, or attitudes that occurs as a result of exposure to environmental stimuli (Bastable, 2003). Learning is an active process in which a person conveys knowledge, skills, and attitudes and incorporates them into his daily life. It is not enough for the teacher to give the person written or verbal information; information alone will not change behaviors. Box 24–1 summarizes some basic principles of learning and provides a quick check for planning teaching sessions. For information about learning theories,

 Go to Chapter 24, **Supplemental Materials: Learning Theories,** on the Electronic Study Guide.

KnowledgeCheck 24–1
- Identify at least three reasons why nurses need to teach clients.
- Define *teaching*.
- Define *learning*.

 Go to Chapter 24, **Knowledge Check Response Sheet and Answers,** on the Electronic Study Guide.

Learning Occurs in Three Domains

People learn in three ways, or *domains:* cognitive, psychomotor, and affective (Bloom & Krathwohl, 1956). You should include each of these domains when writing objectives and planning teaching and evaluation

---

BOX 24–1 Five Rights of Teaching

When you are making a teaching plan, you can use this as a checklist to ensure that you consider each of the five "rights" of teaching in the plan.

Right Time

- Is the learner ready, free of pain and anxiety, and motivated?
- Have you and the learner a trusting relationship?
- Have you set aside sufficient time for the teaching session?

Right Context

- Is the environment quiet, free of distractions, and private?
- Is the environment soothing or stimulating, depending on the desired effect?

Right Goal

- Is the learner actively involved in planning the learning objectives?
- Are you and your client both committed to reaching mutually set goals of learning that achieve the desired behavioral changes?

- Are family or friends included in planning so that they can help follow through on behavioral changes?
- Are the learning objectives realistic and valued by the client; do they reflect the client's lifestyle?

Right Content

- Is the content appropriate for the client's needs?
- Is it new information or reinforcement of information that has already been provided?
- Is the content presented at the learner's level?
- Does the content relate to the learner's life experiences or is it otherwise relevant to the learner?

Right Method

- Do the teaching strategies fit the learning style of the learner?
- Do the strategies fit the client's learning ability?
- Are the teaching strategies varied?

---

strategies, which are discussed later in this chapter. Table 24–1 provides examples of client learning in each of the domains. For a more detailed version of this table, which identifies levels of behavior associated with each domain,

 Go to Chapter 24, **Tables, Boxes, Figures: ESG Table 24–1,** on the Electronic Study Guide.

Cognitive Learning

Cognitive learning includes storing and recalling information in the brain. Ranging from simple to complex processes, it encompasses six levels of behavior: memorization, recall, comprehension and analysis, synthesis, application, and evaluation of ideas (Table 24–1). Strategies and tools for teaching cognitive content include lecture, reading materials, panel discussion, audiovisual materials, programmed instruction, computer-assisted instruction (CAI), and problem-based learning (e.g., case studies and care plans).

Psychomotor Learning

Psychomotor learning involves learning a skill that requires both mental and physical activity. It requires that the learner accept and value the skill (the affective domain) as well know about the skill (the cognitive domain). Strategies and tools used to

teach psychomotor skills include demonstration, audiovisual materials (e.g., videotapes), and printed materials (especially with pictures).

Affective Learning

Affective learning includes changes in feelings, beliefs, attitudes, and values. It is considered the "feeling domain." Levels of affective behavior are shown in Table 24–1. Strategies and tools for promoting affective learning include role modeling, panel discussion, one-to-one counseling and discussion, audiovisual materials (e.g., videotapes, movies), and printed materials.

KnowledgeCheck 24–2
- What are the three domains of learning?
- Give an example of each of the domains of learning.

 Go to Chapter 24, **Knowledge Check Response Sheet and Answers,** on the Electronic Study Guide.

 ## CriticalThinking 24–1
By now, you have probably already learned how to assess a patient's blood pressure (BP).

- Think about how you were taught to perform that *skill*. What would have been the best way for *you* to learn to take a BP? To read a book and look at the pictures? To watch a video?

TABLE 24-1 Bloom's Domains of Learning

Domain and Levels of Behavior	Examples
Cognitive (thinking) Includes memorization, recall, comprehension, and ability to analyze, synthesize, apply, and evaluate ideas.	A client is able to report the names and amounts of the three medications he is taking. A client explains the expected effect of the medication she has been prescribed. A client designs a planned schedule for dressing changes on her leg. A client describes how to distinguish between normal inflammation and signs of infections in a wound. A client recognizes the need for behavioral changes to decrease the chance of recurrence of infection.
Psychomotor (skills) Includes sensory awareness of cues involved in learning, as well as imitation and performance of skills and creation of new skills.	A client identifies that he needs to read directions before starting a project. A client brings personal equipment to a teaching session. A new mother follows the instructor who is demonstrating diapering of her newborn, imitating her movements. A new father is observed diapering his newborn after observing a demonstration. A client independently changes her complex dressing. The wound heals with no signs of infection. A client with limited vision creates a new approach to giving his daily injections.
Affective (feelings) Includes receiving and responding to new ideas, demonstrating commitment to or preference for new ideas, and integrating new ideas into value system.	An adolescent makes eye contact with the nurse as she explains the admission process. A client asks questions about what to expect during a procedure he is to undergo. A parent of a child who has just been admitted to the hospital expresses commitment to staying with her child after the nurse explains the impact of hospitalization. A client who has overcome drug addiction chooses to present his story to high school groups.

Sources: Adapted from Bloom, B. S., Mesia, B. B., & Krathwohl, D. R. (1964). *Taxonomy of educational objectives* (Vol. 1: *The Affective Domain* and Vol. 2: *The Cognitive Domain*). New York: David McKay; Bloom B. S., & Krathwohl, D. R. (1956). *Taxonomy of educational objectives: The classification of educational goals. Handbook I: Cognitive domain.* New York: Longmans, Green.

To have someone tell you how to do it? To have someone demonstrate the skill? Some other way?
- Now think about the *principles* involved with BP (e.g., normal ranges, the physiological regulation of the BP). What, for you, would have been the best way to learn the principles? Read a book? Listen to a lecture? Take a BP on a patient? Work a case involving BP? Some other way?
- From your answers to the two preceding questions, what (if anything) can you conclude about different domains of learning and the kinds of activities to use in teaching and learning in each domain?

Many Factors Affect Client Learning

Learning is complex. Many factors can either enhance or interfere with it. An understanding of the following factors will help you to design effective teaching interventions and promote client learning.

Motivation

Motivation is desire from within. It is created by an idea, a physical need, an emotion, or some other kind of force. Without motivation, little learning can occur.

Motivation is greatest when clients recognize the need for learning, believe it is possible to improve their health, and are interested in the information they are being given. Think about classes you have taken. Have you studied harder in some than in others? What motivated you? Was it because you were intrigued by the information, wanted to earn a good grade, or something else?

Motivation may be based on physical and social needs, the need for task mastery, and health beliefs. In your teaching, try to apply the following tips for motivating learners.

- Conveying your interest in and respect for the learner and the learning process helps to motivate the learner.
- Creating a warm, friendly environment can enhance social needs motivation, as can your enthusiasm.
- You can sometimes motivate clients by helping them identify a physical need. For example, Heather ("Meet Your Patient") may not be aware that her child is at risk for accidents and injury from home hazards. Helping her to understand the normal behavior of a 3-year-old may help her to see the need for child-proofing her home.
- The need for achievement and competence is related to task mastery and self-efficacy. When a person succeeds at a task, he is usually motivated to continue learning. Rewards and incentives can provide this type of motivation.
- The client will be motivated to learn only if she believes that health is important. Heather may understand that a 3-year-old likes to explore and may recognize that there are safety hazards in the home; however, she will not be motivated to learn safety measures if her attitude is that "it is no big deal."

Many of the following factors also provide motivation as well as contributing in other ways to learning.

Readiness

Readiness is the demonstration of behaviors that indicate that the learner is both *motivated* and *able* to learn *at a specific time*. A client is not "ready" for teaching right before scheduled tests or treatments, because anxiety about the testing may make it difficult to focus on the material. So in addition to timing and motivation to learn, readiness includes the physical and emotional ability to learn.

Physical Condition

Physical factors (e.g., pain, strength, coordination, energy, senses, mobility) are one aspect of readiness. You must consider them in your planning. For example:

- Pain interferes with the ability to concentrate on the material being presented.

- The client needs adequate strength, coordination, energy, and mobility to demonstrate psychomotor learning.
- You will need to adapt your teaching and evaluation strategies to accommodate clients with impaired hearing or vision.

Emotions

Emotions are another aspect of readiness. Severe anxiety, stress, or emotional pain interfere with the ability to learn. In addition, the learning itself, and the idea that behaviors must be changed, can create anxiety. However, a mild level of anxiety can enhance learning by providing motivation. For example, a client newly diagnosed with diabetes may not be experiencing any symptoms or complications from the disease. If the client seems uninterested in learning about diabetes, you may be able to motivate him (i.e., create some anxiety) by pointing out the potential and serious complications (e.g., blindness, kidney damage) of uncontrolled diabetes. Provoke anxiety carefully so that the client does not interpret you words as a threat.

Timing

You must present information at a time when the learner is ready to learn. Timing is therefore related to readiness, and it is important in the following ways, as well.

1. People retain information better when they have an opportunity to use it soon after it is presented. For example, a student reads about insulin in her textbook and takes a test on the content 2 weeks later. Another student reads the same information and during the 2 weeks also administers different types of insulin to several patients. The second student will have an advantage at test time.
2. The learner needs enough time to be able to absorb and apply the information. Change the preceding example slightly. The student reads about diabetes, including pathophysiology, medications, and diet, on Monday night and takes the test on Tuesday. The student has not really had time to absorb and apply this complex information.

Active Involvement

Learning is more meaningful when the client is actively engaged in the planning and the learning activities. Learners retain 10% of what they read, but they retain 90% of what they speak and do (London, 1999). Passive listening is not a good way to retain information. Activities that require the use of more than one sense (e.g., the use of slides with lectures) promote learning. Can you think of other examples of learning that involve multiple senses?

Feedback

Feedback is information about the learner's performance. For example, a test grade is feedback, as is saying, "You need to work on that some more," or "You maintained sterile technique." Positive feedback encourages the learner to continue with the educational process. This is especially critical when significant behavioral changes are required. Sometimes you may need to act like a coach, encouraging the learner with frequent feedback and praise and suggesting alternatives. You may sometimes need to point out errors, but do so in a positive way when you can. Never use ridicule, sarcasm, anger, or punishment, because they cause the client to avoid you and detract from learning.

Repetition

The client is more likely to retain information and incorporate it into his life if it is repeated. Each time you repeat the information, the learner comprehends more. This is especially true of learning psychomotor skills. Do you remember the first time you counted a radial pulse? Even that simple skill may be difficult at first. By now it is probably very easy for you.

 CriticalThinking 24–2

Use examples from your own experience, if you can. Do not use examples you have read in the preceding sections.

- Give an example to illustrate the importance of relevance in learning.
- Give an example to illustrate the importance of repetition in learning.
- Give an example to illustrate the importance of timing in learning.

Environment

An ideal learning environment is private, quiet, physically and psychologically comfortable, and free from distractions. Have you ever tried to concentrate on a lecture when the school band was rehearsing outside your window? Or right after lunch when you were sitting in a warm, stuffy room? When you are planning a teaching session, provide good lighting and comfortable seating that is conducive for conversations. Have your teaching materials ready at hand to avoid gaps in the teaching session. If you have an area that is set aside for teaching, try to use inspirational or motivational accessories (e.g., photographs, posters).

A quiet, private space is ideal for teaching, but sometimes there is none available. You can at least try to find a quiet corner, pull the bed curtain shut, or sit close to the client so that you can talk softly

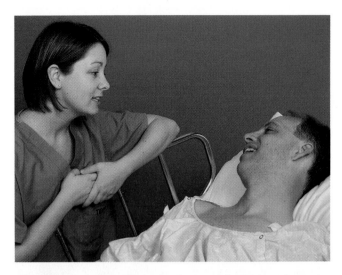

FIGURE 24–1 To provide privacy, sit or stand close to the patient so that you can talk softly.

(Figure 24–1). Make the best of what you have to work with.

Scheduling the Session

Plan for uninterrupted time to allow you to adequately assess and understand the client. The teaching time doesn't need to be long, just uninterrupted. Based on the client's condition (e.g., activity intolerance, attention span), shorter teaching sessions may be best for comprehension and retention. Finding the time to teach can be a challenge, but a moment can be a teaching session, as shown in Box 24–2.

BOX 24–2 Teachable Moments

A student nurse walks into her patient's room. This week in class she has been studying patient teaching. Her instructor has informed the students that she expects them to incorporate teaching into each clinical day. But the student ponders, "I am way too busy to find time to teach. What am I going to do?" Later in the day, she asks the nurse who is co-assigned to her client for suggestions. The nurse questions the student: "Did you take the patient's blood pressure?" When the student answers that she did, the nurse says, "Did you explain why you were doing that and what the BP readings mean?" Again the student says, "Yes." The nurse asks, "When you gave your patient his medications, did you explain why you are giving each one and the common side effects?" The student says, "Yes," and a light dawns! The student begins to understand that almost every patient contact presents an opportunity for teaching and that teaching can be fit into a short time frame.

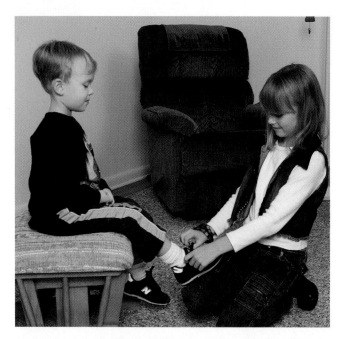

FIGURE 24–2 When teaching psychomotor skills, consider the person's gross and fine motor development.

Amount and Complexity of Content

The more complex or detailed the content, the more difficult it is to learn and retain, as you probably know from your own learning experiences. For example, imagine teaching parents about the need for isolation precautions for their newborn who has just been diagnosed with a rare immune disorder. In comparison, teaching parents of a normal newborn about the recommended immunization schedule would be far less challenging.

In addition, the greater the change, the greater the challenge for both teacher and client. For example, a person who must lose 50 lb, stop smoking, and stop drinking will have a bigger learning challenge than one who has to learn a daily schedule for taking medications.

Communication

Communication is central to the teaching and learning process. Teachers and learners communicate information, perceptions, and feelings to each other. Barriers to communication include language differences, hearing problems, cultural differences, and various environmental issues, such as noise and distraction. Attend carefully to verbal and nonverbal feedback that the client gives; it can tell you whether the learner is attentive and focusing on the learning activities. For more information about communication, see Chapter 18.

CriticalThinking 24–3

A client who has a brain injury needs to learn how to administer insulin. Another learner, who must learn to change a wound dressing, has attention deficit hyperactivity disorder (ADHD).

- How do you think these clients' health status might affect:
  1. Their motivation to learn?
  2. Their ability to be actively involved in the learning?
- What approaches or changes might you need to make in:
  1. The learning environment?
  2. The timing of the teaching session?
  3. The use of repetition?
  4. Your communication?
  5. The amount and complexity of content presented in a session?
  6. Your use of feedback?
  7. The amount of teacher support?

Special Populations

For clients who have special needs (e.g., those with learning disabilities, attention deficit disorder, mental illness, communication disorders, or brain injury) you must plan carefully to ensure that you use appropriate strategies to maximize learning. Consider a variety of teaching approaches—one size does not fit all. For example, you may need to use small, frequent learning sessions or pay special attention to decreasing distracting stimuli in the environment. Or you may need to present content slowly, use repetition, and be satisfied with small amounts of progress. The adaptations you make will depend on the nature of the special need, so if you are not familiar with the patient's condition, you must acquire theoretical knowledge of it.

Developmental Stage

An understanding of intellectual development will help you to gear your teaching strategies and content to the level of the learner. Chapter 9 includes an extensive discussion of intellectual development, including Piaget's theory (1952). When teaching psychomotor skills, you will need to assess the person's fine and gross motor development. For example, a young child may not have adequate fine motor skills to complete a skill such as tying shoes without assistance (Figure 24–2).

Stages of Cognitive Development

Piaget identified three stages of cognitive development that are especially important in client teaching in the cognitive domain:

- *The preoperational stage* (2 to 7 years old), in which the child begins to acquire language skills and find meaning through use of symbols and pictures.

- *The stage of concrete operations* (7 to 11 years old), in which children learn best by manipulating concrete, tangible objects and can classify objects in two or more ways (e.g., identify a shape as a triangle and also as

green). Logical thinking begins, and the child can understand the relationship between numbers and the idea of reversibility. He also can begin to recognize and adapt to the perspective of others.

- *The formal operational stage* (age 11 years or older), in which the person can use abstract thinking and deductive reasoning. The person can relate general concepts to specific situations, consider alternatives, begin to establish values, and try to find meaning in life. Not everyone reaches this stage, including some adults.

Always assess cognitive development. For clients who have not achieved the stage of formal operations, use examples instead of definitions; use concrete rather than abstract terms. Refer to Box 24–3 for some principles that apply especially to adult learners.

When teaching older adults, consider the effects of aging and chronic disease on the person's functioning—the same as you do with other interventions. Allow extra time for teaching, and stop occasionally for rest periods. Assess for sensory deficits (e.g., hearing and vision). Use large print for the visual aids, and repeat information as necessary.

Teaching Children

When you work with children, use strategies to reduce their anxiety and enhance their emotional readiness to learn. For instance, for a child who needs surgery, schedule a tour of the hospital at least one week prior to the admission date, and introduce the child to staff members and other patients of the same age (if possible). Have the child practice breathing exercises or other aspects of tests or treatments that he will be involved in. With the parents' permission, provide the child with an ice cream or other "treat" from the hospital cafeteria, and give the child a coloring book or other item about the upcoming surgery to take home.

If you are teaching a child in the preoperational stage or an adult with limited intellectual development, you will need to simplify the content and use pictures and concrete examples. For example, there is little point in explaining to a toddler the rationale for taking an antibiotic. Instead, tell the child that the medicine will keep her from getting sick; use pictures of a child drinking from a medicine cup, or provide a calendar that the child can mark each time she takes a dose.

Cultural Factors

Awareness of norms, values communication, social structure, time orientation, and cultural identification are important in planning teaching (see Chapter 13 for information about these concepts). If English is not the client's primary language, you may need to use an interpreter. During the planning process, you may need to negotiate with the client to ensure compliance and

BOX 24-3 Principles of Adult Learning

- Adults are more independent and self-directed than children; therefore, they can often identify their own learning needs.
- Adults must recognize the need to learn before they become willing to learn.
- Adults may be afraid of the learning process because of (1) fear of failure, (2) past unsatisfactory experiences with educational processes, (3) not having participated in formal education for many years, or (4) feeling that "being taught" is for children.
- Adults are more motivated to learn if they think they will be able to use the information or skills immediately rather than at some time in the future.
- Adults prefer to be a partner in the learning process—to have some control over what they learn and how they learn it.
- Adults have previous life experiences that can enhance learning. The teacher needs to relate new content to past experiences and knowledge and to have learners use their experiences to solve problems.
- Some older adults may feel threatened by the need to learn new information. They may feel, "I've gotten along just fine all these years without needing to know that; why should I learn it now?" Or they may believe that they are "too old to learn." These attitudes may be defenses to avoid failure or to resist change.

demonstrate respect. Box 24–4 highlights key concepts of culturally competent teaching.

Literacy

Literacy is a greater problem in the United States than many people realize. **Literacy** is defined by the U.S. Department of Education (1999) as the "ability to use print and written information to function in society to achieve one's goals, and to develop one's knowledge and potential." About 20% of adults in the United States (nearly 45 million people) cannot read and write at a level considered necessary for functioning in everyday life. Many, for example, cannot total an entry on a bank deposit slip or locate the time and place of a meeting on a form (National Center for Education Statistics, 1996/2003).

Never assume that your client is literate. Many adults have learned to hide the fact that they cannot read. You can assess their level of literacy by asking them to read some printed material aloud to you. Always check the reading level of materials used for

BOX 24-4 Culturally Competent Teaching

- Inquire or observe interactions among family members to decide who is the decision maker and how decisions are made. Include the family in the planning and teaching.
- Assess for customs or taboos that may conflict with the information you plan to present.
- Observe verbal and nonverbal communication patterns.
- Assess whether the family is past, present, or future oriented.
- Determine whether you should have a same-sex nurse teach a client about personal topics, such as birth control and sexually transmitted infections. Different cultures have different ideas about what is appropriate for discussion between men and women.
- Determine whether the client's values and wishes are in congruence or conflict with the family.
- Respect, accept, and validate the client's beliefs.
- Find sources of information that can help you learn about the culture and its healthcare practices.
- Admit unfamiliarity with the culture, but express willingness to learn.
- Find ways to incorporate the client's current healthcare practices and beliefs into the plan of care unless there is potential for harm.

- Speak slowly and clearly; avoid slurring syllables.
- Do not use slang expressions.
- Use short sentences and concrete rather than abstract words. Present only one idea in each sentence.
- Use pictures and other visual aids to help communicate your meaning.
- Provide teaching materials in the client's language. If you cannot read it, have it translated so that you can judge its appropriateness.
- Avoid using humor; jokes often do not translate well because of subtle meaning changes.
- Obtain feedback carefully. Do not assume that a client who smiles, nods, and says yes really understands what you are teaching. The client may be embarrassed to ask questions or may feel that it will embarrass you.
- Encourage the client to ask questions; stop often to evaluate client understanding.

Sources: Hong, O-S. (2001). Limited English proficiency workers: Health and safety education, *AAOH, 49*(1), 21–26; London, F. (1999). *No time to teach.* Philadelphia: Lippincott; Purnell, L. D., & Paulanka, B. J. (2003). *Transcultural health care: A culturally competent approach* (2nd ed.). Philadelphia: F. A. Davis Company; Spector, R. E. (2004). *Cultural diversity in health and illness* (6th ed.). Upper Saddle River, NJ: Prentice Hall.

---

client teaching. They are sometimes written at too high a reading level, which may make them unusable for clients who are taking on responsibility for self-care. If you are creating written materials, follow these tips (Mayer, 2002):

- Use short sentences and easy words of one or two syllables.
- Use active rather than passive voice. For example, instead of saying, "The pill should be taken every 8 hours," say "Take the pill every 8 hours."
- Use as many drawings and photographs as possible to illustrate your statements.

Barriers to Teaching and Learning

As you gain experience in teaching, you will learn to recognize the factors we have just discussed (e.g., timing, the environment) and to manipulate those that can be changed to enhance the teaching and learning experience. At the same time, take care to avoid factors that act as outright barriers to teaching/learning. The most common barriers to effective teaching and learning are identified in Box 24–5.

KnowledgeCheck 24–3

- List and define six factors that affect the learning process.
- What is one strategy you could use to motivate a client who seems uninterested in learning?
- What are some aspects of the environment that can enhance or interfere with learning?
- What two strategies might you use with a learner who is at a low level of cognitive development?

 Go to Chapter 24, **Knowledge Check Response Sheet and Answers,** on the Electronic Study Guide.

CriticalThinking 24–4

- List some actions you can take to avoid each of the teacher barriers.
- Give an example of each of the barriers to the learner. For "stress of illness," here is one example: A patient is frightened after having a heart attack, worried about the cost of the medical treatment, and worried about not being able to go to work; so he cannot concentrate on the material being presented to him.

Note: These questions may be difficult, depending on your knowledge base and experience. Work with others to answer the questions, as necessary.

Practical Knowledge
knowing how

The teaching process parallels the nursing process. You will assess learning needs and readiness, make educational diagnoses, write learning objectives, plan and implement teaching strategies, and evaluate client learning. Effective client teaching begins with assessment of learning needs.

| Assessment |

A learning assessment will help you to determine the right setting for the teaching, the necessary content to cover, learning goals, and teaching strategies. Your initial assessment consists of general information about the amount of time and resources available for your teaching. Also be clear about your intended audience. For example, with Heather ("Meet Your Patient") assess the following:

- *Learning needs.* To understand her own child's behaviors, Heather needs to learn about normal growth and development and nutritional needs of 3-year-olds. She will need safety and health instructions for the next year, because her child may not return for another checkup until age 4.

- *Client's knowledge level.* You need to identify Heather's current expectations of her toddler as well as her understanding of how the child has developed up to this point. You should also find out what Heather knows about toddler nutrition and language development.

- *Health beliefs and practices.* Determine Heather's (and her daughter's) current healthcare practices as well as trust and investment in the healthcare system. For example, what kinds of meals does she offer the toddler?

- *Physical readiness.* Is Heather able to sit and listen to the information presented? You may need to provide appropriate play materials for her toddler so that she will require less attention from her. Some interruptions are likely, because 3-year-olds have very short attention spans.

- *Emotional readiness.* Heather has expressed concern that her child is so small, which offers you an opportunity to begin the teaching based on her interest in her child's progress and health. However, she may have trouble concentrating if her child is restless or if she has limited time for her appointment.

- *Ability to learn.* During the interview, you can begin to assess Heather's ability to learn, based on her responses to questions. You can also ask her educational level.

BOX 24–5 Barriers to Effective Teaching and Learning

Barriers for the Teacher

- Lack of time
- Lack of preparation to teach
- Lack of space and privacy
- Teaching not seen as a priority (either by the nurse or the organization)
- No third-party reimbursement for teaching
- Frustration with the amount of documentation needed
- Lack of coordination by various healthcare providers

Barriers for the Learner

- The stress of illness
- Physical condition
- Anxiety
- Low literacy
- A negative environmental influence
- Lack of time to learn
- Overwhelming amount of behavioral change needed
- Lack of support and ongoing positive reinforcement
- Lack of willingness to take responsibility
- The complexity of the healthcare system, which can lead to discouragement or abandonment

---

- *Literacy level.* You might ask Heather to read a short statement or paragraph related to the information you're teaching.

- *Neurosensory factors.* By observing Heather's interactions with her toddler, you can assess her vision, hearing, and manual dexterity. Observe her response to visual and auditory clues that are given by her child or healthcare providers. Watching her manipulate a pen, pencil, or toy could help you determine manual dexterity.

- *Learning styles.* Ask Heather how she learns best. Understanding that she probably doesn't have large amounts of time to read or listen, you might give her single-page handouts, videos, or pamphlets instead of books or longer booklets.

For guidelines and questions to ask when conducting a learning assessment,

 Go to Chapter 24, **Assessment Guidelines and Tools, Learning Assessment Guidelines,** in Volume 2.

| Nursing Diagnosis |

Deficient Knowledge is the most frequently used (and perhaps misused) nursing diagnosis for a teaching plan. It may be either a problem or the etiology of a problem.

Deficient Knowledge as Primary Problem

You should use Deficient Knowledge only if you believe that the lack of knowledge is the *primary* problem. Use it to describe conditions in which the patient needs new, additional, or extensive knowledge. Identify the specific knowledge deficit as the problem, and follow with the etiology and related signs and symptoms. For example:

> Deficient Knowledge (diabetic foot care) related to lack of prior experience, as manifested by anxiety and many questions about foot care

Deficient Knowledge as Etiology

Deficient Knowledge is probably most effectively used as the etiology of other nursing diagnoses, such as the following:

- Ineffective Health Maintenance related to Deficient Knowledge of immunizations
- Risk for Impaired Parenting related to Deficient Knowledge of child developmental stages and needs for stimulation
- Ineffective Management of Therapeutic Regimen related to Deficient Knowledge of the procedure for drawing up and injecting insulin
- Noncompliance (with prescribed medications) related to Deficient Knowledge about the side effects and benefits of the antihypertensive medication
- Risk for Imbalanced Nutrition: Less Than Body Requirements related to the pregnant woman's Deficient Knowledge about additional calories and nutrients needed during pregnancy and her fear of "getting fat"

Wellness Diagnoses

Teaching is the primary intervention for wellness diagnoses, such as Effective Breastfeeding, Health-Seeking Behaviors, Readiness for Enhanced Communication, and the more than 10 other NANDA labels beginning with the phrase "Readiness for Enhanced."

Incorrect Uses of Deficient Knowledge

Beware of routine or premature diagnosing. It is easy to see that a patient lacks information, label it as a Deficient Knowledge problem, and try to solve the problem by giving information—which may not be what the patient needs at all. Always look beyond the knowledge deficit to see what problematic *responses* it produces.

Do not use Deficient Knowledge routinely as a problem label for all patients. There are information needs associated with almost every medical and nursing diagnosis. However, you cannot assume that a particular patient needs to be taught that information. For example, a person with a foot ulcer secondary to long-standing diabetes may already know more than you do about foot care. For most nursing diagnoses (e.g., Anxiety, Imbalanced Nutrition), you can merely write a nursing order to provide the informal teaching needed instead of writing a Deficient Knowledge diagnosis.

Do not use Deficient Knowledge for problems involving the client's *ability to learn*. To accurately describe such situations, use non-NANDA diagnoses such as:

- Impaired Ability to Learn related to fear and anxiety
- Impaired Ability to Learn related to delayed cognitive development
- Lack of Motivation to Learn related to feelings of powerlessness

| Planning Outcomes |

Before making a teaching plan, educators contract with the learner for what they want to accomplish together. **Contractual agreements** are agreements between teacher and learner about how to achieve mutually set goals. The contract usually describes the responsibilities of both teacher and learner, time frames for the teaching, content to be included, and expectations of all participants. Learning contracts increase commitment by the learner to reach the teaching and behavioral goals. They are usually informal.

Teaching goals are broad in scope and set down what is expected as the final outcome of the teaching and learning process. They should address all three domains of learning. In contrast, **learning objectives** are single, specific, one-dimensional behaviors that must be completed to accomplish the goal. They are short term and ideally are accomplished in one or two sessions. Similar to patient outcomes in the nursing process, learning objectives/goals should include an action verb, an activity that can be measured or observed, the circumstances of the learner's performance, and how learning will be measured. For example:

> *Goal:* Client will be able to demonstrate ability to perform newborn care in 3 days.
>
> *Learning Objectives:* (1) Client changes infant's diaper, making sure that umbilical cord remains outside the diaper. (2) Client demonstrates bathing baby while maintaining newborn's temperature of greater than 97.5°F.

TABLE 24-2	Active Verbs for Domains of Learning	
Cognitive Domain	**Affective Domain**	**Psychomotor Domain**
Compare	Cry	Adapt
Define	Choose	Apply
Describe	Defend	Arrange
Design	Discuss	Assemble
Differentiate	Display	Begin
Explain	Form (e.g, an opinion)	Change
Give examples	Express	Construct
Identify	Give	Create
List	Help	Demonstrate
Name	Initiate	Draw up (e.g., medication)
Plan	Justify	Inject (e.g., medication)
State	Relate	Manipulate
Summarize	Revise	Move
	Select	Organize
	Share	Show
	Smile	Start
	State a feeling	Take
	Use	Work
	Value	

See Table 24–2 for examples of active verbs for each domain of learning. See Chapter 5 for a review of goals and outcomes.

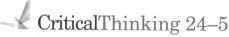 CriticalThinking 24–5

A client has just been diagnosed with diabetes mellitus. He must check and record his blood glucose (using a finger-stick) three times a day. The two of you establish a goal that he will be able to perform glucose testing independently within 1 week. What objectives would you need to write to achieve this goal?

NOC standardized outcomes for Deficient Knowledge depend on the content that needs to be taught. *Nursing Outcomes Classification (NOC)* (Moorhead, Johnson, & Maas, 2004) has identified 30 "Knowledge" outcomes for specific topics, for example, Knowledge: Diabetes Management and Knowledge: Infant Care.

VOL 2 Go to Chapter 24, **Standardized Language, NOC Outcomes for Health Knowledge,** in Volume 2.

If you use Deficient Knowledge as the etiology of another diagnosis (e.g., Imbalanced Nutrition) then you would use NOC outcomes linked to that diagnosis (e.g., Knowledge: Diet, or Nutritional Status).

Individualized goals/outcome statements you might write for a client with a diagnosis of Deficient Knowledge include examples such as the following:

• For Deficient Knowledge (Breastfeeding): After demonstration and teaching, mother will position infant correctly at breast.

• For Deficient Knowledge (Child Physical Safety): After demonstration and explanation, parents will fasten toddler safely and securely in infant car seat.

• For Deficient Knowledge (Diabetes Management): After reading pamphlets, client will explain the relationship of carbohydrate intake and exercise to blood sugar.

As you can see, choice of outcome is directly related to the area in which the client lacks knowledge or information.

The outcomes you choose depend on whether you have used Deficient Knowledge in the problem clause or the etiology clause of the nursing diagnosis. For example, if your nursing diagnosis for Heather ("Meet Your Patient") were Knowledge Deficit (Toddler Nutrition) related to lack of experience and family support, then one outcome might be, "Heather will plan nutritious meals for her child, based upon the Food Guide Pyramid." If, however, your diagnosis for the child *were* Risk for Impaired Nutrition: Less Than Body Requirements related to the mother's Deficient Knowledge about nutrition, then one outcome might be, "Toddler will gain weight so that she is in at least the 10th percentile for weight by September of this year."

| Planning Interventions/Implementation |

In Chapters 5 and 6, you learned about creating a nursing care plan. For clients and families with learning needs, you will create individualized teaching plans. The teaching plan is often one part of the client's complete nursing care plan.

Creating Teaching Plans

The process of creating a teaching plan differs from that of creating a nursing care plan in two key ways: First, in a teaching plan, the interventions are actually teaching strategies. Second, when planning teaching, you need to plan content, sequencing, and the types of instructional materials to be used. Let's apply these aspects of a teaching plan, using the example of Heather in the "Meet Your Patient" scenario. You have assessed the need for anticipatory guidance regarding safety for her 3-year-old. Your nursing diagnosis is Deficient Knowledge (safety for a 3-year-old) related to the mother's inexperience.

- *Teaching strategies* are the method used to present content. For Heather, they might include one-to-one instruction and printed information. (A description of various teaching strategies follows shortly.)
- The *content* of your teaching includes all the information that needs to be learned to reach the desired goal. It can include facts, skills, or emotions. For Heather, the content of your informal teaching might include the following:

  Poison control and prevention—Curiosity and lack of ability to understand danger puts the toddler at greater risk.

  Accident prevention—This would include the need for car seats, increased supervision when exploring, and the use of a helmet when the child rides a tricycle.

  Risk of choking—Foods that are hard to swallow or chunky (e.g., hot dogs) are a concern for a 3-year-old.

  Need for immunizations and physical checkup during the next year.

- *Scheduling and sequencing* refer to how you will organize the information, that is, in what order to present the topics. As a general rule, you should present simple before complex topics and nonthreatening topics before more controversial ones. You must also determine when the teaching session(s) should be scheduled based on client and teacher's needs. When extensive content is involved, it is best to schedule a teaching session in advance; the teacher and learner are then committed and prepared for the session. Using small amounts of time can be effective if teaching is brief and organized.

  You could teach Heather about poison control and accident prevention in the lobby while she and her toddler are waiting for the child to be examined. During the child's examination, you could review immunizations and the need for an annual checkup. At the end of the examination, when discussing the child's nutrition, you might include a discussion of foods that constitute a choking hazard.

- *Instructional materials* are materials and tools that are used to present and reinforce learning. You might give Heather printed handouts about poison control (including the Poison Control Center [PCC] telephone number) and about accident prevention (e.g., how to properly install a child car seat). The child's immunization record would list current immunizations and the schedule for further immunizations may be printed on it. To involve the child, you might include a coloring book about one of the topics.

Go to page 541 for an example of a teaching plan.

Selecting NIC Interventions

NIC standardized interventions related to patient learning depend on the nursing diagnoses you have identified. *Nursing Interventions Classification (NIC)* (Dochterman & Bulechek, 2004) lists 27 patient education interventions from which to choose, depending on the content being taught. Two examples are Health Education and Teaching: Disease Process. To see the entire list,

 Go to Chapter 24, **Standardized Language, NIC Interventions for Patient Education,** in Volume 2.

Selecting Specific Teaching Strategies

Several different types of teaching strategies are currently available. Before selecting one, consider the learner's differences, needs, learning style, and advantages and disadvantages of each method.

Teaching Plan

Client Data

Emily O'Connor is the APN in charge of the student health center on campus at State University. A research project by one of her nursing students last semester revealed that only 35% of women surveyed on campus performed monthly breast self-examination (BSE). Emily has decided to teach students and interested campus staff members about the importance of BSE and the proper technique. To reinforce the content information, Ms O'Connor develops handouts with pictures and charts to make them more visually appealing. She also follows one of the first principles of adult motivation: Provide food, so people who are not a captive audience (as hospitalized patients are) will have an additional reason to attend.

Nursing Diagnosis

Deficient Knowledge (health behaviors) about BSE as evidenced by campus-wide survey results showing that only 35% of women performed monthly BSE.

NOC Outcome	NIC Intervention
Knowledge: Health Behavior (1805)	Teaching: Group (5604)

Teaching Environment:	Overall Strategy/Approach:
1. Provide an environment conducive to learning. Promote relaxation by personal introductions, food and drinks at breaks. *Rationale: When adult learners are in an environment in which they feel comfortable, they are less distracted and more able to learn. An effective atmosphere of adult learning promotes the physical and emotional comfort of the participants, motivates persons to acquire new knowledge, and enhances content retention (Rankin & Stallings, 1996).*	1. Focus on real-world problems. 2. Emphasize application of content to everyday life. 3. Relate content to life experience. 4. Explain how the education will solve a problem. 5. Involve learners in the educational process. 6. Use a variety of methodologies. *Rationale: Utilizes principles of adult learning. Using a variety of methodologies is important because different people learn in different ways.*

Instructional Materials

1. Printed materials (brochures, fact sheets)
Rationale: Print materials at an appropriate reading level for the target audience allow participants to review information on their own wherever they are. While study participants preferred multimedia presentations, post-test scores showed significant improvement regardless of content form (Bader & Strickman-Stein, 2003).

2. Videotape of BSE
Rationale: Women learning by watching a videotape performed BSE more frequently than women who did not see a videotape (Janda, Stanek, Newman, Obermair, & Trimmel, 2002).

3. Flash or other interactive multimedia (animation, narration, and text) on computer, to accompany PowerPoint slides.
Rationale: In one study, participants learning about lung cancer received instruction in five forms, and 71% ranked the Flash presentation as their preferred format for learning (Bader & Strickman-Stein, 2003). Women who participated in an interactive multimedia educational program about breast cancer perceived breast cancer to be a more personally important health issue, learned more and reported less anxiety about cancer screening than did women learning from written materials (Street, VanOrder, Bramson, & Manning, 1998).

➤

Teaching Plan *(continued)*

Learning Objective	Schedule/ Sequence	Content*	Teaching Strategy
By the end of the first educational session, participants will be able to explain why BSE is important	April 1–8	1. Determine date, time, and content of class to be held.	Advertise the educational session by using posters on campus, the campus newspaper, and the daily e-mail newsletter.
	April 9 6:30–7:00 P.M.	2. Social hour. Dessert and beverages. Get acquainted.	
	7:00–7:30 P.M.	3. Identify risk factors for breast cancer.	Lecture with slides
		4. Discuss current treatments for breast cancer.	
		5. Describe how BSE helps with early diagnosis, enhancing chances for cure.	
	7:30–7:50 P.M.	6. Provide thorough instruction on BSE technique.	Videotaped demonstration of BSE
	7:50–8:00 P.M.	7. Promote awareness and incorporate reminders in follow-up contact with participants.	Questions and answers
	8:00–9:00 P.M.	8. Provide optional practice and/or Flash program on BSE.	Set up Flash program on three computers for participants to use before and after the formal class hour.

Rationale: Content is based on the Health Belief Model, designed by the U.S. Public Health Service. It identifies four key factors that promote health-seeking behavior (adapted for this setting): (1) Person perceives she is at risk for disease (breast cancer); (2) Person perceives the disease is harmful and has serious consequences; (3) Person believes the suggested intervention is of value; (4) Person believes treatment (screening) effectiveness is worth overcoming barriers to treatment (screening) (Rankin & Stallings, 1996; The Communication Initiative [TCI], 2003; Clarke-Tasker & Wade, 2002).

Evaluation

Eighteen women attended the session. When Ms O'Connor began the educational session, participants were seated in chairs facing the front of the room, where the screen was set up for a PowerPoint presentation. She distributed the handout materials and provided a short introduction. Before she began teaching, two women asked questions about breast cancer and screening tests. Three women shared stories about friends and family members who had breast biopsies. One had a question about mammograms. During this discussion, the women turned their chairs to face each other and talked among themselves. When there was a lull in the discussion, one of the secretaries said she thought she had a lump and was too scared to do anything about it.

Ms O'Connor realized that learning takes place when participants share stories with facilitation by the group leader. Teaching does not have to be controlled by the facilitator. Even though she had a teaching plan, she was flexible enough to modify the plan to meet participants' needs. She turned off the projector, turned on the lights, and, instead of lecturing, she shared information by answering questions and guiding the discussion.

During this process, Ms O'Connor realized she had made assumptions about the participants' goals for this educational program and their educational needs. She learned that the women who attended came to the program with an understanding of risk factors for breast cancer; they knew that the disease is serious and that interventions are valuable. They wanted to talk about their fears, concerns, and questions; they wanted to separate myths from facts; and they wanted to learn proper technique and how they could remember to do monthly BSE.

After the session, Ms O'Connor realized that she needed to revise her plan and hold a second session in a week or two. Her assumption that a lack of knowledge was responsible for the low number of women performing BSE was not confirmed by discussion with the women. She developed new goals for the second session:

1. By the end of the educational intervention, participants will:
    a. State that questions about breast cancer have been addressed
    b. Share strategies for overcoming barriers to performing BSE
    c. Identify the role anxiety plays as a barrier to BSE
    d. List steps to follow if a lump or other abnormality is identified

2. At the 1-year follow-up point, participants will report that they performed monthly BSE in 10 of the last 12 months.

Sources

Bader, J. L., & Strickman-Stein, N. (2003). Evaluation of new multimedia formats for cancer communications. *Journal of Medical Internet Research, 5*(3), e16.

Clarke-Tasker, V. A., & Wade, R. (2002, May-June). What we thought we knew: African American males' perception of prostate cancer and screening methods [electronic version]. *Association of Black Nursing Faculty Journal.*

The Communication Initiative (TCI). (2003, July 29). *Health belief model.* Retrieved April 20, 2004, from *http://www.comminit.com/ctheories/sid-8180.html*

Janda, M., Stanek, C., Newman, B., Obermair, A., & Trimmel, M. (2002). Impact of videotaped information on frequence and confidence of breast self-examination. *Breast Cancer Research and Treatment, 73*(1), 37–43.

Rankin, S. H., & Stallings, K. D. (2001). *Patient education: Issues, principles, practices* (4th ed.). Philadelphia: Lippincott.

Street, Jr., R. L., VanOrder, A., Bramson, R., & Manning, T. (1998). Preconsultation education promoting breast cancer screenings: Does the choice of media make a difference? *Journal of Cancer Education, 13*(3), 152–161.

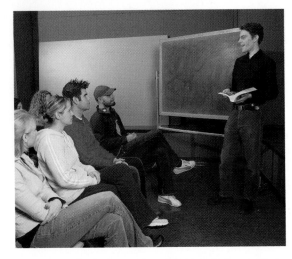

FIGURE 24–3 The advantage of lecturing is that you can teach more than one person at a time.

Lecture

Lecture is a traditional method in which one or more presenters orally share information while a group of learners sits and listens (Figure 24–3). It can be enhanced by including discussion and question-and-answer periods for clarifying content and by use of flip charts, transparencies, posters, and models.

Advantages: Efficient and cost-effective way to impart information, especially to large groups.

Limitations: Does not allow for individualization of teaching. Not effective for teaching in the psychomotor or affective domains. Does not promote retention of material.

Group Discussion

In a group discussion, several participants discuss topics, exchanging information and presenting their points of view. The teacher acts as facilitator to achieve objectives shared with the group at the beginning of the session. Discussions can become lively. Effective group discussion requires an atmosphere of trust that encourages everyone to participate.

Advantages: Learner-centered and effective for teaching in the affective and cognitive domains.

Limitations: The teacher must be comfortable with less structure and with unpredictable responses. Less effective with teaching in the psychomotor domain.

Demonstration and Return Demonstration

In this method, the teacher explains and demonstrates a skill or task. The client then demonstrates comprehension by returning the demonstration. Return demonstrations should be scheduled close to the initial teaching of the skill.

Advantages: Most effective in teaching psychomotor skills (e.g., use of equipment, self-injection, dressing changes). Can be used in small groups if enough equipment is available.

Limitations: Does not work well with large groups. Is time-consuming and labor intensive.

One-to-One Instruction

In one-to-one instruction, one teacher orally presents information to one learner. They mutually formulate objectives at the beginning of the session. Follow-up often includes printed or audiovisual materials. You will often use this method as a nurse.

Advantages: Gives the teacher the opportunity to establish a relationship with a learner, convey interest in his learning needs, and tailor the teaching to the learner's needs as the teaching proceeds. Allows reluctant students to more readily ask questions. Enables the teacher to obtain frequent feedback so that material can be repeated and clarified as needed. Useful for teaching in all three domains: affective, psychomotor, and cognitive.

Limitations: Very labor-intensive and reaches the fewest numbers of learners. May be overwhelming to learners because of the large quantity of information given in a short period of time and therefore may not promote retention. Tends to isolate the learner from others who may share the same learning needs and who could provide support.

Audiovisual Materials

Teachers often use materials that make use of visual illustrations and sound (Figure 24–4). Audiovisual materials may include film, tape, recordings, slides, or computer-generated material. They can be effective supplements to other methods if the teaching session is followed by a question-and-answer session, a discussion of the content, a test, or printed materials to expand understanding. Videotapes of familiar children's

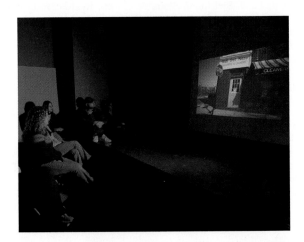

FIGURE 24–4 Audiovisual materials can enhance teaching and learning.

characters, such as Big Bird visiting the doctor or going to the hospital, can be very effective for children.

Advantages: A stimulating method because it engages both sight and hearing. Can be used with large groups.

Limitations: Not as efficient as lecture or reading in terms of the amount of content that can be covered. Can be expensive because it requires special hardware (e.g., projectors, screens) and media (e.g., videotapes), which must be replaced when they become outdated.

Printed Materials

Printed materials may come in the form of fact sheets, discharge instructions, printed pamphlets, or detailed booklets. To make sure the clients comprehend the information, you must provide an opportunity for clients to ask questions after they have read the materials. You will usually use printed materials to supplement other teaching strategies. Printed materials for children include storybooks, coloring books, and activity books with mazes and other games.

When you are creating your own teaching materials, remember the tips for ensuring readability in the "Literacy" section of this chapter. Many standard word processing programs, such as Microsoft Word, allow you to check the reading level of materials you create. For instructions, access the "Help" function and type in "readability." Figure 24–5 is an example of a patient teaching fact sheet written at the level of grade 6.8.

Advantages: Printed materials allow for standardized information to be presented to each client, but with some room for individualization. Clients can read information on their own time; thus, printed materials make efficient use of teacher time. Excellent way to reinforce material taught in lecture, demonstration and return demonstration, or one-to-one instruction.

Limitations: The method assumes literacy, motivation to read materials, and visual acuity. Materials at an average reading level, with words that most people understand, must be available.

Programmed Instruction

Programmed instruction consists of printed material that presents content, questions, and answers, which the learner completes individually. Programmed instruction typically provides feedback for incorrect answers, but you should be available for questions and clarification after the student completes the instruction. Programmed instruction was the precursor to computer-assisted instruction.

Advantages: Allows learners to proceed at their own speed. Requires less teacher time.

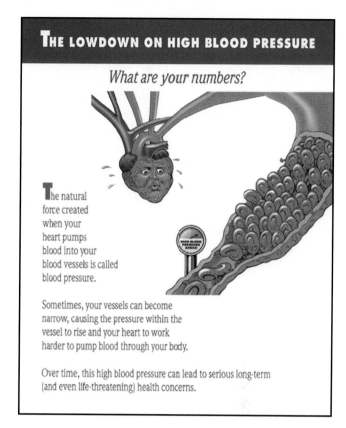

FIGURE 24–5 The reading level of this patient teaching aid is grade 6.8.

Limitations: Printed materials may lack the excitement of audiovisual presentations and group discussions. Requires motivation to complete; works best with independent learners.

Simulation

Simulation is a method that creates an experience that is similar to an actual one but without risks and consequences. Simulation requires the learner to make decisions, solve problems, and review the effects of her actions. Simulations can occur through written case studies as well as models, computer programs, and physical setups (e.g., practicing injections in the nursing lab).

Advantages: Practicing through simulations can increase confidence, evaluate effectiveness of teaching, and trouble-shoot areas of concern before an actual situation arises. Simulation allows nurses to learn new skills without risk to patients.

Limitations: Physical setups may require special equipment and extensive preparation time.

Role-Playing

Role-playing is used primarily with groups to achieve learning in the affective domain. Participants take on

unrehearsed roles without a script to follow. The teacher must develop the situation so that participants can take on and develop understanding of the roles they are given.

Advantages: Similar to simulation, this is a safe method to rehearse real-life situations before being confronted with them. Role-playing is usually even less structured than simulation, although the two can be combined.

Limitations: Requires follow-up discussion to allow learners to air their feelings, attitudes, and observations. Learners must be willing to participate either as observers or role-players. Some people may feel self-conscious when role-playing.

Role Modeling

In role modeling, the teacher teaches by example, demonstrating the behaviors and/or attitudes to be learned. For example, a nurse who is exercising and following a low-calorie diet to attain a healthy weight is a role model for patients who need to lose weight.

Many experienced pediatric nurses find that role modeling using a puppet or a child's own doll or stuffed animal can be helpful in reducing the child's anxiety and enhancing the child's learning. For instance, you can suggest that the child be "the nurse" and "feel Miss Bunny's pulse," or have a puppet "suggest" to a child, "When I get a shot, I say, 'Ouch!' real loud, and then it's all over!"

Advantages: Role modeling allows the learner to identify with the teacher. Can increase motivation and ability to perform a desired behavior.

Limitations: Learners need to be aware and receptive to this type of teaching.

Self-Instruction

Self-instruction is a method in which the learner studies independently using carefully designed materials. Self-study modules are developed with objectives and various types of materials, including workbooks, computer programs, videotapes, and audiotapes with worksheets. Teachers need to be available for questions or feedback at certain points in the process.

Advantages: The opportunity to work at their own pace is appealing to many learners. Frees teachers and students from being tied to a classroom.

Limitations: Requires literacy skills and motivation; can be isolating for those who need frequent feedback and support from others. Requires a great deal of time for the initial preparation of modules.

Distance Learning

With distance learning, teacher and learner are not in the same physical location. Live or taped instructions are sent from the teacher to the learner. Two or more individuals or classrooms may be connected by video or teleconferencing.

Advantages: Allows for teaching to remote or multiple sites at the same time; can link many individuals separated by great distances. Current technology provides the opportunity for interactive teaching rather than a one-way process.

Limitations: Requires good technological skills from the teacher, expensive equipment, and a great deal of time for preparation and organization.

List Serves and Web Sites

Learners can obtain information and support from the Internet through list serves and web sites. Learners can connect with others in similar situations through list serves. Distance learning courses often make use of the Internet.

Advantages: Makes a vast amount of information readily available. Many government or professional organizations have a wealth of information for consumers to assist in self-care and in making healthcare decisions.

Limitations: The teacher has no control over the information on a web site; the information may or may not be accurate. You should evaluate each web site before recommending it to a patient. See Chapter 39 for information about evaluating materials you obtain from a web site.

Computer-Assisted Instruction (CAI)

Computer-assisted instruction (CAI) involves the use of a computer to present information and provide feedback and in this way is similar to programmed learning. CAI may include video or audio clips that enhance learning.

Advantages: This method allows the learners to proceed at their own pace. It usually includes review questions or interactive quizzes that enhance comprehension. Learners can access programs at a time that is convenient for them. CAI provides feedback while the learner progresses through the study module.

Limitations: Learners must have access to a computer, have adequate visual acuity and literacy skills, and have computer skills. Because this method is impersonal, and because personal support facilitates learning, be sure to also plan occasional person-to-person contact with the learner.

Gaming

Gaming requires the learner to participate in an activity that includes competition and has preset rules (e.g., a board game that allows players to move when they answer a question correctly). The teacher serves as a facilitator who sets the ground rules and explains the process as well as keeps the flow going. Games can be created or purchased commercially.

Advantages: Gaming can be used with individuals or groups and can make learning fun. It can be used to introduce new information or reinforce previous learning.

Limitations: Some participants may not enjoy the competitive atmosphere or may have disabilities that preclude participation.

KnowledgeCheck 24–4

- True or false: When a patient has a learning disability, you should use a non-NANDA diagnosis (e.g., Impaired Ability to Learn) to describe the problem.
- True or false: Learning objectives are short term and, ideally, should be accomplished in one or two teaching sessions.
- List and state the advantages and disadvantages of at least six teaching strategies.

 Go to Chapter 24, **Knowledge Check Response Sheet and Answers,** on the Electronic Study Guide.

| Evaluation of Learning |

As with all nursing interventions, you must evaluate not only the outcomes of the teaching—that is, patient learning—but also the teaching plan and how it was implemented. You should evaluate (as you may recall from Chapter 7) the entire nursing process. Was your assessment adequate, or did you fail to notice that the patient was physically uncomfortable and therefore not ready to learn? Was your nursing diagnosis accurate? Were your learning objectives realistic? When evaluating the teaching, consider the type of strategy you used, the timing of the teaching, the content, the amount of information, and the teaching materials. The client is your best source for feedback. He can tell you whether the materials and methods were helpful, uninteresting, and so on.

The following methods are commonly used for outcomes evaluation (client learning).

- *Tests and written exercises* can be used to measure retention and progress toward meeting cognitive objectives. This method requires the learner to be actively involved and have adequate literacy skills.
- *Oral questions / interviews / questionnaires / checklists* allow clients to evaluate their own progress and determine future learning needs. You may obtain more information by talking with the client; however, you may obtain a more honest evaluation by using written questions.
- *Direct observations of client performance* are anecdotal, descriptive notes that you make of the client's performance. They will help you in providing feedback to the client either to reinforce accurate learning or to correct misinformation. Provide feedback as soon as possible after you observe performance.
- *Reports and client records.* Clients and/or families can keep records of performance and results. You can then evaluate the data and give feedback. You can make plans for further teaching when you analyze the data.

Clients will not remember everything you teach them. That is normal. If you start to question your effectiveness as a teacher, think about one of the courses you took last semester. Did you score 100% on every test? How much of the material presented in that course do you remember now? Repetition and practice are necessary for retention.

Documentation of Teaching and Learning

As is true for all nursing interventions (refer to Chapter 16), it is important to document the responses of the client and family to teaching interventions. Documentation also provides legal proof that teaching was done and communicates the information to other health professionals. Document what was taught and the client statements, skills, and behaviors that provide evidence of learning. Informal teaching that occurs during other care activities you may simply record in the nurse's notes. For planned teaching that is done frequently for a particular population of clients, many agencies provide special documentation forms. For an example of a patient education record,

 Go to Chapter 24, **Tables, Boxes, Figures: ESG Figure 24–1,** on the Electronic Study Guide.

| toward evidence-based practice |

Friesen, P., Peplar C., & Hunter, P. (2002). Interactive family learning following a cancer diagnosis. *Oncology Nursing Forum, 29*(6), 981–987.

Clients who were receiving radiotherapy or chemotherapy were followed 5 months post diagnosis. They were interviewed in their homes with family members included. The researchers found that families learned in a process that included gathering, interpreting, and sharing information about living with cancer. Interactive family learning is a mode of learning that can also include support.

Grimes-Holsinger, V. (2002). Comparing the effect of a skills checklist on teaching time required to achieve independence in administration of infusion medication. *Journal of Infusion Nursing 25*(2), 109–120.

This study looked at the effectiveness of a skills checklist as a method to decrease the amount of time required to teach a client to complete a skill independently. The study found that when nurses used the checklist, the client became independent in a shorter time, thereby reducing the number of teaching visits.

Schrecengost, A. (2001). Do humorous preoperative teaching strategies work? *AORN Journal, 74*(4), 683–689.

With early discharge and managed care, time is a critical element. Nurses need to be efficient and effective in pre-

operative teaching. This study sought to evaluate the impact of humor on retention of knowledge presented preoperatively. Researchers studied clients undergoing open heart surgery and receiving teaching about postoperative pulmonary exercises. The differences in results between the control and experimental group were not significant. However, the experimental group that received teaching via cartoons did better on their post test than did the control group.

1. What important point does the third study make that you could use in your teaching?

2. Why do you think it is important to reduce the time required for a client to perform a skill independently?

3. Why do you think it is important to reduce the number of teaching visits?

4. Based on the results of the third study, would you use humor in your teaching plans? Why or why not?

5. Do you feel that humor can be used to enhance a nurse-patient relationship or a teacher-learner relationship? Why or why not?

 Go to Chapter 24, **Toward Evidence-Based Practice Suggested Responses,** on the Electronic Study Guide.

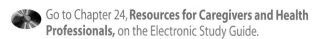 Go to Chapter 24, **Resources for Caregivers and Health Professionals,** on the Electronic Study Guide.

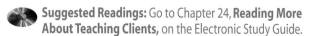 **Suggested Readings:** Go to Chapter 24, **Reading More About Teaching Clients,** on the Electronic Study Guide.

 Bibliography: Go to Volume 2, Bibliography.

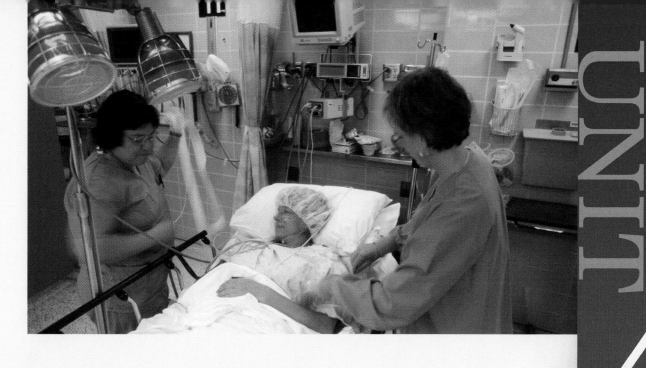

How Nurses

Support Physiological Functioning

25 CHAPTER

Stress
& Adaptation

Learning Outcomes

After completing this chapter, you should be able to:

* Define stress.

* Explain the difference between adaptive and maladaptive coping strategies.

* Explain the relationship between stressors, responses, and adaptation.

* Describe physical changes occurring during the three stages of Selye's general adaptation syndrome (GAS).

* Explain how Selye's local adaptation syndrome (LAS) is different from the GAS.

* Discuss the inflammatory response: What triggers it, and what physiological changes occur?

* Explain how anxiety, fear, and anger relate to stress.

* Provide examples and definitions of specific ego defense mechanisms.

* Describe the effects of prolonged stress and unsuccessful adaptation on the various body systems.

* Compare and contrast crisis and burnout.

* State three ways in which you could assess for each of the following: (1) stressors and risk factors, (2) coping methods and adaptation, (3) physiological responses to stress, (4) emotional and behavioral responses to stresses, (5) cognitive responses to stress, and (6) adequacy of support systems.

* Describe several interventions or activities for preventing and managing stress.

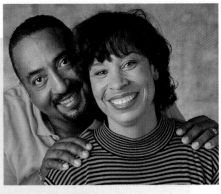

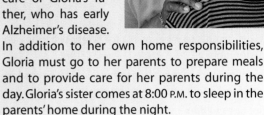

Your Patients

Gloria and her husband, John, live in a residential community from which John commutes to work in a nearby city. Gloria runs an accounting business from their home. They have two teenage boys, who are active in sports, church activities, Boy Scouts, and the school band. The boys need transportation to activities. Gloria and John teach Sunday school and are Boy Scout leaders. Gloria's mother needs knee replacement surgery and so cannot take care of Gloria's father, who has early Alzheimer's disease.

In addition to her own home responsibilities, Gloria must go to her parents to prepare meals and to provide care for her parents during the day. Gloria's sister comes at 8:00 P.M. to sleep in the parents' home during the night.

Theoretical Knowledge
knowing why

Everyone experiences stress as a part of daily life, but we each perceive and respond to stress in our own unique way. Our responses are holistic—that is, physical, psychological, spiritual, and social. As a nurse, you need to understand stress to help your clients cope effectively and adapt to the stressors of illness and caregiving. In addition, you will encounter many stressful situations in your career, so you must develop healthful ways of responding.

WHAT IS STRESS?

Stress is any disturbance in a person's normal balanced state. A **stressor** is a stimulus that the person perceives as a challenge or threat; it disturbs the person's equilibrium by initiating a physical or emotional response. When stress occurs, it produces voluntary and involuntary **coping responses** aimed at restoring equilibrium (balance, or homeostasis). The changes that take place as a result of stress and coping are called **adaptation.** We can also define adaptation as an ongoing effort to maintain external and internal equilibrium.

Stress is not necessarily bad. It can keep you alert and motivate you to function at a higher performance level. For example, when you are preparing for an examination, your desire to succeed can create just enough anxiety to motivate you to study. On the other hand, if you become too anxious, you may be unable to focus on the task.

Types of Stressors

The sources of stress are infinite; however, stressors are commonly categorized in the following ways:

• *Distress/eustress.* **Distress** threatens health, and **eustress** (literally "good stress") is protective. A passionate kiss can produce as strong a stress response as a slap in the face. On the Holmes-Rahe stress scale for example, marriage and divorce receive similarly high scores.

 Go to Chapter 25, **Assessment Guidelines and Tools, the Holmes-Rahe Social Readjustment Scale,** in Volume 2.

• *External/internal.* Stressors may be **external** to the person, for example, death of a family member, a hurricane, or even something as simple as excessive heat in a room. Stressors may also be **internal,** for example, diseases, anxiety, nervous anticipation of an event, or negative self-talk.

• *Developmental/situational.* **Developmental stressors** are those that can be predicted to occur at various stages of a person's life. For example, most young adults face the stress of leaving home and beginning a career, and many middle-aged adults must adjust to aging parents and accepting their own physical changes. In a sense, developmental stressors may be easier to cope with because they are expected and the person has some time to prepare for them. For theoretical knowledge about developmental stages, refer to the theories of Erikson and Havighurst in Chapter 9. Also see Box 25–1 for examples of developmental stressors.

Situational stressors are unpredictable. For example, you cannot predict that you will experience

BOX 25-1   Stressors Throughout the Life Span

The following are common developmental stressors. Not everyone will experience these stressors, however.

Childhood

- Stressors occur primarily in the home
- Absence of parental figures
- Failure of parents to meet needs for safety, security, love and belonging
- Failure of parents to meet basic physiological needs for oxygen, food, elimination, rest, and cleanliness
- School-age children may experience stressors at school or among peers

Adolescence

- Exposure to an expanded environment and a wider circle of friends
- Rapid changes in body appearance
- Need for academic achievement
- Peer pressure
- Maintaining self-esteem while searching for identity
- Decisions about the future in the areas of school, work, and relationships
- Conflicts between standards for behavior and the sex drive
- Decisions about and involvement with drugs

Young Adult

- Separation from family, starting college
- Making the transition from youth to adult responsibilities
- Preparing for careers: graduation from college, learning a trade
- Establishing career goals and planning progress to move up the ladder of success

- Financial stressors around partnerships and providing a home for family
- Parenting children
- Conflicts between responsibilities for work and family or other relationships

Middle Age

- Career challenges continue
- Child rearing continues; marriage of the children; grandparenting
- Dealing with too many responsibilities: e.g., children, work, elderly parents, community activities
- Empty-nest syndrome when the children leave home
- Being "sandwiched" between caring for aging parents as well as children or grandchildren
- "Mid-life crisis" (wanting to escape from one's present life); the person regresses and tries to recapture youth (e.g., by buying a new sports car, making geographic move, taking an exotic vacation, engaging in an affair, daydreaming about the ideal life in retirement)

Older Adults

- Losses of family and friends, resulting in loneliness and isolation
- Changes in physical appearance and functional abilities
- Major life changes (e.g., retirement, loss of life partner)
- Health problems (e.g., chronic diseases) with accompanying discomfort or pain
- The cost of health care
- Learning to live on a fixed, perhaps inadequate, income
- Adjusting to loss of independence

---

an automobile accident, a natural disaster, or an illness. Situational stressors can occur at any life stage and can affect infants, children, and adults equally.

- *Physiological/psychosocial.* **Physiological stressors** are those that affect body structure or function. They may be chemical (e.g., poison, medications), physical or mechanical (e.g., trauma, cold), nutritional (e.g., vitamin deficiency), biological (e.g., viruses, bacteria) or genetic (e.g., inborn errors of metabolism). **Psychosocial stressors** are external stressors that arise from our work, family dynamics, living situation, social relationships, and other aspects of our daily lives. The Holmes-Rahe Scale in Volume 2 contains examples of psychosocial stressors.

KnowledgeCheck 25–1

Refer to the "Meet Your Patient" scenario.

- What are Gloria's stressors? Classify each of them as follows: (1) Are they physiological or psychosocial? (2) Are they developmental or situational?
- What are John's stressors?

 Go to Chapter 25, **Knowledge Check Response Sheet and Answers,** on the Electronic Study Guide.

Models of Stress

Some theorists conceptualize stress as a complex, dynamic, and reciprocal transaction between person and environment. Other theorists view stress solely as a

stimulus that causes psychological or physiological responses that in turn increase vulnerability to disease. This chapter uses the **response-based model** of Hans Selye (1974, 1976), and our distinction between *stressors* and *stress* stems from this model. Selye found that physical, emotional, psychological, and spiritual stressors, or the anticipation of a stressor (as in anxiety), can initiate nonspecific physiological *responses*. Selye defined these responses as stress.

To learn more about the transaction and stimulus models of stress,

 Go to Chapter 25, **Supplemental Materials: Models of Stress,** on the Electronic Study Guide.

 CriticalThinking 25–1

- Make a list of your own stressors in the following areas: work, school, family, and living situation.
- What physiological stressors do you have?

HOW DO COPING AND ADAPTATION RELATE TO STRESS?

Coping strategies are those thinking processes and behaviors a person uses to manage stressors. Some examples are problem solving, daydreaming, making changes in lifestyle (e.g., exercising more, eating less), sleeping, and consulting others for support or advice. Coping strategies can be adaptive or maladaptive.

Adaptive (effective) coping consists of making healthy choices that reduce the negative effects of stress (e.g., exercising to relieve tension). Sometimes the difference between effective and ineffective coping is in the degree to which a technique is used (see the section "Ego Defense Mechanisms" on page 559 for examples).

Maladaptive (ineffective) coping does not promote adaptation. Unhealthful coping choices include overeating, working too much, and substance abuse. Although a maladaptive behavior may temporarily relieve anxiety, it may have other harmful effects. For example, a person who smokes to relieve the tensions of a stressful work situation may experience an immediate decrease in anxiety. However, the person is doing nothing to change or adapt to the stressful situation and, over time, is increasing her risk of respiratory disease.

Three Approaches to Coping Are Commonly Used

People use three approaches to cope with stress, at different times and in various combinations:

1. *Altering the stressor.* In some situations, a person takes actions to remove or change the stressor. For example, Gloria ("Meet Your Patient") might remove one of her stressors by resigning her position as a Scout leader.

2. *Adapting to the stressor.* It is not always possible to remove or change a stressor. Adapting involves changing one's thoughts or behaviors related to the stressor. Gloria cannot change the fact that her father needs care and that her mother needs surgery, but as she gains experience as a caregiver, she may find easier and more efficient ways to care for her parents. This would give her a little more time to relax or attend to other responsibilities.

3. *Avoiding the stressor.* Sometimes, it is healthful to avoid a stressor. For example, you may find that being with a certain person is stressful for you, even though you have tried many times to change the dynamics of the relationship. In that case, it may be best to sever your relationship with the person. In other situations, avoidance may be maladaptive. For example, a woman who discovers a lump in her breast becomes anxious that she may have cancer. She copes with her anxiety by putting it out of her mind and avoids seeing her physician. If the lump is cancerous, it will not be treated at an early stage.

The Outcome of Stress Is Either Adaptation or Disease

Stress results in either adaptation or disease. Successful adaptation allows for normal growth and development and effective responses to changes and challenges in daily life. The outcome depends on the balance between the strength of the stressors and the effectiveness of the person's coping methods (Figure 25–1). In the following equation, **E** is the event (stressor), **R** is the person's response (which is determined in part by past experiences, perception of the stressor, and coping methods used), and **O** is the outcome.

$$\mathbf{E} + \mathbf{R} = \mathbf{O}$$

E		**R**		**O**
stressful event		response (experience, perception, coping methods)		outcome (adaptation or disease)

Some events produce more stress than others. However, a person with good coping skills can usually adapt to a single stressful event, even a very demanding one. But suppose several stressors occur in a short period of time. For example, Gloria ("Meet Your Patient") has many stressors, so her coping abilities may be taxed to the limit. When there are many stressors or when stressors continue for a long period of time, adaptation is more likely to fail.

Personal Factors Influence Adaptation

Fortunately, successful adaptation does not depend entirely on being able to alter or avoid stressors. Various personal factors also influence the outcome:

- *Perception of the stressor.* A person's perception may be realistic or exaggerated. Suppose two women with similar coping skills and support systems both must

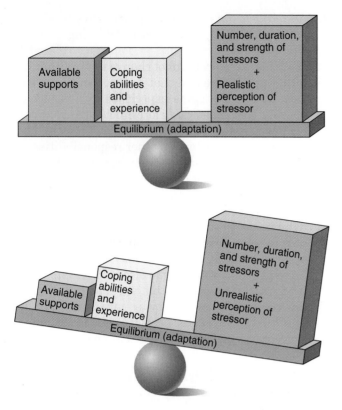

FIGURE 25–1 Adaptation occurs when a person has supports and coping abilities adequate to enable him to deal with the stressors. A realistic perception of the stressful event promotes adaptation, whereas an unrealistic perception makes adaptation more difficult.

have a mastectomy. Mrs. King thinks, "Yes, I am losing a part of my body, but I am more than just a breast. This will be a difficult adjustment, but I am so grateful to be alive." Mrs. Alan thinks, "I will be so ugly. My husband won't want to touch me. I won't be a woman now. This is the worst thing that could ever happen." Which woman do you think is most likely to adapt successfully to this change in her body?

• *Overall health status.* On the one hand, stressors may actually cause a healthy person to engage in constructive adaptive behaviors that improve health. A person who has just discovered that he has hypertension may react by modifying his diet and exercising to lower his blood pressure and prevent complications. On the other hand, a person with severe, chronic arthritis who has been coping for years with pain and immobility may be too overwhelmed and exhausted to take any actions to lower his blood pressure.

• *Support system.* A **support system** may include friends, family, counseling groups, church groups, or other like-minded people who share common interests. A good support system can help a person adapt to stress, provide emotional support, encourage expression of feelings, and help the person solve problems. They may also provide financial and other concrete

types of support, such as a place to live, meal preparation, household help, child care, and transportation.

• *Other personal factors.* Age, developmental level, and life experiences (e.g., observing how others handle stress) all affect a person's response to stress. For example, infants and the very old may lack the physiological reserve to adapt to physical stressors such as temperature extremes, dehydration, or illness.

Even with a positive attitude and good coping skills, excessive amounts of stress can lead to maladaptation and disease. Some people succumb to illness after only a few stressors, whereas others seem to adapt to multiple, intensely difficult stressors. Each person has a different ability to tolerate stress, but everyone has a breaking point at which stress becomes overwhelming.

KnowledgeCheck 25–2

• True or false: The difference between adaptive and maladaptive coping is that maladaptive coping does not relieve stress.

• In addition to avoiding the stressor, what are two other approaches to coping?

• (Complete the sentence.) The outcome of stress (adaptation or disease) depends on the balance between the strength, number, and duration of the stressors and _____.

 Go to Chapter 25, **Knowledge Check Response Sheet and Answers,** on the Electronic Study Guide.

HOW DO PEOPLE RESPOND TO STRESSORS?

Although Selye's (1974, 1976) response-based model acknowledges physical, emotional, psychological, and spiritual *stressors,* his ideas about responses (*stress*) are primarily physiological. As you know, the body has various homeostatic mechanisms for regulating its internal environment to maintain homeostasis. In Selye's theory, physiological responses to stress are described by the general adaptation syndrome (GAS) and the local adaptation syndrome (LAS).

The General Adaptation Syndrome Includes Nonspecific, Systemic Responses

The **general adaptation syndrome (GAS)** is Selye's name for the group of nonspecific responses that all people share in the face of stressors. Regardless of the specific stressor, the responses involve the whole body, especially the autonomic nervous system and the endocrine system. For example, a near-miss automobile accident and kicking the winning field goal at a football game would both produce the same general body responses. The GAS has three stages: (1) the initial alarm stage, (2) resistance (adaptation), and (3) the final stage of either recovery or exhaustion (Figure 25–2).

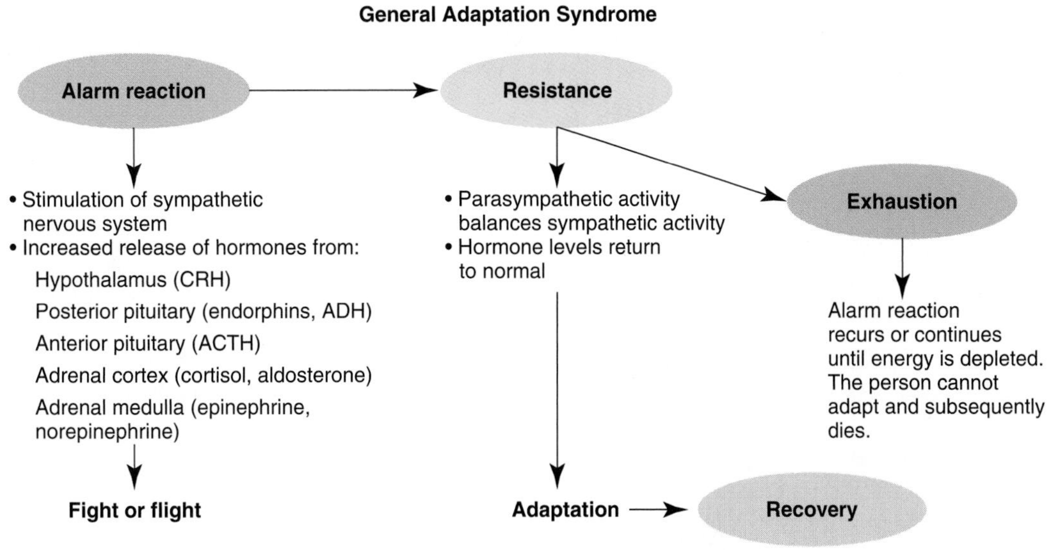

General Adaptation Syndrome

FIGURE 25–2 The stages of Selye's general adaptation syndrome (GAS) are (1) *alarm* (also called "fight or flight"); (2) *resistance* (or adaptation), in which the body enacts physical and psychological adaptive mechanisms to maintain homeostasis; and (3) either *recovery* or *exhaustion* (which usually ends in disease or death).

The Alarm Stage

Imagine yourself in this situation: It is dark. You are alone, walking to your car, when you hear footsteps behind you. You stop and look around and see no one. As you begin walking again, the footsteps return. You walk faster; the footsteps are faster. Stop reading, shut your eyes, and use your imagination. How do you feel? Pay attention to your physical and emotional reactions. If you are not feeling a response to this imaginary situation, think back to a time when something similar happened to you—when something frightened you.

Is your heart pounding?
Are you breathing fast?
Is there a flutter in your stomach?
What is the physical sensation in your muscles?
Do you feel frightened? What are your emotions?
Are you straining to hear the footsteps?
Do you want to run away, or are you "frozen"?
If someone were to walk into the room where you are studying right now, would it startle you?

This scenario should help you to imagine the experience of the alarm stage, during which the body prepares for *"fight or flight."* The alarm stage has two phases, shock and countershock. The **shock phase** begins when the cerebral cortex first perceives a stressor and sends out messages to activate the endocrine and sympathetic nervous systems. Large amounts of epinephrine and various other hormones prepare the body for fight or flight. The shock phase does not last long—usually less than 24 hours, and sometimes only a minute or two. In the **countershock phase,** all the changes produced in the shock phase are reversed, and the person becomes less able to deal with the immediate threat.

Endocrine System Responses

In response to alarm, the following endocrine responses occur:

1. The *hypothalamus* releases corticotropin-releasing hormone (CRH).
2. *CRH,* together with messages from the cerebral cortex, directs the pituitary to release adrenocorticotropic hormone (ACTH) and antidiuretic hormone (ADH).
3. *ACTH* stimulates the adrenal cortex to produce and secrete glucocorticoids (especially cortisol) and mineralocorticoids (especially aldosterone).
   - *Cortisol,* in general, has a glucose-sparing effect. It increases the use of fats and proteins for energy and conserves glucose for use by the brain. Cortisol also has an anti-inflammatory effect. See Figure 25–3 for the effects of cortisol during the alarm reaction of the GAS.
   - *Aldosterone* promotes fluid retention by causing the kidneys to reabsorb more sodium. Thus, it helps to increase fluid volume and maintain or increase blood pressure.
4. *ADH* also promotes fluid retention by increasing the reabsorption of water by kidney tubules. See Figure 25–4 for the effects of aldosterone and ADH.
5. *Endorphins,* secreted by the hypothalamus and posterior pituitary, act like opiates to produce a sense of well-being and reduce pain.
6. *Thyroid-stimulating hormone (TSH)* is secreted by the pituitary gland to increase efficiency of cellular metabolism and fat conversion to energy for cell and muscle needs.

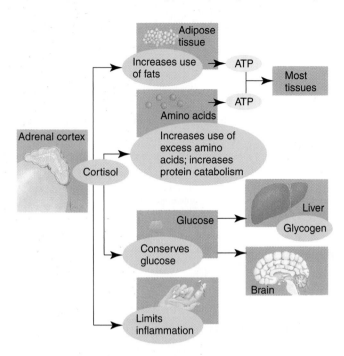

FIGURE 25–3   Functions of cortisol during the alarm stage of the GAS.
Source: Scanlon, V., & Sanders, T. (2003). *Essentials of anatomy and physiology* (4th ed.). Philadelphia: F. A. Davis Company, p. 228.

Sympathetic Nervous System Responses

The cerebral cortex also sends messages via the hypothalamus to stimulate the sympathetic nervous system. The sympathetic nervous system stimulates the adrenal glands to secrete adrenaline (epinephrine) and norepinephrine, which increase mental alertness. This allows the person to assess the situation and aids in a decision to stand and fight or run away in flight. Adrenaline also increases the ability of the muscles to contract and causes the pupils to dilate, producing greater visual fields. See Figure 25–5 for the effects of adrenaline during the alarm reaction of the GAS.

Other Body System Responses in the Alarm Stage

The following are some body system responses that occur in the alarm stage as a result of endocrine and sympathetic nervous system activity. Refer to Figures 25–2 through 25–5 to see how these changes are produced.

- *Cardiovascular system.* The heart rate and contraction force increase. Peripheral and visceral vasoconstriction increases blood flow to vital organs (e.g., brain, lungs) and to muscles preparing for flight. Blood volume and blood pressure also increase, and the blood clots more readily.

- *Respiratory system.* The bronchioles dilate, thereby increasing depth of respiration and tidal volume. This makes oxygen available for diffusion to muscle, brain, and cardiac cells.

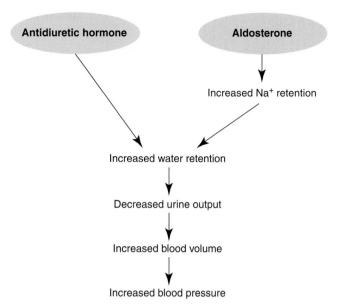

FIGURE 25–4   The release of ADH (from the posterior pituitary) and aldosterone (from the adrenal cortex) leads to sodium and water retention, increases blood volume, and increases blood pressure.

- *Metabolism.* The rate of metabolism increases. The liver converts more glycogen to glucose (*glycogenolysis*), making it available for energy. Except in the brain, the body uses less glucose for energy. The use of amino acids and the mobilization of fats for energy (*lipolysis*) increase.

- *Urinary system.* Blood flow to the kidneys decreases, and they retain more sodium and water. The kidneys secrete renin, which produces *angiotensin*. In turn, angiotensin constricts the arterioles and tends to increase blood pressure.

- *Gastrointestinal system.* Peristalsis and secretions of digestive enzymes decrease. Blood glucose level increases to fuel the energy needed for fight or flight.

- *Musculoskeletal system.* Blood vessels dilate, increasing flow of blood (and thus oxygen and energy) to skeletal muscles.

The Resistance Stage

During the second stage of the GAS, **resistance** (or *adaptation*), the body tries to cope, protect itself against the stressor, and maintain homeostasis. Stabilization involves the use of physiological and psychological coping mechanisms. Psychological defense mechanisms for coping will be discussed shortly. Physical adaptations help the heart rate, blood pressure, cardiac output, respiratory function, and hormone levels return to normal. If the person adapts successfully or if the stress can be confined to a small area (as in the inflammatory response, also discussed shortly), the body regains homeostasis. If the stress is too great (as in serious illness or

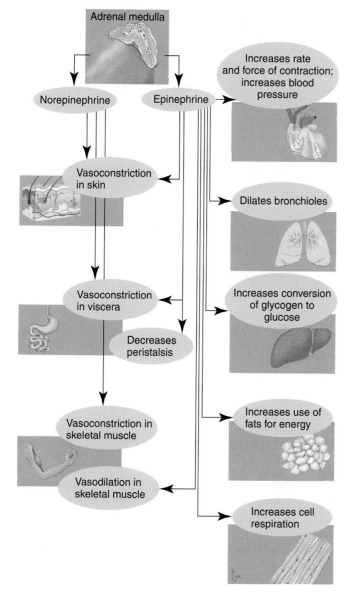

FIGURE 25–5 Functions of epinephrine and norepinephrine during the alarm stage of the GAS. *Source:* Scanlon, V., & Sanders, T. (2003). *Essentials of anatomy and physiology* (4th ed.). Philadelphia: F. A. Davis Company, p. 227.

severe blood loss), defense mechanisms fail, and the person enters the third phase of the GAS.

The Exhaustion or Recovery Stage

If stress continues and adaptive mechanisms become ineffective or are used up, a person enters the final stage, **exhaustion.** Physiological responses in this stage include vasodilation, decreased blood pressure, and increased pulse and respirations. Physical adaptive resources and energy are depleted. The body is unable to defend itself and cannot maintain resistance against the continuing stressors. Exhaustion usually ends in disease or death.

In contrast, if adaptation is successful, the final stage is **recovery.** For example, following a miscarriage, a couple participates in a support group and begins to focus more deeply on their relationship with each other. They are able gradually to resolve their grief.

KnowledgeCheck 25–3

- In general, what is the difference between the alarm stage and the resistance stage of the GAS?
- Name the gland that releases each of the following hormones in response to stress, and name each hormone's function: corticotropin releasing hormone (CRH), antidiuretic hormone (ADH), adrenocorticotropic hormone (ACTH), aldosterone, cortisol, epinephrine, and norepinephrine.
- In the alarm stage of the GAS, what are the effects of the sympathetic nervous system on each of the following: heart, blood vessels in skeletal muscle and to the brain, glycogen stores?
- What is the effect of Selye's resistance stage on the cardiovascular and respiratory systems? On hormone levels?

Go to Chapter 25, **Knowledge Check Response Sheet and Answers,** on the Electronic Study Guide.

The Local Adaptation Syndrome Involves a Specific Local Response

Whereas the GAS is a whole-body response to a stressor, the **local adaptation syndrome (LAS)** is a localized body response; that is, it involves only a specific body part, tissue, or organ. It is a short-term attempt to restore homeostasis. As a nurse, the two most common LAS responses you will deal with are the reflex pain response and the inflammatory response (others include blood clotting and pupil constriction in response to light).

Reflex Pain Response

When you perceive a painful stimulus, especially in one of your limbs, you immediately and unconsciously withdraw from the source of pain. If you've ever accidentally touched a hot stove, you certainly didn't stop to ponder, "Hmmm, I think I will withdraw my hand." You pulled your hand away before you could even think about it. This is a protective **reflex** (an involuntary, predictable response). Pain receptors send sensory impulses to the spinal cord, where they synapse with the spinal motor neurons. The motor impulses travel back to the site of stimulation, causing the flexor muscles in the limb to contract. This is a local, rather than a whole-body, response.

Inflammatory Response

The **inflammatory response** is a local reaction to cell injury, either by pathogens or by physical, chemical, or other agents (Box 25–2). Its mechanisms are the same, regardless of the injuring agent, and produce the classic symptoms of inflammation: pain, heat, swelling, redness, and loss of function. The inflammatory

25-2 Agents Causing Inflammatory Response

The following agents stimulate the inflammatory response by causing cell injury:

- Autoimmune disorders
- Antigen-antibody responses
- Body substances (e.g., digestive enzymes leaking into the abdomen; accumulation of uric acid crystals in joints)
- Chemical injury (e.g., acid or alkali burns)
- Ischemia
- Neoplastic growth (i.e., cancer)
- Pathogens (e.g., bacteria, viruses)
- Physical agents:

  Heat or cold

  Radiation

  Electrothermal injury

  Mechanical trauma (e.g., abrasion, contusion, laceration, puncture, incision, fractures, sprains)

process includes a vascular response, a cellular response, formation of exudate, and healing.

- *Vascular response.* Immediately after injury, blood vessels at the site constrict (narrow) to control bleeding. After the injured cells release histamine, the vessels dilate, increasing blood flow to the area **(hyperemia).** Under the influence of kinins released by the dying cells, the capillaries become more permeable, allowing movement of fluid from capillaries into tissue spaces. The tissue becomes edematous. After leukocytes move into the area, localized blood flow again decreases, to keep them in the area to fight infection.

- *Cellular response.* White blood cells migrate to the site of injury. They phagocytize (engulf) bacteria, other foreign material, and damaged cells and destroy them. Sometimes they form a "wall" around an invading pathogen. The accumulation of dead white cells, digested bacteria, and other cell debris in the presence of infection is called *pus.*

- *Exudate formation.* The fluid and white cells that move from the circulation to the site of injury are called **exudate.** The nature and quantity of exudate depends on the severity of injury and the tissues involved. For example, a surgical incision may ooze serosanguineous (clear or pinkish) exudate for a day or two.

- *Healing.* **Healing** is the replacement of tissue by regeneration or repair. **Regeneration** is replacement of the damaged cells with identical or similar cells.

However, not all cells can regenerate (e.g., some central nervous system neurons and cardiac muscle cells cannot regenerate). Most injuries heal by **repair,** wherein scar tissue replaces the original tissue.

The inflammatory response is adaptive in that it protects the body from infection and promotes healing. However, chronic inflammation, as in arthritis, is itself a stressor.

Do not confuse inflammation with infection. Inflammation is a mechanism for eliminating invading pathogens; therefore, you always see inflammation when there is infection. However, inflammation is stimulated by trauma as well as by pathogens (as in the example of a sprained ankle); thus, it can also occur in the absence of infection.

KnowledgeCheck 25–4

- What are four characteristics of the local adaptation syndrome (LAS)?
- Name two LAS responses.
- What are the classic symptoms of the inflammatory process?

 Go to Chapter 25, **Knowledge Check Response Sheet and Answers,** on the Electronic Study Guide.

Psychological Responses to Stress Include Feelings, Thoughts, and Behaviors

Recall that stress responses are holistic. That means we respond and adapt to stress psychologically as well as physiologically. Psychological responses are both emotional and cognitive, and they include feelings, thoughts, and behaviors. They may be fleeting, as in a flash of anger that is gone in seconds; or long-term, as in the avoidance of relationships by an adult whose needs for love and security were not met as a child. Examples of psychological responses are shown in Box 25–3.

As with physical responses, psychological responses can be adaptive or harmful. For example, Mr. Laslow and Mr. Harvey have both had heart attacks and are both anxious about the future. To relieve his anxiety, Mr. Laslow takes a problem-solving approach, learning about diet, exercise, and lifestyle changes that he must make. Mr. Harvey uses denial; he cannot even accept that he has "really" had a heart attack. He says, "I'm not an invalid. I feel fine. I could follow all those rules and still get hit by a truck and die tomorrow." Both of these responses may relieve the person's anxiety. Which one do you think is more adaptive in the long term?

Anxiety and Fear

As discussed in Chapter 11, **anxiety** is diffuse and not easily defined. NANDA (2003, p. 9) defines it as a "vague, uneasy feeling of discomfort or dread accompanied by an autonomic response (the source often nonspecific or unknown to the individual); a feeling of apprehension

BOX 25-3 Psychological Responses to Stressors

Cognitive Responses

- Difficulty concentrating
- Poor judgment
- Decrease in accuracy (e.g., in counting money)
- Forgetfulness
- Decreased problem-solving ability
- Decreased attention to detail
- Difficulty learning
- Narrowing of focus
- Preoccupation, daydreaming

Emotional Responses

- Anger
- Anxiety
- Depression
- Fear
- Feelings of inadequacy
- Low self-esteem
- Irritability
- Lack of motivation
- Lethargy

Behavioral Responses

- Crying, emotional outbursts
- Dependence
- Poor job performance
- Substance use and abuse
- Sleeplessness (or sleeping too much)
- Change in eating habits (e.g., loss of appetite, overeating)
- Decrease in quality of job performance
- Preoccupation (i.e., daydreaming)
- Illnesses
- Increased absenteeism from work or school
- Increased number of accidents
- Avoiding social situations or relationships
- Rebellion, acting out

---

caused by anticipation of danger." Notice that the response is not to a danger but to the *anticipation* of danger. An anxious person worries; feels nervous, uneasy, and fearful; may be tearful; and often has physical symptoms, such as nausea, trembling, and sweating.

Fear is an emotion or feeling of apprehension from an identified danger, threat, or pain. The danger may be real or imagined. Anxiety and fear produce similar responses; however, some experts differentiate them as follows:

- Fear is a cognitive response, whereas anxiety is an emotional response.
- Fear is related to a present event, whereas anxiety is related to a future (or anticipated) event.
- The source of fear is easily identifiable, whereas the source of anxiety may not be identifiable.
- Fear can result from either a physical or a psychological event; anxiety results from psychological conflict rather than physical threat.

Mild to moderate anxiety may be adaptive because it motivates and mobilizes the person to action. However, severe anxiety consumes energy and interferes with the person's ability to focus on and respond to what is really happening. See Chapter 11 to refresh your theoretical knowledge of anxiety and fear, including levels of anxiety.

Anxiety and fear initiate release of epinephrine, which stimulates the sympathetic nervous system and prepares the person for fight or flight. Therefore, living with anxiety can be physically, emotionally, and spiritually exhausting.

 ## CriticalThinking 25-2

- Read the two following scenarios.
  1. You are a student assigned to a 6-hour day in the clinical area. Each time you have a clinical day coming up, you feel anticipation and look forward to working in the clinical area. However, you do not know what to expect. You think: "What will my patients be like? How will the day go? Do I know enough to handle it? Do I need to practice any procedures?" It is hard to answer these questions until you are actually on the unit and see your patient.
  2. Given the same situation, suppose that when you begin your clinical day, your clinical instructor tells you that he will be in the agency asking questions, supervising, evaluating your performance—and, perhaps from your perspective, making your life miserable.
- In which situation are you most likely to feel fear? Explain your reasoning.

Ego Defense Mechanisms

Just as the body responds physiologically to stressors, it has psychological responses that protect the person from anxiety and assist with adaptation. **Ego defense mechanisms** are unconscious mental mechanisms that make a stressful situation more tolerable

TABLE 25–1 Psychological Defense Mechanisms

Defense Mechanism	Examples	Examples and Consequences of Overuse
Avoidance—unconsciously staying away from events or situations that might open feelings of aggression or anxiety.	"I can't go to the class reunion tonight. I'm too tired; I have to sleep."	The person becomes socially isolated because of the tension he feels when around other people.
Compensation—making up for a perceived inadequacy by developing or emphasizing some other desirable trait.	A small boy who wants to be on the football team instead becomes a great singer.	Use of drugs or alcohol to gain courage to enter a social situation.
Conversion—emotional conflict is changed into physical symptoms that have no physical basis. The symptoms often disappear after the threat is over.	Feeling back pain when it is difficult to continue carrying the pressures of life; developing nausea that causes the person to miss a major exam.	Laryngitis, inability to speak on the anniversary of father's death. Continued anxiety can lead to actual physical disorders, such as gastric ulcers.
Denial—transforming reality by refusing to acknowledge thoughts, feeling, desires, or impulses. This is unconscious; the person is *not* consciously lying. Denial is usually the first defense learned.	A student refuses to acknowledge that he is barely passing anatomy, does not withdraw from the class, and is now failing a nursing course. An alcoholic states, "I can quit any time I want to."	Overuse can lead to repression and dissociative disorders (e.g., dual personalities, selective amnesia).
Displacement—"kicking the dog." Transferring emotions, ideas, or wishes from one original object or situation to a substitute inappropriate person or object that is perceived to be less powerful or threatening.	Husband loses his job, goes home, and yells at his wife. (This mechanism is rarely adaptive.)	In extreme situations, this mechanism leads to verbal and physical abuse.
Dissociation—painful events are separated or dissociated from the conscious mind.	A person who was sexually abused as a child describes the events as though they happened to a sibling.	May result in a dissociative disorder, such as multiple personality disorder.
Identification—a person takes on the ideas, personality, or characteristics of another person, especially someone that the person fears or respects.	Children play cowboy, police, fireman, or mommy.	Assumes mannerisms, wears clothing, and arranges hair and physical appearance to match those of the other person.
Intellectualization—cognitive reasoning is used to block or avoid feelings about a painful incident.	When her husband dies, the wife relieves her pain by thinking, "It's better this way; he was in so much pain." Person says, "I think" rather than, "I feel."	"My husband loves me, so he doesn't like it when another man talks to me; that's why he beats me."
Minimization—not acknowledging or accepting the significance of one's own behavior, making it less important.	"It doesn't matter how much I drink. I never drive when I'm drinking."	Person engages in unhealthy or antisocial behavior; no motivation to change behavior.

by decreasing the inner tension associated with the stressors. Table 25–1 identifies some common psychological defense mechanisms.

When used in small doses, and for mild to moderate anxiety, defense mechanisms can be helpful. When overused, however, they become habits that give us the false illusion that we are coping. If psychological defense mechanisms are inadequate to diminish the threat and restore equilibrium, the person may develop an anxiety disorder.

TABLE **25-1** *(continued)*

Defense Mechanism	Examples	Examples and Consequences of Overuse
Projection—Blaming others. Attributing one's own personality traits, mistakes, emotions, motives, and thoughts to another; "finger pointing."	"The clinical instructor makes me nervous, so I cannot do well." "I forgot to bake cookies because you did not tell me that cookies were due at school today."	Person cannot see his own responsibility for a situation, so he cannot make adaptive behaviors. Person criticizes habits in others that are the same as one's own bad habits.
Rationalization—use of a logical-sounding excuse to cover up or justify true ideas, actions, or feelings. An attempt to preserve self-respect or approval or to conceal a motive for some action by giving a socially acceptable reason. Similar to intellectualization, but uses faulty logic.	"It was God's will that this happened to me." "If I didn't have to work, I would be a better wife."	This mechanism can lead to self-deception.
Reaction formation—similar to compensation, except the person develops the exact opposite trait. The person is aware of her feelings but acts in ways opposite to what she is really feeling.	"It's OK that you forgot my birthday" (when it really is not O.K.)	Overuse can cause failure to resolve internal conflicts.
Regression—using behavior appropriate in an earlier stage of development to overcome feeling of insecurity in a present situation.	Cooks and eats a comfort food (e.g., hot fudge sundae). A 60-year-old divorcee dresses and acts like a teenager.	Can interfere with perception of reality.
Repression—unconscious "burying" or "forgetting" of painful thoughts, feelings, memories, ideas; pushing them from consciousness to unconscious level. A step deeper than denial.	Having no memory of sexual abuse by sibling or father. An adolescent forgets to put out the trash because being "bossed" makes him angry, but he feels guilty if he consciously chooses not to do it.	Flashbacks, traumatic stress syndrome, and amnesia.
Restitution (*undoing*)—making amends for a behavior one thinks is unacceptable, to reduce guilt.	Giving a treat to a child who has been punished for wrongdoing.	May send double messages. Relieves the person of the responsibility for honesty about the situation.
Sublimation—unacceptable drives, traits, or behaviors (often sexual or aggressive) are unconsciously diverted to socially accepted traits.	Anger is expressed by aggression when playing sports. A person who chooses to not have children runs a day-care center.	The "acceptable" behavior might reinforce the negative tendencies, and the person may still show signs of the undesirable trait or behavior. For example, a person indulges in child pornography to obtain sexual gratification.

Source: Neeb, K. (2001). *Fundamentals of mental health nursing* (2nd ed.). Philadelphia: F. A. Davis Company.

Anger and Depression

Anger is a strong, uncomfortable feeling of animosity, hostility, extreme indignation, or displeasure. A person who cannot control stressors may become apprehensive (anxious about what may happen) and may respond with anger. Thus, moderate anger is often a first protective response against anxiety. As anxiety increases and the person recognizes fear, he feels more threatened and may resort to bullying behavior to increase the personal feeling of power, control, and self-esteem.

Anger may be expressed in screaming or shouting, throwing things, or hitting, or more subtly with sarcastic, caustic remarks. Some people attempt to soften their hurtful remarks, or make them more socially acceptable, through the use of humor and joking. When anger involves destructive behaviors such as physical or verbal abuse, it is called **hostility.** When expressed appropriately and clearly (i.e., verbally), anger can be adaptive, because it temporarily releases the person's feelings of tension. When the anger is out in the open, both parties can deal with it. Nevertheless, even verbal expressions of anger can be destructive if the anger continues after the person expresses it.

Depression is sometimes associated with unresolved anger and may result from stress. It is normal to feel depression in response to any loss or a traumatic event, but long-term depression is a cause of concern. Review Chapter 11 for information about depression.

KnowledgeCheck 25–5

- In addition to ego defense mechanisms, name three common emotional responses to stress.
- Explain how mild to moderate anxiety can be adaptive.
- True or false: One difference between anxiety and fear is that the danger in anxiety may be imagined, whereas in fear the danger is real.
- What are ego defense mechanisms?

 Go to Chapter 25, **Knowledge Check Response Sheet and Answers,** on the Electronic Study Guide.

Spiritual Responses to Stress Are Multifaceted

Spiritual responses to stress are multifaceted. Many people depend on a higher power or religious community for support when coping with stress. Some search for a larger meaning in the illness or other stressor. Others may view stress as a test, or a punishment, or a challenge.

Often, a first response during the alarm stage is to pray or ask for help. Prayer, meditation, and religious affiliation can also help during the second stage (adaptation). In the final stage, spiritual resources may be exhausted, leaving the person feeling abandoned, helpless, and hopeless. If your own spiritual life is healthy, you will be better equipped to support patients who are experiencing spiritual challenges. For more information about spiritual responses to stress, see Chapter 14.

WHAT HAPPENS WHEN ADAPTATION FAILS?

Living with continual stress strains adaptive mechanisms. This strain can lead to exhaustion and disease, which in turn can lead to more stress. Once established,

this type of positive feedback loop is difficult to break. Three types of disorders that can develop when adaptation fails are stress-induced organic responses, somatoform disorders, and psychological disorders.

Stress-Induced Organic Responses

As a result of repeated central nervous system stimulation and frequent elevation of certain hormones, continual stress brings about long-term changes in various body systems. People who use maladaptive coping strategies (e.g., overeating, substance abuse) create additional stress on the body, further contributing to disease.

- *Cardiovascular system.* Continued secretion of epinephrine may cause cardiovascular disorders including angina, myocardial infarction, cardiomegaly, and congestive heart failure, all of which lead to decreased cardiac output. As cardiac output decreases, less oxygen circulates to meet cellular metabolic demands, and the body experiences fatigue. Prolonged secretion of epinephrine and renin result in vasoconstriction, causing hypertension. ADH, aldosterone, ACTH, and cortisol create electrolyte imbalance and retention of sodium and water, thus promoting peripheral edema.

- *Endocrine system.* Continuing high levels of blood glucose and insulin can cause diabetes. Metabolic disorders of hyperthyroidism or hypothyroidism can result as persistent demands for thyroid hormone production cause a rebound failure of the gland.

- *Immune system.* Stress reduces the ability of the body's immune cells to differentiate between self and nonself. Thus, the immune cells begin to attack body tissues, producing autoimmune illness. Common autoimmune illnesses include rheumatoid arthritis, lupus, cancer, and allergies. In addition, studies of patients with HIV suggest that stress increases viral replication and suppresses the immune system (Robinson, Mathews, & Witek-Janusek, 2000).

- *Gastrointestinal system.* The gastrointestinal system may respond to central nervous system stimulation with constipation or diarrhea, gastroesophageal reflux, colitis, or irritable bowel syndrome. Continued secretion of hydrochloric acid produces gastric hyperacidity and erosion of the gastrointestinal tract.

- *Musculoskeletal system.* Constant readiness for fight or flight produces muscle tension and pain in various body sites. Tension headache and temporomandibular joint pain result from prolonged muscle tension in the head, neck, and spine.

- *Respiratory system.* Epinephrine and circulating hormones dilate the bronchial tubes and increase the rate of respiration. Hyperventilation can produce symptoms of alkalosis, including dizziness, tingling

hands and feet, and anxiety. Distress in the respiratory system can exacerbate existing asthma, hay fever, and allergies.

Somatoform Disorders

Somatoform disorders are conditions characterized by the presence of physical symptoms with no known organic cause. They are believed to result from unconscious denial, repression, and displacement of anxiety. Certain people seem predisposed to somatoform disorders—for instance, those who do not handle anxiety well and those who are dependent, emotionally needy, frustrated, and resentful (Neeb, 2001). The physical symptoms allow the person to avoid a situation that, if confronted, would provoke extreme anxiety. The following are examples of somatoform disorders:

- **Hypochondriasis.** The person is preoccupied with the idea that he is or will become seriously ill. The person is abnormally concerned with his health and interprets his real or imagined symptoms unrealistically, fearing that they will get worse or become incurable.
- **Somatization.** In this disorder, anxiety and emotional turmoil are expressed in physical symptoms, loss of physical function, pain that changes location often, and depression. The patient is unable to control the symptoms and behaviors.
- **Somatoform pain disorder.** This is emotional pain that manifests physically. Pain is the patient's main concern. The level of pain the person states is inconsistent with the physical condition—that is, no physical cause can be found for the pain. The pain does not change location.
- **Malingering.** Malingering is different from the other disorders because it is a *conscious* effort to escape unpleasant situations. The patient merely pretends to have the symptoms.

KnowledgeCheck 25–6

- Name and describe three stress-induced organic or systemic responses to stress.
- Name and describe at least three somatoform disorders.

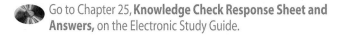 Go to Chapter 25, **Knowledge Check Response Sheet and Answers,** on the Electronic Study Guide.

Stress-Induced Psychological Responses

Even if coping mechanisms are effective initially, with long-term stress, exhaustion sets in, and the mechanisms begin to fail. The person may then try maladaptive ways to cope. As work and personal relationships deteriorate, the person loses self-esteem. Prolonged stress can eventually result in crisis and burnout. More severe responses include psychiatric illnesses, such as anxiety disorders, clinical depression, and post-traumatic stress disorder (PTSD). Anxiety and depression were discussed in Chapter 11. We discuss crisis, burnout, and PTSD next.

Crisis

A **crisis** exists when (1) an event in a person's life drastically changes the person's routine and he perceives it as a threat to self, and (2) the person's usual coping methods are ineffective, resulting in high levels of anxiety and inability to function adequately. Such events are often sudden and unexpected (e.g., serious illness or death of a loved one, serious financial losses, an automobile accident, rape, and natural disasters).

Keep in mind that each person has a different tolerance for stress and that an event that creates a crisis for one may be just a minor nuisance for another. Nevertheless, most experts agree that people experiencing crisis go through five phases (Neeb, 2001; Stuart & Sundeen, 1999).

1. *Precrisis.* In response to the event and the anxiety, the person uses her usual coping strategies. The person has no symptoms, denies any stress, and may even report a feeling of well-being.
2. *Impact.* If the usual strategies are not effective, anxiety and confusion increase. The person may have trouble organizing her personal life. The person may feel the stress but minimize its severity.
3. *Crisis.* The person experiences more anxiety and tries new ways of coping, such as withdrawal, rationalization, and projection (refer to Table 25–1). The person recognizes the problem but denies that it is out of control.
4. *Adaptive.* The person redefines the threat and perceives the crisis in a realistic way. She begins to think rationally and does some positive problem solving, regains some self-esteem and is able to begin socializing again. Adaptation is more likely if the person can use effective coping strategies and if situational supports are available.
5. *Postcrisis.* The aftermath of a crisis may have both positive and negative effects on functioning. The person may have developed better ways of coping with stress. Or, she may be critical, hostile, and depressed, and she may use maladaptive strategies (e.g., overeating or substance abuse) to deal with what has happened.

People in crisis are at risk for physical and emotional harm, so intervention is essential (see "Crisis Intervention" on page 572).

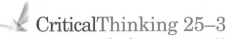

CriticalThinking 25–3

Suppose you are the charge nurse on a 30-bed surgical unit. In addition, you must assume care of three patients because another nurse called in sick. It is a normal, busy day with seven postoperative patients and eight discharges. In addition, a patient went into cardiac arrhythmia and was transferred to the coronary care unit. Because the sick nurse was supposed to work a 12-hour shift and no replacement has been found, you are told you must stay and work 4 hours overtime. You had plans to have dinner with your spouse this evening because it is your anniversary. Now you will surely not be home before 8:00 P.M., and you will be exhausted.

- What would be the stressors for you in this situation?
- What thoughts and feelings would you have?
- What physical responses would you probably notice?
- What are some psychological responses that you would use to help you adapt and cope with this day?
- How would you probably react if the same thing happens on the following day?

Burnout

Burnout occurs when nurses and other professionals cannot cope effectively with the physical and emotional demands of the workplace. Examples of stressors specific to nursing include the following:

- Dealing with difficult personalities (e.g., patient, supervisors, physicians)
- Working 12-hour shifts with minimal breaks for food, water, or rest
- Frequent rotating shifts that upset the circadian rhythm of the body and lower the immune system response
- Mandatory overtime
- Being "floated" to an unfamiliar unit (e.g., a maternity nurse may be "floated" to an orthopedic unit)
- Workload: low staffing ratio (one nurse to many patients)
- Frustration with patients (e.g., who do not follow therapeutic routines)
- Need to constantly anticipate patients' needs and cope with the unexpected
- Feeling helpless against patient's disease process or lack of healing
- Dealing with death and dying
- Lack of rewards (both intrinsic and extrinsic)
- Lack of participation in decision making
- Inability to delegate responsibilities
- Organizational philosophy that conflicts with personal philosophy

Excessive demands by an employer serve as a catalyst for burnout. In some situations, the nurse receives no respect and little support from the employer or co-workers. Filled with feelings of injustice for treatment received, the nurse may respond with anger and frustration, feel overwhelmed and helpless, and suffer low self-esteem and depression. The nurse who burns out may develop a physical illness or a negative attitude or may use maladaptive coping techniques such as smoking, substance abuse, or distancing from patients— "going through the motions" but not really interacting with patients in a meaningful way. Many nurses in such situations give up and leave nursing. You will find suggestions for preventing burnout later in the chapter.

Post-Traumatic Stress Disorder

Post-traumatic stress disorder (PTSD) is a specific response to a violent, traumatizing event, such as an earthquake or other natural disaster, or to physical or emotional abuse, such as rape, torture, or war experience. The victim experiences anxiety and flashbacks that may last for months or years. Other symptoms include social withdrawal, feelings of low self-esteem, changes in existing relationships, difficulty forming new relationships, irritability and outbursts of anger for no obvious reason, depression, and chemical abuse or dependence.

Counseling and special intervention are needed to help the person cope with and recover from the impact of the traumatic event.

KnowledgeCheck 25–7

Define *crisis, burnout,* and *post-traumatic stress disorder.*

 Go to Chapter 25, **Knowledge Check Response Sheet and Answers,** on the Electronic Study Guide.

Practical Knowledge
knowing how

People under stress may not be thinking clearly, so it is important to intervene to relieve their immediate anxiety as much as possible, demonstrate empathy, and develop rapport before beginning an assessment. Focus the patient by asking short, direct questions and then proceeding to open-ended questions that will provide you with as much information as possible (see Chapter 18).

| Assessment |

Assessment should explore subjective and objective data about the person's stressors, risk factors, coping and adaptation, support systems, and stress responses

(psychosocial and physiological). For a stress scale and guidelines for assessing all of these factors.

 Go to Chapter 25, **Assessment Guidelines and Tools, the Holmes-Rahe Social Readjustment Scale** and **Assessing for Stress: Questions to Ask,** in Volume 2.

Assess Stressors, Risk Factors, and Coping and Adaptation

Data about the patient's stressors and risk factors should help you to (1) determine whether the client has a realistic or an exaggerated perception of the stressors, (2) identify factors that increase risk for future stress, and (3) identify interventions to reduce current stress and to provide anticipatory guidance to prevent future stress. You might begin gathering this data by having the client complete a stress inventory, such as the Holmes-Rahe Scale. Then follow up with questions such as those in "Assessment Guidelines and Tools" in Volume 2. You will also find questions to help you obtain information about the patient's coping methods and adaptation in those guidelines.

Assess Responses to Stress

When assessing responses to stress, recall that stress responses are holistic. Therefore, you will need to assess physiological, emotional, cognitive, and behavioral indicators of stress. For examples of questions to ask,

 Go to Chapter 25, **Assessment Guidelines and Tools, Assessing for Stress: Questions to Ask,** in Volume 2.

Assessing Physiological Responses

Because the GAS is nonspecific, you must obtain data from all body systems (for physical examination techniques, see Chapter 19). A check of vital signs for elevations in pulse, respiration, and blood pressure will indicate whether the fight-or-flight response is present. In your general survey, or overview, of the patient, you should note hygiene, grooming, facial expression, and ability to make eye contact. Box 25–4 summarizes physiological responses that indicate stress. If coping is successful, clinical signs and symptoms of stress may not be present.

Assessing Emotional and Behavioral Responses

Assess for the emotional and behavioral responses to stress that are described in Box 25–3. As the client answers questions, note posture, facial expression, body tension, and other nonverbal behaviors. Also note mood and affect. Does the client seem angry, anxious, or depressed? Check the client's records, observe for and ask the client about destructive behaviors (e.g.,

---

BOX 25–4 Physiological Responses to Stressors

- Dilated pupils
- Muscle tension
- Stiff neck
- Headaches
- Nail biting
- Skin pallor
- Skin lesions (e.g., eczema)
- Diaphoresis, sweaty palms
- Dry mouth
- Nausea
- Weight or appetite changes
- Increased blood glucose
- Increased heart rate
- Cardiac dysrhythmias
- Hyperventilation
- Chest pain
- Water retention
- Increased urinary frequency or decreased urinary output
- Diarrhea or constipation
- Flatulence

---

drug abuse, anger). The client may or may not be aware that the feelings or behaviors are related to stress.

Assessing Cognitive Responses

You can assess the client's cognitive functioning as you assess other functional areas. See Box 25–3 to review examples of cognitive responses. Notice whether the person has difficulty focusing and responding to your questions. When you ask the client to describe and rate the intensity of the stressors, you can begin to assess whether he perceives the stressors realistically or in an exaggerated way. The client's responses concerning any coping strategies will give you an idea of his problem-solving abilities.

Assess Support Systems

Recall that support systems such as family, friends, and co-workers can be important to the success of a client's coping strategies. Conversely, these people may be affected by the same stressors or by the client's response to them. For these reasons, you should determine the supports available and their ability to assist the client—that is, do the significant

BOX 25-5 Nursing Diagnoses Associated with Stress

Physical Domain

Constipation

Delayed Growth and Development

Diarrhea

Disturbed Energy Field

Disturbed Sleep Pattern

Fatigue

Imbalanced Nutrition (can be More Than or Less Than Body Requirements)

Nausea

Pain (e.g., backache)

Risk for Imbalanced Fluid Volume

Risk for Injury

Sleep Deprivation

Behavioral Domain

Ineffective Health Maintenance

Ineffective Therapeutic Regimen Management

Cognitive Domain

Disturbed Thought Processes

Impaired Memory

Emotional Domain

Anxiety

Decisional Conflict

Defensive Coping

Fear

Grieving (Anticipatory or Dysfunctional)

Impaired Adjustment

Ineffective Coping

Ineffective Denial

Low Self-Esteem (Chronic or Situational)

Interpersonal Relationships Domain

Caregiver Role Strain

Compromised or Disabled Family Coping

Impaired Parenting

Impaired Social Interaction

Ineffective Community Coping

Interrupted Family Processes

Post-Trauma Syndrome

Relocation Stress Syndrome

Social Isolation

Spiritual Domain

Hopelessness

Spiritual Distress

---

others have the sensitivity and skills to be supportive? For examples of questions to ask,

VOL 2   Go to Chapter 25, **Assessment Guidelines and Tools, Assessing for Stress: Questions to Ask,** in Volume 2.

CriticalThinking 25–4

Review the scenario of Gloria and John ("Meet Your Patient"). How much does it really tell you about the clients' situation?

- Which aspect of stress do you have the most information about: their stressors, their coping methods and adaptation, their responses to stress, or their support systems?
- What facts do you have about either Gloria's or John's physiological responses to their multiple stressors? What can you infer that their responses might be?
- What facts do you have about the clients' emotional and behavioral responses to their stressors?
- What information do you have about how well they are adapting to stress?
- What data do you have about their support systems? What information do you need?

| Nursing Diagnosis |

Stress is nonspecific, so there is almost no limit to the number of nursing diagnoses that could be stress-induced. It is important to correctly identify the etiology so that you can choose interventions to remove or modify the stressor. For example, if you believe a patient's diarrhea is being caused by stress, you would intervene by modifying the stressor, helping the patient to perceive the stressor differently, and so on. If, instead, the diarrhea were being caused by a gastrointestinal virus, your interventions would not have been helpful. Box 25–5 lists nursing diagnoses commonly associated with stress.

KnowledgeCheck 25–8

- How might you identify and assess Gloria and John's stressors ("Meet Your Patients")?
- List three questions you could ask to find out how Gloria is coping and adapting to stress.
- List three questions you could ask to assess Gloria's physiological responses to stress. What observations might you also make?

- List three questions you could ask to assess Gloria's emotional and behavioral responses to stress.
- How might you determine whether stress is affecting Gloria's cognitive functioning?
- You know that Gloria's sister is providing some support. How could you find out more about the extent of Gloria and John's support system?

 Go to Chapter 25, **Knowledge Check Response Sheet and Answers,** on the Electronic Study Guide.

| Planning Outcomes/Evaluation |

NOC standardized outcomes are outcomes that, if achieved, demonstrate resolution of the problem stated by the nursing diagnosis. For example, if you make a diagnosis of Anxiety related to client's perception that he will not be able to fulfill family responsibilities, you might use the NOC outcome, Anxiety Control. For a list of NOC outcomes,

 Go to Chapter 25, **Standardized Language, Outcomes and Interventions for Stress-Related Nursing Diagnosis,** in Volume 2.

Individualized goal or outcome statements are also specific to each nursing diagnosis. Broad, general goals for clients experiencing stress are to (1) reduce the strength and duration of the stressor, (2) relieve or remove responses to stress, and (3) use effective coping mechanisms. Examples of specific outcome statements you might write include the following:

- Reports (or physical exam reveals) reduction in physical symptoms of stress.
- Less physical tension is observed in facial expression and other muscle groups.
- Verbalizes increased feelings of control in the stressful situation.
- Identifies and uses available support systems (e.g., family, community agency).
- Uses problem-solving and anxiety-reducing techniques.
- Describes decreased feeling of anxiety.
- Demonstrates relaxation and stress-reducing strategies.

| Planning Interventions/Implementation |

NIC standardized interventions for stress may be linked to either the problem or the etiology of the nursing diagnosis. Using the preceding example of Anxiety related to client's perception that he will not be able to fulfill family responsibilities, some interventions may focus on supporting the client's ability to fulfill family roles; others may focus on general techniques for relieving anxiety (e.g., Aromatherapy, Calming Technique). For other NIC interventions,

 Go to Chapter 25, **Standardized Language, Outcomes and Interventions for Stress-Related Nursing Diagnoses,** in Volume 2.

Specific nursing activities will be individualized on the basis of the patient's needs and the etiologies of the nursing diagnoses. As you implement stress-reduction interventions, it is essential to consider compliance. Will the patient adhere to or cooperate with therapeutic suggestions? Does the person wish to use complementary or alternative care measures? How open is she to deviating from traditional Western therapies? Confer and collaborate with patients to determine what will fit most comfortably into their lifestyle. Those are the interventions that will be most effective.

Most stress-relieving interventions work by one or more of the following:

1. Removing or modifying the stressor(s)
2. Supporting coping abilities (e.g., changing the person's perception of the stressor)
3. Treating the person's responses to stress (i.e., symptoms)

As you read through the following interventions, see whether you can identify the rationale for the action. Is it 1, 2, or 3?

Health Promotion Activities

People cannot always control the occurrence of a stressful event, and there are no high-tech treatments for coping with stress. However, a healthy lifestyle can prevent some stressors and improve the ability to cope with others. Chapter 41 provides an in-depth discussion of wellness promotion. The following suggestions are a brief guide to a healthy lifestyle.

Nutrition

Nutrition is important for maintaining physical homeostasis and resisting stress. For example, adequate nutrition is essential to maintain the integrity of the immune system; and proteins are needed for tissue building and healing. In addition, overweight and malnutrition are stressors that may lead to illness. See Chapter 26 for detailed information about nutrition. To summarize, you should advise clients to:

- Maintain a normal body weight.
- Limit the intake of fat (especially animal fat) to no more than 30% of daily calories.
- Limit the intake of sugar and salt.
- Eat more fish and poultry and less red meat.

- Eat smaller, more frequent meals to aid digestion.
- Consume 25 grams of fiber (fruits, vegetables, and whole grains) daily to promote bowel elimination.
- Consume no more than two alcoholic beverages per day.

Exercise

Regular exercise promotes physical homeostasis by improving muscle tone and controlling weight. It also improves the functioning of the heart and lungs and reduces the risk of cardiovascular disease. Exercise also improves emotional homeostasis by promoting relaxation and reducing tension. During exercise, **endogenous** opioids are released, creating a feeling of well-being.

- To achieve health benefits, the client needs to exercise for at least 30 minutes most, if not all, days of the week (Thompson & Manore, 2004).
- Advise clients who are obese, chronically ill, or who have always been sedentary to consult a primary caregiver before beginning a new exercise program.
- Suggest that the client identify a variety of physical activities that he enjoys (e.g., swimming, bicycling, walking, sports) and, if possible, schedule regular sessions with one or more exercise "buddies." These strategies help the client adhere to the exercise routine.

Sleep and Rest

Sleep and rest restore energy levels, allow the body to repair itself, and promote mental relaxation. Most people need 7 or 8 hours of sleep a day; however, the amount of sleep varies among individuals. Stress, pain, and illness may interfere with the ability to sleep, so some clients may need help identifying and implementing techniques for relaxing and going to sleep (see Chapter 33 for more information on sleep).

Leisure Activities

As compared to exercise, which not everyone enjoys, leisure activities are any activities that provide joy and satisfaction. They may involve physical activity (after all, many people do enjoy exercising), or they may be sedentary activities, such as reading, painting, and even watching television. Leisure activities are a form of rest and, as such, are restorative.

Time Management

People who manage their time efficiently and organize their life routines feel more in control and, therefore,

less stressed. If clients feel overwhelmed, you can help them to prioritize tasks and make "to do" lists. It is also important that they learn to delegate responsibilities and set boundaries on the use of time. A working couple with three children may need to assign each child mealtime tasks, such as setting the table, drying the dishes, and so forth. Or they may need to limit the amount of time they spend cooking, reserving elaborate meals for weekends.

Time management also includes saying no. Out of a need to be liked or a strong sense of responsibility to others, people sometimes try to make everyone happy by agreeing to all requests for assistance: from spouse, children, parents, friends, church, school, and the community. You can prompt clients to identify how much they can realistically accomplish—what is essential to do, and what would be "nice" to do. Help clients to work out a balance between their responsibilities to self and their responsibilities to others.

Avoiding Maladaptive Behaviors

Some people use maladaptive behaviors as a response to stress. For others, the behaviors themselves become stressors. Advise clients to avoid the following unhealthful behaviors:

Drinking more than two alcoholic beverages per day
Consuming excess caffeine (e.g., coffee, tea, colas)
Eating large quantities of nutrient-poor food, such as sweets
Smoking or chewing tobacco
Using illegal street drugs
Abusing over-the-counter medications
Avoiding social interaction

KnowledgeCheck 25–9

Name and discuss at least four aspects of a healthy lifestyle that can help prevent or relieve stress.

 Go to Chapter 25, **Knowledge Check Response Sheet and Answers,** on the Electronic Study Guide.

Relieving Anxiety

Because anxiety is a common response to illness, medical tests, and treatments, you will use anxiety-relief interventions every day of your professional life. For example, when you tell clients what to expect before you perform a procedure or ask them to take deep breaths during a painful treatment, you lessen anxiety. If you have developed a therapeutic, trusting relationship, your very presence will help to ease the patient's anxiety. You will find specific interventions for anxiety in Chapter 11, and many of the interventions in the following sections provide anxiety relief as well.

| toward evidence-based practice |

Blau, G., Tatum, D. S., & Ward-Cook, K. (2003). Correlates of work exhaustion for medical technologists. *Journal of Allied Health, 32*(3), 148–157.

Researchers studied 196 medical technologists over a 4-year period to determine whether work-related demands and resources were related to subsequent work exhaustion. They found that several variables were related to work exhaustion:

- Increased levels of perceived interference of work with family
- Heavy task load
- Lower organizational support

They found that distributive justice (fairness) served as a support to help decrease the effects of work exhaustion and lack of organizational support.

DePew, C. L., Gordon, M., Yoder, L. H., & Goodwin, C. W. (1999). The relationship of burnout, stress, and hardiness in nurses in a military medical center: A replicated descriptive study. *Journal of Burn Care Rehabilitation, 20*(6), 515–522.

Researchers studied 49 registered nurses working in seven special care units, using the following written instruments: a tedium and burnout scale, the nursing stress scale, and a scale to test hardiness. They found that hardiness alone accounted for 35% of burnout variance—meaning that lack of hardiness is a predictor of burnout. Among nurses who scored high in hardiness, adding more stress did not significantly increase burnout.

Gilbar, O. (1998). Relationship between burnout and a sense of coherence in health social workers. *Social Work in Health Care, 26*(3), 39–49.

In a study of 81 social workers working in the fields of physical illness, mental illness, and the disabled, researchers found that health social workers who had a strong sense of group coherence experienced less burnout than those with a weak sense of coherence.

Leiter, M. P., Harvie, P., & Frizzell, C. (1998). The correspondence of patient satisfaction and nurse burnout. *Social Science in Medicine, 47*(10), 1611–1617.

Researchers conducted a survey of 711 nurses and 605 patients. They found that patients on units where nurses found their work meaningful were more satisfied with all aspects of their hospital stay (e.g., nursing care, physician care, information provided). Patients on units where nurses felt more exhausted or more frequently expressed the intent to quit were less satisfied with the various component of their care. Also, nurse cynicism was associated with lower patient satisfaction with their interactions with nursing staff.

McGowan, B. (2001, July 4–10). Self-reported stress and its effects on nurses. *Nursing Standard, 15*(42), 33–38.

A random sample of 72 nurses working in a children's hospital in Belfast, Northern Ireland, completed the Nurse Stress Index questionnaire. Results indicated that as stress levels rose, job satisfaction fell. The only significant (negative) contribution to job satisfaction scores was stress resulting from a perceived lack of organizational support and involvement. Researchers concluded job satisfaction was negatively affected by stress and that the main sources of stress were shortage of resources and time, management's lack of appreciation, and initiating change.

Which of the preceding studies provides some support for the following statements made in your text? Explain why you chose that study, and describe any reservation you might have about the amount of support it provides.

1. Filled with feelings of injustice for treatment received, the nurse may respond with anger and frustration…. The nurse who burns out may develop a physical illness, a negative attitude … and distancing from patients—"going through the motions," but not really interacting with patients in a meaningful way.

2. Burnout occurs when nurses and other professionals cannot cope effectively with the physical and emotional demands of the workplace. Examples of stressors specific to nursing include the following:

- Working 12-hour shifts with minimal breaks for food, water, or rest
- Mandatory overtime
- Being "floated" to an unfamiliar unit (e.g., a maternity nurse may be "floated" to an orthopedic unit)
- Workload: low staffing ratio of one nurse to many patients
- The nurse may receive no respect and little support from the employer or co-workers.

3. Fortunately, successful adaptation does not depend entirely on being able to avoid stressors. Various personal factors also influence the outcome … [including] overall health status. Stressors may actually cause a healthy person to engage in constructive adaptive behaviors that improve health…. Some people succumb to only a few stressors, whereas others seem to adapt to multiple, intensely difficult stressors.

4. A good support system can help a person adapt to stress in a healthy manner.

 Go to Chapter 25, **Toward Evidence-Based Practice Suggested Responses,** on the Electronic Study Guide.

Anger Management

Anger is a common response to stress. However, clients usually do not openly say, "I am angry." In fact, they may not even recognize that they are angry. Instead, they engage in angry behaviors. For example, they may become hypercritical of family members or caregivers, become verbally abusive, or become demanding. By now you have probably heard stories from nurses about the client who is "on the call light constantly." Unfortunately, such behaviors often provoke anger in others—even nurses. Be aware of how you are responding to angry clients. Are you relieving your own stress, or are you relieving the client's stress? If you respond angrily to relieve your own stress, you may provoke further anger in the client and even escalate the situation to the point of violence. For other tips on managing anger,

 Go to Chapter 25, **Technique 25–1: Dealing with Angry Patients,** in Volume 2.

Stress Management Techniques

It is important to teach your clients about relaxation and other stress management techniques. Most such techniques focus on discharging tension or simplifying one's life to modify stressors or control stress responses. **Relaxation** is a state of reduced physical and mental arousal. It is an important intervention because it generally reverses some stress responses. By elongating muscle fibers, relaxation reduces neural impulses sent to the brain. Other physical responses include increased peripheral skin temperatures and decreases in activity of the brain with alpha wave activity (see Chapter 33), activity in other body systems, blood pressure, heart rate, and respiratory rate and oxygen consumption.

Many of the techniques in this section are complementary or alternative therapies that require special training, and which are discussed in detail in other chapters. For 101 other suggestions for coping with stress,

 Go to Chapter 25, **Tables, Boxes, Figures: ESG Box 25–1,** on the Electronic Study Guide.

- *Exercise* reduces stress because it releases tension held in muscles, improves muscle tone and posture, expresses emotions, and stimulates the secretion of endorphins, thus creating a feeling of well-being and relaxation.
- *Relaxation techniques* involve teaching the patient to relax individual muscle groups. **Progressive relaxation** in a quiet meditation state or lying in bed, relaxing and contracting muscle groups is much less

traumatic and damaging to fragile joints and muscles than active exercise. Therefore it may be used even by people who are not in good health. **Passive relaxation,** in which the person relaxes the muscle groups without first contracting them, is even less traumatic and requires even less energy.

- *Meditation* involves heightening one's attention or awareness. Regular meditation increases harmony between mind, body, and spirit, thereby reducing anxiety and giving the person control. See Chapter 40 for further information. For a script to lead a client through a guided meditation to reduce stress,

 Go to Chapter 25, **Tables, Boxes, Figures: ESG Box 25–2,** on the Electronic Study Guide.

- *Visualization or imagery* techniques are often used to complement the effects of relaxation techniques. They are explained in Chapters 30 and 40.
- *Biofeedback* techniques use electronic instruments to measure neuromuscular and autonomic nervous system activity and provide information about those responses to the person. The immediate feedback helps the person become aware of and learn how to voluntarily control certain physiological responses, such as those produced by stress (Olson, 1987). Biofeedback practitioners require special training, and most are credentialed in biofeedback.
- *Acupuncture* involves insertion of a needle into "meridian points" to regulate the flow of energy or life force throughout the body. It can modify pain perception and restore normal physiological functions (e.g., decrease the heart rate). Special training is required to use this intervention (see Chapter 30).
- *Chiropractic adjustment* involves manual realignment of the vertebrae. Misalignment of the vertebrae is thought to lead to loss of function and to illness. Realignment is performed to free energy, release muscle tension, and improve body function and health. Chiropractors undergo special education and training before they are qualified to perform adjustments. See Chapter 40 for more information.
- *Reiki and therapeutic touch* are focused on energy modulation. Healing energy is channeled through a practitioner's hands to improve well-being. See Chapters 30 and 40 for more information.
- *Massage,* through manipulation of the soft tissues, relaxes muscles, releases body tension, improves circulation, and allows energy and blood to flow through muscles and soft tissues more readily. See Chapters 30 and 40 for more information. For instructions on how to give a back rub,

 Go to Chapter 33, **Procedure 33–1: Giving a Back Massage,** in Volume 2.

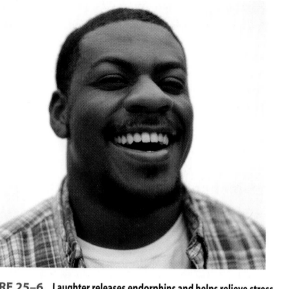

FIGURE 25–6 Laughter releases endorphins and helps relieve stress.

- *Reflexology* is the application of pressure to specific points on the feet, hands, or ears, which are thought to correspond with certain organs of the body. The goal is to relieve blockage, promote the flow of energy, and reduce tension—thus, reflexology may be helpful in treating stress-related illnesses. See Chapter 40 for more information.

The following are simpler activities you can recommend to most clients to aid in relaxation and stress reduction:

- *Humor.* Reading and telling jokes, viewing funny movies or stand-up routines, and simply appreciating the humor of situations all help release tension and anger and increase coping abilities (Phipps, 2002; Johnson, 2002). Laughter (as in Figure 25–6) releases endorphins and relieves feelings of stress (Cousins, 1979).
- *Listening to music.* Music soothes and relaxes when its vibrations are in harmony with body frequencies. Listening to tranquil music can also relax the mind.
- *Engaging in art activities.* Painting, working with clay, and engaging in other art activities help to express emotions and release endorphins.
- *Dance and sports,* like other forms of exercise, release pent-up physical tension and emotions.
- *Journal writing* helps the person to reflect on experiences and express emotions. The catharsis of journal writing often provides insights into causes of stress and ways to modify stressors.

Changing Perception of Stressors or Self

Recall that altering one's perception is one way to improve adaptation to stress. For clients who have an

complementary and alternative modalities (CAM)

Critical Care Uses

Keegan, L. (2003). Therapies to reduce stress and anxiety. *Critical Care Nursing Clinics of North America, 15*(3), 321–327.
This article reports on the successful use of alternative and complementary therapies as adjunct therapies to help decrease stress for critical care patients. Therapies included in the report are aromatherapy, hydrotherapy, humor, imagery, massage, music, and relaxation.

Sneed, N. V., Olson, M., Bubolz, B., & Finch, N. (2001). Influences of a relaxation intervention on perceived stress and power spectral analysis of heart rate variability. *Progress in Cardiovascular Nursing, 16*(2), 57–64, 79.
This study was designed to determine whether electrocardiographic monitoring can detect changes in sympathetic and parasympathetic dominance following a relaxation intervention called therapeutic touch (TT). Thirty healthy subjects and three TT practitioners were monitored by continuous electrocardiographic monitoring (Holter) before (15 minutes), during, and after (15 minutes) TT was administered.

Therapeutic touch produced no detectable change in most subjects. However, four subjects experienced exaggerated parasympathetic responses to the TT. Researchers concluded that further research is needed to determine why some subjects may have greater change in autonomic tone in response to TT. This information would enable practitioners to predict who will demonstrate physiological response to relaxation interventions.

unrealistic perception of the stressor and can imagine only negative outcomes, a technique called **cognitive restructuring** may be helpful. Using this technique, you help the clients to recognize their negative focus and to restructure their thinking in more positive and realistic ways. For example, you might encourage a working mother with demanding parents to take a single positive step, such as saying no to someone at least once a day.

You can also help clients to identify positive aspects of themselves and their coping abilities. This promotes self-esteem and helps them to recognize and use the resources they have for coping with their stressors. **Positive self-talk** is another method for increasing self-esteem. Each time you hear negative self-talk, stop the client, and ask him to rephrase the statement so that it is positive.

Identifying and Using Support Systems

You can facilitate successful adaptation by helping clients to identify and contact people and groups who offer various supports (e.g., listening, encouragement, advice, problem solving, help with household tasks, financial support). Be aware of the groups available in your community (e.g., Weight Watchers, Alcoholics Anonymous, Parents Without Partners, Reach for Recovery). You may need to teach socialization skills to clients who are socially isolated so that they can begin to build a support system.

Providing Spiritual Support

In addition to helping clients obtain spiritual support from church groups and clergy, you can help to strengthen the client spiritually. You may wish to:

- Pray for or with clients, if they desire. Prayer can help reduce their feelings of powerlessness and loneliness.
- Help clients to define their values and set boundaries that honor themselves and uphold those values.
- Teach clients to silently recite an affirming mantra (e.g., on inhalation, say, "I am free." Exhale and say, "Stress, leave me.")

For other ways to provide spiritual support, see Chapter 14.

Crisis Intervention

As an entry-level nurse in acute and ambulatory care settings, you are more likely to see patients in the first three phases of crisis and not be present for the adaptive and postcrisis stages. The goals of crisis intervention at an entry level of practice include the following (Brammer & MacDonald, 1998; Neeb, 2001):

1. Assess the situation.
2. Ensure safety.
3. Defuse the situation.
4. Decrease the person's anxiety.
5. Determine the problem.
6. Decide on the type of help needed.
7. Return the person to precrisis level of functioning.

For further information,

 Go to Chapter 25, **Technique 25–2, Crisis Intervention Guidelines,** in Volume 2.

Crisis centers often rely on telephone counseling ("hotlines"). If telephone counseling is not adequate, or if observations of the home environment are needed, home visits may be necessary.

KnowledgeCheck 25–10

- Describe at least five specific interventions for dealing with an angry person.
- What is cognitive restructuring?
- What is the purpose of positive self-talk?
- List the seven steps of crisis intervention.
- Why is relaxation an important stress intervention?

 Go to Chapter 25, **Knowledge Check Response Sheet and Answers,** on the Electronic Study Guide.

Stress Management in the Workplace

You will need to pay attention to your feelings, your body, and your personal responses to stress. If you notice that you are eating constantly, yelling at your children, not sleeping well, and so on, check your body. Do you feel tired? Are the muscles in your face and shoulders tense? If so, you need to start managing your stress. You can manage workplace stress and help prevent burnout by following the advice you give your patients. For examples,

 Go to Chapter 25, **Tables, Boxes, Figures: ESG Box 25–1,** on the Electronic Study Guide.

When stressors arise from the workplace, the following actions are especially important:

- Have realistic expectations of yourself and others. Don't be overcritical, most people, including you, are doing the best they can.
- Ask for help. Some nurses feel that they must know everything, but asking for help does not indicate weakness. It can even make others feel good by giving them the opportunity to practice collegiality.
- Support colleagues who need help with tasks or with their feelings. This adds to the overall good feeling on a unit.
- Accept the things that you cannot change. Complaining and negative talk add to your own stress and that of others. Get involved in constructive efforts to change policies (e.g., regarding staffing, overtime, safety practices, and so on). If you cannot effect the changes, and if you cannot accept things as they are, you may need to think about leaving the organization rather than subjecting yourself to continual stress.
- Join and support professional organizations, such as the American Nurses Association (ANA), that address workplace issues.
- Obtain counseling for severe stress.

Making Referrals

This chapter has presented many assessments and interventions for reducing stress. Remember, though,

that you are not yet an expert nurse and that no one is an expert in all areas. It is important not to "get in over your head" with clients who under stress. You can help by recognizing your limitations and by referring the client to the appropriate professionals as needed (e.g., a spiritual leader, a counselor, a social worker, a practitioner of complementary therapies, a physician, a psychologist, or a psychiatrist).

 CriticalThinking 25–5

Sally is an RN seeking employment at a local nursing home. She left her previous employer because of stress and frustration with agency policy, for which the bottom line was financial gain rather than patient care. What can Sally do to help ensure that she will not have the same problem in the new agency?

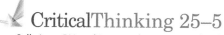 Go to Chapter 25, **Resources for Caregivers and Health Professionals,** on the Electronic Study Guide.

 Suggested Readings: Go to Chapter 25, **Reading More About Stress and Adaptation,** on the Electronic Study Guide.

 Bibliography: Go to Volume 2, Bibliography.

26 Nutrition

Learning Outcomes

After completing this chapter, you should be able to:

* Identify the types, functions, metabolism, and major food sources of (1) the energy nutrients, (2) vitamins, (3) minerals, and (4) water.

* Differentiate among the various sources of nutritional information (e.g., USDA dietary guidelines, food guide pyramids).

* Calculate a client's basal metabolic rate.

* Identify the primary nutritional considerations of various developmental stages.

* Discuss how each of the following affects and is affected by nutritional status: lifestyle choices, vegetarianism, dieting for weight loss, culture and religion, disease processes, and functional limitations.

* Describe the special diets discussed in this chapter.

* Describe tools and techniques for gathering subjective data about nutritional status.

* Compare the effectiveness of various anthropometric measurements.

* Explain the significance of body mass index.

* List at least five physical assessment findings that indicate nutritional imbalance.

* Identify laboratory values that are indicators of nutritional status.

* Discuss the need for and advisability of vitamin and mineral supplementation.

* Describe nursing interventions for patients with special needs: Impaired Swallowing, NPO, older adults, and Self-Care Deficit (Feeding).

* Identify and discuss six nursing interventions for Imbalanced Nutrition: Less Than Body Requirements and for Imbalanced Nutrition: More Than Body Requirements.

* Safely provide enteral and parenteral nutrition for patients.

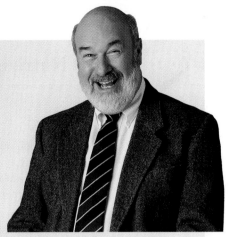

Your Patients

As part of a class assignment you are to assist a local business with their wellness program. You will be completing health risk appraisals and gathering the following data on each of the employees: height, weight, medical and nutritional history, and lifestyle practices. Today you will screen two employees, and then each will have blood drawn for a complete blood count (CBC), comprehensive metabolic panel, and lipid panel:

- Isaac Schwartz, a 50-year-old accountant, works long hours. He describes a sedentary lifestyle, no tobacco use, infrequent alcohol use, no medical problems, and a nutritional history of skipping meals and daily consumption of restaurant food. You measure his height and weight as 69 inches tall and 245 lb.
- Sujing Lee, a 29-year-old project manager, regularly works 65 hours per week. Sujing is 30 weeks pregnant. She does not smoke or drink and has never been hospitalized or had surgery. She has gained a total of 25 lb since becoming

pregnant. Her diet consists mainly of traditional Chinese food. She eats three meals a day and always brings lunch from home. Lately she has felt "tired all the time." At the screening she weighs 126 lb and measures 63 inches tall.

At the end of your clinical day, you need to compile a report on the clients you have seen. How would you interpret the data on height, weight, and nutrition? What, if any, additional information do you need to help you evaluate their nutritional status? In this chapter you will read about dietary recommendations, energy balance, and nutritional concerns across the lifespan. You will gain the theoretical knowledge to answer these questions, as well as practical knowledge about managing nutritional problems.

Theoretical Knowledge
knowing why

Low-fat, sugar-free, reduced-calorie, low-sodium, calcium-enriched . . . these are just a few of the hundreds of claims on packaged foods available today. At home, a barrage of TV and print media ads hypes nutritional supplements, weight-loss pills, and new diets, while the news carries conflicting reports on the benefits and dangers of phytochemicals, antioxidants, and trans-fatty acids. With so many options and so much advice available, it's no wonder that many people are confused about what to eat. You can help by providing accurate, current, and individualized nutritional counseling.

Nutrition is the study of food and how it affects the human body and influences health. Because good nutrition is essential to wellness and because poor nutrition contributes to disease, clients need clear and appropriate nutritional information. Before you can provide effective counseling, you need to know about the nutrients found in foods, as well as how the body

metabolizes food for energy. In addition to these topics, this chapter also explores principles of energy balance and factors that influence nutritional status.

WHAT ARE THE ENERGY NUTRIENTS?

The cells and tissues of the body depend for their functioning on building blocks called **nutrients.** Any one food may contain a variety of nutrients; for instance, cheese contains carbohydrates, protein, lipids, vitamins, and minerals. Some nutrients supply the body with energy, whereas others, called *micronutrients,* help manufacture, repair, and maintain cells. In this section, we discuss the three classes of nutrients that provide the body with energy: carbohydrates, proteins, and lipids. Table 26–1 lists the sources of and requirements for these nutrients.

The body requires a constant supply of energy. Physiological mechanisms constantly convert stores of more complex forms of chemical energy into usable energy, which is then carried to individual cells. The term **metabolism** encompasses all the ways in which the body changes and uses nutrients. Two types of

TABLE **26-1** Energy Nutrients

Nutrient	Sources	Enzymes Involved in Digestion	Requirements
Carbohydrates	*Simple sugars* occur mainly in corn syrup, honey, milk, table sugar, molasses, sugar cane, sugar beets, and fruits. *Complex carbohydrates* occur in vegetables, breads, cereals, pasta, grains, and legumes.	Salivary amylase (mouth) Ptyalin (mouth and stomach) Pancreatic amylopsin Intestinal: sucrase, lactase, maltase	There is debate about the amount of carbohydrate needed in the diet. Many popular diet plans alter carbohydrate intake: the Atkins diet is a low-carbohydrate plan, whereas the Pritikin and Ornish diets recommend high intake of complex carbohydrates. Body size and activity level affect the amount of carbohydrate used by the body. The 2002 DRIs specify that adults should get 45–65% of their calories from CHO, or 130 grams per day (g/d).
Proteins	*Complete proteins* come mostly from animal sources: meat, poultry, fish, eggs, and milk products. *Incomplete proteins* are supplied by plant sources (e.g., grains nuts, legumes, seeds, vegetables). They can be combined to make complete proteins.	Stomach: pepsin Pancreas: trypsin, chymotrypsin, carboxypeptidase Intestine: aminopeptidase, dipeptidase	Protein needs depend on age, body size, and physical state. Needs are increased during growth periods, such as childhood and pregnancy. The average adult needs about 1 gram of protein per kilogram of body weight per day. The 2002 DRIs specify that adults should get 10–35% of their calories from protein, or 0.8 g/kg of body weight (46–56 g/d for an "average" person).
Lipids	*Saturated fats* occur in pork, beef, poultry, seafood, egg yolk, and dairy; coconut oil and palm oil. *Unsaturated fats (from plants)* occur in olives, olive oil, vegetable oils (peanut, soybean, cottonsead, corn, safflower), nuts, and avocados. *Essential fatty acids (linoleic acid [omega-6] and alpha-linolenic acid [omega-3])* occur in polyunsaturated vetetable oils and in fatty fish (e.g., salmon). *Trans fats* occur in hydrogenated oils, some margarines, packaged baked goods, and many processed foods.	Lingual: lipase Gastric: lipase, tributyrinase Bile salts Pancreate lipase (steapsin)	There is debate about the appropriate amount of fat in the diet. The American Heart Association recommends that people obtain less than 30% of their calories from fat; less than 10% of calories should come from saturated fats. Clients with increased risk for heart disease may need stricter control. The 2002 DRIs specify that adults should get 20–35% of their calories from fat; children, 25–40%.

metabolic reaction, anabolism and catabolism, occur continually and are adjusted according to the needs of the body. **Anabolism** involves the formation of larger molecules from smaller ones. For example, if protein is needed for tissue repair, amino acids are recombined to form proteins. This process requires energy. **Catabolism** involves the breakdown of larger molecules into smaller components. One of the results of this separation is the release of energy. Most metabolic reactions, including metabolism of nutrients, are catalyzed by enzymes; each is specific and catalyzes only one type of reaction.

Carbohydrates

Carbohydrates (CHO) are the primary energy source for the body. **Simple carbohydrates,** commonly called *sugars,* are named according to the number of sugar (or *saccharide*) units making up their chemical structure (Figure 26–1). **Monosaccharides** (simple sugars) consist of a single unit; **disaccharides** are molecules made up of two saccharides. **Complex carbohydrates** consist of long chains of saccharides, called **polysaccharides. Dietary fiber,** a polysaccharide, is the indigestible "fibrous skeleton" of plant foods. Humans do not have the enzymes to digest fiber; thus, it provides no usable glucose.

Carbohydrates perform several functions:

1. *Supply energy for muscle and organ function.* Carbohydrates, which are more easily and quickly digested than proteins and lipids, fuel strenuous short-term skeleton muscle activity and provide nearly all the energy for the brain. Human beings store glucose in liver and skeletal muscle tissue as **glycogen.** Glycogen is converted back into glucose to meet energy needs. This process is called **glycogenolysis.** If carbohydrates are not available, proteins and lipids (fats) can also be used for energy.

2. *"Spare protein."* If glycogen stores are low (for instance, in a person who is undernourished), physical activity causes the breakdown of body stores of protein **(gluconeogenesis)** and lipids (fats) to use for energy. Unfortunately, when proteins are used for energy, they are then not available for their primary functions of tissue growth, maintenance, and repair. Fats are converted directly into an alternative fuel called **ketones;** ketones raise the acidity of the blood and can lead to acid-base imbalance.

3. *Other physiological functions.* Carbohydrates enhance insulin secretion, increase satiety (feeling of fullness and satisfaction), and improve absorption of sodium and excretion of calcium. **Insulin** is a pancreatic hormone that promotes the movement of glucose into the cells for use.

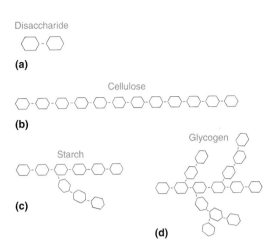

FIGURE 26–1 Carbohydrates. Each hexagon represents a 6-carbon simple sugar, such as glucose. *A,* A disaccharide, such as maltose. *B,* Cellulose, a polysaccharide. *C,* Starch, a polysaccharide. *D,* Glycogen, a polysaccharide.

Refer to Table 26–1: How many servings of carbohydrates did you eat yesterday? How many were simple carbohydrates? How many were complex carbohydrates?

Proteins

Proteins are complex molecules made up of *amino acids.* Every amino acid consists of a central carbon atom connected to a hydrogen atom, an acid, an *amine* (a region of the molecule containing nitrogen) and a side chain. Only the side chain varies from one amino acid to another (Figure 26–2). Just 20 different amino acids are the building blocks of most of the proteins in the human (Table 26–2). The **essential amino acids** are significant in our diets because the body cannot manufacture them. They must be supplied by food or nutritional supplements. In contrast, the body can synthesize the 10 **nonessential amino acids.** Therefore, we do not need to obtain them from food.

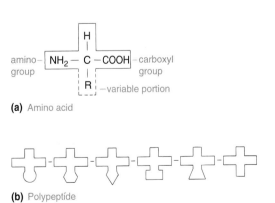

FIGURE 26–2 Amino acids. *A,* The structural formula of an amino acid. The "R" represents the variable portion of the molecule. *B,* A polypeptide. Several amino acids, represented by different shapes, are linked by peptide bonds.

TABLE 26-2   Amino Acids

Type	Description	Examples
Essential	Must be obtained from the diet; cannot be made in the body	Arginine*, histidine, isoleucine, leucine, lysine, methionine, phenylalanine, threonine, tryptophan, and valine
Nonessential	Easily synthesized by the body	Alanine, aspargine, aspartic acid, cysteine, glutamic acid, glutamine, glycine, proline, serine, and tyrosine

*Considered by some to be "semiessential" because it cannot be synthesized at a rate that will support growth. Therefore, it is essential for children, but not for most adults.

Sources: Grodner, M., Anderson, S., & DeYoung, S. (2000). Foundations and clinical applications of nutrition: A nursing approach (2nd ed.). St Louis: Mosby; Guyton, A. C., & Hall, J. E. (2000). Textbook of medical physiology (10th ed.). Philadelphia: W. B. Saunders; Thompson, J., & Manore, M. (2005). Nutrition and health: An applied approach. San Francisco: Benjamin Cummings; Williams, S. R. (1995). Basic nutrition and diet therapy (10th ed.). St Louis: Mosby.

For protein synthesis to occur, every amino acid necessary to build that protein must be available. **Complete protein** foods contain all of the essential amino acids necessary for protein synthesis. These usually come from animal sources. **Incomplete protein** foods (e.g., nuts, grains) do not provide all of the essential amino acids. However, by combining two incomplete proteins, a complete protein can be made. For instance, peanut butter on whole-grain bread constitutes a complete protein. Protein complementing allows for a healthful vegetarian diet.

Refer to Table 26–1: How many servings of protein did you eat yesterday? How many were complete proteins? How many were incomplete proteins? Do you think that protein foods accounted for more than 10% of your food intake yesterday?

Protein Metabolism and Storage

Although protein digestion begins in the stomach, most protein digestion occurs in the small intestine, where enzymes break it down into amino acids (see Table 26–1). The body continually breaks down and resynthesizes protein into tissues, adjusting as needed to maintain overall protein balance. The body also maintains a balance between tissue protein and plasma protein. When amino acids are catabolized, the nitrogen-containing part is converted to ammonia (NH_3) and excreted in the urine as urea. Therefore, nitrogen balance reflects how well body tissues are being maintained.

Nitrogen balance occurs when intake and output of nitrogen are equal. A **positive nitrogen balance** exists when nitrogen intake exceeds output, making a pool of amino acids available for growth, pregnancy, and tissue maintenance and repair.

Negative nitrogen balance exists when nitrogen intake is lower than nitrogen loss. This occurs in illness, injury (e.g., burns), and malnutrition. Which patient ("Meet Your Patients") is probably in positive nitrogen balance?

Functions of Protein

Dietary proteins perform the following functions:

1. *Tissue building.* Protein is the structural material of every cell in the body. In fact, except for water, protein makes up the biggest part of the body. It is essential for growth, maintenance, and repair of body cells and tissues.
2. *Metabolism.* **Enzymes,** which facilitate cellular reactions throughout the body, are proteins. For example, proteins are precursors to digestive enzymes and hormones (e.g., thyroxine). In addition, proteins combine with iron to form hemoglobin, the oxygen carrier in red blood cells.
3. *Immune system function.* Lymphocytes (special white blood cells) and antibodies (components of our immune system that defend against foreign invaders) are proteins.
4. *Fluid balance.* Because they attract water, proteins in cells and the bloodstream help regulate fluid balance.
5. *Acid-base balance.* Blood proteins function as buffers, helping to regulate acid-base balance.
6. *Secondary energy source.* As noted earlier, proteins can be broken down to provide energy when stores of the other energy nutrients are inadequate (Thompson & Manore, 2005).

Individual protein needs vary according to age, sex, weight, and health. Most North Americans eat

BOX 26-1 Types of Lipids

Glycerol molecules (bonded to) Fatty acid molecules		
Glycerides		
Monoglycerides	1	1
Diglycerides	1	2
Triglycerides	1	3
Sterols	0	0
Phospholipids	1	2 + a phosphate group

more protein than they need, especially in the form of meat. There is no health benefit from eating more than the recommended amount of protein. In fact, there may be health risks in eating diets high in animal protein, which (1) adds saturated fat to the diet, increasing the risk for certain cancers and coronary artery disease; and (2) has been associated with kidney stones and calcium loss through the urinary system.

Lipids

Lipids are organic (carbon-containing) substances that are insoluble in water. They are made up of carbon, hydrogen, and oxygen—the same basic elements that make up carbohydrates. The term *lipid* comes from *lipos,* the Greek word for "fat." Technically speaking, however, only lipids that are solid at room temperature are called **fats,** whereas those that are liquid at room temperature are called **oils.** For example, butter is a fat even when it is melted, because it would be solid at room temperature.

People in developed countries typically eat a diet relatively high in fat. In the United States, about 45% of our total kcals come from fat. Fat is an essential nutrient, but certain types, when overconsumed, can also be a health hazard.

Lipid metabolism occurs in the small intestine, where bile and pancreatic enzymes begin splitting the fatty acids from their glycerol backbone. Lipids are stored as adipose tissue. Because lipids are insoluble in water, and because blood is primarily water, lipid absorption requires a solvent carrier.

Types and Sources of Lipids

The three types of lipids found in foods are glycerides, sterols, and phospholipids (Box 26–1). **Glycerides** (also called **true fats**) consist of one molecule of glycerol attached to one, two, or three fatty acid chains (Figure 26–3). *Glycerol* is an alcohol composed of three

carbon atoms. *Fatty acids* are long chains of carbon and hydrogen atoms ending in an acid. Most glycerides found in foods are *triglycerides,* which are compounds consisting of a glycerol molecule attached to three fatty acids.

Sterols are lipids, but they are not made of fatty acids. They consist of rings of carbon and hydrogen. The most important sterol in the body is **cholesterol,** a waxlike substance needed for the formation of cell membranes, vitamin D, estrogen, and testosterone. Cholesterol is synthesized in the liver, and it is also found in the fatty portion of animal foods.

Phospholipids (which contain a phosphate group) are soluble in water. They are a key component of **lipoproteins,** which consist of phospholipids and a protein. Because they are water soluble, lipoproteins are the major transport vehicles for lipids in the bloodstream. By "wrapping" triglycerides with water-soluble phosphates and proteins, lipoproteins deliver these substances to body cells.

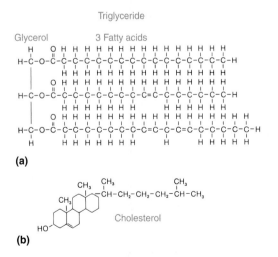

FIGURE 26–3 Lipids. *A,* a triglyderide made of one glycerol and three fatty acids. *B,* The steroid cholesterol. The hexagons represent rings of carbon and hydrogen.

TABLE 26–3 Dietary Fats

Type of Fat	Sources	Effect on Blood Cholesterol
Monounsaturated	Olives; olive oil, canola oil, peanut oil; cashews, almonds, peanuts, and most other nuts; avocados	Lowers LDL Raises HDL
Polyunsaturated	Corn, soybean, safflower, and cottonseed oils; fish	Lowers LDL Raises HDL
Saturated	Whole milk, butter, cheese, and ice cream; red meat; chocolate; coconuts, coconut milk, and coconut oil	Raises LDL Raises HDL
Trans-fatty acids	Most margarines; vegetable shortening; partially hydrogenated vegetable oil; deep-fried chips; many fast foods; most commercial baked goods	Raises LDL

- **Low-density lipoproteins (LDL)** transport cholesterol to body cells. Diets high in saturated fats increase LDLs circulating in the bloodstream and may result in fatty deposits on vessel walls, causing cardiovascular disease. As a result, LDL is often known as the "bad cholesterol."

- **High-density lipoproteins (HDL)** remove cholesterol from the bloodstream, returning it to the liver, where it is used to produce bile; thus, a high blood level of HDL is considered protective against cardiovascular disease. It is often known as the "good cholesterol."

Saturated and Unsaturated Fatty Acids

Fatty acids are classified as either saturated or unsaturated. **Saturation** means that a substance is holding all that it is capable of holding (e.g., think of a wound dressing saturated with blood). In **saturated fatty acids,** every carbon atom is fully bound to (or "saturated" with) hydrogen. The molecules pack tightly together at room temperature and are dense, solid, and heavy. A fat made up mostly of saturated fatty acids is called a **saturated fat.**

Animal fats are the primary source of saturated fats in the North American diet; however, many processed foods contain saturated fats. In addition, saturated fats called **trans-fatty acids** are found in many margarines and other processed foods containing *hydrogenated vegetable oils.* In the process of *hydrogenation,* food manufacturers add hydrogen to polyunsaturated plant oils, such as corn oil, to break the double carbon bonds and straighten out the molecules. This process both solidifies the fat and protects it against rancidity; however, many researchers consider trans-fatty acids to be even more harmful to health than saturated fats of animal origin (Severson & Burke, 2003). Saturated fats have been shown to increase blood cholesterol levels.

An **unsaturated fatty acid** is one that is not completely filled with all the hydrogen it can hold. Therefore, it is lighter and less dense. Fats made up primarily of unsaturated fatty acids are called **unsaturated fats.** Molecules of **monounsaturated fats** have one unfilled spot where hydrogen is not attached. **Polyunsaturated fatty acids** contain two or more unfilled spots for hydrogen. At the spot(s) where the molecule does not have a hydrogen attached, it becomes kinked and does not pack together. This is why these fats are liquid at room temperature. Replacing saturated fats in the diet with mono- and polyunsaturated fats reduces the risk of heart disease and stroke.

Refer to Table 26–3: How many servings of fat did you eat yesterday? How many were saturated fats; how many were unsaturated?

Essential and Nonessential Fatty Acids

As with proteins, a fatty acid is considered **essential** if (1) the body cannot manufacture it and (2) its absence creates a deficiency disease. The essential fatty acids are **linoleic acid (omega-6)** and **alpha-linolenic acid (omega-3).** Omega-6 fatty acid is found mainly in polyunsaturated vegetable oils. Omega-3 fatty acid can be obtained in adequate amounts by eating fatty fish twice a week (Wardlaw, Hampl, & DiSilvestro, 2004).

Functions of Lipids

Lipids perform the following functions:

1. *Supply essential nutrients.* Food fats supply the essential fatty acids and aid in the absorption of fat-soluble vitamins.
2. *Energy source.* Although carbohydrates are the primary energy source during strenuous physical activity, our bodies burn fat for energy when we are engaging in sustained light activity, such as walking or gardening, and when we are at rest. The body also burns fat for energy when glycogen stores are exhausted.
3. *Flavor and satiety.* The lipid content of food gives it its creamy taste and texture and promotes our sense of satiety. Fats are digested more slowly than carbohydrates, so stomach emptying time is slower.
4. *Other functions.* Body fat provides thermal insulation, protects vital organs, and enables accurate nerve-impulse transmission. In addition, lipids are a component of every cell membrane and are essential to cell metabolism.
5. *Cholesterol functions.* Cholesterol is a component of every cell in the body, where it lends suppleness and support. It is also a component of bile, which helps digest fats, and serves as a precursor to all steroid hormones, including sex hormones. When lipid metabolism is "disordered," cholesterol contributes to atherosclerosis.

 CriticalThinking 26–1

Review the information you collected on the two employees ("Meet Your Patients").

- What conclusions, if any, can you make about their intake of carbohydrates, protein, and lipids?
- How might you gather additional data on their intake of the energy nutrients?

WHAT ARE THE MICRONUTRIENTS?

Vitamins and minerals are called **micronutrients** because they are required by the body only in very small amounts. Although they provide no energy, they are critical in regulating a variety of body functions.

Vitamins

Vitamins are organic substances that are necessary for metabolism or preventing a particular deficiency disease. Because the body cannot make vitamins, they must be supplied by the foods we eat. Vitamins are critical in building and maintaining body tissues, supporting our immune system so we can fight disease,

and ensuring healthy vision. They also help our bodies to break down and use the energy found in carbohydrates, proteins, and lipids (Thompson & Manore, 2005). Vitamins are especially critical during periods of rapid growth, pregnancy, lactation, and convalescence. Some evidence supports the claim that certain vitamins prevent chronic illness (Institute of Medicine, 2000).

Table 26–4 summarizes information about vitamins, including specific functions and recommended dietary allowances (RDAs). RDAs represent the daily dietary intake that is adequate to meet the needs of 97 to 98% of all healthy individuals in a group, such as men, women, or infants (National Academy of Sciences, 2001).

The **fat-soluble vitamins** are A, D, E, and K. They are found in fatty foods, such as butter, fish, and poultry. They are stored primarily in the liver and adipose tissues, although vitamin E is deposited in all body tissue. Because the body can store these vitamins, we do not need to consume them every day; however, diets extremely low in fat and disorders affecting fat digestion and absorption can lead to deficiency of fat-soluble vitamins. In contrast, because they are not readily excreted, excessive supplementation with the fat-soluble vitamins can lead to toxicity. Vitamin D is unique in that the body can synthesize it from a cholesterol compound in the skin when we receive adequate exposure to sunlight. However, adequate exposure is not possible in winter months for anyone living at a latitude of 40° or more north or south of the equator.

The **water-soluble vitamins** include vitamin C and the B-complex vitamins: thiamine, riboflavin, niacin, pyridoxine (vitamin B_6), folic acid, pantothenic acid, biotin, and cyanocobalamin (vitamin B_{12}). Because these vitamins are soluble in water, excess amounts are regularly excreted by the kidneys in the urine. Thus, toxicity is rare except in people with renal disease. However, because excess amounts are excreted, the body cannot store these vitamins; so they need to be consumed every day. Inadequate intake is much more likely to lead to deficiency in water-soluble vitamins than to deficiency in fat-soluble vitamins.

Minerals

Minerals are inorganic elements found in nature. They occur in foods either naturally or as additives, as well as in supplements. **Major minerals (macrominerals)** are minerals that the body needs in amounts of 100 mg/day or greater. **Trace minerals** are essential, but in a lower concentration. In the United States, calcium deficiency is one of the most common mineral

deficiencies. See Table 26–5 for information about selected minerals.

Minerals assist in fluid regulation, nerve impulse transmission, and energy production; they are essential to the health of bones and blood and help rid the body of harmful by-products of metabolism (Thompson & Manore, 2005). Evidence also shows that minerals play key roles in disease prevention and treatment. For example:

1. Adequate *calcium* intake throughout the life span decreases the likelihood of osteoporosis (a condition marked by porous bones).
2. *Iron* deficiency causes anemia, the most common nutritional problem worldwide.
3. *Magnesium* may decrease the risk of hypertension and coronary artery disease in women.

Minerals are absorbed mostly in the large intestine. If the body is deficient in a mineral, it absorbs more; if the body has enough, it absorbs less and excretes more in the feces. Minerals interact with other minerals, vitamins, and other substances to accomplish absorption and metabolism and perform their functions. For example, iron absorption is enhanced in the presence of vitamin C, and vitamin D deficiency inhibits calcium absorption.

WHY IS WATER AN ESSENTIAL NUTRIENT?

Water is made up of hydrogen and oxygen. Water makes up about half of total body weight (55–65% in men and 50–55% in women). Men have greater muscle mass; muscle contains a relatively large amount of water. Water is distributed in two body compartments. **Intracellular fluid** is the water contained within each living cell. It makes up about 40% of the total body weight. **Extracellular fluid** is external to the cell membrane (e.g., in the fluid portion of blood and lymph and in the gastrointestinal tract); it accounts for 20% of body weight. Water is critical to the body because its functions are essential to life:

1. *Solvent.* Water is the basic solvent for the body's chemical processes.
2. *Transport.* Circulating as blood, water serves as a medium for transporting oxygen, nutrients, and metabolic wastes.
3. *Body structure and form.* Water "fills in the spaces" in body tissues (e.g., in muscle).
4. *Temperature.* Water helps maintain body temperature. When body temperature rises, evaporation of sweat helps cool the body.

The amount of water a person requires varies according to the environmental humidity and temperature, activity level, age, and metabolic needs. The average adult needs to drink about 2.5 to 3 liters of water per day. We also obtain water in the foods we eat. What foods can you think of that are high in water content?

Overall fluid balance is maintained when fluid intake in liquids, foods, and metabolic reactions matches fluid output through urine, feces, respiration, and sweat. Fluid and electrolyte balance is discussed in Chapter 36.

KnowledgeCheck 26–1

* What is the body's most usable energy source?
* Which nutrient's primary function is growth and repair of tissue?
* Identify five functions of adipose tissue (body fat).
* Which type of vitamin requires daily consumption to maintain appropriate levels?
* What distinguishes a major mineral from a trace mineral?
* Identify at least four functions of water.

 Go to Chapter 26, **Knowledge Check Response Sheet and Answers,** on the Electronic Study Guide.

WHAT ARE SOME RELIABLE SOURCES OF NUTRITION INFORMATION?

For the body to function at an optimal level, nutrients must be supplied in specific amounts. Nutrition information sources are of two types: standards and guides. **Standards** are a reference for nutrient intake thought to meet the nutritional needs of most healthy population groups. They are not intended to indicate individual requirements or therapeutic needs. Rather, they list nutrient amounts in measurements, such as grams and milligrams. **Food guides** are more practical tools that you can use in educating patients and families. They specify the number of servings of foods and food groups needed daily, so nonprofessionals can use them in making healthful meal choices. In general, standards and guides provide recommendations to healthy individuals but they are not sensitive to the needs of people experiencing metabolic or other medical problems.

Dietary Reference Intakes (DRIs)

The National Academy of Sciences, in a collaborative effort by the United States and Canada, has established standards, the **Dietary Reference Intakes (DRIs),** to promote the consumption of healthful nutrient levels. For carbohydrates and lipids, the *acceptable macronutrient distribution range (AMDR)* is used. To view the DRIs and AMDRs for males and females in various age groups,

 Go to Chapter 26, **Reading More About Nutrition, Supplemental Materials, Dietary Reference Intakes: Vitamins, Dietary Reference Intakes: Macronutrients,** and **Dietary Reference Intakes: Elements,** on the Electronic Study Guide.

TABLE 26–4 Vitamins: Adult Dietary Reference Intakes (DRIs)[*]

Vitamin	Function	RDA[†]	Sources	Effects of Deficiency	Symptoms of Excess
			Fat-Soluble Vitamins		
A	• Night and color vision • Cellular growth and maturity • Maintaining healthy skin and mucous membranes • Growth of skeletal and soft tissues • Reproduction	700–900 mcg/d	Fish liver oil, liver, butter, cream, egg yolk, yellow fruit, green leafy vegetables, fortified milk	Night blindness, xerosis, xerophthalmia, keratomalacia, skin lesions	GI upset, headache, blurred vision, poor muscle coordination, fetal defects
D	• Regulates blood calcium levels • Regulates rate of deposit and resorption of calcium in bone	5–10 mcg/d(AI)	Fish liver oil, fish, fortified milk, sunlight exposure	Bone and muscle pain, weakness, softening of bone, fractures, rickets	Fatigue, weakness, loss of appetite, headache, mental confusion, mental retardation in infants
E	• Antioxidant • Protects red blood cells and muscle tissue cells	15 mg/d	Vegetable oils, nuts, milk, eggs, muscle meats, fish, wheat and rice germ, green leafy vegetables	Hyporeflexia, ataxia, hemolytic anemia, myopathy	Insufficient blood clotting, impaired immune system
K	• Synthesis of clotting factors • Bone development	75–90 mcg/d(AI)	Green leafy vegetables, liver (Intestinal bacteria synthesize a form of vitamin K, so deficiency is unlikely.)	Increased bleeding	Jaundice and hemolytic anemia in infants
			Water-Soluble Vitamins		
Thiamin	• Cellular metabolism (producing energy from glucose and storing energy as fat) • Nervous system function • Gastrointestinal system function • Cardiovascular system function	1–1.2 mg/d	Whole grain, enriched cereal, beef, pork, liver, peas, beans, nuts	Peripheral neuritis, loss of muscle strength, depression, memory loss, anorexia, constipation, dyspnea, decreased alertness and reflexes, fatigue, irritability, beriberi	Unlikely; readily excreted
Riboflavin	• Cellular metabolism • Antioxidant • Tissue health and growth	1–1.3 mg/d	Milk, cheese, eggs, green vegetables, whole grain, enriched grains, bread, organ meats, poultry, fish	Tissue inflammation and breakdown: Sore throat, stomatitis, swollen tongue, facial dermatitis, anemia; poor wound healing	Unlikely; readily excreted

TABLE 26-4 Vitamins: Adult Dietary Reference Intakes (DRIs)* *(continued)*

Vitamin	Function	RDA†	Sources	Effects of Deficiency	Symptoms of Excess
Niacin	Cellular metabolism to produce energy	14–16 mg/d	Enriched breads and cereals, chicken, tuna, liver, peanuts, dairy products	Weakness, poor appetite, indigestion, dermatitis, diarrhea, headache, dizziness, insomnia. Chronic: CNS damage (confusion, neuritis, dementia), pellagra	Facial flushing, itching, nausea, liver damage
B_6 (Pyridoxine)	• Protein (and some carbohydrate) metabolism • RBC production • Neurotransmitter synthesis	1.3–1.5 mg/d	Meats, poultry, fish, beans, nuts, seeds, dairy products, enriched cereals	Rash, stomatitis, seizure, peripheral neuritis, depression	Irreversible nerve damage (i.e., extremity numbness, walking difficulties)
Pantothenic acid	• Cell metabolism of fat and cholesterol • Amino acid activation • Heme formation	5 mg/d (AI)	Occurs widely in most foods. Best sources: meats, whole grain cereals, legumes	Deficiency is unknown	Unlikely; readily excreted
Folacin (folate, folic acid)	• Cellular metabolism • Neurotransmitter synthesis • Cell division • DNA synthesis • Hemoglobin formation	400 mcg/d	Green leafy vegetables, asparagus, liver, yeast, eggs, beans, fruits, enriched cereals	Megaloblastic anemia, neural tube defects	Increased seizure activity, hives, respiratory distress, itching, rash
B_{12} (cyanocobalamin)	• Metabolic reactions • Maintain myelin sheath • Hemoglobin synthesis	2.4 mcg/d	Dairy products, meat, poultry, fish, liver, milk, cheese, eggs	Pernicious anemia, irreversible nerve damage, memory loss, dementia	Unlikely; readily excreted
C	• Collagen synthesis • "Cementing" substance for capillary walls • Antioxidant • Iron absorption • Immune function	75–90 mg/d	Citrus fruits, tomatoes, potatoes, green vegetables, cauliflower	Anemia, tissue bleeding, easy bone fracture, gingivitis, petechiae, poor wound healing, joint pain, scurvy	Stomach inflammation, diarrhea, oxalate kidney stones

*Dietary Reference Intakes (DRIs) represent:
  • Recommended Dietary Allowances (RDAs)—Intake set to meet the needs of 97–98% of individuals in a group
  • Adequate Intakes (AIs)—Believed to cover the needs of all individuals in the group.
  • Upper Intake Levels (UIs)—The maximum daily intake likely to pose no risk of adverse affects.
Values in table are RDAs unless marked (AI).

†RDAs are usually less than adult values for infants and children, more for pregnant women, and highest for lactating women. RDAs for some vitamins (e.g., vitamin A) are higher for older adults and higher for men than for women.

 Go to Chapter 26, **Supplemental Materials, Dietary Reference Intakes: Vitamins,** on the Electronic Study Guide.

Sources: Dietary reference intakes for energy, carbohydrate, fiber, fat, fatty acids, cholesterol, protein, and amino acids. (2002). Washington, DC: The National Academies Press. Also available at www.nap.edu, retrieved February 27, 2004. Guyton, A. C., & Hall, J. E. (2000) *Textbook of medical physiology* (10th ed.). St Louis: Mosby; Scanlon, V. C., & Sanders, T. (2003). *Essentials of anatomy and physiology* (4th ed.). Philadelphia: F. A. Davis Company.

TABLE 26–5 Minerals: Adult Dietary Reference Intakes[*]

Mineral	Function	RDA[†]	Sources	Effects of Deficiency	Symptoms of Excess
			Macrominerals		
Calcium (Ca)	Bone and teeth formation, blood clotting, nerve conduction, muscle contraction, cellular metabolism, heart action	1000–1300 mg/d (AI)	Dairy products, sardines, green leafy vegetables, broccoli, whole grains, egg yolks, legumes, nuts, fortified products	Bone loss, tetany, rickets, osteoporosis	Kidney stones, constipation, intestinal gas
Magnesium (Mg)	Aids thyroid hormone secretion, maintains normal basal metabolic rate, activates enzymes for carbohydrate and protein metabolism, nerve and muscle function, cardiac function	240–420 mg/d	Whole grains, nuts, legumes, green leafy vegetables, lima beans, broccoli, squash, potatoes	Tremor, spasm, convulsions, weakness, muscle pain, poor cardiac function	Weakness, nausea, malaise
Phosphorus (P)	Bone and tooth strength, overall metabolism, formation of enzymes, acid-base balance	700–1250 mg/d	Dairy products, beef, pork, beans, sardines, eggs, chicken, wheat bran, chocolate	Bone loss Poor growth	Tetany, convulsions
Potassium (K)	Intracellular fluid control, acid-base balance, nerve transmission, muscle contraction, glycogen formation, protein synthesis, energy metabolism, blood pressure regulation	No RDA established. Range for adults is about 2000–3500 mg/d	Unprocessed foods, especially fruits, many vegetables, meats, potatoes, avocados, legumes, milk, molasses, shellfish, dates, figs	Muscle weakness (including weakness of heart and respiratory muscles), weak pulse, fatigue, abdominal distention (Rarely occurs as a result of inadequate dietary intake. More likely due to losses from prolonged vomiting, diarrhea, or some diuretic drugs.)	Cardiac dysrhythmias, cardiac arrest, weakness, abdominal cramps, diarrhea, anxiety, paresthesia
Sodium (Na)	Water balance, acid-base balance, muscle action, nerve transmission	No stated RDA. Limit to ≤ 2.4 g/d	Table salt (NaCl), milk, meat, eggs, baking soda, baking powder, celery, spinach, carrots, beets	Dizziness, abdominal cramping, nausea, vomiting, diarrhea, tachycardia, convulsions, coma (rarely occurs except in heavy exercise and sweating)	Thirst, fever, dry and sticky tongue and mucous membranes, restlessness, irritability, convulsions

➤

TABLE 26-5 Minerals: Adult Dietary Reference Intakes[*] *(continued)*

Mineral	Function	RDA[†]	Sources	Effects of Deficiency	Symptoms of Excess
		Trace Minerals			
Copper	Aids in iron metabolism, works with many enzymes in protein metabolism and hormone synthesis	700–900 mcg/d	Liver, seafood, cocoa, legumes, nuts, whole grains	Rarely occurs: anemia, low WBC count, poor growth	Vomiting, nervous system disorders
Fluoride	Increases resistance to dental caries	3–4 mg/d (AI)	Fluorinated water, toothpaste, dental treatment, seaweed, fish, tea	Increased dental caries	Stomach upset, staining of teeth, bone pain
Iodine	Synthesis of the thyroid hormone, thyroxine	150 mcg/d	Iodized salt, saltwater fish, dairy products, enriched white bread	Goiter, poor infancy growth, cretinism, hypothyroidism	Skin lesions, thyroid malfunction
Iron	Synthesis of hemoglobin, general metabolism (e.g., of glucose), antibody production, drug detoxification in the liver	8–18 mg/d	Meats, eggs, spinach, seafood, broccoli, peas, bran, enriched breads, fortified cereals	Small, pale RBCs, anemia	Hemochromatosis
Zinc	Cofactor for many enzymes involved in growth, insulin storage immunity, alcohol metabolism, sexual development and reproduction	8–11 mg/d	Primarily meats and seafood; also legumes, peas, and whole grains	Skin rash, diarrhea, decreased appetite, hair loss, poor growth and development, poor wound healing	Reduced copper absorption, diarrhea, cramps, depressed immune function

[*]Dietary Reference Intakes (DRIs) represent:
  • Recommended Dietary Allowances (RDAs)—Intake set to meet the needs of 97–98% of individuals in a group.
  • Adequate Intakes (AIs)—Believed to cover the needs of all individuals in the group.
  • Upper Intake Levels (UIs)—The maximum daily intake likely to pose no risk of adverse affects.
Values in table are RDAs unless marked (AI).

[†]RDAs are usually less than adult values for infants and children, more for pregnant women, and highest for lactating women. RDAs for some minerals are higher for older adults and different for men and women.

 Go to Chapter 26, **Supplemental Materials, Dietary Reference Intakes: Elements,** on the Electronic Study Guide.

Sources: Dietary reference intakes for energy, carbohydrate, fiber, fat, fatty acids, cholesterol, protein, and amino acids. (2002). Washington, DC: The National Academies Press. Also available at www.nap.edu, retrieved February 27, 2004. Guyton, A. C., & Hall, J. E. (2000). *Textbook of medical physiology* (10th ed.). St Louis: Mosby; Scanlon, V. C., & Sanders, T. (2003). *Essentials of anatomy and physiology* (4th ed.). Philadelphia: F. A. Davis Company.

The DRIs are a revision of the older **Recommended Dietary Allowances (RDAs)** for vitamins and minerals, protein, and total kcals that are thought to meet the needs of 97 to 98% of individuals in a group. For vitamins and minerals, the DRI tables include RDAs and **Adequate Intakes (AIs),** intakes adequate to meet the needs of all individuals in a group.

 The National Academy of Sciences (NAS) government web site, **www.nap.edu,** offers files you can download.

BOX 26-2 Dietary Guidelines for Americans 2005— Key Points

- Consume a variety of nutrient-rich foods daily.
- Adopt a balanced eating pattern (e.g., the USDA Food Guide) to meet recommended intakes.
- Limit the intake of saturated fats, trans fats, and cholesterol. Keep fat intake below 20 to 35% of total calories. Most fats should come from foods such as fish, nuts, and vegetable oils.
- Limit your intake of added sugars, salt, and alcohol.
- Achieve and maintain a healthy weight.
- Be physically active each day.
- Balance calorie intake with increase or decrease in activity.
- Choose a variety of fruits and vegetables each day.
- Choose fiber-rich fruit, vegetables, and whole grains often. At least half the grains should come from whole grains.
- Cook, chill, and store foods to keep them safe from microorganisms.
- Clean hands, food contact surfaces, and fruits and vegetables. Do not wash or rinse meat and poultry. (Also see Chapter 21 for food safety.)

Source: Abstracted from U.S. Department of Agriculture. (2005). *Dietary guidelines for Americans 2005.* Retrieved April 26, 2005, from www.healthierus.gov/dietaryguidelines

USDA Dietary Guidelines

In 1980 the United States Department of Agriculture (USDA) developed dietary guidelines for Americans. Box 26–2 presents current guidelines to help people evaluate their food habits and work toward general improvement in their diet. The guidelines do not specify daily amounts of food and nutrients.

Canada's Food Guide for Healthy Eating

Canada's Food Guide to Healthy Eating (Figure 26–4) advises choosing a variety of foods from each of four groups. A high and low number is given for each group, and people are advised to choose their total amount of food based on age, body size, activity level, gender, pregnancy, and lactation. The specified range of servings furnishes 1000 to 1400 kcals.

USDA Food Guide Pyramid

In 1992, the USDA introduced a diet-teaching tool called the Food Guide Pyramid. A new tool, called MyPyramid (Figure 26–5), replaced the old pyramid in 2005. Based on USDA dietary guidelines, it illustrates healthful daily food choices. MyPyramid stresses the following concepts for healthy eating:

- *Activity.* The steps are a reminder of the importance of daily physical activity.
- *Moderation.* The wider base represents foods with little or no solid fats or added sugars. The narrower top area stands for foods with more solid fats and sugars, which should be eaten less often.
- *Personalization.* The person on the steps of the pyramid symbolizes the need to individualize diet choices (one size does *not* fit all). To find the kinds and amounts of food you need to eat each day, based on personal factors,

 Go to the **MyPyramid web site at http://www.MyPyramid.gov**

- *Proportionality.* Notice that the food group bands are of different widths. The widths are a general guide to how much food you should choose from each group. For example, the "Oils" group is a very thin area, and the "Grains" area is very large. This gives you a general idea that you should eat many more servings of grains than of oils.
- *Variety.* Six different colors represent the food groups. This illustrates the importance of variety in your diet; you need foods from all groups each day.
- *Gradual improvement.* The slogan, "Steps to a Healthier You," suggests that you can benefit from taking even small steps to improve your diet and lifestyle.

For information about serving sizes and nutrients provided by each food group, see Table 26–6 on page 590.

You can find several other food guide pyramids, as well. For a Vegetarian Diet Pyramid, see Figure 26–6 on page 591. For Asian, Latin, Vegetarian, and Mediterranean Diet Pyramids,

 Go to the **Oldways Preservation and Exchange Trust web site at www.oldwayspt.org**

and follow the "Traditional Diet Pyramids" Link.

For a Food Guide Pyramid for People Over 70 Years,

 Go to the **Tufts University Friedman School of Nutrition Science and Policy web site at http://nutrition.tufts.edu/consumer/pyramid.html**

For the Diabetes Food Pyramid,

 Go to the **American Diabetes Association web site at http://www.diabetes.org/nutrition-and-recipes/nutrition/foodpyramid.jsp**

FIGURE 26–4 **Canada's Food Guide for Healthy Eating.** *Source:* From *Canada's Food Guide to Healthy Eating,* Health Canada, 1992. Reproduced with the permission of the Minister of Public Works and Government Services: Canada, 2004.

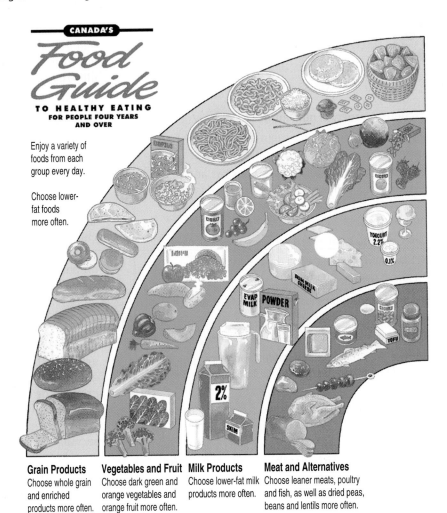

Enjoy a variety of foods from each group every day.

Choose lower-fat foods more often.

Grain Products
Choose whole grain and enriched products more often.

Vegetables and Fruit
Choose dark green and orange vegetables and orange fruit more often.

Milk Products
Choose lower-fat milk products more often.

Meat and Alternatives
Choose leaner meats, poultry and fish, as well as dried peas, beans and lentils more often.

Different People Need Different Amounts of Food

The amount of food you need every day from the four food groups and other foods depends on your age, body size, activity level, whether you are male or female, and if you are pregnant or breast-feeding. That's why the Food Guide gives a lower and higher number of servings for each food group. For example, young children can choose the lower number of servings, while male teenagers can go to the higher number. Most other people can choose servings somewhere in between.

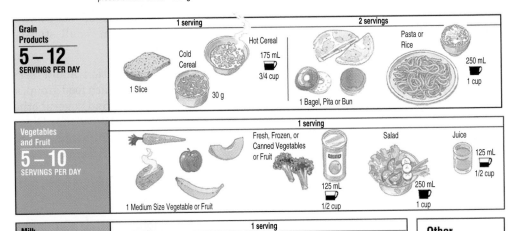

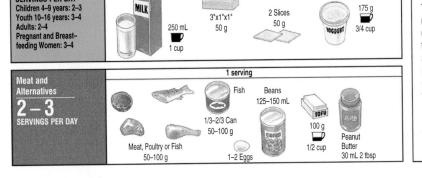

Other Foods

Taste and enjoyment can also come from other foods and beverages that are not part of the 4 food groups. Some of these foods are higher in fat or Calories, so use these foods in moderation.

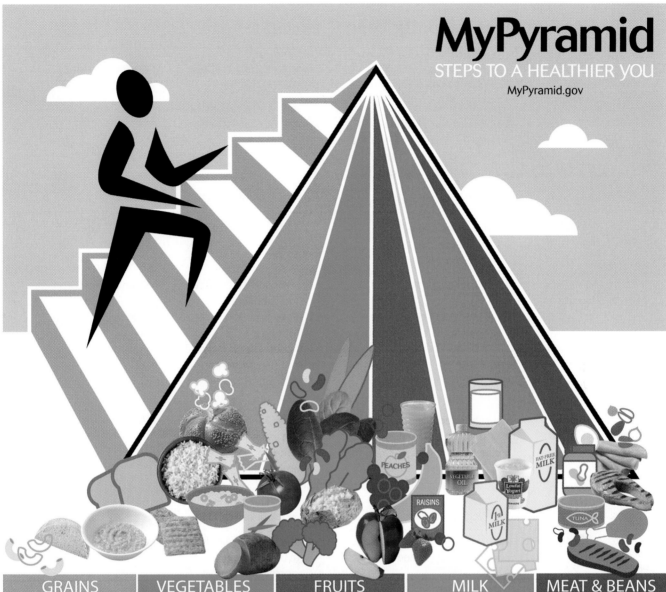

MyPyramid
STEPS TO A HEALTHIER YOU
MyPyramid.gov

GRAINS	VEGETABLES	FRUITS	MILK	MEAT & BEANS
Make half your grains whole	Vary your veggies	Focus on fruits	Get your calcium-rich foods	Go lean with protein
Eat at least 3 oz. of whole-grain cereals, breads, crackers, rice, or pasta every day 1 oz. is about 1 slice of bread, about 1 cup of breakfast cereal, or 1/2 cup of cooked rice, cereal, or pasta	Eat more dark-green veggies like broccoli, spinach, and other dark leafy greens Eat more orange vegetables like carrots and sweetpotatoes Eat more dry beans and peas like pinto beans, kidney beans, lentils	Eat a variety of fruit Choose fresh, frozen, canned, or dried fruit Go easy on fruit juices	Go low-fat or fat-free when you choose milk, yogurt, and other milk products If you don't or can't consume milk, choose lactose-free products or other calcium sources such as fortified foods and beverages	Choose low-fat or lean meats and poultry Bake it, broil it, or grill it Vary your protein routine – choose more fish, beans, peas, nuts, and seeds

For a 2,000-calorie diet, you need the amounts below from each food group. To find the amounts that are right for you, go to MyPyramid.gov.

Eat 6 oz. every day	Eat 2½ cups every day	Eat 2 cups every day	Get 3 cups every day; for kids aged 2 to 8, it's 2 cups	Eat 5½ oz. every day

Find your balance between food and physical activity

- Be sure to stay within your daily calorie needs.
- Be physically active for at least 30 minutes most days of the week.
- About 60 minutes a day of physical activity may be needed to prevent weight gain.
- For sustaining weight loss, at least 60 to 90 minutes a day of physical activity may be required.
- Children and teenagers should be physically active for 60 minutes every day, or most days.

Know the limits on fats, sugars, and salt (sodium)

- Make most of your fat sources from fish, nuts, and vegetable oils.
- Limit solid fats like butter, margarine, shortening, and lard, as well as foods that contain these.
- Check the Nutrition Facts label to keep saturated fats, *trans* fats, and sodium low.
- Choose food and beverages low in added sugars. Added sugars contribute calories with few, if any, nutrients.

MyPyramid.gov
STEPS TO A HEALTHIER YOU

U.S. Department of Agriculture
Center for Nutrition Policy and Promotion
April 2005
CNPP-14

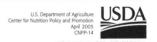

FIGURE 26–5 **USDA MyPyramid: Steps to a Healthier You.** *Source:* U.S. Department of Agriculture (2005).

TABLE 26–6   Serving Sizes for Daily Food Choices

Food Group	What Counts as a Serving	Recommendations for Improving the Diet[*]	Major Nutrients Provided
Fats, oils, sweets	No serving sizes are given. Amounts consumed should be determined by individual energy needs, and these foods should not replace any from other groups	Use canola, peanut, and olive oil instead of margarine and butter	Essential fatty acids
Milk, yogurt, and cheese	1 cup (8 oz) milk or yogurt $1\frac{1}{2}$ oz natural cheese 2 oz processed cheese 2 cups cottage cheese 1 cup custard/pudding	Use nonfat or low-fat dairy products	Protein, calcium, riboflavin, potassium, zinc, iron, fats
Meat, poultry, fish, dry beans, eggs, nuts	2–3 oz cooked meat, poultry or fish 1 to $1\frac{1}{2}$ cups cooked dry beans (e.g., navy beans, lima beans) 4 Tbsp peanut butter 3 oz tofu 2–3 eggs $\frac{1}{2}$ to 1 cup nuts	• Eat lean meat; cut off fat before cooking • Use soy products as meat substitutes • Eat 2 servings of fatty fish (salmon, tuna, herring, swordfish) per week	Protein, niacin, iron, vitamin B_6, zinc, thiamin, vitamin B_{12} (only in animal foods)
Vegetable group	$\frac{1}{2}$ cup chopped raw or cooked vegetables (e.g., broccoli, green beans, potatoes, squash, carrots) 1 cup raw leafy vegetables (e.g., turnip greens, cabbage, lettuce, broccoli) $\frac{3}{4}$ cup vegetable juice	• Include 1 serving of a green leafy vegetable daily • Eat one good source of vitamin A daily (green or orange vegetables such as carrots, sweet potatoes, spinach, broccoli, or red cabbage)	Vitamin A, vitamin C, folate, magnesium, fiber
Fruit group	$\frac{1}{4}$ cup dried fruit $\frac{1}{2}$ cup chopped, cooked or canned fruit $\frac{3}{4}$ cup fruit juice 1 medium apple, banana, orange 1 melon wedge	• Eat fresh fruit; avoid fruit with added sugar • Choose 1 or 2 sources of vitamin C daily (oranges, grapefruit, cantaloupe, strawberries, or citrus fruit juice)	Vitamin C, potassium (bananas, apricots), fiber
Breads, cereals, rice, and pasta	1 slice of bread 1 oz of ready-to-eat cereal $\frac{1}{2}$ to $\frac{3}{4}$ cup cooked cereal, rice, or pasta	• Use whole-grain breads and pasta • Eat oatmeal or bran cereal each day • Eat at least $\frac{1}{2}$ cup of dried beans, peas, or lentils daily	Starch, thiamin, riboflavin (if enriched), iron, niacin, folate, magnesium, fiber (especially in whole grains)

[*]Suggestions in this column are *not* from the MyPyramid food guide. They offer information for choosing the most nutritious foods within a group.

Source: Adapted from the U.S. Department of Agriculture, revised edition of the former *Basic Four Food Groups Guide* (1994).

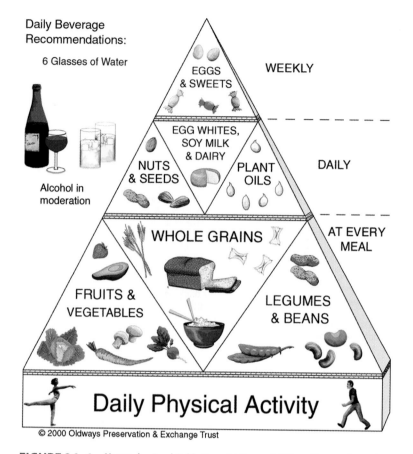

The Traditional Healthy Vegetarian Diet Pyramid

Daily Beverage Recommendations:

6 Glasses of Water

Alcohol in moderation

EGGS & SWEETS — WEEKLY

EGG WHITES, SOY MILK & DAIRY

NUTS & SEEDS

PLANT OILS — DAILY

WHOLE GRAINS — AT EVERY MEAL

FRUITS & VEGETABLES

LEGUMES & BEANS

Daily Physical Activity

© 2000 Oldways Preservation & Exchange Trust

Diet Characteristics

Dietary data from vegetarians across the world that enjoyed the lowest recorded rates of chronic diseases and the highest adult life expectancy show a pattern similar to the one illustrated in the list below. The healthfulness of this pattern is corroborated by epidemiological and experimental nutrition.

1. Multiple daily servings of foods from the three Fruits and Vegetables, Whole Grains, Legumes, and Beans mini-pyramids.
2. Daily servings from the three Nuts and Seeds, Plant Oils, and Egg Whites, Soy Milks and Dairy mini-pyramids.
3. Occasional or small-quantity servings from the Eggs and Sweets mini-pyramid.
4. Attention to consuming a variety of foods from all seven mini-pyramids.
5. Daily consumption of enough water throughout the day to assure good health.
6. Regular physical activity at a level which promotes healthy weight, fitness, and well-being.
7. Reliance upon whole foods and minimally processed foods in preference to highly-processed foods.
8. Moderate regular intake of alcoholic beverages such as wine, beer, or spirits (optional).
9. Daily consumption of unrefined plant oils.
10. Dietary supplements as necessary, based upon factors such as age, sex, and lifestyle, with special attention to those avoiding dairy and/or eggs (Vitamins D and B_{12}).

FIGURE 26–6 Vegetarian Food Guide Pyramid. *Source:* © Oldways Preservation and Exchange Trust. www.oldways.org

Nutrition Facts Panels

You are probably familiar with the **Nutrition Facts panel** shown in Figure 26–7, because the United States Food and Drug Administration (FDA) requires this label on all packaged foods sold in the United States. The Nutrition Facts panel contains important information about serving size, number of servings per package, total calories and calories from fat per serving, a list of the key nutrients in the food, and the *percent daily values* (%DV) for the nutrients listed on the panel. The %DV identifies the percentage that a serving of the food contributes to a consumer's overall intake of the nutrient listed.

KnowledgeCheck 26–2

- What are the DRIs?
- List the current USDA dietary guidelines.

 Go to Chapter 26, **Knowledge Check Response Sheet and Answers,** on the Electronic Study Guide.

CriticalThinking 26–2

How might you use the various sources of nutritional information to evaluate the nutritional status of the clients introduced in the "Meet Your Patients" scenario?

WHAT MUST I KNOW ABOUT ENERGY BALANCE?

The energy in carbohydrates, proteins, and lipids is measured in terms of **calories,** or, more precisely, **kilocalories (kcal).** A kcal is the amount of heat required to raise the temperature of 1 kg of water 1° centigrade. To maintain a stable weight, the kcal we consume must equal the kcal we burn. Any deviation results in weight loss or weight gain. Below is the amount of energy liberated from the metabolism of 1 gram of energy nutrients:

- Carbohydrates = 4 kcal/g
- Protein = 4 kcal/g
- Fat = 9 kcal/g

The Food Label at a Glance

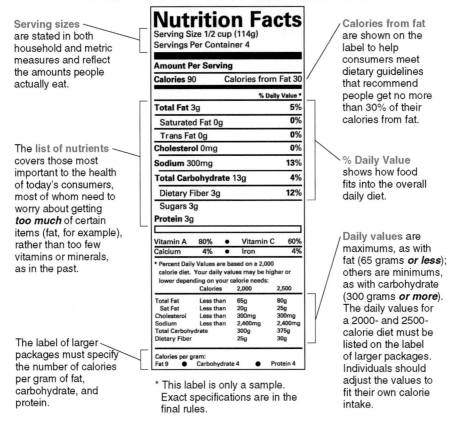

Serving sizes are stated in both household and metric measures and reflect the amounts people actually eat.

The list of nutrients covers those most important to the health of today's consumers, most of whom need to worry about getting **too much** of certain items (fat, for example), rather than too few vitamins or minerals, as in the past.

The label of larger packages must specify the number of calories per gram of fat, carbohydrate, and protein.

Calories from fat are shown on the label to help consumers meet dietary guidelines that recommend people get no more than 30% of their calories from fat.

% Daily Value shows how food fits into the overall daily diet.

Daily values are maximums, as with fat (65 grams **or less**); others are minimums, as with carbohydrate (300 grams **or more**). The daily values for a 2000- and 2500-calorie diet must be listed on the label of larger packages. Individuals should adjust the values to fit their own calorie intake.

Nutrition Facts
Serving Size 1/2 cup (114g)
Servings Per Container 4

Amount Per Serving

Calories 90   Calories from Fat 30

% Daily Value *

Total Fat 3g	5%
Saturated Fat 0g	0%
Trans Fat 0g	0%
Cholesterol 0mg	0%
Sodium 300mg	13%
Total Carbohydrate 13g	4%
Dietary Fiber 3g	12%
Sugars 3g	
Protein 3g	

Vitamin A	80%	Vitamin C	60%
Calcium	4%	Iron	4%

* Percent Daily Values are based on a 2,000 calorie diet. Your daily values may be higher or lower depending on your calorie needs:

		Calories	2,000	2,500
Total Fat	Less than		65g	80g
Sat Fat	Less than		20g	25g
Cholesterol	Less than		300mg	300mg
Sodium	Less than		2,400mg	2,400mg
Total Carbohydrate			300g	375g
Dietary Fiber			25g	30g

Calories per gram:
Fat 9   •   Carbohydrate 4   •   Protein 4

* This label is only a sample. Exact specifications are in the final rules.

FIGURE 26–7   **A Nutrition Facts panel.** *Source:* U.S. Food and Drug Administration (2003).

KnowledgeCheck 26–3

Imagine that you have just eaten a food consisting of 4 grams of protein, 18 grams of carbohydrate, and 1 gram of fat.

- What would your total kcal intake be?
- What percentage of your kcal are from carbohydrates? Protein? Fat?

 Go to Chapter 26, **Knowledge Check Response Sheet and Answers,** on the Electronic Study Guide.

A diet of too few kcal is likely also to lack essential nutrients. People who are undernourished may experience weakened immunity, stunted growth, and hormonal disruption. Too many kcal cause obesity, which increases the risk for chronic diseases such as diabetes, arteriosclerosis, hypertension, hyperlipidemia, and cancers. In determining total energy (kcal) needs, consider two factors: the client's basal metabolic rate (BMR) and the duration and intensity of daily physical activity.

What Is Basal Metabolic Rate?

The **basal metabolic rate (BMR)** is a measure of the energy required by resting tissue to maintain basic function. *Direct measurement* of BMR requires use of a calorimeter: an insulated unit that measures temperature changes of water that are produced by exposure to a fasting individual at rest. Although it is very accurate, it is rarely used because most institutions do not have calorimeters and because the test requires a controlled environment and a 12-hour fast. Direct measurement of BMR is used primarily by researchers. *Indirect calculation* of BMR, sometimes called the resting energy expenditure (REE), includes the following:

- Measuring oxygen uptake per unit of time. This can be done in an exercise lab.
- Serum thyroxine levels (a blood test).
- A formula for calculating BMR when precise measurement is not required (Box 26–3).

Factors Affecting Basal Metabolic Rate

When interpreting test results, consider the following factors that influence BMR:

- *Body composition.* Lean body tissue has greater metabolic activity than fat and bones. This explains why women, who have on average more adipose tissue than men, also have lower BMRs.
- *Growth periods.* BMR increases during periods of growth, such as the first 5 years of life, adolescence, pregnancy, and lactation.
- *Body temperature.* The BMR increases 7% for each 1°F (0.83°C) rise in body temperature.

26-3 Calculating Basal Metabolic Rate (BMR)

Women:	0.9 kcal/kg of body weight per hour
Men:	1.0 kcal/kg body weight/hour

Example: Isaac Schwartz ("Meet Your Patients") weighs 245 lb. 1 kilogram = 2.2 pounds. Divide 245 by 2.2 to convert pounds to kilograms:

$$245 \div 2.2 = 111.3$$

Now complete the calculation:

$$1.0 \times 111.3 \times 24 \text{ hours} = 2671.2$$

- *Environmental temperature.* Cold weather, especially temperatures below freezing, causes a slight rise in the BMR to generate body heat and maintain normal body temperature.
- *Disease processes.* Diseases involving increased cellular activity, such as cancer, anemia, cardiac failure, hypertension, and asthma, result in BMR elevation. For the same reason, systemic injury (e.g., severe burns) increases BMR.
- *Prolonged physical exertion.* Metabolic demands are also elevated during prolonged physical exertion (e.g., chopping wood, running).

How Do I Calculate a Client's Total Energy Needs?

The amount of energy required varies according to the intensity of the activity (Table 26–7). A person's total daily energy requirement is the number of kilocalories necessary to replace those used for basic metabolism plus those used in physical activities. The following are simple estimates based on activity level and age:

- Sedentary women and older adults need 1600 kcal/day.
- Children, teenage girls, active women, and most men need 2200 kcal/day.
- Teenage boys, active men, and very active women need 2800 kcal/day.

However, these estimates have limited applicability. For instance, is a woman who works a desk job but walks for 30 minutes a day sedentary, active, or somewhere in between? To calculate energy use more precisely, you need to know the person's physical activity, including the intensity and duration of the activity. For each pound of body weight, a person needs the following per day:

Sedentary and:
Underweight	13 kcal
Normal weight	13 kcal
Overweight	9 to 11 kcal

Moderately active and:
Underweight	18 kcal
Normal weight	16 kcal
Overweight	13 kcal

Active and:
Underweight	18 to 23 kcal
Normal weight	18 kcal
Overweight	16 kcal

Heightened emotional states may also increase energy needs, not because they directly increase metabolic activity, but because they increase muscular activity in the form of muscle tension, restlessness, and agitated movements.

26-7 Levels of Physical Activity: Energy Expended and Examples*

Intensity Level	Light	Light to Moderate	Moderate	High
Energy Expended	120–150 kcal/hour	150–300 kcal/hour	300–420 kcal/hour	420–700+kcal/hour
Examples of Activities	Dressing Showering Shaving Rocking Writing Typing Standing	Housework (e.g., sweeping) Light gardening Mowing lawn (motorized) Painting Walking 2–3 mph Bicycling 5½ mph Canoeing 2–3 mph	Digging Mowing lawn (manually) Walking 3½–4 mph Ballet Ballroom dancing Golf (no cart) Tennis (doubles)	Shoveling snow Walking 5 mph Climbing Bicycling 15–25 mph Cross-country skiing Jogging 5 mph Swimming Aerobic dancing

*Precise energy use varies with body weight. For example, an individual weighing 200 lb burns about 740 calories per hour during aerobic dance, whereas an individual weighing 125 lb burns about 470 during the same activity.

KnowledgeCheck 26–4

You have already calculated the expected BMR for Mr. Schwartz ("Meet Your Patients") for a 24-hour period.

- If Mr. Schwartz describes himself as working at a desk 8 to 10 hours per day, lawn mowing manually every other week during the summer, and playing an occasional game of golf, how would you classify his general activity level?
- After interviewing Mr. Schwartz, you estimate his average kcal intake to be approximately 3000 kcal per day. Determine whether his kcal intake is sufficient or insufficient to maintain his present activity level.

 Go to Chapter 26, **Knowledge Check Response Sheet and Answers,** on the Electronic Study Guide.

What Are Some Body Weight Standards?

Weight standards have been established to correlate weight with good health and longevity and to help determine a client's ideal body weight. The **general weight guide** uses a formula to determine a reasonable weight based on height:

Men: 106 lb (47.7 kg) for the first 5 ft (150 cm), then add 6 lb/in. (2.7 kg/2.5 cm)
Women: 100 lb (45 kg) for the first 5 ft (150 cm), then add 5 lb/in. (2.25 kg/2.5 cm)

Various **height-weight tables** have been developed over the years. For an example,

 Go to Chapter 26, **Tables, Boxes, Figures: ESG Table 26–1,** on the Electronic Study Guide.

Such tables are based on statistical estimates and often include variations for age, gender, and body frame. Use standards and standardized tables with caution because they are based on limited samples and may create unrealistic expectations, especially at the low weight ranges. Consider the following example. You have two male clients; each weighs 200 lb. Mike is 72 inches tall, works out vigorously 5 days per week, and has 18% body fat. Jim is 72 inches tall, rarely exercises, and has 35% body fat. Which of these clients requires more kcal to maintain his present weight? Which of these clients is at lower risk for cardiovascular disease?

If you answered Mike, you are correct. Although both men have the same height and weight, Mike has more lean body mass. He will burn kcal more rapidly and be able to eat more without gaining weight. When attempting to determine a client's overall fitness, you must consider body composition.

Body composition analysis attempts to quantify lean body mass versus percent body fat. Lean body mass includes muscle, bone, and connective tissue. Lean tissue weighs more than fat; thus, a person who engages in regular weight-bearing exercise and is physically fit may actually weigh more than an individual of similar appearance who is sedentary and unfit. Various methods to assess body composition, known as *anthropometric measurements,* are presented in the "Assessment" section, beginning on page 602.

 CriticalThinking 26–3

Examine your dietary intake for the next 3 days to determine how balanced your diet is. Use the following format and record all intake.

	Day 1	Day 2	Day 3
Breakfast			
Lunch			
Dinner			
Snacks			

- How does your diet compare to the USDA Food Guide Pyramid or Canada's Food Guide in terms of:
  a. Servings of bread, cereal, rice, and pasta? _____
  b. Servings of vegetables? _____
  c. Servings of fruits? _____
  d. Servings of milk, yogurt, and cheese? _____
  e. Servings of meat, poultry, fish, dry beans, eggs, and nuts? _____
  f. Servings of fats, oil, and sweets? _____
- From what you have learned from this activity, what habits could you change in patterns of eating in order to achieve optimal nutrition?

WHAT FACTORS AFFECT NUTRITION?

Several modifiable and nonmodifiable factors influence nutritional needs and choices. The most influential factors are development, knowledge, lifestyle, culture, disease processes, and functional limitations.

Developmental Stage

At specific developmental stages, nutritional needs and eating patterns vary according to physiologic growth, activity level, metabolic processes, disease prevention, and other factors.

Infants to One Year

An infant grows most rapidly during the first year of life. Birth weight triples during the first year, and length increases 50%. Nutritional needs per unit of body weight are greater than at any other time. The infant needs adequate protein for tissue building and enough carbohydrates to furnish energy and "spare"

the protein. Fetal iron stores are depleted at 4 to 6 months, so intake of iron becomes important. The infant needs calcium for bone growth and development of teeth, calcium and vitamin C for iron absorption, and vitamin D for calcium regulation.

Compared to adults, infants have a higher metabolic rate and greater water loss through the skin, which comprises a greater proportion of the body. These factors, along with immature kidneys, mean that infants need proportionately more fluid than adults. To meet nutritional and fluid needs, the infant requires 80 to 100 mL of breast milk or formula per kg of body weight per day.

The only safe choices for meeting fluid and nutrient needs in the first months of life are breast milk and commercially prepared formulas. Breast milk is the ideal food for infants because it is matched to their nutritional requirements. In addition, it enhances maturation of the infant's immune system and provides passive immunity against a number of infections. Breastfed infants also have a reduced exposure to foreign dietary antigens and a reduced risk of subsequent allergies (Oddy, 2002).

When breastfeeding is contraindicated or the mother chooses not to breastfeed, numerous commercial formulas are available. The most commonly used formula is modified cow's milk available in powder, liquid concentrate, or ready-to-use liquid. Other types include iron-fortified, soy, and hypoallergenic formulas. The American Academy of Pediatrics (1999) recommends that all formulas contain between 4 and 12 mg/L of iron. Infants under 1 year old should not receive regular cow's milk because it may cause gastrointestinal bleeding and may place too much strain on the infant's kidneys. It may also be associated with later development of type I diabetes (American Academy of Pediatrics, 1994). Honey and corn syrup should not be used as a source of carbohydrates in preparing infant formula. They are potential sources of botulism toxin, which can be fatal in children under 1 year old (Williams & Schlenker, 2003).

At 4 to 6 months, infants may be started on solid foods, beginning with infant rice cereal, preferably iron-fortified. They progress to eating table food by 1 year of age. If solid foods are begun too early, they may trigger allergies. Vitamin supplements may be prescribed for both breastfed and bottle-fed infants; iron supplements are usually prescribed at age 6 months.

Toddlers and Preschoolers

Toddlers grow more slowly in comparison to infants and have fewer energy demands. Toddlers require about 900 to 1800 kcal and 1250 mL of fluid per day, depending on body weight. As the gastrointestinal system matures, they are able to eat most foods and adjust to the adult pattern of three meals a day. By age 3, most children have all of their deciduous teeth and can chew adult food.

Deficiencies in iron, calcium, and vitamins A and C are common during this period. It is important that the parent offer a variety of foods to provide these essential nutrients. This can be a challenge, because toddlers assert their autonomy and manipulate their parents by refusing foods offered. They may take a long time to eat or refuse to eat at all. Parents should not turn mealtime into a battle of wills or use foods to punish or reward; such reactions may affect the child's attitude toward food. To encourage the child to eat, you may offer parents the following suggestions:

- Keep only nutritious foods in the house to avoid battles over nutrient-poor snacks.
- Serve foods in a "child-friendly" way; for example, arrange tortillas, cheese, tomato slices, and beans in a smiling face.
- Allow the child to "graze" throughout the day on healthful foods rather than insisting that she sit through formal meals at the table.
- Avoid "combined" foods, such as casseroles and stews.
- Limit consumption of sweet desserts.
- Do not use dessert as a reward for eating other foods (e.g., "You can't have cookies until you eat your meat").

Preschoolers are similar to toddlers in their growth and nutritional needs; however, their eating patterns typically improve. They begin to form responses to specific foods, such as refusing all green vegetables or drinking less milk. They often refuse casseroles and foods with sauces. They might also eat only one particular food for several days. Because they are active, preschoolers require nutritious between-meal snacks. Lifelong food habits are developed during this stage, so encourage families to widen the variety of foods offered to preschoolers and to investigate the diet provided by their child's day care or preschool.

School-Age Children

In the school-age period, growth and body changes occur gradually. Permanent teeth erupt, and the digestive system matures. School-age children need about 2400 kcal and 1750 mL of fluid per day. An adequate supply of vitamins and minerals is critical, because the body is still growing and preparing for the demands of adolescence.

Parental control over food intake declines because advertising influences the child's food choices. The child eats away from home and may buy junk food with his lunch money. Even if the child brings lunch from home, he may trade his food or not eat lunch at all. Parents should encourage their children to eat breakfast to provide nutrients and energy to fuel problem-solving skills, memory, and sports and playground

Early Warning Signs of an Eating Disorder

Food Behaviors

- Skips meals
- Takes only tiny portions
- Will not eat in front of others
- Always has an excuse not to eat
- Usually has a diet soda or coffee in hand
- Eats only food that is low in fat

Appearance and Body Image Behaviors

- Wears baggy clothes
- Complains of being fat
- Obsesses about clothing size
- Spends lots of time inspecting self in the mirror

Exercise Behaviors

- Exercises excessively and compulsively
- May tire easily
- Pushes self beyond normal expectations

Social Behaviors

- Tries to please everyone and withdraws if unsuccessful
- Tries to care for everyone but self
- Tries to control what and where family eats
- Relationships tend to be superficial or dependent

activities. Poor eating habits may lead to obesity. Leading causes of childhood obesity include the following:

- Routine consumption of high-fat, high-sugar fast foods, nutrient-poor foods, and high-kcal snacks and beverages
- Loss of family mealtime
- Eating in front of a TV or computer
- Lack of regular physical activity to burn the kcal consumed

Adolescents

The onset of puberty marks the beginning of adolescence, a time of dramatic growth and development of the reproductive system. Boys experience an increase in muscle tissue and bone length and density. At menstruation, girls experience fat deposition. The needs of the adolescent body for energy, vitamins, and minerals approaches that of the infant. In particular, adolescents need protein, calcium, iron, and B and D vitamins.

Boys, in particular, seem to eat constantly. Adolescents have active lifestyles and snack often, preferring ready-to-eat, eat-on-the-run foods, such as chips, cookies, ice cream, and fast foods. Unfortunately, most such foods have little nutrient value. Adolescents are responsible for their own food decisions, so the best approach for parents is to keep only healthful snack foods (e.g., cheese, fruit, raw vegetables) in the home.

For girls, the need for nutrients conflicts with intense social pressure to be slim, resulting in a dramatic rise in eating disorders in this age group. **Anorexia nervosa** is a psychiatric disorder characterized by self-starvation. **Bulimia nervosa** refers to binge eating (eating an excessive amount of food in a short period of time) followed by self-induced vomiting or laxative abuse to purge food. According to the National Association of Anorexia Nervosa and Associated Disorders (2003), more than half of teenage girls either are or think they should be on a diet. Serious medical and psychological complications arise from excessive kcal restriction in adolescence, including cardiac, renal, liver, and metabolic disorders, as well as decreased bone density and an increased risk for fractures. Thus, you will need to recognize the early warning signs of eating disorders, such as the behavior changes described in Box 26–4.

Adults

Young adults continue to require adequate amounts of protein, vitamins, and minerals, but not at the same levels as in adolescence. Calcium, folic acid, and iron continue to be critical, especially in women, for bone and reproductive health. Maintaining unhealthful behaviors developed earlier, such as limited physical activity, begins to cause repercussions in adulthood.

The BMR of middle adults decreases, potentially causing weight gain if dietary intake and activity level are unchanged. Individuals may begin to experience chronic illnesses such as diabetes, hypertension, obesity, and hyperlipidemia, often as a result of poor lifestyle choices and heredity. Dietary modification and exercise are essential to control these diseases.

Older Adults

Nutritional needs of older adults vary only slightly from middle adulthood. Lean body mass, physical activity, and BMR decrease, resulting in slightly reduced energy requirements. As bone density decreases, calcium requirements increase, especially in women at risk for *osteoporosis*. Complex carbohydrates, especially fruits and vegetables, are important in older adults to maintain bowel function, and adequate fluid is important to prevent dehydration. However, it is common for older adults to lose interest in eating and for the thirst sensation to decrease.

TABLE 26-8 Daily Food Requirements for Adults Over Age 70

Food Group	Adults ≥ 70 years
Supplement of calcium, vitamin D, and vitamin B$_{12}$	As prescribed. Not everyone needs supplements. People should consult their healthcare providers.
Fats, oils, and sweets	Use sparingly
Milk, yogurt, and cheese group	3 or more servings
Meat, poultry, fish, dry beans, eggs, and nut group	2 or more servings
Vegetable group	3 or more servings
Fruit group	2 or more servings
Bread, fortified cereals, rice, and pasta group	6 or more servings
Water equivalents	8 or more servings

Sources: Russell, R., Rasmussen, H., & Lichtenstein, A. (1999). Modified food guide pyramid for people over seventy years of age. *Journal of Nutrition, 129*(3), 751–753; Friedman School of Nutrition Science & Policy. (1995–2004). Guide to the modified pyramid for older adults. Retrieved July 12, 2004, from http://nutrition.tufts.edu/consumer/pyramid.html

For older adults with chronic diseases, primary care providers often prescribe diets low in salt, simple sugars, or fat. Unfortunately, the ability to taste and smell diminishes with age, and many clients find these diets unappealing. Other sensory changes, such as diminished vision or hearing, limit mobility and interaction, making it more difficult to purchase and prepare food. Tooth loss and gum disease limit chewing ability, forcing many older adults to eat only soft food. Arthritic hands may have difficulty preparing and eating food, and when they are no longer able to drive, many older adults must rely on local markets, where food choices may be limited. Lack of money may also significantly limit food choices. Physical problems may also affect nutrition, including gastroesophageal reflux, decreased gastric secretions, decreased intestinal peristalsis, and glucose intolerance.

With advancing age, older adults face many losses. As a result, depression and social isolation are common. Both negatively affect appetite. **Adult failure to thrive** is a complex disorder seen in many institutionalized older adults. It is characterized by weight loss, decreased activity and interaction, and increasing frailty.

See Table 26–8 for dietary requirements for adults older than 70 years. This table is based on the modified food pyramid for older adults developed by Tufts University (Russell, Rasmussen, & Lichtenstein, 1999). Notice that the main difference is that older adults require smaller quantities of most foods. In general, they require slightly more of the milk/yogurt/cheese group and slightly less of all other groups, especially the breads/cereal group. Older adults should be sure to consume at least eight glasses of water or other fluids (e.g., soups) to help prevent constipation and dehydration. They should choose primarily green leafy vegetables and brightly-colored fruits. Also note that older adults may need supplements of calcium, vitamin D, and vitamin B$_{12}$.

Pregnant and Lactating Women

Nutritional requirements increase dramatically during pregnancy as the mother provides for the nutritional needs of the fetus. Folic acid intake is critical in the first trimester of pregnancy (the first 13 weeks) to prevent neural tube defects. Adequate protein and calcium are important for growing muscle, brain, and bone tissues; iron is essential to maintain maternal and fetal blood supplies and stores during pregnancy. It is almost impossible to consume the recommended amount of dietary iron, so supplements are commonly prescribed, as are supplements of folic acid and calcium. Pregnant women need about 300 additional kcal per day in the second and third trimesters of pregnancy.

Women need 500 additional kcal per day when breastfeeding. They continue to need additional protein and calcium, as well as increased fluid intake to make adequate amounts of breast milk. Needs vary based on the size of the baby and the frequency of breastfeeding. The quantity of the breast milk depends

on an adequate supply of fluids and nutrients. However, the nutritional quality of the milk remains the same even if dietary intake is not adequate. For more information on nutrition in pregnancy and lactation, consult a maternal-newborn nursing textbook.

KnowledgeCheck 26–5

- Why is breast milk an ideal food source for infants?
- Why are the infant's nutritional needs per unit of body weight greater than at any other time?
- Why is it sometimes a challenge to meet the nutritional needs of toddlers?
- What is the challenge in meeting the nutritional needs of school-age children?
- Which age group experiences a growth spurt second only to that of infants?
- Why are energy (kcal) requirements less for older adults?

 Go to Chapter 26, **Knowledge Check Response Sheet and Answers,** on the Electronic Study Guide.

 CriticalThinking 26–4

Make a list of all the food products you have seen advertised on television and in magazines. What implications does this have for the nutritional status of the public?

Lifestyle Choices

Nutrition-related lifestyle choices include the following:

- *Dietary patterns.* Obviously, consuming more kcal than are expended in activity results in weight gain; however, the type of food consumed is equally important to health. Whole foods, such as fresh fruits and vegetables, whole grains, and legumes, promote health, whereas foods high in simple sugars, saturated and trans fats, and sodium increase the risk for health problems.

- *Oral contraceptive use.* This method of family planning lowers the serum level of vitamin C and several B vitamins. Women with marginal nutrient intake may need vitamin supplements.

- *Using food to cope.* If used often, poor coping patterns, such as reacting to stress by skipping meals, binge eating, or consuming too much of a single food (e.g., snack foods or chocolate) can result in poor nutrition.

- *Smoking.* Smoking can reduce vitamin C levels by as much as 30% (Geronimus et al., 1993). If the person cannot quit smoking, a vitamin C supplement may help compensate.

- *Alcohol.* A 12-oz beer contains 150 kcal; a juice-based cocktail contains about 160 kcal. This can add many unnecessary kcal to the regular diet. In addition, alcohol significantly decreases the rate of fat metabolism, contributing to obesity. Excessive alcohol

use interferes with adequate nutrition by (1) replacing the food in the person's diet, (2) depressing the appetite, (3) decreasing the absorption of nutrients by its toxic effects on intestinal mucosa, and (4) impairing the storage of nutrients. People who use alcohol heavily need multivitamin supplements, especially B vitamins and folic acid.

Vegetarianism

All vegetarian diets exclude red meat and poultry, but beyond this distinction is a wide spectrum of diets. **Semi-vegetarians** are the most inclusive, allowing fish, eggs, and dairy products as well as plant-based foods. **Ovo-lacto vegetarians** are somewhat more strict; they eat eggs and dairy products, but not fish. **Lacto-vegetarians** consume only dairy and plant-based foods. **Vegans** eat only foods of plant origin, and a **fruitarian** diet includes only fruits, nuts, honey, and vegetable oils. Soy beans, soy milk, tofu, and processed protein products can be used by all but fruitarians to enhance the nutritional value of the diet.

People choose vegetarian diets for a number of reasons. As noted in Chapter 14, some religions prohibit consumption of animal flesh or foods of animal origin. Ethical considerations related to humane treatment of animals cause some people to adopt a vegetarian diet. However, in the last few decades many people have adopted a vegetarian diet simply as a health choice, noting the abundant research indicating that vegetarianism reduces the risk of disease and promotes wellness by limiting fat intake.

Although ovo-lacto vegetarians have no higher rate of nutrient deficiencies than the meat-eating population, they must choose foods carefully to include enough of the following nutrients:

- *Vitamin B$_{12}$* is not found in foods of plant origin; it is found in animal products, such as eggs and milk products. Vegans must consume foods fortified with B$_{12}$ or take B$_{12}$ supplements. Long-standing B$_{12}$ deficiency can result in severe and irreversible neurologic impairment.

- *Protein* may be inadequate, especially in vegan children who do not care for the taste of soy milk, tofu, and other soy-based meat substitutes. For adults, a varied diet that meets normal nutrient and energy needs is also likely to supply adequate amounts of essential amino acids. Complementary proteins should be eaten throughout the day, but careful meal-by-meal balance of amino acids is usually not necessary. Review Table 26–2 and Proteins on pages 577 and 578.

- *Iron* reserves are harder for vegans to maintain because the iron from plant foods is not absorbed as well as that from animal sources. Remember, though, that it's easier to absorb dietary iron when it

is eaten with foods that contain vitamin C, so eating fruit or vegetables containing vitamin C with meals helps to compensate.

- *Vitamin D* may be inadequately supplied by vegetarian diets, so vitamin-D fortified foods (e.g., soy and dairy milk are usually vitamin D fortified) should be included. Adequate sun exposure also helps to compensate for lack of dietary intake.
- Vegans, fruitarians, and others who limit animal foods usually need to supplement the diet with vitamin B_{12}, vitamin D, calcium, iron, and zinc. This is especially important for children and women who are pregnant or lactating.

In addition to following the information contained in the Vegetarian Food Pyramid (see Figure 26–6), to ensure adequate nutrients it may be wise for vegetarians to consult a qualified nutrition professional, especially during periods of growth, breastfeeding, pregnancy, or recovery from illness. For recommended servings of vegetarian food groups,

 Go to Chapter 26, **Tables, Boxes, Figures: ESG Table 26–2,** on the Electronic Study Guide.

Dieting for Weight Loss

In 2003, one popular Internet bookseller offered no fewer than 36,655 books on weight-loss diets! Many diets, including the DASH diet, the American Heart Association diet, and others, are nutritionally sound, but many others are "fad diets," claiming to produce speedy, effortless, almost miraculous, weight loss. You can recognize fad diets by the following characteristics. They:

- Promise quick and dramatic weight loss, which is usually achieved only temporarily because it results from loss of body fluids.
- Limit the range of foods from which the dieter can select (e.g., only fruits and vegetables for the first week), leading to an imbalance in nutrients.
- Often recommend purchase of supplements and/or special packaged meals; in many cases, these are brands that they endorse or actually produce.
- Include no practical strategies that help dieters permanently change eating and activity patterns.

As soon as they achieve their weight-loss goal, fad dieters typically revert to former eating habits and regain the weight. In contrast, more moderate calorie-restriction diets, such as the American Heart Association diet:

- Describe food selection and preparation tips and other behavior modifications that can lead to slow, sustained weight loss.
- Promote a diet that includes a variety of food choices and a balance of nutrients.

- Encourage physical activity as a cornerstone of weight loss.
- Emphasize self-monitoring, cognitive strategies, and behavior modification.

Ethnicity, Culture, and Religious Practices

As described in Chapters 13 and 14, religion and culture can have a major impact on diet and lifestyle. The following are examples:

- Language barriers may make it difficult for a client to understand nutritional information. For those patients, simple visual aids may be useful.
- Ethnic/cultural food choices often reflect the foods that were plentiful in the region of origin (e.g., fish in coastal communities, coffee and cocoa beans in equatorial regions), as well as foods that were readily grown in the native soil (e.g., rice in warm wetlands, potatoes in colder climates).
- Other diet choices reflect a concern for food preservation: for instance, people from various geographic regions eat salted meats and dried fruits and cook with fiery spices to combat microbes.
- Certain religions may require fasting or abstaining from certain foods. For example, Roman Catholics fast on Ash Wednesday and Good Friday; Kosher dietary laws prohibit eating pork and shellfish.

Traditional diets of many cultures are healthful and should not be discouraged; in fact, contemporary adaptations made to these diets may compromise their nutritional quality. Examples of adapted traditional diets are the Asian, Latin, and Mediterranean Diet Pyramids, mentioned earlier.

Disease Processes and Functional Limitations

Chronic diseases (e.g., diabetes mellitus, gastrointestinal disorders) can alter nutrient intake, digestion, absorption, use, and excretion. Any illness, especially when accompanied by fever, increases the need for protein, water, and kcal to meet the demands of increased metabolic rate. Traumatic injury (e.g., burns, surgery) requires extra protein and vitamin C for wound healing and tissue rebuilding. People with long-term insufficient kcal intake (e.g., patients with cancer) also suffer from **protein-calorie malnutrition,** which is characterized by weight loss and muscle and fat wasting. A variety of other physical and psychological disorders and/or their treatments can adversely affect a client's nutrition:

- *Appetite.* A poor appetite results in decreased intake of food and therefore of nutrients. It is a common problem in alcoholism. Almost all oral medications

BOX 26–5

Medications with a High Incidence of Nausea

- Acetylsalicylic acid (aspirin)
- Antibiotics
- Anticonvulsants (dilantin)
- Antidepressants
- Anti-inflammatory agents
- Antineoplastic agents (chemotherapy)
- Asthma medications (especially theophylline)
- Birth control pills
- Fluoride supplements
- Opioids
- Potassium chloride
- Vitamin and mineral supplements

have the potential to cause nausea or vomiting, thereby decreasing appetite. Box 26–5 lists medications with a high incidence of nausea. Some medications directly decrease appetite, for example, aspirin, diphenhydramine (Benadryl), and lithium carbonate (Lithobid).

- *Cognitive function.* A person with a developmental delay, severe mental illness, confusion, or memory loss may be unable to remember what, when, or whether she has eaten.

- *Ability to obtain food.* Paralysis or hemiplegia (e.g., from a stroke) can cause functional limitations that affect mobility and, hence, the ability to shop for food. Social factors also limit the ability to gather or procure food. People with limited income may be forced to choose between buying food, medication, or household utilities. Homeless people and others in extreme poverty are often reduced to eating from trash cans and dumpsters or consuming nonfoods, such as paper, grass, and clay.

- *Ability to prepare food.* Preparing food takes time and energy. A person with severe dyspnea from chronic obstructive pulmonary disease (COPD), for example, may not have the stamina to prepare a nutritious meal. Instead, she may eat prepared foods that are high in sodium content. Fatigue is also caused by advanced chronic disease, severe anemia, pregnancy, depression, or excess work.

- *Chewing.* Decayed or missing teeth and ill-fitting dentures make chewing difficult. The person often resorts to eating only soft foods, many of which lack fiber.

- *Swallowing.* Acute disorders affecting the throat, such as pharyngitis, make swallowing painful. Cancer

of the larynx or esophageal strictures also makes swallowing painful and frequently leads to avoiding food.

- *Stomach function.* Heartburn, indigestion, and other stomach disorders are common. People may eat only bland foods or avoid certain foods to prevent the pain or burning that follow eating.

- *Peristalsis.* Peristalsis is the wavelike action that propels food through the intestinal tract. Bowel inflammation or infection, diverticuli (outpouchings of the intestine), or tumors may increase peristalsis, thereby decreasing absorption of nutrients. In addition, high stress levels may either speed or slow transit time.

- *Enzyme secretions.* Liver, gallbladder, or pancreas problems affect the secretion of enzymes involved in digesting foods. Nearly 50 million Americans lack the enzyme needed to digest milk. About 75% of African Americans and Native Americans are lactose intolerant; incidence is 90% among Asian Americans (National Institute of Diabetes and Digestive and Kidney Diseases, 2003).

In addition to the direct effects of diseases and disorders, nutrition may be affected by the drugs and therapies used to treat them. For example, chemotherapy and radiation therapy may cause oral ulcers, intestinal bleeding, or diarrhea—which interfere with eating and absorbing nutrients from food. Certain drugs alter nutrient metabolism, and others increase or decrease nutrient excretion. Some drugs affect specific nutrients. For example, acetylsalicylic acid (aspirin) decreases folate levels and increases excretion of vitamin C; laxatives may cause calcium and potassium depletion; and thiazide diuretics decrease the absorption of vitamin B_{12}.

KnowledgeCheck 26–6

- List at least three nutrients that may be more difficult to supply through a vegetarian diet.
- When selecting a program for weight loss, what factors should a person consider?
- Why should you encourage clients from various cultures to follow their traditional diets?
- Describe the effects on nutrition of (1) smoking and (2) heavy alcohol use.

 Go to Chapter 26, **Knowledge Check Response Sheet and Answers,** on the Electronic Study Guide,.

WHAT ARE SPECIAL DIETS?

Many people must follow a modified diet to assist in managing their illness. In addition, all inpatients at healthcare facilities must have a diet ordered by their primary care provider. The following are the most commonly prescribed modified diets.

Regular Diet

A regular diet, also called the "house diet," is appropriate for clients without special nutritional needs. This diet is a balanced meal plan that supplies 2000 kcal per day. Many facilities provide vegetarian and ethnic variations (Asian menu, Kosher, and so on). Inpatients choose each meal from a list of menu choices.

Have you ever eaten "hospital food"? Or have you heard someone complain that "hospital food is bland and unimaginative"? There is some justification for that complaint. House diets must accommodate the varied tastes of all patients, so they are usually lightly seasoned. Selections are limited to avoid unpopular items (e.g., brussels sprouts) and restrict fatty, fried, or gassy foods, which many patients tolerate poorly. However, you should refrain from making negative comments to patients about the food.

NPO

NPO means no food or fluid (including water) by mouth. This may be ordered prior to surgery or an invasive procedure to limit the risk of aspiration. Common orders are "NPO after midnight," or "NPO 8 hours prior to procedure." Most well-nourished, well-hydrated patients easily tolerate short-term NPO status. However, no one can tolerate prolonged periods of NPO. Intravenous fluids may be given to provide hydration, and clients who must remain NPO for a lengthy period need enteral or parenteral nutrition to prevent malnutrition.

Diets Modified by Consistency

Patients undergoing surgery, bowel procedures, or acute illness may need, for a short period of time, a diet modified by consistency. Long-term consistency modification is required for patients with chronic health concerns that affect their ability to chew or swallow (e.g., Impaired Dentition and Impaired Swallowing).

- A **clear liquid diet** provides fluids to prevent dehydration and supplies some simple carbohydrates to help meet energy needs. Items included in a clear liquid diet include water, tea, coffee, broth, clear juice (usually apple, grape, or cranberry juice), popsicles, carbonated beverages, and gelatin. Clear liquids do not supply adequate calories, protein, and other nutrients, so timely progression to more nutritious diets is recommended. If clear liquids are required for more than 3 days, commercial clear liquid supplements are usually prescribed.

- A **full liquid diet** contains all the liquids included in the clear liquid diet plus any food items that are liquid at room temperature: soups, milk, milk shakes, puddings, custards, juices, some hot cereals, and yogurt. It is difficult to obtain a balanced diet on a full liquid plan, so it should be used for a short time only. If it is needed for a longer time, it should be planned by a professional dietitian. High calorie, high-protein supplements are often added.

- A **mechanical soft diet** is the diet of choice for people with chewing difficulties resulting from missing teeth, jaw problems, or extensive fatigue. A soft diet includes all items on the full liquid diet plus soft vegetables and fruits, breads, pastries, eggs, cheese, and chopped, ground, or shredded meat. Many food items can be added to this diet by cooking them extensively or blending or grinding to alter their texture. This diet can supply a full range of nutrients but is quite low in fiber. As a result, constipation is a risk.

- A **pureed diet** is a blended diet. Any food item may be eaten; however, the consistency must be altered by blending. Often liquids are added to the food to create a texture that may be scooped onto serving plates.

Diets Modified for Disease

Some health conditions require modification of dietary intake. The following are the most common diets:

- *Calorie-restricted.* Used for clients who must lose weight.

- *Sodium-restricted.* Used for clients with blood pressure or fluid balance problems.

- *Fat-restricted.* Used for clients with elevated cholesterol or triglyceride levels; may also be ordered for general weight loss.

- *Diabetic.* Used to manage calories and carbohydrate intake for clients with diabetes mellitus.

- *Renal diet.* Used to manage electrolytes and fluid for clients with renal insufficiency.

- *Protein-controlled diet.* Used to manage liver and kidney disease.

- *Antigen-avoidance diets.* Used for clients allergic to or intolerant of certain foods, such as a gluten-free diet for clients with celiac disease.

- *Calorie-protein push.* Used when there is a need to heal wounds, maintain or increase weight, or promote growth. If the person cannot consume enough calories by adding fats and proteins to his regular diet, high calorie-high protein supplements may be used.

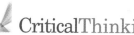

CriticalThinking 26–5

Analyze the following diets. Which nutrients are missing or difficult to obtain from these diets?

- Clear liquid
- Full liquid

Practical Knowledge
knowing how

Nutrition is a basic human need. But more than a physical necessity, it has emotional associations as well. We eat when we are hungry, but we also eat for pleasure, because the food tastes good! Food has become a part of most social events and activities. A certain food may symbolize one's cultural or religious affiliation or even be a political statement (e.g., refusal to eat lettuce in support of migrant workers). It is wise to keep in mind that food has different meanings to different people and that personal beliefs, habits, and preferences are as important as nutritional knowledge in determining what a person eats.

Good nutrition not only is essential for health, but also is a key aspect of disease management. In the rest of this chapter, we will look at assessing nutritional status and diagnosing and planning care for a variety of nutrition problems. In addition, we will discuss specifically the care of patients who are underweight/undernourished or overweight/obese.

| Assessment |

The nutrition component of the overall health history provides information for identifying nutrition-related problems. It includes subjective data about the client's dietary history and related factors. For the components of a nutritional history,

 Go to Chapter 26, **Assessment Guidelines and Tools, Nutritional History,** in Volume 2.

You can obtain a dietary history during any routine assessment. When you take a **dietary history,** whether you use a form or an interview, you collect general knowledge of the client's basic eating habits, food attitudes and preferences, cultural factors, and use of dietary supplements. A dietary history creates a picture of the client's food habits and eating behaviors. To collect detailed data on what the client is actually eating, ask him to keep a **food diary.** The following are three types of food diaries:

- A **24-hour recall** requires the client to name all food eaten within a day. Simply ask questions such as "Yesterday, what did you eat for breakfast/lunch/dinner/snacks?" A 24-hour recall is simple, requires no equipment, and can be used as often as required. However, accuracy of the data may be questionable, because some people have difficulty remembering everything they ate the previous day, and any single day may be atypical. Sometimes, a family member can help the client recall intake more accurately.

- A **food frequency questionnaire** asks the client to identify the number of times per day, week, or month a particular food group is eaten (e.g., fruits, red meats). You can modify the questions according to the client's specific issues. Food frequency questionnaires provide a more global image of the client's nutritional intake than the 24-hour recall; however, accuracy is still a problem.

- A **food record** is the most accurate food diary. It provides information on the quantity as well as the types of foods eaten. You ask the client in advance to keep a record of measured and weighed amounts of all foods he eats in a 3-day period. From the detailed information collected, you can analyze the total kcal and nutrient content for the recorded period. Although the food record provides meaningful results, it requires a high level of cognitive and psychomotor functioning that not all clients have. It also requires commitment to the process for 3 days, which may be difficult for some people.

How Do I Screen Clients for Nutritional Problems?

Nutritional screening is performed to determine deficiencies or excesses in the diet. The degree of screening performed depends on the client's condition or concerns. Cursory screening consists of evaluation of height, weight, and body mass index coupled with a brief dietary history. Clients who are found to be at risk for nutritional problems should be further evaluated. Three screening methods commonly used include the subjective global assessment, the Mini Nutritional Assessment, and the Nutrition Screening Initiative.

 Go to Chapter 26, **Assessment Guidelines and Tools, Assessing for Nutritional Problems,** in Volume 2.

How Can I Assess Body Composition?

When assessing body composition, you use **anthropometric measurements.** These are noninvasive physical examination techniques to determine body dimensions. Simple examples are height and weight; other examples are discussed in the following sections. Anthropometric measurements are used to assess growth rate in children and to indirectly assess adults' protein and fat stores. To obtain accurate data, you must use standardized equipment and procedures and compare the data to existing reference standards for men and women.

Skinfold Measurement

The client's skinfold thickness reveals information about current nutritional status as well as long-term

BOX 26–6 Calculating Body Mass Index (BMI)

BMI = weight in kilograms ÷ (height in meters)^2

Example:
Robert weighs 165 lb. Convert his weight to kilograms:

$$165 ÷ 2.2 = 75 \text{ kg}$$

He is 71 inches tall. Convert his height to meters.

$$1 \text{ meter} = 39.37 \text{ inches}.$$

Divide 71 inches by 39.37 inches; he is 1.8 meters tall (rounded off)

His BMI is 75 kg ÷ $(1.8)^2$ = 23

The normal BMI for adults ranges from 18.5 to 24.9.

Classification of Body Mass Index Values

Classification	BMI (kg/m2)	Risk of Comorbidities
Underweight	< 18.5	Low
Normal weight	18.5–24.9	Average
Pre-obese	25.0–29.9	Mildly increased
Class I obesity	30.0–34.9	Moderate
Class II obesity	35.0–39.9	Severe
Class III obesity	≥40.0	Very severe

changes in subcutaneous adipose tissue stores. Use a caliper to obtain the most accurate measurement. For instructions on taking skinfold measurement,

 Go to Chapter 26, **Technique 26–1: Measuring Triceps Skinfold,** in Volume 2.

The most reliable location is the triceps for children and women and the subscapular area in men. The combined measurements of triceps skinfold and mid-upper arm circumference yield a better estimate of muscle and fat areas than a single measurement.

Circumferences

Another method of examining the percentage of body fat is to use girth or circumference measurements. *Mid-upper arm circumference* is routinely measured as part of screening. For people who are obese, *abdominal*

circumference is the preferred measurement. *Waist-to-hip ratio (WHR)* measures evaluate obesity by assessing abdominal fat. A WHR of greater than 1 in men and greater than 0.8 in women indicates obesity. A high level of abdominal fat is associated with increased risk for hypertension, diabetes, hyperlipidemia, and cardiovascular disease. For specific instructions on measuring abdominal circumference and mid-upper arm circumference,

 Go to Chapter 26, **Technique 26–2: Measuring Circumferences to Evaluate Body Composition,** in Volume 2.

Body Mass Index

Body mass index (BMI) can be precisely measured using scanning devices that measure *bioelectrical impedance*—the conduction of a harmless electrical charge through the client's body. Lean tissue readily conducts the charge, whereas adipose tissue does not. You will usually estimate BMI roughly by using the calculation formula in Box 26–6. You may also consult tables with precalculated values based on height and weight. For an example of a height-weight table,

 Go to Chapter 19, **Procedure 19–1: Performing the General Survey,** in Volume 2.

The normal BMI for adults ranges from 18.5 to 24.9. The usefulness of BMI values is limited for athletes because of their highly developed muscle mass, and for pregnant and postpartal women because their increased weight is normal. In addition, BMI values have not been specifically calculated for people over age 65. Despite these limitations, BMI is useful in identifying underweight and obese individuals.

KnowledgeCheck 26–7

- What is the most accurate type of food diary?
- Compare and contrast four nutritional screening approaches.
- Identify three nutritional risk factors.

 Go to Chapter 26, **Knowledge Check Response Sheet and Answers,** on the Electronic Study Guide.

CriticalThinking 26–6

Calculate your WHR.
Use Box 26–6 in this volume to calculate your BMI. Evaluate the result.

- How useful is this data?
- Do you feel you need to pursue a program of weight loss? Why?

Imaging Techniques

Imaging techniques are not widely used to evaluate lean body mass because they are quite expensive to perform. These methods include the following:

- *Dual-energy x-ray absorptiometry (DEXA).* DEXA is used to assess bone mineral content and density. Because lean tissue has different absorptive properties than adipose tissue, this technique shows promise for wider use because it is quick and noninvasive.
- *Computed tomography (CT).* CT scans measure volume rather than actual body tissue composition. They can provide information about the quantity of adipose tissue, particularly in body cavities.
- *Magnetic resonance imaging (MRI).* MRI is an excellent noninvasive method for directly assessing body composition. The cost and availability of the machinery, however, make it impractical for day-to-day evaluation of clients.

Underwater Weighing

Hydrodensitometry, or underwater weighing, is another method of determining body composition. It requires total submersion of the patient in a tank of water. Because fat readily floats, the person's buoyancy will vary depending on his percentage of body fat. This method is considered the gold standard for body composition measures. However, clinical applications of this method are limited because it is impractical to use with children, the elderly, or individuals who are severely ill.

KnowledgeCheck 26–8

- What are the most reliable locations for skinfold measurement?
- What are the implications of an increased WHR?

 Go to Chapter 26, **Knowledge Check Response Sheet and Answers,** on the Electronic Study Guide.

What Physical Examination Findings Are Cues to Nutrient Imbalance?

You should correlate physical examination with other assessment findings, such as nutritional and medical history, dietary intake, anthropometric measurements, and laboratory findings. For guidelines in performing a nutrition-focused physical examination,

 Go to Chapter 26, **Assessment Guidelines and Tools, Nutrition-Focused Physical Examination,** in Volume 2.

Refer to Chapter 19 as needed for a review of physical examination techniques.

What Are the Signs of Severe Malnutrition?

Malnutrition is a condition of impaired development or function caused by a long-term deficiency, excess, or imbalance in energy and/or nutrient intake. Symptoms of undernutrition due to insufficient food are reduced physical activity, weight loss, and reduced height. Other diseases develop as a result of specific vitamin and mineral deficiency, such as beriberi (neurological deficits), scurvy (delayed wound healing and poor bone growth), and pellagra (diarrhea and dementia). See Tables 26–4 and 26–5, on pages 582–583 and 585–586, respectively, for specific signs of vitamin and mineral excesses and deficits.

Malnutrition is most common among children, older adults, and people with chronic illnesses such as cancer, HIV, and COPD. To assess for malnutrition in children, compare weight, height, and head circumference to the standards (norms) for the child's age. Other indicators in children include the presence of iron deficiency anemia and, in adolescents, a delay of stages of sexual maturation (Matarese & Gottschlich, 1998).

KnowledgeCheck 26–9

- Identify at least 10 physical examination findings that would lead you to suspect nutritional problems.
- What factors would lead to poor wound healing?

 Go to Chapter 26, **Knowledge Check Response Sheet and Answers,** on the Electronic Study Guide.

Tests Reflecting Nutritional Status: Norms

diagnostic testing

• Blood sugar	70 mg/dL to 110 mg/dL Capillary blood sugar is frequently assessed at the bedside. A simple fingerstick is required. Serum blood glucose levels are assessed by drawing a venous blood sample. The level is measured in the laboratory.
• Serum albumin	3.5–5 g/dL
• Pre-albumin	15–36 mg/dL
• Globulin	2.3–3.4 g/dL
• Blood urea nitrogen (BUN)	8–20 mg/dL
Elderly slightly higher	
Children	5–18 mg/dL
• Creatinine	0.5–1.2 mg/dL
• Hemoglobin	
Male	14–18 g/dL
Female	12–16 g/dL
Pregnant female	11 g/dL

What Laboratory Values Indicate Nutritional Status?

Various laboratory or biochemical indicators provide information about nutritional status. These include blood glucose, serum protein level and associated indices, total lymphocyte count, and hemoglobin (see Diagnostic Testing box).

Blood Glucose

The blood glucose level indicates the amount of fuel available for cellular energy. A homeostatic mechanism regulates the concentration of glucose in the blood. Levels above the normal set point trigger the release of insulin, which causes the glucose to move into body cells and to be stored in the liver and muscles. A level falling below the normal set point triggers the release of glucagons, leading to the release of glucose from storage.

Hypoglycemia (blood glucose of less than 70 mg/dL) limits the fuel supply to the body, resulting in symptoms ranging from weakness to coma. Often the cause is insufficient food intake, excessive physical exertion, or a disproportionate amount of hypoglycemic agents.

Hyperglycemia (blood glucose greater than 109 mg/dL fasting or greater than 126 mg/dL at random) is a sign of diabetes mellitus, an endocrine problem, which may develop as a result of either insufficient insulin production or resistance to the existing supply of insulin. A high blood glucose level does not mean that there is more fuel available for cellular energy, though. A characteristic of diabetes is that although there is more than enough glucose in the blood, it cannot enter and be used by the cells. Repeated blood glucose measures are required before making a diagnosis of diabetes mellitus because glucose levels may be temporarily elevated as a result of excessive carbohydrate intake or emotional and physical stressors.

A temporary rise in blood sugar may produce weakness or fatigue. Prolonged elevations lead to weight loss, blurred vision, ketosis (incomplete metabolism of fat due to inability to use carbohydrates as fuel), renal failure, and peripheral neuropathy (damage to nerves due to prolonged exposure to high glucose levels).

VOL 2 — Go to Chapter 26, **Procedure 26–1: Checking Fingerstick (Capillary) Blood Glucose Levels,** in Volume 2.

See the Critical Aspects box on page 612 for a summary.

Serum Protein Levels and Indices

Protein molecules dissolve in blood to form plasma proteins. Tissue proteins are a combination of albumin and globulin, so serum protein levels are indicators of protein stores.

- **Albumin** is synthesized in the liver and constitutes 60% of total body protein. Low levels of albumin are associated with malnutrition, malabsorption, acute and chronic liver disease, and repeated loss of protein through burns, wounds, or other sources. The half-life of albumin is 18 to 21 days. As a result, there is a lag in detecting nutritional problems based on serum albumin.

- **Pre-albumin** level fluctuates daily and is considered a better marker of acute change.

- **Transferrin** is a protein that binds with iron. Because it has a half-life of only 8 to 9 days, it allows for faster detection of protein depletion than does measuring albumin. Transferrin can be measured directly or indirectly (by a total iron-binding capacity test, or TIBC). It also reflects iron status. In a person with iron deficiency, the TIBC will be increased; in a person with anemia, the TIBC will be decreased.

Other markers are used to monitor protein metabolism:

- **Urea** is formed in the liver as an end product of protein metabolism and is excreted through the kidneys. As such, the serum blood urea nitrogen (BUN) level is an indicator of liver and kidney function. An elevated BUN level is seen with impaired kidney function, dehydration, excessive protein breakdown (often seen with diabetes mellitus, hyperthyroidism, or starvation) or excessive dietary protein intake. Low levels are seen with impaired liver function, fluid overload, and low protein intake.

- **Creatinine,** an end product of skeletal muscle metabolism, is excreted through the kidney and is an excellent indicator of renal function. Increased levels may indicate impaired kidney function or loss of muscle mass.

- **Lymphocytes,** or white blood cells (WBC), are the body's first line of defense against microorganisms. For a detailed discussion of the role of WBCs in infection control, as well as a discussion on the types of WBCs and their normal values, see Chapter 20. A decrease in total lymphocytes, known as **leukopenia,** is associated with malnutrition, protein deficiency, alcoholism, bone marrow depression, and anemia.

- **Hemoglobin** is composed of **heme,** an iron-rich compound, and **globulin,** a serum protein. Adequate iron intake is required to produce heme. Therefore, a low hemoglobin may indicate inadequate iron intake or chronic blood loss. Globulin forms the backbone of hemoglobin as well as antibodies, glycoproteins, lipoproteins, clotting factors, and a variety of key enzymes. A decreased globulin level indicates insufficient protein intake or excessive protein loss.

Delegating Nutritional Assessment

You may safely delegate to nursing assistants or other UAPs the measurement of weight, height, and intake and output; other nursing staff (e.g., licensed practical nurses) can collect a nutritional history. However, the registered nurse (RN) is responsible for reviewing and interpreting these findings. When delegating these tasks, you must also tell the UAP or LPN how often the measurements are to be made. Review Chapter 7 for making delegation decisions.

KnowledgeCheck 26–10

- What are the likely causes of hyperglycemia?
- Why is it important to identify the serum albumin level?

 Go to Chapter 26, **Knowledge Check Response Sheet and Answers,** on the Electronic Study Guide.

CriticalThinking 26–7

The Mini Nutritional Assessment (MNA) in Volume 2 is completed for a 70-year-old woman and yields the following results:
Part I Screening = 8
Part II Assessment = 10

- What would her Malnutrition Indicator Score be, and what does this indicate?
- What type of physical assessment findings would support this score?
- What type of anthropometric findings would support this score?
- What type of laboratory values would support this score?

| Nursing Diagnosis |

For clients who have no symptoms of or risk factors for nutrition problems, use the diagnostic label Readiness for Enhanced Nutrition. NANDA defines this as "pattern of nutrient intake that is sufficient for meeting metabolic needs and can be strengthened" (2005, p. 128).

Nutrition as the Problem

You can use the following four NANDA labels to describe general nutrition problems:

- Imbalanced Nutrition: Less Than Body Requirements
- Imbalanced Nutrition: More Than Body Requirements
- Risk for Imbalanced Nutrition: More Than Body Requirements
- Self-Care Deficit (Feeding)

As you have learned, nutrition problems have many causes. Etiologies for undernutrition include eating disorders, difficulties with chewing, vomiting, alcoholism, food intolerances, metabolic disorders, digestive disorders, and absorption disorders. For overnutrition, etiologies include overeating, lack of exercise, and metabolic

or endocrine disorders. The following nursing diagnoses may also contribute to nutrition problems: Diarrhea, Health-Seeking Behaviors (Nutrition), Impaired Swallowing, Nausea, Noncompliance (with prescribed diet), and Deficient Knowledge (nutrition).

The following is an example of a nutrition nursing diagnosis statement:

> Imbalanced Nutrition: Less Than Body Requirements related to difficulty chewing and Impaired Swallowing

Nutrition as the Etiology

Nutritional problems can also be the etiology of problems in other functional areas, for example:

- Ineffective Breastfeeding related to inadequate milk production 2° insufficient intake of calories and fluids
- Constipation related to insufficient intake of fluids and fiber
- Diarrhea related to excessive intake of alcohol and/or sugar
- Risk for Infection related to inadequate intake of calories and protein
- Impaired (or Risk for Impaired) Skin Integrity related to inadequate intake of protein and/or vitamin A
- Disturbed Sleep Pattern related to excessive caffeine intake or to eating fatty and spicy foods near bedtime
- Impaired Social Interaction related to low self-esteem 2° obesity

| Planning Outcomes/Evaluation |

The overall *Healthy People 2010* nutrition goal for the United States population is to "promote health and reduce chronic disease associated with diet and weight" (U.S. Department of Health and Human Services, 2000). For specific objectives related to that goal,

 Go to Chapter 26, **Tables, Boxes, Figures: ESG Box 26–1,** on the Electronic Study Guide.

NOC standardized outcomes directly linked to nutritional problems include the following: Nutritional Status, Nutritional Status: Food and Fluid Intake, Nutritional Status: Nutrient Intake, and Weight Control.

You would choose other NOC outcomes based on the patient's nursing diagnosis. For example, for Situational Low Self-Esteem related to obesity, you might use Self-Esteem; for Noncompliance (prescribed diet), you could use Adherence Behavior, Compliance Behavior, or Treatment Behavior: Illness/Injury.

Individualized goals/outcome statements you might write for a patient with nutrition-related problems include the following:

- Loses 1 lb per week until ideal weight is attained.

- After one teaching session, uses the Food Guide Pyramid to describe a healthy diet.
- Follows the prescribed modified diet that, at a minimum, meets the DRIs.
- Eats a variety of foods that provide a balanced diet.
- Achieves appropriate BMI (height-weight) range within 6 weeks.

| Planning Interventions/Implementation |

NIC standardized interventions directly linked to nutrition problems include the broad interventions of Nutrition Management, Nutrition Therapy, Nutritional Counseling, and Nutritional Monitoring. These interventions could probably be used for most nutrition problems, regardless of the etiologies. The other 13 interventions grouped under Nutritional Support address specific etiologies (e.g., Swallowing Therapy).

 Go to Chapter 26, **Standardized Language, NOC Outcomes and NIC Interventions Related to Nutrition,** in Volume 2.

Individualized nursing actions are determined by the patient's nursing diagnosis. They may include, for example, counseling regarding vitamin and mineral supplementation, teaching clients on a limited budget how to buy nutritious foods, supporting special nutritional needs, and assisting clients with meals.

Vitamin and Mineral Supplementation

Do you take a vitamin tablet every day? Do you know anyone who takes megadoses of vitamin C to prevent a cold? Or zinc to cure one? Noncredentialed nutrition "experts" recommend, and sell, megadoses of the entire alphabet of vitamin and mineral supplements to prevent cancer and heart attacks, improve your sex life, prevent aging, and work other miracles. However, conservative health professionals may scoff at supplements, insisting that a nutritious diet supplies all the micronutrients you need. Somewhere in the middle, most likely, lies the truth. A growing body of research suggest that certain supplements provide health benefits. Remember, too, that RDAs are for "average" needs. Individual needs for micronutrients vary. During periods of increased nutrient demands, it may be difficult to get enough nutrients from diet alone. For example, folic acid and iron supplements are important for pregnant women.

NIC Intervention—Nutritional Counseling

When teaching clients about supplements, keep the following principles in mind:

1. Dietary supplements may be appropriate for people whose diet does not provide the recommended intake of specific vitamins. With a few exceptions, there is little evidence to suggest that people will be harmed by taking vitamin supplements in appropriate amounts (U.S. Preventive Services Task Force [USPSTF], 2003).

2. Individual needs vary, and those needs should determine the specific nutrients and amounts used. For example:
   - Newborn infants are given a vitamin K injection to prevent hemorrhaging because they do not yet have bacterial flora in the gut to synthesize the vitamin.
   - Breastfed infants may need a vitamin D supplement (but not other vitamins) if the mother does not have an adequate diet or if the baby does not receive enough exposure to sunlight.
   - Vegetarians who eat little or no animal products may need a vitamin D supplement.
   - The USPSTF recommends folic acid supplementation for people taking methotrexate.
   - All women who are capable of becoming pregnant should obtain 400 micrograms daily from fortified foods or supplements, in addition to the naturally occurring folate they eat in foods.
   - Most adults older than 50 years should obtain vitamin B_{12} from fortified foods or supplements.
   - People who do not eat dairy products need supplemental calcium.

3. Food is the best source of nutrients. Supplements do not replace the need to eat a nutritious diet. Vitamins need carbohydrate, protein, and fat to do their work. Specific supplements for certain individual situations are more effective if the person also has an adequate diet.

4. Read supplement labels carefully. They provide information about toxicity levels, dosage, and side effects.

5. Encourage patients to ask their primary care provider's advice before taking vitamins.

6. Advise patients to follow the dosages recommended in the DRIs or RDAs.

7. Be certain that any health claims made for a supplement are based on sound research.

8. The long-term effects of most nutritional supplements have yet to be fully researched.

The same principles apply with regard to mineral supplementation. Supplements of specific minerals may be needed during growth periods (i.e., pregnancy, lactation, and adolescence), but as a rule healthy adults eating balanced diets do not need supplements. People who require mineral supplementation include those who refuse dairy products (and therefore lack calcium), and those with clinical problems such as iron-deficiency anemia, zinc deficiency (e.g., in alcoholism and long-term low-calorie diets), and treatment with certain diuretics (e.g., for hypertension).

Nutritious Foods on a Limited Budget

Many studies document hunger and malnutrition among the poor in the United States. When your clients cannot afford to buy food, you should teach them about available assistance and make appropriate referrals to programs such as the following:

• *Food Stamp Program.* For households with income below the program's "poverty limit," this federal program issues coupons that can be used to buy food to cover the household's needs.

• *Commodity Distribution Program.* The federal government buys certain surplus food items to support certain agricultural products. These include both perishable and nonperishable commodities, which are distributed to persons in need. Examples include peanut butter and cheese.

• *Supplemental Food Program for Women, Infants, and Children (WIC).* This federal program provides free food to low-income women who are pregnant or breast-feeding and to children under age 5. Typical foods that are available are milk, eggs, cheese, cereals, juice, and infant formulas. They are intended to supplement the diet with protein, iron, and vitamins. They are not meant to supply all necessary food for the household.

• *National school lunch and breakfast programs.* These programs subsidize schools that provide free or reduced-rate breakfasts and/or lunches to poor children. All students, then, pay slightly less than the full cost of the meal. Lunches must supply about one-third of the child's RDA for energy and nutrients.

NIC Intervention—Teaching: Individual

You can help your clients to use their food dollars creatively by teaching them to follow the suggestions in the accompanying Self-Care box.

Supporting Special Nutritional Needs

Patients with special needs, such as patients with Impaired Swallowing, patients who are NPO, and older adults, may require specific nutrition interventions.

Impaired Swallowing

The NANDA diagnosis Impaired Swallowing may be caused by mechanical obstruction (e.g., tumor), neuromuscular impairment (e.g., facial paralysis), stroke, cerebral palsy, or a host of other anatomical or physiological defects. Nutritional support for patients with Impaired Swallowing includes activities from the NIC intervention Swallowing Therapy (Dochterman & Bulechek, 2004, pp. 697–698) For a list of these activities,

VOL 2 Go to Chapter 26, **Technique 26–3: Interventions for Patients with Impaired Swallowing,** in Volume 2.

self-care

Teaching Your Patients to Buy Nutritious Foods on a Limited Budget

• Plan ahead. (1) Look at the supermarket advertisements in the paper or in their fliers, and plan meals around the sale items that are also the most nutrient-dense. (2) Make a list of the foods you need. This will help you to control impulse buying and extra trips to the store.

• Buy wisely. (1) Buy "generic" instead of more expensive and widely advertised brands. (2) Watch for sales of nutrient-dense items. Stock up on and freeze them for later use if you do not need them right away. (3) Buy in quantity—if it results in real savings and if you can use that amount of food before it spoils. (4) Limit "convenience" foods (e.g., frozen dinners); they are expensive and often high in fat and sodium. (5) Buy foods when they are in season; for example, fresh tomatoes are less expensive, and better tasting, in the summer than in the winter.

• Substitute dairy products, beans and lentils, and peanut butter for more expensive meat. Substitute powdered milk for whole milk.

• Buy inexpensive cuts of meat; avoid processed "lunchmeats" and hot dogs.

• If transportation is not a problem, buy fresh foods at farmers' markets, at consumer co-ops, and from neighbors who have gardens.

• Purchase oatmeal and cream of wheat instead of cold, sugared cereals.

• Buy frozen concentrated fruit juices instead of juice in plastic jugs and cardboard boxes.

• Avoid eating at fast-food restaurants. Meals are more expensive and less nutritious than those you can prepare at home.

• Avoid shopping at convenience stores. Items are usually more expensive than in supermarkets.

• Read the nutrition facts panels on prepared foods to be sure you obtain the most nutrition for the money.

Patients Who Are NPO

Patients who cannot have oral food and fluids require comfort measures. Intravenous fluids for hydration may also include small amounts of glucose, but certainly not enough to meet body needs. Provide or assist the patient with oral hygiene. If allowed, provide ice chips, hard candy, chewing gum, or sips of water

for rinsing the mouth. Advise family or visitors not to eat or drink around the patient, and try to schedule other activities for the patient at mealtimes.

Older Adults

Nutritional problems of older adults are similar to those for adults of all ages, but the incidence of problems may be higher among older adults. The following interventions are appropriate for patients of any age who experience the problems.

- *Self-Care Deficit: Feeding.* You will find interventions in the section "Assisting Patients with Meals," following.

- *Loss of appetite; diminished sense of smell and taste.* Refer to the section "Improving the Patient's Appetite."

- *Decreased income.* Refer to the Self-Care box. In addition, for older adults in the United States, two types of food programs are available for you to recommend. Everyone over age 60, regardless of income, can eat hot noon meals at a community center (under the Congregate Meals Programs). Those who are ill or disabled can receive meals at home under the Home Delivered Meals Program. Socially needy persons (e.g., someone who is homeless) are given priority.

- *Nutritional deficiencies.* Advise clients to eat nutrient-dense foods and to eat essential foods first. Because the sense of taste is decreased, older adults may prefer concentrated sweets; and because they may also have a poor appetite, once they eat sweets they may not be hungry enough to eat other foods.

- *Gastroesophageal reflux.* Advise clients to not eat just before bedtime and to elevate the head of the bed 30 to 40°. It is also important to avoid overeating, avoid bending over, and take their prescribed medications. They should also avoid fruit juices, fatty foods, chocolate, alcohol, and smoking; all of these stimulate reflux. If overweight, the client should lose weight.

- *Decreased gastric secretions.* People with this problem should eat regularly scheduled meals, chew their food thoroughly, and take prescribed medications. They should be certain to eat foods rich in vitamin D to ensure calcium absorption.

- *Glucose intolerance.* Obviously, patients with glucose intolerance should avoid concentrated, refined sugars (e.g., candy, ice cream, desserts), unless they have been told to use it to treat hypoglycemia. Complex carbohydrates (e.g., cereals, vegetables) are better tolerated. Smaller, more frequent meals may also be necessary.

- *Decreased intestinal peristalsis.* To prevent constipation, advise patients to eat a diet high in fiber, including a minimum of five servings of fresh fruits and vegetables every day (prunes and prune juice are often effective); exercise regularly; drink at least 8 glasses of water or other fluids per day; and eat meals on a regular schedule.

Assisting Patients with Meals

Some patients are at risk for nutritional deficits as a result of a Self-Care Deficit (Feeding), which may be caused by loss of cognitive, musculoskeletal, or neuro-muscular function; weakness; pain; or environmental barriers. An important intervention for such patients is to assist them with eating (NIC interventions are Feeding and Self-Care Assistance: Feeding). Nursing activities include the following:

- Assess for functional deficits that contribute to the Self-Care Deficit.

- Assess intake for nutritional adequacy.

- Demonstrate the use of assistive devices and alternative methods for eating and drinking.

- Refer the patient and family to an agency that can help them obtain a home health aide.

- Collaborate with occupational and physical therapists in planning care.

- Serve one food at a time; serve small amounts.

- Assist the patient to eat and drink only as necessary; encourage independence.

- Serve finger foods (e.g., fruit, bread) to promote independence.

- Provide privacy during meals if the patient is embarrassed; to further maintain dignity, use a napkin, not a bib, over the patient's clothes.

- Allow the patient to determine in which order he will eat the foods.

- Sit down while feeding the patient; do not rush.

- Have casual conversation with the patient while feeding him to make mealtime more pleasant and relaxed.

- If the patient can feed himself, prepare the food on the tray for him (e.g., cut the meat, peel an orange, open the milk and butter containers).

For additional guidelines,

 Go to Chapter 26, **Technique 26–4: Assisting Patients with Meals,** in Volume 2.

WHAT ARE OVERWEIGHT AND OBESITY?

The BMI is a commonly used tool to define weight status. A client with a BMI greater than 25 but less than 29.9 is considered **overweight.** In contrast, **obesity** is a BMI of 30 or higher.

| Nursing Diagnosis |

NANDA diagnoses define the overweight or obesity problem in the following ways:

- *Imbalanced Nutrition: More Than Body Requirements* is used when a person consumes nutrients in excess of metabolic needs. The defining characteristics are

(1) triceps skinfold greater than 15 mm in men and 25 mm in women, or (2) weight 20% over ideal for height and frame.

- *Risk for Imbalanced Nutrition: More Than Body Requirements* identifies the potential for an individual to experience intake of nutrients in excess of metabolic needs.

Etiologies of those NANDA diagnoses include the following:

- Consuming more kcal than needed for activity, gender, height, and weight.
- Reducing activity level without modifying food intake.
- Genetic predisposition to obesity. For example, low BMR and excess adipose tissue distribution are common in certain ethnic groups.
- Ineffective coping mechanisms—for instance, the use of binge eating to reduce anxiety or relieve boredom.
- Cultural influences—some cultural norms encourage excess weight, particularly as an indication of wealth.
- Decreased levels of thyroid hormone can lower BMR, causing weight gain.
- Ineffective Health Maintenance—for example, high-fat diet, inactivity, and avoidance of health assistance.
- Impaired Physical Mobility, which limits physical activity and decreases energy expenditure.

Being overweight may contribute to the development of other nursing diagnoses. Excess weight, and especially obesity, makes activity more difficult; therefore, over time, the person becomes more sedentary, and the body becomes deconditioned (weakened). The following are examples:

- Activity Intolerance related to deconditioned state secondary to long-term sedentary lifestyle
- Decreased Cardiac Output related to prolonged deconditioned state
- Constipation related to inadequate physical activity
- Risk for Injury (and/or Risk for Falls) related to deconditioned state and generalized weakness
- Social Isolation related to poor self-image secondary to excess weight

| Planning Outcomes/Evaluation |

The NOC standardized outcome for evaluating weight is Weight Control. If it becomes necessary to monitor nutritional status, you could use the labels of Nutritional Status: Food and Fluid Intake and Nutritional Status: Nutrient Intake.

Individualized goals/outcome statements include the following examples:

- States pertinent factors contributing to weight gain.

- Claims ownership and responsibility for current eating patterns.
- Designs dietary modifications to meet individual long-term goal of weight control.
- Accomplishes desired weight loss in a reasonable time frame (1 to 2 lb/wk).
- Incorporates appropriate physical activities requiring energy expenditure into daily life.

| Planning Interventions/Implementation |

For the *NIC standardized interventions* for overweight and obese clients,

 Go to Chapter 26, **Standardized Language, NOC Outcomes and NIC Interventions for Overweight/Obesity and Underweight/Malnutrition,** in Volume 2.

Individualized nursing activities include the following:

- Suggest keeping a food diary for a number of days. Analyzing the diary will provide valuable information on intake and circumstances that trigger eating. It may help to identify behavioral or coping issues. Keep in mind that many patients eat less than usual when they are keeping a food diary.
- Weigh the client weekly under the same conditions. Weekly weights allow the client to monitor his progress and can motivate the client to follow the weight-loss regimen.
- Instruct the client regarding adequate intake. Lifestyle changes must be permanent for the client to maintain weight loss. For the client, the first step is to learn about a balanced diet and the kcal content of foods.
- Encourage the client to adopt an exercise program. Increased physical activity will not only burn off excess stores of fat but also increase the body's resting metabolic rate. Individuals should begin gradually with low-impact activities, such as walking for 20 minutes several times a week.
- Fat substitutes are available to improve flavor and texture of low-fat foods while reducing total dietary fat. Recall that fats contain 9 kcal per gram, so reducing fat intake is an important part of most weight-loss diets. Fat substitutes are not absorbed; therefore, they contribute few kcal. The American Heart Association (2004) states that fat substitutes, used appropriately, can provide flexibility in diet planning. Although the USDA (FDA) considers fat substitutes to be safe, long-term benefits and risks are not yet known. In addition, it is not unusual for people to experience diarrhea and stomach cramps when using fat substitutes.

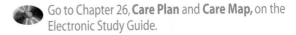 Go to Chapter 26, **Care Plan** and **Care Map,** on the Electronic Study Guide.

WHAT ARE UNDERWEIGHT AND UNDERNUTRITION?

A person becomes underweight when he consumes fewer kcal than needed based on his activity, gender, height, and weight. Consuming too few kcal may result in serious undernutrition; that is, insufficient intake of protein, fat, vitamins, and minerals. The causes of underweight status may be psychological, social, economic, or physiological. A person can also be malnourished with regard to specific nutrients without being underweight.

Eating disorders are a growing problem in North America. Both anorexia and bulimia can result in hair loss, low blood pressure, generalized weakness, amenorrhea, osteoporosis, brain damage, and even death. Other problems arising from being underweight include decreased resistance to infection and cold intolerance.

| Nursing Diagnosis |

Nursing diagnoses you may use for clients who are underweight or undernourished include the following:

- Imbalanced Nutrition: Less Than Body Requirements—intake of nutrients is insufficient to meet metabolic needs.

- Risk for Imbalanced Nutrition: Less Than Body Requirements. This diagnosis is appropriate for clients who are at risk for insufficient intake of nutrients to meet metabolic needs. Note that this is not a NANDA diagnosis.

- Adult Failure to Thrive—progressive functional deterioration of a physical and cognitive nature. The person has no appetite, is apathetic, and consumes less than 75% of normal requirements at each or most meals.

The following nursing diagnoses may be the etiology of the underweight condition:

- Impaired Dentition may be used if dental caries, dental fractures, or missing teeth affect the ability to chew food.

- Impaired Swallowing may influence intake if an individual has pain with swallowing or chokes and/or coughs with swallowing attempts.

- Impaired Oral Mucous Membrane (e.g., stomatitis, ulcers) limits dietary intake because of pain and altered sense of taste.

- Diarrhea (frequent, loose, liquid stools) prevents absorption of nutrients.

- Chronic Confusion and cognitive decline create problems with reasoning and responding appropriately to stimuli. The person may forget to eat or forget how to prepare and eat food.

The following nursing diagnoses may result from an underweight or malnourished condition:

- Risk for Delayed Development is considered when there is a 25% or more delay in the development of cognitive, language, or motor skills due to poor nutritional intake.

- Risk for Infection may be appropriate for a client in a debilitated state due to inadequate nutrition.

- Risk for Impaired Skin Integrity results from inadequate intake of food and fluids and from excessive weight loss.

| Planning Outcomes/Evaluation |

The NOC standardized outcome for assessing weight is Weight Control. If it becomes necessary to monitor nutritional status, you could use the labels of Nutritional Status: Food and Fluid Intake and Nutritional Status: Nutrient Intake.

Individualized goals/outcome statements include the following:

- Progressively gains weight toward desired goal.

- Verbalizes willingness to follow diet.

- Body mass and weight are within normal limits.

- Laboratory values (e.g., albumin, CBC) are within normal limits.

- Recognizes factors contributing to underweight.

| Planning Interventions/Implementation |

For the *NIC standardized interventions* for undernutrition,

 Go to Chapter 26, **Standardized Language, NOC Outcomes and NIC Interventions for Overweight/Obesity and Underweight/Malnutrition,** in Volume 2.

Individualized nursing activities for clients who are underweight or undernourished include the following:

- Assess for recent changes in physiological status (e.g., pain, fatigue, illness, and immobility).

- Offer high-calorie and high-protein (nutrient-dense) foods. Serve these foods when the person is most likely to be hungry. Avoid food with little nutritional value; when intake is limited, it is essential that it not be wasted on "empty" calories.

- Consult with a dietitian on strategies to increase the nutritional content of foods.

- Weigh the client regularly under the same conditions. Weigh the client one to two times per week if nutritional status is severely jeopardized to assess the effectiveness of the therapeutic plan.

- Offer high-protein supplements. Offer nutritious high-protein supplements between meals to increase intake of protein and calories. It may be easier for the client to drink a small amount of a supplement than to eat enough food to supply equivalent nutrients.

Procedure 26–1: Checking Fingerstick (Capillary) Blood Glucose Levels

- Have the patient wash hands with warm soap and water. Some agency policies may still require that you cleanse the patient's finger with an alcohol prep pad.

- Check the reagent test strips for expiration date.

- Engage the sterile lancet, hold it perpendicular to the skin, and puncture the skin.

- Wipe off the first drop of blood; then allow contact between the drop of blood and the test patch.

- Place the correct reagent strip into the blood glucose meter.

- After the indicated amount of time, read the blood glucose level indicated on the digital display.

(Most meters include instructions from the manufacturer. Follow the instructions.)

Procedure 26–2: Inserting Nasogastric and Nasoenteric Tubes

- Place the patient in a sitting or high-Fowler's position.

- Measure the length of the nasogastric tube by measuring from the tip of the nose to the earlobe to the xiphoid process. For nasoenteric tubes, add 8 to 10 cm (3 to 4 in.) to this measurement.

- Lubricate the tube with water-soluble lubricant.

- Have the patient hyperextend the neck.

- Insert the tube gently through the nostril.

- When the patient begins to gag, instruct him to tilt the head forward, drink water, and swallow.

- Withdraw the tube immediately if respiratory distress occurs during insertion.

- Confirm tube placement by testing the pH of the aspirate, by auscultation, and/or by x-ray film.

- Tape the tube in place.

Procedure 26–3: Administering Feedings Through Gastric and Enteric Tubes

- Check medical order for the type of formula, rate, route, and frequency of feeding.

- Verify tube placement before administering the feeding.

- Elevate the head of the bed at least 30° while administering the feedings and for an hour after administration.

- Check residual volume before feeding.

  For continuous feeding: Check gastric residual volume every 4 to 6 hours. If the residual is 10% greater than the formula flow rate for 1 hour (or alternatively, a total of 150 mL), hold the feeding for 1 hour and recheck. Notify the physician if the residual is still not within normal limits.
  For gastrostomy, percutaneous endoscopic gastrostomy (PEG) tubes, and jejunostomy tubes: (1) Check residual volume every 4 hours. (2) Residual volumes are not checked for jejunostomy tubes.

- Flush the tubing with 30 mL of water every 4 hours and before and after medication administration.

- Change the tube feeding administration set every 24 hours.

Procedure 26–4: Removing a Nasogastric or Nasoenteric Tube

- Assist the patient to a sitting or high-Fowler's position.

- Clear the tube of secretions by injecting 10 mL of air through the main lumen.

- Have the patient hold his breath, and gently, but quickly, withdraw the tube.

- Discard the equipment.

- Suggest community resources (e.g., Meals on Wheels). Additional assistance may be needed to improve access to food.

The following sections discuss more fully nursing interventions for improving the appetite, as well as alternative feeding methods.

Improving the Patient's Appetite

Illness, with its accompanying pain, anxiety, and medications, often causes appetite loss. This is especially true for institutionalized patients, who have little control over food choices and preparation. You will need to make an effort to see that hospitalized patients eat the food that is served. It is not enough merely to order meals and deliver the trays. The following measures may help improve appetite and intake, and subsequently, nutritional status:

- Offer frequent, small meals. Even distribution of foods throughout the day helps prevent gastric distention and improves appetite by keeping the patient from being overwhelmed with a large amount of food.

- Restrict liquid intake with meals to prevent gastric distention or feeling full before the patient consumes sufficient nutrients.

- Keep the patient environment neat and clean and free of unpleasant sights, odors, and medical equipment. These often trigger loss of appetite.
- Provide or assist with good oral hygiene.
- Provide a pleasant eating environment.
- Serve foods attractively; arrange the tray so the person can easily reach the food.
- Position the person comfortably for mealtime.
- Find out what the person likes to eat, and encourage family and friends to bring foods from home.
- Control pain around the clock, and avoid painful treatments prior to meals.

Alternative Feeding Methods

If a patient cannot meet his nutritional needs through an enhanced diet and measures to stimulate the appetite, you may need to use an alternative feeding method. Feeding can occur through the intestinal tract as enteral nutrition, or intravenously as parenteral nutrition.

What Is Enteral Nutrition?

Enteral nutrition (*tube feeding*) refers to the delivery of liquid nutrition into the upper intestinal tract via a tube. Tube feeding may be used in addition to or instead of oral intake. It is the preferred method of feeding for a patient who has a functioning intestinal tract but needs nutritional support (e.g., patients with high metabolic needs, such as those with trauma, burns, or severe malnutrition; neurological disorders that affect swallowing; anorexia nervosa; prematurity (infants); failure to thrive; or specific bowel diseases). Tube feeding may be a short- or long-term therapy.

Studies indicate that enteral feedings are preferred to parenteral (i.e., intravenous) nutrition because they reduce incidence of sepsis and maintain intestinal structure and function (Guenter, Ericson, & Jones, 1997). However, there are some risks associated with enteral feedings. If enteral formula is aspirated into the lungs, it can lead to infection, pneumonia, abscess formation, and adult respiratory distress syndrome (ARDS). The high glucose content of enteral formulas provides a medium for bacterial growth. Other complications include diarrhea, alterations in drug absorption and metabolism, and various metabolic disturbances.

Types of Feeding Tubes

Short-term enteric feedings (less than 6 weeks) are usually delivered through a **nasogastric (NG)** tube or a nasoeneteric (NE) tube. As a nurse, you may be asked to place a nasogastric, or small-bore, feeding tube. The tube is inserted through one side of the nose, passed through the nasopharynx into the esophagus, and finally into the stomach. Placing the tube through

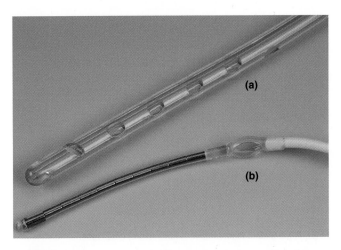

FIGURE 26–8 *A,* Nasogastric tubes may be used for drainage of the stomach or feeding. Smaller gauge tubes are preferred for feeding. *B,* Weighted nasoenteric tube.

the mouth is an option, but this method is more likely to trigger gagging or unconscious chewing on the tube.

VOL 2 Go to Chapter 26, **Procedure 26–2: Inserting Nasogastric and Nasoenteric Tubes,** in Volume 2.

The Critical Aspects box on page 612 provides a summary of the procedure.

A **nasoenteric (NE) tube** is longer than an NG tube, extending through the nose down into the duodenum or jejunuem. As with an NG tube, a small, flexible tube is preferred for feeding. An NE tube may be used instead of an NG tube for patients at risk for aspiration. This includes patients who have a decreased level of consciousness, absent or diminished gag reflex, or severe gastroesophageal reflux.

The **lumen** (inside diameter) of a feeding tube is measured using the **French (Fr) scale:** The larger the lumen, the larger the diameter. Most feeding tubes for adults are 8 to 12 Fr and 90 to 108 cm (36 to 43 in.) long (Figure 26–8a). Each Fr unit is about 0.33 mm, so a 12 Fr tube is about 4 mm in diameter. Large-bore NG tubes (greater than 12 Fr) are occasionally used for feeding. However, they are less flexible and are more commonly used if stomach drainage is required.

For long-term feedings, a **percutaneous gastrostomy tube (PEG)** or **jejunostomy tube** is preferred (Figure 26–9). These are placed surgically or laparoscopically through the skin and the abdominal wall into the stomach or jejunum. The surgical incision is sometimes sutured tightly around the tube to hold it in place and prevent leakage. You must use surgical asepsis to care for a new incision. However, once the incision heals, you can remove and reinsert the tube for each feeding. Once the tube is in place, it is the most comfortable of all of the feeding tubes. Historically, a PEG was reserved for clients needing long-term nutritional support. However, that trend is

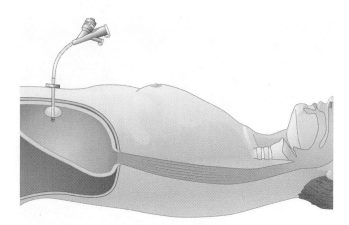

FIGURE 26–9 A percutaneous gastrostomy (PEG) tube.

changing. Patient comfort and improved technology leading to ease of insertion have made PEG an option even for short-term use.

The focus of this chapter is on use of enteral tubes as a route for feeding; however, they are inserted for other reasons:

- Lavage of the stomach (e.g., when there is bleeding and in cases of poisoning or medication overdose).
- Collecting a specimen of stomach contents for laboratory tests
- After surgery, to prevent nausea, vomiting, and gastric distention

Checking Feeding Tube Placement

NG and NE feeding tubes are placed without direct visualization. Therefore, you must check the location of the tip of the feeding tube before infusing an enteral feeding. Failure to verify placement could be disastrous because it may result in infusion of formula into the lungs. *Radiographic verification* is the most reliable method for confirming tube placement. All feeding tubes contain markings that may be detected by radiographic films. Radiography is often used to confirm initial tube placement; however, it is too expensive to use for ongoing verification of placement. Furthermore, even if the tube is placed correctly in the stomach (or intestine) on insertion, it may later move upward, so you must check placement before every feeding, or once a shift for continuous feedings. Other methods to verify the tube location include the following:

- *Aspiration of stomach contents.* Gastric contents are normally greenish-brown; intestinal contents, yellow-green due to the influence of bile.
- *Measuring the pH (acidity) of the aspirate.* Because of the action of hydrochloric acid in the stomach, gastric contents have an acidic pH. Stomach contents normally measure a pH of 1 to 4. However, if the client is receiving medications to control stomach acidity, such as antacids, H_2 blockers, or proton pump inhibitors, the pH may be as high as 6.

- *Injecting air into the feeding tube.* If the tube is in the stomach, injecting 5 to 30 mL of air produces a gurgling sound audible by listening with a stethoscope over the stomach. If the tube has been inadvertently placed in the lungs, you will not hear gurgling. This is the least reliable method for checking placement of an NG or NE tube.

For guidelines for checking enteral tube placement,

 Go to Chapter 26, **Technique 26–5: Checking Feeding Tube Placement,** in Volume 2.

KnowledgeCheck 26–11

- When is enteral nutrition the preferred alternative feeding?
- Identify and describe the types of enteral nutrition tubes.
- List four tube placement verification techniques.

 Go to Chapter 26, **Knowledge Check Response Sheet and Answers,** on the Electronic Study Guide.

Administering Enteral Feedings

In a few institutions, enteral feeding formulas are blended in the kitchen, but most use one of the many commercially prepared products. The type of product selected depends on the patient's health condition. Products vary in nutritional components and caloric concentration. Box 26–7 describes the main types of enteral feeding preparations.

Feeding Schedules **Continuous feedings** provide a constant flow of formula and an even distribution of nutrition throughout the day. For example, an infusion of 50 mL/hr for 24 hours of a 1 kcal/mL formula provides 1200 kcal per day. Continuous infusions are administered, usually via small-bore NG or NE tube or PEG, to patients in debilitated states who require intensive nutritional support. Feedings may be interrupted for periodic instillation of medications or flushing with water.

- *Pump-controlled infusions* are recommended for jejunal feedings and for gastrostomy feedings given by continuous infusion to decrease gastroesophageal reflux (American Gastrointestinal Association, 1995). A feeding pump ensures a steady flow rate.
- *Gravity feedings* can also be used, but the rate of delivery is not precise, and they increase the risk of gastroesophageal reflux, diarrhea, and aspiration. You regulate the drip rate by adjusting a clamp on the tubing clamp, much the same as adjusting an IV rate.

Cyclic feedings are administered regularly; however, the infusion time is less than 24 hours per day. Nocturnal feedings are a form of cyclic feedings. The patient is able to eat meals and participate in activities throughout the day but receives an infusion of enteral formula at night while at rest. Another variant is a 20-hour infusion. A 4-hour break allows time

26-7 Types of Enteral Feeding Solutions

- *"Basic" feeding formulas* are used for clients who have no significant nutritional deficits but are unable to eat or eat sufficiently. They provide 1 kcal per mL of solution, and meet the needs of most patients. A standard formula contains 12–20% of kcal in protein, 45–60% of kcal in carbohydrates, and 30–40% of kcal from fats. They also contain vitamins and minerals. They are usually lactose-free and contain complex forms of carbohydrates, fats, and proteins. Therefore, they require digestion and absorption.

- *High-protein formulas* are for clients who have substantial need for protein, such as those with burns, open wounds, or malnutrition.

- *"Elemental" formulas* do not contain complex proteins; instead, they contain amino acids or peptides. They are reserved for patients with severe small bowel absorptive dysfunction. These formulas are fiber-free and highly osmotic. Their use is controversial.

- *Diabetic formulas* are for clients who require tube feedings to meet nutritional needs but have type I or type II DM. These formulas control carbohydrate intake.

- *Renal formulas* are for clients who require tube feedings to meet nutritional needs but have renal failure or renal insufficiency as a comorbidity. These formulas limit potassium, sodium, and nitrogen intake.

- *Pulmonary formulas* provide 55% of the calories as fat so that less CO_2 is produced per unit of oxygen consumed. They are used, for example, for patients with lung disease.

- *Fiber-containing formulas.* Because fiber has a potential protective effect for multiple disease states, including diverticulosis, colon cancer, diabetes, and heart disease, fiber-containing formulas may be used for patients in long-term care facilities or patients who require enteral feedings for a prolonged period of time.

>75% but <90%, give 100 mL of formula after each meal.

>50% but <75%, give 200 mL of formula after each meal.

>25% but <50%, give 300 mL of formula after each meal.

0 to 25% of the ordered diet, give 400 mL of formula.

Intermittent feedings are sometimes given by **bolus,** if the patient can tolerate this method. In this method, you use a syringe to deliver 300 to 400 mL of formula through the tube over a 5- to 10-minute period. This is the easiest method to teach family members for home care, and it frees the patient from mechanical devices that limit activity. But because the fluid is given more rapidly by this method, it increases the risk for aspiration and for stomach distention. You can use it only with gastric tubes, never with intestinal tubes.

Feeding Systems May Be Open or Closed   An **open system** is exposed to the environment. One example is to open cans of formula and use a syringe to inject the formula into the tube; alternatively, you can pour it into a reservoir (e.g., a plastic bag). You should flush and clean the system after each delivery. Most agencies require that an open-system feeding not hang for more than 4 hours.

A **closed system** is a prefilled system (e.g., a bag or a bottle) that functions much like IV fluid. The container is spiked by tubing that is attached to the feeding pump or run through a manually controlled drip chamber. Closed systems decrease the risk of contamination. A prefilled closed-system container can safely hang for 24 to 36 hours if you use sterile technique. You can measure out the specified amount in the drip chamber, allowing the remainder of the container to be used later in the day.

Administer feedings at room temperature, and be sure to check the expiration date of any feedings prior to starting an infusion. For complete instructions,

 Go to Chapter 26, **Procedure 26–3: Administering Feedings Through Gastric and Enteric Tubes,** in Volume 2.

In this volume, the Critical Aspects box on page 612 summarizes this procedure.

Monitoring Patients Receiving Enteral Nutrition

For patients receiving enteral nutrition, you will need to monitor tube placement, skin condition, laboratory values (especially blood glucose, BUN, and electrolytes), feeding residual, and gastrointestinal status. For guidelines,

 Go to Chapter 26, **Technique 26–6: Monitoring Patients Receiving Enteral Nutrition,** in Volume 2.

for the feeding pump to be disconnected for hygiene and other activities.

Intermittent feedings are given to supplement oral intake or for patients who desire greater mobility to take part in activities, such as physical therapy. Feedings are given on a regular or periodic basis several times a day, usually over 30 to 60 minutes. An example of an order for a *regular feeding* is, "Give 250 to 500 mL of enteral nutrition every 4 to 6 hours." *Periodic feedings* are often based on oral intake. Consider the following periodic feeding order:

If the client consumes 90 to 100% of the ordered diet, give no additional feeding.

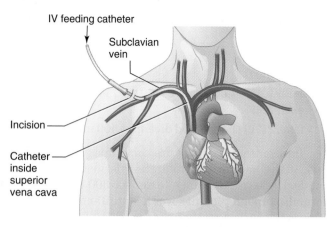

IV feeding catheter

Subclavian vein

Incision

Catheter inside superior vena cava

FIGURE 26–10 The subclavian vein is the site of choice for parenteral nutrition.

Removing Feeding Tubes

When a patient's condition has stabilized and she no longer requires enteral nutrition, the feeding tube may be removed. For the steps to follow,

 Go to Chapter 26, **Procedure 26–4: Removing a Nasogastric or Nasoenteric Tube,** in Volume 2.

See the Critical Aspects box on page 612 for a summary of the procedure. A PEG tube is usually clamped if feedings are no longer required.

CriticalThinking 26–8

Your client has dementia and is frequently agitated. She has been progressively losing weight. An interdisciplinary team (IDT) recommended enteral nutrition due to poor oral intake; however, the client has repeatedly pulled out her NG tube and had an episode of aspiration pneumonia last month. What recommendations might you consider at the next IDT meeting?

What Is Parenteral Nutrition?

Parenteral nutrition is the delivery of nutrition intravenously through a central venous catheter (CVC). This is the preferred method of feeding for clients who cannot be nourished through the gastrointestinal tract. IV nutrition may be partial or total. *Partial parenteral nutrition* is used with clients who are able to meet some of their nutritional needs through oral intake. Clients with shortened small bowel secondary to injury or disease often use parenteral nutrition in addition to oral intake to meet caloric and nutrient needs. *Total parenteral nutrition (TPN)* is used for clients who are severely malnourished, have extensive burns or trauma, or have conditions that require resting the gastrointestinal system. Because TPN solutions are hypertonic, they must be administered in a large, high-flow vein. The subclavian vein is the site of choice (see Figure 26–10). High blood flow through the vessel causes rapid dilution of the concentrated TPN and thereby prevents vessel damage.

Home Nutritional Support

Clients frequently administer enteral and parenteral nutrition at home. To assist the client or caregiver with the management of home nutritional therapy, teach the following aspects.

- *Formula.* Review the type of formula the patient should receive. Enteral or IV solutions are clearly marked with their contents. Emphasize that the caregiver double-check that the correct solution is being used and that the expiration date and time have not been reached before administering any feeding.

- *Administration.* Carefully review how to administer the feeding. Emphasize the need for hand washing before hanging the infusion. If TPN is administered at home, be sure that the client or caregiver is aware of proper technique. After a period of time, the client may be able to tolerate delivering 1 to 3 L of PN at night. The rate must be increased at the beginning and decreased when ending the delivery. This allows the client more mobility during the day.

- *Access device.* Review the care required for the access device, including site care, dressing changes, and flushing.

- *Storage.* Stored enteral and parenteral nutrion must be refrigerated to prevent bacterial contamination.

- *Monitoring.* Instruct the client or caregiver to report a rise in temperature, weight loss, change in bowel movements, decrease in urine output, or change in condition.

- *Follow-up.* Arrange for the client to be regularly weighed and assessed to monitor the adequacy of the feedings. Often clients weigh at home and report to the primary care provider's office for ongoing monitoring of progress and review of lab work.

TPN solutions contain 10 to 50% concentrations of dextrose in water along with amino acids. They also contain vitamins, minerals, and trace elements. Standard TPN formulas are available at many healthcare facilities; however, TPN can be modified to meet individual needs. Lipid emulsions containing essential fatty acids and triglycerides must also be administered weekly for clients who rely completely on parenteral nutrition.

TPN solutions are prepared in liter batches under strict aseptic conditions. Its high nutrient concentration makes TPN an excellent feeding alternative; however, it also makes the solution ideal for bacterial growth. To decrease the risk of infection, TPN bottles should hang for no more than 12 hours (some agency policies specify 24 hours). Use surgical aseptic technique when changing the dressing for the central line, as well as when changing solution and tubing. To decrease the risk of

contamination, do not use the TPN infusion line for administering any other medicines or solutions.

Because TPN solutions are high in glucose, you should begin the infusion slowly (usually less than 30 to 60 mL/hr) to prevent hyperglycemia. Most TPN infusions contain insulin to aid in the absorption of the glucose. Additional insulin is supplied based on results of blood sugar monitoring. If an infusion falls behind schedule, do not increase the rate in an attempt to catch up (this can cause osmotic diuresis and dehydration). When TPN is discontinued, you must do it gradually (perhaps over as many as 48 hours) to prevent a sudden drop in blood sugar.

Monitor patients receiving parenteral nutrition for the following:

- *Tube insertion site.* Because the catheter is inserted into a central vessel, infection at the site can lead rapidly to sepsis.

- *Weight.* Weight is measured to assess the adequacy of the IV nutrition and adjust formula as needed.
- *Glucose.* Formulas contain a high concentration of glucose; you may need to give insulin.
- *Diuresis and dehydration* can occur if hypertonic dextrose is infused too rapidly.
- *Lab values* (electrolytes, blood sugar, albumin, BUN, and creatinine) are a guide for formula adjustment.

Patients may receive enteral or parenteral nutrition in the home as well as in the hospital or institution. The Home Care box reviews teaching related to alternative feeding methods in the home. You should review these topics with the patient or caregiver. For further guidelines,

 Go to Chapter 26, **Technique 26–7: Monitoring Patients Who Are Receiving Total Parenteral Nutrition,** in Volume 2.

| toward evidence-based practice |

Breitkopf, C. R., & Berenson, A. B. (2004). Correlates of weight loss behaviors among low-income African-American, Caucasian, and Latina women. *Obstetrics & Gynecology, 103* (2), 231–239.

A total of 1709 African American, Caucasian, and Latina women aged 12–58 years attending a federally funded family planning clinic reported their weight loss behaviors during the previous 30-day period. Approximately 60% (999) had a BMI greater than 25. A total of 35.3% (603) of women reported dieting during the 30-day period, whereas 43.7% (746) exercised. Only 14.8% (253) of the sample reported both dieting and exercising. Another 15.1% (258) used diet pills, and 4.3% (69) purged. The use of exercise as a weight loss strategy was inversely related to the number of pregnancies a woman had experienced. Women with a smoking history, currently or in the past, were more likely than nonsmokers to report purging. African Americans were least likely to report dieting or exercising. Exposure to family members using diet pills, dieting, or purging was associated with increased odds of performing these behaviors.

Neumark-Sztainer, D., Sherwood, N. E., French, S. A., & Jeffery, R. W. (1999). Weight control behaviors among adult men and women: Cause for concern? *Obesity Research, 7*(2), 179–188.

A total of 714 women and 229 men participated in a community-based weight gain prevention program by completing surveys about their weight control behaviors annually for 3 years. Women were more likely than men to report weight control behaviors, with particularly strong associations found between gender and "history of dieting" (odds ratio = 8.1) and "participation in an organized weight loss program" (odds ratio = 11.7). Among both genders, exercise was the most frequently reported specific weight loss practice (66% of women and 53% of men), followed by decreasing fat intake (62% of women and 48% of men). A total of 22% of the women and 17% of the men reported unhealthy dietary behaviors, such as diet pills, purging, or laxative use.

---

1. Based on these two studies, what conclusions, if any, can you make about weight loss strategies?

2. What effect does this data have on your thoughts about how to teach weight loss?

 Go to Chapter 26, **Toward Evidence-Based Practice Suggested Responses,** on the Electronic Study Guide.

 Go to Chapter 26, **Resources for Caregivers and Health Professionals,** on the Electronic Study Guide.

 Suggested Readings: Go to Chapter 26, **Reading More About Nutrition,** on the Electronic Study Guide.

 Bibliography: Go to Volume 2, Bibliography.

27 | Urinary Elimination

Learning Outcomes

After completing this chapter, you should be able to:

✳ Describe the normal structure and function of the organs in the urinary system.

✳ Describe the processes of urine formation and elimination.

✳ Discuss factors that affect urinary elimination.

✳ Describe the contents of a nursing assessment and physical examination focused on urinary elimination.

✳ Accurately measure urine output.

✳ Describe procedures for collecting various types of urine specimens.

✳ List and describe diagnostic tests used in identification of urinary elimination problems.

✳ Discuss common elimination problems: urinary tract infection, urinary retention, and urinary incontinence.

✳ Identify nursing diagnoses associated with altered urinary elimination.

✳ Describe nursing interventions that promote normal urination.

✳ Provide care for clients experiencing urinary problems.

✳ Perform urinary catheterizations following accepted procedures.

✳ Discuss nursing care appropriate for clients who have a urinary diversion.

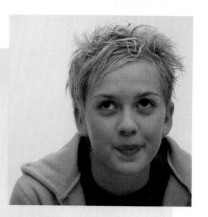

MEET Your Patient

During your assigned clinical experience at University Hospital, the RN asks you to complete the admission process for Jessica, a 22-year-old university student who is complaining of frequent, painful urination. As you interview her, Jessica becomes embarrassed. "It's really hard to talk about this. Do you really need all these details?" she inquires. Then, she asks to use the bathroom. You ask her to give you a midstream clean-catch urine sample while she is in the restroom. When she returns, she gives you a small specimen of pink-colored, strong-smelling urine. "I feel like I have to go so bad and then I hardly have any urine. It's a little bloody, and I'm not having my period," she states.

You close the door and interview Jessica in private about her usual urination pattern and current symptoms. Your calm approach and straightforward manner put her at ease. She confides that she has recently become sexually active and that her symptoms began after spending the weekend

with her new partner. You take her vital signs: oral temperature 99.4°F (37.4°C), radial pulse 88 bpm, respiratory rate 20, and blood pressure 108/72 mm Hg.

After you report your assessment data to the RN, the emergency department (ED) physician asks you to perform a dipstick urinalysis on the urine sample and to send the urine sample to the lab for culture and sensitivity. He asks you: "Well, what do you think we need to do next?" How would you answer his question?

As you gain theoretical and practical knowledge in this chapter, we will return to this case study to discuss how you might answer the physician's question and support Jessica's recovery. You will also have the opportunity to evaluate your feelings about giving care that patients may regard as highly personal or even embarrassing.

Theoretical Knowledge
knowing why

A variety of factors, including personal hygiene, age, nutrition, stress, sexual activity, and medications, play a role in urinary health. That's why it is vitally important that you take a holistic approach to patients who have altered urinary elimination patterns. Such an approach requires theoretical knowledge of normal urinary physiology, factors that influence urinary elimination, and common alterations in urinary function.

HOW DOES THE URINARY SYSTEM WORK?

To understand problems affecting the urinary system, you'll need to first understand how the urinary system functions in a healthy individual. The organs of the urinary system include the kidneys, ureters, bladder, and urethra (Figure 27–1).

The Kidneys Filter and Regulate

The kidneys filter metabolic wastes, toxins, excess ions, and water from the bloodstream and excrete them as urine. If kidney function is impaired, these substances reach toxic levels and begin to poison the body's cells. The kidneys also help to regulate blood volume, blood pressure, electrolyte levels, and acid-base balance by selectively reabsorbing water and other substances. Secondary functions of the kidneys are to produce erythropoietin, secrete the enzyme renin, and activate vitamin D_3 (calcitrol). The kidneys are located against the posterior abdominal wall behind the peritoneum (they are **retroperitoneal**). The average kidney weighs about 5 ounces and is the shape of a kidney bean (see Figure 27–1).

The outer layer, or **cortex,** of the kidney is composed of millions of microscopic functional units called *nephrons* (Figure 27–2). The inner layer, or **medulla,** consists of 8 to 10 wedge-shaped cones called the *renal pyramids*. The renal pyramids are made up of bundles of collecting tubules. The innermost area is the **renal**

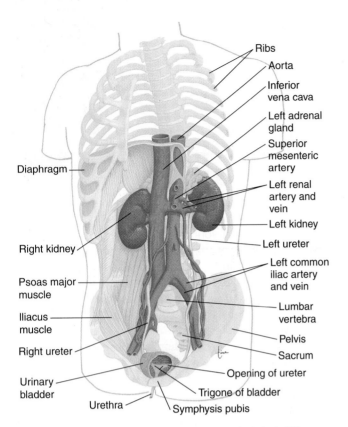

FIGURE 27–1 The organs of the urinary system include the kidneys, ureters, bladder, and urethra.

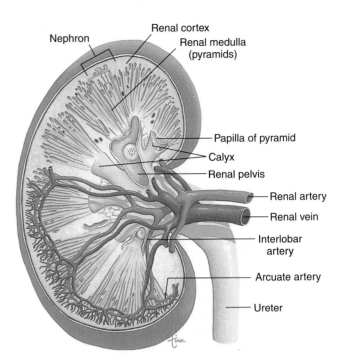

FIGURE 27–2 A cross-section of the kidney, showing the renal cortex, medulla, pyramids, and calyces.

pelvis. Funnel-shaped extensions known as **calyces** (singular: **calyx**) enclose the central portion of each renal pyramid and direct urine into the renal pelvis.

The Nephrons Form Urine

The **nephron** is the basic structural and functional unit of the kidney (Figure 27–2). There are about 1 million nephrons in each kidney. Each nephron consists of:

1. A double-walled hollow capsule, the **Bowman's capsule,** enclosing a **glomerulus,** a knotty ball of capillaries
2. A series of filtrating tubules
3. A collecting duct

Together, these structures act as a microscopic filter, controlling the excretion and retention of fluids and solutes according to the body's moment-by-moment needs. Urine is formed by filtration, reabsorption, and secretion, discussed next.

For a detailed view of a nephron,

 Go to Chapter 27, **Tables, Boxes, Figures: ESG Figure 27–1,** on the Electronic Study Guide.

Glomerular Filtration

Figure 27–3 summarizes the process of urine formation. The first step, **filtration,** occurs in the glomeruli.

The renal arteries bring blood to the kidneys and into the glomeruli. Blood pressure forces plasma, dissolved substances, and small proteins out of the porous glomeruli into Bowman's capsule to form a liquid called **filtrate.** The **glomerular filtration rate** is the amount of filtrate formed by the kidneys in 1 minute. The average is 100 to 125 mL per minute.

Unless the glomerular capillaries are inflamed or damaged, large molecules such as blood cells and blood proteins are too large to filter across their walls. Glomerular filtrate resembles blood plasma, except that it contains much less protein and no blood cells.

Tubular Reabsorption

The filtrate moves from Bowman's capsule into a highly twisted tubule (*proximal convoluted tubule,* Figure 27–3). As the filtrate journeys through the tubule, 99% is reabsorbed into the peritubular capillaries. Approximately 1% of filtrate returns, as urine, to the *collecting tubule,* which transports it into the ureters. Wastes and toxins that remain in the blood after filtration are actively transported into the filtrate (reabsorbed) in the *distal* and *collecting tubules.* These are also the sites of water and sodium reabsorption under the control of antidiuretic hormone (ADH) and aldosterone.

When the amount of fluid in the body decreases (e.g., because of low intake or blood loss), the posterior pituitary gland secretes more ADH. This causes the distal and collecting tubules to reabsorb more water into the blood. At the same time, the adrenal cortex secretes more aldosterone, which increases the reabsorption of

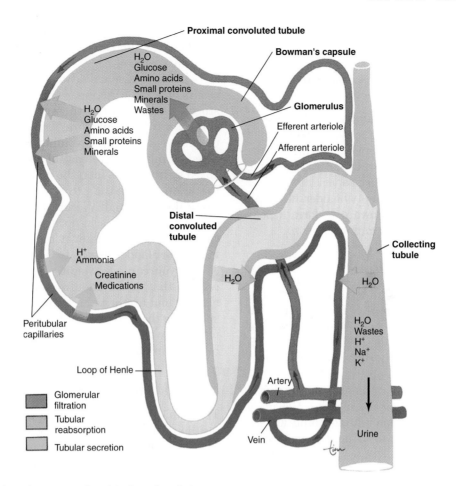

FIGURE 27–3 A schematic representation of the formation of urine.

sodium, and water follows sodium back into the blood. ADH and aldosterone thus have the effect of maintaining normal blood volume and blood pressure.

When the amount of water in the body increases (e.g., as in ingestion of excessive fluids), ADH is suppressed and the opposite effect occurs. Urine becomes dilute and water continues to be eliminated until its concentration returns to normal (Scanlon & Sanders, 2003).

Tubular Secretion

Some substances are actively secreted from the blood in the peritubular capillaries into the renal filtrate. For example, metabolic waste products, such as ammonia and creatinine, and some medications are secreted into the filtrate and then eliminated in urine. In addition, the kidneys help maintain the normal pH of blood by secreting hydrogen ions (H^+).

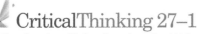

CriticalThinking 27–1

If a client is suffering from impaired kidney function, what signs and symptoms might you expect to see?

The Ureters Transport Urine

The remaining organs of the urinary system transport or store the urine once it is formed. From the collecting tubules, urine travels into the renal pelvis and enters the ureter. Each kidney has one ureter, approximately 26 to 30 cm (10 to 12 in.) long and 1.25 cm (0.5 in.) in diameter (see Figure 27–1). The ureters contract in peristaltic waves to move urine toward the bladder. At the opening between the ureter and the bladder is a flap of mucous membrane that acts as a one-way valve, allowing urine to enter the bladder but preventing backflow (**reflux**) into the ureter.

The Urinary Bladder Stores Urine

The urinary bladder (see Figure 27–1) is a sac-like organ that receives urine from the ureters and stores it until discharged from the body. The wall of the bladder consists of four layers:

1. An innermost mucous membrane seals off the remaining layers from exposure to urine.
2. A layer of connective tissue supports the mucous membrane.

3. Three layers of longitudinal and circular smooth muscle fibers are collectively called the **detrusor muscle.**

4. An outermost layer of fibrous connective tissue covers the detrusor layer.

When the bladder is empty, it shrivels and its elastic wall becomes heavily folded. As it receives newly formed urine, it expands and the wall becomes smooth. An average, normal bladder can store 500 mL (one pint) of urine, but it may distend when needed to a capacity twice that amount. You cannot palpate an empty bladder, but a full or distended bladder extends upward to form a pear shape that you can feel in the suprapubic region.

The Urethra Transports Urine

The urethra transports urine from the bladder to the body exterior. In females, the urethra is about 3 to 4 cm (1.5 in.) long and is anchored to the anterior wall of the vagina by connective tissue; it opens at the **urinary meatus** between the clitoris and vaginal opening. In males the urethra extends about 20 cm (8 in.) from the bladder to the urinary meatus at the distal end of the penis. As it leaves the bladder, the male urethra passes through a surrounding gland known as the **prostate.** In addition to urine, the male urethra also carries semen.

Because the female urethra is so short, women are especially prone to urinary tract infection from microorganisms residing in the vagina and rectum. The mucous membrane of the urethra (in both men and women) is continuous with the bladder and the ureters. Therefore, infection in the urethra can easily spread through the bladder and up into the kidneys.

KnowledgeCheck 27–1
- Identify the major structures of the urinary system.
- What are the functions of the kidneys?
- Briefly describe how urine is formed.
- What role do the ureters, bladder, and urethra play in urinary elimination?

 Go to Chapter 27, **Knowledge Check Response Sheet and Answers,** on the Electronic Study Guide.

HOW DOES URINARY ELIMINATION OCCUR?

Where the bladder connects to the urethra is a thickening of smooth muscle called the **internal urethral sphincter.** When closed, the internal sphincter keeps urine in the bladder from entering the urethra. When the bladder contains 200 to 450 mL of urine (50 to 200 mL in children), the distention activates stretch receptors in the bladder wall. The stretch receptors send sensory impulses to the *voiding reflex center* in the spinal cord, triggering motor impulses that cause the detrusor muscle to contract and the internal sphincter to relax. The internal urethral sphincter is not under voluntary control.

Voiding (also called **urination** or **micturition**) occurs when contraction of the detrusor muscle pushes stored urine through the relaxed internal urethral sphincter into the urethra. This triggers the conscious urge to void. However, voiding may be voluntarily delayed by inhibiting release of a second, **external urethral sphincter.** When the person is ready to urinate, the brain signals the external sphincter to relax, and urine flows through the urethra. Further contraction of the detrusor muscle normally forces out any urine remaining in the bladder. After the detrusor muscle relaxes, the bladder begins to fill with urine again.

As you can see, voiding and control of urination require that, in addition to normal functioning of the bladder and urethra, the brain, spinal cord, and nerves supplying the bladder and urethra be intact. The person must be aware of the need to urinate and able to respond by either inhibiting the reflex or by going to the toilet.

Normal Urination Patterns

The kidneys produce urine at a rate of about 60 mL per hour, or 1500 mL per day. However, output may fluctuate by 1000 mL to 2000 mL depending on various factors discussed in the next section. Most people void about five or six times per day—normally on awakening, after each meal, and just prior to bedtime.

Characteristics of Normal Urine

Specific gravity is a measure of dissolved solutes in a solution. As the concentration of solutes increases, specific gravity increases. The specific gravity of distilled water is 1.000 because there are no dissolved solutes. The normal specific gravity range for urine is 1.002 to 1.028. As fluid intake increases, urine becomes dilute and lighter in color and may even become almost colorless as specific gravity approaches 1.000. In contrast, if fluid intake is low or there have been fluid losses, as with diarrhea or vomiting, the urine darkens and the specific gravity rises. Characteristics of urine are discussed in depth later in this chapter. Also,

 Go to Chapter 27, **Diagnostic Testing, Urinalysis,** in Volume 2.

CriticalThinking 27–2
- How does Jessica's ("Meet Your Patient") urinary elimination pattern differ from normal?
- What would you expect to find if you measured her specific gravity?
- Jessica's symptoms suggest a urinary tract infection. How might this be related to the fact that she has recently become sexually active?

WHAT FACTORS AFFECT URINARY ELIMINATION?

Given the complex structure and physiology of the urinary organs, it isn't surprising that many variables affect their function.

Developmental Factors

Developmental factors affect urine volume and frequency and control of voiding.

Infants and Children

A newborn's kidneys produce 15 to 60 mL of urine per kilogram of body weight per day. Newborns do not concentrate urine well and, therefore, may void up to 25 times during the first 24 hours of life. Normal specific gravity of their urine is 1.008. Over the first weeks of life, the urine gradually becomes more concentrated, and the well-hydrated infant produces eight to ten wet diapers a day (Polan & Taylor, 2003). Infants do not have voluntary control of voiding because neuromuscular functioning is immature.

The timing of toilet training is highly variable and is influenced by family and culture, as well as the presence of older children who can act as role models. In the United States, most parents begin toilet training when their child is between 18 and 24 months of age. This timing can vary widely among cultures. For example, it is not unusual for Chinese children to be completely toilet-trained by their first birthday. Before toilet training can occur, toddlers must be able to control the external urethral sphincter, sense the urge to void, communicate their need to use the toilet, and remove their clothing. Full control over urination is usually established by age 3 but may occur as late as age 5. Daytime dryness usually occurs before toddlers can go without a diaper all night.

Occasional wetting (**enuresis**) is entirely normal in children, even in the early school years, especially when the child is intensely involved in a game, test, or other absorbing activity. Such events should be accepted calmly and not punished. **Nocturnal enuresis,** or bed-wetting, is considered normal until well after toilet training has been firmly established and should not be considered a problem until age 6.

Older Adults

The size and functioning of the kidneys begin to decrease at about age 50, and by age 80 only about two-thirds of the functioning nephrons remain. This results in a decline in filtration rate, which affects the ability to dilute and concentrate urine, but does not normally create problems unless an illness alters fluid balance. For example, when older adults lose fluids and electrolytes through vomiting and diarrhea, it is difficult for their kidneys to maintain acid-base and electrolyte balances. Chronic diseases such as arteriosclerosis, common in older adults, can reduce blood flow and impair renal function. Decreased kidney function places older adults at risk for drug toxicity, as well (see Chapter 23).

The potential volume of the bladder decreases because of a loss of elasticity in the bladder wall; thus, older adults need to urinate more frequently, such as during the night (**nocturnal frequency**), and during car trips. In women, childbearing may have weakened the pelvic muscles, whereas in older men, the prostate gland may be enlarged; either of these conditions can lead to leakage of urine. Loss of elasticity and muscle tone also decreases the ability of the bladder to empty completely. Retention of urine after voiding then increases the risk for bladder infections.

Personal, Sociocultural, and Environmental Factors

Many people put off voiding while they are working, watching TV, or busy with other tasks. Delaying urination promotes urinary stasis and can lead to bladder infections. Other situations can inhibit voiding, as well. A person who is anxious and tense cannot relax the abdominal and perineal muscles and the external urethral sphincter. It is then difficult to void, as in the following situations:

- *Lack of time.* Most people find it difficult to void when they feel rushed; therefore, when helping patients to void, make sure you have scheduled enough time for them to relax fully.
- *Lack of privacy.* Many people require privacy for voiding and if they are in a restaurant or other unfamiliar environment, they may be embarrassed even to ask for directions to a bathroom. Some hospitalized clients may also avoid asking for assistance to the bathroom.
- *Loss of dignity.* In Chapter 10, we talked about the loss of dignity that hospitalized patients experience. Patients who need assistance with toileting may be especially vulnerable to such feelings, especially if they require catheterization or a bedpan. It is important, therefore, to acknowledge such feelings and encourage the patient to participate in other aspects of self-care, such as bathing and dressing.
- *Cultural influences.* Some patients will state personal, cultural, or religious requirements for toileting assistance to be provided by a person of the same gender, or they will wait until a visit from a family member before acknowledging their need for help with voiding.

Nutrition, Hydration, and Activity Level

Substances that contain caffeine, such as coffee, tea, cola, and chocolate, act as diuretics and increase urine production. Consuming large amounts of alcohol

BOX 27-1 Diuretics

Thiazide Diuretics

Thiazide diuretics are used to treat high blood pressure by reducing the amount of sodium and water in the body. They also dilate blood vessels, thereby lowering blood pressure. In the United States, numerous thiazide diuretics are available. Below are several that are widely used:

- Aquatensen (methyclothiazide)
- Diulo, Mykrox (metolazone)
- Diuril (chlorothiazide)
- Esidrix (hydrochlorothiazide)
- Hydro-chlor, HydroDIURIL, Microzide, Oretic (hydro-chlorothiazide)
- Hygroton or Thalitone (chlorthalidone)
- Naturetin (bendroflumethiazide)

In Canada, numerous thiazide diuretics are available. Below are several that are widely used:

- Apo-Chlorthalidone, Hygroton, Novo-Thalidone, Uri-don (chlorthalidone)
- Apo-Hydro, Diuchlor H, HydroDIURIL, Neo-Codema, Novo-Hydrazide (hydrochlorothiazide)
- Duretic (methyclothiazide),
- Naturetin (bendroflumethiazide)

Potassium-Sparing Diuretics

Potassium-sparing diuretics reduce the amount of water in the body. Unlike other diuretic medicines, these medicines do not cause potassium loss. Commonly used brand names in the United States include the following:

- Aldactone (spironolactone)
- Dyrenium (triamterene)
- Midamor (amiloride)

Commonly used brand names in Canada include the following:

- Aldactone (spironolactone)
- Dyrenium (triamterene)

- Midamor (amiloride)
- Novospiroton (spironolactone)

Loop-Acting Diuretics

Loop-acting diuretics cause the kidneys to excrete more urine by reabsorbing less water. This reduces the amount of water in the body and lowers blood pressure.

Commonly used brand names in the United States include the following:

- Bumex (bumetanide)
- Demadex (torsemide)
- Edecrin (ethacrynic acid)
- Lasix (furosemide)

Commonly used brand names in Canada include the following:

- Apo-Furosemide (furosemide)
- Edecrin (ethacrynic acid)
- Furoside, Lasix, Novosemide, or Uritol (furosemide)

Medications That Have Significant Interactions with Diuretics

- Digoxin
- Certain antidepressants, especially when taking thiazide or loop-acting diuretics
- Other medicines for high blood pressure
- Lithium
- Cyclosporine (an immunosuppressant), especially when the patient is taking a potassium-sparing diuretic

Common Side Effects of Diuretics

- Weakness
- Muscle cramps
- Skin rash
- Increased sensitivity to sunlight (with thiazide diuretics)
- Dizziness or lightheadedness
- Joint pain

---

impairs the release of antidiuretic hormone (ADH), resulting in increased production of urine. In contrast, a diet high in salt causes water retention and decreases urine production.

The kidneys also "spare" water when a person is dehydrated, such as after heavy exercise or simply when fluid intake is inadequate. This causes the urine to be concentrated and low in volume. During lengthy sessions of physical activity, especially in hot weather, the body loses sodium and other electrolytes rapidly through sweat; for this reason, a nutrient-balanced sports beverage may be more beneficial than plain

water in helping to prevent dehydration (Thompson & Manore, 2005). For most adults, pale to clear urine indicates adequate hydration.

KnowledgeCheck 27–2

- What quantity of urine in the bladder will stimulate the urge to void?
- Identify at least three methods for determining whether hydration is adequate and urine output is within normal limits.

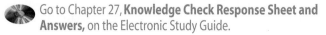 Go to Chapter 27, **Knowledge Check Response Sheet and Answers,** on the Electronic Study Guide.

BOX 27-2 Medications Associated with Urinary Retention

Class	Examples
Antihistamines	chlorpheniramine (Chlortrimeton), loratadine (Claritin)
Tricyclic antidepressants	amitriptyline (Elavil), desipramine (Norpramin)
MAO inhibitors	phenelzine (Nardil), tranylcypromine (Parnate)
Antispasmodics	dicyclomine (Bentyl)
Antiparkinsonism medications	benztropine mesylate (Cogentin), levodopa
Beta-adrenergic blockers	propranolol (Inderal), naldolol (Corgard)

Medications

Various medications affect urination. *Phenazopyridine hydrochloride (Pyridium)*, a bladder analgesic, turns the urine a deep orange-red color. *Diuretics*, sometimes called "water pills," treat blood pressure, fluid retention, and edema by increasing elimination of urine. Diuretics are classifed as thiazide, potassium-sparing, or loop-acting diuretics. See Box 27–1. In contrast, a number of medications have a side effect of urinary retention. They inhibit the free flow of urine due to *anticholinergic effects* (e.g., medications given to relieve bladder spasms). See Box 27–2 for a listing of the most common medications associated with urinary retention.

Still other medications are **nephrotoxic** (damaging to the kidneys). These include some antibiotics, such as gentamicin (Garamycin) and amphotericin B (Amphotec, a fungicide), and high doses or long-term use of aspirin and ibuprofen (Motrin).

Surgery and Anesthesia

Reproductive and urinary tract surgeries can affect urine solutes, normal urine characteristics, and the ability to pass urine normally. Manipulation of the urinary tract frequently leads to trauma, bleeding, or the introduction of bacteria into a normally sterile tract. Swelling after diagnostic or invasive procedures and childbirth may cause urinary retention.

Surgery in the pubic area, vagina, or rectum is associated with a high incidence of trauma to the urinary organs, lower abdominal swelling, loss of pelvic muscle control, and increased pressure on the kidneys, ureters, or bladder. Surgery on the reproductive organs, such as hysterectomy in women or transurethral resection of the prostate in men, usually requires the use of an indwelling catheter (tube) for draining the bladder postoperatively. The urine may be red or pink-tinged after any invasive urinary tract surgery or procedure.

Anesthetic agents can decrease blood pressure and glomerular filtration, thus decreasing urine formation. Spinal anesthesia decreases the patient's awareness of the need to void, which may lead to bladder distention.

Pathological Conditions

Disorders of the urinary system that affect urinary elimination include the following:

- Infection or inflammation of the bladder, ureters, or kidneys
- **Renal calculi** (kidney stones) or tumors, which obstruct the normal flow of urine
- In older men, **hypertrophy** (excessive growth) of the prostate gland due to benign or cancerous lesions, which interferes with flow of urine from the bladder into the urethra

Diseases involving other systems can indirectly affect urinary function. For example:

- Cardiovascular and metabolic disorders decrease blood flow through the glomeruli and thus impair filtration and urine production.
- Any condition that affects the nervous system controlling the urinary system organs will impair urinary elimination. After a stroke or spinal cord injury, for example, some patients may lose bladder control.
- **Neurogenic bladder** occurs as a result of impaired neurological function. The person cannot perceive bladder fullness nor control the urinary sphincters. The bladder becomes flaccid or spastic, causing frequent involuntary loss of urine.
- Systemic infection, especially when accompanied by a high fever, causes the kidneys to reabsorb and retain water.
- Mobility and communication problems may cause inability to get to the bathroom in time or inability to communicate the need for assistance. This may result in urination in inappropriate settings or at inappropriate times.

- Cognitive changes that alter perception of the urge to void or severe psychiatric concerns that alter perception or ability to manage activities of daily living may lead to "accidents."

KnowledgeCheck 27–3

- What common medications increase the amount of urine voided?
- What types of medications are associated with urinary retention?
- What types of conditions or surgeries are associated with a high incidence of altered urination?

 Go to Chapter 27, **Knowledge Check Response Sheet and Answers,** on the Electronic Study Guide.

Practical Knowledge
knowing how

As a nurse, you will monitor and assist clients with urinary elimination, teach them about body function, and work collaboratively with the healthcare team to facilitate normal urinary function. In the remainder of the chapter we will discuss these activities. Also see the Nursing Care Plan and the Care Map.

| Assessment |

To assess urinary elimination, you will use data from the nursing history, physical examination, and diagnostic and laboratory reports.

Nursing History

Because urination patterns vary among individuals, you will need a nursing history to determine what is normal for a particular client. As you interview the client, pay attention to her reaction to your questions. Many people are embarrassed about discussing urination. Tailor your assessment to the client's needs, and use language that makes the client comfortable.

For a set of interview questions,

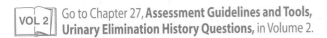 Go to Chapter 27, **Assessment Guidelines and Tools, Urinary Elimination History Questions,** in Volume 2.

For clients with a urinary diversion, you should also gather data on the client's usual care of the stoma, use of appliances, and adjustment to the ostomy.

Physical Assessment

Physical assessment for urinary elimination includes examination of the kidneys, bladder, urethra, and skin surrounding the genitals, as appropriate. For a

complete discussion of physical examination of the genitourinary system,

 Go to Chapter 19, **Procedure 19-17: Assessing the Male Genitourinary System,** and **Procedure 19-18: Assessing the Female Genitourinary System,** in Volume 2.

KnowledgeCheck 27–4

- What should you discuss with your client when performing a nursing history focused on urinary elimination?
- What are the key elements of a physical assessment for a client with urination problems?

 Go to Chapter 27, **Knowledge Check Response Sheet and Answers,** on the Electronic Study Guide.

 CriticalThinking 27–3

In the "Meet Your Patient" scenario, some assessment findings were given for Jessica, the university student. If you performed the preceding urinary tract assessments, what findings might you expect?

Assessing the Urine

In addition to observations already mentioned, assessment of the urine includes measuring urine output and conducting a variety of bedside tests.

Measuring Urine Output

Measuring urine output is part of a comprehensive plan to monitor a client's fluid status. Recall that the kidneys produce urine at a rate of approximately 60 mL per hour, or 1500 mL per day. However, urinary output fluctuates depending on the quantity of fluids the patient drinks and on other factors, such as the ability of the heart to circulate the blood, adequate kidney functioning, and the ability of the patient to void the urine. You must know both the intake and the output (I&O), as well as relevant physical conditions, to interpret the meaning of the patient data. For example, if urine output is low, you cannot assume that the patient's kidneys are not working properly. If his intake is also low, he may be dehydrated. But what does it mean if his intake is high and his output low? Yes, this could mean his kidneys are not working well. However, it could also mean that his kidneys are producing urine but that he has urinary retention because of something that is obstructing flow.

To measure fluid intake, record all fluids the patient drinks or receives intravenously. Include foods that become liquid at room temperature (e.g., ice cream), ice chips (record the fluid as half the volume of the ice chips), and tube feedings. For a full discussion of measuring intake, go to Chapter 36. See Chapter 16, Figure 16–6, for an example of a form to document the I&O.

Nursing Care Plan

Client Data

Desmond Washington, a 69-year-old man, comes to the clinic 4 weeks after having a prostatectomy for prostate cancer. He was discharged from the hospital on postoperative day 4 and went home with an indwelling urinary catheter. The catheter was removed at his last visit, 19 days after surgery.

Mr. Washington is meticulously groomed. He is friendly, greeting other patients in the clinic and chatting with the clinic personnel. When his nurse brings him to an exam room and asks how he feels, he says, "I saw the sun come up today. I appreciate that more now. The good Lord has given me a new lease on life, and I intend to use it!" His nurse continues, "That's great, Mr. Washington. How have you been doing since the catheter was removed?" Mr. Washington's smile fades. He lowers his voice and says, "You know, I think that's the worst part of this whole thing. I hate wearing these diapers—they make me feel, well, like an old man. I'm certainly not ready for this."

The nurse continues, "Do you have *any* control of your urine?" Mr Washington explains, "I may go for hours and stay dry, and then it seems for no reason, I wet myself. Take yesterday, for example. I was sitting on the sofa watching the ballgame when someone came to the door. I got up to answer the door, and all of a sudden, I felt wet. I didn't even have anything to drink so I could make it through the afternoon and stay dry. And if I cough? Forget it. Niagara Falls. Can something be done so I can hold my urine again?"

Nursing Diagnosis

Stress Urinary Incontinence related to disruption of the urinary sphincter and related pelvic muscles by surgery as evidenced by client report of involuntary loss of urine with increased intraabdominal pressure.

NOC Outcomes

Urinary Continence (#0502)
Urinary Elimination (#0503)

Individualized Goals/Expected Outcomes

By the next visit, Mr. Washington will:
1. Describe three things he can do that will help regain urinary continence.
2. Explain three interventions to cope with leaked urine.
3. Report that he is drinking adequate amounts of fluids during the day.

➤

Nursing Care Plan *(continued)*

Nursing Interventions/Activities	Rationale
NIC Interventions Urinary Elimination Management (#0590) Urinary Incontinence Care (#0610) **Nursing Activities** 1. Obtain midstream voided urine specimen for urinalysis.	Urinary tract infection can cause or worsen incontinence (Urinary Continence Guideline Panel [UCGP], 1992).
2. Identify factors that contribute to Mr. Washington's incontinence by using an incontinence diary.	Identifying activities or other factors that cause loss of urine control can guide specific interventions. A diary facilitates monitoring over time and can identify patterns that could otherwise be missed (UCGP, 1992; Dowling-Castronovo & Bradway, 2003).
3. Teach pelvic floor muscle exercises (PFME).	PFME strengthen pelvic muscles and enhance sphincter control. They have been shown to increase urinary continence without side effects in men who have undergone prostatectomy (UCGP, 1992; VanKampen, et al., 2000; Hay-Smith, 2000).
4. Use biofeedback when needed in conjunction with PFME training to help Mr. Washington isolate pelvic floor muscles.	Biofeedback allows clients to receive auditory or visual (or both) cues when the proper muscles are contracted, so they learn what the proper muscle contraction feels like. Biofeedback also allows the nurse or therapist to objectively measure strength of contractions (UCGP, 1992; Hunter, Moore, Cody, & Glazener, 2004).
5. Teach timed voiding. Have Mr. Washington void on a schedule of every 2 hours.	Voiding on a schedule of every 2 hours can reduce the amount of urine in the bladder, thus reducing the likelihood of leakage with activities of daily living (UCGP, 1992; Burgio, Stutzman, & Engel, 1989; Wyman, 2003).
6. Explain the need to drink adequate fluids and *not* limit fluids in an effort to prevent incontinence. Help Mr. Washington identify ways to drink a minimum of 1500 mL/day.	Adequate fluid intake is important to maintain dilute urine, which is less irritating to the bladder; to maintain systemic hydration; and to reduce the risk for constipation, which can contribute to urinary incontinence (UCGP, 1992; Dowling-Castronovo & Bradway, 2003).

Nursing Interventions/Activities	Rationale
7. Assist client in selecting appropriate absorbent products that collect urine for temporary management while continence management is ongoing.	Proper absorbent garments and pads can collect and trap urine, keep skin clean and dry, reduce odor, and minimize the risk of soiling accidents (UCGP, 1992).
8. Help client develop a personal hygiene routine that will maintain skin integrity.	Proper hygiene will reduce the risk of skin irritation and infection. Use warm (not hot) water, and pat (don't scrub) the perineal area. A barrier cream will repel fluid and protect the skin from urine.
9. Offer referral to support group.	Support groups provide a sense of community and enhance problem-solving skills of members. Mr. Washington may feel less embarrassment when he discovers that others share his problems.
10. Explain that urinary incontinence is common after prostatectomy, but that it may be only temporary.	Urinary incontinence can be a troubling complication of prostatectomy for many men. Fortunately, it usually resolves with active management within 6 to 12 months of surgery.

➤

Nursing Care Plan *(continued)*

There are many treatment recommendations that are not supported by research. Anecdotally, they may work for some clients. These include reducing caffeine consumption; eliminating bladder irritants, such as artificial sweeteners, spicy foods, and citrus from the diet; losing weight; and quitting smoking. In addition, it is important for nurses to understand that the pathophysiology of urinary incontinence is different in men and women and that interventions that are successful in women may or may not be equally successful in men.

Evaluation

At the end of the visit, Mr. Washington said, "I didn't know there were things I could do about the leaking urine. Before surgery, all I cared about was getting rid of the cancer. I don't need a support group—maybe I'll lead one!" Mr. Washington had been placing folded paper towels in his underwear to collect urine because he thought absorbent products were too expensive, but with guidance from his nurse, he identified products that would fit in his budget. He liked that they would not be visible through his clothing.

At Mr. Washington's next visit, the nurse will review the initial collaborative goals and stated outcomes and perform a client assessment to determine whether the goals were reached in the stated time frame.

Mr. Washington currently has a positive attitude and is focused on "beating" his cancer first and on managing complications of surgery second. As time passes, incontinence may persist and may become more frustrating for him once he is fully recovered from surgery. Mr. Washington initially declined referral to a support group, but he may be more interested in joining one in the future for help dealing with long-term consequences of prostatectomy.

References

Burgio, K. L., Stutzman, R. E., & Engel, B. T. (1989). Behavioral training for post-prostatectomy urinary incontinence. *Journal of Urology, 141*(2), 303–306.

Dowling-Castronovo, A., & Bradway, C. (2003). Urinary incontinence. In M. Mezey, T. Fulmer, I. Abraham, & D. A. Zwicker (Ed.), *Geriatric nursing protocols for best practice,* pp. 83–98. New York: Springer Publishing Company.

Hay-Smith, J. (2000, November/December). Pelvic floor re-education. *Evidence Based Medicine, 5,* 183.

Hunter, K. F., Moore, K. N., Cody, D. J., & Glazener, C. M. (2004). Conservative management for postprostatectomy urinary incontinence (Cochrane Review). In *The Cochrane Library.* Chichester, UK: John Wiley & Sons, Ltd.

Urinary Continence Guideline Panel (UCGP). (1992). *Urinary incontinence in adults.* Rockville, MD: Agency for Healthcare Policy and Research, Public Health Service, U.S. Department of Health and Human Services.

VanKampen, M., DeWeerdt, W., VanPoppel, H., DeRidder, D., Feys, H., & Baert, L. (2000, January 8). Effect of pelvic-floor re-education on duration and degree of incontinence after radical prostatectomy: A randomised controlled trial. *The Lancet, 355,* 98–102.

Wyman, J. F. (2003, March). Treatment of urinary incontinence in men and older women. *American Journal of Nursing, 103*(3), 26–35.

Care Map

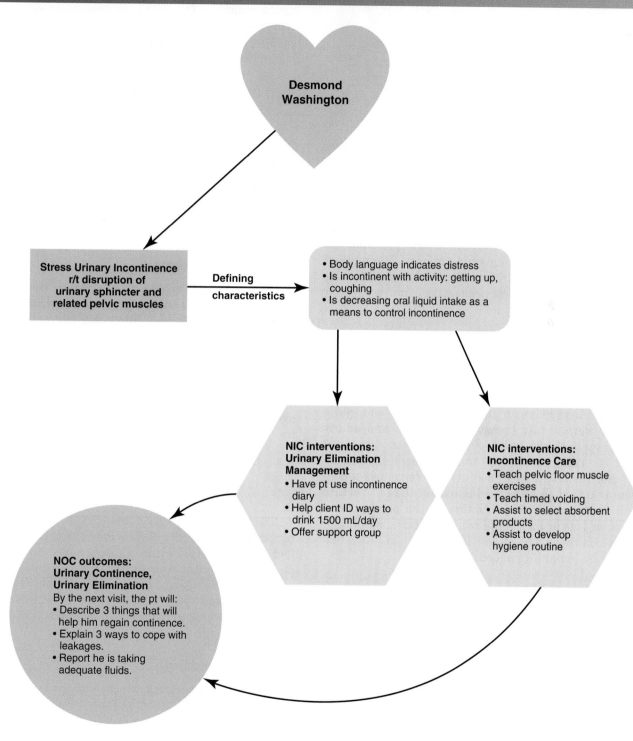

Desmond Washington

Stress Urinary Incontinence r/t disruption of urinary sphincter and related pelvic muscles

Defining characteristics

- Body language indicates distress
- Is incontinent with activity: getting up, coughing
- Is decreasing oral liquid intake as a means to control incontinence

NIC interventions: Urinary Elimination Management
- Have pt use incontinence diary
- Help client ID ways to drink 1500 mL/day
- Offer support group

NIC interventions: Incontinence Care
- Teach pelvic floor muscle exercises
- Teach timed voiding
- Assist to select absorbent products
- Assist to develop hygiene routine

NOC outcomes: Urinary Continence, Urinary Elimination
By the next visit, the pt will:
- Describe 3 things that will help him regain continence.
- Explain 3 ways to cope with leakages.
- Report he is taking adequate fluids.

Key:

- Nursing diagnosis
- Defining characteristics
- NIC interventions and nursing activities
- NOC outcomes

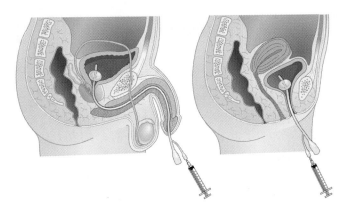

FIGURE 27–4 An indwelling catheter may be used for patients who are unable to void because of inflammation or disease or who require continual observation of urine flow.

Observe universal precautions when handling urine to prevent exposure to body fluids. Always wear disposable procedure gloves, and avoid splashing the urine and contaminating your uniform. The method you use to measure urine is dictated in part by the amount of help the client needs with urination.

Voided Urine

Many ambulatory clients need no assistance with urination. Be sure to inform them that their intake and output (I&O) is being monitored, and explain how they can help. Place a specimen "hat" under the toilet seat to collect urine, or have male clients void into a urinal. Periodically measure the output and empty the urine into the toilet. For clients who can assist with recording the I&O, provide a bedside clipboard.

For the client with mobility problems, use a bedpan or urinal to collect urine output. Use a fracture pan for clients with a fracture of the pelvis, lower back, or legs or for clients who have casts, splints, or braces on their legs. Male clients may void into a urinal while remaining in bed.

 Go to Chapter 28, **Procedure 28–2: Placing and Removing a Bedpan,** in Volume 2.

For complete instructions for measuring urine output from a bedpan or urinal,

 Go to Chapter 27, **Technique 27–1: Measuring Voided Urine and Obtaining a Specimen,** in Volume 2.

Urine from a Catheter

An *indwelling catheter*, also known as a Foley or a retention catheter, is a flexible plastic tube that is inserted through the urethra into the bladder. It is held in place by a balloon that is inflated in the bladder above the detrusor muscle (Figure 27–4). Catheter insertion and ongoing care are discussed in the "Planning Interventions/Implementation" section of this chapter.

You will usually measure urine output from the indwelling catheter at the end of each shift unless otherwise ordered. Clients who require close monitoring of I&O will have a special collection bag with a measuring chamber. Often this is used to assess hourly urine output.

For complete instructions for measuring urine from a catheter,

 Go to Chapter 27, **Technique 27–2: Measuring Urine from an Indwelling Catheter,** in Volume 2.

Obtaining Samples for Urine Studies

Many disorders of the urinary system can be assessed by examining urine. You will perform some of these tests at the bedside. For others, you will collect a specimen that is analyzed in the lab. The various types of urine samples are discussed below.

Freshly Voided Specimen

To collect a freshly voided sample, collect the urine in the same manner as when you are measuring intake and output. Pour the urine into a specimen container labeled with the patient's name, the date, and the time of collection. Many facilities require packaging the container in a moisture-proof specimen-handling bag. Follow agency policy on additional packaging. Transport the specimen to the lab as soon as possible (according to agency policies). If there is a delay in getting the specimen to the lab, most agencies recommend refrigeration.

 Go to Chapter 27, **Technique 27–1: Measuring Voided Urine and Obtaining a Specimen,** in Volume 2.

For infants and very young children, you will apply a special collection device over the genitals to collect the specimen. While wearing procedure gloves, cleanse the genital area and allow the skin to dry. Remove the covering over the adhesive strips on the collection bag, and apply the bag over the genitals. When the child urinates, remove the collection bag and place the entire bag in a specimen container.

Clean-Catch Specimen

Many diagnostic tests require a clean-catch urine specimen. The client must cleanse the genitalia before voiding and collect the sample in midstream because the initial flow of urine may contain organisms from the urethral meatus or distal urethra. A midstream sample is free of these contaminants. The Critical Aspects box on page 645 summarizes key steps in collecting a clean-catch sample. For the complete procedure,

 Go to Chapter 27, **Procedure 27–1: Collecting a Clean-Catch Urine Specimen,** in Volume 2.

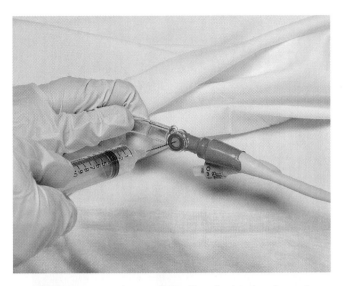

FIGURE 27–5   Inserting a sterile needle and syringe into the specimen port to obtain a sterile specimen from an indwelling catheter.

Sterile Urine Specimen

You can obtain a sterile urine specimen by inserting a catheter into the bladder or by withdrawing a sample from an indwelling catheter. Never take the specimen from the collection bag because that urine may be several hours old.

To obtain a specimen from an indwelling catheter, insert a needle into the specimen port of the catheter and withdraw urine. Never disconnect the catheter from the drainage tube to obtain a sample. Interrupting the system creates a portal of entry for pathogens, thereby increasing the risk of contamination. If the urine is not flowing briskly, you may need to clamp the catheter for 15 to 30 minutes to allow a fresh sample to collect in the tubing. Figure 27–5 illustrates how to obtain a sterile specimen from an indwelling catheter. For a discussion of the steps involved,

 Go to Chapter 27, **Technique 27–3: Obtaining a Sterile Urine Specimen from a Catheter,** in Volume 2.

24-Hour Urine Collection

A 24-hour urine collection may be ordered to evaluate some disorders. You must use a large collection container and collect all urine voided in the 24-hour time period. Occasionally you will be asked to collect each voiding in a separate container. To begin collection, have the patient void and record the time. Discard this first voiding, but collect all urine for the next 24 hours. Be sure to inform the patient and all staff about the collection. Post signs in prominent locations, such as the client's bathroom or entry door, to remind staff of the ongoing test. Also,

 Go to Chapter 27, **Technique 27–4: Collecting a 24-Hour Urine Specimen,** in Volume 2.

Terms Associated with Urination

Acute renal failure (ARF): An acute rise in the serum creatinine level of 25% or more. May be caused by inadequate blood flow to the kidney, injury to the kidney glomeruli or tubules, or obstruction of kidney outflow.

Anuria: The absence of urine. This term is used when urine output is less than 100 mL in 24 hours.

Dysuria: Painful or difficult urination. May be associated with infection or partial obstruction of the urinary tract as well as medications that trigger urinary retention.

End-stage renal disease (ESRD): A permanent rise in serum creatinine levels associated with loss of kidney function that must be treated with dialysis or transplantation. Also known as chronic renal failure (CRF).

Frequency: The need to urinate at short intervals.

Hematuria: Blood in the urine. May be due to trauma, kidney stones, infection, or menstruation.

Oliguria: Urine output of less than 400 mL in 24 hours.

Nephropathy: A broad term meaning disease of the kidney.

Nephrotoxic: A substance that damages kidney tissue. Some antibiotics (gentamycin, tobramycin, and amikacin), nonsteroidal anti-inflammatory drugs, lead, and contrast media have the potential to be nephrotoxic.

Nocturia: Frequent urination after going to bed. May be caused by excessive fluid intake as well as a variety of urinary tract and cardiovascular problems.

Polyuria: Excessive urination. May be caused by excessive hydration, diabetes mellitus, diabetes insipidus, or kidney disease.

Proteinuria: The presence of protein in the urine. May be a sign of infection or kidney disease.

Pyuria: Pus in the urine. May be caused by lesions or infection in the urinary tract.

Urgency: A sudden, almost uncontrollable need to urinate.

Routine Urinalysis

A routine urinalysis (UA) is one of the most commonly ordered laboratory tests. It is used as an overall screening test as well as an aid to diagnosing renal, hepatic, and other diseases. Urinalysis requires a freshly voided sample.

Urinalysis techniques include "dipstick" testing and/or microscopic analysis. Dipstick testing is commonly performed at the bedside; microscopic examination is done in the lab. Box 27–3 contains several

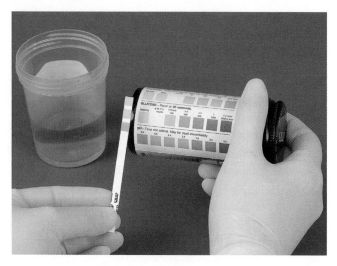

FIGURE 27–6 Commercial testing kits contain a reagent for a specific substance. A chemical reaction with the urine causes a color change that you interpret using a color chart.

terms used to describe urine characteristics and quantity. For the expected findings and common variants of urinalysis,

 Go to Chapter 27, **Diagnostic Testing, Urinalysis,** in Volume 2.

Bedside Testing (Dipstick)

Dipstick testing can determine pH and specific gravity and the presence of protein, glucose, ketones, and occult blood in the urine. Commercially prepared kits contain a reagent designed to detect a specific substance (e.g., glucose). The reagent may be a paper test strip, a fluid, or a tablet. When contacted by the urine, a chemical reaction causes a color change that you compare to a color chart (Figure 27–6). You will need good lighting to evaluate the test strip results. Read the kit label to be certain that you are using the correct reagent and that the kit is not past the expiration date. Follow the manufacturer's directions regarding the amount of urine needed and the time needed for the reagent to develop. For guidelines for dipstick testing,

 Go to Chapter 27, **Technique 27–5: Dipstick Testing of Urine,** in Volume 2.

You may delegate bedside urine testing to unlicensed assistive personnel (UAP) if you know that he has the knowledge and skill to perform the procedure. Ask the UAP to report the test results to you and to save the urine sample in case you should need to repeat the test.

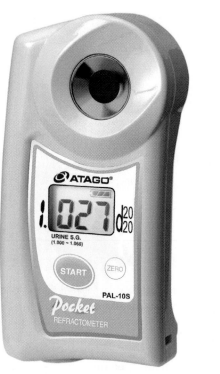
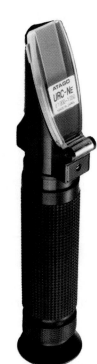

FIGURE 27–7 A refractometer indicates urine concentration by measuring the extent to which a beam of light is refracted ("bent") when passed through the urine. (Courtesy of atago USA, Inc., customerservice@atago-usa.com)

Specific Gravity

Specific gravity, an indicator of urine concentration, can be measured with a reagent strip. However, when you need to be precise and accurate, you should use a refractometer. Specific gravity is usually tested in the laboratory, but it is a nursing responsibility in some settings. For guidelines when testing urine specific gravity,

 Go to Chapter 27, **Technique 27–6: Measuring Specific Gravity of Urine,** in Volume 2.

A **refractometer** (Figure 27–7) measures the extent to which a beam of light changes direction when it passes through the urine (the *refractive index*). If the concentration of solids is high, the light is refracted more. The method is quick and easy to perform and requires only a few drops of urine. An older testing method used the **urinometer (hydrometer),** which is based on the principle that a body will float in liquid when the concentration of dissolved substances is high and sink when the liquid is more dilute. A refractometer is more precise, requires a much smaller specimen, is more compact, and poses less risk of spills and exposure to body fluids than does the urinometer. Some of the older glass urinometers may, in addition, have mercury in their base, posing a risk for environmental contamination should they break (see Chapter 21).

KnowledgeCheck 27–5

- Explain how to collect a clean-catch urine specimen.
- You are caring for a patient on a hospital unit from 7:00 A.M. to 12 noon. Based on the following information, calculate the I&O and comment on your findings.

> Receiving IV fluid at 125 mL/hr
> 8:00 A.M. breakfast—4 oz juice, toast, scrambled eggs, 8 oz coffee
> 9:30 A.M.—3 oz water
> 7:00 A.M. to 12 noon—wound drainage: 360 mL
> 7:00 A.M. to 12 noon—urine output per indwelling catheter: 180 mL

 Go to Chapter 27, **Knowledge Check Response Sheet and Answers,** on the Electronic Study Guide.

CriticalThinking 27–4

- Why do you think the first voided urine is discarded at the start of a 24-hour urine collection?
- Below are the dipstick findings you obtained on the clean-catch specimen from Jessica ("Meet Your Patient").

Feature	Result
pH	8.0
Specific gravity	1.030
Protein	Negative
Glucose	Negative
RBCs	Trace
Nitrite	+1
WBCs	+2
Bilirubin	Negative
Ketones	Negative
Urobilinogen	Negative

a. Identify the abnormal findings.
b. What would you expect the findings of her urine culture and sensitivity to demonstrate?

Blood Studies

Blood urea nitrogen and creatinine levels are commonly measured to assess renal function and hydration. For normal ranges,

 Go to Chapter 27, **Diagnostic Testing, Blood Studies: BUN and Creatinine,** in Volume 2.

Common Diagnostic Procedures

A variety of diagnostic procedures may be performed on the urinary tract. These procedures are conducted in the operating room, procedures suite, or radiology department. Typically nurses are responsible for preparing the client for the procedure, delivering aftercare, and sometimes assisting the physician. For a discussion of urinary system studies and the nursing responsibilities associated with them,

 Go to Chapter 27, **Diagnostic Testing, Studies of the Urinary System,** in Volume 2.

| Nursing Diagnosis |

Urinary elimination problems are described by several nursing and medical diagnoses. NANDA diagnoses specific to urinary elimination include the following:

- Impaired Urinary Elimination
- Urinary Incontinence (Functional, Reflex, Stress, Total, Urge)
- Risk for Urge Urinary Incontinence
- Urinary Retention
- Readiness for Enhanced Urinary Elimination
- Risk for Infection (Urinary Tract)

Urinary problems may also be the etiology of other nursing diagnoses, such as the following:

- Anxiety related to urinary urgency and recent episode of incontinence
- Body Image Disturbance secondary to new urostomy
- Risk for Impaired Skin Integrity related to exposure to urine secondary to incontinence
- Acute Pain related to bladder spasms and urinary tract infection
- Social Isolation related to frequent periods of incontinence
- Toileting Self-Care Deficit related to impaired cognition secondary to recent cerebrovascular accident

Common urinary elimination problems, including urinary tract infection, retention, incontinence, and urinary diversions are discussed at length in the remainder of this section.

Urinary Tract Infections

Normally urine is free of bacteria, viruses, and fungi. A urinary tract infection (UTI) occurs when microorganisms, usually *Escherichia coli (E. coli),* which normally lives in the colon, enter the urethra and begin to multiply. An infection limited to the urethra is called **urethritis. Cystitis** occurs when bacteria travel up

BOX 27–4 Signs and Symptoms of Urinary Tract Infection

Urinary Frequency	Bladder spasms
Urgency	Edema
Foul-smelling urine	Chills
Pyuria	Fever
Dysuria	Back pain
Hematuria	Nausea and vomiting

the urethra into the bladder, causing a bladder infection. If not treated promptly, the infection may progress superiorly (upward) to the ureters or kidneys (**pyelonephritis**).

Several biological safeguards are in place in the urinary system to prevent UTIs. One-way valves at the junction of the ureters and bladder help prevent urine from backing up toward the kidneys. In addition, the flow of urine during urination helps wash bacteria out of the body. In men, the prostate gland produces secretions that slow bacterial growth. But despite these safeguards, infections still occur.

Risk Factors for Urinary Tract Infection

People who are more prone to UTIs include the following:

- *Sexually active women.* During sexual activity, perineal pathogens may enter the urethra. Because a woman's urethra is short, pathogens can gain rapid access to the bladder.

- *Women who use spermicidal contraceptive gel.* Spermicides reduce normal flora in the vagina, allowing pathogens to multiply unrestricted.

- *Older women.* The loss of estrogen associated with menopause leads to drying of the mucosa in the vagina and urethra and a decrease in protective normal flora.

- *Men with an enlarged prostate.* An enlarged prostate may develop as a result of aging or cancerous changes. Pressure from the prostate creates difficulty emptying the bladder, resulting in stagnant urine, which provides an excellent medium for the growth of bacteria.

- *People with kidney stones.* Kidney stones (*renal calculi*) obstruct the flow of urine, creating stagnation, and irritate the urinary tract as they are passed.

- *Anyone who has an indwelling catheter.* A catheter provides a pathway for bacteria to migrate up into the urinary system.

- *People who have diabetes mellitus.* Glucose in the urine provides nutrients for bacteria to multiply.

- *People who have a history of UTIs.* Anyone with a previous UTI is more likely to experience a recurrence (National Kidney and Urologic Diseases Information Clearinghouse, 2004).

Recognizing and Treating Urinary Tract Infections

The presence of bacteria in a symptomatic patient is used in the medical diagnosis of UTI. To assist in the diagnosis of UTI, assess for the signs and symptoms in Box 27–4. You will also need to collect a midstream clean-catch urine specimen.

Antibiotics are used to treat UTI. The length and type of treatment depends on the location and severity of infection. In general, a bladder infection may be treated for 1 to 5 days with oral antibiotics. In contrast, pyelonephritis (kidney infection) may require IV antibiotics for several days followed by a 7- to 14-day course of oral antibiotics.

 CriticalThinking 27–5

As you may have concluded, Jessica ("Meet Your Patient") has a UTI. What additional history questions would you like to ask Jessica?

Urinary Retention

Urinary retention is an inability to empty the bladder completely. Etiologies include obstruction, inflammation and swelling, neurological problems, medications, and anxiety.

- *Obstruction.* Among men, an enlarged prostate is the most common cause of obstruction in the lower urinary tract. Other obstructions include stones lodged in the urethra, strictures or scars from previous injury, tumors or blood clots in the urinary system, and fecal impaction. Impacted stool distends the rectum and causes forward pressure on the urethra, interfering with the flow of urine out of the bladder.

- *Inflammation and swelling.* Obstruction may also occur as a result of inflammation and swelling, for example, from infection or surgery in the pelvic region. Swelling narrows the diameter of the urethra so that urine cannot flow freely.

- *Neurological problems.* Recall that voiding requires that the brain, spinal cord, and nerves supplying the bladder and urethra must be intact. Conditions that affect innervation of the bladder include spinal cord tumors or injury, herniated disk, and viral infections involving perineal nerves (e.g., genital herpes).

- *Medications.* Anesthesia and other medications can also cause temporary problems with urination. Box 27–2 provides examples of medications with anticholinergic or alpha-adrenergic effects that may impede urine flow.
- *Anxiety.* Painful urination may produce anxiety and lead to voluntary withholding of urination.

Urinary Incontinence

Urinary incontinence (UI) is a lack of voluntary control over urination. Over 20 million Americans have urinary incontinence. Incontinence affects people of all ages and social and economic levels. It affects both sexes, but women are twice as likely as men to have this condition. Among adult women, 15 to 30% experience UI. Among those age 60 or older, the incidence is even higher. In addition, at least half of the 1.5 million Americans who live in nursing homes are incontinent. Overall, institutions spend at least $5.2 billion on incontinence supplies and services (Newman & Palmer, 2003). The total number of people affected by incontinence is presumed to be far greater than current estimates, because incontinence is a disorder that is often not discussed.

In healthy adults, episodes of incontinence occur rarely, usually in response to an extreme situation, such as being unable to find a restroom on a lengthy car trip. Incontinence is not a normal change that occurs with aging. This myth is pervasive and often leads older adults to avoid seeking treatment. Many people do not mention leakage of urine to healthcare providers because they are embarrassed or believe that nothing can be done. Unfortunately this acceptance may lead to restriction of activities and ultimately to loneliness, depression, and isolation (Fultz & Herzog, 2001).

In men, UI is most often related to benign prostatic hyperplasia (enlarged prostate) or to prostatectomy. In women, it is often related to childbirth, specifically to vaginal delivery. Incidence is even higher among those who required episiotomy or forceps- or vacuum-assisted birth. Other risk factors for UI are perimenopausal status, high body mass index, diabetes, and current cigarette smoking.

Types of Urinary Incontinence

The Agency for Healthcare Research and Quality guidelines (Fantl et al., 1996) identified the following seven types of UI:

- **Urge incontinence** is the involuntary loss of urine associated with a strong urge to void. It is often referred to as overactive bladder.
- **Stress incontinence** is an involuntary loss of urine with increased intraabdominal pressure. NANDA specifies "loss of less than 50 mL of urine" (2003, p. 96). Etiological factors include pregnancy, child-

birth, obesity, chronic constipation, and straining at stool. Activities that produce the symptom include exercise, laughing, sneezing, coughing, and lifting.
- **Mixed incontinence** is a combination of urge and stress incontinence.
- **Overflow incontinence** is the loss of urine in combination with a distended bladder. Causes of overflow incontinence include fecal impaction, neurological disorders, and enlarged prostate.
- **Functional incontinence** is the involuntary loss of urine in the absence of urinary system injuries or nervous system problems. NANDA (2003, p. 94) defines functional incontinence as the "inability of usually continent person to reach the toilet in time to avoid unintentional loss of urine." Etiologies include confusion, disorientation, or mobility problems.
- **Transient incontinence** is a short-term incontinence that is expected to resolve spontaneously. Causes include UTI and medications, especially diuretics.
- **Unconscious (reflex) incontinence** is loss of urine when the person does not realize the bladder is full and has no urge to void. Central nervous system disorders and multisystem problems are common causes. NANDA defines Reflex Urinary Incontinence as the "involuntary loss of urine at somewhat predictable intervals when a specific bladder volume is reached" (2003, p. 95). NANDA adds specific causes: tissue damage from radiation, cystitis, bladder inflammation, or radical pelvic surgery.

Enuresis, which tends to be familial, is involuntary urination after about 5 to 6 years of age, when control is usually established. It is more common in boys than girls, and the precise cause is not fully understood. **Nocturnal enuresis** (bed-wetting) is common in preschoolers and should not be considered a problem until after age 6. Enuresis is *primary* if bladder training was never achieved; *secondary* if control was established and then lost (Riley, 1997). Enuresis has been associated with stress (e.g., marital discord), UTI, allergies, abnormal electroencephalographic patterns, sleep disorders, and small bladder capacity; however, the cause is not always apparent.

Treatments for Urinary Incontinence

Medications and surgery are multidisciplinary approaches that may be used to manage UI. Medications include topical estrogen for women who have UI associated with urogenital atrophy, and anticholinergic drugs such as oxybutynin (Ditropan) and tolterodine (Detrol), which inhibit involuntary bladder contractions. Surgical treatment, such as bladder suspension and prostate resection, are an option for some patients. Independent nursing interventions (e.g., teaching Kegel exercises) are discussed later in this chapter.

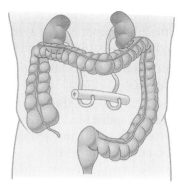

FIGURE 27–8 An ileal conduit is the most common urinary diversion.

Conditions Requiring Urinary Diversions

A **urinary diversion,** or **urostomy,** is a surgically created opening for elimination of urine. Urostomies are used to treat patients who have conditions such as birth defects, cancer, trauma, or disease of the urinary system. A patient with a urinary diversion does not eliminate urine via the urethra. Instead, urine bypasses the bladder and is expelled through the **stoma** or **ostomy.** The patient no longer has voluntary control of urination. Urine constantly flows through the stoma and is collected in a pouch that the patient wears. Risks associated with urinary diversions are primarily infection and permanent kidney damage, which can occur from hydronephrosis (distention of the kidneys with urine, which results from obstruction of the ureter).

The following are three types of urinary diversions:

- A **cutaneous ureterostomy** reroutes the ureter(s) directly to the surface of the abdomen, forming a small stoma. It may be unilateral or bilateral. This procedure has limited use because it provides a pathway for pathogens on the skin to directly enter the kidney. The stomas are small and difficult to fit with a collection appliance.

- An **ileal conduit** (also known as a **Bricker's loop** or **ileal loop**) is the most common type of urinary diversion (Figure 27–8). A small piece of ileum is removed with blood and nerve supply intact. The remainder of the ileum is reconnected to prevent disruption of flow through the bowel. The free segment of ileum is sutured closed at one end, and the other end is brought out to the abdominal wall to create a stoma. The result is a small pouch into which the ureters are implanted. Urine, along with mucus from the ileum, drains continuously from the stoma. This procedure is preferable to a cutaneous ureterostomy because the mucous membrane lining the ileum protects the kidneys from ascending infection. In addition, the ileum creates a stoma that is easier to fit with an appliance.

- A **continent urostomy** (Figure 27–9), also known as an **ileal bladder conduit,** or **Kock pouch,** is a variation of the ileal conduit. Urine drains from the

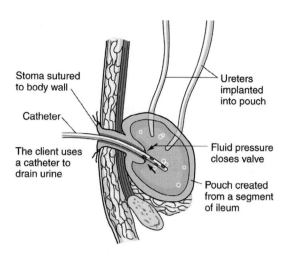

FIGURE 27–9 A continent urostomy allows the client to manage urine without the need to wear an ostomy appliance.

ureters into a surgically created ileal pouch. The stoma created on the abdomen contains a nipple valve to keep urine from leaking. Rather than having urine flow constantly, the patient with an ileal bladder conduit inserts a catheter into the stoma to drain urine through the valve. A second valve prevents reflux of urine back into the kidneys.

 CriticalThinking 27–6

What types of challenges or problems do you think a patient with a urinary diversion might experience?

| Planning Outcomes/Evaluation |

The general goal related to urinary elimination is that patients will comfortably void approximately 1500 mL of light yellow urine in 24 hours. Because normal urine elimination patterns vary, the frequency and amount of urine are based on the individual's pattern, food and fluid intake, medications, and other factors.

NOC standardized outcomes for urinary problems, regardless of the specific problem, are the following: Kidney Function, Urinary Continence, Urinary Elimination, and Tissue Integrity: Skin & Mucous Membranes (because urinary elimination problems often place the patient at Risk for Impaired Skin Integrity).

Individualized goals/outcome statements you might use to evaluate the effectiveness of interventions for urinary problems include the following:

- Will resume his normal urination pattern by (date).
- Will discuss his feelings about his urostomy.
- Will have no visible blood in urine after 2 days on antibiotics.
- Responds to the urge to void in a timely manner.
- After voiding, states he feels he has emptied his bladder completely.
- Postvoiding residual volume is less than 150 mL.

| Planning Interventions/Implementation |

For *NIC standardized interventions* for patients with urinary elimination nursing diagnoses,

 Go to Chapter 27, **Standardized Language, NIC Interventions for Urinary Problems,** in Volume 2.

You should select nursing activities to meet individual needs and address problem etiologies.

Specific nursing activities for patients with elimination problems fall into the following categories: promoting normal urination, preventing urinary tract infection, managing urinary retention, managing urinary incontinence, and caring for patients who have urinary diversions. The rest of this chapter discusses those activities.

Promoting Normal Urination

As a nurse, you should have a repertoire of independent nursing activities for promoting normal urination. These include providing privacy, positioning, scheduling elimination, providing and monitoring fluid and nutrition, and assisting with hygiene.

Provide Privacy

Although urination is a normal physiological process, most people consider it a very private matter. Taking a matter-of-fact approach confirms to patients that you are comfortable with this aspect of care. Provide privacy when discussing or providing care related to urination. Excuse visitors from the room, draw the dividing curtains in shared rooms, and close the door to the room. Whenever possible, give the patient time alone to void. Do not, for example, hover outside the bathroom door asking, "Are you OK?" or "Are you finished?" However, if the client is very weak, you may need to remain with him.

Assist with Positioning

Most men stand to void and may have difficulty voiding in other positions. Whenever possible, assist the client to the bathroom to use the toilet and allow him to assume his preferred position. Alternatively, provide a bedside commode or urinal for the client to use. To place a urinal, position the patient in a semi-Fowler's position with the legs slightly spread. Place the urinal on the bed between the patient's legs, and insert his penis in the urinal.

Women generally find an upright seated or squatting position to be the most comfortable position for voiding. If a female patient must remain in bed, provide a bedpan. Place her in a semi-Fowler's position to urinate unless contraindicated. Raise the siderails or provide an overhead trapeze so that the patient will have grip holds to maneuver herself onto and off the bedpan. If the patient is very weak, you may need an assistant to help you position her on the bedpan, and you may need to stay with her to help her maintain her position on the bedpan. For the steps involved,

 Go to Chapter 28, **Procedure 28-2: Placing and Removing a Bedpan,** in Volume 2.

Also see the Critical Aspects box in Chapter 28 of this volume.

Facilitate Toileting Routines

Most patients void on awakening, after meals, and prior to bedtime. Some patients have routines with regularly scheduled toileting times. Identify your patient's pattern, and stick to it as much as possible. If you anticipate a change in pattern, inform the patient. For example, if the patient is to receive a diuretic, explain that he will need to urinate more often. Similarly if the patient is scheduled for a diagnostic procedure or activity, inform him ahead of time so that he may void before the activity begins.

Provide assistance to all patients who have mobility problems and those who use the bedpan. Discuss with all UAPs the need to offer assistance so that patients experience minimal delays.

Promote Adequate Fluids and Nutrition

Patients should drink eight to ten large glasses (about 3000 mL) of fluid daily unless health problems limit their fluid intake. Adequate hydration promotes urinary tract function and flushes the system of waste products. Unfortunately, many people do not meet the recommended intake. Water is the preferred fluid because soda, coffee, and tea often contain caffeine or additives that may cause diuresis. However, the amount of fluid is more important than the type. If the patient will not or cannot drink water, provide the fluid he prefers. Other suggestions include the following:

- For patients with limited mobility, keep water or other liquids in easy reach.
- You may need to remind young children or patients with cognitive or psychiatric disorders to drink fluids.
- For patients who have increased fluid needs, provide goals for intake, and remind them frequently to drink.
- Many foods have substantial fluid content. If the patient requires additional fluid for hydration, consider adding soup and watery foods, such as watermelon, to the diet. In contrast, if the patient requires fluid restriction, you will have to calculate these foods into the fluid balance.

Teaching Your Client About Preventing UTI

- Drink at least 8 to 10 glasses of fluid per day to keep urine dilute and to flush bacteria from the urinary tract. Water is best.

- Urinate when you first feel the urge. Do not postpone urination regularly, because bacteria can multiply in stagnant urine.

- Always wipe from front to back after urination or defecation.

- Wear cotton underwear, because nylon or other synthetic fabrics prevent evaporation of moisture. Also avoid tight-fitting clothing. Bacteria and other microorganisms grow well in a warm, moist environment.

- Urinate after having intercourse to flush away bacteria that might have entered the urethra.

- If you have a history of UTI, avoid using the diaphragm, spermicidal contraceptive gel, or unlubricated or spermicidal condoms.

- If you have a history of UTI, avoid bubble baths and baking-soda baths.

- Promptly report any symptoms of UTI to your healthcare provider.

Assist with Hygiene

Urine is irritating to the skin. Therefore, perineal cleansing is an integral part of toileting hygiene. Many ill patients are unable to do this for themselves, so you will need to provide perineal care. If the patient can ambulate to the bathroom, you will merely need to assist with her usual cleansing routines. You may assist the patient by pouring warm soapy water over the genitals while she is seated on the toilet, the bedside commode, or on the bedpan. Be sure to rinse with warm water, because soap may be drying to the genital mucosa. Also offer a moist washcloth or towelette for washing hands after toileting. For further information,

Go to Chapter 22, **Procedure 22-4: Providing Perineal Care,** in Volume 2.

KnowledgeCheck 27–6

- Identify activities that promote normal urination patterns.
- Write at least two nursing diagnostic statements that would be appropriate for Jessica in the "Meet Your Patient" scenario.

Go to Chapter 27, **Knowledge Check Response Sheet and Answers,** on the Electronic Study Guide.

Teaching Prevention of Urinary Tract Infection

An important part of UTI treatment is prevention of future infection. The accompanying Self-Care box presents the teaching points that you should include in your sessions with patients at risk for UTI or recovering from a UTI.

Managing Urinary Retention

Clients with a mechanical obstruction to urine flow are treated by surgical removal or repair of the obstruction (e.g., resection of the prostate gland, removal of bladder calculi). For clients who have loss of bladder tone, collaboratively, you may (1) administer cholinergic medications, such as bethanechol chloride (Urecholine), which promote bladder emptying by stimulating contraction of the detrusor muscle; (2) use **Credé's maneuver** (apply manual pressure over the bladder to promote emptying); and (3) perform urinary catheterization. Independent nursing measures to assess and promote urination include the following:

- Monitor intake and output.
- Assess for risk factors for urinary retention (e.g., prostatic hypertrophy, pelvic surgery and medications with anticholinergic side effects, such as diazepam [Valium], some antidepressants, and diphenhydramine [Benadryl].
- Inspect and palpate for bladder distention.
- Place the patient in as normal a voiding position as possible.
- Provide privacy.
- Run water nearby, or place the patient's hands in warm water.
- Pour water over the perineum, or assist the patient to take a warm sitz bath.
- Measure post-voiding residual urine (see the following section).

Catheterization

Urinary catheterization is the introduction of a pliable tube (catheter) into the bladder to allow drainage of urine. Urinary catherization is performed to:

- Obtain a sterile urine specimen.
- Empty the bladder for surgical or diagnostic purposes.
- Prevent or treat bladder overdistention and urinary retention (e.g., after surgery) when other measures fail.
- Measure the urine that remains in the bladder after the patient voids. This is commonly referred to as **post-void residual volume** and is measured as part of the diagnostic workup for a patient with urinary retention or incontinence.

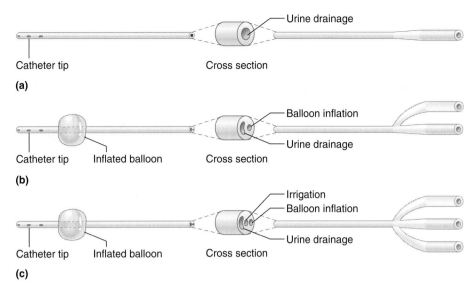

FIGURE 27–10 Types of catheters. *A,* A single-lumen catheter is used to obtain a urine sample or immediately drain the bladder. *B,* A double-lumen catheter is the most commonly used indwelling catheter. *C,* A triple-lumen catheter is inserted when the patient requires irrigation of the bladder.

Observe strict sterile technique when inserting and caring for a urinary catheter because the risk for infection is high. The catheter provides a connection between the external environment and a normally sterile system. Additionally, when the patient has an indwelling catheter, microorganisms are no longer flushed from the urethra through voiding. In fact, an indwelling urinary catheter is the most common cause of nosocomial infections.

Catheterization can injure the urethra if the catheter is too large, is forced through strictures, or is inserted at an incorrect angle. For male patients, when inserting a catheter you must elevate the penis so that it is perpendicular to the body; this straightens the normally curved urethra, helping to prevent trauma. Catheters must be well lubricated on insertion to prevent damaging the delicate mucosa of the urethra.

Patients with spinal cord injuries or neurological disorders use intermittent catheterization to drain the bladder and limit the risk of infection. Many actually perform **intermittent self-catheterization,** although caregivers may assist. Although you will use sterile technique for catheterization, most patients who self-catheterize use clean technique. In spite of this difference, intermittent catheterization carries a substantially lower risk of infection than does an indwelling catheter (Johansson, Athlin, Frykholm, Bolinder, & Larsson, 2002; Ord, Lunn, & Reynard, 2003; Pomfret, 2000). See the accompanying Self-Care box on page 642.

Types of Catheters

Urinary catheters are usually made of rubber or plastic, but silicone, latex, or polyvinyl chloride (PVC) may also be used. PVC catheters are good for long-term use (up to 6 weeks) because they soften and conform to the urethra. For even longer periods of use (e.g., up to 3 months), silicone may be used because it helps prevent encrustation around the urinary meatus. Some catheters have a lubricant and/or antimicrobial coating to help prevent infection. Always check for latex and iodine allergies before performing a catheterization.

Catheters are sized by the diameter of the lumen; the larger the number, the larger the lumen. For example, #8 and #10 French catheters are used for children; they are smaller in diameter than the #14 and #16 French catheters typically used for adults. Men usually need a larger size (e.g., #18 Fr) than women. Catheters also come in different lengths: a 22 cm catheter is appropriate for women, whereas for males you will need a 40 cm catheter.

A **straight catheter** is a single-lumen tube that is inserted for immediate drainage of the bladder (e.g., to obtain a sterile urine specimen, to measure postvoid residual volume, or to relieve temporary bladder distention). After the bladder is empty or the sample obtained, the catheter is removed and the patient resumes voiding independently.

An **indwelling catheter,** also known as a *Foley* or *retention catheter,* is used for continuous bladder drainage (e.g., when the bladder must be kept empty or when continuous urine measurement is needed). It is usually a double-lumen tube: one lumen is used for urine drainage, and the second lumen is used to inflate a balloon near the tip of the catheter. The inflated balloon holds the catheter in place at the neck of the bladder. The balloon is sized according to the volume of fluid used to inflate it. For most patients you will use a 5 mL balloon; for children 3 mL; and for achieving hemostasis after a prostatectomy, a 30 mL balloon. A triple-lumen indwelling catheter is used when the patient requires intermittent or continuous bladder irrigation. Figure 27–10 illustrates the different types of catheters.

Teaching Your Client About Clean Intermittent Self-Catheterization (CISC)

The goals of intermittent self-catheterization are to (1) completely empty the bladder and (2) prevent urinary tract infections. Assess the patient's physical ability to reach the urethra and manipulate the equipment. Teach the patient:

- The basic location of urological landmarks (e.g., the urethra). Demonstrate to a female patient that her urethra is located between her clitoris and vagina. A woman may use a mirror. Patients who cannot see their urethra may be taught to locate it by touch.

- That some CISC catheters can be reused; some are disposable.

- To catheterize as often as needed—perhaps every 2 to 3 hours at first.

- To discard a reuseable catheter when it becomes difficult to clean or difficult to insert. A CISC catheter may be reused for 2 to 4 weeks.

- To soak the catheter in a white vinegar solution once a week to control odor and remove mucus deposits.

- To contact a healthcare provider if symptoms of UTI occur (e.g., urine contains sediment or becomes cloudy, or burning on urination or a fever occurs).

- To contact a healthcare provider if there is bleeding, pain, or difficulty passing the catheter.

- To drink 2000 to 3000 mL of fluid each day to ensure a quantity of urine adequate to flush the bladder.

Procedure for Men

1. Try to void before catheterization. If you are unable to void or if the amount is less than 100 mL (or the amount specified by your healthcare provider), then insert the catheter.

2. Assemble the catheter, lubricant, and drainage receptacle.

3. Thoroughly wash your hands with soap and water; cleanse the penis and the urethral opening.

4. Lubricate the catheter to 6 inches (15 cm).

5. Stand over the toilet or assume a comfortable position (e.g., sitting on the toilet).

6. Hold the penis perpendicular (at a right angle) to the body.

7. Gently insert and advance the catheter.

8. When you meet resistance, at the level of the prostate, take deep breaths to try to relax, and advance the catheter.

9. When urine flow starts, advance the catheter 1 inch (2.5 cm) more; return the penis to its natural position; hold the catheter in place until the urine flow stops and bladder is empty.

10. Withdraw the catheter slowly in small increments to be sure the entire bladder empties.

11. Wash catheter with soap and water. If it is reusable, rinse and dry it well; if it is disposable, discard it immediately.

12. Store catheters in a clean, dry, secure place.

13. Record the amount of urine obtained.

Procedure for Women

1. Try to void before catheterization. If you are unable to void or if amount is less than 100 mL (or the amount specified by your healthcare provider), then insert catheter.

2. Assemble the catheter, lubricant, and drainage receptacle; a good light is important for women.

3. Thoroughly wash hands with soap and water; cleanse the labia and urethra with soap and water or with a moist towelette; rinse. Cleanse and rinse from front to back.

4. Lubricate the catheter to about 1 inch (2.5 cm).

5. Assume a comfortable position. Some women perform CISC standing up with one foot on the toilet.

6. Locate the urethral opening; it is between the clitoris and the vagina.

7. Spread the vaginal lips with the second and fourth finger; use the middle finger to feel for the urethral opening.

8. Gently insert the catheter into the opening, guiding it upward toward the umbilicus (bellybutton).

9. When urine flows, advance the catheter another 1 inch (2.5 cm); hold it in place until the urine stops and the bladder is empty.

10. Withdraw the catheter slowly, in small increments, to be sure the entire bladder empties.

11. Wash catheter with soap and water. If it is reusable, rinse and dry it well; if it is disposable, discard it immediately.

12. Store catheters in a clean, dry, secure place.

13. Record the amount of urine obtained.

Source: Knowles, D.R. (2002, October 28). Medical encyclopedia: clean intermittent self-catheterization. Review provided by VeriMed Healthcare Network. Accessed July 9, 2004, from http://www.nlm.nih.gov/medlineplus/print/ency/article/003972.htm

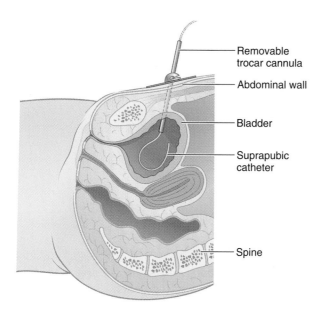

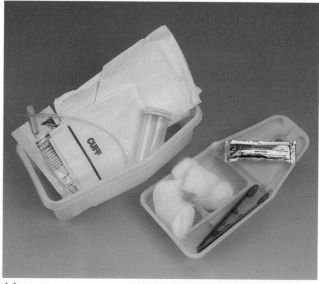

(a)

FIGURE 27–11 A suprapubic catheter drains urine from a surgically created opening into the bladder, bypassing the urethra.

A **suprapubic catheter** is used for continuous urine drainage when the urethra must be bypassed (e.g., after gynecological surgery or where there is prostatic obstruction). A suprapubic catheter is inserted through an incision above the symphysis pubis (Figure 27–11). It is often sutured in place but may occasionally be a double-lumen catheter held in place by a balloon.

Supplies for Catheterization

The supplies used for inserting an indwelling catheter are usually prepackaged (Figure 27–12). Included in the kit are sterile gloves, swabs or cotton balls, a solution for cleansing the urethral meatus, sterile lubricant, a sterile indwelling catheter, a syringe filled with sterile water to inflate the retention balloon, drainage tubing, and a drainage collection bag. Kits contain the most common catheter sizes, usually #12, #14, or #16 French. Pediatric kits contain #8 or #10 French catheters. Many facilities also have prepackaged kits for straight (single-lumen) catheterization. Instead of a drainage collection bag, these have a drainage basin for collecting urine. Both types of kit may also contain a sterile urine cup for collecting a sterile specimen.

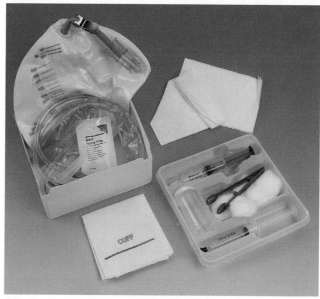

(b)

FIGURE 27–12 Supplies for catheter insertion usually come in a prepackaged kit. *A,* Straight catheter kit. *B,* Indwelling catheter kit.

KnowledgeCheck 27–7

- Describe the difference between a catheter used for straight catheterization and one used for ongoing drainage.
- Why is intermittent catheterization preferred for patients who must be catheterized over lengthy periods of time?

 Go to Chapter 27, **Knowledge Check Response Sheet and Answers,** on the Electronic Study Guide.

Urinary Catheter Insertion

To insert a urinary catheter, you will need to gather the appropriate supplies and prepare the patient. Explain to the patient the reason for the catheter insertion, the expected length of time the catheter will be needed, and the sensations he is likely to have. Most patients experience a sensation of pressure and some discomfort (but not pain) when a catheter is inserted. Explain that when the catheter is inserted it may feel as though he is voiding, but that the urine is going into the tube, not on the bed. If there is swelling or bleeding in the urinary tract, insertion may be painful.

Most patients are embarrassed by this procedure. A professional approach, along with draping and other privacy measures, helps relieve distress. As you are draping the patient, offer to answer any further questions he may have.

Use a dorsal recumbent position for both men and women. For female patients, make sure to lower the

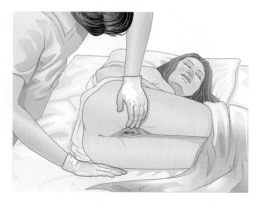
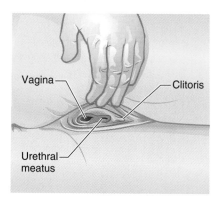

FIGURE 27–13 For women who cannot assume a dorsal recumbent position, you can use the side-lying position and lift the superior buttock to expose the urethral meatus.

knee gatch of the bed so that you can easily visualize the urinary meatus. You may need to place a firm cushion under the patient's buttocks to prevent her sinking into a soft mattress and obscuring visibility of the meatus. For women who are unable to assume a dorsal recumbent position, consider Sims' position or a lateral position (Figure 27–13).

 Go to Chapter 27, **Procedure 27–2: Inserting a Urinary Catheter,** in Volume 2.

The accompanying Critical Aspects box provides an overview.

Caring for the Patient with an Indwelling Catheter

The following are nursing goals when providing care for a patient with an indwelling catheter:

- *Prevent urinary tract infection.* An indwelling catheter is connected to a drainage tube and collection bag, which constitute a closed system. This means that it cannot be opened at any point. This minimizes the chance for pathogens to enter the system and infect the urinary tract.
- *Maintain free flow of urine.* Maintaining free flow of urine prevents backflow of urine into the bladder, which can cause bladder distention and injury. Stasis of urine also provides a medium for growth of microorganisms.
- *Prevent transmission of infection.* When providing catheter care, observe universal precautions.
- *Promote normal urine production.* Adequate urine production flushes pathogens out of the bladder, provides natural irrigation of the tubing, and prevents stasis of urine.
- *Maintain skin and mucosal integrity.* Secure the tubing to the leg to prevent traction on the bladder. Provide hygiene care so that the perineal skin and mucosa do not become irritated by feces encrustation of the catheter.

For a comprehensive list of nursing activities to help you meet the preceding goals,

 Go to Chapter 27, **Technique 27–7: Caring for a Patient with an Indwelling Catheter,** in Volume 2.

Catheter and Bladder Irrigation

You may perform an irrigation to maintain patency of a urinary catheter, to wash out the bladder, or to instill medications into the bladder. An *intermittent irrigation* is most commonly used for medication instillation, whereas a *continuous irrigation* is used to maintain patency when blood, clots, or debris are anticipated. Routine intermittent irrigations (e.g., every shift, every week) are sometimes ordered to ensure patency; however, these should be avoided and irrigation done only as necessary.

A client requiring a continuous irrigation should have a triple-lumen catheter in place: one lumen for injecting water into the balloon when the catheter is inserted, another for the irrigating solution to flow into the bladder, and a third for the solution and urine to flow out of the bladder. A double-lumen catheter system may need to be opened for irrigation and, therefore, creates a high risk for infection. Although "open" irrigation was used in the past, it is no longer recommended.

 Go to Chapter 27, **Procedure 27–3: Intermittent Bladder or Catheter Irrigation,** and **Procedure 27–4: Continuous Bladder Irrigation,** in Volume 2.

The Critical Aspects box on page 645 provides overviews of these procedures.

Removing an Indwelling Catheter

Removing a urinary catheter is a simple task, but you must monitor patients carefully afterward. Gather the necessary supplies, and tell the patient what you are about to do, what she will feel, and that you will need to monitor her urination after removal. Explain that this procedure is usually painless.

VOL 2 For steps to follow in *all* procedures, refer to the inside back cover of Volume 2.

critical aspects of procedures 27–1 through 27–5

Procedure 27–1: Collecting a Clean-Catch Urine Specimen

- Don clean procedure gloves.

- Wash the perineum or the end of the penis first with soap and water, then with antiseptic solution. (For women, wash from front to back; for men, use a circular motion from urethra outward.)

- Have the patient begin voiding. After the stream begins, collect a 30 to 60 mL specimen.

- Maintain sterility: Do not touch the inside of the container or the container lid.

- Place lid on container, label the container, and transport it to the lab in a timely manner.

Procedure 27–2: Inserting a Urinary Catheter

- Take an extra pair of sterile gloves and an extra sterile catheter into the room.

- Be sure that you have good lighting, especially for female patients. Take a procedure lamp to the bedside if necessary.

- Work on the right side of the bed if you are right-handed; the left side, if you are left-handed.

- Drape the patient for privacy.

- Perform perineal care before the procedure; wash your hands; open the kit.

- Don sterile gloves and maintain sterile technique while manipulating kit supplies and performing the procedure.

- Once you have touched the patient with your non-dominant hand, do not remove that hand from the patient.

- Lubricate the catheter tip before insertion.

- Insert the catheter 5 to 7.5 cm (2 to 3 in.) for women, 17 to 22.5 cm (7 to 9 in.) for men, until urine flows.

- Drain the bladder; collect needed samples; measure urine, and connect drainage bag as needed.

Procedure 27–3: Intermittent Bladder or Catheter Irrigation

- Establish a sterile field under the specimen removal port or the irrigation port on a three-way catheter.

- Because of the risk of infection, never disconnect the drainage tubing from the catheter.

- Use sterile irrigation solution, warmed to room temperature.

- Instill the irrigation solution slowly.

- Repeat the process as necessary.

Procedure 27–4: Continuous Bladder Irrigation

- Drape the patient, exposing the irrigation port of the indwelling catheter.

- Using aseptic technique, insert the connecting tubing into the irrigation solution container.

- Prime the tubing, removing all the air.

- Don clean procedure gloves.

- Pinch the irrigation port of the catheter; remove any plug, and connect the irrigation tubing to the port.

- Regulate the flow of the irrigant appropriately.

- Monitor for urine output.

Procedure 27–5: Applying an External (Condom) Catheter

- Application of a condom (external) catheter is a clean procedure.

- The penis should be clean and dry prior to catheter application.

- When applying the condom, stabilize the penis with your nondominant hand.

- Leave a gap of 2.5 to 5 cm (1 to 2 in.) between the condom and the tip of the penis to prevent skin irritation.

- It is important to use only the tape supplied in the application kit to secure the catheter.

  For condom catheters that contain adhesive material on the inside of the condom, grasp the penis and gently compress the condom onto the shaft.

- Be certain that the tubing from the end of the catheter to the bedside drainage (or leg) bag is free from kinks.

home care

Managing Incontinence

- Routinely ask clients and families about incontinence. Patients and families often do not raise the issue.

- Phrase the question indirectly. Patients are likely to answer no if you ask directly, "Are you incontinent?" For example, ask: "Do you wear a pad to keep your clothes dry?" "Do you ever wet your clothing?" "Do you sometimes not make it to the toilet in time?"

- Ask where the toilet is and whether the patient can get there easily. For example, must he go upstairs?

- In a two-story house with a toilet on only one floor, place a commode on the other floor in the room where the patient spends most of his time. With a written prescription, Medicare may reimburse this expense.

- For some patients, a commode should be placed by the bedside on a large, absorbent, washable mat (to absorb any urine that leaks).

- Teach behavioral techniques for incontinence management.

- Because most home caregivers are middle-aged or older women, they may have continence problems of their own. Teach them pelvic muscle exercises and the best techniques for lifting and turning the patient in bed.

Source: Lewis, L. (2003). Managing incontinence at home. *American Journal of Nursing, 3*(suppl.), 41.

Ask the patient to notify you the first time she voids. The catheter may have caused some edema of the urethra, which will interfere with voiding at first. Therefore, you must assess regularly for bladder distention until normal voiding is reestablished. The same is true for patients who have had rectal, perineal, or lower abdominal surgery, which also creates perineal edema.

If a catheter is in place for several weeks and the urine has been draining continuously, the bladder does not stretch and contract as it does in normal voiding. Therefore, the muscle loses tone and the patient may require bladder retraining. Agencies have differing procedures for this; however, one method is to begin clamping the catheter for certain periods of time (e.g., 1 to 4 hours) to allow the bladder to fill, and then release the clamp to allow urine to drain from the bladder. This should stimulate the bladder muscle and improve tone.

For guidelines to follow when removing a retention catheter,

 Go to Chapter 27, **Technique 27–8: Removing a Retention Catheter,** in Volume 2.

After removing the catheter, note and record the time and amount of the first voiding and the appearance of the urine. Compare the patient's intake to her output for the next 8 to 12 hours, and palpate the bladder for distention.

KnowledgeCheck 27–8

- What actions should you take before inserting a catheter?
- When caring for a client with an indwelling catheter, you notice sandy particles around the urethral meatus. What should you do?
- How often should the urine collection bag be emptied?

 Go to Chapter 27, **Knowledge Check Response Sheet and Answers,** on the Electronic Study Guide.

CriticalThinking 27–7

You are caring for a patient who had an indwelling catheter removed 12 hours ago. The patient has not voided. What action should you take?

Managing Urinary Incontinence

Because urinary incontinence is so prevalent, you are likely to be called on to treat it frequently in your practice. Most incontinence is managed with skin care and behavioral interventions, but medications are sometimes used. Refer to the accompanying Home Care box.

For a comprehensive list of nursing interventions for managing urinary incontinence,

 Go to Chapter 27, **Technique 27–9: Managing Urinary Incontinence,** in Volume 2.

Perineal Skin Care

Normal urine is acidic. When it remains in contact with the skin, it becomes alkaline, causing encrustations to collect on the skin. The skin then becomes macerated and excoriated. It is essential to keep the skin, clothing, and bedding clean and dry. Barrier creams may be used for irritated skin; antifungals may be prescribed (e.g., nystatin [Mycostatin]) for fungus growth.

Behavioral Interventions

Nurses have taken the lead in investigating incontinence and treatment options. However, despite their interest in researching it, practicing nurses are not claiming UI as a basic nursing care issue, and there is little evidence to suggest they are using the guidelines that have been developed. That is unfortunate, because aggressive nursing intervention can help to improve patients' quality of life, capacity for physical activity, and self-esteem. It can also help to reduce the cost of health care. Think of this as an opportunity for you to improve practice!

Recent guidelines outline five categories of nonpharmacological treatment options that nurses commonly provide independently: lifestyle modification, bladder training, pelvic floor muscle rehabilitation, anti-incontinence devices, and supportive interventions (Wyman, 2003). These therapies have been proven to be effective for most patients.

- *Lifestyle modification.* Lifestyle modifications involve dietary changes, increased fluid intake, weight management, smoking cessation, avoidance of constipation, and physical activity that does not include high-impact exercise.

- *Bladder training.* The goal of bladder training is to enable the patient to hold increasingly greater volumes of urine in the bladder and to increase the interval between voidings. This involves patient teaching, scheduled voiding, and self-monitoring using a voiding diary. In addition to teaching the mechanisms of urination, teach distraction and relaxation strategies to help inhibit the urge to void. Other techniques include deep breathing and guided imagery.

- *Scheduled voiding* is a form of bladder training involving timed voiding and habit retraining. The client must be mentally and physically capable of self-toileting. Initially the patient may be scheduled to attempt voiding every 2 hours or even more often. As a pattern develops and the person gains greater control, the length of time between voiding may be increased. Scheduled voiding is usually combined with other techniques, including lifestyle adjustments and pelvic muscle exercises.

- *Pelvic floor muscle rehabilitation.* Pelvic floor muscle exercises (PFME) are a mainstay of UI treatment for women. PFME strengthen perineal muscles and help to prevent and treat stress, urge, and mixed UI. **Kegel exercises** are the most commonly used. See the accompanying Self-Care box for guidelines in teaching your patients about Kegel exercises. Cure rates of UI, based on patient diaries, range from 16 to 27%, and improvement rates vary from 48 to 80.7% with PFME alone. To be successful, the patient must do the exercises correctly and practice them daily. A period of 6 to 12 months may be required before treatment is effective.

- *Vaginal weight training* is another form of PFME. The woman inserts a small cone-shaped weight in the vagina for two 15-minute periods per day. The woman must contract the pelvic floor muscles to keep the weight in her vagina. Some women prefer this form of PFME because it helps them identify the correct muscles for contraction. However, this method has not been shown to produce better outcomes than Kegel exercises.

- *Biofeedback* has been advocated by some women as an adjunct to PFME. Small electrodes are attached to the skin on the perineum. The electrodes detect a

Teaching Your Patient About Pelvic Floor-Muscle Exercises (PFME)

Teach patients the following routine to strengthen pelvic floor muscles:

- Imagine that you are urinating and wish to stop the flow; also tighten your rectum as though you were trying to keep from passing gas. The muscles you contract to interrupt flow are the pelvic floor muscles. (*Note:* Caution the patient against doing Kegel exercises while actually urinating because this may cause backflow of urine.)

- You should feel your rectum tighten. Women may also feel the vagina tighten. However, your abdomen should *not* tighten—check by placing your hand lightly on your abdomen. Also, do not contract the thigh and gluteal muscles.

- Hold each contraction for 5 to 10 seconds and then rest for 5 to 10 seconds. Some people may be able to hold for only 3 seconds at first. Count, "one-and-two-and-three . . ." Keep contraction and relaxation times equal; that is, if you hold a contraction for 5 seconds, rest 5 seconds before the next contraction.

- A recommended daily exercise routine is to perform 40 to 60 PFME divided into two to four sets of 15 exercises each time. Do one set sitting, one standing, and one lying down. Do not do all 40 to 60 exercises at one time; spread them out through the day.

- One way to remember to perform your exercises it to associate them with an activity. For example, do a Kegel at every stoplight or stop sign when you are in the car. Or do a Kegel every time you go to the bathroom—but not while you are urinating.

pelvic floor contraction and provide feedback to the patient about the strength of the contraction and the accuracy of the movement. An offshoot of biofeedback is *electrical stimulation.* A small electrical current is delivered through vaginal, rectal, or surface electrodes that triggers an involuntary contraction of the pelvic floor. Two or three 15- to 30-minute sessions are typically performed each day.

- *Supportive interventions.* Supportive interventions focus on helping the patient reach the toilet and perform toileting self-care. Bedside commodes, raised toilet seats, bedpans, and urinals all make it easier to urinate independently. Gait and strength training

also improve the person's ability to reach the toilet in time. When continence cannot be achieved, absorbent products with waterproof coverings are available. Provide meticulous skin care when these products are used. Under no circumstances should you refer to these as "diapers." To do so is disrespectful of the patient's dignity.

 CriticalThinking 27–8

How do you feel about instructing patients about PFME? Do you think a woman should always provide this instruction? Explain your thinking.

Anti-incontinence Devices

Anti-incontinence devices are designed to reduce the incidence of UI or provide a pathway for urine flow. They include the following:

- A *pessary,* or intravaginal support device. This is inserted into the vagina to prevent pelvic organ prolapse, which may trigger UI. An *incontinence pessary* is inserted into the vagina to support the bladder neck.
- An external occlusive device that is removed prior to voiding. For women, a urethral meatus covering is used. For men, a penis clamp is common.
- An internal urethral meatus plug, which may be used by men and women. This is a disposable, single-use device, typically used for activities that cause stress incontinence.
- A valved catheter that allows urine to be drained on a schedule.
- An indwelling urethral catheter. This is used as a last resort to control the flow of urine and protect the perineal skin.
- A bed alarm, which will waken the patient if incontinence occurs.
- An external collection device. Condom catheters are most commonly used.

When anti-incontinence devices are used, it is important to observe for vaginal or urinary tract infection, blood in the urine, and vaginal erosion.

 Go to Chapter 27, **Procedure 27–5: Applying an External (Condom) Catheter,** in Volume 2.

See also the Critical Aspects box on page 645.

Pharmacological and Surgical Interventions

Although it is not the treatment of choice, some forms of incontinence may respond to pharmacological treatment. Estrogen may be prescribed for postmenopausal

women when incontinence is secondary to atrophic vaginitis. For urge incontinence, medication may be used to relax the detrusor muscle and increase bladder capacity (e.g., anticholinergics, smooth-muscle relaxants, calcium-channel blockers, and antidepressants). For stress incontinence, drugs may be given to improve urethral sphincter muscle functioning (e.g., the decongestant phenylpropanolamine [Triaminic]).

When incontinence is caused by cystocele, rectocele, or an enlarged prostate gland, surgical techniques may be appropriate (e.g., bladder neck suspension to create a normal angle between the bladder and urethra, and prostatectomy).

Managing Enuresis

Teach parents that occasional wetting (called *enuresis*) is entirely normal in children even in the early school years, especially when the child is intensely involved in a game, test, or another absorbing activity. They should accept such events calmly and not punish the child.

For *nocturnal enuresis,* or bed-wetting, medications may be prescribed. However, a variety of other solutions can be tried, such as the following:

- Limit fluid intake in the evening.
- Wake the child to urinate just before the parents retire.
- Use a bed alarm that wakens the child when wetting occurs. Over time, this conditioning may be effective; however, once the alarm is removed, the child may relapse into enuresis.
- Reassure parents that in many cases, loving acceptance and passage of time provide the cure.
- If bed-wetting persists into the school-age years, the child should receive a thorough medical evaluation to rule out underlying disease processes.
- Parents should plan to bathe the child in the morning rather than at bedtime to minimize urine odor.

Young children may feel anxious about using the bathroom in a clinic, hospital, or any unfamiliar environment. They may be especially anxious about using a bedpan. Also, be aware that the stress of an illness or hospitalization may cause a child to regress in his ability to toilet independently. You may need to schedule regular trips to the bathroom and to watch for nonverbal cues that the child needs to void.

 CriticalThinking 27–9

What treatment options for incontinence have you seen used in your clinical experience? What options do you believe should be used more frequently? Less frequently? Explain your thinking.

Caring for a Patient with a Urinary Diversion

A patient with a urinary diversion requires physical and psychological care. Initially you will care for the ostomy. However, the goal is for the patient to become comfortable with his changed body and to assume self-care.

Patients experience a variety of reactions to the stoma. Patients with continent ostomies are usually more comfortable with their stoma. Your attitude and willingness to discuss the body changes associated with an ostomy will help your patient begin his adjustment. In many communities, the local ostomy association has counselors available to visit patients, discuss the psychological changes associated with a urinary diversion, and help them with physical care of the stoma. Most counselors are adept because they too have ostomies. They are able to share practical and personal information with patients based on their own experience with similar challenges. To find the local chapter, consult your phone book, or

 Go to the **United Ostomy Association website at www.uoa.org**

Nursing care of a patient with a urinary diversion should begin with a thorough assessment. A healthy stoma ranges in color from deep pink to brick red, regardless of skin color, and is shiny and moist at all times. A pale, dusky, or black stoma often indicates inadequate blood supply. Immediately document and report such findings to the surgeon. Assess the skin surrounding the stoma for signs of irritation, such as redness, tenderness, skin breakdown, and/or drainage. When the normally acid urine remains in contact with the skin, it becomes alkaline. Encrustations collect on the skin, and the skin becomes macerated and excoriated. A moisture-proof skin barrier is usually placed around the stoma to protect surrounding skin. More extensive discussion about stoma care is covered in Chapter 28.

 Go to Chapter 28, **Procedure 28-5: Changing an Ostomy Appliance,** in Volume 2.

For guidelines for caring for a patient with a urinary diversion,

 Go to Chapter 27, **Technique 27–10: Caring for Patients with Urinary Diversions,** in Volume 2.

 Go to Chapter 27, **Resources for Caregivers and Health Professionals,** on the Electronic Study Guide.

 Suggested Readings: Go to Chapter 27, **Reading More About Urinary Elimination,** on the Electronic Study Guide.

 Bibliography: Go to Volume 2, Bibliography.

| toward evidence-based practice |

Cooper, G. & Watt, E. (2003). An exploration of acute care nurses' approach to assessment and management of people with urinary incontinence. *Journal of Wound, Ostomy, & Continence Nursing, 30*(6), 305–313.

Using an exploratory descriptive design, 33 registered nurses from medical and surgical areas of an adult acute-care hospital in Melbourne, Australia, participated in a study to examine knowledge of urinary incontinence. Each nurse was given a questionnaire with five scenarios, each representing typical stories relating to different types of urinary incontinence. The participants' responses were analyzed for themes, and findings were presented back to the participants to check their validity. The results of this study suggest that acute care nurses have limited ability to assess and manage varying types of urinary incontinence because of limited knowledge, but other contributing factors are lack of time, lack of support, and a culture that fails to promote independent practice.

---

1. For each of these roles, discuss the implications of the study findings.
   - Student nurse
   - Patient with incontinence
   - Nurse educator
   - Nurse administrator
   - Health policy analyst predicting costs of care

2. Discuss in small groups how to improve care of patients with incontinence at the sites used by your class for clinical days. Identify actions that you might take at the clinical sites.

 Go to Chapter 27, **Toward Evidence-Based Practice Suggested Responses,** on the Electronic Study Guide.

28 CHAPTER

Bowel Elimination

Learning Outcomes

After completing this chapter, you should be able to:

* Identify the basic structures and functions of the gastrointestinal system.

* Discuss factors that affect bowel elimination.

* Describe normal bowel elimination.

* Differentiate among the various types of bowel diversions.

* Discuss common bowel elimination problems.

* Identify appropriate nursing history questions to assess bowel elimination problems.

* Perform a physical examination focused on bowel elimination.

* List and describe diagnostic tests used to identify bowel elimination problems.

* State nursing diagnoses associated with altered bowel elimination.

* Describe nursing interventions that promote normal bowel elimination.

* Provide care for clients experiencing alterations in bowel elimination.

* Discuss nursing care associated with the use of bowel diversions.

Your Patient

MEET

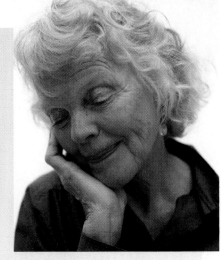

You are assigned to care for Mrs. Zeno, a frail 96-year-old woman who broke her hip last month after a fall at home. Mrs. Zeno was hospitalized for surgical repair of her hip but is now in a skilled nursing facility (SNF) for rehabilitation. The UAP informs you that Mrs. Zeno has eaten poorly for the past week, eating only 25 to 40% of her meals and refusing the protein supplements that were added to her diet. Mrs. Zeno tells you she would like to go home: "I have my routine and the foods I like. I think I'd be better there." As you review the chart in preparation for clinical, you note that she has not had a bowel movement (BM) for 3 days. Her last BM was small and very hard.

What additional assessments should you perform? What, if anything, is of concern about her bowel pattern? What actions should you take with Mrs. Zeno?

In this chapter we discuss bowel function and common disorders associated with bowel elimination. You will gain theoretical and practical knowledge to help you answer those questions and provide care for clients with bowel elimination concerns.

Theoretical Knowledge
knowing why

Bowel elimination is a normal process by which we eliminate waste products from our bodies. To understand bowel elimination, you will need knowledge of the anatomy and physiology of the gastrointestinal tract.

WHAT ARE THE ANATOMICAL STRUCTURES OF THE GASTROINTESTINAL TRACT?

The gastrointestinal (GI) tract is a smooth-muscle tube approximately 5 m (15 ft) long, running through the body from the mouth to the anus. Its major functions are to digest and absorb the nutrients present in food and to eliminate food waste products as feces (Figure 28–1). Feces consist primarily of bacteria, insoluble fiber, and other material that was not absorbed during passage through the GI tract. The structures of the GI tract are the mouth, esophagus, stomach, small intestine, large intestine, rectum, and anus.

The Mouth

Mechanical digestion begins in the mouth with **mastication,** or chewing. Food is torn into small pieces, mashed, moistened with saliva, and formed into a bolus that is then swallowed into the esophagus. The mouth contains glands that secrete enzymes, such as ptyalin and salivary amylase, which begin the digestion of carbohydrates.

The Esophagus

The bolus of food travels through the esophagus to the stomach. The esophagus is a tube of smooth muscle, which alternately contracts and relaxes in waves of **peristalsis** to push the bolus toward the stomach. The bolus travels the length of the esophagus (about 25 cm, or 10 in.) in about 15 seconds. The *cardiac sphincter* (also called the *gastroesophageal sphincter*) relaxes to allow food to pass into the stomach. When the cardiac sphincter is constricted, it prevents acidic stomach contents from flowing back into the esophagus.

The Stomach

The stomach is a distensible sac that extends from the esophagus to the small intestine. The stomach stores food while it churns and mixes it, providing further mechanical breakdown. Chemical digestion continues in the stomach, which secretes hydrochloric acid (HCl), a protein-digesting enzyme called *pepsin,* and *gastric lipase,* an enzyme that begins the digestion of lipids. The stomach lining also secretes a mucus coating that

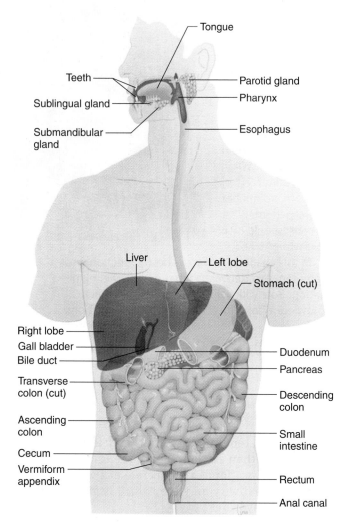

FIGURE 28–1 **The gastrointestinal tract extends from mouth to anus. The major functions of the gastrointestinal system are to digest and absorb the nutrients in the food we eat and to eliminate food waste products as feces.** *Source:* Scanlon, V., & Sanders, T. (2003). *Essentials of anatomy and physiology* (4th ed.). Philadelphia: F. A. Davis Company, p. 351. Used with permission.

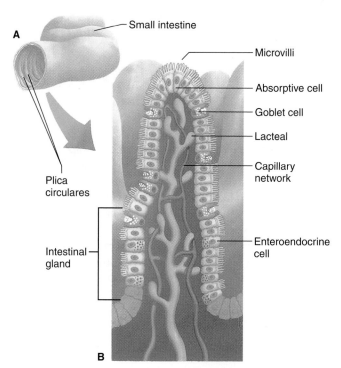

FIGURE 28–2 **The small intestine is highly folded, providing a vast surface area for absorption of nutrients. The microvilli form a brush border, which is the site of most nutrient absorption. A, Section through the small intestine showing the plica circulares (circular folds) of the mucosa and submucosa. B, Microscopic view of a villus showing the internal structure.** *Source:* Scanlon, V., & Sanders, T. (2003). *Essentials of anatomy and physiology* (4th ed.). Philadelphia: F. A. Davis Company, p. 364. Used with permission.

protects the stomach from being corroded by HCl. Food remains in the stomach an average of 4 hours. Food leaves the stomach as a liquid called **chyme.**

The Small Intestine

The small intestine is a convoluted tube that connects the stomach and the large intestine. About 2.5 cm (1 in.) in diameter and approximately 6 m (20 ft) long if fully extended, it occupies the majority of the abdominal cavity. Most digestion and absorption of food occurs in the small intestine, with the aid of enzymes from the pancreas and bile from the gallbladder. Chyme travels slowly, by peristalsis, through the small intestine, and peristalsis halts periodically to allow for absorption. The small intestine consists of three segments: the duodenum, jejunum, and the ileum.

- The **duodenum** is the first section of small intestine—a C-shaped tube that branches off from the stomach. It is about 30 to 60 cm (1 to 2 ft) long. The duodenum processes chyme by mixing it and adding enzymes. The bile duct and main pancreatic duct both enter the small intestine at the level of the duodenum, providing bile from the liver and gallbladder to digest lipids, and pancreatic enzymes to digest lipids, proteins, and carbohydrates.

- The **jejunum** is the coiled midsection of the small intestine. It is about 1.8 to 2.4 m (6 to 8 ft) long and forms the connection between the duodenum and ileum. Its major function is to absorb carbohydrates and proteins.

- The **ileum** joins the small and large intestine. It is responsible for absorption of fats, bile salts, and some vitamins, minerals, and water; however, nutrients are absorbed mainly in the duodenum and jejunum.

We noted earlier that the total length of the small intestine, if it were stretched out, is approximately 6 m (20 ft), but in our bodies it is much shorter because it is folded to provide a vast surface area for absorption. The inner wall of the small intestine is covered by millions of tiny fingerlike projections called **villi** (Figure 28–2).

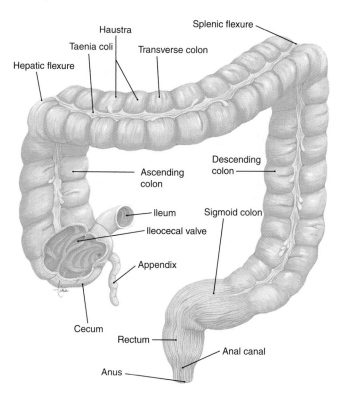

The villi are covered with even tinier projections called **microvilli.** The combination of folds, villi, and microvilli increase the surface area of the small intestine greatly, facilitating absorption of nutrients.

The Large Intestine

The **large intestine,** also known as the **colon,** is larger in diameter than the small intestine (6.3 cm, or 2.5 in.) but shorter in length—about 1.5 to 1.8 meters (5 to 6 feet). It extends from the ileum of the small intestine to the anus. It contains seven segments: the cecum, ascending colon, transverse colon, descending colon, sigmoid colon, rectum, and anus (Figure 28–3).

Undigested food entering the first portion of the large intestine, the **cecum,** consists mostly of cellulose and water. The connection of the ileum to the cecum is controlled by the **ileocecal valve.** Under most conditions, the valve prevents backflow of chyme from the colon into the small intestine. The **appendix** is a small, fingerlike appendage off the cecum. It is believed to be a **vestigial organ**—one whose significance has diminished over time—however, it is lined with lymphatic tissue and may play a role in immune function.

The next three segments, the **ascending, transverse,** and **descending colon,** ring the small intestine. The **sigmoid colon** is a final, small segment of bowel that twists medially and downward to connect with the rectum and anus.

The colon secretes mucus, which facilitates smooth passage of stool, and absorbs water, some vitamins, and minerals. Approximately 80% of the fluid that enters the colon is reabsorbed along its passage. Normal flora in the colon aid in the digestive process. These bacteria are responsible for producing vitamin K and several of the B vitamins.

The large intestine has two sets of muscles that give it a puckered appearance. Longitudinal muscles, known as **taenia coli,** run lengthwise along the colon surface. Tension in these muscles gathers up the colon into pouched segments known as **haustra** all along its length (see Figure 28–3). In addition, the colon wall contains circular muscles that, together with the taenia coli, cause the colon to expand and contract in length and width to achieve haustral churning, peristalsis, and mass peristalsis.

- **Haustral churning** moves digestive contents around within each haustra. This action promotes reabsorption of water.
- **Persitalsis** continues throughout the length of the large intestine, where it propels intestinal contents toward the rectum and anus.
- **Mass peristalsis** is a powerful contraction along a lengthy segment of bowel. It is facilitated by the **gastrocolic reflex,** which is triggered by food entering the stomach and small intestine. Mass movements usually occur only one to three times each day, and they are responsible for most of the propulsion of the contents in the transverse and sigmoid colon.

The Rectum and Anus

The **rectum** is approximately 15 cm (6 in.) long and is continuous with the **anus,** the last 2.5 cm (1 in.) of the colon. A highly vascular folded tube, the rectum is free of waste products until just before defecation.

The anus has two ringlike muscles that function as sphincters. The **internal sphincter** involuntarily relaxes and opens when stool is present in the rectum. The **external sphincter** is under voluntary control. Voluntary relaxation of the external sphincter allows stool to be expelled from the body (Figure 28–4). The anus is highly vascular. Chronic pressure on the veins within the anal canal, as with prolonged sitting or retained feces, can cause **hemorrhoids** (distended blood vessels within or protruding from the anus).

KnowledgeCheck 28–1

- What are the major functions of the small intestine and large intestine?
- How do the rectum and anus control elimination of feces from the body?

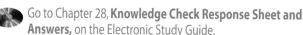
Go to Chapter 28, **Knowledge Check Response Sheet and Answers,** on the Electronic Study Guide.

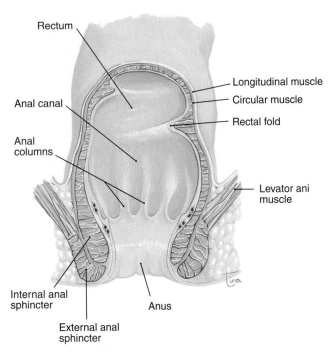

Rectum

Anal canal

Anal
columns

Internal anal
sphincter

External anal
sphincter

Longitudinal muscle

Circular muscle

Rectal fold

Levator ani
muscle

Anus

FIGURE 28–4   Internal and external anal sphincters shown in a frontal section through the lower rectum and anal canal. *Source:* Scanlon, V., & Sanders, T. (2003). *Essentials of anatomy and physiology* (4th ed.). Philadelphia: F. A. Davis Company, p. 364. Used with permission.

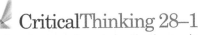

CriticalThinking 28–1

Based on your knowledge that hemorrhoids are dilated blood vessels in the anal canal, what symptoms would you expect a patient with hemorrhoids to exhibit?

HOW DOES THE BOWEL ELIMINATE WASTE?

As you have learned, reabsorbtion of water from chyme in the large intestine produces a semisolid mass known as **feces.** Feces is a mixture of fiber and undigested food, shed epithelial cells, inorganic material (e.g., calcium and phosphates), bacteria, and water. Small amounts of fat may be present. Gas, or **flatus,** which is produced during digestion, may also be present.

The Process of Defecation

The process by which the bowel eliminates waste is called **defecation.** When fecal material reaches the rectum, distention stimulates stretch receptors to initiate contraction of the sigmoid colon and rectal muscles, along with relaxation of the internal anal sphincter. At the same time, sensory impulses transmitted to the central nervous system (CNS) produce a conscious urge to defecate. We respond to this signal by voluntarily contracting our diaphragmatic and abdominal

muscles to increase downward pressure, while at the same time relaxing the external anal sphincter. These actions allow feces to be propelled through the anus. If we ignore the signal to defecate, the reflexive contractions ease for a few minutes, until mass peristalsis occurs again.

A person can increase the pressure to expel feces by contracting the abdominal muscles while maintaining a closed airway. This is called the **Valsalva maneuver.** Although it assists with the passage of stool, clients with heart disease, glaucoma, increased intracranial pressure, or a new surgical wound should be cautioned to avoid the Valsalva maneuver because it raises blood pressure, increases pressure within the abdominal cavity, and is associated with an increased risk for cardiac arrhythmias.

Normal Defecation Patterns

Many grocery stores, pharmacies, and even convenience stores have half an aisle or more of products devoted to bowel function. Some products promote bowel movements (BMs), and others treat diarrhea. All claim to return the consumer to "regularity." The sheer volume of products suggests that bowel function problems are common. Nevertheless, many people avoid the topic of bowel elimination—it is not typically something they chat about with their neighbors. As a result, many patients have unanswered questions about their bowel function and may turn to you for information.

Part of the confusion about bowel function is that there is a wide range of "normal." The frequency of BMs may range from several times per day to once a week. As long as the person passes stools without excessive urgency (needing to rush to the toilet), with minimal effort and no straining, without blood loss, and without the use of laxatives, you can regard bowel function as normal.

Normally stool is approximately 75% water and 25% solid when expelled. This combination yields a soft, formed semisolid. If passage through the colon is slowed, more water is reabsorbed from the feces. The result is the formation of dry, hard stool that requires more effort to pass. If transit time through the colon is faster than normal, less water is reabsorbed, and stools are watery.

Feces is usually brown in color because **bile salts,** which aid in the digestion of fat, are excreted in the feces. Bile is normally golden yellow, but the action of bacteria in the GI tract change the color to brown. Bacteria are also responsible for the odor of feces.

Flatus, or gas, is formed in the digestive process. Some is swallowed air that accompanies the intake of food. A small portion diffuses from blood into the GI tract. However, most of the gas is created by bacterial fermentation in the colon. Flatus is a mixture of

nitrogen, carbon dioxide, hydrogen, methane, and hydrogen sulfide.

CriticalThinking 28–2

- Based on your knowledge of normal bowel function, how would you describe Mrs. Zeno's ("Meet Your Patient") bowel function? Is it normal or abnormal?
- What additional information, if any, do you need to know to answer this question?

WHAT FACTORS AFFECT BOWEL ELIMINATION?

As you know from the preceding discussion, there is a wide range of acceptable frequency for BMs. Each person develops a pattern that is based on several factors.

Developmental Stage

Bowel elimination patterns change throughout the life span. During the first 2 days of life, the newborn passes meconium through the anus. **Meconium** is green-black in color, tarry, and sticky and results from swallowed amniotic fluid. Stools transition to a yellow-green color over the next few days. After that, the appearance of the feces depends largely on the type of feeding the infant receives. Breastfed babies pass golden yellow stools, whereas formula-fed babies pass tan stools. Initially babies defecate frequently, usually after each feeding. The stools tend to be watery while the large intestine is still immature. Gradually normal flora develop in the colon, and stools become firmer and less frequent.

The ability to control defecation typically develops at about 2 to 3 years of age. Toilet training requires neural and muscular control as well as conscious effort. The child must be aware of the urge to defecate, be able to maintain closure of the external anal sphincter while getting to the toilet, and be able to remove clothing. When toddlers become engrossed in play, they sometimes ignore the need to move their bowels, and soiling is common. As children mature, they gradually learn to gain more control over defecation. In fact, school-age children and adolescents often delay defecation until they have come home or have completed an activity.

The bowel pattern set in childhood normally continues into late adulthood if the client consumes adequate fiber and fluid and engages in regular physical activity. However, peristalsis, intestinal smooth muscle tone, perineal muscle tone, and sphincter control normally decrease with aging. These physiological processes can contribute to bowel elimination problems among older adults, especially if they decrease their activity and fiber intake.

BOX 28–1 High-Fiber Foods

- Apples with skin
- Bran cereal
- Broccoli, cauliflower, and other cruciferous vegetables
- Cabbage
- Carrots
- Cherries
- Corn
- Dried beans, peas, and legumes
- Dried fruits
- Flaxseed
- Greens such as chard, kale, collards, and turnip greens
- Oatmeal
- Oranges
- Pears with skin
- Plums with skin
- Popcorn
- Potato with skin
- Prunes
- Raisins
- Strawberries
- Whole-grain cereal products

Personal and Sociocultural Factors

Privacy is important to most people, as is sufficient time to have a bowel movement without feeling the need to hurry. Clients working in fast-paced jobs may have difficulty even consciously recognizing the need to defecate, and some habitually ignore the need, promoting bowel dysfunction. Parents and caregivers of infants and toddlers may postpone their own toileting needs because of fear of leaving the children alone. Some clients are acutely embarrassed by the thought that anyone might realize they are having a bowel movement and will wait until they are entirely alone before even entering the bathroom.

Have you ever heard the following phrase: "He puts his stress in his gut"? Stress has a major influence on motility of the GI tract. It may cause diarrhea or constipation, and it is a primary risk factor in the development of *irritable bowel syndrome,* a disorder associated with bloating, pain, and altered bowel function.

Nutrition, Hydration, and Activity Level

Nutrition, hydration, and activity all relate to bowel function.

- *Fiber.* As noted earlier, regular intake of food promotes peristalsis. People who eat on a regular schedule are likely to develop a regular pattern of defecation. Irregular eating creates irregular bowel elimination. The type of food eaten is also important. High-fiber foods (Box 28–1) promote peristalsis

and defecation by increasing bulk. Bulky foods absorb fluids and increase stool mass. The increased mass stretches bowel walls, initiating peristalsis and the defecation reflex.

Other foods have specific effects in the bowel. For example, the active bacteria in yogurt stimulate peristalsis, while at the same time promoting healing of intestinal infections. Low-fiber foods, such as pasta and other simple carbohydrates and lean meats, slow peristalsis. Foods like broccoli, onions, and beans lead to excess gas in many people. Spicy foods may also cause gas, as well as more frequent bowel movements.

Dietary supplements can also affect bowel function. For example, calcium supplements cause constipation in many clients, whereas magnesium loosens stools. Supplemental vitamin C softens stools and, in high doses, may cause diarrhea in sensitive clients.

- *Fluids.* A minimum of 6 to 8 glasses (1400 to 2000 mL) of fluid per day is required to promote healthful bowel function. Inadequate fluid intake or excessive fluid loss, as in diarrhea or vomiting, slows peristalsis and leads to dry, hard stools that are difficult to pass. Excessive fluid intake (especially beverages with high sugar content) may lead to rapid passage through the colon and soft or watery stools. Different types of fluids have varying effects on sensitive individuals. For instance, consuming large amounts of milk may cause constipation in some people. Coffee promotes peristalsis in many clients and may even cause loose stools in sensitive clients.

- *Activity.* Physical activity seems to stimulate peristalsis and bowel elimination. In addition, sedentary people are likely to have weaker abdominal muscles. Clients with health concerns that limit activity (e.g., such as shortness of breath, pain, or required bedrest) often experience constipation.

Medications and Procedures

Many medications may affect peristalsis. All oral medicines have the potential to affect the function of the GI tract. Examples include the following:

- *Antacids,* often used for heartburn, neutralize stomach acid but may slow peristalsis.

- *Aspirin and other nonsteroidal anti-inflammatory drugs (NSAIDs),* such as ibuprofen, irritate the stomach. Repeated use can lead to ulceration of the stomach or duodenum.

- *Antibiotics* given to combat infection decrease the normal flora in the colon. The result is often diarrhea. Bacterial populations can be maintained with supplements of probiotics (e.g., acidophilus) or daily consumption of yogurt.

- *Iron,* a common mineral supplement, is available as an over-the-counter (OTC) medication and is often prescribed for the treatment of anemia. Iron has an astringent effect on the bowel and is notorious for causing constipation.

- *Pain medications,* particularly opioids (narcotics), slow peristalsis and are associated with a high incidence of constipation.

- *Antimotility drugs,* such as diphenoxylate (Lomotil) may be used to treat diarrhea. They work by slowing peristalsis.

- *Laxatives* are used to treat constipation. In general, laxatives work by stimulating peristalsis (see Box 28–2, page 667). They come in many forms and are frequently abused by people who self-medicate with OTC drugs.

Clients undergoing anesthesia and surgery often experience sluggish bowel elimination. The delay in bowel elimination may be caused by a variety of circumstances:

- *Anesthesia.* General anesthesia (which renders the patient unconscious) and analgesics (administered preoperatively and postoperatively for pain) slow bowel motility. Spinal anesthesia and epidural anesthesia are less likely to cause this effect.

- *Stress.* Regardless of the type of anesthesia, most clients find surgery a stressful event. As you may recall from Chapter 25, if stress activates the general adaptation syndrome (GAS), autonomic nervous system and endocrine responses ensue. Among those responses is a slowing of peristalsis.

- *Manipulation of the bowel during surgery.* Abdominal or pelvic surgery in which the bowel is manipulated may result in a **paralytic ileus,** a cessation of bowel peristalsis. Although peristalsis halts, the bowel continues to produce secretions. Without peristalsis, secretions remain stagnant, causing distention and discomfort. To decrease the complications of paralytic ileus, patients who have had bowel surgery typically have a nasogastric (NG) tube with low constant or intermittent suction. The NG tube removes secretions until peristalsis returns. To review insertion of an NG tube or management of a patient with an NG tube,

 Go to Chapter 26, **Procedure 26-2: Insertion of a Nasogastric Tube,** in Volume 2.

- *Decreased mobility.* After surgery, patients often experience discomfort that affects mobility. This further hinders GI motility and increases the risk for constipation.

- *Perineal surgery.* Patients who have had surgical interventions involving the perineal region may fear pain or that their sutures will "tear" or "break" during

bowel elimination, and therefore they resist the urge to evacuate their bowel.

• *Anal sphincter surgery.* Patients who have had surgery that disrupts the anal sphincter may experience uncontrolled drainage after surgery.

Pregnancy

In early pregnancy, many women experience fluid loss due to "morning sickness"—periods of nausea and vomiting—which, despite the name, may occur at any time of day. As the pregnancy progresses, the growing uterus crowds and displaces the intestines, and the increased level of progesterone slows intestinal motility. As a result, pregnant women often experience constipation, decreased appetite, and irregular food intake. In addition, the increasing pressure of the uterus and the increased blood volume of normal pregnancy increase the woman's risk for hemorrhoids.

KnowledgeCheck 28–2

• What is a normal defecation pattern?
• Identify the factors that affect bowel elimination.

 Go to Chapter 28, **Knowledge Check Response Sheet and Answers,** on the Electronic Study Guide.

 CriticalThinking 28–3

• Review the case of Mrs. Zeno ("Meet Your Patient"). What factors may be affecting her bowel elimination?
• What additional information do you need?

Pathological Conditions

Several disorders affect bowel function. Among them are neurological disorders that affect innervation of the lower GI tract, cognitive conditions that limit the ability to sense the urge to defecate, pain or immobility that leads to sluggish peristalsis, and pathological conditions of the GI tract. Constipation and diarrhea are discussed in the "Nursing Diagnosis" section of the chapter. Other common disorders are food allergies, food intolerances, and diverticulosis.

• *Food allergies.* The National Institute of Allergy and Infectious Diseases (NIAID) characterizes a **food allergy** as a true immune system reaction prompted by the presence in the body of an allergenic food (NIAID, 2003). Some common food allergens include dairy products, egg whites, shellfish, wheat, peanuts, citrus fruits, and soy. Immune responses to foods manifest as a variety of symptoms ranging from a mild rash to anaphylactic shock. Common GI symptoms suggesting food allergy include constipation, diarrhea, a burnlike rash around the anus, abdominal discomfort, bloating, excessive gas, and intestinal bleeding (Sears & Sears, 1999).

• *Food intolerances.* In contrast to a food allergy, a **food intolerance** is specifically linked to the GI system. It produces such symptoms as GI discomfort, pain, gas, bloating, diarrhea, or constipation after the person consumes the food. An example is *lactose intolerance,* a deficiency of the enzyme lactase, which is responsible for the breakdown of milk sugar (lactose). Such symptoms can mimic those of a food allergy, but food intolerances are not caused by immune responses.

• *Diverticulosis.* When the colon must repeatedly move highly compacted fecal material, over time the longitudinal and circular muscles enlarge. This increases force on the mucosal tissues, causing them to "balloon" out between the muscles and to form pouches in which fecal matter becomes trapped. The development of these saclike outpouchings of mucosa through the muscle layers of the colon wall is a condition called **diverticulosis.** In some cases, the pouches become infected, a condition called **diverticulitis,** and antibiotics or surgery is required. People whose diets are low in fiber or consist mainly of refined foods are especially at risk for diverticulosis.

Bowel Diversions

A **bowel diversion** is a surgically created opening for elimination of digestive waste products. The procedure is performed for clients with a variety of conditions, including cancer, ulcerations, trauma, or inadequate blood supply. A client with a bowel diversion does not eliminate via the anus. Instead, the **effluent** (output) is expelled through a surgically created opening in the abdominal wall, called a **stoma** or **ostomy.** The effluent may range from liquid to solid, depending on the part of the bowel that is being diverted. A bowel diversion close to the ileocecal valve (between the small and large intestine) will have a constant flow of liquid effluent. In contrast, a bowel diversion close to the rectum will have effluent that resembles feces (Figure 28–5).

Bowel diversions may be temporary or permanent. *Temporary bowel diversions* are common after surgical interventions for benign conditions of the bowel. They allow healing of the distal portion of the bowel. Once adequate healing has occurred, surgical **reanastomosis** (reconnection) of the bowel is performed, and the patient once again has BMs from the anus. *Permanent bowel diversions* are performed if the bowel is necrotic (dead) or cannot be salvaged because of severe disease or trauma.

Ileostomy

An **ileostomy** brings a portion of the ileum through a surgical opening in the abdomen, bypassing the large intestine entirely. Drainage at this level is liquid and

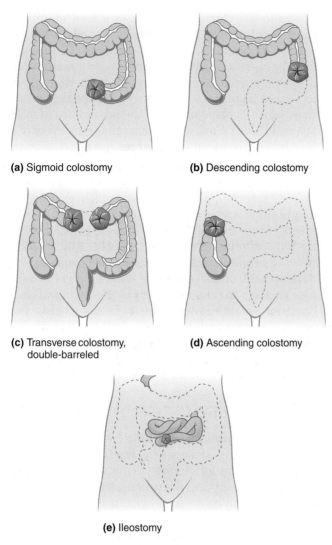

(a) Sigmoid colostomy

(b) Descending colostomy

(c) Transverse colostomy, double-barreled

(d) Ascending colostomy

(e) Ileostomy

FIGURE 28–5 **Location of various bowel diversion ostomies. Shaded areas indicate sections of the bowel that are removed or being "rested." The closer the colostomy is to the ascending colon ("higher"), the more liquid and continuous the drainage will be.** *A,* Sigmoid colostomy. *B,* Descending colostomy. *C,* Transverse colostomy. *D,* Ascending colostomy. *E,* Ileostomy.

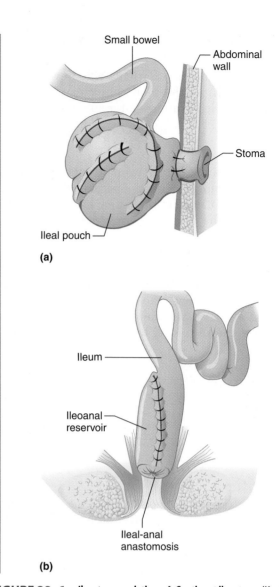

(a)

(b)

FIGURE 28–6 **Ileostomy variations.** *A,* **Continent ileostomy (Kock pouch).** *B,* **Ileoanal reservoir.**

continuous. The patient must wear an ostomy appliance at all times to collect the drainage. Two variations of an ileostomy are designed to control drainage more effectively and to cause less body image disturbance. However, many clients are not candidates for these procedures because of their underlying disease.

- A **Kock pouch,** or continent ileostomy, creates an internal pouch, or reservoir, to collect ileal drainage (Figure 28–6A). To drain the pouch, the patient inserts a tube through the external stoma into the pouch several times per day. This alternative avoids continuous drainage and allows the patient to be free of an ostomy appliance.

- A **total colectomy with ileaoanal reservoir** removes the colon, creates a pouch from the ileum, and connects the ileum to the rectum (Figure 28–6B).

The patient evacuates the bowel on the commode in the usual manner. Although this procedure should result in continence of bowel elimination, the feces will still be liquid.

Colostomy

A **colostomy** brings a portion of the colon through a surgical opening in the abdomen. The location of the colostomy determines the consistency of the feces eliminated, as well as the need to wear an ostomy appliance (see Figure 28–5). The closer the colostomy is to the ascending colon, the more liquid and continuous the drainage will be. In contrast, a colostomy close to the sigmoid colon will produce solid feces. Colostomies near the rectum, such as sigmoid colostomies, can often be controlled by diet and irrigation. As a result, the client may not need to wear an ostomy appliance to collect drainage.

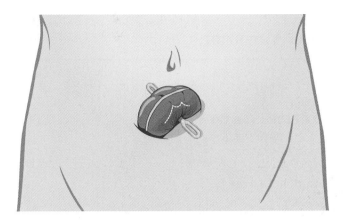

FIGURE 28–7   A loop colostomy.

A colostomy created in the transverse colon is usually temporary and may be either a double-barreled or loop colostomy. A **double-barrelled colostomy** (Figure 28–5C) has two separate stomas that externalize the bowel on both sides of the portion that has been removed. The proximal stoma is the functioning end that drains fecal material. The distal stoma may drain mucus and is sometimes called a mucus fistula. A **loop colostomy** (Figure 28–7) consists of a segment of bowel brought out to the abdominal wall. The posterior wall of the bowel remains intact, but a plastic rod is wedged under the bowel to keep it from slipping back into the abdomen. The anterior wall is incised, and the mucosal surface is left visible and open to air. It, too, has a functioning proximal end and limited drainage from the distal end.

KnowledgeCheck 28–3

* What changes in bowel elimination are associated with constipation? With diarrhea?
* Why are bowel diversions performed?
* What determines the nature of the effluent from a bowel diversion?

 Go to Chapter 28, **Knowledge Check Response Sheet and Answers,** on the Electronic Study Guide

Practical Knowledge
knowing how

As a nurse, you will monitor and assist clients with bowel elimination, teach about bowel function, and work collaboratively with the healthcare team to facilitate normal bowel function in well and ill clients. In the remainder of the chapter we will discuss these activities.

| Assessment |

To assess bowel elimination, you must obtain a nursing history, perform a physical examination focused on elimination, and review diagnostic and laboratory data associated with bowel function and elimination.

Nursing History

Because bowel patterns vary, you will need a nursing history to determine what is normal for each client. As you interview clients, pay attention to their reactions to your questions. Many people are embarrassed by discussion about bowel function. Tailor your assessment to the client's needs, and use language that makes the client comfortable. The following items should be part of your assessment:

* Normal bowel pattern
* Appearance of stool
* Changes in bowel habits or stool appearance
* History of elimination problems
* Use of bowel elimination aids, including diet, exercise, medications, and remedies

For a list of questions that you may use to assess each of these areas,

 Go to Chapter 28, **Assessment Guidelines and Tools, Focused Assessment: Bowel Elimation,** in Volume 2.

For clients with a bowel diversion, you will also gather data on the client's usual care of the stoma, use of appliances, and adjustment to the ostomy. Table 28–1 describes characteristics of normal and abnormal stool.

Physical Assessment

Physical assessment for bowel elimination includes examination of the abdomen, rectum, and anus. Observe the size, shape, and contour of the abdomen, and listen to bowel sounds. You might also palpate the anus and rectum for the presence of stool or masses.

 Go to Chapter 28, **Assessment Guidelines and Tools, Focused Assessment: Bowel Elimination,** in Volume 2. Also go to Chapter 19, **Procedure 19–14: Assessment of the Abdomen** and **Procedure 19–19: Assessment of the Rectum and Anus,** in Volume 2.

Normal bowel sounds are high-pitched, with approximately 5 to 35 gurgles every minute. *Hyperactive bowel sounds* are very high-pitched and more frequent than normal. They may occur with small bowel obstruction and inflammatory disorders. *Hypoactive bowel sounds* are low-pitched, infrequent, and quiet. A decrease in bowel sounds indicates decreased peristalsis. If after listening for 3 to 5 minutes you hear no bowel sounds, you can describe them as *absent*. Absent bowel sounds may occur after abdominal surgery and indicate a paralytic ileus.

TABLE 28-1 Normal Characteristics of Feces and Variations

Normal	Variations

Frequency
Number of BMs per day varies
Infants:
    Bottle-fed, 1–3 per day
    Breastfed, 4–6 per day
Adults: Daily or 2–3 per week
	Hypermotility:
	    Infants: > 6 stools per day
	    Adults: > 3 stools per day
	Hypomotility:
	    Infants: < every 1 or 2 days
	    Adults: < once a week

Color Infants: yellow Adults: brown	Bile pigment gives feces its brown color. Infant stools are yellow because of their rapid passage. White or clay-colored stool may indicate absence of bile (e.g., as in bile duct obstruction) or use of some antacids. Light brown stool may indicate diet high in milk products and low in meat. Pale, fatty stool may indicate malabsorption of fat. Black, tarry stool (**melena**) may indicate use of iron medications or upper GI bleeding; eating large quantities of red meat, spinach, and dark green vegetables may cause feces to be almost black. Red stool may indicate bleeding in lower intestinal tract. Stool darkens the longer it is left standing after defecation.
Quantity Adults: about 150 g per day	Quantity varies with amount of food eaten, from 100 to 400 g per day.
Shape Approximately the diameter of the rectum: about 2.5 cm (1 in.) in diameter; tubular shape	Narrow, pencil-shaped stool may indicate intestinal obstruction or constriction, or rapid peristalsis Small, marble-shaped stool may indicate slow peristalsis, with longer time in the large intestine.
Consistency Formed, soft, moist	Consistency is related to gastric motility and is affected by food and fluid intake. Hard stool indicates constipation. The more time spent in the large intestine, the more water is reabsorbed, and the harder the stool. May also indicate dehydration. Liquid stool may indicate diarrhea; rapid peristalsis (e.g., from infection).
Odor Pungent; affected by foods eaten	Normal odor is created by putrefaction and fermentation in the lower GI tract. Odor is also influenced by the pH of the stool, which is normally neutral or slightly alkaline. Strong, foul odors may indicate blood in the stool, especially in the upper GI tract, or infection.

KnowledgeCheck 28–4

- What should you discuss with your client when performing a nursing history focused on bowel elimination?
- Describe the physical assessment you would perform for a client with constipation.

 Go to Chapter 28, **Knowledge Check Response Sheet and Answers,** on the Electronic Study Guide.

Diagnostic Tests

Several diagnostic tests may be performed to assess for bowel elimination problems. They may be classified as direct or indirect visualization studies or laboratory studies.

Direct Visualization Studies

Direct visualization studies are used for diagnostic and treatment purposes. They are conducted by a

gastroenterologist. For a description of the most common tests,

 Go to Chapter 28, **Laboratory and Diagnostic Testing, Direct Visualization Studies of the Gastrointestinal Tract,** in Volume 2.

The nurse's role during these studies is to prepare the patient for the test, function as an assistant, and/or provide aftercare. You will assist the patient to the appropriate position, monitor the patient's tolerance of the procedure, provide pain medication or sedation to keep the patient comfortable during the exam, and provide reassurance to the patient as the test proceeds.

 CriticalThinking 28–4

A client asks you why he must perform a bowel prep with a strong laxative before having a colonoscopy. How might you reply?

Indirect Visualization Studies

Indirect visualization studies are radiographic views of the lower GI tract. The simplest of the tests is an abdominal flat plate, an anterior to posterior x-ray view of the abdomen used to detect gallstones, fecal impaction, and distended bowel. For a description of this and other relevant diagnostic studies,

 Go to Chapter 28, **Laboratory and Diagnostic Testing, Indirect Visualization Studies of the Gastrointestinal Tract,** in Volume 2.

Laboratory Studies

Stool specimens may be analyzed to detect blood, infection, or parasite infestation. The client must void first and then defecate in a clean, dry bedpan, bedside commode, or a special container (half hat) placed under the toilet seat. A small sample is obtained and sent to the laboratory for analysis or analyzed at the bedside. To obtain a specimen from an infant or young child, you will collect freshly passed feces from a diaper.

Handling Stool Specimens

Wear clean gloves when you handle the container or manipulate stool specimens. Use tongue blades to transfer the stool specimen to the container provided by the lab. Do not contaminate the outside of the specimen container. In most cases you will need approximately 2.5 cm (1 in.) of formed stool or 20 to 30 mL of liquid stool. If blood, mucus, or purulent material is present, be sure to include this with the sample. Transport the specimen to the laboratory as soon as possible. If that is not possible, consult the laboratory for appropriate storage. Usually you will need to refrigerate the specimen until it can be received in the lab.

Fecal Occult Blood Test

You may be called on to assess stool for the presence of blood. Blood may be visible to the eye or **occult** (hidden). You can perform the test for occult blood at the bedside, although some institutional policies require it to be done in the laboratory. The test is called a *guaiac test, Hemoccult,* or *fecal occult blood test.* It requires use of a special reagent that detects the presence of **peroxidase,** an enzyme present in hemoglobin. Only a small smear of stool is required. The Critical Aspects box on page 662 presents highlights. For the complete procedure,

 Go to Chapter 28, **Procedure 28–1: Testing Stool for Occult Blood,** in Volume 2.

For home testing, the patient should restrict certain types of food for 3 days before stool testing; for example, red meat, chicken, fish, horseradish, and some raw fruits and vegetables may result in a false-positive reading. The patient should not take salicylates (e.g., aspirin), steroids, iron preparations, or anticoagulants for 7 days before the test, because they, too, can produce a false-positive result. Ingestion of vitamin C can produce a false-negative result (American College of Physicians, 1997). The test should not be done if a woman is having her menstrual period or if the person has bleeding hemorrhoids or hematuria. Complying with these restrictions may not always be possible in clinical settings, though.

Assessing for Pinworms

Pinworms (an intestinal parasite) are small, white, threadlike worms that live in the cecum. They come to the anal area to deposit eggs during the night and migrate back up through the rectum during the day. In assessing a child, you can spread the buttocks while the child is sleeping and examine the anus to see whether any pinworms are visible to the naked eye. You can test for the presence of the eggs with tape. In the morning, as soon as the patient awakens, press clear cellophane tape against the anal opening. Remove the tape immediately, and place it on a slide. You may also need to do perianal swabs for microscopic study. The test may need to be repeated on consecutive days.

 Go to Chapter 28, **Technique 28–1: Testing for Pinworms,** in Volume 2.

For steps to follow in *all* procedures, refer to the inside back cover of Volume 2.

Procedure 28-1: Testing Stool for Occult Blood

- Use a clean, dry collection container.

- Take care that the sample is not contaminated by urine or menstrual blood.

- Be careful not to contaminate the outside of the collection container with feces.

- Test two small stool samples from separate areas of the large sample.

- Spread each sample thinly, one at a time, onto the "windows" of the Hemoccult slide.

- Place the correct number and size of drops of developer solution into the "windows" of the opposite side on the Hemoccult slide.

- Record a positive result if the slide windows turn blue.

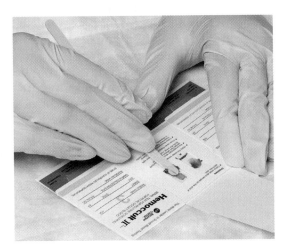

Procedure 28- 2: Placing and Removing a Bedpan

- Determine whether the patient will need to use a regular bedpan or a fracture pan.

- Don clean procedure gloves.

- Help the patient to achieve a position on the bedpan that will be most helpful in facilitating urinary or bowel elimination. Place the patient in semi-Fowler's position whenever possible. Modify the position based on the patient's condition.

- Provide clean washcloths and towels for the patient to perform personal hygiene when elimination is complete. Assist if the patient cannot perform these tasks independently.

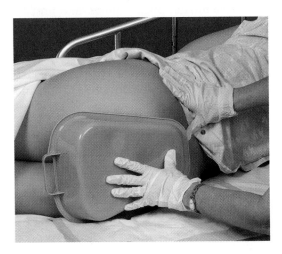

Procedure 28-3: Administering an Enema

- Determine the patient's ability to retain the enema solution.

- If the patient is immobile, have a bedpan or bedside commode available.

- Warm the solution.

- Lubricate the tip of the enema tubing generously.

- Insert the tubing only about 7.5 to 10 cm (3 to 4 in.) into the rectum.

- Hold the container at the correct height above the level of the hips.

- Instill the solution at a slow rate.

- Encourage the patient to take slow, deep breaths and hold the solution for 5 to 15 minutes, depending on the type of enema.

- Assess the patient for cramping or inability to retain the solution.

- Document the results.

Procedure 28-4: Removing Stool Digitally

- Trim and file your fingernails if they are long. Nails should not extend over the end of the fingertips.

- Obtain baseline vital signs and determine whether the patient has a history of cardiac problems or other contraindications.

Procedure 28–4: *(continued)*

- Determine whether the procedure will be accompanied by suppository insertion or enema administration (e.g., will an oil-retention enema be given first?)

- Use only one or two fingers, and remove stool in small pieces.

- Allow the patient periods of rest, and monitor for signs of vagal nerve stimulation.

- Teach the patient lifestyle changes necessary to prevent stool retention.

Procedure 28-5: Changing an Ostomy Appliance

- Change the pouch every 3 to 5 days. Frequency will also depend on the type of stoma, the equipment used (e.g., one- or two-piece pouch), the effluent, the patient's preference, and the climate (i.e., change more frequently during the summer).

- Empty the old pouch prior to removing it, if possible.

- Remove the wafer or pouch slowly and gently, pulling down from the top with one hand while holding counter-tension with the other.

- Assess the stoma and the peristomal skin area for abnormalities (e.g., discoloration, swelling, redness, irritation, excoriation, bleeding).

- Use a measuring guide to determine the size of the stoma.

- Trace the size of the opening onto the back of the wafer, and cut the wafer opening about 2 to 3 mm ($\frac{1}{16}$ to $\frac{1}{8}$ inch) larger.

- Apply the new wafer with gentle pressure.

Note: Some pouches come with the wafer attached, some without. These instructions assume that the wafer is attached.

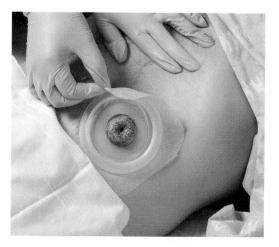

Procedure 28-6: Irrigating a Colostomy

- Determine the patient's normal bowel pattern before surgery.

- Use 500 to 1000 mL, preferably 1000 mL, of warm tap water, priming the tubing prior to irrigation.

- Position the patient in front of or on the toilet or bedside commode. If the patient is immobile, place her in left side-lying (Sims') position, and use a bedpan.

- Remove the existing colostomy appliance. Examine the stoma and periostomal skin.

- Place the irrigation sleeve over the stoma.

- Lubricate the cone at the end of the irrigation tubing. Through the top of the irrigation sleeve, gently insert the cone into the stoma.

- Open the clamp, and begin the irrigation.

- When the irrigation is complete, clamp the top of the sleeve. Allow approximately 30 minutes for evacuation.

- Remove the sleeve, and rinse, dry, and store it. Apply a new colostomy appliance.

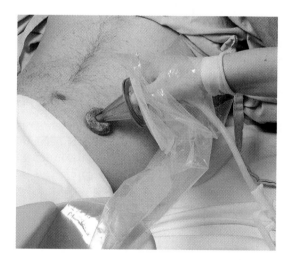

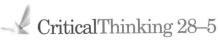

CriticalThinking 28–5

You are reviewing a client's chart and note that the client was tested for fecal occult blood. The results are as follows:

3/10 negative for occult blood
3/11 no BM
3/12 no BM
3/13 no BM
3/14 positive for occult blood
3/15 negative for occult blood
3/16 negative for occult blood

What can you conclude? What questions do these findings raise?

| Nursing Diagnosis |

Common nursing diagnoses related to bowel elimination include the following:

- *Bowel Incontinence* is a change in normal bowel habits characterized by involuntary passage of stool. *Subjective defining characteristics* include inability to recognize the urge to defecate or inability to feel rectal fullness. *Objective data* include constant dribbling of soft stool, fecal odor, fecal staining of clothing or bedding, and inability to delay defecation.

    Etiologies include high abdominal or intestinal pressure, chronic diarrhea, colorectal lesions, dietary habits, decline in muscle tone, immobility (inability to get to the bathroom), inaccessiblity of bathroom facilities, impaction, impaired cognition, laxative abuse, loss of rectal sphincter control, and motor nerve damage.

- *Constipation.* Because frequency of bowel elimination varies, constipation is usually defined as a decrease in the frequency of bowel movements resulting in the passage of hard stool. Stools become dry and hard when peristalsis slows and too much water is reabsorbed from the fecal mass. *Subjective defining characteristics* include abdominal pain, a feeling of rectal fullness, straining or pain with defecation, and some rectal bleeding. Unrelieved constipation may eventually result in a **fecal impaction,** in which dry, hard stools lodged in the rectum cannot be passed.

    Etiologies include abdominal muscle weakness, ignoring the urge to defecate, insufficient physical activity, depression, emotional stress, changes in eating patterns, and insufficient fiber or fluid intake. Habitual laxative use may also cause constipation as the colon becomes responsive only to the stimulating effect of the laxative.

- *Risk for Constipation* is an appropriate diagnosis for clients at increased risk because of bedrest, medications such as opioids, or surgery. Use this diagnosis for a client with a condition or taking medications known to decrease peristalsis. *Risk factors* include abdominal muscle weakness, habitually ignoring the urge to defecate, insufficient intake of fluid and fiber, dehydration, and certain medications (e.g., anticholinergics, calcium channel blockers).

- *Perceived Constipation* is an appropriate diagnosis for a client who makes a self-diagnosis of constipation and uses laxatives, suppositories, or enemas to ensure a daily bowel movement. *Etiologies* may include cultural and family health beliefs and impaired thought processes.

- *Diarrhea* is the passage of loose, unformed or watery stools. *Defining characteristics* include abdominal pain, cramping, and urgency; at least three loose, liquid stools per day; and hyperactive bowel sounds. The patient may also experience bloating, fever, and blood in the stools, depending on the cause of the diarrhea. Persistent diarrhea threatens fluid and electrolyte balance, especially in young children and older adults.

    Etiologies include high stress levels, anxiety, medication effects, alcohol abuse, laxative abuse, radiation, tube feedings, infections or inflammatory processes, malabsorption, and parasites. The most common cause is GI infection; however, diarrhea may occur with a chronic disease, such as celiac disease or irritable bowel syndrome.

- *Toileting Self-Care Deficit* is impaired ability to perform or complete own toileting activities. You can use this diagnosis for patients who cannot manipulate their clothing for toileting, carry out proper toilet hygiene, flush the toilet, get to the toilet or commode, or sit on or rise from the toilet or commode. *Etiologies* of this diagnosis include impaired mobility, pain, cognitive impairment, musculoskeletal or neuromuscular impairment, weakness, developmental disability, and lack of motivation. Strictly speaking, this is not a bowel problem. Bowel function may be normal, but the person simply cannot manage toileting.

Bowel elimination problems may also form the etiology of other nursing diagnoses and collaborative problems. Examples include the following:

- Social isolation r/t embarrassment secondary to bowel incontinence

- Potential Complication: electrolyte imbalance secondary to diarrhea (older adults, very young children, and infants are at especially high risk)

- Impaired Skin Integrity r/t irritating effects of feces secondary to diarrhea

- Anxiety r/t perceived need for a daily bowel movement

- Disturbed Body Image r/t bowel diversion

CriticalThinking 28–6

- What data do you have about Mrs. Zeno's ("Meet Your Patient") bowel function?
- What else would you like to know about her bowel function (what other symptoms often accompany these cues)?
- Which NANDA nursing diagnosis best describes this cue cluster?
- In addition to this nursing diagnosis, what other data in the scenario might also be contributing to her infrequent BMs?
- From the scenario data, how would you describe the etiology of Mrs. Zeno's problem?
- What questions do you still have about the etiology?

| Planning Outcomes/Evaluation |

The general bowel elimination goal is that the patient will have soft, formed bowel movements regularly.

For *associated NOC standardized outcomes* for bowel elimination diagnoses,

VOL 2   Go to Chapter 28, **Standardized Language, Selected Standardized Outcomes and Interventions for Bowel Elimination Diagnoses,** in Volume 2.

When bowel elimination is the etiology, choose outcomes linked to the problem side of the diagnosis. For example, for Impaired Skin Integrity r/t irritating effects of diarrhea stool, the NOC outcomes might fall within Tissue Integrity: Skin and Mucous Membranes.

Individualized goals/outcome statements depend on the nursing diagnosis. Because normal bowel elimination patterns are individualized, regularity is based on the individual's pattern. Examples include: the following:

- Will resume his normal bowel pattern by (date).
- Will discuss his feelings about his colostomy.

| Planning Interventions/Implementation |

Bowel elimination is a normal physiological function. However, discussing it often causes embarrassment. Some people associate uncleanliness with bowel elimination. Others are very focused on the regularity of their bowel movements. For these reasons, it is important for you to convey an attitude of acceptance and display professionalism when providing care for patients with problems of bowel elimination.

For *NIC standardized interventions and activities* for patients with bowel elimination problems,

VOL 2   Go to Chapter 28, **Standardized Language, Selected Standardized Outcomes and Interventions for Bowel Elimination Diagnoses,** in Volume 2.

Specific nursing activities to promote normal bowel function and relieve elimination problems are in the next section.

Promoting Normal or Regular Defecation

Promoting regular defecation entails a number of independent nursing activities. These include providing privacy, positioning, timing, providing hydration and nutrition, and promoting exercise.

Privacy

Try this exercise. Imagine that your class assignment for today is to stand in front of the classroom and describe to the class your normal pattern of defecation, including frequency, appearance, and other characteristics of the stool. How would you feel about that? Would you do it?

Although defecation is a normal physiological function, most patients consider it a very private matter. Provide privacy for your patient when discussing or providing care related to bowel elimination. Taking a matter-of-fact approach will confirm to patients that you are comfortable with this aspect of care. When assisting a client with bowel elimination, excuse visitors from the room, draw the dividing curtains in shared rooms, and close the door to the room. Many patients are embarrassed by the odor of bowel movements and therefore may ignore the urge to defecate. Using an aromatic spray or other odor-reducing product may help to reduce embarrassment.

Positioning

An upright seated or squatting position is the most comfortable for defecation and decreases the need to strain. When possible, assist the patient to the bathroom to use the toilet. An alternative is to place a bedside commode next to the bed for patients who are unable to ambulate to the bathroom. If the patient must remain in bed, place the client in a semi-Fowler's position to use the bedpan. Patients who are unable to assume this position because of surgery, trauma, or other medical conditions must use supine or side-lying positions. These positions are unnatural for bowel elimination and place the client at risk for constipation.

Raise the siderails or provide an overhead trapeze so that the patient can grip them to maneuver on and off the bedpan. If the patient is extremely weak, you may need an assistant to help you position him on the bedpan. In addition, you may need to remain with the person while he uses the bedpan to help him maintain position on the bedpan. The Critical Aspects box on page 662 provides highlights of this procedure. For the complete procedure,

 VOL 2   Go to Chapter 28, **Procedure 28–2: Placing and Removing a Bedpan,** in Volume 2.

Timing of Defecation

Recall that food entering the duodenum triggers mass peristalsis. As a result, the urge to defecate often occurs after meals. Advise patients not to ignore this urge, because doing so may result in constipation. For patients who are ambulatory, allow some free time after meals to use the restroom. For those who cannot toilet independently, provide assistance ambulating to the bathroom or using the bedpan. Discuss with the UAPs with whom you work the need to offer assistance without waiting to be asked, so that patients experience minimal delays.

Fluids and Nutrition

Teach clients the importance of fluids and a balanced diet in promoting soft, formed, regular bowel movements. The diet should be rich in fresh fruits and vegetables, whole-grain foods, legumes, and water, yet low in simple sugars, carbonated beverages, and processed foods. Adequate dietary fiber is essential. Encourage a daily intake of 25 to 30 grams of fiber to provide bulk, attract water into the stool, and promote peristalsis. Unfortunately, a typical modern diet is low in fiber, often as low as 5 to 8 grams per day. Box 28–1 provides a list of high-fiber foods.

An intake of eight to ten 8-ounce glasses of fluid daily (2000 to 2400 mL) is recommended to keep stool soft and aid in production of mucus to lubricate the colon. Indeed, a high-fiber diet that is inadequate in fluid can result in constipation. Water is the preferred fluid because soda, coffee, and tea often contain caffeine or additives that promote diuresis. However, because the diuretic effect of these fluids is minimal, they are acceptable for clients who simply will not drink enough plain water.

Exercise

Physical activity increases peristalsis and promotes defecation. Encourage patients to exercise three to five times per week and to engage in daily walking or light activity. Assist hospitalized or institutionalized patients to ambulate as soon as their condition permits. Even limited activity, such as getting out of bed or walking 10 feet, decreases the risk for constipation.

Provide range-of-motion (ROM) exercises for patients who must remain on bedrest. Even passive ROM exercises (the joints are moved through ROM by the nurse) promote peristalsis. Chapter 31 provides additional information about activity and ROM exercises.

For clients who can assist with exercise, the following exercises promote abdominal and perineal strength:

- *Thigh strengthening.* Have the client slowly bring one knee up to his chest, briefly hold it, then lower

the leg to the bed. Repeat this pattern alternating legs. Encourage the client to perform this exercise several times per hour while he is awake.
- *Abdominal tightening.* Have the client tighten and hold the abdominal muscles for a count of 5 and then relax. This exercise works the abdominal muscles used during defecation.

KnowledgeCheck 28–5

Identify at least five independent nursing actions that you can take to encourage regular elimination in a well client.

  Go to Chapter 28, **Knowledge Check Response Sheet and Answers,** on the Electronic Study Guide.

CriticalThinking 28–7

How could you facilitate regular bowel elimination for Mrs. Zeno ("Meet Your Patient")? What information do you need?

Managing Diarrhea

Diarrhea may occur as a result of contaminated food, a viral infection, or dietary change, or as a side effect of a medication. Patients with diarrhea are at risk for fluid and electrolyte imbalance. Water and potassium loss are the primary concerns. Infants, young children, and the frail elderly are most vulnerable and may require hospitalization and intravenous fluid replacement therapy. Ideally, oral liquids replace the lost fluid and potassium.

Nursing interventions focus on treating the diarrhea itself, as well as its associated problems (cramping, fluid and electrolyte imbalances, and Impaired Skin Integrity):

- Monitor frequency, amount, color, and consistency of stools to determine severity of diarrhea.
- Monitor intake and output, body weight, and vital signs to assess for fluid losses.
- Assess skin turgor and mucous membranes for evidence of fluid imbalance.
- Monitor serum electrolyte levels to detect imbalances.
- Assess the perineal area for alterations in skin integrity. Clients with diarrhea may experience perianal irritation and excoriation.
- Provide assistance with hygiene to protect the skin.
- Encourage your patient to sip liquids often to replace the losses.
- Avoid a sudden large intake of fluid or food, because this may trigger mass peristalsis.
- Teach the client about or provide a clear liquid diet, including electrolyte replacement fluids, (e.g., Pedialyte or sports drinks that have been diluted by 50%

or more). Clear broth and gelatin are also good choices.

- If your client has an appetite, advise a BRAT diet: bananas, (white) rice, applesauce, toast. These foods are easy to digest, provide calories for energy, and help offset potassium loss.

- Highly spiced foods or large quantities of raw fruits and vegetables may cause diarrhea in some patients. Tell patients to keep track of foods that trigger this response and to eat them in moderation.

- Several medications, especially antibiotics, may also cause diarrhea. A change in medications may be required to manage diarrhea. Plain yogurt consumed daily may help to prevent this response.

Antidiarrheal medications are not recommended for acute diarrhea. In many cases, diarrhea is a response to infection or unusual foods and serves as a mechanism to rid the body of the pathogens or troublesome food. Although antidiarrheal medications are available without a prescription, caution patients to avoid using them unless instructed by their healthcare provider. Medication is usually reserved for use with chronic diarrhea—diarrhea that has persisted for more than 1 month—which is often due to a disease state.

Opiates (e.g., paregoric) and opiate derivatives (e.g., loperamide [Imodium]) are the primary antidiarrheal drugs prescribed. Although they slow peristalsis and inhibit diarrhea, they may cause drowsiness; advise patients, especially older patients, to use them with caution. Pepto-Bismol (bismuth subsalicylate) is a readily available OTC medication that is useful with traveler's diarrhea because it has antimicrobial and antisecretory properties.

Managing Constipation

Clients most likely to experience constipation are those who (1) have decreased activity or are on bedrest, (2) are receiving opioids or other medications that slow peristalsis, and (3) have decreased fluid and fiber intake. The strategies to prevent and treat constipation are identical to the activities that promote regular bowel elimination. They include the following:

- Increase the intake of high-fiber foods.
- Increase fluid intake.
- Increase physical activity.
- Provide privacy for using the toilet.
- Assist the patient to a seated or squatting position whenever possible. A semi-Fowler's position is preferred for a client on bedrest.
- Allow the patient uninterrupted time to use the toilet especially after meals, when mass peristalsis occurs.

BOX 28-2 **Types of Laxatives**

- *Stool softeners* cause moisture and fat to penetrate the stool, thereby softening it and making it easier to pass. Example: docusate sodium (DSS or Colace)

- *Osmotic laxatives* work by drawing water into the bowel from surrounding tissue. Examples: polyethylene glycol (Miralax), lactulose

- *Lubricant laxatives* coat the GI tract with a thin waterproof layer. Mineral oil is an example. Because the lubricant coats the entire GI tract, it may interfere with the absorption of nutrients. Mineral oil is potentially dangerous in debilitated patients. Inhaled droplets can lead to a form of pneumonia.

- *Stimulant laxatives* are bowel irritants. They irritate the intestinal wall, stimulating intense peristalsis. Examples: senna and bisacodyl (Dulcolax)

- *Bulking agents* are high in fiber. They must be combined with sufficient fluid intake to be effective. The fiber attracts fluid into the colon, and the bulk of the stool stimulates the urge to evacuate. Examples: Metamucil, Citrucel, Psyllium, Fibercon

- *Combination laxatives* are laxatives that contain more than one type of laxative ingredient. The most common type is a combination stimulant laxative and stool softener.

When lifestyle modifications are ineffective in preventing and treating constipation, medications may be given. Box 28–2 discusses the types of laxatives available. Bulking agents are actually fiber in a nonfood source. These are the preferred medications for treating constipation. Many laxatives are readily available OTC and are used by clients to treat actual or perceived constipation. Habitual laxative use, except for bulking agents, may cause reliance on medication for bowel elimination and, ironically, may lead to further constipation. See the Self-Care box, on page 668, on laxative use for key points to discuss with clients about managing constipation.

Managing Fecal Impaction

Fecal impaction is the presence of a hardened fecal mass in the rectum. The impaction often blocks the passage of normal stool and sets up a vicious cycle of furthering hardening of stool. Liquid stool may leak, seeping around the hardened mass, and the patient may report feelings of fullness, bloating, constipation, diminished appetite, and a change in bowel habits. You can detect fecal impaction by digital examination of the rectum. To treat a fecal impaction, you will use enemas or digital removal of stool. Once the impaction

Teaching Your Patient About Laxative Use

Discuss the following topics with clients who have concerns about the frequency of their bowel movements or ask about laxatives.

The frequency of BMs may range from several times per day to once per week. As long as stools are passed without excessive urgency, with minimal effort and no straining, and without the use of laxatives, bowel function may be regarded as normal.

To maintain normal bowel function:

- Eat a well-balanced diet that includes whole grains, fresh fruits, and vegetables.
- Drink eight to ten glasses of fluid per day.
- Engage in daily exercise to stimulate peristalsis.
- Set aside uninterrupted time after breakfast or dinner for using the toilet.
- Do not ignore the urge to defecate.
- Whenever there is a significant or prolonged change in bowel habits, report this to your healthcare provider.

If you are experiencing constipation, choose bulking agents, such as Metamucil or psyllium, to treat the problem rather than other over-the-counter laxatives. Be sure to drink plenty of water when using bulking agents.

has been removed, establish a bowel regimen to prevent recurrence of impactions.

Enemas

An enema is the introduction of solution into the rectum to soften feces, distend the colon, and stimulate peristalsis and evacuation of feces. Some enema solutions are chosen because they irritate the mucosa of the rectum and sigmoid colon and assist with forceful evacuation of stool.

Types of Enemas

Enemas may be classified as cleansing, retention, or return-flow. The primary care provider generally orders the specific type to administer to a patient.

Cleansing Enemas

Cleansing enemas promote removal of feces from the colon. They may be used to:

- Treat severe constipation or impaction.

- Clear the colon in preparation for visualization procedures, such as colonoscopy.
- Empty the colon when starting a bowel training program.

Historically, cleansing enemas were used prior to surgical procedures and childbirth to prevent the escape of feces. That use is very limited now; they are used only before surgeries of the lower GI tract and for some pelvic surgeries.

Cleansing enema solutions include hypotonic solutions and hypertonic solutions. With *hypotonic solutions* (saline, tap water, and soap) you introduce a large volume (500 to 1000 mL for adults, 100 to 250 mL for infants) of fluid into the rectum. The volume causes intestinal distention and leads to rapid evacuation of stool. Large-volume solutions may be contraindicated in patients who have weakened intestinal walls.

In contrast, *hypertonic solutions* are usually smaller in volume (70 to 120 mL, or 3 to 4 ounces, for adults). The hypertonic solution attracts water into the colon, causing distention and stimulating peristalsis and defecation. Hypertonic solutions may be contraindicated for patients who tend to retain sodium or water (e.g., those with renal failure and congestive heart failure). Table 28–2 summarizes information about enema solutions.

A cleansing enema may be given "high" or "low." A "low" enema is given by standard procedure. A "high" enema attempts to clear as much of the large intestine as possible. With a "high" enema, the client receives initial instillation of the fluid in the left lateral position. The client then moves to the dorsal recumbent position and then the right lateral position for the remainder of the instillation. This turning process allows the fluid to follow the shape of the large intestine.

Retention Enemas

Retention enemas introduce a solution into the colon that is meant to be retained for a prolonged period. Consequently the volume is small, usually 90 to 120 mL. The following are the most common forms of retention enemas.

- *Oil-retention enemas* instill 90 to 120 mL of oil into the rectum to soften stool and lubricate the rectum. This type of enema may be used to assist a client to pass hard stool or prior to digital removal of stool. It may also be used in conjunction with a cleansing enema. The oil-retention enema is given at least 1 hour prior to the cleansing enema.

 Go to Chapter 28, **Technique 28–2: Administering an Oil-Retention Enema,** in Volume 2.

- *Carminative enemas* instill 60 to 150 mL of solution into the rectum to help expel flatus and relieve

TABLE 28-2 Solutions Commonly Used in Enemas

Solution	Examples	Action	Time until BM	Adverse Effects
Hypotonic	500–1000 mL of tap water	Large volume distends the colon, thereby stimulating peristalsis; water also softens stool	15 minutes	Fluid and electrolyte imbalance, especially water intoxication, is possible if enema is not expelled
Isotonic	500–1000 mL of normal saline (0.9% NaCl solution)	Large volume distends the colon, thereby stimulating peristalsis; some softening of stool also occurs	15 minutes	Fluid and electrolyte imbalance, especially sodium retention
Hypertonic	90–120 mL of sodium phosphate (Fleets); available as a commercially prepared solution	Attracts water into the colon, thereby causing distention	Rapid acting: 5–10 minutes	Sodium retention
Oil	90–120 mL of mineral oil, cottonseed oil, or olive oil; available as a commercially prepared solution	Softens the feces, lubricates the rectum	Varies widely. An oil-retention enema is often given 1–3 hours before a cleansing enema is administered.	

bloating and distention. This procedure is used after abdominal or pelvic surgery when peristalsis is slow to return and the client experiences pressure from gas. Solutions may be commercially prepared or prepared on the unit. A common carminative enema is the "MGW" enema; a mixture of magnesium sulfate, glycerin, and water in a ratio of 1:2:3 (e.g., 15 mL magnesium sulfate, 30 mL of glycerin, and 45 mL of water).

- *Medicated enemas* may be used to instill antibiotics to treat infections in the rectum or anus or to introduce anthelminthic agents for treatment of intestinal worms and parasites.
- *Nutritive enemas* administer fluid and nutrition through the rectum for patients who are dehydrated and frail. They are most commonly used in hospice care as a means to provide hydration for dying patients.

Return-Flow Enemas

A return-flow enema, known as a *Harris flush,* may be ordered to help a patient expel flatus and relieve abdominal distention. Approximately 100 to 200 mL (for adults) of tap water or saline is instilled into the rectum. The rectal tube and solution container are then lowered below the level of the rectum to encourage return flow of the solution. This process is repeated several times, or until distention is relieved. If the solution becomes thick, discard it and begin again with new solution.

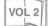 Go to Chapter 28, **Technique 28–3: Administering a Return-Flow Enema,** in Volume 2.

Administering an Enema

Before administering an enema, explain the purpose of the enema and what the patient can expect. For example, the patient will probably experience some cramping with a large-volume enema. Reassure the patient that you will be immediately available to help her to the restroom or onto the bedpan.

Responses to an enema are governed by the height of the solution container, the speed of flow, the concentration of the solution, and the resistance of the rectum. Hypotonic and isotonic solutions are easier to retain. Hypertonic solutions are irritating to the intestinal mucosa and cause a rapid evacuation. Muscle tone and history of constipation or other bowel disorders determine the resistance of the rectum. A client with a long history of constipation is more likely to be able to tolerate a large-volume enema, because the rectum and colon have become distended over time.

Because of gravity, the higher the solution container, the faster the solution flows into the bowel. As a rule, place the solution container no higher than 30 cm (12 in.) above the rectum (7.5 cm or 3 in., for children). This allows for a steady flow of solution that is easily tolerated. Rapid instillation will cause rapid distention of the bowel and intense cramping. Slower instillation will be more comfortable for the client and allow him to retain the fluid for a period of time to soften the stool. The Critical Aspects box on page 662 reviews the procedure. For detailed instructions,

 Go to Chapter 28, **Procedure 28–3: Administering an Enema,** in Volume 2.

KnowledgeCheck 28–6
- Identify the types of enemas available for use.
- How do hypotonic and isotonic enemas differ from hypertonic enemas?
- What actions can you take to make the patient more comfortable when he receives an enema?

 Go to Chapter 28, **Knowledge Check Response Sheet and Answers,** on the Electronic Study Guide.

Digital Removal of Stool

If fecal impaction does not respond to use of stool softeners and enemas, you will need to digitally remove feces from the rectum. Digital removal is accomplished by breaking up the hardened mass into pieces and manually extracting the pieces. You may administer an oil-retention enema at least 30 minutes prior to digital removal to soften the stool and decrease the patient's discomfort during the procedure.

Aside from discomfort, the pressure generated in the rectum may stimulate the vagus nerve, slowing the heart rate. For that reason, you must have an order from the primary care provider. The Critical Aspects box on page 662 summarizes the procedure. For complete steps,

 Go to Chapter 28, **Procedure 28–4: Removing Stool Digitally,** in Volume 2.

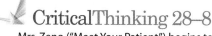 CriticalThinking 28–8

Mrs. Zeno ("Meet Your Patient") begins to pass liquid stool. What actions should you take? Explain your reasoning.

Managing Flatulence

Recall that flatus is a natural by-product of digestion. When gas is excessive or leads to complaints of abdominal distention, cramping, or discomfort, it is known as **flatulence.** Some people develop flatulence after eating gas-producing foods, such as beans, cabbage, cauliflower, onions, or highly spiced foods. For others, flatulence occurs when fiber intake is increased. Clients with irritable bowel syndrome experience a constellation of symptoms that include flatulence. Constipation is often accompanied by flatulence because digestive by-products undergo prolonged fermentation in the colon. You can help clients manage flatulence by teaching them the following:

- Be aware of and avoid foods that trigger flatulence.
- Follow self-care strategies (identified earlier) for maintaining regular bowel movements.
- For patients who have had surgery with gaseous anesthesia, encourage them to ambulate and perform bed exercises to stimulate peristalsis and the passage of gas.

In severe cases, you may need to insert a rectal tube to aid in the elimination of flatus. For a description,

 Go to Chapter 28, **Technique 28–4: Inserting a Rectal Tube,** in Volume 2.

Managing Bowel Incontinence

Bowel incontinence is the inability to control the discharge of feces and flatulence. Physiological conditions causing bowel incontinence include neurological conditions that affect innervation of the rectum and anus, uncontrolled diarrhea, impaction resulting in leakage of stool, and cognitive changes that alter perception of the urge to defecate. Clients who have severe psychiatric problems may be incontinent because of altered perception or inability to manage activities of daily living. Bowel incontinence is also created by functional limitations—for example, when a client recognizes the need to have a BM but cannot get to the toilet independently or in time to defecate in the toilet. Illnesses that limit mobility often lead to incontinence.

Bowel incontinence may be embarrassing. As clients worry about future episodes, anxiety escalates. In addition, clients with bowel incontinence are at risk for Impaired Skin Integrity. Refer to the Nursing Care Plan on page 673 for a patient with fecal incontinence; see also the care map that accompanies the care plan. In general, nursing interventions include the following:

- Monitor pattern of BMs.
- Provide the bedpan or assist the patient to the bathroom at regular intervals and at times BMs are most likely to occur.
- Change clothing and/or bed linens as soon as possible to prevent skin irritation and embarrassment.
- Provide prompt hygiene care after any episodes of incontinence.
- Monitor skin for evidence of breakdown. Use moisture-barrier cream if redness or irritation is

noted. Consider use of a fecal incontinence pouch for skin protection (discussed in the following section).

- Review diet, fluid intake, activity, and medicines. Work with the primary care provider to alter the above factors to encourage regular bowel movements.
- Consider a bowel training program.
- You may use incontinence pads or barrier pads to prevent fecal drainage from soiling clothing and linens. Never place the plastic side of the pad next to the patient's body.
- Never refer to incontinence pads as "diapers" when caring for adults or children who have been toilet-trained. This inappropriate reference may cause embarrassment and lower the patient's self-esteem.

Fecal Incontinence Pouch

A fecal incontinence pouch may be used for patients with incontinence to protect perianal skin or to collect large samples of feces. The pouch collects fecal drainage, keeping feces away from the skin. This is a commonly used approach for clients with uncontrolled diarrhea.

A variety of pouch systems may be used. Most frequently, a moisture-proof barrier is applied around the anus, and a plastic pouch is secured to the barrier. The equipment may be the same as that used for patients with an ostomy. (Ostomy care is discussed later in the chapter.) You will need to assess the system regularly to ensure that no leaks have occurred and to empty contents. Empty the fecal pouch when it is one-third to one-half full to prevent the pouch from getting too heavy. Pay close attention to the perianal skin as you perform your assessment. You may need to use moisture-barrier cream on the surrounding skin. You will usually change the fecal pouch at least every 72 hours and whenever there is evidence of leakage.

Bowel Training

A bowel training program assists the patient to have regular, soft, formed stools. It is appropriate for clients who have chronic constipation, impaction, or bowel incontinence. Elements of a bowel training program include the following:

- Plan the program with the patient and caregiver.
- Gradually increase fiber in the diet while monitoring consistency of the stool.
- Increase fluid intake to at least eight glasses of water per day, if not contraindicated.
- Initiate a designated uninterrupted time for defecation: usually after meals, especially in the morning.
- Provide privacy for the patient during the designated time.
- Develop a staged treatment plan if constipation develops. Usually, additional fiber is added as a first

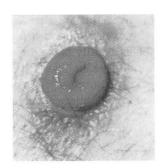

FIGURE 28–8 **A healthy stoma is deep pink to brick red and is shiny and moist.**

measure. A stool softener is next, followed by a suppository such as bisacodyl (Dulcolax).

- Regularly modify the plan based on the patient's response.

KnowledgeCheck 28–7

- What are the major patient care concerns associated with bowel incontinence?
- What are the elements of a bowel training program?

 Go to Chapter 28, **Knowledge Check Response Sheet and Answers,** on the Electronic Study Guide.

Caring for a Patient with a Bowel Diversion

Patients experience a variety of reactions to a bowel diversion, and each person has unique physical and psychological needs. Initially you will care for the ostomy, but the goal is for the patient to assume self-care.

Assessing a Stoma

You should begin care with a thorough assessment of the stoma. A healthy stoma (Figure 28–8) ranges in color from deep pink to brick red, regardless of the patient's skin color, and is shiny and moist. Pallor or a dusky blue color indicates ischemia, and a brown-black color indicates necrosis.

Immediately after surgery, the stoma will be swollen and enlarged. As the inflammation subsides and healing occurs, the stoma will shrink. By 6 to 8 weeks, it will be at its permanent size. Stoma size varies according to the size of the person and the part of the bowel that was externalized (see Figure 28–5). An ileostomy stoma is generally smaller than a colostomy stoma. The stoma will protrude above the level of the abdomen by approximately 1.3 to 2.5 cm (0.5 to 1 in.).

Output from an ileostomy stoma is liquid and contains digestive enzymes. An ostomy further in the GI tract will have more solid output and fewer enzymes. Presence of enzymes in the effluent increases the likelihood of skin breakdown. Assess the skin surrounding

Nursing Care Plan *(continued)*

NIC Interventions/Activities	Rationale
NIC Interventions Bowel Management #0430 Bowel Training #0440 **Nursing Activities** 1. Conduct a comprehensive assessment of all factors related to fecal incontinence and impaired bowel elimination.	Fecal incontinence has multiple possible causes. The best nursing interventions are those based on client assessment (Norton & Chelvanayagam, 2000). Constipation is attributed to immobility, weak straining ability, use of constipating drugs, neurological disorders, lack of dietary fiber, and poor fluid intake (Schnelle & Leung, 2004; Scarlett, 2004).
2. During physical examination, inspect the perianal skin for possible causes of fecal incontinence or skin irritation resulting from exposure to liquid stool.	Congenital abnormalities and hemorrhoids can lead to incontinence. Skin tags can make cleansing difficult and lead to minor soiling that is difficult to distinguish from actual fecal incontinence (Norton & Chelvanayagam, 2000).
3. Inquire about Mrs. Grimaldi's access to the bathroom and toileting facilities at home and work. Provide regular toileting assistance as long as the client needs it during her hospitalization.	A lack of convenient access to the toilet can precipitate fecal incontinence (Doughty, 1996; Schnelle & Leung, 2004).
4. Work with Mrs. Grimaldi to establish a bowel reeducation program, starting with bowel cleansing.	Cleansing is indicated for any client with rectal impaction or palpable stool in the descending or sigmoid colon. Cleansing with manual disimpaction, laxatives, and/or enema allows hardened stool to pass from the colon and removes any potential blockages to stool elimination (Doughty, 1996; Schnelle & Leung, 2004; Scarlett, 2004).
5. Normalize stool consistency by ensuring that Mrs. Grimaldi drinks 30 mL/kg per day and by gradually increasing dietary fiber with bran or with bulking agents. Mrs. Grimaldi is drinking only about 1200 mL of fluid per day. If she weighs 125 lb (56.7 kg), she would need to drink 1700 mL of fluid per day.	Increasing fluid intake is one of the easiest ways to normalize stool consistency in clients with constipation. Increasing dietary fiber improves stool consistency and reduces fecal incontinence (Bliss et al., 2001; Korula, 2002). Bulk should be added to the diet slowly to reduce the risk that the client will develop bloating, gas, or diarrhea. Dosing of bulking agents can be increased weekly until desired results are achieved; the results are more important than the amount of fiber ingested (Doughty, 1996).

Nursing Interventions/Activities	Rationale
6. Teach Mrs. Grimaldi about how her body works to produce stool, ways to gently signal the body to defecate, the importance of responding to the urge to defecate, and how immobility, medications, and dehydration can cause constipation.	Gaining knowledge about bodily functions allows clients to be active participants in their care. Addressing causes of constipation can reduce the risk of recurrence (Schnelle & Leung, 2004).

Evaluation

Review initial outcomes and goals. Reassess daily Mrs. Grimaldi's progress toward stated discharge goals.

The day before Mrs. Grimaldi's discharge, she had no palpable stool on physical exam, and she no longer needed the intravenous analgesics; her PCA pump was discontinued. She was drinking approximately 20 mL/kg per day of fluids, she had begun taking 2 tablespoons of psyllium dissolved in water every morning, and she had a bowel movement each of the previous 2 days with stool of normal consistency for the first time in more than a month. She was able to state the actions she would take at home: continue the bulk supplements, try to increase her fluid intake to 30 mL/kg per day, use nonconstipating analgesics, and increase her mobility each day. The nurse charted that the goals were met.

References

Bliss, D. Z., Jung, H. J., Savik, K., Lowry, A., LeMoine, M., Jensen, L., et al. (2001). Supplementation with dietary fiber improves fecal incontinence. *Nursing Research, 50,* 203–213.

Dochterman, J. M., & Bulechek, G. M. (Eds.). (2004). *Nursing interventions classification (NIC)* (4th ed.). St Louis: Mosby.

Doughty, D. (1996). A physiologic approach to bowel training. *Journal of Wound, Ostomy, and Continence Nursing, 23,* 46–56.

Korula, J. (2002). Dietary fibre supplementation with psyllium or gum arabic reduced faecal incontinence in community-living adults. *Evidence Based Medicine, 7,* 20.

Moorhead, S., Johnson, M., & Mass, M. (Eds.). (2004). *Nursing outcomes classification (NOC)* (3rd ed.). St Louis: Mosby.

Norton, C., & Chelvanayagam, S. (2000). A nursing assessment tool for adults with fecal incontinence. *Journal of Wound, Ostomy, and Continence Nursing, 27,* 279–291.

Scarlett, Y. (2004). Medical management of fecal incontinence. *Gastroenterology, 126,* S55–S63.

Schnelle, J. F., & Leung, F. W. (2004). Urinary and fecal incontinence in nursing homes. *Gastroenterology, 126,* S41–S47.

Care Map

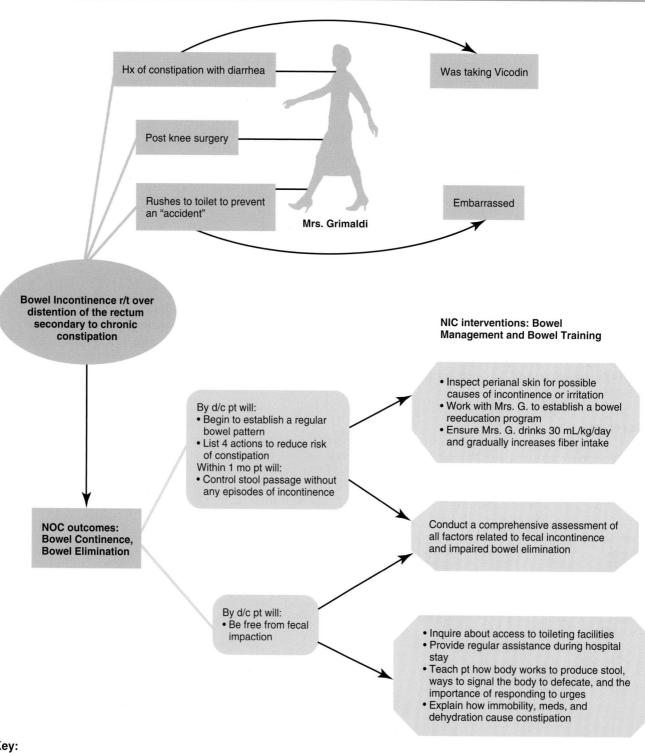

Hx of constipation with diarrhea

Was taking Vicodin

Post knee surgery

Rushes to toilet to prevent an "accident"

Embarrassed

Mrs. Grimaldi

Bowel Incontinence r/t over distention of the rectum secondary to chronic constipation

NIC interventions: Bowel Management and Bowel Training

By d/c pt will:
• Begin to establish a regular bowel pattern
• List 4 actions to reduce risk of constipation
Within 1 mo pt will:
• Control stool passage without any episodes of incontinence

• Inspect perianal skin for possible causes of incontinence or irritation
• Work with Mrs. G. to establish a bowel reeducation program
• Ensure Mrs. G. drinks 30 mL/kg/day and gradually increases fiber intake

NOC outcomes: Bowel Continence, Bowel Elimination

Conduct a comprehensive assessment of all factors related to fecal incontinence and impaired bowel elimination

By d/c pt will:
• Be free from fecal impaction

• Inquire about access to toileting facilities
• Provide regular assistance during hospital stay
• Teach pt how body works to produce stool, ways to signal the body to defecate, and the importance of responding to urges
• Explain how immobility, meds, and dehydration cause constipation

Key:

Data

Nursing diagnosis

NOC outcomes

Other outcomes

NIC interventions and nursing actions

BOX 28-3 Dietary Changes Associated with an Ostomy

Note: These are only suggestions. Each person must, by trial and error, discover what works best for him.

General Guidelines for Patients

- Initially you may be asked to follow a bland, low-residue or soft diet for a month or two, to prevent obstructions and GI upsets. Advance the diet by adding one new food at a time.
- Eat three or more meals daily at regular times.
- People with ostomies may require additional fluid to compensate for the loss of the large intestine.
- Avoid chewing gum, as it may cause you to swallow air, causing a noisy stoma.
- Avoid foods that cause gas, odor, blockage, or loose stools. Introduce them into your diet one at a time and be aware of their effects.

Foods That May Cause Gas or Odor

- Asparagus
- Cabbage
- Beans
- Broccoli
- Cauliflower
- Radishes
- Brussels sprouts
- Peas
- Melons
- Carbonated beverages
- Beer
- Eggs
- Fish
- Garlic
- Onions

Foods That May Help Control Odor or Gas

- Yogurt
- Parsley
- Cranberry juice
- Buttermilk

High-fiber Foods That May Cause Blockage

You can eat some of these foods (e.g., mushrooms, shrimp) if you cut them into small pieces and chew them very thoroughly. As long as blockage does not occur, these foods should not necessarily be avoided, but used carefully.

- Raw or minimally cooked fruits and vegetables (e.g., coleslaw, Chinese stir-fried vegetables, oranges, apple skins)
- Stringy foods (e.g., celery, coconut, spinach, bean sprouts, green beans, orange pulp)
- Foods with tough skins (e.g., corn, dried fruits, pears, tomatoes)
- Foods with seeds (e.g., raspberries)
- Mushrooms, nuts
- Shrimp, lobster

Foods That May Cause Loose Stools

- Fried foods
- Highly seasoned foods
- Beer
- Raw vegetables
- Onions
- Licorice
- Raw fruits
- Baked beans
- Large meals
- Milk
- Chocolate
- Caffeine

Note: Never restrict fluids in an effort to control diarrhea.

Foods That May Alleviate Diarrhea

- Bananas
- Applesauce
- Cheese
- Creamy peanut butter
- Starchy foods (e.g., boiled rice, bread, potatoes)

Sources: United Ostomy Association. Retrieved 4/21/04 from *http://www.uoa.org.* Whitney, E. N., Cataldo, C. G., & Rolfes, S. R. (1998). *Understanding normal and clinical nutrition* (5th ed.). Belmont, CA: Wadsworth Publishing Company.

| toward evidence-based practice |

Schnelle, J. F., & Leung, F. W. (2004). Urinary and fecal incontinence in nursing homes. *Gastroenterology, 126*(1 Suppl 2), S41–S47.

At least 50% of nursing home residents experience urinary and fecal incontinence due to immobility and dementia. Approximately half of incontinent residents show immediate improvement when provided with consistent toileting assistance. The effects of toileting assistance on the frequency of fecal incontinence are less dramatic than those reported for urinary incontinence, primarily because of constipation.

Garrigues, V., Galvez, C., Ortiz, V., Ponce, M., Nos, P., & Ponce, J. (2004). Prevalence of constipation: Agreement among several criteria and evaluation of the diagnostic accuracy of qualifying symptoms and self-reported definition in a population-based survey in Spain. *American Journal of Epidemiology, 159*(5), 520–526.

Researchers conducted a cross-sectional survey in 1999 to estimate the prevalence of chronic constipation and to evaluate the diagnostic accuracy of the symptoms and the self-reported definition of constipation. They developed a 21-item questionnaire and mailed it to a random sample of 489 subjects, aged 18 to 65 years, in Spain. A total of 349 subjects (71%) responded to the questionnaire. The prevalence of self-reported constipation was 29.5%. Female gender was identified as a risk factor for constipation; fiber intake and physical exercise were found to be protective factors.

---

1. Imagine that you are managing a nursing home where there is an incontinence rate of 70%. You wish to hire another UAP and begin educating the nurses and UAPs there about ways to manage incontinence among the residents. Which article would you use to help justify this addition to your budget? How would you use it?

2. Based on these two articles, what three nursing interventions would you insist that your staff institute in a standardized care plan for promoting normal bowel function? Give rationale for each.

 Go to Chapter 29, **Toward Evidence-Based Practice Suggested Responses,** on the Electronic Study Guide.

 Go to Chapter 28, **Resources for Caregivers and Health Professionals,** on the Electronic Study Guide.

 Suggested Readings: Go to Chapter 28, **Reading More About Bowel Elimination,** on the Electronic Study Guide.

 Bibliography: Go to Volume 2, Bibliography.

Sensory Perception

Learning Outcomes

After completing this chapter, you should be able to:

* Identify the components of the sensory experience.

* Compare and contrast sensory deprivation and sensory overload.

* List factors placing clients at risk for altered sensory perception.

* Discuss the hazards of sensory deficits in vision, hearing, taste, smell, touch, and proprioception.

* Identify factors that affect sensory stimulation.

* Assess clients for signs and symptoms of altered sensory perception.

* State nursing diagnoses and outcomes appropriate for clients with problems of sensory perception.

* Describe nursing interventions to prevent sensory deprivation and sensory overload.

* Discuss strategies to enhance communication with clients with sensory deficits.

MEET Your Patients

At a clinical post-conference, your instructor presents the following cases:

- Joshua is a 28-year-old patient in the intensive care unit (ICU). He had a car accident 3 weeks ago and has had several surgeries to repair a fractured femur, ruptured spleen, and intracranial bleeding. He was on a ventilator for 10 days and has had numerous invasive procedures. The nurses report that he is very confused and has been hallucinating.
- Richard is a 90-year-old man who has been a resident at a skilled nursing facility for 10 years. He has no visitors, never leaves his room, has no television or radio in the room, and no longer speaks. He does not respond to verbal or tactile stimulation. He lies

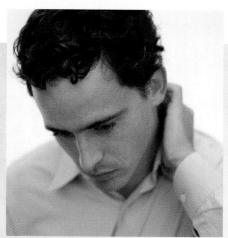

in bed in a fetal position. When staff try to move him, he moans and howls.

Your instructor asks you to consider how these patients are similar and how their care might overlap. It seems hard to imagine that these patients could have much in common. What similarities can you see? As you read this chapter, follow these cases and other examples illustrating the effects of altered sensory or perceptual function.

Theoretical Knowledge
knowing why

We experience the world through our senses. Vision, hearing, smell, taste, touch, and our sense of our body in space all help us to interpret and interact with our environment in a meaningful way. To grow, develop, and function, we must be able to sense this input and respond.

Many patients who are being treated for one condition also have a preexisting sensory deficit (e.g., a client whom you are teaching self-injection for diabetes may also be blind). Others develop alterations in sensory function as a result of their illness or of medications they are taking. This chapter will help you provide care for such patients.

COMPONENTS OF THE SENSORY EXPERIENCE

Our senses give us information about our environment and what is happening inside our body. The purpose of sensation is to allow the body to respond to changing situations and maintain homeostasis. A sensory experience involves four components: stimulus, reception, perception, and an arousal mechanism. A **stimulus** may be a sight, sound, taste, pain, or anything that stimulates a nerve receptor. The brain must receive and process it to make it meaningful.

Reception

Reception is the process of receiving stimuli from nerve endings in the skin and body. A receptor converts a stimulus to a nerve impulse and transmits the impulse along sensory neurons to the central nervous system. Some receptors remain activated for as long as the stimulus is applied. However, most receptors *adapt* to stimuli; that is, their response declines with time. Adaptation explains why, over time, you become unaware of an unpleasant smell or the persistent hum of an air conditioner.

Receptors usually respond to only one type of stimulus. For example, taste buds in the mouth detect sweet, sour, salty, or bitter, whereas receptors in the retina detect light rays. The following are examples of the many types of sensory receptors in the body:

- *Mechanoreceptors* in the skin and hair follicles detect touch, pressure, and vibration.
- *Hair cells,* the receptors for hearing, which are located in the cochlea of the ear, detect sound waves. In the vestibular apparatus of the ear, receptors for equilibrium and balance detect acceleration of the body and position of the head.

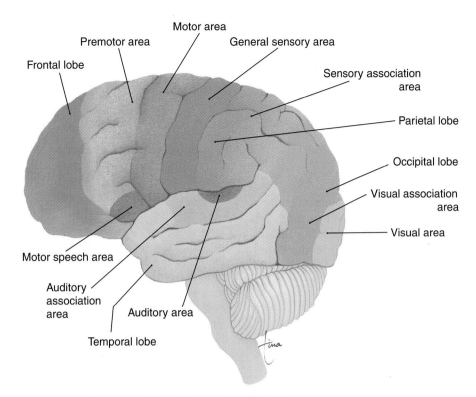

Motor area

Premotor area   General sensory area

Frontal lobe

Sensory association area

Parietal lobe

Occipital lobe

Visual association area

Visual area

Motor speech area

Auditory association area

Auditory area

Temporal lobe

FIGURE 29-1   Special sensory areas of the brain receive and interpret stimuli from the senses.

- *Thermoreceptors* in the skin detect variations in temperature.
- *Proprioceptors* in the skin, muscles, tendons, ligaments, and joint capsules coordinate input to enable us to sense the position of our body in space (proprioception).
- *Photoreceptors* located in the retina of the eyes detect visible light.
- *Chemoreceptors* for taste are located in our taste buds. Chemoreceptors for smell *(olfactory receptors)* are located in the epithelium of the nasal cavity.

Perception

Perception is the ability to interpret the impulses transmitted from the receptors and give meaning to the stimuli. After the receptors generate nerve impulses, the impulses travel along neural pathways to the spinal cord and brain. They are then relayed to specialized locations in the brain where perception of the stimuli occurs (Figure 29–1). For example, vision is perceived in the occipital lobes, hearing in the temporal lobes, and touch in the somatosensory area. Perception requires functioning of the sensory receptors, the reticular activating system, neural pathways, and brain.

Perception occurs when the person becomes conscious of the stimulus and receives the information. It would not be possible to process all the stimuli that constantly bombard us. The brain discards about 99% of all sensory information as irrelevant and unimportant.

For example, you are usually unaware of your clothing touching your body. However, if you focus on it, you can feel it.

Perception of a stimulus is affected by several factors:

- *Location* of the receptors and pathway activated
- *Number* of receptors activated
- *Frequency* of action potentials generated (which varies according to the intensity of the stimulus)
- *Changes* in location, number, and frequency

Past experiences, knowledge, and attitude also influence perception.

Arousal Mechanism

For the central nervous system to perceive, interpret, and react to incoming stimuli, it must be alert. The **reticular activating system (RAS),** located in the brainstem, controls consciousness and alertness. The neurons of the RAS make connections between the spinal cord, cerebellum, thalamus, and cerebral cortex, relaying visual, auditory, and other stimuli that help keep us awake and alert. Without such stimuli, the central nervous system (CNS) becomes lethargic, and the person may lose consciousness. Anesthesia, sedatives, opioids, and some other drugs depress the RAS, as does a darkened, quiet environment. Not surprisingly, as you will learn in Chapter 33, sleep is regulated by the RAS.

As we discussed earlier, the brain adapts to constant stimuli, such as a ticking clock. Thus, to maintain arousal, some variation in stimuli is required, such as different pieces of music or an ever-changing view. The level of stimuli needed to maintain arousal varies: Some people feel optimally alert in bright, noisy, fast-paced environments, whereas others prefer much lower levels of stimulation.

Responding to Sensations

Humans respond to sensations when they are alert and receptive to stimulation. For example, a fatigued new mother may wake up to the soft cry of her infant yet sleep through the persistent ringing of the doorbell. The response to a stimulus is based on the following factors:

- *Intensity.* An intense stimulus excites more receptors, leading to a greater response. For example, a bright, glaring light can cause you to squint and shield your eyes, whereas a dim light may cause little reaction.

- *Contrast.* Contrast is also stimulating. Imagine being outside in cold, windy weather. If you enter an unheated garage, you instantly feel warmer because the building blocks the wind. If you then go inside to a room with a blazing fireplace, you will need to take off layers of clothing rapidly because the contrast in temperature will make you feel hot.

- *Adaptation.* Often we take stimuli for granted. Have you ever taken a vacation to a remote place? Suddenly you notice the stars, quiet surroundings, and the smell of the flowers. At home you have become accustomed to your surroundings and fail to notice these things. But in a different setting, they become noticeable. Now recall your first clinical experience. Did you notice the noise and activity on the unit? Nurses become accustomed to the noise, lights, and activity and are able to "tune them out." Unfortunately, these stimuli are all new to patients, so they notice them and may have difficulty resting.

- *Previous experience.* Prior experience with a stimulus affects ongoing responses to the same stimulus. Have you ever seen a patient scrunch her eyes, grit her teeth, or turn away from an injection before you are even ready to give it? This may mean that she has had a prior negative experience with injections.

KnowledgeCheck 29–1
- What is the difference between reception and perception?
- What are the four components of a sensory experience?
- What is the role of the reticular activating system in the sensory experience?

 Go to Chapter 29, **Knowledge Check Response Sheet and Answers,** on the Electronic Study Guide.

FACTORS AFFECTING SENSORY FUNCTION

Among the many factors affecting sensory function are developmental stage, culture, health status, medications, stress level, personality, and lifestyle.

Developmental Variations

People have differing sensory perceptual abilities at different stages of life. In addition, the need for and use of sensory stimulation differs throughout life. Without adequate sensory stimulation, children may have developmental delays.

Newborns can track objects and respond to light, but their vision is far less acute than that of older children and adults. Newborn hearing is especially acute at low frequencies. Newborns can also discriminate between different tastes, and they prefer sweet over sour. They react to odors and seem to be able to discriminate between the smell of their own mother's breast milk and that of another woman. The sense of touch is keenly present at birth; the face, hands, and soles of the feet are the most sensitive (Polan & Taylor, 2003).

Infants require sensory stimulation to grow and develop. Tactile stimulation through cuddling, feeding, and soothing creates a bond between infant and caregiver, provides comfort and pleasure, and teaches the infant about the external environment. Exposure to voices, music, and ambient noise develops the auditory nervous system. By 1 year of age, the child can discriminate between different sounds and often recognize the source. Lights, colors, and contrast allow the infant to observe the world in which she lives.

In early childhood, visual acuity improves; full depth perception is achieved during the preschool period. Hearing is usually fully developed in young children; however, they may experience reversible hearing loss as a result of frequent ear infections and cerumen impaction. In contrast to toddlers, who often lose their balance when walking, older children are sure and steady on their feet.

The *school-age years and adolescence* are associated with increasing social interaction and formal education. These experiences provide a wealth of sensory stimulation.

By early *adulthood* senses are at their peak, unless they are affected by illness or injury. As the adult ages, all of the senses are affected. Table 29–1 discusses sensory changes associated with aging. Sensory decline with aging may cause withdrawal, depression, social isolation, and hallucinations.

Culture

Culture affects the nature, type, and amount of interaction and stimulation that people feel comfortable

TABLE 29-1	Sensory Function Changes with Aging

Sense	Changes Associated with Aging
Vision	Visual changes with aging include presbyopia (decreased ability to focus on close objects), decreased ability to adapt to light and dark, decreased peripheral vision, decreased tear production, and increased density of the lens.
Hearing	Hearing changes with aging include presbycusis (hearing loss of high-frequency tones) and decreased speech discrimination.
Taste	Taste buds atrophy, decreasing the ability to perceive tastes, especially sweet.
Smell	Atrophy of the olfactory bulb decreases the ability to perceive smell.
Touch	Cutaneous changes with aging decrease the ability to perceive light touch, pain, and temperature variations.
Kinesthesia	Kinesthetic changes include a decrease in muscle fibers and diminished conduction speed of nerve fibers, resulting in slowed reaction time, decreased speed and power of muscle contractions, and impaired balance.

with. Cultural values affect the amount of eye contact, distance between people, and touch people prefer. Compare the day-to-day experience of an older adult living in a remote farming community to someone living in an extended family home in the center of a large city. The amount of stimulation deemed normal would be very different for each of these people.

Assess your clients' cultural needs. For example, you may think your hospitalized patient needs quiet time alone to rest. However, if he is accustomed to being surrounded by a large family, he may actually rest better in the midst of what you perceive to be chaos. Also, use touch advisedly. For some people it is comforting; for others, it may be offensive.

Illness and Medications

Many illnesses can affect sensory reception and perception. Neurological disorders, such as multiple sclerosis, slow the transmission of nerve impulses. Diseases that affect circulation (e.g., atherosclerosis) may impair function of the sensory receptors as well as the brain, thereby altering perception and response. Some diseases affect specific sensory organs. For example, diabetic retinopathy is the leading case of blindness among adults aged 20 to 74. Hypertension, too, can damage the retina of the eyes.

Several **medications** affect sensory function. For example, aspirin and furosemide (Lasix) become ototoxic if taken for a long period of time and impair function of the auditory nerve. CNS depressants, such as opioid analgesics and sedatives, blunt reception and perception of stimuli.

Stress

Have you ever been under a lot of stress? How did it feel? When you are under stress, do you find yourself looking for or avoiding stimuli? Obviously stress provides added stimulation. As a result, a person who is bored may add stress. By setting a goal, such as running a marathon, the person undertakes a series of activities to reach that goal. In that regard, stress provides sensory stimulation at a time when the person may have been experiencing deprivation.

However, stress can cause too much stimulation. Physical illness, pain, hospitalization, tests, and surgery are all stressors that can lead to sensory overload—more stimuli than the person can handle. Jason ("Meet Your Patient") has been under tremendous physical and emotional stress as a result of his injuries and surgeries. His situation is one in which you might want to decrease unnecessary stimuli (e.g., noise, lights, too many visitors).

Personality and Lifestyle

Are you the kind of person who likes to have people around all the time? Do you thrive on noise and action? Or are you the kind of person who loves to curl up with a book and a cup of tea? Your clients also vary in their personality and lifestyle. Some people, by nature, like excitement, change, and stimulation; others prefer a more predictable and quiet life. Clients are at risk for sensory alterations if their previous level of stimuli does not match their current level. Health problems, a change of environment, or loss of a partner can each create changes in stimuli.

BOX 29-1 Signs of Sensory Deprivation and Sensory Overload

Sensory Deprivation	Sensory Overload
Irritability	Irritability
Confusion	Confusion
Reduced attention span	Reduced attention span
Decreased problem-solving ability	Decreased problem-solving ability
Drowsiness	Drowsiness (due to insomnia)
Depression	Muscle tension
Preoccupation with somatic complaints (e.g., heart palpitations)	Anxiety
	Inability to concentrate
Delusions (misinterpretations of external stimuli)	Decreased ability to perform tasks
Hallucinations (seeing, hearing, feeling, tasting, or smelling something that is not there)	Restlessness
	Disorientation

KnowledgeCheck 29–2

- Identify the major factors that affect sensory function.
- Compare and contrast the sensory changes in childhood with those in older adulthood.

 Go to Chapter 29, **Knowledge Check Response Sheet and Answers,** on the Electronic Study Guide.

SENSORY ALTERATIONS

Human beings are constantly striving to achieve **sensoristasis,** a state of optimum arousal. Sensory alterations occur when the body experiences limited stimulation (sensory deprivation), excessive stimulation (sensory overload), or meaningless stimulation.

Sensory Deprivation

Sensory deprivation is a state of RAS depression caused by a lack of meaningful stimuli. When environmental stimuli are deficient, the remaining stimuli, such as distant noises, minor pain, and cold extremities can become overly noticeable or distorted, filling in the "sensory gap" and causing the patient a level of distress that is out of proportion to the stimulus. Sensory deprivation can be caused by environmental conditions or by interference with the reception or perception of stimuli. Clinical manifestations include problems with perception, cognition, and emotion (Box 29–1).

Clients at risk for sensory deprivation include those who:

- Have impaired sensory reception (e.g., patients with neurological injury, dementia, depression, sleep deprivation, or sensory losses; and patients receiving CNS depressants).
- Cannot transmit or process stimuli (e.g., nerve or brain injury).

- Have restricted mobility.
- Have sensory (e.g., vision, hearing) deficits.
- Are confined to a nonstimulating, monotonous environment. Examples include children in orphanages, people in prison, homebound disabled and older people, patients in nursing homes and other institutions, and hospitalized patients in isolation, seclusion, or private rooms.
- Are from a different culture (because of inability to interpret received cues).

As you might expect, interventions for sensory deprivation focus on providing stimuli and supporting sensory perceptual function. They are discussed in more detail in the "Practical Knowledge" section of this chapter.

Sensory Overload

Sensory overload develops when either environmental or internal stimuli—or a combination of both—exceed a higher level than the client's sensory system can effectively process. This sometimes occurs in clients who, because of neurological or psychiatric disorders, are unable to adapt to continuing, nonmeaningful stimuli. Some clinical manifestations of sensory overload are similar to those of sensory deprivation (see Box 29–1).

Hospitalized patients often experience sensory overload due to physical discomfort in combination with anxiety, separation from loved ones, and the experience of being in the unfamiliar hospital environment. Medications that stimulate the CNS may also contribute to overload, as will substances such as caffeine and over-the-counter weight-loss pills. In addition, physical conditions that activate the CNS (e.g., hyperthyroidism) also contribute to sensory overload.

Patients at risk for sensory overload are those in an environment with excessive stimuli or more stimuli than is usual for that person. For example, a patient who lives alone in a rural environment might experience sensory overload on a busy medical-surgical unit.

KnowledgeCheck 29–3

- How does sensory deprivation occur?
- Identify five manifestations of sensory deprivation.
- How does sensory overload occur?
- Identify five manifestations of sensory overload.

  Go to Chapter 29, **Knowledge Check Response Sheet and Answers,** on the Electronic Study Guide.

CriticalThinking 29–1

Review the stories of Joshua and Richard ("Meet Your Patients"). How are these patients similar? For each patient, what factors may have contributed to his current concerns?

Sensory Deficits

Sensory deficits may stem from impaired reception, perception, or both. Of the six basic sensory deficits discussed here, impaired vision and hearing are the ones you are most likely to encounter in nursing practice. Drawing on your personal experience, think how many people you know who wear glasses or contact lenses or who wear a hearing aid. How many do you know whose vision or hearing is not completely corrected by such aids? You can see that sensory deficits are common.

A sudden onset of a deficit is unnerving and may lead to disorientation and anxiety. Gradual changes allow the person to adapt, often without even realizing it. The patient who has progressively lost hearing may, over time, keep turning up the sound on his radio and telephone and not realize that others find the sound blaring.

When there is a deficit in one sense, the other senses may become sharper to compensate. Six sensory deficits are discussed in the following sections.

Impaired Vision

Vision occurs when light rays that focus on the retina trigger a nerve impulse that is transmitted to the visual area of the brain in the occipital region. Visual deficits may result from trauma or disease of the eye, microvascular problems, or CNS disorders. Common causes of visual deficits include refractive errors, orbital trauma, cataracts, glaucoma, diabetic or hypertensive retinopathy, or loss of visual fields after stroke. Box 29–2 describes several common visual deficits. Changes in vision affect all aspects of daily living and may severely limit mobility and interaction. See Chapter 19 for detailed assessment of the eye and Figure 19–4 for an illustration of structures of the eye.

BOX 29–2 Common Visual Deficits

- **Myopia,** or nearsightedness, means that the patient is able to see close objects well but not distant objects. For example, a person with 20/200 vision can see an object from 20 feet away that a person with normal sight could see from a distance of 200 feet.

- **Hyperopia,** or farsightedness, implies that the eye sees distant objects well. A person with hyperopia may have 20/10 vision—he can see an object from 20 feet that a normal eye can see from 10 feet, however, near vision is impaired.

- **Presbyopia** is a change in vision associated with aging. The lens becomes less elastic and less able to accommodate to near objects. If you're over 40 years of age, there's a good chance you may be experiencing this problem.

- **Astigmatism** is caused by an irregular curvature of the cornea or lens that scatters light rays and blurs the image on the retina. The person has blurred vision with distortion.

- **Cataracts** are a clouding of the lens, resulting in blurred vision.

- **Glaucoma** is a type of vision loss caused by increased pressure in the anterior cavity of the eyeball that distorts the shape of the cornea and shifts the position of the lens. It can eventually lead to blindness.

- **Macular degeneration** is the loss of central vision due to damage to the *macula lutea,* the central portion of the retina. The leading cause of visual impairment in U.S. residents older than age 50, it is characterized by slow, progressive loss of central and near vision. It is usually present in both eyes.

- **Strabismus** (crossed eyes), in which one eye deviates from a fixed image, can cause permanent vision loss.

Impaired Hearing

Hearing occurs when sound waves entering the ear canal are converted to vibrations and transferred from the middle ear to the inner ear. Vibrations cause the hair cells in the cochlea to bend, generating impulses that are carried by cranial nerve VIII to the brain. The auditory area in the brain is located in the temporal lobes. The auditory area interprets the sound and allows you to determine from which direction the noise is coming. See Chapter 19, Figure 19–6 for an illustration of the structures of the ear.

Hearing deficits may result from injury or disease in structures of the ear, the nerves, or the brain. Box 29–3 presents information on hearing loss. Inability to hear decreases the ability to communicate and thus hampers social interaction. It may interfere with a patient's ability to understand instructions from healthcare professionals and create a safety hazard due to inability to hear warnings.

BOX 29-3 Common Hearing Deficits

- **Conduction deafness** results when one of the structures that transmits vibrations is affected. It may be a temporary or permanent condition caused by infection of the middle ear, a punctured tympanic membrane, or arthritis of the auditory bones.

- **Nerve deafness** occurs when there is damage to cranial nerve VIII or the receptors in the cochlea. It may result from ototoxic medications (e.g., gentamycin) or viral infections that affect cranial nerve VIII. Chronic exposure to loud noise may also lead to nerve and receptor impairment.

- **Presbycusis** is a progressive sensorineural loss associated with aging. It results from deterioration of the hair cells in the cochlea. Presbycusis leads to diminished ability to hear high-pitched sounds and to distinguish sounds in a noisy environment.

- **Central deafness** results from damage to the auditory areas in the temporal lobes. Tumor, trauma, meningitis, or CVA (cerebrovascular accident, i.e., stroke) in the temporal lobe may cause this.

- **Tinnitus** is a term used to describe ringing in the ears. Most tinnitus comes from damage to the microscopic endings of the nerve in the inner ear, for example, trauma, turbulent blood flow, hypertension, ear infection, medications, otosclerosis, or arthritic changes of the bones of the ear.

- **Impacted cerumen** is a condition in which earwax becomes tightly packed in the ear canal, blocking the canal. Patients with impacted cerumen may experience a feeling or fullness or pain, decreased hearing, or tinnitus.

- **Otosclerosis** is a hardening of the bones of the middle ear, especially the stapes. The stapes becomes fixed and leads to poor sound transmission to the inner ear. The cause of this disorder is unknown.

- **Otitis media** is a middle ear infection. It is a common childhood illness that may be caused by viruses or bacteria.

BOX 29-4 The Effects of Medications on Taste

Numerous medications affect the sense of taste. A study presented at the 2004 American Chemical Society Meeting (Zervakis & Schiffman, 2004) found that most prescription medications are foul-tasting and may have a profound affect on the sense of taste. In a test of 62 prescription medications, "bitter, sour, and metallic" described all the medications. Medications with the highest incidence of taste disturbance include the following:

- Antibiotics
- Anticonvulsants, such as phenytoin (Dilantin) and carbamazepine (Tegretol)
- Antihistamines and decongestants
- Antihypertensive and cardiac medications
- Chemotherapy agents
- Lithium carbonate (Lithobid)
- Antipsychotics
- Antidepressants
- Statins
- Muscle relaxants

Impaired Taste

Taste imparts flavor and interest to food. Taste deficits may decrease the pleasure associated with eating; weight loss and malnutrition may result.

Taste depends on the functioning of the taste buds on the tongue and, to a lesser extent, on the soft palate. Four types of taste buds exist: sweet, sour, salty, and bitter. A proposed fifth taste bud, glutamate, can detect savory flavors. The buds for sweet and salty tastes are primarily on the tip of the tongue; for sour taste, on the two lateral sides of the tongue; and for bitter taste, primarily on the posterior tongue and the soft palate. When stimulated, taste buds generate nerve impulses that travel along the facial and glossopharyngeal nerves (cranial nerves VII and IX, respectively) to the taste area in the parietal-temporal cortex. Foods stimulate different combinations of taste buds. That stimulation, together with the sense of smell, produces the vast number of tastes we can perceive.

Impaired taste most commonly results from **xerostomia** (excessively dry mouth), which may be due to the effect of medications, decreased saliva production, inadequate fluid intake, poor nutrition, or poor oral hygiene. In addition, loss of the sense of smell commonly causes loss of taste. Other causes of taste deficits include the common cold; infections of the nose, sinuses, mouth, or salivary glands; smoking; vitamin B_{12} or zinc deficiency; injury to the mouth, nose, or head; and medications. Box 29–4 discusses the effect of medications on taste.

Impaired Smell

The sense of smell is triggered when chemoreceptors in the upper nasal cavities detect vaporized chemicals. Chemoreceptors generate impulses carried by the olfactory nerve (cranial nerve I) into the olfactory area in the temporal lobes. Vaporized molecules can be detected from a far distance, so the sense of smell can serve as an early warning system for detection of smoke and noxious chemicals.

complementary and alternative modalities (CAM)

Essential Oils

Aromatherapy is the use of naturally extracted aromatic essences from plants to balance, harmonize and promote the health of body, mind and spirit. It is a natural, non-invasive treatment system designed to affect the whole person, not just the symptom or disease. It is thought to work by promoting the body's natural ability to balance, regulate, heal, and maintain itself.

The following are the top 10 essential oils used in aromatherapy:

- **Eucalyptus, *Eucalyptus globulus* or *Eucalyptus radiata*.** Helpful in treating respiratory problems, such as coughs, colds, and asthma. Also helps to boost the immune system, and relieve muscle tension.

- **Ylang Ylang, *Cananga odorata*.** Helps one to relax, and can reduce muscle tension. Good antidepressant.

- **Geranium, *Pelargonium graveolens*.** Helps to balance hormones in women, good for balancing the skin. Can be both relaxing and uplifting, as well as antidepressant.

- **Peppermint, *Mentha piperita*.** Useful in treating headaches, muscle aches, digestive disorders such as slow digestion, indigestion, and flatulence.

- **Lavender, *Lavandula angustifolia*.** Relaxing, and also useful in treating wounds, burns, and skin care.

- **Lemon, *Citrus limon*.** Very uplifting, yet relaxing. Helpful in treating wounds, infections, and house cleaning and deodorizing.

- **Clary sage, *Salvia sclarea*.** Natural pain killer, helpful in treating muscular aches and pains. Very relaxing, and can help with insomnia. Also very helpful in balancing hormones.

- **Tea tree, *Melaleuca alternifolia*.** A natural anti-fungal oil, good for treating all sorts of fungal infections including vaginal yeast infections, jock itch, athlete's foot, and ringworm. Also helps to boost the immune system.

- **Roman chamomile, *Anthemus nobilis*.** Very relaxing, and can help with sleeplessness and anxiety. Also good for muscle aches and tension. Useful in treating wounds and infection.

- **Rosemary, *Rosmarinus officinalis*.** Very stimulating and uplifting, good to help mental stimulation as well as to stimulate the immune system. Very good for muscle aches and tension. Stimulating to the digestive system.

The sense of smell is vital to the sense of taste. Recall the last time you had a cold or stuffed up nose. When the sense of smell is lost **(anosmia),** food does not taste the same. Patients who are unable to smell food lose their appetite, and nutritional deficits may result. Permanent anosmia may develop following cranial nerve damage, a tumor, or atherosclerosis. It may also be inherited and nonpathological. Zinc deficiency, heavy smoking, cocaine use, rhinitis, and sinusitis can cause reversible anosmia.

Nurses may make therapeutic use of a patient's sense of smell. **Aromatherapy,** the use of odors for therapeutic effect, has become the most widely practiced complementary therapy among nurses in the United States (Buckle, 2001). See the accompanying CAM box; also see Chapter 40 for more information about aromatherapy. Olfaction has been shown to play a role in memory, mood, and safety. See the Toward Evidence-Based Practice box for discussion of current research on smell, memory, and mood.

Impaired Tactile Perception

Touch is crucial to growth and development. It provides pleasure, warns us of injury, and communicates information about the external environment. The study in Box 29–5 investigated the effect of touch on nurses, examining how touch may decrease nurses' anxiety. The implication is that touch may affect nurses' ability to provide care for others.

The dermis of the skin contains receptors for the cutaneous sensations of light touch, pressure, heat, cold, and pain. Information from these receptors is transmitted to the sensory areas in the parietal lobes. The number of cutaneous receptors determines the sensitivity of an area and the amount of space devoted to that region in the sensory cortex area. The hands and face have the most receptors and therefore the most space in the sensory cortex.

A person's ability to perceive touch is often measured in terms of *two-point discrimination*, that is, the ability to perceive as distinct two close but separate points pressed against the skin. On the lips and fingertips, a person can normally distinguish between points less than 4 mm apart, whereas on the torso, normal two-point discrimination is over 2 cm.

Loss of tactile sensitivity can be caused by a cerebrovascular accident (stroke), brain or spinal tumor or injury, or peripheral nerve damage caused by diabetes, Guillain-Barré syndrome, or chronic alcoholism.

| toward evidence-based practice |

Herz, R.S. (2004). A naturalistic analysis of autobiographical memories triggered by olfactory visual and auditory stimuli. *Chemical Senses, 29*(3), 217–224.

Researchers at Brown University compared the effect of presenting information on three memory cue items (campfire, freshly cut grass, popcorn) in olfactory, visual, and auditory form. Results revealed that memories recalled by odors were significantly more emotional and vivid than those recalled by the same cue presented by sight or sound. However, no differences were detected in the content of the subjects' memories. Analysis revealed that age, gender, and culture did not affect results.

Moss, M., Cook, J., Wesnes, K., & Duckett, P. (2003). Aromas of rosemary and lavender essential oils differentially affect cognition and mood in healthy adults. *International Journal of Neuroscience, 113*(1), 15–38.

Researchers randomly assigned 144 participants to one of three independent groups to assess the olfactory impact of the essential oils of lavender and rosemary on cognitive performance and mood in healthy volunteers. With the participant seated in a cubicle, mood was assessed with a visual analog questionnaire. The cubicle was then infused with either lavender, rosemary, or no odor, and participants were asked to complete a computerized cognitive assessment battery. On completion of the test, mood was assessed again using the same visual analog questionnaire. Participants were deceived as to the true aim of the study until the testing was completed.

Results indicated that lavender produced a significant decline in performance of working memory and impaired reaction times for both memory- and attention-based tasks compared to controls. In contrast, rosemary produced a significant improvement in overall quality of memory but also impaired speed of memory compared to controls.

Following the completion of the cognitive assessment test, both the control and lavender groups were significantly less alert than the rosemary group; however, the control group was significantly less content than both the rosemary and lavender groups.

---

1. What implications, if any, do these studies have for nursing care?

2. What has been your experience with aromatherapy? Would you consider using it in the clinical setting? Why or why not?

 Go to Chapter 29, **Toward Evidence-Based Practice Suggested Responses,** on the Electronic Study Guide.

BOX 29–5   The Effect of Touch on Nurses

McElligott, D., Holz, M. B., Carollo, L., Somerville, S., Baggett, M., Kuzniewski. S., & Shi, Q. (2003). A pilot feasibility study of the effects of touch therapy on nurses. *Journal of the New York State Nurses Association, 34*(1), 16–24.

This pilot study examined the effect of touch therapy on relaxation and anxiety in staff nurses in a prospective, randomized, blinded clinical trial, with a convenience sample of 24 nurses working 12-hour shifts.

Quantitative Phase of the Study

- Intervention: touch (massage) therapy
- Outcome variables:

    Relaxation, measured by physiological parameters

    Anxiety, measured by a visual analog scale

- Results:

    Both groups demonstrated decreased anxiety.

    The experimental (massage) group showed greater differences between pre-and post-treatment anxiety scores.

The mean change in physiological parameters between groups was not significant.

Qualitative Phase of the Study

Each participant was interviewed at the completion of the study. Themes derived from the interviews included the following:

- Importance of touch in nursing care
- Stress reduction
- Increased self-awareness
- Need for self-care
- New understanding of the mind-body connection

Discussion

Massage therapy was associated with subjective reports of decreased anxiety. However, relaxation was not demonstrated by physiological measures. Participants qualitatively verified the importance of touch in nursing and self-care.

CriticalThinking 29–2

- Why do you think a person with impaired tactile perception is at risk for injury?
- Speculate as to the possible nature of injuries that might occur.

Impaired Kinesthetic Sense

Kinesthesia, or muscle sense, is a complex process involving **propioceptors** that detect stretch in muscles to create a mental picture of how the body is positioned. Conscious muscle sense is perceived in the parietal lobes. Unconscious muscle sense occurs in the cerebellum, which coordinates movement.

Problems of the inner ear commonly impair kinesthesia. The vestibular apparatus of the inner ear has hair cells that detect rotation or acceleration of the body and thus are essential for kinesthesia. Because the vestibular cell nuclei also receive input from neurons involved in vision, a mismatch between the position or acceleration of the head and the visual field can result in motion sickness. This is why it is not advisable to read a book or map while riding in a car traveling on a winding road.

Parkinson's disease, other neurological disorders, tumors, cerebrovascular accident, and even certain medications can impair kinesthesia. Kinesthetic deficits place the patient at risk for balance and coordination problems and falls. Box 29–6 highlights activities that enhance proprioception.

KnowledgeCheck 29–4

- Discuss the difference between myopia and hyperopia.
- What is the difference between conduction deafness and nerve deafness?
- Identify three factors that may impair the sense of taste.
- How is the sense of smell triggered?
- What areas of the body have the greatest number of tactile receptors?
- What type of health concerns may be generated by kinesthetic deficits?

Go to Chapter 29, **Knowledge Check Response Sheet and Answers,** on the Electronic Study Guide.

 CriticalThinking 29–3

Imagine that you are experiencing sensory deficits. Which deficits would you find most challenging?

Practical Knowledge
knowing how

As a nurse, you should always consider your client's sensory perceptual status. Sensory deficits and excess or inadequate stimulation have a significant influence

---

BOX 29–6 **Activities to Enhance Proprioception**

Kinesthesia, or muscle sense, is enhanced by activities that tone muscles and increase coordination. These activities are helpful for individuals of any age. Examples include the following:

- Rhythmic movement (e.g., tai chi, dance, yoga)
- Aerobic activities, such as walking, running, or bicycling
- Strength training, such as weight-bearing exercise or use of light weights
- Flexibility activities, such as stretching
- Balance conditioning with eyes open and closed
- Putting joints through full range of motion, especially rotational movements

---

on quality of life and may be especially troublesome for institutionalized clients.

| Assessment |

Assessment of sensory perception includes the following items (see Chapter 19):

- Factors affecting sensory perception
- Mental status
- Recent changes in sensory stimulation
- Use of sensory aids
- The client's environment
- The support network
- Focused examination of vision, hearing, taste, smell, touch, and balance

Nursing History

In your nursing interview, you will assess the client's usual and current state of sensory function, as well as gather a history of sensory problems and use of sensory aids. In addition to interviewing the client and family, assess the environment and patient situation for factors that may alter sensory function. This section provides a brief overview of each of those items. For complete guidelines,

 Go to Chapter 29, **Assessment Guidelines and Tools, Nursing History: Sensory Perceptual Status,** in Volume 2.

Assess Changes in Sensory Function

To assess changes in sensory function, you will need to obtain a history of the client's usual sensory function

as well as information about the client's current status. For a list of questions you can use for this purpose,

 Go to Chapter 29, **Assessment Guidelines and Tools, Nursing History: Sensory Perceptual Status,** in Volume 2.

Assess Risk Factors for Impaired Sensory Perception

You should perform a comprehensive assessment for any client at increased risk for sensory alterations: older adults, clients with limited mobility, clients who are bedbound or homebound, clients in intensive care units, and clients with known sensory deficits, especially if the change has been acute. Routinely assess developmental level, health status, medications, stress and coping mechanisms, personality, and lifestyle.

Assess Mental Status

Sensory alterations may trigger changes in mental status, and altered mental status can interfere with sensory perception. A check of mental status includes assessment of behavior, appearance, response to stimuli, speech, memory, and judgment. Normal findings include an ability to express and explain realistic thoughts with clear speech, follow directions, listen, answer questions, and recall significant past events. For a guide for assessing mental status,

 Go to Chapter 19, **Technique 19–6,** in Volume 2.

You can assess many of those factors as you interact with the client. For example, if you have asked the client the questions covered in the previous section, you have already formed an impression about his appearance, speech, ability to express himself, and other facets of mental status. In addition, you must specifically assess the client's level of orientation. Chapter 19 presents additional discussion of mental status screening and orientation. See Table 19–5 for a tool for describing level of consciousness.

Assess Use of Sensory Aids

Sensory aids are devices that assist with sensory function. They include glasses, contact lenses, hearing aids, canes, and walkers. For sample interview questions,

 Go to Chapter 29, **Assessment Guidelines and Tools, Nursing History: Sensory Perceptual Status,** in Volume 2.

Assess the Environment

The environment is an important source of stimulation. Consider how different the environment is for Joshua and Richard ("Meet Your Patients"). Joshua is in a crowded space with lights and noise 24 hours per day. He has had a number of invasive procedures and is most likely receiving pain medication. In contrast, Richard is in a quiet room with little exposure to light, noise, or touch. As Joshua's and Richard's situations demonstrate, a healthcare environment can have too much or too little stimuli. As part of your assessment, assess how the client is responding to the conditions of the environment.

- *Compare your data about the client's personality and lifestyle with the current environmental situation.* In healthcare facilities, patients are subjected to lights, noises, and odors that cause them anxiety. They may hear others who are crying out in pain. For most, the environment is substantially different from anything they are used to. A patient from a small, quiet environment may become overwhelmed and develop sensory overload in a hospital setting. Even a client used to a rapid-paced lifestyle may experience overload if he is also subjected to pain, nausea, dizziness, or other manifestations of illness. In contrast, a client used to an active life may find the hospital setting boring.
- *Assess the effect of the environment on sensory deficits.* For example, for a patient with age-related hearing changes, the background noise of the healthcare environment may make it difficult to hear voices. A patient with visual deficits or impaired balance will often modify his home environment to allow optimal function; however, when the patient is in an institution, these aids are no longer present. To assist the patient, you must determine which environmental factors make his deficits worse and which situations help to compensate.

Assess the Support Network

For a client with a sensory deficit, his support network may serve as a buffer or a hindrance. For example, an older adult with macular degeneration has progressive loss of vision. If he lives alone, the effect of the visual loss will be quite different from what it would be if he lived with an extended family. Support persons may help the client to adapt to deficits by assuming chores that the client can no longer perform or by providing comfort to the client so that he is less distressed by the sensory losses.

A support network can also be influential when clients are experiencing sensory deprivation or overload. Recall that Richard ("Meet Your Patients") has no visitors. What influence do you think frequent visits by family members would have on Richard? If you say that Richard would receive more stimulation and may not be sensory deprived, you are correct. Family members can also help clients who are confused from sensory alterations by reorienting and calming the client.

Physical Examination

Physical assessment of sensory function requires assessment of the six senses.

 Go to Chapter 19, **Procedure 19–16: Assessing the Sensory-Neurological System, Procedure 19–6: Assessing the Eyes,** and **Procedure 19–7: Assessing the Ears and Hearing,** in Volume 2.

For a bedside assessment that you can use to easily assess sensory function,

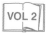 Go to Chapter 29, **Assessment Guidelines and Tools, Bedside Assessment of Sensory Function,** in Volume 2.

KnowledgeCheck 29–5

- Identify six areas that you should assess for a client with known or suspected sensory alterations.
- What factors must be evaluated when it is known that a client uses a sensory aid?
- Identify at least two ways that you can assess vision and hearing deficits at the bedside.

 Go to Chapter 29, **Knowledge Check Response Sheet and Answers,** on the Electronic Study Guide.

CriticalThinking 29–4

How would you assess Joshua and Richard ("Meet Your Patients") for sensory alterations? You may need to review the "Meet Your Patients" scenario at the beginning of this chapter to answer this question.

| Nursing Diagnosis |

NANDA International (2005) identifies the following diagnostic labels for use with sensory-perceptual problems:

- *Disturbed Sensory Perception (specify): Visual, auditory, kinesthetic, gustatory, tactile, olfactory* is a change in the amount or patterning of incoming stimuli accompanied by a diminished, exaggerated, distorted, or impaired response to such stimuli. Use this diagnosis when there is excessive or insufficient environmental stimuli or when the patient has altered sensory reception, transmission, and/or integration; biochemical or electrolyte imbalances; or psychological stress.

- *Acute Confusion* is the abrupt onset of a cluster of global, transient changes and disturbances in attention, cognition, psychomotor activity, level of consciousness, and/or sleep/wake cycle. This diagnosis may be used for clients experiencing delirium, severe pain, sleep deprivation, dementia, or intoxication associated with alcohol or drug use.

- *Chronic Confusion* is the irreversible, long-standing, and/or progressive deterioration of intellect and personality characterized by decreased ability to interpret environmental stimuli and decreased capacity for intellectual thought processes. It is manifested by disturbances of memory, orientation, and behavior. This diagnosis may be used for clients with Alzheimer's disease, Korsakoff's psychosis, multi-infarct dementia, cerebrovascular accident, and head injury.

- *Impaired Environmental Interpretation Syndrome* is a consistent lack of orientation to person, place, time, or circumstances over more than 3 to 6 months, necessitating a protective environment. This diagnosis includes, but is broader than, Chronic Confusion. It also includes Impaired Memory and inability to reason and concentrate. It often accompanies depression, Huntington's disease, and dementia.

- *Impaired Memory* is the inability to remember or recall bits of information or behavioral skills. Impaired memory may be attributed to pathophysiological or situational causes; it may be either temporary or permanent. Impaired memory may be seen with fluid and electrolyte imbalance, excessive environmental disturbances, certain medications, or age-related changes.

- *Risk for Peripheral Vascular Dysfunction* can be used when the patient is at risk for disruption in circulation, sensation, or motion of an extremity. Risk factors include trauma, orthopedic surgery, vascular obstruction, burns, immobilization, and mechanical compression (e.g., from a tourniquet, cast, or restraint).

- *Unilateral Neglect* is a lack of awareness and attention to one side of the body. It is manifested by consistent inattention to stimuli on the affected side and may be caused by neurological illness or trauma, one-sided blindness, and effects of other disturbed perceptual abilities.

Disturbed Sensory Perception may also be the etiology of other nursing diagnoses. Examples include the following:

- Risk for Falls related to visual impairment
- Risk for Injury related to reduced tactile sensation
- Self-Care Deficit: Total, related to kinesthetic impairment
- Impaired Home Maintenance Management related to visual impairment
- Deficient Diversional Activity related to reluctance to be in social situations because of hearing impairment
- Imbalanced Nutrition: Less Than Body Requirements related to loss of appetite secondary to impaired taste

- Anxiety related to history of unsteady gait and falls
- Social isolation related to embarrassment about Impaired Memory

| Planning Outcomes/Evaluation |

For *NOC standardized outcomes* associated with sensory perception diagnoses,

Go to Chapter 29, **Standardized Language, Selected NOC Outcomes and NIC Interventions for Sensory Perceptual Nursing Diagnoses,** in Volume 2.

Individualized goals/outcomes statements you might write for a client with Disturbed Sensory Perception include the following:

- Compensates for visual impairment by maximizing the use of touch and hearing.
- Verbalizes the importance of eating nutritious foods, despite the fact that they "taste funny."
- Demonstrates proper use of her hearing aid.
- Participates in at least one unit activity daily.

As always, use the goals and outcomes you write to evaluate the client's responses to nursing interventions. The outcomes focus your data collection; comparing the new data against the outcomes allows you to determine patient progress.

| Planning Interventions/Implementation |

For *NIC standardized interventions* associated with sensory perception nursing diagnoses,

Go to Chapter 29, **Standardized Language, Selected NOC Outcomes and NIC Interventions for Sensory Perceptual Nursing Diagnoses,** in Volume 2.

Specific nursing activities to address sensory perception problems are based on the nursing diagnosis chosen, especially on its etiology. Common nursing activities are discussed in the following sections.

Promoting Optimal Sensory Function

Optimal sensory function requires periodic health screening along with early identification and treatment of health problems. Comprehensive health care is the ideal approach, because sensory problems are often related to other health disorders. For example, to protect his vision, a client with hypertension needs to have periodic eye examinations as well as to control his blood pressure. See the Self-Care box on page 693 for information to teach your clients about self-care to promote their vision and hearing. For additional information on health promotion and health screening, see Chapter 41.

Preventing Sensory Deprivation

As a nurse, you are responsible for interventions to prevent sensory deprivation. If your assessment indicates that the client is at risk for sensory deprivation, include that information in the nursing care plan, along with specific strategies for prevention. Be sure to communicate this information to unlicensed assistive personnel (UAPs) so they can participate in this aspect of care.

- Help the patient with glasses or a hearing aid to apply the assistive device whenever she is not sleeping or resting. This will allow the patient to receive stimuli. Make sure glasses are clean and in good repair. Check that the hearing aid has working batteries and the sound is set at the appropriate level.
- Make regular contact with the patient. Introduce yourself, and address the patient by name. If the patient is disoriented, provide information at each visit. For example, "Good morning, Mr. Booker. My name is Elsa. I am the registered nurse taking care of you this morning. It is a few minutes after eight in the morning. I'm going to take your blood pressure and get you ready for breakfast."
- Explain all procedures and care you provide to the client. This will decrease anxiety, help orient confused clients, and allow for more stimulation.
- Include the use of touch in your care of the client. You may want to hold a client's hand while talking or provide a back rub with morning and bedtime care. Adjust the amount of touch you provide according to the client's reaction. Gentle hand massage may be effective in calming agitated clients.
- Provide continuity of care by assigning the same personnel whenever possible.
- Hang a message board in the room. Ask family members to post photos, cards, or notes.
- Hang a calendar in the room, along with a schedule of activities. A large clock on the wall is also helpful.
- Provide visual stimulation through artwork on the walls, colorful pajamas and robes, pictures, or flowers.
- A television or radio in the room may provide meaningful stimulation. Teach assistive personnel to choose appropriate music and programs for the client. Inappropriate choices (e.g., cartoons with laugh tracks) offer meaningless stimulation and may lead to sensory deprivation.
- Unless the patient objects, open curtains during the daytime to allow sunlight to enter the room. Avoid keeping the patient in a dark room, except to promote sleep.
- Encourage clients to have some form of social interaction. Encourage long-term care clients to participate in scheduled activities. Assist acute-care clients

Teaching Your Client About Sensory Perceptual Health

Vision

- Work with your primary healthcare provider to control conditions such as hypertension and diabetes.

- Have regular eye examinations and vision screening: every 2 to 4 years if you are aged 40 through 64; every 1 to 2 years if you: (1) have a family history of glaucoma or serious eye injury, (2) are of African ancestry, (3) are taking steroids, or (4) are over 65 years of age.

- Have your prescriptions for glasses or contact lenses reviewed at each screening and updated if needed.

- Call your healthcare provider for prompt examination if you have eye pain, discharge, a change in vision, or bleeding.

- Be sure that visual screening is done at your child's elementary school. If not, consult your pediatrician or other care provider. Your infants or preschoolers should be screened at their routine office visits.

- If you are pregnant, obtain early and adequate prenatal care to prevent danger of premature birth and exposure of the newborn to high-volume oxygen.

- Keep sharp or pointed tools (e.g., scissors) out of reach of infants, toddlers, and preschoolers.

- Teach children to walk carefully when carrying pointed tools or other objects.

- Teach children to stay away from projectile activities, such as lawn-mowing.

- Keep the child away from firearms and fireworks.

- Insist that your child use eye protection when playing sports such as tennis or baseball.

- Insist that children wear helmets when skating or riding bicycles and that teenagers wear helmets when riding motorcycles.

- For children who wear glasses, be sure the lenses are made of shatterproof safety glass.

Hearing

- If you are pregnant, obtain early prenatal care, avoid ototoxic drugs, and be sure you are tested for syphilis and rubella (German measles). Avoid anyone you suspect may have rubella.

- Auditory screening is often performed in elementary school; however, most adults do not have their hearing regularly screened. If you work in an area with a high noise level, you should have your hearing checked regularly. Early detection may prevent hearing loss.

- Children with frequent ear infections require evaluation to determine whether hearing loss has occurred.

- Middle and older adults may begin to experience difficulty distinguishing voices in a crowd or hearing the television or radio. These are indications of hearing loss and should be evaluated; you may need a hearing aid.

- Hearing loss is not a "natural part of aging."

Taste

Dental health is an important aspect of maintaining taste. Decayed teeth, gum disease, and other disorders of the mouth may affect the ability to taste. Have your teeth cleaned and examined at least yearly. You may need additional dental work to promote oral health.

---

out of bed for meals or visits from family and friends. Staff members can visit at intervals or encourage clients to leave their rooms.

- Teach patients to provide their own stimulation by counting, singing, reading, or reciting poetry.

- Develop alternative methods of communication when interacting with clients with aphasia or who speak another language. Communication boards, a magic slate, pictures, or writing may be helpful.

- Encourage family members to bring in familiar objects from home.

- Consider using pet therapy. Many facilities have resident pets or can arrange to have pets visit. A singing bird may delight a bedbound resident. In long-term care facilities, resident cats often favor

bedbound clients for their frequent naps. Pet therapy increases socialization, decreases loneliness, and decreases blood pressure (Hooker, Freeman, & Stewart, 2002).

- Carefully monitor the use of sedating medications that may contribute to sensory deprivation.

- Collaborate with other healthcare team members in caring for clients with sensory deprivation. Music therapy, activities, physical therapy, speech therapy, nutritional therapy, and occupational therapy may all be valuable in the care of the client.

- Stimulate the senses with smells such as fruits and flowers. Pleasant smells may stimulate appetite.

- When at all possible, avoid isolating the patient. Ensure that any patient in isolation receives adequate

stimulation from nurses, family members, or assistive personnel.

Ideally you will use these activities to prevent sensory deprivation. However, these same activities are also used in the care of clients who have been diagnosed with sensory deprivation.

 CriticalThinking 29–5

Which of the strategies to treat sensory deprivation would be most appropriate for Richard ("Meet Your Patients")?

Preventing Sensory Overload

Sensory overload is sometimes an unfortunate outcome of hospitalization. To prevent or treat sensory overload, consider the following strategies.

- Introduce yourself when meeting the client. Address the client by name.
- Minimize unnecessary light and noise. Instruct assistive personnel to be aware of appropriate noise and light levels, especially at night.
- Use radio and TV appropriately. Choose programs to meet the client's interests. Do not leave the TV or radio on 24 hours a day.
- Establish a schedule for care. Plan care to provide uninterrupted periods of sleep and rest. A schedule will prevent unnecessary interruptions during rest periods and will provide the client with advance notice of what to expect during the day. Instruct assistive personnel in the importance of allowing the patient adequate rest and the need to avoid interruptions.
- Speak in a moderate tone of voice, using a calm and confident manner.
- Do not speak about the client to others in his presence.
- Control pain and nausea with ordered medications.
- If possible, provide a private room and limit visitors. Reduce unessential tasks by other health team members.
- Teach clients about stress reduction techniques. Relaxation tapes that promote visualization and deep-breathing techniques are available. Tapes with soothing music are also suitable.
- Reduce noxious odors by promptly emptying commodes and bedpans, removing meal trays, using deodorant sprays, and keeping wounds covered.
- Provide a calm presence. Observe for the client's reaction to environmental stimuli. Remove annoying or bothersome stimuli if possible.
- Consider the use of earplugs for the client.

 CriticalThinking 29–6

Review the scenario of Joshua, the young ICU patient with sensory overload ("Meet Your Patients").

- Which sensory overload strategies would be most appropriate for an ICU patient?
- Which would be least likely to be successful or not feasible based on the setting?

Provide rationale for your choices. You may need to visit an ICU or talk with classmates who have been to ICU to answer this question.

Caring for Clients with Sensory Deficits

Regardless of the primary medical diagnosis, when a client has a sensory deficit you may need to modify your approach to the client or alter the environment. The specific interventions depend on the type of deficit (i.e., visual, hearing, olfactory, taste, tactile, kinesthetic, and altered mental status). Describe the sensory deficits on the nursing care plan, along with strategies to deal with them. For example, if the patient recovering from an abdominal surgery has no vision out of his left eye, nursing orders should specify to approach the patient from the right.

Interventions for Disturbed Sensory Perception (Visual)

Visual deficits range from minor problems, such as the need for corrective lenses, to complete blindness. Surgical procedures of the eye may cause temporary visual problems. Problems that limit movement of the head may limit peripheral vision but have no effect on central vision. To provide care for the client with visual deficits, you will need to fully describe the scope of the deficit on the care plan.

For the client with sight, your interventions focus on enhancing vision:

- Place eyeglasses within easy reach.
- Make sure eyeglasses are clean, in good repair, and of the proper prescription. For information on caring for contact lenses, see Chapter 22. Also,

 Go to Chapter 22, **Procedure 22–12,** in Volume 2.

- Provide sufficient light, but avoid glare by using soft, diffuse lighting.
- Provide sunglasses, visors, or hats with brims when the patient is outdoors.
- A magnifying lens or large-print books and magazines may be helpful for clients with presbyopia.
- A client with significant visual impairment should be evaluated for ability to drive. Many people resist

giving up driving privileges, because this severely limits their lifestyle. However, poor vision places the driver, passengers, pedestrians, and other drivers at risk for harm.

If the client uses a seeing-eye dog, do not distract the dog. A seeing-eye dog in a harness is working and should be approached only with the owner's permission. For suggestions for communicating with a client who is blind or has limited sight,

 Go to Chapter 29, **Technique 29–1: Communicating with Visually Impaired Clients,** in Volume 2.

Interventions for Disturbed Sensory Perception (Auditory)

A hearing impairment can limit communication and place the client at risk for social isolation. In addition, clients with impaired hearing are unable to receive warnings. This places them at risk for injury (e.g., they may not hear a fire alarm). Your nursing interventions should focus on supporting auditory function, improving communication, and creating a safer environment.

Supporting Auditory Function

If the client has a hearing aid, check to make sure that it is working properly, the batteries are functional, and the sound is adjusted to a comfortable level for the client. Encourage your client to wear her hearing aid as much as possible. A significant number of people with hearing impairment do not wear hearing aids. To review care of a hearing aid,

 Go to Chapter 22, **Technique 22–3,** in Volume 2.

Closed-caption television allows the client to read the dialogue and continue to enjoy his favorite shows or stay current with the news. For telephones, consider sound amplification or conversion to text-telephone service. Some clients may also be candidates for hearing aid dog service.

Cerumen impaction is a common cause of conduction hearing loss. Regular inspection of the ear canals will detect this problem. See the accompanying Critical Aspects box for key information on otic irrigation for cerumen impaction. For the complete steps,

 Go to Chapter 29, **Procedure 29–1: Performing Otic Irrigation,** in Volume 2.

Improving Communication

For a client with hearing impairment, provide written instructions to ensure that she understands the

---

critical aspects of procedure 29–1

Otic Irrigation

 For steps to follow in *all* procedures, refer to inside back cover of Volume 2.

- Warm the irrigating solution to body temperature.
- Assist the patient into a sitting or lying position, with the head tilted away from the affected ear.
- Straighten the ear canal by pulling up and back on the pinna. For a young child, pull down and back to straighten the canal.
- Instruct the patient to notify you if he experiences any pain or dizziness during the irrigation.
- Place the tip of the nozzle (or syringe) into the entrance of the ear canal, and direct the stream of irrigating solution gently along the top of the ear canal toward the back of the client's head.
- Continue irrigating until the canal is clean.

---

teaching and instructions. For additional suggestions for communicating with hearing-impaired persons,

 Go to Chapter 29, **Technique 29–2: Communicating with Hearing-Impaired Clients,** in Volume 2.

Promoting Safety

Suggest that your client modify her home environment. For example, install blinking lights that alert the person to an incoming phone call or the ring of a doorbell. Blinking alarm clocks, burglar alarms, and smoke detectors are also available. For institutionalized patients, keep background noise to a minimum, and keep a call bell within easy reach of the patient.

KnowledgeCheck 29–6

- Identify three safety measures that may be used with clients with visual impairment.
- Identify three safety measures that may be used with clients with hearing impairment.

 Go to Chapter 29, **Knowledge Check Response Sheet and Answers,** on the Electronic Study Guide.

Interventions for Disturbed Sensory Perception (Olfactory)

An impaired sense of smell diminishes taste and denies the client the pleasure of enjoying food. This often leads to weight loss. Home safety issues are also a concern for the client who cannot smell. Measures to

Sensory Deficits—Safety and Health Measures

To promote safety and health, instruct clients in the following points:

Visual Deficits

- Do not use throw rugs on the floors.
- Keep spaces uncluttered.
- Do not rearrange furniture.

Hearing Deficits

- Install blinking lights that alert the person to an incoming call or the ring of a doorbell.
- Install blinking alarm clocks, burglar alarms, and smoke detectors.

Olfactory Deficits

- Have gas appliances regularly inspected and maintained to prevent gas leaks.
- Check smoke detectors and replace batteries regularly.
- If you cannot detect food spoilage by smell or taste, date foods and inspect them for any evidence of spoilage. Spoilage usually causes changes in the color and consistency of canned, fresh, or leftover foods.

Gustatory Deficits

- Perform frequent oral hygiene to encourage appetite and enhance the sense of taste.
- Enhance the meal experience by concentrating on the visual appeal of the meal, the plates, and the dinner table.
- Avoid bland, overcooked food. Use spices liberally unless they are contraindicated.
- Vary food texture, color, and temperature to provide more interest.

Tactile Deficits

- Use a bath thermometer to monitor water temperature and prevent burns.
- Change position frequently to relieve pressure on bony prominences.
- Use properly fitting shoes and socks.
- Immediately report any signs of circulatory impairment (e.g., declining motor function, cool temperature, gray-blue coloration).
- Inspect daily for open areas, cuts, abrasions, or areas of redness.

---

protect the client with olfactory impairment are found in the accompanying Home Care box.

Interventions for Disturbed Sensory Perception (Gustatory)

Many people find great pleasure in life from the different tastes of food. Without the gustatory sense, a client may eat less and be at risk for nutritional deficits and weight loss. If the client has lost weight, be sure to check the fit of any dentures or dental appliances. Weight changes may affect their fit and make it even harder to eat.

For hospitalized clients, provide frequent oral hygiene. Assess for sores or open areas in the mouth. These require prompt treatment because they may become infected and further deteriorate the sense of taste. Teach clients to eat foods separately or drink water between bites to distinguish the taste of the food more readily. Seasonings, salt substitutes, spices, or lemon may improve the taste of foods and encourage the client's appetite. For home care suggestions, refer to the Home Care box.

Interventions for Disturbed Sensory Perception (Tactile)

Clients with peripheral vascular disease, spinal cord injury, diabetes, cerebrovascular accident, trauma, or

fractures are at risk for diminished tactile sensation. These clients may not notice a cut or wound in an area with limited sensation. For institutionalized patients, inspect the affected area daily. Look for open areas, cuts, abrasions, or areas of erythema. Any of these findings requires care. Also see the Home Care box.

If the patient consents, you can stimulate the sense of touch by brushing his hair, giving a back rub, or touching him when giving care. You may need to use firm pressure for him to feel the touch. Frequent turning and positioning may also help. Some patients are overly sensitive to touch. In those instances, you must minimize irritating stimuli: Use a bed cradle, and keep bed linens loose to keep them off the skin as much as possible.

Interventions for Confused Clients

Confusion can be temporary or permanent. Confusion is an aspect of both delirium and dementia. **Delirium** is an acute, reversible state of confusion caused by medications and a variety of physiological processes, such as hypoxia, metabolic disturbances, infection, or sensory alterations. It may be accompanied by changes in the level of consciousness. In contrast, **dementia** is a chronic and progressive deterioration in mental function caused by physical changes in the brain.

Your nursing care should promote reorientation and decrease anxiety. Following are several techniques that may be useful. Notice that several are the same as the interventions for preventing sensory deficit.

- Introduce yourself each time you meet with the client. Wear a readable (large, plain type) name tag to reinforce your introduction.
- State the client's name each time you interact with him.
- Identify the day, date, and time as you interact with the client. Provide calendars and clocks that are easily visible.
- Provide visual clues to time, such as opening the drapes during the day and closing them at night.
- Face the client when you communicate.
- Take an unhurried approach to communication. Speak calmly, simply, and directly, and allow adequate time for the client to answer any questions you raise.
- Use short sentences with few words: "It's bath time," rather than, "Let's go have a bath and get you all nice and clean for visitors."
- Do not offer too many choices. Doing so confuses the patient.
- A person with dementia is often anxious, worried, and fearful. Find ways to make the person feel more secure and comfortable before you begin focusing on the content of your communication. For example, gently hold or pat the patient's hand.
- Try to respond to the person's feelings instead of the content of his words. This helps to reassure the person. For example, if a woman is constantly searching for her husband, don't say, "Your husband is not here." Rather, say, "You must miss your husband," or "Tell me about your husband."
- Realize that the person is probably distressed and is doing the best he can. Be affectionate, reassuring, and calm, even when things make no sense.
- If the person has difficulty finding the right word, supply it for him unless it upsets him. This helps keep him from becoming frustrated.
- If you do not understand what the patient is trying to say, ask him to point to it or describe it (e.g., "What does a zishmer look like?").
- Place personal objects, photos, and mementos in the client's immediate environment. Discuss the personal objects with the client.
- Establish a routine for care. Assign the same caregivers each day.

- Provide simple explanations for all care and treatments.
- Consider using alternative therapy, such as music therapy.
- Encourage the patient to participate in familiar activities.
- Maintain a safe environment. For example, store medications away from the patient's reach, keep doors and windows closed securely to prevent wandering, and use bed or chair monitors.

Interventions for Unconscious Clients

The unconscious client is unable to interact with you but requires reality orientation nevertheless. In addition to some of the preceding suggestions, you should include the patient's support persons in the care. Teach them the necessary strategies. Also incorporate more touch into the plan of care.

Safety measures are a priority for unconscious clients. Keep the bed in low position when you are not at the bedside, and keep the siderails up. If the patient's blink reflex is absent or her eyes do not close totally, you may need to give frequent eye care to keep secretions from collecting along the lid margins. The eyes may be patched to prevent corneal drying, and lubricating eye drops may be ordered.

KnowledgeCheck 29–7

- What are the major concerns associated with loss of smell and taste?
- What safety measures should be taught to a client with tactile impairment?
- How can you best assist a client who is confused?

 Go to Chapter 29, **Knowledge Check Response Sheet and Answers,** on the Electronic Study Guide.

 CriticalThinking 29–7

What types of interventions would be most appropriate for Joshua and Richard ("Meet Your Patients")—that is, interventions for sensory deficits, sensory deprivation, sensory overload, or confusion?

 Go to Chapter 29, **Resources for Caregivers and Health Professionals,** on the Electronic Study Guide.

 Suggested Readings: Go to Chapter 29, **Reading More About Sensory Perception,** on the Electronic Study Guide.

 **Bibliography:** Go to Volume 2, Bibliography.

30 Pain Management

Learning Outcomes

After completing this chapter, you should be able to:

* Define pain.

* Classify pain according to origin, cause, duration, and quality.

* Describe the physiological changes that occur with pain.

* Discuss two physiological mechanisms involved in pain modulation.

* Discuss factors that influence pain.

* Identify the effect of unrelieved pain on each of the body systems.

* Discuss nonpharmacological pain relief measures.

* Describe pharmacological measures, including nonopioid analgesics, opioid analgesics, and adjuvant analgesics.

* Describe chemical and surgical pain relief measures.

* Explain why pain should be considered the fifth vital sign.

* Identify the steps involved in creating a pain management program for a client.

* Write an individualized goal for a client with a nursing diagnosis of Acute Pain.

* Explain how to use a patient-controlled analgesia (PCA) system.

* Describe a method for evaluating a pain management program.

Your Patient

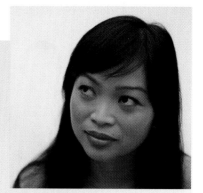

As a special experience, your instructor has arranged for you to spend a half-day in the intensive care unit (ICU). As you enter the ICU, you are a little apprehensive. Your patient today is a 23-year-old Asian woman who was in an automobile accident yesterday and sustained chest and abdominal injuries. You walk into the room with your clinical instructor to meet your patient, Miss Eunice Chu Ling. She was taken to the operating room during the night to have her spleen removed. She is intu-bated (has an endo-tracheal tube in her airway that is con-nected to a ventilator), has an intravenous line running, and a chest tube on the left side that is draining bloody fluid. Her parents and siblings are in the room sitting rigidly in the chairs smiling at you. Miss Chu Ling is awake and grimacing. You want to ask her if is she is in pain, but she cannot speak.

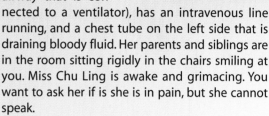

Theoretical Knowledge
knowing why

Many of us enter nursing to relieve suffering and promote healing. Pain is one of the most distressing symptoms we deal with, yet it is the most frequent reason people seek medical attention (Joint Commission on Accreditation of Healthcare Organizations [JCAHO], 2000). Nurses are often considered the "cornerstone of pain management" (Wright & Bell, 2001); thus, it is crucial that you gain solid theoretical knowledge of what pain is and why it occurs.

WHAT IS PAIN?

The International Association for the Study of Pain (IASP) and the American Pain Society define pain as "an unpleasant sensory or emotional experience associated with actual or potential tissue damage, or described in terms of such damage" (APS, 1992, p. 16; Mersky & Bogduk, 1994, p. 971). Although this definition provides an excellent foundation for our discussion of pain, as a nurse, you will also need to understand the holistic dimensions of the pain experience.

Pain can cause sleep loss, irritability, cognitive impairment, functional impairment, and immobility, and thus it can be destructive to the patient and family. Although we usually think of pain in this negative context, pain is also protective, warning us of potential injury to the body. Recall the last time you touched a hot object with your bare hand. Undoubtedly you quickly pulled your hand away when you felt discomfort. Without the ability to sense pain, you might have developed a burn. Pain can also prompt us to change our actions: After we have been sitting at the computer for a while, muscle pain may prompt us to get up and stretch or go out for a walk; or the gastrointestinal discomfort we experience after overeating may remind us to eat more moderately in the future.

Pain is also a multidimensional experience, affecting and being affected by nearly every other aspect of life. For instance, severe back pain can affect a client's job performance, engagement in social activities, sexual intimacy, sleep and rest, ability to exercise, and ability to perform activities of daily living. These factors, in turn, can affect the client's level of and response to pain.

Margo McCaffery, a nursing expert on pain, describes pain as "whatever the person says it is, and existing whenever the person says it does" (1989, p. 17). In other words, pain is a subjective experience. Unlike a pulse or blood pressure, you cannot measure pain objectively. In addition, your expectations of your patients' pain will be influenced by your own values, ideals, and life experiences. However, as McCaffery's definition indicates, you will need to put aside your personal beliefs about pain and focus on the *patient's* experience.

You will be able to manage pain more effectively if you can classify the type of pain the patient is experiencing. Pain can be classified by the site of pain, cause of pain, duration, or other qualities.

Origin of Pain

Cutaneous or **superficial pain** arises in the skin or the subcutaneous tissue. If you have ever touched a

699

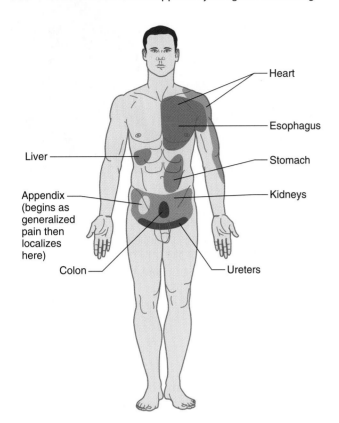

FIGURE 30–1   Most common areas of referred pain.

hot object or received a paper cut, you have experienced superficial pain. Although the injury is superficial, it may cause significant short-term pain.

Visceral pain is caused by the stimulation of deep internal pain receptors. It is most often experienced in the abdominal cavity, cranium, or thorax. Visceral pain may vary from local, achy discomfort to more widespread, intermittent, and crampy pain. The description of the quality and extent of the pain often serves as a strong clue to the cause. Menstrual cramps, labor pain, gastrointestinal infections, bowel disorders, and organ cancers all produce visceral pain.

Deep somatic pain originates in the ligaments, tendons, nerves, blood vessels, and bones. Deep somatic pain is more diffuse than cutaneous pain and tends to last longer. A fracture or sprain, arthritis, and bone cancer can cause deep somatic pain.

Radiating pain starts at the source but extends to other locations. For instance, the pain of a severe sore throat may extend to the ears and head. Or the pain of an episode of gastroesophageal reflux ("heartburn") may radiate outward from the sternum to involve the entire upper thorax.

Referred pain occurs in an area that is distant from the original site. For example, the pain from a heart attack may be experienced down the left arm, through the back, or into the jaw. See Figure 30–1 for other examples of referred pain.

Phantom pain is pain that is perceived to originate from an area that has been surgically removed.

Patients with amputated limbs may still perceive that the limb exists and experience burning, itching, and deep pain in that area.

Psychogenic pain refers to pain that is believed to arise from the mind. The patient perceives the pain despite the fact that no physical cause can be identified. Psychogenic pain can be just as severe as pain from a physical cause. See the discussion of somatoform pain disorder in Chapter 25.

Cause of Pain

Physical pain is either nociceptive or neuropathic. These two types of pain differ in the way they affect the patient as well as in how they are treated.

Nociceptive pain is the most common type of pain experienced. It occurs when pain receptors, which are called **nociceptors,** respond to stimuli that are potentially damaging. Nociceptive pain may occur as a result of trauma, surgery, or inflammation.

Neuropathic pain is a complex and often chronic pain that arises when injury to one or more nerves results in repeated transmission of pain signals even in the absence of painful stimuli. The nerve injury may originate from any of a variety of conditions, such as poorly controlled diabetes, a stroke, a tumor, or a viral infection. Some medications, such as chemotherapy, can trigger nerve injuries that may cause neuropathic pain even after the medication is discontinued. It is estimated that 20 to 40% of patients referred to pain clinics suffer from neuropathic pain (Verhaak, 1998).

Duration of Pain

Acute pain has a short duration and is generally rapid in onset. It varies in intensity and may last up to 6 months. This type of pain is most frequently associated with injury or surgery. It is protective in that it indicates potential or actual tissue damage. Although acute pain may absorb a patient's physical and emotional energy for a short time, it is helpful for the patient to know that it will generally disappear as the tissues heal.

Chronic pain is pain that has lasted 6 months or longer and often interferes with daily activities. It can be related to a progressive disorder, or it can occur when there is no current tissue injury, as in neuropathic pain. Patients with chronic pain may experience periods of remission and exacerbation. Unlike acute pain, chronic pain is often viewed as meaningless and may lead to withdrawal, depression, anger, frustration, and dependence. Next to incurability, chronic pain is the most feared aspect of contracting cancer or another progressive disease.

Intractable pain is both chronic and highly resistant to relief. This type of pain is especially frustrating

for the patient and care provider. It should be approached with multiple methods of pain relief.

Quality of Pain

The words patients use to describe the quality of their pain help care providers to determine the probable cause and most effective treatment. Patients may describe pain quality with a variety of adjectives, such as *sharp* or *dull, aching, throbbing, stabbing, burning, ripping, searing,* or *tingling.* They may refer to its periodicity as *episodic, intermittent,* or *constant.* Patients also use a variety of terms to convey the intensity of their pain, such as *mild, distracting, moderate, severe,* or *intolerable.*

KnowledgeCheck 30–1

How would you classify the pain that the following patients are experiencing?

- A patient with metastatic cancer
- A patient with back pain that was the result of an automobile injury a year ago
- A patient who had bowel surgery yesterday
- A patient with a broken leg
- A patient who just had his leg amputated but feels as though the leg is still there
- You just received a paper cut while turning the pages of a book

 Go to Chapter 30, **Knowledge Check Response Sheet and Answers,** on the Electronic Study Guide.

 ## CriticalThinking 30–1

How would you expect a patient with neuropathic pain to appear?

WHAT HAPPENS WHEN SOMEONE HAS PAIN?

Review the story of Eunice Chu Ling in the "Meet Your Patient" scenario. Eunice has been in an auto accident that caused severe injuries. She has had surgery and is connected to a variety of monitoring and invasive devices. She is awake but cannot speak. However, through the maze of equipment you can see that she is grimacing. Consider these aspects of Eunice's experience as we explore the physiology of pain.

Transduction

Pain-sensitive nociceptors are found in the skin, subcutaneous tissue, joints, walls of the arteries, and most internal organs. The skin has the highest density of nociceptors, and the internal organs the least. Eunice's injuries, surgery, and procedures have stimulated nociceptors throughout her body. In a process

called **transduction,** nociceptors become activated by the perception of potentially damaging mechanical, thermal, and chemical stimuli.

- *Mechanical stimuli* are external forces that result in pressure or friction against the body. Eunice's injuries are predominantly of this type. They involve stretching of tissue in joints and body cavities related to bleeding and swelling, and compression of body tissues caused by the force of the accident. Other types of mechanical stimuli are surgical incisions, friction or skin shearing that occurs from sliding down in bed, or pressure from a mechanical device, such as a cast or brace.
- *Thermal stimuli* result from exposure to extreme heat or cold. If you've ever touched a hot object and rapidly pulled away or suffered an earache when outdoors without a hat on a frigid day, you have experienced pain from thermal stimuli.
- *Chemical stimuli* can be internal or external. Lemon juice or any acidic substance on an open area in the skin causes sharp, sudden pain. This is an example of pain from *external* chemical stimuli. In contrast, the chest pain experienced during a myocardial infarction (heart attack) is caused by *internal* chemical stimuli; specifically, the chemical changes that result from tissue ischemia.

In the "Meet Your Patient" scenario, the physical evidence suggesting that Eunice may be in pain includes bruising, swelling, surgical incisions, and her tubes and IV. However, many tissue injuries reveal no physical, external clues. This is especially true of injuries caused by internal chemical stimuli. This is one reason why it is important to believe the patient's report of pain.

Tissue damage prompts the release of substances such as bradykinin, histamine, and prostaglandins, which perpetuate the activation of nociceptors in the surrounding tissues. Bradykinin is also a powerful vasodilator that triggers a release of inflammatory chemicals that cause the injured area to become red, swollen, and tender. Inflammation is the single greatest cause of pain.

Transmission

Peripheral nerves carry the pain message to the dorsal horn of the spinal cord in a process known as **transmission** (Figure 30–2). Pain messages are conducted to the spinal cord along either of two types of fibers:

- **A-delta fibers** are large-diameter myelinated fibers that transmit impulses at 6 to 30 meters per second. These fibers transmit *fast pain* impulses from acute, focused mechanical and thermal stimuli. For instance, when you bump your knee, the initial sharp pain is carried by A-delta fibers. Pleasurable

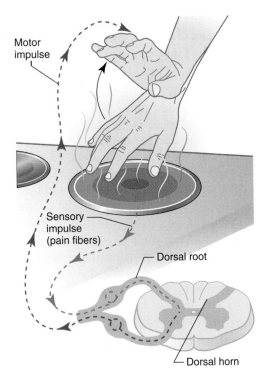

Motor impulse

Sensory impulse (pain fibers)

Dorsal root

Dorsal horn

FIGURE 30–2 After nociceptors are activated, pain is transmitted along A-delta fibers or C fibers to the dorsal horn of the spinal cord. From there, the pain message is sent to the brain for perception.

stimuli to skin receptors, such as from massage, also stimulate A-delta fibers.

• **C fibers** are smaller unmyelinated fibers that transmit *slow pain* impulses, that is, dull, diffuse pain impulses that travel at a slow rate. C fibers conduct pain from mechanical, thermal, and chemical stimuli. If you bump your knee, the lingering ache in the tissue will be carried by C fibers.

At the dorsal horn, A-delta fibers synapse with long fiber neurons that cross the spinal cord and transmit the message directly to the brain. In contrast, C fiber impulses synapse with shorter fiber neurons that pass through several synapses before reaching the brain. Communication of pain impulses across any of these synapses requires chemicals called neurotransmitters, one of the most important of which is *substance P*. Once transmitted, some pain messages enter the reticular formation of the brain stem. However, most pain impulses are transmitted to the thalamus of the brain. An integrating center, the thalamus directs the impulses to three regions of the brain: (1) the somatosensory cortex perceives and interprets physical sensations; (2) the limbic system is involved in emotional reactions to stimuli; and (3) the frontal cortex is involved in thought and reason. The person now perceives pain.

Pain Perception

Perception involves the recognition and definition of pain in the frontal cortex. The point at which the brain recognizes and defines a stimulus as pain is called the **pain threshold.** The number and intensity of stimuli necessary to produce pain, as well as the duration and characteristics of the pain produced, vary from patient to patient. Although the pain threshold usually remains fairly constant for an individual over time, repeated experience with pain can reduce a patient's threshold.

Pain tolerance is the duration or intensity of pain that a person is willing to endure. This not only varies from person to person but also for the same person in different situations. For example, a mother donating a kidney to her child may not complain of a great deal of postoperative pain. Yet if this same person had a kidney removed because it was cancerous, her pain tolerance may be completely different. Extreme sensitivity to pain is called **hyperalgesia.**

Pain Modulation

In a process called **modulation,** pain signals can be either facilitated or inhibited, and the perception of pain can be thereby changed. Two mechanisms allow for modulation of pain: the endogenous analgesia system and the gate-control mechanism.

In the **endogenous analgesia system,** neurons in the brain stem activate descending nerve fibers that conduct impulses back to the spinal cord. These impulses trigger the release of endogenous opioids and other substances to block the continuing pain impulses and provide pain relief. *Endogenous opioids* are naturally occurring analgesic neurotransmitters that inhibit the transmission of pain impulses and the release of substance P. The three neurotransmitters are: enkephalins, dynorphins, and beta endorphins. Endogenous opioids bind to opiate receptor sites in the central and peripheral nervous system at four receptor sites, designated as mu (μ), kappa (κ), delta (δ), and sigma (σ). These sites are also involved in reception when patients take pain medicines. Each of the receptor sites has a different affinity for various medications. In addition, nonpharmacologic measures such as exercise, meditation, visualization, and music therapy can prompt the release of endogenous opioids.

Pain impulses can also be modulated at the spinal level. In 1965, Melzack and Wall introduced the **gate-control theory of pain modulation,** which states that somatic signals from nonpainful sources can inhibit signals of pain (Germann & Stanfield, 2002). As slow-pain impulses travel along C fibers from the periphery to the brain, they encounter a "gate" involving interneurons in the spinal cord. Blocking this gate with competing impulses can inhibit the transmission of pain impulses. Imagine that you've just hit your arm against a hard surface. Almost without thinking, you reach down and rub the area. Your massage stimulates skin receptors. These send sensory impulses

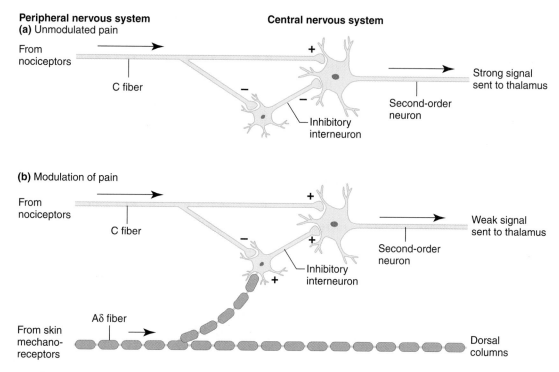

FIGURE 30–3 The gate-control theory of pain modulation. (*A*), Normally, C fibers carrying slow-pain signals block inhibitory interneurons and transmit their signals across the synapse unimpeded. (*B*), A-delta fibers carrying pleasurable signals (e.g., from touch), excite inhibitory interneurons, which then block the transmission of slow-pain signals (+ equals transmission, − equals no transmission).

along fast A-delta fibers, which quickly excite inhibitory interneurons at the "gate." These interneurons in turn block some of the pain signals being carried along the slower C fibers (Figure 30–3). In addition to massage and other forms of pressure, heat and cold, and electrical stimulation such as transcutaneous electrical nerve stimulation (TENS) can activate the A-delta fibers and reduce pain.

Descending impulses from the brain, including impulses related to mood or emotion, are also thought to open or close the gate. For this reason, medications for depression are sometimes used for patients with chronic pain. Nonmedication therapies, such as meditation, exercise, relaxation techniques, and laughter, may also compete with C fiber impulses and block the gate. These strategies are discussed later in this chapter. In summary, on a purely physiological basis, pain is simply transduction, transmission, perception, and modulation. However, as we discuss next, our experience of pain involves far more than these four processes.

KnowledgeCheck 30–2

- What must occur to generate pain?
- What are the four physiological steps involved in the pain process?

 Go to Chapter 30, **Knowledge Check Response Sheet and Answers,** on the Electronic Study Guide.

CriticalThinking 30–2

Based on what you have learned about pain modulation, what nursing interventions might help Eunice ("Meet Your Patient") be more comfortable?

WHAT FACTORS INFLUENCE PAIN?

Think back to the last time you experienced significant pain. Was it obvious to others that you were in pain? Were you demonstrative? Quiet? Withdrawn? Did you moan or cry out? Now recall Eunice Chu Ling's reaction. What accounts for these different responses to pain?

Pain is universal, yet each person experiences and responds to pain differently. This uniqueness gives you a hint about its nature: Pain is a complex phenomenon that influences and is influenced by emotions, age, sociocultural factors, and communication and cognitive impairments.

Emotions

The most common emotions associated with pain are fear, guilt, anger, helplessness, and loneliness. Imagine how Eunice Chu Ling must be feeling. She has had a traumatic accident, undergone surgery, and is now a

patient in the ICU, intubated and unable to talk. How do you think she might feel, and how might her feelings affect and be affected by her pain?

Undoubtedly Eunice is experiencing fear. She has been in a serious accident and can't even ask questions about what is going on. In addition, she may be feeling any of a variety of specific fears. Some patients fear that their pain means that their illness or injury is life-threatening. Others fear their pain will eventually become intolerable. Many patients fear that if they ask for pain medication, they will be judged as weak. Still others fear that if they accept pain medication, they will become addicted to it. When such fears remain unresolved, they can prolong or increase the patient's pain.

In addition to fear, Eunice is also probably experiencing confusion and helplessness. Depending on her role in the accident, she may also feel angry or guilty. Fortunately, family members have come to visit, but when they leave and she is by herself, Eunice may experience loneliness or even a sense of abandonment. You can easily see that people in pain do not experience one single emotional reaction to the experience. Instead, a flood of feelings may overwhelm them, and these emotions in turn may escalate their pain. Often patients get in a vicious cycle: Illness and pain trigger emotional reactions, and the emotional reactions exacerbate the pain.

As you learned in Chapter 11, anxiety and depression are mood disorders. Anxiety is most commonly associated with acute pain, but the anticipation of pain may also trigger anxiety. Waiting for surgery or a procedure that you know will be painful offers plenty of time to think about the unpleasantness and to become anxious. In contrast, depression is most often linked with chronic pain, especially intractable pain.

A person's emotional response to pain is affected by previous pain experiences. Often patients who have had numerous painful experiences are more anxious about the prospect of experiencing pain and are more sensitive to pain. This is especially troublesome for children and adults who require a series of surgeries for their medical condition. Conversely, patients who have had good pain relief in the past are usually more relaxed and will initiate appropriate requests for assistance.

Rarely is pain purely physical or emotional. Instead it is usually a combination of both. Interventions to relieve pain may alleviate feelings of fear and helplessness, and interventions addressing these emotions, such as reflective listening and gentle touch, often aid in pain relief.

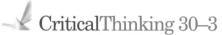

CriticalThinking 30–3

Imagine being in a situation similar to Eunice Chu Ling. What emotions might you experience?

Developmental Stage

The behavior people exhibit with pain is strongly influenced by their stage of development. Newborns have the same sensitivity to pain as older infants and children, and preterm infants may have a greater sensitivity (McCaffery & Pasero, 1999). Infants and small children usually respond to pain by crying loudly. The most common kind of pain that children experience is acute pain resulting from injury, illness, or necessary medical procedures.

Research suggests that infants' and children's memories of painful experiences can influence later behavior. For example, in a study of pain experienced with routine vaccinations, it was found that boys who had been circumcised and not received anesthesia cried longer and had higher pain scores than those who had not been circumcised (Taddio, Katz, Hersich, & Koren, 1997).

You can assess pain in children through self-report, behavioral observation, or physiological measures. Be sure to consult the parents about the child's stress signals and reaction to pain. See the "Assessment" section in this chapter for specific tools to help assess a child's pain. Also,

VOL 2 | Go to Chapter 30, **Assessment Guidelines and Tools,** in Volume 2.

Persons over age 60 experience about twice as many painful experiences as those under 60. Many older adults falsely believe that pain and suffering come with age, so they may not complain about pain. Often their discomfort is evident only in nonverbal cues, such as grimacing, withdrawal, or decreased activity.

Sociocultural Factors

We learn behaviors associated with pain through interaction with family and social support groups. Beliefs about the value of expressing pain or minimizing it are often tied to culture. As you care for clients of various backgrounds, you may notice patterns of behavior. For example, some Latino patients may gain comfort from crying or moaning when they are in pain, whereas some patients of northern European descent may value silence. Be careful, however, not to assume that patients will react according to responses you have seen in others of the same ethnic or cultural group, because each patient is unique.

Three words—*pain, hurt,* and *ache*—seem to be used across many cultures to describe pain (McCaffery & Pasero, 1999). For this reason, many pain assessment tools can be successfully translated into various languages (Box 30–1). If you work in an area where there are many non-English-speaking patients, you

BOX 30-1 **Pain in Several Languages**

Language	Pain	Where?
Spanish	dolor	donde?
French	douleur	ou?
Italian	dolore	dove?
German	Schmerz	wo?

may benefit from pain assessment tools that have been translated into the languages you are most likely to encounter.

The people who are around patients in pain may also have culturally determined responses to the experience. Recall how Eunice Chu Ling's family is responding. Although you may think it odd that they are smiling, they may be doing so because they want to make a favorable connection with you, the nurse, because you will be responsible for providing care to Eunice. As a nurse, you will be around many people in pain and will see a wide variety of responses. Avoid reaching hasty conclusions about the meaning of those responses.

Nursing has its own culture. Most nurses respond compassionately to those in pain. However, if you fail to recognize that pain is a unique multidimensional experience, you may misjudge a patient's reaction to injury, surgery, or other discomforts.

Communication and Cognitive Impairments

One of your greatest challenges as a nurse will be caring for patients in pain who have impaired cognition or communication (e.g., patients who have suffered stroke or dementia, who are intubated, or have limited command of the local language). These patients are unable to express their needs verbally and are at risk for underassessment of pain and inadequate pain relief. You will need to consider their behavioral cues as a form of self-report. Common nonverbal cues of pain include decreased activity, grimacing, frowning, crying, moaning, and irritability.

Less obvious indicators you may see in cognitively impaired patients include the following ("The Management of Persistent Pain," 2002):

- Facial expressions (e.g., a sad or frightened expression, rapid eye blinking)

- Vocalizations (e.g., noisy breathing, profanity, verbally abusive language)

- Changes in physical activity (e.g., fidgeting, increased pacing or rocking, disruptive behavior)

- Changes in routines (e.g., refusing food, difficulty sleeping)

- Mental status changes (e.g., increased confusion)

Physiological cues include elevated blood pressure and pulse. Be aware, however, that the absence of these cues does not automatically mean that pain is absent.

Cognitively impaired patients may be able to use a pain scale (a tool to measure pain), but you must allow sufficient time for the patient to respond. If the nonverbal person has a caregiver, request assistance from her, because she may be able to best interpret the patient's needs. Intubated patients may be able to write or point to a pain scale. Remember, if a procedure or a disease process would be painful to you, it will most likely be painful for any patient.

KnowledgeCheck 30–3

- What are the most common emotional responses to pain?
- What factors influence behavioral responses to pain?

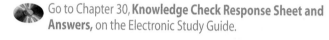 Go to Chapter 30, **Knowledge Check Response Sheet and Answers,** on the Electronic Study Guide.

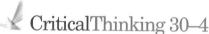 CriticalThinking 30–4

Eunice Chu Ling is unable to communicate verbally because of her intubation. She is grimacing in pain. After you medicate her for pain, how would you determine whether her pain has been relieved?

HOW DOES THE BODY REACT TO PAIN?

Our bodily reactions to pain are influenced primarily by the stage of the pain experience, as well as the intensity, the duration, and quality of the pain.

Pain triggers a variety of changes in the body. At the onset of acute pain, the body reacts automatically by activating the sympathetic nervous system. As discussed in Chapter 25, this fight-or-flight (stress) response is protective. It minimizes blood loss, maintains perfusion to vital organs, prevents and fights infections, and promotes healing.

If the pain continues, the body adapts, and the parasympathetic nervous system takes over. However, the actual pain receptors continue to transmit the pain message so that the person remains aware of the tissue damage. Again, this is largely protective; for example, the pain that you feel for several days after you sprain your ankle reminds you to stay off it until it is fully healed.

The severity and duration of the pain significantly affect how the person continues to respond to it. Often the person is able to ignore mild pain, but pain that is severe and unrelieved can consume his thoughts and change his daily living patterns. Box 30–2 identifies common pain responses.

BOX 30-2   Common Pain Responses

Physiological (Involuntary) Responses

Sympathetic Responses (Acute Pain)

- Increased systolic blood pressure
- Increased heart rate and force of contraction
- Increased respiratory rate
- Dilated blood vessels to the brain, increased alertness
- Dilated pupils
- Rapid speech

Parasympathetic Responses (Deep or Prolonged Pain)

- Decreased systolic blood pressure, possible syncope
- Decreased pulse rate
- Changeable breathing patterns
- Withdrawal
- Constricted pupils
- Slow, monotonous speech

Behavioral Responses (Voluntary)

- Withdrawing from painful stimuli
- Moaning
- Facial grimacing
- Crying
- Agitation
- Guarding the painful area

Psychological (Affective) Responses

- Anxiety
- Depression
- Anger
- Fear
- Exhaustion
- Hopelessness
- Irritability

Unrelieved Pain

Unrelieved pain can produce harmful effects in many body systems.

- *Endocrine system.* Ongoing pain triggers release of excessive amounts of hormones, including adrenocorticotropic hormone (ACTH), cortisol, antidiuretic hormone (ADH), growth hormone (GH), catecholamines, and glucagon. Insulin and testosterone levels decrease. These hormone shifts activate carbohydrate, protein, and fat catabolism (breakdown), hyperglycemia, and poor glucose use. The inflammatory process, combined with these endocrine and metabolic changes, can result in weight loss, tachycardia, fever, increased respiratory rate, and even death.

- *Cardiovascular system.* Unrelieved pain leads to hypercoagulation and an increase in heart rate, blood pressure, cardiac workload, and oxygen demand. The combination of hypercoagulation and increased cardiac workload may lead to unstable angina (chest pain), intracoronary thrombosis (clot formation in the vessels that supply the heart), and myocardial ischemia and infarction (heart attack).

- *Musculoskeletal system.* Unrelieved pain causes impaired muscle function, fatigue, and immobility. Pain that is poorly controlled can prevent the patient from performing activities of daily living and engaging in physical therapy.

- *Respiratory system.* Pain causes splinting, the voluntary limiting of thoracic and abdominal movement in an effort to reduce pain. Splinting reduces tidal volume (air exchanged with each breath) and increases inspiratory and expiratory pressures. These changes can result in complications such as pneumonia and atelectasis.

- *Genitourinary system.* Unrelieved pain causes release of excessive amounts of catecholamines, aldosterone, ADH, cortisol, angiotension II, and prostaglandins. These hormones lead to decreased urinary output, urinary retention, fluid overload, hypokalemia, hypertension, and increased cardiac output.

- *Gastrointestinal (GI) system.* In response to pain, intestinal secretions and smooth muscle tone increase, and gastric emptying and motility decrease.

KnowledgeCheck 30–4

- What are the effects of untreated pain on each of the body systems?
- How might untreated pain affect the progress of a patient recovering from major illness?

 Go to Chapter 30, **Knowledge Check Response Sheet and Answers,** on the Electronic Study Guide.

Practical Knowledge
knowing how

As we discussed earlier, a person's *pain threshold* is the point at which that person perceives a stimulus as painful, whereas *pain tolerance* is the amount of pain a person is willing to endure. Both differ greatly from person to person. You should regularly assess for pain

and accept the patient's report of pain. Increases in pain may indicate a need for more aggressive pain management or may indicate a change in condition. The patient in pain deserves a thorough assessment.

| Assessment |

To treat pain effectively, you must first understand the patient's perception of pain. To do this, begin with a pain history. Taking a pain history is the most effective way to perform an assessment. Each agency will have different assessment forms for this history. For a list of questions that are typically asked,

 Go to Chapter 30, **Assessment Guidelines and Tools, Taking a Pain History,** in Volume 2.

Pain, the Fifth Vital Sign

To raise awareness of pain and emphasize pain relief, the American Pain Society recommends assessing for pain as the fifth vital sign. This means that you should ask patients to rate their pain intensity whenever you take a full set of vital signs. By simply raising the question with each vital signs check, you will prompt your clients to report pain more often. Also, teach unlicensed assistive personnel (UAPs) to ask patients about their pain when taking vital signs and to report their findings to you (Slaughter, Pasero, & Manworren, 2002). Box 30–3 provides the clinical approach to pain assessment recommended by the Agency for Health Care Policy and Research (AHCPR).

Donovan and Miaskowski (1992) recommend that you perform pain assessments routinely, but not limited to:

- On admission to a healthcare facility
- Before and after each potentially painful procedure or treatment
- When the patient is at rest, as well as when involved in a nursing activity
- Before you implement a pain management intervention, such as administering an analgesic drug, and 30 minutes after the intervention
- With each check of vital signs, if the pain is an actual or potential problem
- When the patient complains of pain

Assessing Pain in Children

With children, art and play are effective ways to assess the child's understanding of pain and the pain management plan. Choose age-appropriate toys to engage the child in acting out feelings. Sometimes this indirect method is more effective than directly asking the child. Remember, most children are very fearful about injections and may deny pain if they think that

---

BOX 30-3   Recommended Clinical Approach to Pain Assessment—Agency for Healthcare Policy and Research

Ask about pain regularly. *Assess* pain systematically.

Believe the patient and family in their reports of pain and what relieves it.

Choose pain control options appropriate for the patient, family, and setting.

Deliver interventions in a timely, logical, coordinated fashion.

Empower patients and their families.

Enable patients to control their course to the greatest extent possible.

Source: Agency for Healthcare Policy and Research, Public Health Service, U.S. Department of Health and Human Services. (1994). AHCPR Publication # 94-0592. Rockville, MD: Author.

---

describing their pain will lead to an injection. You can also use a pain-rating scale consisting of simple illustrations of faces. For an example,

 Go to Chapter 30, **Assessment Guidelines and Tools, Using Pain Scales,** in Volume 2.

How Do I Assess for Nonverbal Signs of Pain?

In addition to the patient's verbal report of pain, you must recognize other responses that may signal pain. (See Box 30–2 for common responses to pain.) Pay attention to the patient's physical signs and symptoms. Is the blood pressure or pulse elevated? Does the client appear ashen? These are signs of sympathetic nervous system stimulation. You will see these signs if the pain is acute. If the pain is unresolved or chronic, the blood pressure and pulse may be lower than normal, and the patient may report feeling faint. These are signs of parasympathetic nervous system stimulation.

When assessing for nonverbal signs of pain, keep the following guidelines in mind:

- *Changes in vital signs generally last only a short time.* The body seeks equilibrium; thus, after more than an hour, the vital signs typically return to what they were previously even though the patient may still be in pain. Continuous, severe pain may elevate the vital signs again from time to time, but they rarely remain elevated. Normal vital signs do *not* mean that the patient is free of pain.

- *Patients may be in pain even if they don't "act like" they are.* Too often, nurses expect patients to "act like" they are in pain. Unfortunately it has been well documented that healthcare professionals fail to assess pain and tend to underrate the pain the patient is experiencing (Gloth, 2001; JCAHO, 2000; McCaffery & Pasero, 1999). They expect to see frowning or crying. Patients who use laughter, distraction, or even sleep to cope with their pain are often undertreated. To assess pain accurately, you must ask your patients and then believe them.

- *Use an interpreter if the patient speaks a different language.* Ask the interpreter to explain to the patient that it is important to manage pain and that you will be using a pain scale regularly to assess the patient's pain. Have the interpreter write out the explanation and directions for the pain scale so that you can refer to these when you assess your patient. With written directions, patients can simply point to a face or numeric line to tell you about their pain when no one is present to translate.

- *Some patients feel that they are being "bad" if they express pain or that they are being "weak" by admitting it.* Such patients may withdraw or become stoic. It is important that you establish a trusting relationship with these patients. Convey your concern, and acknowledge that they are experiencing pain. A trusting relationship will allow your patients to be free to verbalize thoughts and feelings.

- *Remember to assess for depression* (see Chapter 11). Depression is often overlooked in the patient in pain. The control of depression greatly facilitates pain management. If depression is not treated aggressively, efforts to manage the pain may not be successful (Gloth, 2001). Avoid the misconception, however, that pain itself is the cause of the depression and that controlling the pain will eliminate the depression. This is rarely the case.

How Do I Use Pain Scales?

To help you assess the intensity of the pain as well as any changes in the pain, you can choose from among a variety of pain scales. Select a pain scale by considering the patient's level of education, language skills, eyesight, and developmental level. Once you choose a particular pain scale for a patient, use it consistently to prevent confusion and allow for comparison. To see some pain scales you might use,

 Go to Chapter 30, **Assessment Guidelines and Tools, Using Pain Scales,** in Volume 2.

KnowledgeCheck 30–5

- How often should you assess the patient for pain, if pain is a potential problem for the patient?

- What are some of the common pain scales used?
- Who should determine if the patient is in pain?

 Go to Chapter 30, **Knowledge Check Response Sheet and Answers,** on the Electronic Study Guide.

 ## CriticalThinking 30–5

What pain rating scale would you use to assess Eunice ("Meet Your Patient")? Why?

| Nursing Diagnosis |

When writing a pain nursing diagnosis, specify the location of the pain and any etiological or precipitating factors that you are aware of. Also identify any knowledge deficits, fear of addiction, or any other fears or beliefs that may interfere with effective pain management. Focusing on the specific nature of pain enables you to choose the most useful interventions. For example:

> Acute Pain (headache) related to changes of position and secondary to increased intracranial pressure

The following NANDA labels are commonly used when pain is the focus of the problem:

- *Acute Pain* for pain with an anticipated or actual duration of less than 6 months.

- *Chronic Pain* for pain with an anticipated or actual duration of more than 6 months.

Notice that NANDA uses only duration, not speed of onset or severity, to differentiate between Acute Pain and Chronic Pain.

Pain affects many areas of functioning. Therefore, it is often the etiology of other nursing diagnoses, such as the following:

- Self-Care Deficit (Bathing/Dressing/Grooming) related to pain in hands secondary to arthritis

- Sleep Deprivation related to chronic back pain of more than a year's duration

- Impaired Walking related to hip pain secondary to joint deterioration

- Ineffective Airway Clearance related to ineffective cough secondary to postsurgical incisional pain

- Ineffective Coping related to overwhelming nature of painful uterine contractions during labor as manifested by crying, moaning, thrashing about in bed

- Impaired Home Maintenance (difficulty cleaning, shopping, and so forth) related to unremitting pain (headache)

- Ineffective Sexuality Pattern related to pain in joints

| Planning Outcomes |

The overall objective when working with a client in pain is to prevent pain whenever possible or, if it is present, to reduce or eliminate pain.

Associated NOC standardized outcomes include the following:

- For Acute Pain: Comfort Level, Pain Control, Pain: Disruptive Effects, and Pain Level.
- For Chronic Pain, use the outcomes for Acute Pain and add the following: Depression Control, Depression Level, and Pain: Psychological Response.

Individualized goals/outcome statements you might write for a client with pain include the following:

- By day 2 post-op, will require only oral analgesics.
- Within 15 minutes of PCA injection, reports pain is <3 on a 1–10 scale.
- Reports that chronic pain does not prevent her from performing activities of daily living.
- Pain Control: Uses pain diary (4: Often demonstrated) (NOC)

Use the goals set in the planning outcomes phase to evaluate the pain relief obtained from nursing and medical interventions.

| Planning Interventions/Implementation |

When planning care, remember that each situation is unique. For example, one terminally ill patient may request complete relief of pain even if this leads to heavy sedation. Yet another patient with the same diagnosis and prognosis may prefer that the pain be decreased to a manageable level so that he may interact with his family or complete any unfinished business. The patient and family must be part of the pain management program. Generally the most effective and least invasive method of pain control is preferable. Remember to include nonpharmacological interventions.

Although overall care of the patient depends on the cause of the pain and on the patient's unique situation, there are nursing interventions and activities that address pain, regardless of its cause.

NIC standardized interventions for Acute Pain include Analgesic Administration, Conscious Sedation, Medication Management, Pain Management, and Patient-Controlled Analgesia (PCA) Assistance.

NIC standardized interventions for Chronic Pain include Behavior Modification, Cognitive Restructuring, Coping Enhancement, Mood Management, Pain Management, and Patient Contracting.

Specific nursing activities (including focused assessments) for clients with Acute Pain and Chronic Pain include the following:

- Actively listen to the patient's reports of pain.

BOX 30-4 Pain Management Tasks That May Be Delegated to Unlicensed Assistive Personnel

Unlicensed assistive personnel (UAPs) may assist you in caring for patients with pain. However, you may *never* delegate the responsibility to assess the patient's pain, monitor the patient's response to pain management strategies, or evaluate the pain management plan. The following tasks may be delegated:

- Repositioning, using pillows for support
- Back rub or massage
- Providing darkness and quiet in the room for sleep
- Straightening sheets
- Mouth care
- Soft music of the patient's preference
- Using distraction (talking or setting up a favorite game for the patient)

- Support the patient in maintaining an active role in her treatment by including her as part of the pain management team.
- Provide prescribed analgesics to the patient in a prompt manner.
- Assess for response to analgesics and nonpharmacological measures, including level of sedation. Make assessments approximately 30 to 60 minutes after the administration of an oral medicine. Injectable medications work quickly, and you should adjust the assessment time accordingly.
- Alter the treatment if the pain is not adequately relieved.
- Provide interventions to manage the side effects of medications.
- Reduce anxiety and fear by offering explanations about care and medications, by allowing the patient to be in control of his pain management, and by providing positive encouragement.
- Consult with the healthcare team about complex pain management issues.
- Delegate appropriate pain management strategies to UAP. See Box 30–4 for a list of strategies that may be delegated to UAP.

Nonpharmacological Pain Relief Measures

The Agency for Healthcare Research and Quality (AHRQ) guidelines recommend the use of alternative

nonpharmacological measures to complement analgesic medications (AHRQ, 2000). This practice has become increasingly common since the 1990s, and it is now estimated that four out of every ten Americans use at least one complementary therapy (Eliopoulos, 1999) when confronted with pain or stress. Nonpharmacological therapies offer an alternative for people with mild pain who do not wish to take potent drugs for pain relief. For many patients, they are satisfying and empowering. However, they should be used as an adjunct to pharmacological therapies for patients with moderate to severe pain.

Cutaneous Stimulation

Cutaneous stimulation (stimulation of the skin) is a method of pain relief based on the gate-control theory of pain. As we discussed earlier, skin stimulation sends impulses along the large sensory fibers, which in turn excite inhibitory interneurons in the spinal cord to "close the gate." This process diminishes the patient's perception of pain. Cutaneous stimulation works best on pain that is localized and not diffuse.

- A **transcutaneous electrical nerve stimulator (TENS)** is a battery-powered device about the size of a pager that is worn externally. TENS units consist of electrode pads, connecting wire, and the stimulator. The pads are directly applied to the painful area. Once activated, the unit stimulates A-delta sensory fibers. A TENS unit can be worn intermittently or for long periods of time, depending on the patient's pain.

- **Percutaneous electrical stimulation (PENS)** combines a TENS unit with percutaneously placed (through the skin) needle probes to stimulate peripheral sensory nerves. PENS is effective in short-term management of acute and chronic pain. PENS therapy in some patients promotes physical activity, increases the sense of well-being, reduces the use of nonopioid medication, and improves sleep.

- **Acupuncture** is the application of extremely fine needles to specific sites in the body. It is believed to stimulate the endogenous analgesia system. Acupuncture is well documented to provide relief from dental pain and has been used extensively after surgery and chemotherapy to treat nausea. Of all the complementary therapeutic approaches, acupuncture enjoys the most credibility in the medical community (Kaptchuk, 2002). There have been some reports in which acupuncture has led to lightheadedness, which may be a concern for patients who are at risk for falls. These patients should be assessed carefully after the treatment.

- **Acupressure** has evolved from the ancient art of acupuncture. Instead of needles, fingertips provide firm, gentle pressure over various pressure points.

This process may have a calming effect through the release of endorphins. Patients can be readily taught key points to stimulate so that they can self-administer acupressure at any time.

- **Massage** decreases pain by providing cutaneous stimulation and relaxing the muscles. *Effleurage,* or the use of slow, long, guiding strokes, is used for obstetrical patients during labor and as back rubs for postsurgical patients. Massage requires little effort from the patient and may improve sleep. For most patients, superficial massage is soothing and relaxing, both mentally and physically. However, some patients do not like to be touched, and you should always obtain verbal permission for a massage. Massage has been shown to increase the flow of body fluids and toxins, which increases the workload of the kidneys and liver (Eliopoulos, 1999).

- The **application of heat and cold** can soothe pain. Examples include heating pads, hot and cold compresses, warm and cold sitz baths, and warm baths. The application of cold causes vasoconstriction and can help prevent swelling and bleeding. Cold can be especially effective in reducing the amount of pain that occurs during procedures. Apply a cold pack to the site before and after a procedure to reduce pain. Heat promotes circulation, which speeds healing. Use caution with these methods, however, because the skin may be injured by either extreme of temperature. Also, because the addition of moisture to heat or cold amplifies the intensity of the treatment, take extra precautions when applying moist heat or cold. Strategies for using heat and cold include:

    Avoid direct contact with the heating or cooling device. Cover the hot or cold pack with a washcloth, towel, or fitted sleeve.

    Apply heat or cold intermittently, for no more than 15 minutes at a time, to avoid tissue injury.

    Check the skin frequently for extreme redness, blistering, cyanosis (blue color), or blanching (white color). If any of these occur, discontinue the treatment immediately, and notify the physician.

- **Contralateral stimulation** involves stimulating the skin in an area opposite to the painful site. Stimulation may be in the form of scratching, rubbing, or applying heat or cold. For example, a patient experiencing pain in the right arm has lotion applied and rubbed into the left arm. This is especially helpful if the affected area is painful to touch, under bandages, or in a cast. It has provided some relief to patients who have phantom pain following an amputation.

Immobilization

Immobilizing a painful body part (e.g., with splints) may offer some relief. It is particularly helpful with

arthritic joints. When this is done, however, you must take great care to remove the splints at regular intervals so that the patient can exercise the area to prevent further injury. Patients in severe pain have the tendency to immobilize a painful area automatically by limiting its use.

Cognitive-Behavioral Interventions

Cognitive-behavioral therapy attempts to alter patterns of negative thoughts and to encourage more adaptive thoughts, emotions, and actions. It is used to decrease depression and anxiety, both of which may play a role in pain. These techniques help patients to deal with their pain by fostering a sense of control over their illness and decreasing feelings of helplessness. Be sure to obtain the patient's permission before using these methods, because the patient may experience psychological or spiritual distress if she considers them inconsistent with her belief system.

- **Distraction** is a method of drawing the patient's attention away from the pain and focusing on something other than the pain. Distraction is based on the belief that the brain can process only so much information at one time. When distraction works, the patient has only a peripheral awareness of pain. You may have responded to this strategy in the past. Have you ever had a headache or muscle pain go away when you become busy with other activities?

    Distraction is useful with all ages, but it should not be used in place of analgesics. Distraction can be visual, tactile, intellectual, or auditory. The distraction that is most effective varies. For some patients, *visual* tactics, such as watching a football game on TV, serve as distraction. *Tactile* distraction includes activities such as massage, hugging a favorite toy, holding a loved one, or stroking a pet. Examples of *intellectual* distraction include becoming engrossed in a crossword puzzle or playing a challenging game. *Auditory* distraction in the form of music therapy has been shown to reduce anxiety during childbirth and appears to improve mood and pain tolerance. Music should not be limited to adults; it can be used for infants and children as well.

    Although distraction can be used for severe pain, it is most effective for mild to moderate pain and for brief periods of time (e.g., for a short procedure such as an injection or infusion). Some patients experience an increase in pain and may become fatigued and irritable when they are no longer distracted.

- **Relaxation techniques** reduce pain in a variety of medical conditions, especially in chronic pain (AHCPR, 1994). In **sequential muscle relaxation**

(SMR), or progressive relaxation, the person sits comfortably and tenses a group of muscles for 15 seconds and then relaxes the muscle while breathing out. After a brief rest, this sequence is repeated using another set of muscles. Patients often start at the facial muscles and work downward to the feet.

- **Guided imagery** uses auditory and imaginary processes to affect emotions and help calm and relax. Guided imagery is used to control acute and chronic pain, both physical and psychological; however, it is more effective for chronic pain. Guided imagery audiotapes can help patients use their imagination to create images of temporary escape that will elicit a sense of well-being. For a script for a guided imagery session,

 Go to Chapter 25, **Supplemental Materials,** on the Electronic Study Guide.

- **Hypnosis** involves the induction of a deeply relaxed state. Once the person is in this state, the hypnotist offers therapeutic suggestions to provide relief of symptoms. For example, the hypnotist may suggest to a patient with arthritis that the pain can be turned down like the volume of a radio (Vicker & Zollman, 1999). Special training in hypnotherapy is required.

- **Therapeutic touch** was developed by nurses and derived from the ancient practice of laying on of hands. Despite its name, therapeutic touch does not require physical contact. It focuses on the use of the hands to direct energy fields surrounding the body. Although research studies on its effect are not consistent, some patients become relaxed and require less pain medication after a session of therapeutic touch (Krieger, 1999).

- **Humor** has positive effects on a patient's physical and emotional health. For most people, laughter is positive and indicates mental well-being. Humor may boost the immune system, as well. It is especially helpful when used before a painful procedure because it lessens anxiety and serves as a form of distraction. Some institutions have humor carts and even humor rooms containing humorous videos, books, and playful items, such as bubbles, fingerpaints, and puppets. Humor is helpful for both children and adults, but it must always be in good taste and age-appropriate. Involve the patient in choosing the humor material, because what one person considers very funny another person may not.

 CriticalThinking 30–6

What has been your experience with using nonpharmacolgical pain relief measures to manage your own pain? How would you incorporate these methods into your nursing practice?

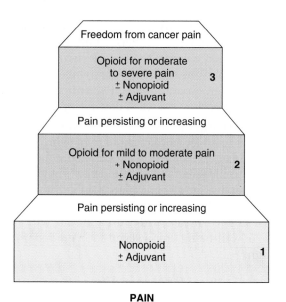

PAIN

FIGURE 30–4 The WHO three-step analgesic ladder. Developed by the World Health Organization (WHO). (1990). Cancer pain relief and palliative care: Report of a WHO expert committee. WHO Tech Rep series, No. 804. Geneva, Switzerland: Author. Used with permission.

Pharmacological Pain Relief Measures

Analgesics are classified into three groups: nonopioids, opioids, and adjuvants. Many health practitioners use the World Health Organization's (WHO) three-step ladder to assist in the selection and titration of an analgesic (Figure 30–4). Each step in the ladder represents severity of pain, by which the analgesic selection is determined. Choice of treatment is based on the level of pain the patient is experiencing. Patients in severe pain should start at the third step. Titration is accomplished according to the patient's response. Monitoring should be regular and continuous. If the patient's pain is not controlled, adjust by moving up the pain ladder. To apply the ladder correctly, you need to know the interactions and side effects of all the drugs recommended on each step.

Administer analgesics at regular times throughout the day if the patient has pain that will last throughout the day. First, determine the dosage that relieves pain at the patient's desired level, then observe how long the first dose lasts. Administer the next dose before the last dose wears off. This around-the-clock (ATC) dosing prevents the patient from experiencing severe pain several times a day and is believed to be better than PRN (as needed) dosing for pain. Explain to the patient that ATC dosing will keep pain at an acceptable level throughout the day and allow the patient to function at an optimal level.

Nonopioid Analgesics

Nonopioid analgesics include a variety of medications that relieve mild to moderate pain. Many also reduce

BOX 30–5 Commonly Used Nonopioid Analgesics

Chemical Name	Brand Name
Acetaminophen	Tylenol
Acetylsalicylic acid (aspirin)	Excedrin, Bayer, others
Celecoxib	Celebrex
Diclofenac	Voltaren, Cataflam
Etodolac	Lodine
Ibuprofen	Motrin, Advil, others
Indomethacin	Indocin
Ketoprofen	Oruvail
Nabumetone	Relafen
Naproxen	Naprosyn, Aleve, Anaprox

inflammation and fever. Several of these medications, including acetaminophen (Tylenol), aspirin, and ibuprofen (Motrin), are available over the counter. All may be used for acute and chronic pain. Most have an onset of action within 1 hour. Box 30–5 features a number of commonly used nonopioid analgesics.

The analgesic properties of acetaminophen and aspirin are often underestimated. Research indicates that 650 mg of aspirin or acetaminophen may relieve as much pain as 50 mg of oral meperidine or 3 to 5 mg of oxycodone, both of which are narcotic analgesics.

Nonopioid analgesics are often compounded with opioids. This allows for a lower dose of opioid to be administered and reduces the incidence of side effects. However, combining two nonsteroidal anti-inflammatory drugs (NSAIDs) is not recommended because it increases the risks of side effects and may not be more effective. However, taking a small daily dose (81 mg) of aspirin to prevent myocardial infarction does not seem to be a risk for patients taking other NSAIDs.

Nonsteroidal Anti-inflammatory Drugs (NSAIDs)

The largest group of nonopioid analgesics is made up of nonsteroidal anti-inflammatory drugs (NSAIDs). These include aspirin and ibuprofen, as well as several others. NSAIDs act primarily in the peripheral tissues by interfering with the production of prostaglandins. As you may recall, prostaglandins sensitize pain receptors and are involved with inflammation. One of the most common side effects of NSAIDs is gastric irritation. Taking the medication with food, lowering the dose, or using enteric-coated pills can reduce the incidence of this side effect. Newer NSAIDs have been developed that are less irritating to the GI tract. These medications markedly decrease the risk of gastric irritation and bleeding; however, they are expensive and available only by prescription. NSAIDs should be used with caution in patients with impaired blood

clotting, renal disease, and gastrointestinal bleeding or ulcers.

Aspirin is a unique NSAID. In addition to reducing inflammation, fever, and pain, it can inhibit platelet aggregation (clumping), the first step in clot formation. Myocardial infarction (heart attack), stroke, and thrombophlebitis (a clot in the peripheral veins) are all associated with platelet aggregation. Because of this property, low-dose aspirin (usually 81 mg) is given to decrease risk of these disorders. Regular use of aspirin will prolong clotting time. Patients who use aspirin should be told that they will bruise easily and will bleed more if cut.

Acetaminophen

Unlike most nonopioid analgesics, acetaminophen has very little anti-inflammatory effect. Instead it has analgesic and fever-reducing properties. It has fewer side effects and is probably the safest of the nonopioids. It does not affect platelet function, rarely causes gastrointestinal problems, and can be used in patients who are allergic to aspirin or other NSAIDs. However, even in recommended doses (up to a maximum of 4000 mg daily), it can cause severe hepatotoxicity (liver toxicity) in patients who consume alcohol and in patients with liver disease.

KnowledgeCheck 30–6

- How do NSAIDs induce pain relief?
- What is the main side effect of NSAIDs?
- In which patients are NSAIDs contraindicated?

 Go to Chapter 30, **Knowledge Check Response Sheet and Answers,** on the Electronic Study Guide.

Opioid Analgesics

Opioids are natural and synthetic compounds that relieve intense pain by binding to opiate receptors and activating endogenous pain suppression in the central nervous system. Although the opiate receptors include mu, delta, kappa, and sigma receptors, the mu receptors are most effective in relieving pain.

Some people may have concerns about using opioids because of fears of respiratory depression, drug tolerance, drug dependence, and addiction. Respiratory depression is rare and can be treated with naloxone (Narcan), an opioid antagonist. **Tolerance** to opioids can occur, but increasing the dose or changing the route of administration can correct that problem. There is no ceiling on the analgesic effects of opioids (Davis, 2000). **Physical dependence** leads to withdrawal symptoms when the drug is removed abruptly; it can be prevented by decreasing the dose slowly over time. **Psychological dependence,** commonly called *addiction,* occurs in less than 1% of patients even after long-term prescribed use of opioids for pain.

Thus, fear of addiction should not prevent patients from receiving opioids for appropriate pain relief.

Most opioids share the same general side effects. The most common are nausea, vomiting, constipation, and drowsiness. Some side effects, such as drowsiness and nausea, improve after a few doses. Large doses may lead to respiratory depression and hypotension. Always assess the patient for level of alertness and respiratory status *before* you administer the drug. Excessive sedation will precede respiratory depression. Other side effects of opioids include difficulty with urination, dry mouth, sweating, tachycardia, palpitations, constipation, bradycardia, rashes, urticaria (hives), or pruritus (itching). You should look up in a drug guide the specific opioid you will be administering for side effects of that particular drug. See Box 30–6 for strategies to prevent common side effects. Constipation is the most prevalent side effect you will treat.

Most patients experience some degree of sedation at the beginning of opioid therapy or when the dose is increased. Monitor postoperative patients who receive opioids for sedation and respiratory depression every 1 to 2 hours during the first 12 to 24 hours after surgery. For an example of a sedation scale,

 Go to Chapter 30, **Assessment Guidelines and Tools, Sedation Rating Scale,** in Volume 2.

Mu Agonists

Mu agonists stimulate Mu receptors and are used for acute, chronic, and cancer pain. They include codeine, morphine, hydromorphine (Dilaudid), fentanyl, methadone, and oxycodone.

Mu agonists are excellent medications for **breakthrough pain**—pain that "breaks through" relief provided by analgesics. Breakthrough analgesia refers to a rescue or extra dose. Drugs used for breakthrough pain should have a rapid onset and short duration. Whenever possible, use the same drug as that given for ongoing pain relief. There is no maximum daily dose limit and no "ceiling" to the level of analgesia from these drugs. You can steadily increase the dose to relieve pain.

Agonist-Antagonists

Another group of opioids are the **agonist-antagonists.** These medications stimulate some opioid receptors but block others. Commonly used medications include mixed agonist-antagonists, such as pentazocine (Talwin) and nalbuphine (Nubain), and partial agonists, such as buprenorphine (Buprenex). These medications are appropriate for acute moderate to severe pain. However, they are inappropriate for severe escalating pain

BOX 30-6 Preventing and Treating Side Effects from Opioids

Before deciding to add another medication to treat a side effect, consider changing the dose or frequency of the current opioid or changing to another opioid.

Side Effect: Constipation

- Add more fruits, vegetables, and fiber to the diet (start on postoperative patients as soon as possible).
- Increase exercise routine. Even walking short distances will help.
- Increase oral fluid intake to eight 8-ounce glasses of water per day.
- If needed, administer stool softeners.
- If above are not effective, administer a mild laxative.
- If constipation continues, soften stool with glycerin suppository and follow up with soapsuds enema.

Side Effect: Nausea and Vomiting

- Reduce opioid dose by combining nonopioid or adjuvant drugs.
- Teach patients that nausea will usually subside after several doses.
- Premedicate or medicate consecutively with an antiemetic. Be aware that this may increase sedation, depending on the antiemetic chosen.
- Teach relaxation techniques.

Side Effect: Pruritus

- Reduce opioid dose by combining with nonopioid or adjuvant drugs.
- Use cool packs, lotion, or topical anesthetics.

- Administer antihistamines, such as Benadryl. Be aware that this may increase sedation.
- Teach the patient that he can generally expect to develop a tolerance to pruritus.
- Use distraction techniques, which frequently work well.

Side Effect: Respiratory Depression

- Assess the patient's respiratory status *before* administering the opioid and frequently afterward.
- Reduce the opioid dose by combining with nonopioid or adjuvant drugs.
- Reduce the opioid dose by 25% when you observe signs of oversedation.
- If the patient is not responsive or only minimally responsive, stop the opioid and administer an antagonist, such as naloxone (Narcan).

Side Effect: Drowsiness

- Assess the patient to ensure that the drowsiness is due to opioid administration and not from another cause.
- Teach the patient that drowsiness will generally subside after a few days as she develops tolerance.
- If analgesia is adequate, reduce the opioid by 25%.
- Discontinue all other nonessential CNS depressant medications.
- During the daytime, offer simple stimulants, such as caffeine.
- Offer a lower dose more frequently to decrease peak concentration.
- Consider another opioid or route of administration.

---

and are not recommended as first-line drugs in any kind of pain (AHCPR, 1992). The reasons are that there is a limit to the analgesia they can provide and that they must be administered parenterally. Agonist-antagonists should not be given to patients taking mu agonists (e.g., morphine) because they may act as antagonists at the mu receptor sites and reduce or reverse the analgesia from the mu agonist.

KnowledgeCheck 30–7

- What are the most common side effects of opioids?
- Identify at least three things that you should monitor when administering opioids.
- What is the risk of addiction to opioids?

 Go to Chapter 30, **Knowledge Check Response Sheet and Answers,** on the Electronic Study Guide.

Routes of Administration for Opioid Analgesics

Use the safest and least invasive route to administer opioids. Below is an overview of administration routes.

- *Oral.* This route is convenient, is safe, and generally produces steady analgesic levels. It is the preferred route of administration unless rapid onset of analgesia is desired. The oral route can be used to provide relief for mild to severe pain. It includes medications that are swallowed but also includes sublingual, transmucosal, buccal, and gingival routes. Oral patient-controlled analgesia (oral PCA) is being used in some hospitals to eliminate the delay between the patient's request for medication and the nurse's administration of it.

- *Nasal.* The intranasal route of administration of drugs has been used for centuries. A rich supply of

blood in this area provides the drug easy access to systemic circulation. The mixed agonist-antagonist opioid butorphanol and the mu agonist sufentanil can be administered intranasally. One drawback to this route is that it may cause burning or stinging.

- *Transdermal.* The transdermal route delivers a continuous release of drug for up to 72 hours. It is a convenient alternative for a patient who requires constant opioid treatment for pain. Fentanyl (Duragesic) is commonly given as a transdermal patch. Use it with care on patients who are febrile, because their increased temperature will increase absorption of the drug. This route is effective for ongoing pain relief but does not provide immediate relief.

- *Rectal.* Suppositories are an excellent alternative to the oral route. This route is effective when the patient is vomiting, has a gastrointestinal obstruction, or is at risk for aspiration if oral medications are used. This route may be contraindicated in patients with neutropenia or thrombopenia because of the potential to cause rectal bleeding while inserting the suppository.

- *Subcutaneous.* The subcutaneous route may be used for intermittent injections and continuous administration of opioids. Continuous subcutaneous infusion (CSCI) of opioids is gaining popularity. CSCI is appropriate for people who cannot tolerate oral opioids or who have dose-limiting side effects from oral administration (e.g., nausea) and who also have limited venous access. Absorption and distribution vary based on the placement site chosen. Hydromorphine and morphine are the drugs most commonly used. Frequently, CSCI of opioids is used for chronic cancer pain. It is better absorbed, is safer, and provides more continuous relief than the intramuscular (IM) route. Small portable medication pumps allow the patient to be mobile. However, some patients find this method painful and time-consuming. You will need to teach patients and their families how to use the pumps, needles, syringes, and other equipment. Because of the small volume of drug (2 to 3 mL per hour) that can be absorbed, two sites may be needed if higher doses are required.

- *Intramuscular (IM).* IM injections are painful, the onset of action is slow, and absorption is unreliable. Consequently, this is not the preferred route of administration of pain medication. With repeated administration, sterile abscesses and fibrotic tissue can result. Nevertheless, this route is often used for short-term pain relief postoperatively. This route should be avoided in children, because they often refuse pain medication to avoid having an injection.

- *Intravenous (IV).* The IV route produces immediate pain relief and is desirable for acute or escalating pain. It is most commonly used for short-term therapy and for hospitalized patients who can be monitored. It is, however, also used for patients with cancer pain and pain from other causes in the home care setting who are unable to tolerate oral opioids. Methods of IV delivery include continuous infusions, bolus, and patient-controlled analgesia (PCA). Patients on a continuous infusion can deliver a bolus for breakthrough pain or procedures such as wound care. Drawbacks to this route include the need for venous access and the need to maintain a patent line. Patients who previously used oral opioids may find the IV equipment cumbersome but they typically report less pain and fewer side effects than with the oral route.

- *Patient-controlled analgesia (PCA).* PCA pumps are an effective and safe way to deliver opioids by IV, epidural, or subcutaneous routes. They provide excellent pain relief and give the patient a sense of control over the pain. The system consists of a programmable infusion pump, a syringe, IV tubing, and a trigger that the patient presses to self-administer a dose. The success of the pump depends on programming a dose that can be administered frequently enough to effectively manage the patient's pain. Some providers order a low continuous rate of infusion as a base that can be supplemented with patient-initiated doses. Most PCA pumps can be programmed with 1- or 4-hour maximum medication limits. If the patient reaches the limit set, the pump will automatically trigger a "lockout" even if the patient keeps pressing the button. Patients need to be educated about this lockout feature; they may not activate the pump enough because they fear overdosing. If you are educating the patient in the use of the PCA pump in the postoperative period, make sure the patient is alert enough to understand the directions and has been given a hearing aid or glasses, if needed, before you offer your explanation. Because of the potential to overdose the patient, only nurses who are trained in PCAs should set up the pump and the program. As a safeguard, another nurse should double-check the setup prior to patient use. Encourage patients to administer a dose before potentially painful activities, such as walking or physical therapy. PCA pumps are contraindicated in patients with cognitive impairment that limits their ability to understand directions. The accompanying Critical Aspects box summarizes the key points involved in use of the PCA.

For detailed instruction on use of a PCA pump,

VOL 2   Go to Chapter 30, **Procedure 30–1: Connecting a Patient-Controlled Analgesia Pump,** in Volume 2.

- *Intraspinal analgesics.* Intraspinal analgesia requires placement of a catheter in the subarachnoid space (for intrathecal analgesia) or the epidural space by an anesthesiologist or a certified registered nurse anesthetist (CRNA). The epidural space is generally preferred because it poses less risk of complications

Connecting a Patient-Controlled Analgesia Pump

- Determine patient's baseline vital signs, cognitive status, and pain level.

- Determine (calculate as needed): the initial bolus (loading) dose, the basal rate, the demand dose, the lockout interval between each dose, and the 1-hour or 4-hour lockout dose limit.

- Prime the connecting tubing.

- Insert into the pump the device containing the medication.

- Lock the pump, and turn it on.

- Set the pump for the loading dose (if ordered), basal rate, demand dose, lockout interval, and the 1-hour or 4-hour lockout dose limit.

- Connect the tubing into the patient's maintenance IV line.

- Start infusing the medication (loading, then basal, dose).

- Put the button that controls dosing within reach of the patient.

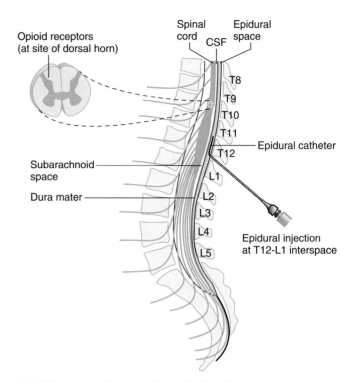

FIGURE 30–5 Placement of an epidural needle and catheter.

(Figure 30–5). Placement of the catheter, as well as the type and concentration of medication, determines the area affected by the medication. Higher doses are needed for epidural than for intrathecal administration.

Usually, two types of drugs are administered through these catheters: opioids and local anesthetics. Opioids can be delivered by PCA, bolus, or continuous infusions. Continuous infusion provides stable, consistent pain relief. The most commonly used opioids for epidural administration are morphine sulfate (Duramorph), fentanyl citrate (Sublimaze), and sufentanil citrate (Sufenta). Local anesthetics are frequently combined with the opioids to reduce the total amount of drug necessary to produce analgesia. Risks of epidural analgesia include dural puncture, infection, hematoma, and nerve damage. For nursing care activities associated with caring for a client with an epidural catheter for pain management,

 Go to Chapter 30, **Technique 30–1: Caring for a Patient with an Epidural Catheter,** in Volume 2.

 CriticalThinking 30–7

- What routes of opioid administration have you seen in your clinical rotation?
- What types of pain relief and side effects have you observed?
- What routes of administration would you like to see? Why?

Equianalgesia

Equianalgesia refers to the approximately equal analgesia that a variety of opioids will provide. Equianalgesic dose calculations provide a starting point when changing from one opioid to another or from one route of administration to another. These doses are approximate and vary according to the number of doses and variety of opioids the patient has received and according to the needs of the patient. Table 30–1 presents information on equianalgesia among opioids.

Adjuvant Analgesics

Adjuvant analgesics may be used as a primary therapy for mild pain or in conjunction with opioids for moderate to severe pain. Drugs in this category include anticonvulsants, antidepressants, local anesthetics, topical agents, psychostimulants, muscle relaxants, neuroleptics, corticosteroids, and others. Adjuvant analgesics reduce the amount of opioid the patient requires. They are especially useful if the patient experiences significant side effects from escalating doses of opioids. Adjuvant analgesics are frequently used in managing neuropathic pain, in which they may be the primary treatment or may be used in conjunction with opioids.

Chemical Pain Relief Measures

Nerve blocks are a type of regional anesthesia. An anesthetic agent is injected into or around the nerve that supplies sensation to a specific part of the body. Most nerve blocks affect a network of nerves called a

TABLE 30-1 Equianalgesic Doses of Opioid Analgesics

Analgesic	Oral/Rectal Dose (mg)	Parenteral Dose (mg)
morphine	30–60	10
hydromorphine (Dilaudid)	7.5–8	1.5
oxycodone	20	Not available
methadone	See below	See below
levorphanol (Levo-Dromoran)	4 for acute pain, 1 for chronic pain	2 for acute pain, 1 for chronic pain
fentanyl	Not available	0.1 (100 mcg)
fentanyl (transdermal)	See below	See below
meperidine (Demerol) (not recommended)*	300	75
codeine (not recommended)**	200	120
hydrocodone	20	Not available
propoxyphene	Not recommended	Not available

- For morphine, the ratio of oral to intravenous dose is 60:10 for opioid-naive patients, 30:10 for others.
- Oxycodone may be used chronically for severe pain only when it is not combined with aspirin or acetaminophen.
- Methadone is an excellent choice for opioid rotation. Calculate the equianalgesic dose using the following method, then reduce the calculated dose by 25–50% to determine the starting dose. The following table shows the ratio of PO morphine to PO methadone.

Oral Morphine Dose	Ratio of Oral Morphine to Oral Methadone
< 90 mg morphine sulfate	4:1 (e.g, 60 mg morphine sulfate: 15 mg methadone)
91–300 mg morphine sulfate	8:1
301–600 mg morphine sulfate	12:1

- Levorphanol has a long half-life and begins to accumulate on days 2 to 3.
- Transdermal fentanyl (fentanyl patch) administered via 50 mcg/hr patch = morphine 100 mg orally per 24 hr = 16 mg orally q4hr = 1.4 mg/hr intravenously.

*Meperidine should be used only for very short-term moderate pain. It is very short-acting (the dose must be repeated at least every 3 hours) and rapidly accumulates neurotoxic metabolites.

**For codeine, dosing is limited by the potential toxicities of the acetaminophen with which it is combined. It should be used for short-term moderate pain only.

How to use an equianalgesic table such as this one: To switch routes of administration, read across rows; to switch opioids, read up and down columns.

Source: Pocket Guide to Pain Management. 2004. Distributed by Tufts-New England Medical Center Pain Clinic. Used with permission.

plexus. Nerve blocks may be used for short-term pain relief for surgical procedures or for long-term management of chronic pain.

Local anesthesia is the injection of local anesthetics into body tissues. Short-acting agents, such as lidocaine, and long-acting agents, such as marcaine, may be used. Local anesthetics are injected into subcutaneous tissue for minor surgical procedures. They may also be injected into joints and muscle for pain relief. New research is investigating the use of pumps to administer local anesthetics at surgical sites for postoperative pain relief.

Topical anesthesia involves applying an agent that contains cocaine, lidocaine, or benzocaine directly to the skin, mucous membranes, wounds, or burns. Topical anesthesia is quickly absorbed and provides pain relief for mild to moderate pain. Many topical anesthetic agents are available over the counter. Sunburn relief agents, gel products for tooth and gum pain, and first aid sprays are forms of topical anesthetics.

TABLE 30–2   Common Misconceptions Among Patients and Caregivers About Pain

Fallacy	Truth
The caregiver is more objective than the patient about the amount of pain experienced.	The patient's report is the "gold standard," and the patient is the authority.
You should wait until the pain is severe before taking medication.	You should take pain medication early and on a regular basis if pain is severe.
There is a significant danger of addiction to pain medications.	Patients in pain rarely become addicted to their pain medications.
Pain is a normal component of aging.	Pain is a symptom that something is wrong and should be treated.
Complaining of pain will label the person as a "bad patient."	The patient should report pain so that it can be treated.
Patients should have severe pain only if they have major surgery.	Even minor surgery and injury can produce severe pain.
Patients will have visible physical or behavioral signs if they are really in pain.	Even when patients are in severe pain, they may not exhibit physical or behavioral signs.

Surgical Interruption of Pain Conduction Pathways

Surgical interruption of pain conduction pathways results in permanent destruction of nerve pathways and is used as a last resort for intractable pain. **Cordotomy** interrupts pain and temperature sensation below the tract that is severed. This is most frequently done for leg and trunk pain. **Rhizotomy** interrupts the anterior or posterior nerve route that is located between the ganglion and the cord. Anterior interruption is generally used to stop spastic movements that accompany paraplegia, and posterior interruption eliminates pain in the area innervated. This procedure may be safely performed at any level along the spine but is most often used for head and neck pain produced by cancer. **Neurectomy** is used to eliminate intractable localized pain. The pathways of peripheral or cranial nerves are interrupted to block pain transmission. **Sympathectomy** severs the paths to the sympathetic division of the autonomic nervous system. The outcomes of this procedure are improvement in vascular blood supply and the elimination of vasospasm. It is used to treat the pain from vascular disorders, such as Raynaud's disease. These therapies are not widely used due to advances in oral and transdermal opioid therapies.

KnowledgeCheck 30–8

- Identify three types of chemical pain relief measures.
- What type of patient might be suitable for surgical interruption of a pain pathway?

 Go to Chapter 30, **Knowledge Check Response Sheet and Answers,** on the Electronic Study Guide.

Misconceptions That Interfere with Pain Management

Pain exists when the patient says it does. But sometimes patients, caregivers, and clinicians have beliefs about pain or pain management strategies that interfere with the treatment plan. For instance, an older patient may fear that severe pain is a sign of impending death instead of an acute situation that requires treatment. Or a family member may worry that pain medication may make the patient comatose. The beliefs of healthcare providers can also interfere with pain management. For example, nurses and other caregivers sometimes doubt the patient's report of pain because:

- Most people don't have pain from that particular illness or procedure.
- There is no obvious, physical cause for the pain.
- They are concerned about drug-seeking behavior and patient addiction.

As you care for patients in pain, remain open to the patient's description of pain, and work with the patient and caregivers to provide pain control. Table 30–2 highlights some of the most common misconceptions about pain.

Managing Pain in Older Patients

Pain management among older patients is especially difficult. Most older adults have at least one chronic condition and take multiple medications. On average, a 70-year-old takes seven different medications. Adding analgesics to an already complex medication regimen increases the likelihood of drug interactions. In addition, drug distribution is altered in older patients because of changes in blood flow to the organs, protein binding, and the difference in body composition. Older adults are at great risk for undertreatment of pain because they and their caregivers may be reluctant to administer analgesics for fear of producing confusion, excessive sedation, drug interactions, and respiratory depression. At the same time, there is a risk of overtreatment due to the higher peak effect and longer duration of pain relief that they experience as a result of changes associated with aging (AHCPR, 1992).

 CriticalThinking 30–8

- Which groups of patients are most at risk for inadequate pain management?
- What can you do to assist each group?
- How do past pain experiences affect present pain experience?

Managing Pain in Patients with Substance Abuse or Active Addiction

It is important to differentiate between physical dependence, which is expected and treatable, and addiction. Addiction is a state of psychological dependence in which the person craves the medication and will place herself in harm's way or demonstrate self-destructive behavior to obtain the drug. The appropriate use of opioids for pain relief rarely leads to addiction. In fact, the rate of opioid addiction among hospitalized patients is less than 1%.

Although addiction from the therapeutic use of opioids is uncommon, substance abuse is a dominant feature of our society and is seen among individuals from all backgrounds. Healthcare professionals often fail to recognize substance abuse unless they actively screen for it. To provide a foundation for good management, you should take a substance abuse history for all patients. This history should include information on alcohol intake because patients whose tolerance for alcohol is high may require a higher dose of opioids. Behavior that may indicate substance abuse or addiction include the following:

- Repeated requests for frequent injections of an opioid, even though the surgery was several days ago
- Refusal to try oral medication
- Continued high opioid dose, even though surgery or acute illness has passed

If you observe these signs, assess the patient carefully because the signs may also indicate untreated withdrawal or increased pain due to complications. When dealing with clients with active addiction, try to assume a nonjudgmental approach.

Although it is certainly important to recognize opioid addiction, you must be careful not to undertreat pain in patients whom you know to abuse substances. There is ample evidence that healthcare professionals mistakenly assume a patient's request for more or different medications to be an indication of addiction. When this happens, the nurse then fails to explore the possibility that the patient's pain is being undertreated. Patients with addictive disease should have the same quality of pain management as all other patients. As a nurse, you will be in a position to help maintain the balance between providing adequate pain relief and protecting against inappropriate drug use (Nichols, 2003).

 CriticalThinking 30–9

You are preparing to give your patient a bath. When you remove his bath equipment from under the bedside table, you find illegal drugs mixed in with the patient's bath equipment. What would you do?

Pain Relief from Placebos

A placebo is defined as "any medication or procedure, including surgery, that produces an effect in a patient because of its implicit or explicit intent, not because of its specific physical or chemical properties" (McCaffery & Pasero, 1999, p. 36). Placebos are usually tablets containing sugar, saline, or water. Why placebos can relieve pain is not well understood. Theories include operant conditioning, faith, anxiety reduction, and endorphin release. They are used with informed consent as controls in clinical trials to test the results of a new medication. Although this may be an appropriate use, placebos do not have a useful place in pain management for the following reasons:

- If the patient responds to a placebo, it does not mean that the patient did not have pain. In classic studies done in the 1950s, 36% of patients demonstrated adequate pain relief from a placebo injection the day after abdominal surgery (Evans, 1974). However, there is no way to determine in advance which patients will experience pain relief; therefore, you risk inadequately treating the patient.
- Even in the same patient, placebos may be effective at one time and not at another.
- Ethically, the most important reason for not using placebos is that their use involves deceit. To use a placebo, the clinician must lie to the client. If

discovered, and it frequently is, the patient's trust in healthcare professionals will be diminished, if not destroyed.

Teaching the Patient and Family About Pain

Patients and caregivers tend to cope more effectively when they are well informed. Because pain is a barrier to learning, be sure to include the patient's family in your teaching. If the patient is discharged from the facility with a prescription for opioids, the family should be taught how to monitor for excessive sedation and to call the healthcare provider for assistance if the patient is not receiving adequate pain relief. The following items should be discussed with the patient and family:

- The cause of the pain, if it is known
- The normal duration of the pain, if known (e.g., postoperative pain generally decreases every day as tissues heal)
- How to use the selected pain scale; ask for a demonstration of use
- The overall pain management plan
- Facts about the analgesic chosen—dose, interval, and route of administration
- If opioids are prescribed, explanation that the risk of addiction is extremely low
- Nonpharmacological ways to treat pain
- Side effects to observe for
- The need to alter the treatment plan if relief is not achieved
- How to contact the healthcare team regarding side effects, change in condition, or ineffective pain management

Documentation

Thoroughly document the pain management plan and the patient's responses. Documentation may be narrative, in either nursing or interdisciplinary notes, or recorded on a pain management flowsheet. Although documentation varies from facility to facility, it typically reflects the entire spectrum of the nursing process:

- The expected outcome for pain management
- The patient's pain level at the present time
- The patient's response to any intervention for pain
- Any adverse reactions that may have resulted from the analgesic
- Planned interventions to improve the pain relief if needed

Typically, pain management flowsheets contain a column for time, pain ratings, and analgesic used, including dose and route, vital signs, and side effects. Pain management flowsheets are tailored to the patient population, the type of pain being monitored, and the clinical setting. For example, the pain flowsheet for a patient on an IV PCA pump will be more complex than a pain flowsheet for a patient on oral medications at home. Written records are important because typically pain recall is poor and patients often underestimate their pain. If pain is not adequately documented, there is no way to prove that it was accurately assessed. This may seriously interfere with care and have legal implications (JCAHO, 2000).

| Evaluation |

Evaluation is critical to a pain management program. Compare your findings with the expected outcomes to determine whether the pain management strategy is effective. Questions to ask include the following:

- Are the patient's pain scores consistently at or better than the desired level? Are they improving?
- What is the quality of the patient's life, according to the patient's standards?

In addition to evaluating the extent to which the pain was relieved, you need to determine which interventions were or were not effective, as well as any adverse reactions to these interventions. Close examination of the patient's pain diary should provide most of the data you need for evaluation. For a sample of a client diary,

 Go to Chapter 30, **Assessment Guidelines and Tools, Client Pain Relief Diary,** in Volume 2.

It is important to reassess the patient's pain regularly. An increase in pain may be a sign of inadequate pain management, but it may also be a sign of developing complications. Before implementing a change in the treatment plan, you should determine whether the pain management plan was carried out correctly. If the decision of the healthcare team is to make a change, remember to evaluate again the effect of this change. Do not assume that your intervention will provide adequate pain relief.

NURSING PROCESS IN ACTION

Mary Jean Thompson, 30 years old, was admitted to the hospital with severe abdominal pain and underwent an appendectomy yesterday. The physician has ordered Demerol 75 mg IM q4hr PRN for pain. Ms Thompson finds the injections painful and waits until she rates her pain a 9 or 10 on a scale of 0 to 10

before requesting an injection. Even after the medication, her pain never drops below a 7 on a scale of 0 to 10 and she is unwilling to turn or ambulate due to the pain.

When you perform your assessment, she tells you she does not want to be sedated. "I hate that groggy, drugged feeling. I'm willing to have some pain to avoid that." After you discuss the importance of pain management to aid in healing and ability to participate in activities and therapy, Ms Thompson states that she would like to have a pain score of 3 to 4 today.

Nursing Diagnosis: Acute Pain (surgical incision) related to possible inadequate analgesia (drug and dosing) because of reluctance to have IM injection, as manifested by not requesting medication until her pain is at a score of 10

Expected Outcome	Nursing Interventions	Rationales
On a scale of 0 to 10, the patient will verbalize pain relief at a score of 3 or below while in bed and 4 or below while ambulating at all times.	Assess and document the patient's verbal and nonverbal expressions of pain relief with each check of vital signs, with every procedure and ambulation, and when the patient is at rest.	Assessment is necessary to determine the effectiveness of the prescribed medications. Assessment and documentation are legal responsibilities for the nurse as well.
	Discuss with the ordering physician the need to modify orders if pain relief measures are ineffective. Recommend PCA.	Ineffective pain management will cause the patient increased stress and can lead to further complications because the patient will be unwilling to move.
	When you obtain new pain orders for a PCA morphine pump, educate the patient about the pump.	PCA requires a patient's understanding and knowledge to be effective.
	Provide nonpharmacological interventions, such as a back rub or other techniques described in this chapter, before rest or sleep, with any exacerbation of pain, and after painful procedures such as ambulation.	Nonpharmacological interventions are synergetic and enhance the relief the opioid gives.
The patient will demonstrate pain relief by participating in ambulation and turning within 24 hours.	Teach the patient to press the PCA pump prior to activities.	Peak blood levels enable the patient to ambulate, cough and deep-breathe, and perform activities of daily living.

Care Map

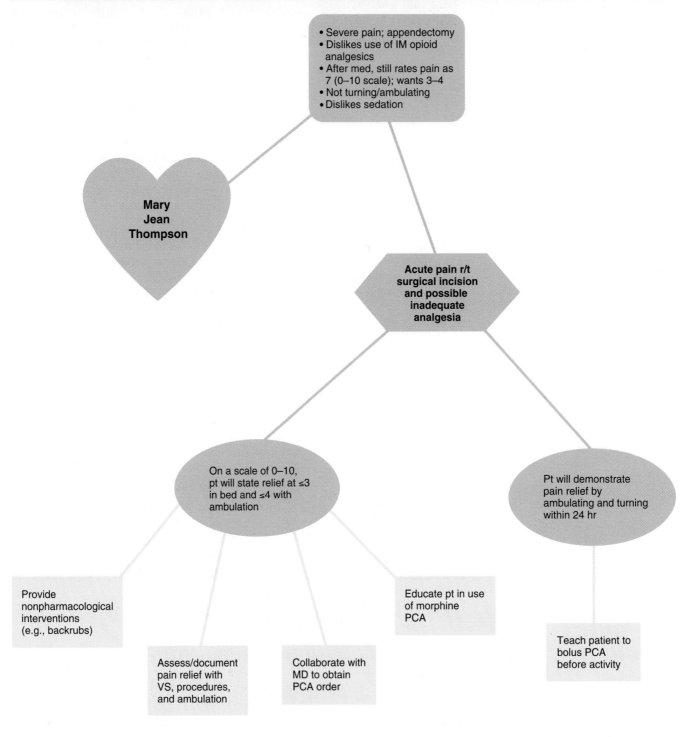

• Severe pain; appendectomy
• Dislikes use of IM opioid analgesics
• After med, still rates pain as 7 (0–10 scale); wants 3–4
• Not turning/ambulating
• Dislikes sedation

Mary Jean Thompson

Acute pain r/t surgical incision and possible inadequate analgesia

On a scale of 0–10, pt will state relief at ≤3 in bed and ≤4 with ambulation

Pt will demonstrate pain relief by ambulating and turning within 24 hr

Provide nonpharmacological interventions (e.g., backrubs)

Assess/document pain relief with VS, procedures, and ambulation

Collaborate with MD to obtain PCA order

Educate pt in use of morphine PCA

Teach patient to bolus PCA before activity

Key:

▨ Data
▨ Nursing diagnosis
▨ Outcomes
▨ Nursing activities

| toward evidence-based practice |

The following studies illustrate the difficulty associated with caring for patients in pain. However, both studies illustrate the importance of the role nurses play in treating pain.

Eifried, S. (2003). Bearing witness to suffering: The lived experience of nursing students. *Journal of Nursing Education, 42*(2), 59–67.

This interpretive phenomenological study explored the lived experience of nursing students as they care for patients who are suffering. Thirteen students were interviewed and wrote narratives about their clinical experience of caring for someone suffering. A key aspect of the students' experiences was their struggle to understand the role of the nurse in relation to suffering. Students' perceived that they were "bearing witness" to an intense emotional experience. Other themes included grappling with suffering, struggling with the indescribable, getting through, being with suffering patients, embodying the experience of suffering, seeing possibilities in suffering, and being aware of their own vulnerability. Students were concerned about their ability to learn and sustain a call to care as they progressed through this experience. The authors conclude that there is a need to include suffering as a curriculum point and to develop a caring community to support students and nurses.

Soderhamn, O., & Idvall, E. (2003). Nurses' influence on quality of care in postoperative pain management: A phenomenological study. *International Journal of Nursing Practice, 9*(1), 26–32.

This phenomenological study explored the influence of nurses on postoperative pain management of patients with complex postoperative situations. Fifteen situations were analyzed. It was found that quality pain management depended on three nursing actions: recognition of an unsatisfactory situation, personal involvement of the nurse in the care of the client, and a desire to provide a positive outcome for the patient. The most crucial aspect appeared to be the nurse's exercising influence on the patient situation to change the treatment plan.

---

1. Based on the information provided in these two studies, what information do you need to prepare for caring for patients who are suffering or in pain? What types of nursing knowledge are necessary?

2. How might you foster a caring community to support students and nurses?

 Go to Chapter 30, **Toward Evidence-Based Practice Suggested Responses,** on the Electronic Study Guide.

 Go to Chapter 30, **Resources for Caregivers and Health Professionals,** on the Electronic Study Guide.

 Suggested Readings: Go to Chapter 30, **Reading More About Pain Management,** on the Electronic Study Guide.

 Bibliography: Go to Volume 2, Bibliography.

Activity
& Exercise

Learning Outcomes

After completing this chapter, you should be able to:

✳ Discuss the physiology of movement.

✳ Use proper body mechanics when providing patient care.

✳ Describe the five forms of exercise discussed in this chapter.

✳ Compare the effects of exercise and immobility on the body.

✳ Discuss factors that affect body alignment and activity.

✳ Identify patients who are at risk for immobility concerns or activity intolerance.

✳ Develop a plan of care for patients with decreased activity tolerance.

✳ Implement care related to a patient's mobility problems.

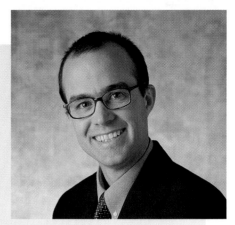

MEET Your Patients

You are attending a health promotion series at the local hospital. For the next 4 weeks, the topic is exercise. In the group you meet the following people:

- Phillip Flanders is a 40-year-old accountant. He works long hours at a desk job and often feels tired. He has never been involved in a regular exercise program. Many of his friends have suggested that he begin exercising to improve his energy and health. Phillip would like to learn about the benefits of exercise and how to start an exercise program.
- Peter Phan is 28 years old. He runs 35 miles per week and plays tennis at least twice per week. He has had several injuries that have caused him to miss exercise. Peter would like to learn what he can do to prevent injuries.

- Helen Jillian is 72 years old. She has hypertension and high cholesterol levels for which she takes four medications. She is 61 inches tall and weighs 290 pounds. Recently, she began having chest pain. She was given nitroglycerin for the chest pain and told to enroll in this class and the CardioFit program at the hospital. She does not understand why she is being asked to do these things because activity seems to trigger her chest pain.

In this chapter you will find answers to each of these patient questions about activity and exercise. In addition, you will learn more about assisting patients with mobility problems.

Theoretical Knowledge
knowing why

Before the rise of civilization, humans spent much of their time hunting and gathering food. Men hunted for game, and women gathered roots, fruits, and other edible plants. People's very survival depended on physical activity, such as moving and lifting. Later, the shift to agriculture freed most people from having to hunt and gather for food, but they did have to grow food for themselves and others. Farming was hard work that kept people active all day long. Today, with modern distribution systems and the Internet, people expend little to no energy to obtain food. In addition, more occupations now place people in front of a desk or a computer screen for long periods of time. Even popular leisure activities, such as watching television or playing video games, are sedentary.

To get enough exercise, most people need to make a conscious effort to build exercise and activity into their lives. Although exercise videos and equipment sell well, the level of fitness in the United States is declining. Nearly half of people aged 12 to 21 do not engage in regular, vigorous activity, and more than 60% of adults do not achieve the recommended daily 30 minutes or more of moderate-intensity physical activity. Another 25% of adults are not active at all. The incidence of inactivity increases with age and is more common among women and people with lower income and less education (United States Department of Health and Human Services, 2001).

PHYSIOLOGY OF MOVEMENT

Activity and exercise require body movement (**mobility**). Mobility depends on the successful interaction between the skeleton, the muscles, and the nervous system.

Skeletal System

The skeletal system includes bones, cartilage, ligaments, and tendons. The skeleton forms the framework of the body, protects the internal organs, produces blood cells, and stores mineral salts (e.g., calcium) and fat.

Bones consist of a hard outer shell with a spongy interior (Figure 31–1). There are 206 bones in the human body. Some bones are long (such as the femur and humerus), some short (phalanges and metacarpals), some flat (sternum and cranial bones), and some are irregularly shaped (vertebrae and tarsal bones). The short, flat, and irregular bones contain red bone marrow that produces red blood cells.

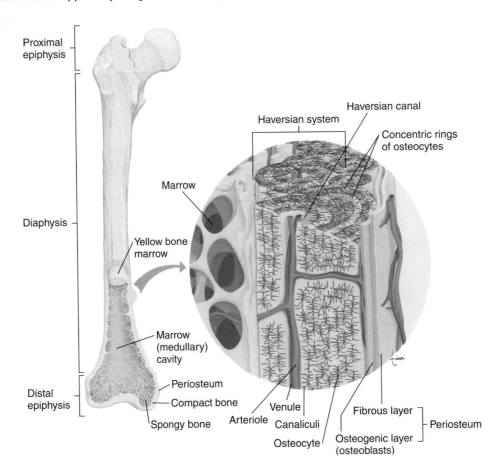

Proximal epiphysis

Haversian system

Haversian canal

Concentric rings of osteocytes

Marrow

Diaphysis

Yellow bone marrow

Marrow (medullary) cavity

Distal epiphysis

Periosteum

Compact bone

Spongy bone

Venule

Arteriole

Canaliculi

Osteocyte

Fibrous layer

Osteogenic layer (osteoblasts)

Periosteum

FIGURE 31–1 **Bone is complex living tissue.**

Bones feel strong and tough, so it is easy to forget that they are composed of living tissue that is constantly building and remodeling. **Osteoclasts** are specialized cells that function as housekeepers in the bone by breaking down old or damaged tissue. **Osteoblasts** repair damaged bone and build new bone to keep the skeleton strong. A delicate balance exists between the actions of the osteoblasts and the osteoclasts.

When two bones come close together **(articulate),** a joint is formed. Body movement occurs at the joints. Joints are classified based on the amount of movement they permit:

- **Synarthroses** are immovable joints (e.g., the sutures between the cranial bones). In youth, these joints have some flexibility to allow growth, but they gradually become rigid.
- **Amphiarthroses** allow for limited movement. Examples are the joints between the vertebrae and pubic bones.
- **Diarthroses,** or **synovial joints,** are freely movable because of the amount of space between the articulating bones. Synovial joints are filled with **synovial fluid,** and the joint surfaces of the articulating bones are covered with smooth **articular cartilage**

(connective tissue found in the joints and skeleton). The synovial fluid and articular cartilage prevent friction as the bones move. Figure 31–2 illustrates terms that are commonly used to describe movement at the synovial joints. Table 31–1 identifies the types of movable joints in the body.

Cartilage, ligaments, and tendons serve as the interface between the skeleton and the muscles. **Ligaments** are fibrous tissues that connect most movable joints. Ligaments are flexible to allow freedom of movement, but strong and tough so they do not yield under force of movement. **Tendons** are fibrous connective tissues that attach muscles to the bone. **Muscles** span a joint and attach by tendons to two different bones.

Muscles

Muscles comprise 40 to 50% of body weight. When they contract, they cause movement. The type of movement depends on the type of muscle: skeletal, smooth, or cardiac.

- *Skeletal muscle* moves the skeleton.
- *Smooth muscle,* found in the digestive tract and other hollow structures, such as the bladder and

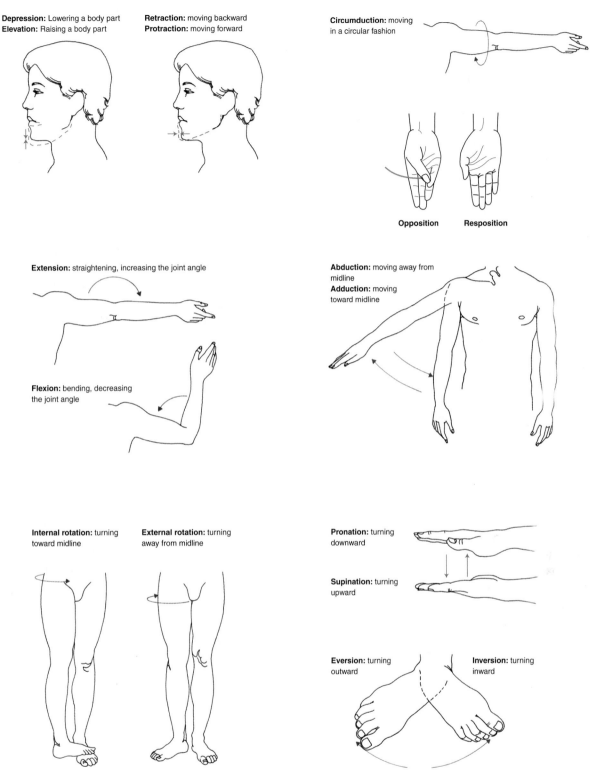

FIGURE 31–2   Terms that are commonly used to describe movement.

blood vessels, produces movement of food through the digestive tract, urine through the urinary tract, and blood through the circulatory system.

- *Cardiac muscle* is a unique form of muscle that has the ability to contract spontaneously. It is responsible for the beating of the heart.

Muscles attach to bone at two points: (1) at the *point of origin,* to the more stationary bone, and (2) at the *point of insertion,* to the more movable bone. The "belly" (thickest part) of the muscle lies between these two points. When a skeletal muscle contracts, it shortens, thus causing one bone to move at the joint.

TABLE 31-1   Types of Synovial Joints

Type	Description	Examples
Ball-and-socket	A rounded head (ball) fits into a cuplike structure (socket) to allow movement in all planes in addition to rotation.	Shoulder and hip joints
Condyloid	An oval-shaped bone fits into an elliptical cavity to allow movement in two planes at right angles to each other.	Wrist
Gliding	Two flat plane surfaces move past each other.	Intervertebral joints
Hinge	A convex surface fits into a cavity, allowing flexion and extension.	Knee and elbow
Pivot	The joint is formed by a ringlike object that turns on a pivot. Motion is limited to rotation.	The atlas and axis
Saddle	One bone surface is concave in one direction and convex in the other. The other surface has the opposite construction so that the bones fit together. Movement is possible in two planes at right angles to each other.	Carpal-metacarpal joint of the thumb

Muscles work in pairs. For example, the biceps brachii contracts to flex the forearm (bend the elbow joint). When the biceps contracts, the opposing muscle, the triceps brachii, relaxes. Similarly, contraction of the triceps is associated with relaxation of the biceps (Figure 31–3).

Nervous System

The nervous system controls the movement of the musculoskeletal system. Motor nerves are classified as follows.

- The *autonomic nervous system* consists of the sympathetic and parasympathetic nervous systems, which innervate involuntary muscles, such as the heart, blood vessels, and glands.

- The *somatic nervous system* innervates the voluntary skeletal muscles.

When you make a conscious decision to bend your elbow, the thought originates in the motor area of your cerebral cortex. The upper motor efferent nerves communicate with the lower motor neurons that conduct impulses to the muscles. When the muscle receives sufficient stimuli, it contracts the biceps as the triceps relaxes and moves the elbow. Movement also occurs through reflex mechanisms. Common reflexes include the knee-jerk reflex and corneal reflex. Reflexes are discussed at length in Chapter 19.

A muscle contraction, whether conscious or reflexive, stimulates afferent nerves that convey information to the cerebral cortex and the cerebellum. This information helps control and coordinate movements.

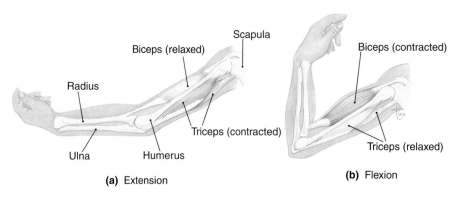

FIGURE 31–3   Antagonistic muscles. A, Extension of the forearm. B, Flexion of the forearm.

Lateral (side) spinal column

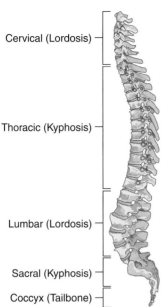

Cervical (Lordosis)

Thoracic (Kyphosis)

Lumbar (Lordosis)

Sacral (Kyphosis)

Coccyx (Tailbone)

FIGURE 31–4 **There are four natural curves to the spine.**

KnowledgeCheck 31–1

- Name three purposes of the skeletal system.
- Define the following movements: abduction, adduction, flexion, extension, circumduction, internal rotation, supination, and pronation.
- Identify three types of muscle.
- How do the muscles and the nerves interact?

 Go to Chapter 31, **Knowledge Check Response Sheet and Answers,** on the Electronic Study Guide.

BODY MECHANICS

Body mechanics is a term used to describe the way we move our body. You should always use good body mechanics and teach good body mechanics to patients as part of your health promotion and disease prevention efforts. Body mechanics includes four components: body alignment, balance, coordination, and joint mobility. In addition, nurses can follow a number of guiding principles to teach proper body mechanics.

Body Alignment

Body alignment, or posture, is an important aspect of body mechanics. Proper posture places the spine in a neutral (resting) position. There are four natural curves to the spine (Figure 31–4). Proper posture maintains these natural curves because it allows movement to occur with less stress and fatigue; the bones are aligned, and the muscles, joints, and ligaments can work at peak efficiency. Good posture also helps contribute to the normal functioning of the nervous system.

Tips to Maintain Proper Posture

- Avoid standing in one position for a lengthy period. If you cannot change positions, elevate one foot on a stool or box, and alternate foot placement frequently.
- Do not lock your knees when standing upright.
- Keep your stomach muscles tight to support your back.
- Do not bend forward at the waist or neck when you are working in a low position.
- When you are seated at your desk, work at a comfortable height.
- Do not wear high-heeled or platform shoes for long periods of time.
- Do not slump when you sit.
- Sit close to your work.
- Use a chair that supports your back in a slightly arched position.
- Sit with your feet flat on the floor and your knees below your hips.
- Sleep on a mattress that is firm but not extremely hard.
- To get out of bed, roll to one side, place your feet on the ground, and push up with your arms.

Most posture problems result from a combination of the following:

- Accidents, injuries, and falls
- Careless sitting, standing, or sleeping habits
- Excessive weight
- Foot problems or improper shoes
- Negative self-image
- Occupational stress
- Poor sleep support (mattress)
- Poorly designed work space
- Visual difficulties
- Weak muscles or muscle imbalance

The accompanying Self-Care box provides tips on how to maintain proper posture.

Balance

The body achieves balance when it is in alignment. For your body to be balanced, your line of gravity

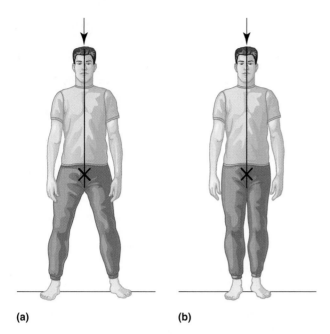

(a) (b)

FIGURE 31–5 *A,* With a wide stance, the center of gravity is closer to the base of support. *B,* With a narrow stance, the body is less stable.

must pass through your center of gravity, and your center of gravity must be close to your base of support. The **line of gravity** is an imaginary vertical line drawn from the top of the head through the center of gravity. The **center of gravity** is the point around which mass is distributed. In the human body, the center of gravity is below the umbilicus at the top of the pelvis. The **base of support** is what holds the body up. The feet provide the base of support.

To place your center of gravity closest to your base of support, stand with your head erect, buttocks pulled in, stomach muscles tight, chest high, shoulders pulled back, and feet wide (Figure 31–5). Use a wide stance, with feet apart and one foot forward when standing for a long period of time. The broader the base of support, the lower the center of gravity, and the easier it is to maintain balance.

Coordination

Smooth movement requires coordination between the nervous system and the musculoskeletal system. Voluntary movement is initiated in the cerebral cortex. However, the cerebellum coordinates movements. As you may recall, *proprioception*—the awareness of posture, movement, and position sense—is largely controlled by the cerebellum. The basal ganglia, located deep in the cerebrum, assists with coordination of movement. Damage to the motor cortex, cerebellum, or basal ganglia affects coordination of movement. For example, a stroke affecting the motor cortex alters gait and changes posture.

Joint Mobility

Joint movement allows us to sit, stand, bend, walk, and perform other activities. **Range of motion (ROM)** is the maxium movement possible at a joint. **Active range of motion** is defined as the movement of the joint through the entire ROM by the individual. Full ROM is part of being physically fit; for that reason, stretching exercises are included in a comprehensive exercise program. **Passive ROM** is a nursing activity that will be discussed later in this chapter. It involves moving joints through their ROM when the patient is unable to do so for himself.

Body Mechanics Guidelines

Principles of body mechanics are the rules that allow you to move your body without causing injury. Historically, nurses have used body mechanics guidelines as the cornerstone of safe practice for moving and lifting patients. However, patient characteristics and condition, as well as the patient care environment, make it difficult to rely on body mechanics alone to prevent injury (Nelson, Fragala, & Menzel, 2003). The American Nurses Association (ANA, 2004) has launched a national campaign titled "Handle With Care" to reduce the risk of back and musculoskeletal injuries among nurses. This campaign emphasizes the use of assistive devices to decrease the risk of injury and recommends virtually no manual lifting. Over the next few years, you will see an increasing presence of assistive devices in clinical facilities to meet this goal. In the interim, continue to use good body mechanics as you move and lift patients. Use the following guidelines as you provide care and teach your patients about safe body movement.

- *Stand in good alignment* (erect posture).
- *Use a wide base of support* (feet spread apart).
- *Minimize bending and twisting.* These movements increase the stress on the back. Instead, face the object or person, and bend at the hips or squat.
- *Squat to lift heavy objects from the floor* (squatting lowers your center of gravity). Push against the strong hip and thigh muscles to raise yourself to a standing position. Avoid bending at the waist.
- *Keep objects close to your body when you lift, move, or carry them.* The closer an object is to your center of gravity, the greater your stability and the less strain on your back.
- *Use both hands and arms when you lift, move, or carry heavy objects.*
- *Raise the height of the bed and bedside table to waist level* when you are working with a patient.
- *When possible, keep your elbows bent when you carry an object.*

- *Use the muscles in your legs as the power for lifting.* Bend your knees, keep your back straight, and lift smoothly. Repeat the same movements for setting the object down.
- *Do not stand on tiptoes to reach an object.* If you must use a ladder or stepstool to reach an object, make sure it is stable and adequate to position your body close to the object.
- *Push, slide, or pull heavy objects* whenever possible, rather than lift them.
- *Make sure you have a good grip on the patients or objects you are moving before attempting to move them.*
- *Work with smooth and even movements.* Avoid sudden or jerky motions.
- *Get help to move a heavy object or patient.* Assess the object or patient you are going to lift. If you have any doubt that you can do it safely by yourself, get help from a co-worker.

KnowledgeCheck 31–2

- Identify the four components of body mechanics.
- Give at least five guidelines for good body mechanics.

 Go to Chapter 31, **Knowledge Check Response Sheet and Answers,** on the Electronic Study Guide.

 CriticalThinking 31–1

While you are attending the health promotion class, Helen Jillian ("Meet Your Patients") develops chest pain and must be assisted to a wheelchair for transport to the emergency department. The instructor asks you to assist Ms Jillian.
- Based on what you know about body mechanics, how would you be able to assist Ms Jillian?
- What additional information do you need to know?

EXERCISE

Physical activity involves movement and energy expenditure by the skeletal muscles. **Exercise** involves physical activity, which requires contraction and relaxation of muscle. As a result, exercise increases muscle tone and strength. Generally, we think of exercise as structured and repetitive physical activity done to improve or maintain physical fitness. The surgeon general of the United States recommends 30 minutes or more of moderate-intensity physical activity on all, or most, days of the week (United States Department of Health and Human Services, 2001).

Types of Exercise

Exercise may be classified according to the type of muscle contraction it involves and according to whether it uses oxygen for energy.

Isometric exercises involve muscle contraction without motion. They are usually performed against an immovable surface or object, for example, pressing the hand against the wall. The muscles of the arm contract, but the wall does not move. Each position is held for 6 to 8 seconds and repeated 5 to 10 times. Isometric training is effective for developing total strength of a particular muscle or group of muscles. It is often used for rehabilitation because the exact area of muscle weakness can be isolated and strengthening can be administered at the proper joint angle. This kind of training requires no special equipment, and there is little chance of injury. Bedridden patients can use this form of exercise to maintain or regain muscle strength.

Isotonic exercise involves movement of the joint during the muscle contraction. A classic example of an isotonic exercise is weight training with free weights. As the weight is moved throughout the range of motion, the muscle shortens and lengthens. Calisthenics, such as chin-ups, push-ups, and sit-ups, all of which use body weight as the resistance force, are also isotonic exercises.

Isokinetic exercise utilizes machines that control the speed of contraction within the range of motion. Isokinetic exercise combines the best features of both isometrics and weight training by providing resistance at a constant, preset speed while the muscle moves through the full range of motion. Specialized machines available at health clubs and physical therapy departments are used for this form of exercise.

Aerobic exercise acquires energy from metabolic pathways that use oxygen—the amount of oxygen taken into the body meets or exceeds the amount of oxygen required to perform the activity. Aerobic exercise uses large muscle groups, can be maintained continuously, and is rhythmic in nature. It increases the heart and respiratory rate, thereby providing exercise for the cardiovascular system while simultaneously exercising the skeletal muscles. Jogging, brisk walking, and cycling are common forms of aerobic exercise.

Anaerobic exercise occurs when the amount of oxygen taken into the body does not meet the amount of oxygen required to perform the activity. Therefore, the muscles must obtain energy from metabolic pathways that do not use oxygen. Rapid, intense exercise, such as lifting heavy objects or sprinting, are examples of anaerobic exercise.

Exercise Program Guidelines

A well-rounded exercise program focuses on flexibility, resistance training, and aerobic conditioning. You must consider each of these factors when designing or evaluating an exercise program.

- *Flexibility training* is important for overall fitness. Stretching before exercise helps warm up the muscles

BOX 31-1 Tests for Determining Exercise Intensity

Target Heart Rate Method

In the target heart rate method, the target heart rate (THR) is calculated from an estimate of maximum heart rate. The estimated maximum heart rate is calculated by the following formula:

$$\text{Maximum heart rate} = 220 - \text{age}$$

The THR is calculated as a percentage of the maximum heart rate. Most persons can exercise at 60 to 80% of the maximum heart rate.

For example, consider a 50-year-old woman. Her maximum heart rate is 170 beats per minute. To exercise at 75% intensity, her target heart rate is 128 beats per minute.

$$\text{Maximum heart rate} = 220 - 50 = 170$$

$$\text{THR} = 0.75 \times 170 = 128$$

The person's heart rate during exercise should be 128 beats per minute, excluding warm-up and cool-down.

Talk Test

The talk test evaluates exercise intensity based on the person's ability to talk while exercising. Short phrases interspersed with breaths or feeling like you can "just respond" is considered an appropriate level to exercise. If you are too short of breath to answer, the level of intensity is too high. An ability to carry on a conversation indicates that you are not exercising hard enough.

Borg Rate of Perceived Exertion Scale

The rate of perceived exertion scale is very easy to use. The person who is exercising selects the rating based on how difficult the exercise feels to the person at that time. Verbal descriptions are provided for comparisons across individuals and tasks:

No exertion at all

Very, very light

Very light

Light

Somewhat hard

Hard

Very hard

Extremely hard

Extremely hard is associated with exercise that corresponds to almost 100% of maximum heart rate. *Somewhat hard* corresponds with 75% of maximum heart; this is the level you should encourage for most individuals.

Sources: Borg, G. (1998). *Borg's perceived exertion and pain scales.* Stockholm, Sweden: Human Kinetics; Foster, C. (2004). 'Talk test' measures exercise intensity. *Medicine & Science in Sports & Exercise, 36* (9), 1632–1636.

---

and prevents injury during exercise. Stretching after exercise cools the muscles and limits post-exercise stiffness. As we get older, joints and muscles become stiffer. A regular flexibility program helps maintain mobility as aging occurs.

- *Resistance training,* which involves movement against resistance, increases muscular strength and endurance. Perhaps the most common type of resistance training is weight lifting. When a person is exercising for strength, the goal is to increase the amount of resistance with each exercise (i.e., lift more weight). When a person is exercising for endurance, the goal is to increase the number of repetitions with each exercise (i.e., lift the weight a greater number of times).

- *Aerobic conditioning* affects fitness and body composition. Components of aerobic conditioning include intensity, duration, frequency, and mode. **Intensity** is how hard one is exercising. Box 31–1 describes three common tests used to evaluate exercise intensity. **Duration** is the amount of time one is exercising. The American College of Sports Medicine (ACSM, 2004) guidelines state that exercise intensity

should be maintained for 30 to 45 minutes. The lower the intensity, the longer a person should exercise, and vice versa. The **frequency** of exercise should be 3 to 5 days per week. The **mode** of exercise is the type of activity that is done. Walking, running cycling, cross-country skiing, aerobic dance, rowing, stair climbing, swimming, and skating are examples.

Many people become discouraged because they don't see immediate results from their efforts. However, cellular changes occur long before the person sees changes in weight or shape. Some tips to help develop an exercise program are included in the Self-Care box on page 733.

Benefits of Regular Exercise

Exercising at any intensity, duration, or frequency has health benefits. As most people know, regular physical exercise decreases the risk of cardiovascular disease, especially coronary heart disease, and prevents or delays the development of hypertension. Other improvements, such as increased muscle tone

Teaching Clients How to Set Up an Exercise Program

If you are over 40, smoke or drink, are sedentary, are overweight, or have a chronic health condition, have a medical evaluation before starting an exercise program.

Getting Started

- *Choose a variety of exercises* that you enjoy and feel comfortable doing, such as walking, biking, dancing, or a team sport.

- *Strive for at least 30 minutes* of activity most days of the week.

- *Select your allies.* Exercising with someone else can make it more fun. If you choose to exercise by yourself, pick a friend with whom you can discuss your exercise progress.

- *Vary your routine.* You may be less likely to get bored or injured.

- *Choose a comfortable time of day.*

- *Don't get discouraged.* It can take weeks or months before you notice some of the changes from exercise.

- *Forget "no pain, no gain."* Although a little soreness is normal after you first start exercising, pain isn't. Stop if you hurt.

- *Make exercise fun.* Find fun things to do, such as taking a walk through the park or watching your favorite show while riding a stationary bike.

- *Sign a contract* committing yourself to exercise.

- *Keep a daily log* of your activities.

- *Think about joining a health club.* The cost gives some people an incentive to exercise regularly.

Exercise Tips

- Warm up your muscles for 5 to 10 minutes before your main session of aerobic exercise.

- Maintain your exercise intensity for 30 to 45 minutes.

- Gradually decrease the intensity of your workout (cool down) and then stretch for 5 to 10 minutes at the end of your workout.

- Accumulate physical activity throughout the day. For example:

  Take the stairs instead of the elevator.
  Go for a walk during your coffee break or lunch.
  Walk all or part of the way to work.
  Park your car at the far end of the parking lot.

- Wear good, shock-absorbing footwear. Shoes that do not support your feet will cause stress on leg bones and the back and, over time, lead to injury.

- Alternate easy and hard exercise days, or alternate modes of exercise (e.g., alternate running, swimming, and biking).

- Take a day off periodically. The body needs a chance to rest and allow bones, joints, and muscles to rest and repair.

- To avoid becoming dehydrated, drink at least 8 ounces of fluid before the exercise, and then pause regularly during the exercise for more. If you are thirsty after the exercise session, drink until you feel satiated. Water is still the best choice to drink during and after exercise.

---

and flexibility, occur throughout the body. Box 31–2 presents numerous other benefits. Exercise is associated with an overall decrease in mortality in men and women of all ages and an overall improvement in quality of life (U.S. Department of Health and Human Services, 1996).

Risks Associated with Exercise

Armed with theoretical knowledge, you should be able to teach your clients realistically about the risks associated with exercise and thereby help them to exercise safely.

- *Cardiac injury.* Fear of triggering a cardiac event prevents some people from exercising. It is true that each year approximately 25,000 deaths occur among high-risk individuals after heavy exertion (Astrand, 2003). But statistics also reveal that the risk of having a heart attack during strenuous exercise is 1 in 1 million for a healthy 50-year-old man who does not smoke or have diabetes. The risk decreases further if the person increases his activity gradually.

- *Musculoskeletal injury.* High-impact exercises, such as running or aerobic dance, may pose a risk for injuries to bones, joints, and muscles. However, you can prevent most such injuries by gradually increasing the activity level or varying activities. Walking is an exercise that most people can do without injury. Injury can also occur from lifting weights. Free weights can cause injury if the person lifts too much weight or uses poor body mechanics when lifting. Working with a trainer to learn how to lift properly markedly decreases the risk of injury. In addition, exercise machines provide some degree of control and are less likely to cause injury.

BOX 31-2 Benefits of Regular Exercise

Cardiovascular System

- Improves pumping action of the heart
- Decreases heart rate and blood pressure
- Improves circulation by increasing the number of capillaries
- Improves venous return to the heart
- Increases high-density lipoprotein (HDL) and decreases low-density lipoprotein (LDL) and total cholesterol
- Decreases risk of thrombophlebitis

Respiratory System

- Improves pulmonary circulation
- Improves gas exchange at alveolar-capillary membrane
- Dilates bronchioles to increase ventilation

Musculoskeletal System

- Improves skeletal development in children
- Increases muscle strength
- Improves flexibility
- Increases coordination
- Helps maintain joint structure and function; reduces risk of osteoarthritis
- Improves bone mineral density
- Improves bone mass with aging; reduces risk of osteoporosis
- Reduces risk of falls and helps older adults maintain an independent lifestyle

Nervous System

- Speeds nerve impulse transmission

Endocrine System

- Increases sensitivity to insulin at the receptor sites
- Increases efficiency with metabolic processes
- Improves temperature regulation
- Facilitates weight management

Gastrointestinal System

- Improves appetite
- Improves abdominal muscle tone
- Decreases risk of colon cancer

Urinary System

- Increases efficiency of kidney function

Integumentary System

- Improves skin tone as a result of improved circulation

Immune System

- Reduces susceptibility to minor viral illnesses

Mental Health

- Increases energy
- Releases endorphins, which assist with pain control and stress management
- Increases time spent in stage IV and REM sleep
- Improves self-esteem and body image
- Provides a nonpharmacological way to relieve symptoms of anxiety and depression

---

- *Dehydration.* Dehydration can occur with prolonged exercise, with warm temperatures, or as a result of health problems or medications. During an intense exercise period, the body can lose 2 liters of fluid for every hour of exercise. It is important to drink before, during, and after the exercise period. Water is still the best choice to drink during and after exercise. Some sports drinks have glucose and electrolytes for replacement and quick energy, but water still has been shown to be the best for fluid replacement.

- *Temperature regulation problems. Hyperthermia* can occur when the person exercises in a hot climate. Hyperthermia is often accompanied by dehydration. *Heat exhaustion* is a potentially life-threatening event. Signs of heat exhaustion include lightheadedness, nausea, headache, fatigue, hyperventilation, loss of concentration, and abdominal cramps. Body temperature rises, but the skin is clammy and cold. In contrast, *hypothermia* can occur when the person does not wear proper clothing or is exposed to cool water for an extended period of time. Hypothermia is characterized by fatigue, confusion, and lack of coordination.

The risks associated with exercise are not as great as the risks of avoiding exercise. Advise clients to follow the tips in the Self-Care box to exercise safely and help prevent injury.

KnowledgeCheck 31–3

- Identify and describe four types of exercise.
- State the components of an exercise program

 Go to Chapter 31, **Knowledge Check Response Sheet and Answers,** on the Electronic Study Guide.

CriticalThinking 31–2

- How would you address Helen Jillian's ("Meet Your Patients") concerns about the risks associated with her engaging in an exercise program?
- Peter Phan ("Meet Your Patients") has experienced a number of injuries as a result of his exercise. Based on your knowledge of exercise, what questions would you like to ask Peter about his exercise program?

FACTORS AFFECTING MOBILITY AND ACTIVITY

Factors influencing activity and exercise include developmental stage, nutrition, lifestyle, attitudes, external factors, diseases, and physical abnormalities. These factors are discussed in the next sections.

Developmental Stage

Neuromuscular development is related to age. A newborn can move his extremities and turn his head from side to side, but he is unable to get from place to place. As the child matures, motor skills and coordination develop. With increasing abilities, the range of possible activities also increases. Unfortunately, children in the United States are becoming more sedentary, and the incidence of obesity continues to rise. For example, 41% of schools offered daily physical education classes for school-age children in 1991. By 1996 the number had declined to 25%. In addition, only 19% of all high school students were physically active for 20 minutes or more in physical education classes every day during the school week. Changes in the economy and a shortage of teachers are expected to lead to further drops in school-based physical education programs (U.S. Department of Health and Human Services, 1996).

Adulthood carries additional demands. Young adults often must balance the responsibilities of school, work, relationships, and family. By middle adulthood, the demands of aging parents, growing children, and work have created an inactive generation that is at increased risk for chronic health problems. The expected physiological changes associated with growing older make it harder to start or maintain an exercise program. Table 31–2 discusses neuromuscular development across the life span and associated nursing considerations.

Nutrition

In the United States, obesity is a major health problem. Obesity often leads to type II diabetes mellitus, atherosclerosis, hypertension, sleep apnea, and some respiratory difficulties. Fast food in super-sized portions, as well as the ready availability of convenience foods high in saturated fat and simple carbohydrates, plays a major role in the obesity problem. Although the obese person has plenty of calories available to expend on exercise, movement becomes more difficult as body size increases. In contrast, people with chronic disease may be in negative nitrogen balance—that is, they do not have adequate protein stores available to maintain or repair body tissue. They experience muscle wasting and fatigue, which lead to decreased activity levels.

Lifestyle

Over the last century, manual labor has declined and work environments have become increasingly sedentary. As a result, individuals need to look toward leisure time for exercise and fitness activities. This requires "making time" for exercise. Personal values about exercise and fitness determine when, or whether, exercise becomes part of a person's routine.

Some people love to exercise. Others see it as pure drudgery or as "something I have to do." A person's culture and support system define what exercise the person is likely to accept. For example, swimming requires wearing a bathing suit. People raised in the Amish culture value modesty and may not choose swimming as a form of exercise. Walking, which allows the person to dress in modest garb, would be an acceptable form of exercise for Amish people. Culture also determines what the person deems attractive. If a plump wife symbolizes that the husband provides well for his family, a man may discourage his wife from starting an exercise program.

Stress

How is your stress level? You may want to turn back to Chapter 25 and evaluate your stress using the questionnaire provided there. A high stress level can produce fatigue. Although you may view exercise as one more thing you don't have time for, exercise is energizing and can be used to relieve stress. For example, taking a brisk 20-minute walk during a study break may allow you to continue working for several more hours. You can also use this technique when caring for patients. Hospitalized patients and family members often experience a lot of stress. Helping the patient take a walk to the courtyard, or instructing family members how to handle the wheelchair so they can take a walk around the block, will help lessen some of the strain.

External Factors

External factors affecting exercise include weather, pollution, neighborhood conditions, finances, and support systems. Weather has a strong influence on activity

TABLE 31-2   The Influence of Developmental Stage on Activity and Exercise

Activity	Nursing Considerations
Infant	
• By the age of 5 months, an infant can roll from abdomen to back. • By 6 months, an infant can turn from back to abdomen. • At 7 months, most infants can sit alone. • Around 9 months, an infant can crawl. • By 10 months, the child can move from a prone to sitting position. • At 11 months, the infant can "cruise" (walk holding onto furniture). • Many infants attempt their first independent steps by 12 months.	• Assess for developmental milestones. • Emphasize variations in reaching milestones. • Emphasize to caregivers the importance of monitoring for safety as the infant becomes mobile.
Toddler	
• By age 3, the toddler can balance on one foot, jump on both feet, walk up steps using both feet, and run. • The toddler can ride a tricycle, put simple puzzles together, build a tower of six to eight blocks, turn knobs, and open lids.	• Teach the importance of providing supervision and a safe environment. • Encourage parents to set limits to protect the child as he begins to explore his world.
Preschool	
• By age 5, most children can stand on one foot for 10 seconds, skip, jump, and hop on one foot or both feet together. Most can climb play structures with ease.	• With the child's increasing mobility, the risk for injury increases. • Encourage daily active play.
School Age	
• By age 8, improved fine-motor skills allow the child to begin to write, learn to knit or crochet, and/or take up a musical instrument. • By age 9, motor development approaches that of an adult. • As fine-motor skills improve, children are able to do more sedentary activities, such as playing video games and using the computer.	• Continue to encourage daily physical activity and exercise.
Adolescent	
• The adolescent reaches adult height and about 90% of peak bone density by the end of adolescence.	• Emphasize the importance of eating a healthy diet, exercising regularly, and avoiding junk food.
Adult	
• The adult often must balance work and family obligations. • For most, activity levels begin to decline in middle age.	• Teach clients about the value of exercise and activity to promote health and prevent disease.
Older Adult	
• Physiological changes associated with aging include: Decreased muscle strength Decreased body mass Decreased bone mass Decreased joint mobility Increased fat deposits	• Assess for ability to perform ADLs and IADLs. • Teach about the importance of exercise and nutrition to promote health and prevent disease. • Monitor gait, balance, posture, and change in height. • Assess risk for falls.

TABLE
3

Disorder:
anemia, a
    Bed
disorders
pregnanc
bed rest,
caused b
discussed

Knowl

* In whic
  cerns t
* What t
* What a
* What i

Go t
Ans

C

* Your te
  calciur
  teachir
  measu
* Phillip
  in a rec
  most o
  weight
  disease
  exercis
  dations
  start ar

HAZARI

Most peo
ness, dise
Even sho
you've ev
bed, you l
your pre-
prolonged
changes i
chological
others are

Effect o

Even one
weak, bec
the first
causes si
soleus, an
sion of th
leads to 7
week. Im
stiff. The

level. Cold, damp weather encourages people to stay inside, whereas warm, sunny weather makes it fun to go outside and exercise. Encourage patients to choose a variety of activities that they enjoy so they can exercise regardless of the weather. Pollution has a similar effect on exercise. When air quality is poor, encourage indoor activities.

Neighborhood conditions, such as crime or lack of parks, influence attitudes about outside activities. Mall walking is an example of a successful way to incorporate exercise into daily patterns when neighborhood conditions do not encourage activity. Lack of money may make it difficult to join a gym and engage in some sports (e.g., skiing, golfing). However, many activities, such as walking, are inexpensive.

The support system is perhaps the most influential external factor. Family and friends who encourage activity will help you find ways to exercise. Those who are themselves sedentary may discourage you.

Diseases and Abnormalities

Diseases and abnormalities in various body systems can negatively influence body alignment, balance, coordination, and joint mobility. In the next sections, we describe some disorders that affect activity and exercise.

Congenital Abnormalities of the Musculoskeletal System

The following are common congenital abnormalities that affect appearance, motor function, and mobility:

* *Syndactylism* is the fusion of two or more fingers or toes. Most cases involving the hands are treated surgically at an early age to limit the effect on fine-motor development.
* *Developmental dysplasia of the hip (DDH)* is an abnormality of the development of the femur, acetabulum, or both. It is usually present at birth but can occur anytime in infancy. The incidence of DDH is about 1 in 1000 live births. Clinical examination is the most important tool to recognize this defect.
* *Foot deformities* occur in about 4% of all newborns. Serial casts or surgery may be used to correct the defect and preserve function.
* *Scoliosis* is a lateral curvature of the spine. Scoliosis can result from congenital bone disorders, neuromuscular impairment, or trauma, but 65% of cases have no known cause and are termed *idiopathic scoliosis.* Idiopathic scoliosis is classified as infantile, juvenile, or adolescent depending on the age of onset.

Nursing responsibilities for all of these disorders include early detection and referral for additional treatment, parent counseling, and careful attention to positioning and transfers.

Diseases Related to Bone Formation or Metabolism

Bone formation abnormalities may be congenital, related to dietary deficiencies, or the result of bone disease. *Osteogenesis imperfecta (OI)* is a congenital disorder of bone and connective tissue that is characterized by brittle bones that fracture easily. Infants with OI are often born with fractures and continue to fracture with minimal trauma or even spontaneously. Prompt recognition and treatment of fractures helps prevent deformities. *Achondroplasia,* or dwarfism, occurs when the bones ossify (harden) prematurely. *Paget's disease* is a metabolic bone disease in which increased bone loss results in pain, pathological fractures, and deformities. This disorder usually affects the skull, vertebrae, femur, and pelvis.

Vitamin D and calcium are needed to form and maintain bone. Deficiencies lead to porous bones. In children, prolonged deficiencies can cause the long bones of the legs to become bowed, retard growth, and lead to frequent fractures. Teach patients to consume a balanced diet that meets the minimum recommendations for vitamins and minerals.

Nursing responsibilities for patients with bone formation abnormalities include collaborative treatments, patient education to promote mobility, providing comfort, and lifting and transferring patients safely.

Diseases Affecting Joint Mobility

Diseases of the joints may be degenerative or inflammatory. The most prevalent type of degenerative joint disease is *osteoarthritis (OA).* OA involves a loss of articular cartilage in the joint, with pain and stiffness as the primary symptoms. Patients may also have decreased range of motion and **crepitus,** a creaking or grating sound, with joint motion. Symptoms are aggravated by weight bearing and joint use and are relieved by resting the affected joints. OA is more common in women, older adults, and people who are overweight.

Rheumatoid arthritis (RA) is a systemic autoimmune disease involving chronic inflammation of the joints and surrounding connective tissue. RA causes joint pain, deformity, and loss of function; patients may also experience fever, fatigue, weakness, and weight loss. RA occurs most frequently in the fingers, wrists, elbows, ankles, and knees. RA occurs in 1 to 2% of the population, with a greater incidence in women. Symptoms may appear as early as 30 years of age, but most patients are over 70. Unlike OA, RA does not improve with rest. Pain is worst when the person arises from bed. Pain and joint deformities may so severely affect mobility that patients cannot care for themselves.

Ankylosing spondylitis is a chronic inflammatory joint disease characterized by stiffening and fusion of the spine and sacroiliac joints. The inflammation occurs

TABLE 31

TABLE **31-3**   Range of Motion at the Joints *(continued)*

Joint	Normal Range	Illustration
Abduction—Spread the fingers apart.	20°	
Adduction—Bring the fingers together.	20°	
Thumb (Saddle Joint)		
Flexion—Move the thumb across the palm of the hand toward the 5th finger.	90°	
Extension—Move the thumb laterally away from the fingers.	90°	
Opposition—Touch the thumb to the top of each finger of the same hand	N/A	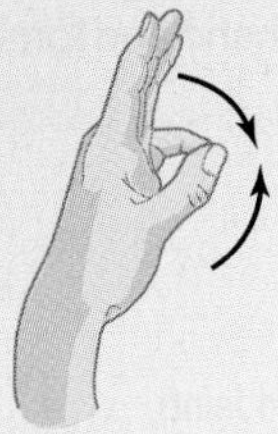
Hip (Ball-and-Socket Joint)		
Flexion—Move the leg forward and up.	Knee extended 90°	
Extension—Move the leg back down beside the other.	Knee flexed 120°	
Hyperextension—Move the leg back behind the body.	30–50°	
Abduction—Move the leg laterally.	45–50°	
Adduction—Sweep the leg inward across the midline.	20–30° beyond the other leg	

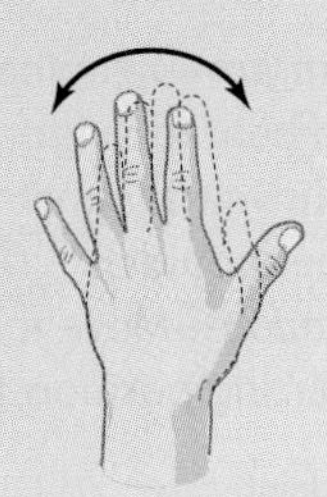

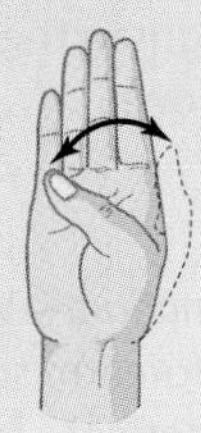

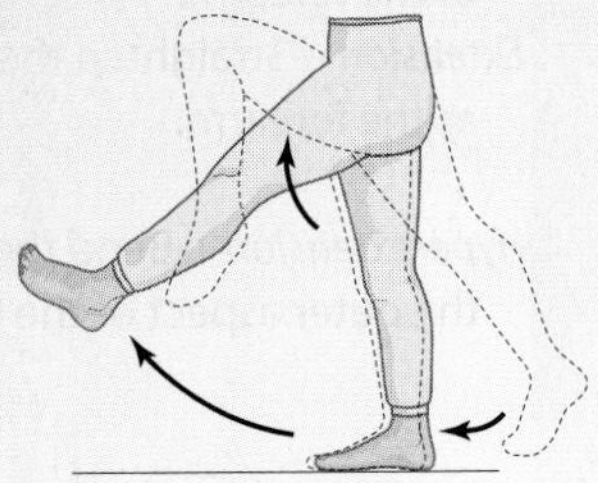

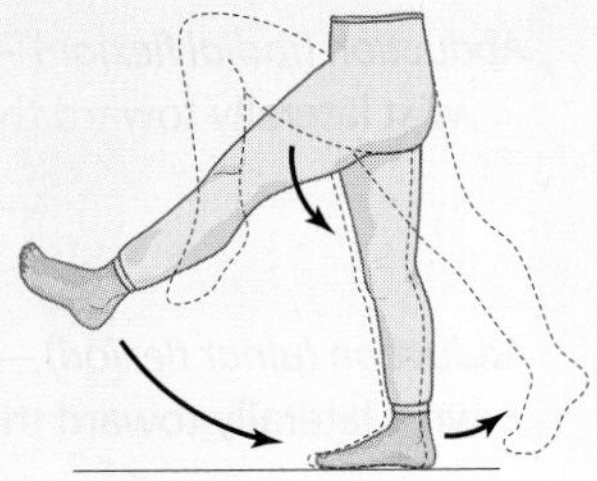

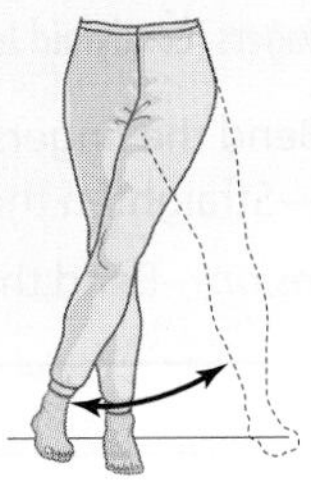

(Left column — partial text, cut off at page margin:)

where the
into the b
adults, eq
toms incl
creased ra
bar curve
causing ky

Gout i
uric acid.
small whi
neous tiss
verely lim

Nursi
problems
ing comfo
ity is seve
with activ

Problems

Osteoporos
occurs whe
teoblasts.
ishes, and
bone mass
of life. Aft
ence a rap
men, a gra
they becon
tures of th
may occur

The be
Teach ado
ride, and c
gram they
older wom
help decre
ask their
mineral lo

Osteo
after bone
pensive to
nent disal
that are ir
of the bod
multiply r
function.
and severe
patients w
laborative
treatment

Trauma

Trauma ca
One of the
ture, or a
fracture in

TABLE 31-3 *(continued)*

Joint	Normal Range	Illustration
Circumduction—Circle the leg, keeping the knee straight.	360°	
Internal rotation—Turn the foot and leg inward toward the other leg.	90°	
External rotation—Turn the foot and leg outward, pointing the toes as far as possible away from the other leg.	90°	
Knee (Hinge Joint)		
Flexion—Bend at the knee, bringing the heel back toward the buttocks.	120–130°	
Extension—Straighten the knee, returning the leg to its original position.	120–130°	
Ankle (Hinge Joint)		
Extension (plantar flexion)—Point the toes and foot downward.	45–50°	
Flexion (dorsiflexion)—Pull the toes and foot upward.	20°	
Foot (Gliding Joint)		
Eversion—Turn the sole of the foot laterally.	5°	
Inversion—Turn the sole of the foot medially.	5°	
Toes (Hinge, Except Intertarsal Joints, Which Are Gliding Joints)		
Flexion—Curl the toes downward.	35–60°	

TABLE 31-3 Range of Motion at the Joints *(continued)*

Joint	Normal Range	Illustration
Extension—Straighten the toes. *Abduction*—Spread the toes apart. *Adduction*—Bring the toes together.	35–60° 0–15° 0–15°	
Trunk		
Flexion—At the waist, bend forward toward the toes. *Extension*—Straighten the trunk from the flexed position. *Hyperextension*—Bend the trunk backward.	70–90° 70–90° 20–30°	
Lateral flexion—Bend the trunk to the side.	20–40°	
Rotation—Turn the upper body from side to side (twist at the waist).	30–45°	

Gait

The way a person moves communicates a lot about his general state of health, mood, and risk for falls. Gait is divided into two phases: stance and swing. In the *stance phase,* the heel of one foot strikes the ground while the opposite foot pushes off and leaves the ground. In the *swing phase,* the leg from behind moves in front of the body. When the right leg is in stance mode, the left leg is in swing mode (see Volume 2, page 302). To assess gait you need to observe the patient walking. Normal gait includes the following features:

- Head is erect, and gaze forward.
- Heel strikes the ground before the toe.
- Opposite arm moves forward at the same time.
- Feet are dorsiflexed in the swing phase.
- Gait is coordinated and rhythmic.
- Weight is evenly distributed, with minimal swing from side to side.
- Movement starts and stops with ease.
- Movement is at a moderate pace.

If the patient uses an assistive device, such as a cane, crutch, or walker, pay attention to how the patient uses the device. You may wish to ask the patient to ambulate a short distance with and without the device to determine whether the device is actually providing stability.

Activity Tolerance

To evaluate activity tolerance, assess and record vital signs before and after activity. Select an activity appropriate for the patient. For a patient without obvious health limitations, consider having her run in place for 3 minutes. If the patient shows any signs of distress, stop the exercise, immediately take a set of vital signs, and repeat the vital signs every minute until they have returned to baseline. A wide swing in vital signs or a slow return to baseline indicates limited activity tolerance.

KnowledgeCheck 31–6

- Describe a focused assessment for a patient experiencing mobility concerns.
- Identify the assessment methods (inspection, palpation, percussion, and auscultation) used when performing a physical examination focused on mobility concerns.

 Go to Chapter 31, **Knowledge Check Response Sheet and Answers,** on the Electronic Study Guide.

 CriticalThinking 31–4

Review the "Meet Your Patient" scenario. Which, if any, of the class participants requires a physical examination focused on mobility concerns? Explain your reasoning.

| Nursing Diagnosis |

Nursing diagnoses that specifically address activity and exercise include the following.

Activity Intolerance is a state in which a patient has insufficient physical or psychological energy to carry out daily activities. Subjective defining characteristics include fatigue, weakness, discomfort on exertion, dyspnea, and verbalization of no interest in activity. Objective defining characteristics include changes in heart rate, blood pressure disproportionate to activity, dysrhythmias or evidence of ischemia on electrocardiogram (ECG), and pallor or cyanosis with activity. Etiologies include conditions that affect tissue oxygenation (e.g., chronic obstructive pulmonary disease or cardiac disease) or conditions that produce fatigue, such as depression, prolonged immobility, and sedentary lifestyle.

Impaired Physical Mobility is limitation of independent purposeful movement of the body. Subjective defining characteristics are pain or discomfort with movement. Objective defining characteristics include limited ROM, limitations in fine- or gross-motor movement, lack of coordination with movement, unstable gait, and difficulty performing ADLs. Etiologies include neuromuscular or musculoskeletal impairment, malnutrition, obesity, deconditioning due to sedentary lifestyle, and lack of knowledge about the importance of activity and exercise for maintenance of health.

Impaired Physical Mobility is a broad, general diagnosis. Use the following, more descriptive diagnoses when the patient has specific deficits: Impaired Bed Mobility, Impaired Walking, Impaired Wheelchair Mobility, and Impaired Transfer Ability.

Mobility problems may also be the etiology of other diagnoses. The following are examples:

- Risk for Disuse Syndrome occurs when there is a risk for deterioration of body systems due to musculoskeletal inactivity. Risk factors include prescribed bedrest, severe pain, altered level of consciousness, mechanical immobilization (traction), and paralysis.
- Acute Pain related to musculoskeletal injury.
- Ineffective Health Maintenance related to prescribed bedrest.
- Risk for Injury related to unsteady gait.
- Self-Care Deficit (Bathing/Hygiene, Feeding, Dressing/Grooming, Toileting) related to Impaired Physical Mobility.

| Planning Outcomes/Evaluation |

For *associated NOC standardized outcomes* for mobility diagnoses,

 Go to Chapter 31, **Standardized Language, Selected NOC Outcomes for Energy Maintenance and Mobility,** in Volume 2.

Individualized goals/outcome statements depend on the nursing diagnosis used. Because activity and exercise abilities are individualized, goals must consider the patient's current condition, expected condition changes, lifestyle, and values. Examples:

- Will independently transfer to the wheelchair by [date].
- Will discuss his feelings about his activity restrictions by [date].

| Planning Interventions/Implementation |

Because attitudes about fitness and activity vary widely, mobility is often a difficult topic. Some people are devastated by activity limitations caused by disease or treatment. Others are able to accept these changes. For these reasons, it is important for you to convey an attitude of acceptance about the patient's current activity level and provide care that helps the patient achieve his optimal level of function.

For *NIC standardized interventions and activities* for patients with mobility problems,

 Go to Chapter 31, **Standardized Language, Selected NIC Interventions for Activity and Exercise Management and Immobility Management,** in Volume 2.

Specific nursing activities to promote exercise and mobility include promoting exercise, preventing injury from exercise, positioning patients, moving patients in bed, transferring patients out of bed, performing range-of-motion exercises, and assisting with ambulation.

Promoting Exercise

The following are the most common reasons people fail to develop a regular exercise program. Included are some suggestions for overcoming those objections:

- "I hate to exercise." *Suggestion:* Pick several activities that you enjoy.
- "I burn out on exercise." *Suggestion:* Plan ahead and build in rest days and varied activities.
- "I am self-conscious about going to the gym and don't have the motivation to exercise by myself." *Suggestion:* Find a friend to exercise with, or develop a reward system for yourself if you continue to exercise.
- "I have tried to exercise, but it didn't make a difference." *Suggestion:* Remember, gaining weight and getting out of shape takes time. Reversing these changes also takes time. Give yourself at least 12 weeks to see the effects of an exercise program.
- "I am too busy with work or family." *Suggestion:* Develop a routine that you can do at lunchtime, or exercise with your family.
- "I find exercise boring." *Suggestion:* Change your routine frequently.
- "Exercise hurts." *Suggestion:* Make sure to exercise at your target heart rate, and plan a rest day after every weight-lifting session.
- "I don't have time." *Suggestion:* Schedule your exercise time. If need be, schedule several short 10- to 15-minute sessions throughout the day.

Preventing Injury from Exercise

As previously discussed, the benefits of exercise outweigh any associated risks. Advise clients to follow the tips in the Self-Care box on p. 733 to exercise safely and help prevent injury.

Positioning Patients

Healthy people regularly shift position to maintain comfort. However, many patients are unable to move without assistance. They require a change of position at least every 2 hours to prevent skin breakdown, muscle discomfort, damage to superficial nerves and blood vessels, and contractures.

A firm mattress provides support to the patient's body and makes it easier to turn the patient (because he does not sink down into the mattress). Most hospital

Teaching Your Patient How to Prevent Back Injuries

- Poor posture is one of the main causes of back pain. Make a conscious effort to maintain good posture at all times.
- Use a firm mattress that provides adequate support.
- Sit with your knees slightly lower than your hips.
- If you must stand for a long period of time, flex your hip and raise one foot on a stool or object 6 to 8 inches off the ground. Periodically switch legs.
- Wear comfortable, low-heeled shoes. Avoid high heels as much as possible.
- Avoid restrictive clothing that inhibits your ability to use good body mechanics.
- Follow principles of body mechanics at all times (e.g., use wide base of support, and do not lift with your back).
- Exercise regularly to maintain your optimal weight and strengthen the muscles of your body.
- Include abdominal exercises in your routine. Strong abdominal muscles help support the back.
- Avoid lifting excessive weight.
- Avoid exercises or movements that cause spinal flexion (e.g., toe-touches, sit-ups with knees extended), excessive flexion of the neck (e.g., abdominal crunches with neck curved to chest), or spinal rotation (twisting).

mattresses are firm. However, when you provide home care, you will find mattresses of various types and conditions. To provide additional support, you can place a piece of plywood under a sagging mattress.

A clean, dry bed also makes it easier to turn the patient and decreases the risk of skin maceration or pressure ulcer formation. Bedding should provide coverage and warmth but not be tucked in so tightly as to restrict movement.

Back injuries are the leading cause of injury among nurses. To protect yourself from injury as you move patients, avoid manual lifting as much as possible. Use assistive equipment and devices, as recommended by the ANA (2005), and always make sure you have adequate help. The amount of help you need depends on the size of the patient, the level of assistance the patient can offer, your size and strength, and the equipment or lines attached to the patient. The accompanying Self-Care box describes strategies to decrease your risk of back injury. Also teach these strategies to your patients.

Positioning Devices

Devices used to maintain body alignment, prevent contractures, and promote comfort are briefly discussed in the next sections.

Adjustable Beds

An adjustable bed, often referred to as a hospital bed, assumes a variety of positions. You can elevate or lower the head of the bed, and elevate the foot of the bed. Often the bed breaks, or "gatches," at the knee to keep the patient from sliding down when the head is elevated. You can also adjust the height of the bed. You should raise the bed to waist height when providing care so that you can use proper body mechanics; place the bed in its lowest position before helping a patient get out of bed or if the patient is at risk for falling.

Several types of specialized beds are used in treating and preventing pressure ulcers. These include alternating, low air loss, immersion (air-fluidized), and oscillating beds. The mattresses may be composed of air, water, or gel. Special beds are further discussed in Chapter 34. A circular bed and Stryker frame are used in the care of patients with severe mobility restrictions. Both can rotate a patient from supine to prone. With the advent of low-pressure specialized beds, these types of beds are now in limited use.

Pillows

Pillows are the most common devices used to assist with positioning, provide support, and elevate body parts. They help position a patient by molding to the body and expanding the weight-bearing area. You will need a variety of sizes to position patients who are unconscious, paralyzed, or frail. To obtain the right size, or if pillows are not available, you can use folded blankets or towels. Foam wedge pillows are useful for elevating the upper body when an adjustable bed is not available and for abducting the hips after hip surgery.

Siderails

Most hospital beds are equipped with siderails. The rails may run the full length of each side of the bed or consist of an upper or lower rail on each side. Siderails are designed to ensure patient safety: They serve as a reminder that the patient should call for assistance before getting out of bed and provide a grip for the patient who is able to reposition himself in bed.

Although siderails are designed to protect patients, they can be a source of injury: Patients can get tangled in the railing or fall between the bed and rail, and confused patients may injure themselves trying to climb over the rails. Siderails may also be considered a form of restraint (see Chapter 21), so be sure to discuss their purpose with patients and family.

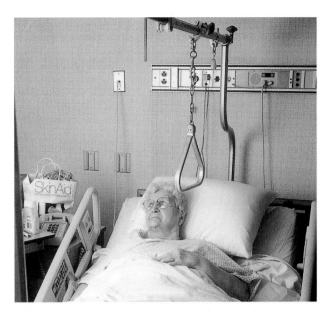

FIGURE 31–6 A trapeze bar provides a grip for the patient to reposition himself independently.

Trapeze Bar

A trapeze bar is a triangular-shaped bar that is attached to an overhead bed frame (Figure 31–6). The patient can use the base of the triangle as a grip bar to move up in bed, turn, and pull up in preparation for getting out of bed or getting on and off the bedpan. Patients can use the trapeze to exercise the upper extremities. Frail patients may not be able to use a trapeze bar because of the amount of effort it requires.

Footboard

When a person is supine, the toes drop, and the feet are in plantar flexion. Able-bodied persons usually shift position throughout the night, so the foot and leg muscles are periodically contracted and relaxed. In contrast, the patient who is unable to move independently will experience a shortening of the gastrocnemius muscle and may have difficulty walking again if prolonged plantar flexion (foot drop) occurs. A footboard is a device placed at the end of the bed to prevent plantar flexion (Figure 31–7). For the footboard to be effective, the heels must be touching it. Each time you turn the patient, you may need to reposition the footboard. High-top sneakers are also useful for preventing foot drop.

Other Positioning Devices

The following are other positioning devices used in the clinical setting.

- *Foot cradles* are metal or plastic devices that are secured at the foot of the bed to hold bedding up off the toes and feet, allowing for free movement.

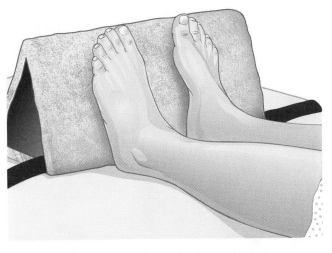

FIGURE 31–7   A footboard is placed at the end of the bed to prevent plantar flexion.

- *Sandbags* are small fabric bags filled with sand. They are used in the same manner as pillows and trochanter rolls; however, they provide firmer support.
- *Trochanter rolls* are made from tightly rolled towels, bath blankets, or foam pads. They are placed snugly adjacent to the hips and thighs to prevent external rotation of the hips. To learn how to make them,

 Go to Chapter 31, **Technique 31–2: Making a Trochanter Roll,** in Volume 2.

- *Hand and wrist splints* may be premanufactured or fashioned from rolled wash cloths. The purpose of splints is to hold the wrist and hand in natural position and prevent claw-hand deformities.

Positioning Techniques

In the next section we briefly describe the various ways to position patients. Table 31–4 illustrates these positions, identifies potential problems associated with them, and offers solutions to prevent the problems. The positions are also described and illustrated in Chapter 19, Table 19-1.

Fowler's Positions

Fowler's position is a semisitting position, in which the head of the bed is elevated 45 to 60°. This position promotes respiratory function by lowering the diaphragm and allowing the greatest chest expansion.

TABLE 31–4   Positioning a Bed-Bound Patient

Position	Potential Problem	Solution
Fowler's	Hyperextension of the neck	Use a small pillow under the head and neck.
	Posterior flexion of the lumbar curvature	Use a firm mattress. Position the patient so that the angle of elevation begins at the hip.
	Dislocation of the shoulders	Position a pillow under the forearms to prevent pull on the shoulders.
	Flexion contracture of the wrist and edema of the hands	Support the hands on pillows in alignment with the forearms.
	Flexion contracture of the fingers and abduction of the thumbs	Use hand splints if appropriate, or provide a large roll in the palm of the hand.
	External rotation of the legs	Place sandbags or rolls alongside the trochanters and upper thighs.
	Hyperextension of the knees	Place a small pillow under the lower legs from the ankles to below the knees. Do this for short periods only; avoid pressure on the popliteal area.
	Foot drop	Use a footboard or high-top sneakers to hold the feet in dorsiflexion.

TABLE 31-4 *(continued)*

Position	Potential Problem	Solution
Lateral 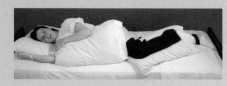	Lateral flexion of the neck	Place a pillow under the head and neck to provide alignment.
	Internal rotation and adduction of the upper shoulder and limited respirations	Place a pillow under the upper arm, and comfortably flex the lower arm.
	Internal rotation and adduction of the femur	Support the upper leg from groin to foot with pillows.
	Twisting of the spine	Align the shoulders with the hips.
	Flexion of the cervical spine	Place a pillow under the head and neck to provide alignment, unless drainage from the mouth is desired.
Prone 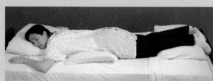	Hyperextension of the lumbar curvature, pressure on the breasts in women or genitals in men, impaired respirations	Place a small pillow under the abdomen.
	Foot drop	Move the patient down in bed so the feet extend over the edge of the mattress, or place a small pillow under the shins so that the toes do not touch the bed.
	Lateral flexion of the neck	Place a pillow under the head and neck to provide alignment, unless drainage from the mouth is desired.
Sims' 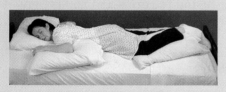	Internal rotation and adduction of the upper shoulder and limited respirations	Place a pillow under the upper arm, and comfortably flex the arm at the elbow.
	Pressure on the shoulder and axilla of the inferior arm	Position the lower arm behind and away from the back.
	Internal rotation and adduction of the femur	Support the upper leg from groin to foot with pillows.
	Twisting of the spine	Align the shoulders with the hips.
	Foot drop	Support the feet in dorsiflexion with sandbags.
	Hyperextension of the neck	Place a pillow under the head and neck to provide alignment.
Supine 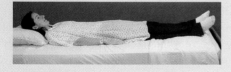	Internal rotation of the shoulders and extension of the elbows	Position the upper arms next to the body. Place pillows under the forearms, and position the wrists in slight pronation.
	Flexion of fingers and abduction of the thumbs	Use hand splints if appropriate, or provide a large roll in the palm of the hand.
	Flexion of the lumbar curvature and hips	Provide a firm mattress, or place a small pillow under the lumbar curvature.
	External rotation of the legs	Place sandbags or rolls alongside the trochanters and upper thighs.
	Hyperextension of the knees	Place a small pillow under the lower legs from the ankles to below the knees.
	Foot drop	Use a footboard or high-top sneakers to hold the feet in dorsiflexion.

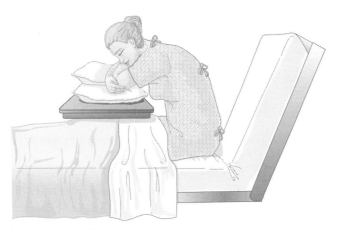

FIGURE 31–8   Orthopneic position is ideal for a patient with shortness of breath.

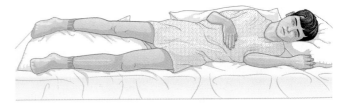

FIGURE 31–9   The oblique position is a modified lateral position that places less pressure on the trochanter.

It is also an ideal position for some patients with cardiac dysfunction. Common variations include **semi-Fowler's position,** in which the head of the bed is elevated only 30° and **high-Fowler's position,** in which the head is elevated 90°.

In **orthopneic position** (Figure 31–8), the head of the bed is elevated 90°, and an overbed table with a pillow on top is positioned in front of the patient. Have the patient lean forward, resting his arms and head on the pillow. This position is helpful for a patient with shortness of breath.

Lateral Positions

The **lateral position** is a side-lying position with the top hip and knee flexed and placed in front of the rest of the body. Lateral position creates pressure on the lower scapula, ilium, and trochanter but relieves pressure from the heels and sacrum. The **lateral recumbent position** is side-lying with legs in a straight line (see Table 19-1). The **oblique position** is an alternative to the lateral position that places less pressure on the trochanter. The patient turns on the side with the top hip and knee flexed; however, the top leg is placed behind the body (Figure 31–9).

Prone Position

In the **prone position,** the patient lies on his stomach with his head turned to one side. This is the only position that allows full extension of the hips and knees. It also allows secretions to drain freely from the mouth and thus is helpful for an unconscious patient. However, this is the most difficult position to move an unconscious or frail patient into, because it requires the greatest amount of manipulation to position the patient appropriately. Prone position creates a significant lordosis (inward curving of the spine in the lower back) and rotation of the neck. Therefore it should not be used for patients with cervical or lumbar

spine problems. You should not use prone position for patients with cardiac or respiratory difficulty because it inhibits chest wall expansion and, therefore, oxygenation. As a rule, you can use this position only for short periods of time.

Sims' Position

Sims' position is a semiprone position. The lower arm is positioned behind the patient, and the upper arm is flexed. The upper leg is more flexed than the lower leg. Sims' position facilitates drainage from the mouth and limits pressure on the trochanter and sacrum. This is an ideal position for administering an enema or a perineal procedure.

Supine Position

In the **supine position,** also known as the **dorsal recumbent position,** the patient lies on his back with head and shoulders elevated on a small pillow. The spine is aligned and the arms and hands comfortably rest at the side.

KnowledgeCheck 31–7

- Describe the following positions: Fowler's, lateral, prone, Sims', and supine.
- What is the advantage of the oblique position versus the lateral position?
- Identify and describe six positioning devices.
- What are three uses for siderails?

 Go to Chapter 31, **Knowledge Check Response Sheet and Answers,** on the Electronic Study Guide.

CriticalThinking 31–5

You are providing care for a young man who is recovering from Guillain-Barré syndrome, a syndrome that produces a reversible paralysis after viral illness. He has been healthy until this present illness. How would you position this patient? Explain your reasoning.

Moving Patients in Bed

To position patients, you must be adept at moving and lifting them in bed. This involves positioning the patient

in the length of the bed, as well as turning her. Before you move a patient, follow these guidelines:

- Identify any activity or movement restrictions.
- Review the patient's medical diagnoses. Identify problems that may affect positioning (e.g., respiratory or cardiac problems).
- Know what equipment (e.g., IVs, drainage devices) must be moved with the patient.
- Assess the size of the patient and her ability to assist with the move.
- Obtain assistance from other staff members, if needed. It is better to get more help than you need rather than not enough help.
- Medicate the patient for pain, if needed.
- Eliminate obstacles from the area around the bed.
- Lock the wheels of the bed.
- Avoid friction on the patient's skin. Cornstarch or powder on the patient or bedding decreases friction. Friction-reducing devices, such as transfer roller sheets, also facilitate movement.
- Use lifting and safety devices at all times.
- Explain to the patient what you are going to do.
- Always use proper body mechanics.

Moving Up in Bed

Frail patients slide down in bed because of gravity and their inability to correct their position. Elevating the head of the bed accentuates the slide and places the patient in an awkward position. If the patient is light in weight or able to provide assistance, you will be able to move her independently. The Critical Aspects box on p. 754 summarizes this procedure. For complete instructions,

 Go to Chapter 31, **Procedure 31-1A: Moving a Patient Up in Bed,** in Volume 2.

Turning in Bed

Turn patients at least every 2 hours to protect their skin and prevent other complications of immobility. For efficient use of time, try to time turning to coincide with moving the patient up in bed. Use pillows and other positioning devices to help the patient maintain the new position. The Critical Aspects box summarizes this procedure. For a complete description,

 Go to Chapter 31, **Procedure 31-1B: Turning a Patient in Bed,** in Volume 2.

Logrolling

Logrolling is a special turning technique used when the patient's spine must be kept in straight alignment.

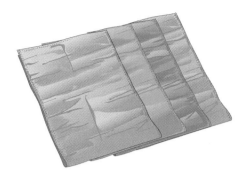

FIGURE 31-10 A transfer roller sheet reduces friction and facilitates movement.

You will need at least two nurses for this procedure, more if the patient is large. Logrolling moves the patient's body as a unit. One nurse is positioned at the level of the patient's head. The other staff members are distributed along the length of the patient. All must move the patient in unison. The Critical Aspects box summarizes this procedure. For a complete description,

 Go to Chapter 31, **Procedure 31-1C: Logrolling a Patient,** in Volume 2.

Friction-Reducing Devices

You can use one of a variety of friction-reducing devices when moving a patient in bed. Transfer roller sheets (Figure 31-10) are thin, low-friction fabric sheets that may be placed beneath the draw sheet to facilitate moving the patient in bed. A scoot sheet is also a thin, low-friction fabric sheet that is positioned under the draw sheet of the patient, but it is attached to a mechanical crank (Figure 31-11). By turning the

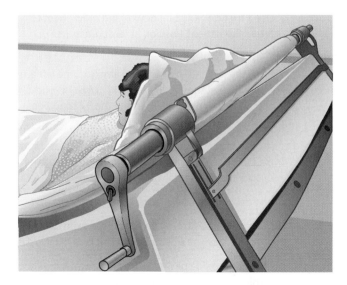

FIGURE 31-11 A scoot sheet allows a single person to move a patient up in bed.

mechanical crank, a single person can move a patient up in bed. Transfer roller sheets are relatively inexpensive and are widely available on clinical units. If one is not available, you can improvise by placing a clean, unused plastic bag under the draw sheet to help you move the patient. The plastic bag reduces drag and facilitates movement. However, unlike the thin fabric of transfer sheets, plastic allows moisture to pool under the patient. Consequently, you should not leave a bag in place under the draw sheet.

Transferring Patients Out of Bed

Stretchers and wheelchairs are used to transport patients between units or to tests or procedures. A stretcher is usually reserved for the patient who is weak, is sedated, or has a condition that does not permit transfer by wheelchair. A wheelchair may be used for transport or as part of an activity program. In addition, you may transfer patients to a stationary chair to increase their general activity level. The Critical Aspects box below summarizes procedures for transferring patients out of bed. For complete procedural steps,

 Go to Chapter 31, **Procedure 31–2A: Transferring a Client from Bed to Stretcher, Procedure 31–2B: Dangling a Patient at the Side of the Bed,** and **Procedure 31–2C: Transferring a Patient from Bed to Chair,** in Volume 2.

In the next sections we discuss devices that are used to facilitate transfers.

---

critical aspects of procedures 31–1 through 31–3

VOL 2 For steps to follow in *all* procedures, refer to the inside back cover of Volume 2.

Procedure 31–1A: Moving a Patient Up in Bed

- Use a friction-reducing device to move the patient if the patient can assist with movement. Use a full body sling if the patient cannot assist.

- Remove the pillow. Have the patient flex her neck, fold her arms across her chest, and place her feet flat on the bed.

- Position a nurse on either side of the patient.

- Use a wide base of support.

- Have the patient, on the count of 3, push off with his heels as you shift your weight forward.

Procedure 31–1B: Turning a Patient in Bed

- Use a friction-reducing device and draw sheet to move the patient. Position at least one nurse on each side of the bed.

- Place the patient's near leg and arm (e.g., the left arm and leg when turning to the right) across his body, and abduct and externally rotate the far shoulder.

- Each nurse places one arm at the level of the patient's shoulders and the other at the level of the patient's hips. Each nurse shifts her weight as both simultaneously roll the patient in the intended direction.

Procedure 31–1C: Logrolling a Patient

- Move the patient as a unit to the opposite side of the bed; raise the siderail on that side.

- Move to the side of the bed that the patient will be turning toward; lower the siderail.

- Each staff member evenly distributes his arms across the patient's length. One nurse is responsible for moving the head and neck as a unit.

- Shift your weight backward as you roll the patient toward you.

Procedure 31–2A: Transferring Patient from Bed to Stretcher

- Move the patient to the side of the bed where the stretcher will be placed.

- Position the stretcher next to the bed, and lock it in place.

- Using the draw sheet, turn the client away from the stretcher.

- Place the transfer board against the patient's back halfway between the bed and stretcher. Position a friction-reducing device over the transfer board. Turn the patient to his back and onto the transfer board with the draw sheet.

- Use the draw sheet to slide the patient across the transfer board onto the stretcher.

Procedure 31–2B: Dangling a Patient at the Side of the Bed

- Place the patient in a supine position, and raise the head of the bed to 90°.

- Apply a gait transfer belt, and place the bed in a low position.

- Stand facing the patient with a wide base of support. Place your foot closest to the head of the bed forward of the other foot.

Procedure 31–2B: (continued)

- Position your hands on each side of the gait transfer belt.

- Rock onto your back foot as you move the patient into a sitting position, and pivot to bring the patient's legs over the side of the bed.

- Stay with the patient as he dangles.

Procedure 31-2C: Transferring a Patient from Bed to Chair

- Have the patient wear nonskid slippers.

- Place the bed in low position, and lock the wheels.

- Assist the patient to dangle at the side of the bed (see Procedure 31-2B).

- Brace your feet and knees against the patient. Bend your hips at the knees, and hold onto the transfer belt.

- If two nurses are available to assist with the transfer, one nurse should be on each side of the patient.

- Instruct the patient to place her arms around you between your shoulders and waist. Ask the patient to stand as you move to an upright position by straightening your legs and hips.

- Instruct the patient to pivot and turn with you toward the chair.

- Have the patient flex her hips and knees as she lowers herself to the chair. Guide her motion while maintaining a firm hold on her.

Procedure 31-3: Assisting with Ambulation

- Have the patient wear nonskid slippers.

- Place the bed in low position, and lock the wheels.

- Assist the patient to dangle at the side of the bed (see Procedure 31-2B).

- If using two nurses each nurse should stand facing the patient on opposite sides of the patient.

- Brace your feet and knees against the patient. Bend your hips at the knees, and hold onto the transfer belt. Pay attention to any known weakness.

- Instruct the patient to place her arms around you between your shoulders and waist (the location depends on the height of the patient and the nurses). Ask the patient to stand as you move to an upright position by straightening your legs and hips.

- Allow the patient to steady herself for a moment.

- One nurse: Stand at the patient's side, placing both hands on the transfer belt. If the patient has weakness on one side, position yourself on the weaker side.

- Two nurses: Each nurse stands at the patient's sides, grasping hold of the transfer belt.

- Slowly guide the patient forward. Observe for signs of fatigue or dizziness.

- If the patient must transport an IV pole, allow the patient to hold onto the pole on the side where you are standing. Assist the patient to advance the pole as you ambulate together.

Transfer Board

A transfer board is a wood or plastic device designed to assist with moving patients. Using a transfer board reduces your risk of injury and promotes a smooth transfer. Place the board under the patient on the side to which he will be moved and use a draw sheet to slide the patient across the board. Transfer boards are also used by patients with long-standing mobility problems to increase their independence. Figure 31–12 is an example of a transfer board used to help a wheelchair-bound patient independently move from bed to chair.

Mechanical Lift

A mechanical lift is a hydraulic device used to transfer patients. Place a fabric sling under the patient, and attach chains or straps from the sling to the lifting device (Figure 31–13). A mechanical lift is especially useful when providing care for obese and immobile patients. Lifts are often used in home care because they allow one person to transfer the patient safely. Most lifts position

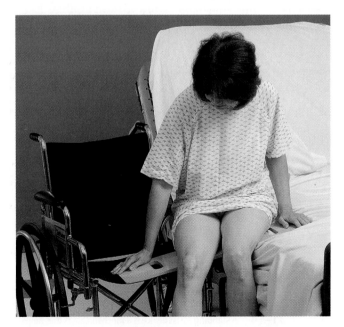

FIGURE 31–12   Transfer boards are used by patients with chronic mobility problems to increase their independence.

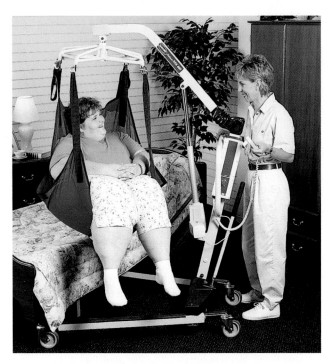

FIGURE 31–13   A mechanical lift is especially useful when providing care to obese and immobile patients.

patients in a seated position and thus are ideal for assisting the patient into a chair. Others suspend the patient in a supine position; they may be used to transfer the patient from bed to stretcher or to suspend the patient while the bed is made. Many such lifts include scales that weigh the patient while he is suspended in the sling. Standing assist devices (Figure 31–14) are mechanical lifts that help the patient move from a sitting to a standing position. A sling is positioned around the back and under the arms of the patient. Specialized chairs and wheelchairs are also available. Each has a mechanical lift in the seat that rises to assist the

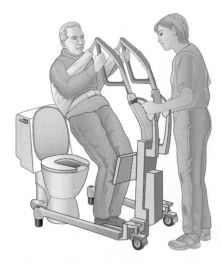

FIGURE 31–14   A standing assist device is a mechanical lift that helps the patient move from a sitting to a standing position.

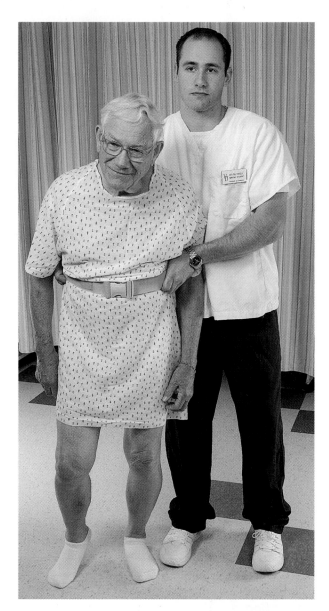

FIGURE 31–15   A transfer belt is placed close to the patient's center of gravity. It may have external grip holds to facilitate transfer or provide a secure mechanism to hold the patient when ambulating.

patient to a standing position. Mechanical lift devices reduce the risk of back and musculoskeletal injury. However, because these devices are expensive, they may not be available at all facilities.

Transfer Belt

A transfer belt is a heavy belt several inches wide, applied around the patient's hips and lower abdomen to facilitate transfer or provide a secure mechanism to hold the patient when ambulating. Place the belt close to the patient's center of gravity. The belt may have external grip holds, or you may grip the entire belt with your hand. Figure 31–15 illustrates the use of a transfer belt.

KnowledgeCheck 31–8

- What criteria determine whether your patient should be logrolled when he is repositioned?
- How often should you turn and reposition a patient?
- Identify the most appropriate device for the following activities:

  Transferring an obese patient from a bed to a stretcher

  Assisting an immobile patient to a recliner chair

  Helping a weak patient from bed to chair

 Go to Chapter 31, **Knowledge Check Response Sheet and Answers,** on the Electronic Study Guide.

Performing Range-of-Motion Exercises

Patients with limited mobility are at risk for developing complications of disuse, such as muscle atrophy and contractures. Range-of-motion exercises limit the complications of immobility. **Active range of motion (AROM)** occurs when the patient independently moves his joints through their range of motion. Patients recovering from illness, injury, or surgery often perform this exercise as a rehabilitation procedure. Performing ADLs and other daily activities exercises most joints. **Passive range of motion (PROM)** is movement of the joints through their range of motion by another person. Both active and passive range of motion improve joint mobility, increase circulation to the area exercised, and help maintain function. However, AROM also improves muscle strength and tone, as well as respiratory and cardiac function. For an explanation of how to perform PROM,

 Go to Chapter 31, **Technique 31–3: Performing Passive Range-of-Motion Exercises,** in Volume 2.

Assisting with Ambulation

Prolonged bedrest is no longer used in the treatment of most disorders. However, as a nurse, you will provide care to patients whose illnesses and injuries curtail their ability to walk and be active. Assisting patients with ambulation includes physical conditioning to prepare the patient for ambulation, as well as assisting the patient to walk.

Physical Conditioning

Patients who have been confined to bed for more than a week or who have sustained major injury require conditioning before they are able to resume walking. Conditioning exercises include the following:

- *Quadriceps and gluteal drills.* The quadriceps muscle group and the gluteal muscles are the largest muscles of the body. To protect your back, use these muscles whenever you lift heavy objects. Patients who are confined to bed can perform isometric muscles to prepare them for walking. Ask the patient to tighten her thigh muscles by pushing downward with her knees and flexing her feet. Hold the position for a count of 5 and then relax. Repeat this process two to three times per hour during the waking hours. To exercise the gluteal muscles, ask the patient to pinch her buttocks together. Repeat this exercise when the patient exercises the quadriceps muscles. Instruct the patient not to hold her breath as she exercises.

- *Arm exercises.* Patients use the arm muscles when getting out of bed and for crutch walking. To help prepare the patient for ambulation, install a trapeze bar. The trapeze bar exercises the biceps muscles. To exercise the triceps muscles, ask the patient to lift his upper body off the mattress by firmly pressing down with the palms. The patient can also do push-ups from a seated position at the side of the bed or from a stationary chair or wheelchair.

- *Dangling.* Dangling is a seated position at the side of the bed. The patient can rest his feet on the floor or a footstool. Use this position to prepare the patient to get up in a chair, to stand, or to ambulate. Patients who have been bedridden frequently become light-headed or develop orthostatic hypotension when first getting up. Dangling allows the patient to experience being upright with limited risk of falling. Do not increase the patient's activity further unless he is comfortable and stable in the dangling position.

- *Daily activities.* Encourage patients to be active in bed and to get out of bed into a chair prior to attempting to walk. ADLs exercise many of the muscle groups the patient needs for ambulation. Getting up to the chair accustoms the patient to an upright posture and is an important predictor of success with ambulation.

 Go to Chapter 31, **Technique 31–4: Assisting with Physical Conditioning Exercises to Prepare for Walking,** Volume 2.

Assisting the Patient to Walk

Before getting the patient out of bed, assess her readiness to walk. Also obtain the appropriate equipment and assistance. When possible, use a transfer belt. Have a chair or additional assistance available on the first few attempts at ambulation. If the patient becomes faint or begins to fall, do not attempt to hold him up by yourself. Instead, protect the patient as you guide him to a seated or lying position. Create a wide base of support, and project forward the hip closest to the patient. Help the patient slide down your leg as you call for help (Figure 31–16). Protect the patient's head as his body descends. The Critical Aspects box on p. 755 summarizes ambulation with one-nurse assist and with two-nurse assist. For the complete procedures,

 Go to Chapter 31, **Procedure 31–3A: Assisting with Ambulation (One Nurse),** and **Procedure 31–3B: Assisting with Ambulation (Two Nurses),** in Volume 2.

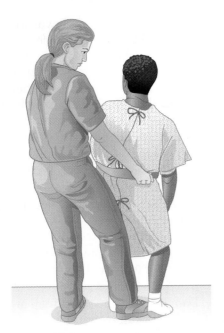

FIGURE 31–16 If the patient begins to fall, the nurse guides the patient gently to the floor or to a chair.

KnowledgeCheck 31–9

- Identify four principles to be followed when performing PROM.
- Describe activities that can promote a patient's readiness for ambulation.
- What action should you take if a patient begins to fall when ambulating?

 Go to Chapter 31, **Knowledge Check Response Sheet and Answers,** on the Electronic Study Guide.

Mechanical Aids for Walking

A variety of aids is available to promote stability and independence when walking. Some aids are intended for short-term use; others will be incorporated into the patient's lifestyle. Some patients consider the use of aids a sign of weakness. As a result, they avoid using the aid and increase their risk of falls. However, most people dread loss of independence, so you can promote the use of walking aids by stressing their importance in helping the person maintain independence. For instructions on sizing canes, walkers, and crutches,

 Go to Chapter 31, **Technique 31–5: Sizing Walking Aids,** in Volume 2.

For instructions on teaching patients to use these aids,

 Go to Chapter 31, **Technique 31–6: Teaching Patients to Use Canes, Walkers, and Crutches,** in Volume 2.

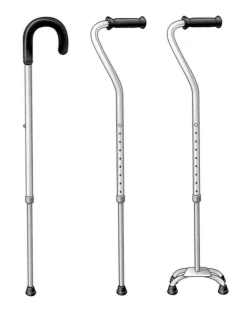

FIGURE 31–17 Three types of canes.

Canes

The following are three basic types of canes used (Figure 31–17):

- *Single-ended cane with a half-circle handle.* This is ideal for the patient who needs minimal support and is able to negotiate stairs.
- *Single-ended cane with a straight handle.* This is ideal for the patient with hand weakness who has good balance.
- *Multiprong canes.* A multiprong cane usually has three or four prongs, and all types have a straight handle. These canes provide a wide base of support and are useful for patients with balance problems.

Cane ends are covered with rubber tips to prevent slipping and improve traction. The length is adjustable. To size a cane, have the patient stand erect, and place the cane tip 20 cm (4 inches) to the side of the foot. The top of the cane should reach to the top of the hip joint so that the patient can hold the cane with her elbow flexed 30°. Instruct patients to do the following:

- Hold the cane on the stronger side.
- Distribute weight evenly between the feet and cane.
- Advance the cane and weaker leg simultaneously, then swing the stronger leg through.
- Avoid leaning over onto the cane.

Walkers

A walker is a lightweight metal frame device with four legs that provides a wide base of support as a patient ambulates. The walker is sized like a cane. It should

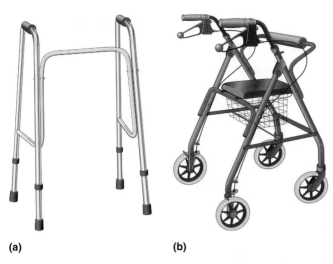

(a)　　　　　　　　　　(b)

FIGURE 31–18 Walkers. *A*, The basic walker is picked up and advanced as the patient steps ahead. *B*, Some walkers have wheels and seats that allow the patient to rest periodically.

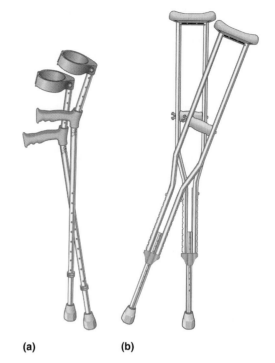

(a)　　　　　　　　　　(b)

FIGURE 31–19 Crutches. *A*, Forearm support crutches. *B*, Axillary crutches.

extend from the floor to the hip joint so that the patient can comfortably hold the walker with 30° flexion of the elbow. When using a basic walker, the patient stands between the back legs of the walker (Figure 31–18*A*). The patient picks up the walker and advances it as he steps ahead. If one leg is impaired, the patient should move that leg forward with the walker. Other forms of walkers are available. Some models have wheels that allow the walker to be rolled forward; others have a seat that allows the patient to rest periodically (Figure 31–18*B*). These walkers are best for patients whose mobility problems are related to fatigue or shortness of breath rather than gait instability.

Braces

Braces support joints and muscles that cannot independently support the body's weight. They are most commonly used in the lower extremities. Physical medicine specialists usually fit the brace. Nursing responsibilities include assisting the patient into and out of the brace and monitoring the condition of the skin under the brace.

Crutches

Crutches are commonly used for rehabilitation of an injured lower extremity. The purpose of using crutches is to limit or eliminate weight bearing on the leg(s) by forcing the user to rely on strength in the arms and shoulders for support. Two forms of crutches are available:

- The *forearm support crutch* is more likely to be used by a patient with permanent limitations. It is usually constructed of lightweight aluminum with a hand hold and a forearm support (Figure 31–19*A*).

- *Axillary crutches* are for both short- and long-term use (Figure 31–19*B*). Properly fitted axillary crutches support the body weight in the hands and arms, not the axilla. For guidelines on how to measure a patient for an axillary crutch,

VOL 2 Go to Chapter 31, **Technique 31–5: Sizing Walking Aids,** in Volume 2.

Crutch walking taxes the arms and hands, so the patient may need exercises for the shoulders, arms, and hands. To build strength in the shoulders and arms, have the patient use a trapeze and lift the hips off the bed with her arms. To develop forearm and hand strength, have the patient squeeze a rubber ball or gripper ball. To strengthen the legs, have the patient perform straight leg raises and isometric tightening of the quadriceps.

When first instructing the patient in crutch use, have the patient stand near a wall with a chair behind her. Help the patient stand and grip the crutches. Ask the patient to sway from side to side on the crutches so that she becomes accustomed to having her arms bear her weight. For guidelines for teaching patients to use crutches,

VOL 2 Go to Chapter 31, **Technique 31–6: Teaching Clients to Use Canes, Walkers, and Crutches,** in Volume 2.

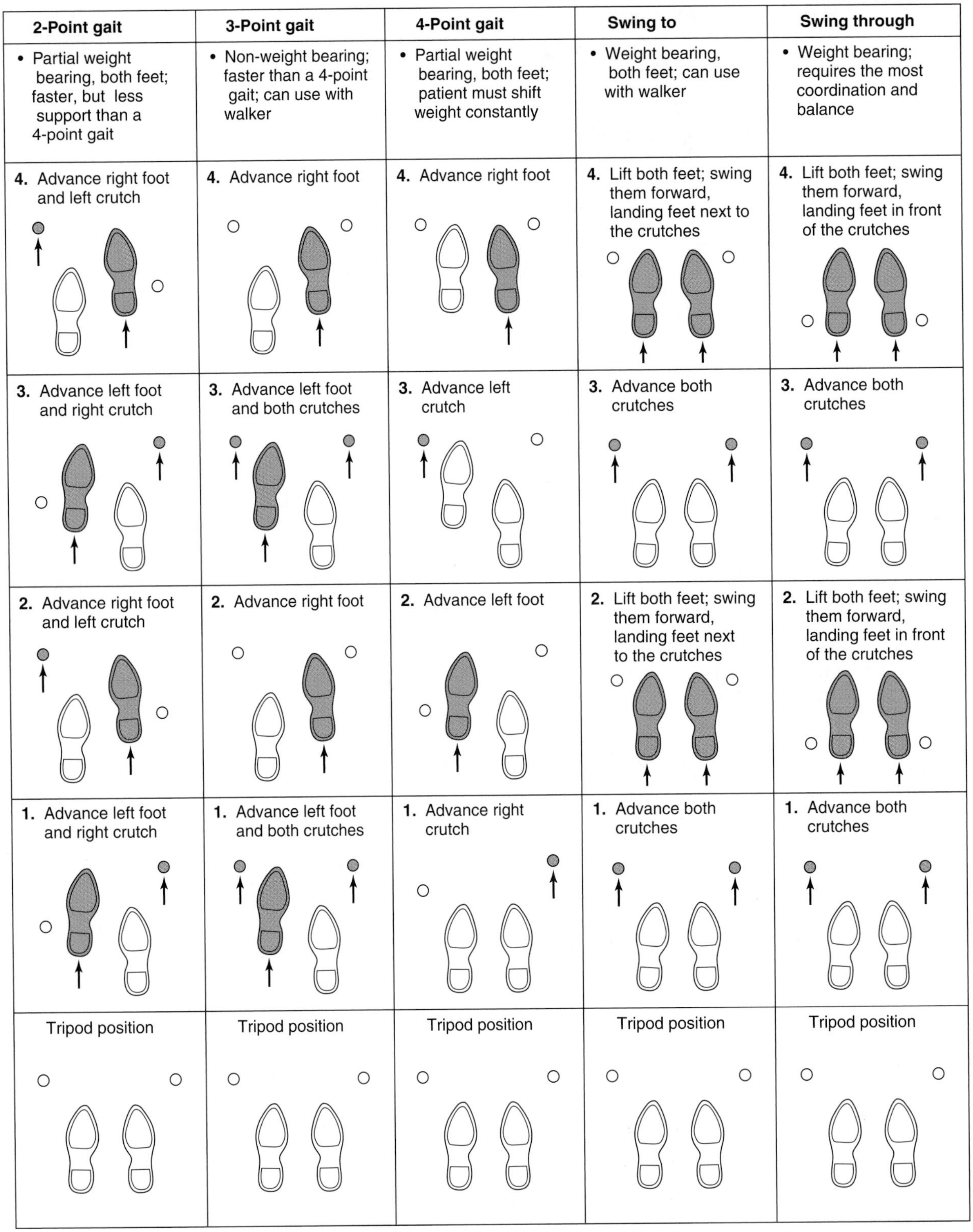

2-Point gait	3-Point gait	4-Point gait	Swing to	Swing through
• Partial weight bearing, both feet; faster, but less support than a 4-point gait	• Non-weight bearing; faster than a 4-point gait; can use with walker	• Partial weight bearing, both feet; patient must shift weight constantly	• Weight bearing, both feet; can use with walker	• Weight bearing; requires the most coordination and balance
4. Advance right foot and left crutch	**4.** Advance right foot	**4.** Advance right foot	**4.** Lift both feet; swing them forward, landing feet next to the crutches	**4.** Lift both feet; swing them forward, landing feet in front of the crutches
3. Advance left foot and right crutch	**3.** Advance left foot and both crutches	**3.** Advance left crutch	**3.** Advance both crutches	**3.** Advance both crutches
2. Advance right foot and left crutch	**2.** Advance right foot	**2.** Advance left foot	**2.** Lift both feet; swing them forward, landing feet next to the crutches	**2.** Lift both feet; swing them forward, landing feet in front of the crutches
1. Advance left foot and right crutch	**1.** Advance left foot and both crutches	**1.** Advance right crutch	**1.** Advance both crutches	**1.** Advance both crutches
Tripod position	Tripod position	Tripod position	Tripod position	Tripod position

FIGURE 31–20   Crutch gaits. The shaded area represents weight bearing. The arrow shows movement.

The basic crutch standing position is known as the tripod position. The crutches are placed to form a triangle with the body. There are five crutch gaits: two-point gait, three-point support, four-point gait, swing-to gait, and swing-through gait. Two-point and four-point gait are used for partial weight bearing, whereas three-point gait is used when weight bearing must be avoided. Swing-to and swing-through are used when weight-bearing is permitted. Figure 31–20 illustrates each of these crutch gaits.

Your instructions for crutch walking should teach the patient how to go up and down stairs. The simplest technique is to instruct the patient to lead with the unaffected leg when going up the stairs and to lead with the affected leg coming down the stairs. Navigating stairs with crutches can be quite dangerous. When possible, have the patient practice this technique before discharge.

KnowledgeCheck 31–10

- What type of cane should a patient with significant balance problems use?
- When are forearm support crutches used?
- Identify five crutch gaits.

 Go to Chapter 31, **Knowledge Check Response Sheet and Answers,** on the Electronic Study Guide.

For a nursing care plan for impaired physical mobility,

 Go to Chapter 31, **Nursing Care Plan,** on the Electronic Study Guide.

 CriticalThinking 31–6

Discuss crutch walking with your peers and family. What instruction would facilitate the best understanding of proper crutch-walking technique?

 Suggested Readings: Go to Chapter 31, **Reading More About Activity and Exercise,** on the Electronic Study Guide.

 Go to Chapter 31, **Resources for Caregivers and Health Professionals,** on the Electronic Study Guide.

 [VOL 2] **Bibliography:** Go to Volume 2, Bibliography.

| toward evidence-based practice |

Simkin, B. S., & Simkin, M. A. (2002). Maximizing the benefits of exercise in the elderly. *Family Practice Recertification, 24*(1), 38–40.

This article stresses the benefits of exercise, such as reducing the risk of cardiovascular disease, improving mobility, and reducing the risk of falls. The authors strongly recommend a physical examination before an older adult begins an exercise program. Additional evaluation, such as stress testing, may be necessary if there is a history of cardiovascular problems or strong family history. For older adults, aerobic activity should be of moderate intensity and low-impact. Nurses should also emphasize to older clients the merits of resistance and flexibility exercises.

Forman, D. E., & Farquhar, W. (2002). Cardiac rehabilitation and secondary prevention programs for elderly cardiac patients. *Clinics in Geriatric Medicine 16*(3), 619–629.

The use of cardiac rehabilitation services for older adults is controversial because of high costs and the need for careful monitoring because of the presence of comorbidities. However, research demonstrates that these services reduce risk factors, increase quality of life, and improve activity tolerance.

---

1. You are in charge of an outpatient geriatric program. Based on these studies, would you institute an exercise program on the unit?

2. Would you allow patients with existing cardiac disease to participate?

 Go to Chapter 31, **Toward Evidence-Based Practice Suggested Responses,** on the Electronic Study Guide.

32 Sexual Health

Learning Outcomes

After completing this chapter, you should be able to:

* Identify the female and male reproductive organs.

* Describe the physical, emotional, social, and spiritual aspects of human sexuality.

* Explain how gender, gender identity, and sexual orientation contribute to expression of sexuality throughout the life cycle.

* Differentiate between typical and atypical forms of sexual expression.

* Explore physical and psychological issues that affect sexuality and sexual functioning.

* Complete a sexual history as part of a comprehensive nursing assessment.

* State nursing diagnoses to describe sexuality problems.

* Explain how sexual health is challenged by high-risk sexual behaviors, sexually transmitted infections (STI), menstrual problems, infertility, negative intimate relationships, sexual harassment, rape, and disorders of the sexual response cycle.

* Provide nursing interventions that enhance sexual well-being.

* Discuss strategies to increase your personal comfort and confidence in providing holistic nursing care.

* Describe approaches for dealing with inappropriate sexual behavior from patients or in the work environment.

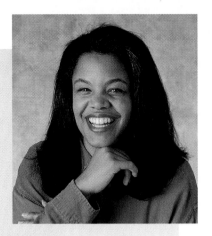

Your Patients

Two days after undergoing a fine-needle aspiration to evaluate a small breast mass, Jocelyn Carter's surgeon informed her that the mass was malignant. He recommended a mastectomy (removal of the breast). Today, she arrives alone at the surgery registration area. You ask how she is feeling, and she tells you that the last week has been a whirlwind of activity. "I had to arrange child care, cancel a business trip, and organize the house so that I could take a few days off to have the surgery. My husband is working overseas this fall, so he couldn't be here to help me. Honestly, I don't know how I'm feeling. I haven't had time to think about it." A few minutes later, as she waits in the surgery holding area, she begins to cry. You hold her hand and ask whether she would like to talk. She asks you, "Do you think my husband will still want me? I'm afraid he will be turned off when he looks at me now."

Gabriel Thomas comes to the outpatient clinic complaining of a throbbing headache for the last 3 days. He explains that he has tried several over-the-counter medicines and has had no relief. You check his blood pressure, and measure the reading at 240/130 mm Hg. When you ask whether he has ever been treated for high blood pressure, he replies, "Are you another one of these people trying to get me to take drugs that will ruin my sex life?"

Frank Thanee, who has heart disease, had a mitral valve replacement 3 days ago. He has been transferred to the cardiology floor for an additional day of hospitalization. His partner, Greg, has spent the last 3 days at the hospital and has just left to check on the apartment and feed their cat. Frank confides that he is worried about his parents' expected visit. "I've never been able to tell them about Greg. They wouldn't be able to understand it, never mind approve. I don't know how to handle this. What do you think I should do?"

Although each of these clients has a different medical diagnosis, all are experiencing a concern related to sexuality. In this chapter we will explore the relationship between health and sexuality, as well as the nurse's role in promoting sexual health.

Theoretical Knowledge
knowing why

When a baby is born, the first question the parents ask is, "Is it a boy or a girl?" In fact, many parents want to know the gender of their baby at the first sonogram, early in the pregnancy. For most parents, this eagerness reflects the fact that their baby's gender will influence their choice of name, clothing, toys, plans to decorate the nursery, and even the ways they handle and communicate with their infant. Such is the power of gender.

However, sexuality encompasses much more than gender. It includes how we perceive ourselves, how we relate to others, and how we express ourselves as sexual beings. Like many people, you may have been socialized to avoid talking openly about sexuality. As a nurse, though, you will find that you must discuss a variety of issues that are vital for clients' optimal wellness.

Some of these discussions may include sexual concerns, dysfunctions, infections, or behaviors. As you gain theoretical knowledge and reflect on the issues of human sexuality, you will be challenged to confront your own biases related to sexuality and to set those aside as you work with your clients. You must meet this challenge to address your clients' sexual health needs in a comfortable and competent manner.

SEXUAL AND REPRODUCTIVE ANATOMY AND PHYSIOLOGY

The reproductive system plays a role in human life that extends far beyond its basic function, to produce children. It influences body image, level of sexual desire, and sense of sexual identity. The first step in exploring human sexuality is to understand the basics of reproductive anatomy and physiology. (For more information to supplement the brief review that follows, consult an anatomy, physiology, or women's health text.)

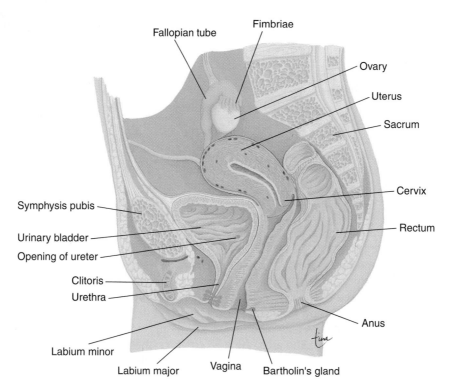

FIGURE 32–1 **The female reproductive system.**

Female Reproductive Organs

The female reproductive system consists of a pair of ovaries and fallopian tubes, the uterus, vagina, and external genital tissues (Figure 32–1). **Ova** (eggs) are produced in the ovaries and travel through the fallopian tubes to the uterus. If fertilization occurs, the embryo embeds in the wall of the uterus for further development. The **vagina** is a muscular tube that receives sperm during sexual intercourse, allows the exit of menstrual flow if fertilization does not occur, and serves as a birth canal at the end of pregnancy.

The external genitalia and the mons pubis are a source of pleasurable sensations. The **mons pubis** is a pad of fatty tissue over the symphysis pubis. It is covered with coarse hair and contains sensitive nerve endings. The external genitalia, or **vulva,** consist of the clitoris, labia majora, labia minora, Bartholin's glands, urinary meatus, and vaginal introitus. The **clitoris** contains erectile tissue, blood vessels, and nerves. It is extremely sensitive and reacts to pleasurable stimuli. The **labia majora** and **labia minora** also respond to touch during sexual activity.

The breasts play an important role in female sexual arousal; in fact, some women can be brought to orgasm solely by caressing the breasts and nipples. The mammary glands, enclosed within the breasts, are also part of the reproductive system. Their role is to produce milk after the birth of an infant.

The Menstrual Cycle

The menstrual cycle governs reproductive ability. The menstrual cycle consists of three phases (Figure 32–2):

1. The **menstrual phase.** Menstruation usually lasts 2 to 8 days. During this phase, the uterus sheds the endometrial lining, and several ovarian follicles develop. Follicle-stimulating hormone (FSH) from the anterior pituitary begins to rise during this phase, leading to a rise in estrogen levels.

2. The **follicular phase.** This next phase is associated with growth of ovarian follicles and regrowth of the endometrium of the uterus. This phase ends with **ovulation,** or release of the ovum from the mature follicle. Luteal hormone (LH) levels from the anterior pituitary rise, as does the estrogen level.

3. The **luteal phase.** In this phase, the ruptured follicle begins to secrete progesterone, which further stimulates growth of the endometrium. If fertilization occurs, the endometrium is ready to support an embryo. If fertilization does not occur, progesterone levels drop, and menses begins.

Male Reproductive Organs

The male reproductive system consists of the testes and a series of ducts and glands that transport sperm. Sperm are produced in the testes and transported through the epididymis, ductus deferens, ejaculatory

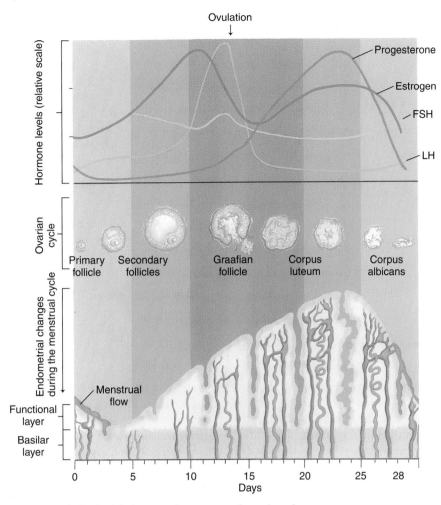

FIGURE 32–2 The menstrual cycle. The levels of the important hormones are shown throughout the cycle. Changes in the ovarian follicle and the relative thickness of the endometrium are also shown.

duct, and urethra (Figure 32–3). Along the path, the reproductive glands (seminal vesicles, prostate, and bulbourethral glands) add secretions that mix with the sperm to produce semen.

The penis functions in the urinary system to transport urine from the bladder to the outside of the body. It has important functions in the reproductive system, as well. Within the penis there are three sections of erectile tissue: the corpus cavernosum and sections of corpus spongiosum above and below the urethra. During sexual arousal these erectile tissues fill with blood, making the penis erect. **Ejaculation** (the expulsion of semen) is brought about by peristalsis of the reproductive ducts and contraction of the prostate and muscles of the pelvic floor. With each ejaculation, approximately 100 million sperm cells are expelled in 2 to 4 mL of semen.

KnowledgeCheck 32–1

- Identify the major structures of the female reproductive system.
- Summarize the three phases of the menstrual cycle.
- Identify the major structures of the male reproductive system.

Go to Chapter 32, **Knowledge Check Response Sheet and Answers,** on the Electronic Study Guide.

SEXUALITY

What do you think of when you see the term *sexuality*? A recent Internet search on the term *sexuality* turned up a hodgepodge of results, including scientific, pornographic, and product-oriented sites. The World Health Organization describes **sexuality** as a "central aspect of being human throughout life and encompasses sex, gender identities and roles, sexual orientation, eroticism, pleasure, intimacy and reproduction" (WHO, 2002). **Sexual identity** is a person's perception of his or her gender, gender identity, gender role, and sexual orientation. All of these are also a part of the person's overall self-concept (see Chapter 11).

What Is Gender?

People often think of *sexuality* as a synonym for *sex*. This is inaccurate. In fact, even the word *sex* has multiple meanings. For example, *sex* is used to describe intimate pleasurable activity (e.g., "We had sex yesterday") or to indicate whether an individual is male or female (e.g., "What sex is your baby?"). In this chapter we use the term **gender** to indicate biological sex

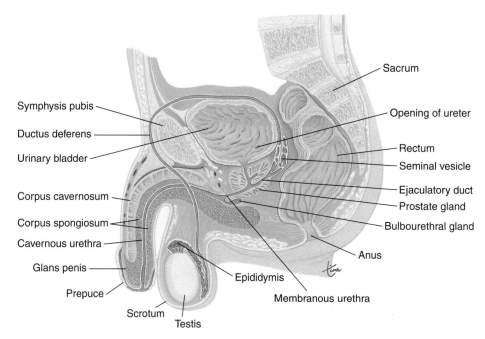

FIGURE 32–3 **The male reproductive system.**

status (male or female) and follow the World Health Organization's definition of sexuality.

Gender is determined at the moment of conception, when an ovum is fertilized by a sperm. The ovum always provides an X chromosome, whereas the sperm may contribute either a second X chromosome, which results in a female, or a Y chromosome, resulting in a male (Figure 32–4).

Gender Roles

Gender roles are the societal norms for gender-appropriate behavior. During the 1950s, television

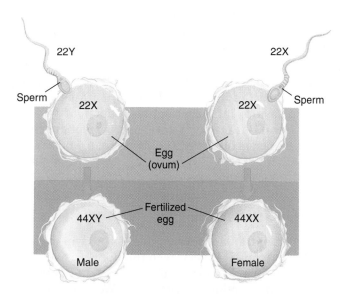

FIGURE 32–4 **The woman provides the X chromosome, and the man may contribute either a second X chromosome, which results in a female offspring, or a Y chromosome, resulting in a male offspring.**

portrayed the father-in-a-suit who went off to work to support his family. Mother, in her apron, spent the day cooking, cleaning, and caring for her perfect children and devoted husband. Even then, many Americans did not identify with this stereotype, and today it may seem laughable. But many of these values remain embedded in our culture. Consider your class structure. How many of your classmates are female? How many are male? Nursing and teaching were among the first professions women assumed outside the home, and women still predominantly comprise them. In contrast, most auto mechanics, plumbers, and politicians are men.

In North America, most people expect men to be strong and to control their feelings, and women to be gentle and to express their feelings. Boys receive positive reinforcement for "masculine" behaviors, such as competitiveness, and may endure teasing if they show passivity. In girls, "feminine" behaviors, such as cooperation, are reinforced, whereas assertiveness may be labeled aggression. But in the past 30 years, more people have defied such stereotypes. Women are successfully performing jobs formerly thought to be "for men only," and men are entering predominantly female professions. Our society's expectations regarding gender roles have expanded.

Today, many parents encourage some **androgyny** in their children. The word *androgyny* is a combination of the Greek words for male, *andro,* and female, *gyn.* By one of its definitions, *androgyny* refers to a blending of traditional masculine and feminine roles. It means that everyone has some skills, traits, and behaviors that may be classified as "masculine" and some that may be "feminine." Androgyny is a positive

trait in that it gives an individual greater adaptability in life situations.

CriticalThinking 32–1

- Provide at least three examples of nonconformity to traditional gender role expectations.
- As a parent, how might you encourage androgyny in your children, if you wished to do so?

Gender Identity

Gender identity, one component of sexual identity, is the image we have about ourselves as a man or woman. It is an internal experience: whether we "feel like" a woman or a man. Usually a little girl sees herself growing up to be a woman, and a young boy sees his future as a man. However, some children form a gender identity that is not the same as their biological gender.

Transgendered (or "differently gendered") is a broad term used to describe people whose gender identity differs in some way from their apparent biological gender. For example, some people think of themselves as female even though they have male genitalia. Longitudinal studies have shown that transgendered persons may be transsexual, intersexed, or cross-dressing; and heterosexual, homosexual, or bisexual (Zucker, 2000).

- A **transsexual** is someone who feels trapped in the body of the opposite gender—for example, a person with the physical appearance and reproductive organs of a woman who "feels" and perceives herself to be a man. It is common for transsexuals to express dissatisfaction with their gender at an early age. They may insist that they will grow up to be the opposite gender. Their preference for dress and play is more typical of the other gender.

- **Preoperative transsexuals** are adults who alter their physical appearance through dress, make-up, and/or the use of hormones so that their external appearance corresponds to their gender identity. After extensive counseling and successfully living in the opposite gender role for 1 to 3 years, they may decide to undergo surgery to reconstruct their external genitalia and remove the reproductive organs of the biological birth gender. After sex reassignment surgery, the **postoperative transsexual** individual legally changes gender. Healthcare settings may have policies regarding room assignment based on the gender of the occupants. For the transsexual or transgender person, private rooms are best.

- **Intersexed** people are born with ambiguous sexual organs (ITPeople, 2004). For example, the person may have female internal organs (ovaries, a uterus), but an external penis. An older term for this is

hermaphrodite. Initially, a developing embryo is in an undifferentiated sexual state—neither male nor female. At about the 7th week of gestation, the sex chromosomes direct the gonads to differentiate into either testes or ovaries. A mutation of any of the genes involved in sexual differentiation or an alteration in hormonal secretion may result in gender alterations. Parents must then face the difficult decision whether to assign a sex and have the child undergo surgery to change the physical appearance or to delay assignment and allow the child to choose at a later time.

- A **cross-dresser** (or **transvestite**) is a person who occasionally or frequently wears the clothes of the opposite sex. Often the person carries out this behavior in secret. Cross-dressers may be heterosexual, homosexual, or bisexual (see the next section, "What Is Sexual Orientation?"). The majority of research on transvestites has focused on men who choose to dress as women, but women also cross-dress.

KnowledgeCheck 32–2

- How is gender determined?
- Distinguish gender, gender role, and gender identity.
- What is androgyny?

 Go to Chapter 32, **Knowledge Check Response Sheet and Answers,** on the Electronic Study Guide.

CriticalThinking 32–2

Do you believe that androgyny is a positive attribute? Explain your thinking.

What Is Sexual Orientation?

Sexual orientation refers to the general tendency of a person to feel sexually attracted to people of a certain gender. Because most people in North America are thought to be **heterosexual** (attracted to members of the opposite sex), heterosexuality is the predominant cultural expectation. However, in the mid-20th century, the research of Alfred C. Kinsey indicated that a population's sexual orientation falls on a bell curve, with the majority of people experiencing at least some attraction to people of the same gender. Kinsey theorized that society influences people to sublimate homosexual feelings and choose exclusively heterosexual relationships. Kinsey's work, which was faulted by opponents for lacking objectivity, was followed by the work of Fritz Klein, who described sexual orientation as an ongoing dynamic process, with people's gender-based inclinations changing over time.

In truth, we do not fully understand what makes up sexual orientation or how it develops. Some theories

hold that it evolves as a result of early learning experiences; others, that it is biologically determined. With increasing research on the biological aspects of sexual orientation, more professionals are concluding that people come to "recognize" the object of their sexual desire rather than "choose" or "prefer" it. Therefore, "sexual orientation" is probably a more accurate term than "sexual preference."

- **Heterosexuality.** As just noted, **heterosexuals** are people who are sexually and emotionally attracted to members of the opposite sex. This segment of the population may be referred to as *straight*. Many major religious traditions reinforce heterosexual behaviors and gender roles. Although some heterosexuals have had same-gender sexual experiences during childhood, adolescence, or adulthood, they still consider themselves heterosexual and have committed relationships with members of the opposite sex.

- **Homosexuality.** For **homosexuals,** the focus of sexual attraction is a person of the same gender. Homosexuals may be referred to as *gay* men and *lesbian* women. According to Rodgers (2001) about 5 to 10% of men and 2 to 4% of women are homosexual. As with heterosexuals, some may be in transient relationships, whereas others maintain loving, long-term relationships.

  Because homosexuality is not an aspect of the dominant culture and is prohibited by some religions, there has been significant discrimination against homosexuals. It can be difficult for gays and lesbians to share this aspect of their life with employers, colleagues, family, and friends. The term "coming out" refers to that time when the person acknowledges to both self and others that he or she is homosexual and is ready to accept the social and emotional consequences of this admission. Of note, the *Diagnostic and Statistical Manual of Mental Disorders* of the American Psychiatric Association (2000) does not classify homosexuality as a psychiatric disorder.

- **Bisexuality.** A person who is **bisexual** is sexually and emotionally attracted to both males and females. This group is perhaps least understood and least accepted by both the heterosexual and homosexual communities. They are less likely to be found in long-term monogamous relationships, because in such a relationship they would more likely be identified as *either* heterosexual or homosexual. However, significant numbers of bisexuals maintain relatively stable and happy marriages because of their sustained sexual attraction to and friendship with their spouse and the importance they place on parenting. Survival of the marriage depends on the partner's acceptance of the bisexual spouse's sexual orientation and extramarital sexual relationships, if any.

KnowledgeCheck 32–3
- What are the majority and minority sexual orientations in our culture?
- What is meant by transgender?

Go to Chapter 32, **Knowledge Check Response Sheet and Answers,** on the Electronic Study Guide.

CriticalThinking 32–3
- What sexual orientations are you comfortable working with?
- Would you have difficulty working with a transsexual or other transgendered client?

How Does Sexuality Develop?

We are sexual beings from birth to death. Expression of our sexuality evolves through the life span. For additional discussion on sexuality and development stages, see Chapter 9.

Birth Through Preschool

Beginning at the moment of birth, parents, caregivers, and others respond to the infant with preconceived thoughts of what that gender role entails. The first 2 years of life can be highly sensual; as infants are nursed, stroked, bathed, and massaged, they develop their first attachment experience through bonding with the mother or other caregiver (Figure 32–5). It is not unusual for this age group to fondle their genitals and enjoy being nude. This is part of their exploration of their bodies, and parents should not overreact. By age 3, most children recognize gender differences and know the names of body parts. Toddlers are interested in their bodies and curious to see the genitals of others.

By age 5, children mimic adults by holding hands or hugging. Adults, who find these actions amusing or endearing, frequently reinforce such behaviors. Young children also may practice getting married, playing house, or playing doctor. It is not unusual for preschool children to masturbate and ask questions about "where babies come from." Parents should give factual answers without going beyond what the child asks.

School Age

The school-age child strongly identifies with the same-sex parent and has mostly same-sex friends. Through interaction at home, school, and other activities, children gain awareness of gender roles and emerging gender identity.

From age 8 to 12, the child is in transition between childhood and puberty. Secondary sex characteristics become apparent. In females, breast buds form, and pubic hair appears. For a significant number

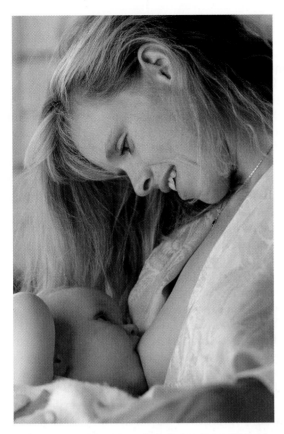

FIGURE 32–5 By being stroked, fed, bathed, and massaged, infants develop their first attachment experience through bonding with mother or other caregiver.

of girls, **menarche** (beginning of menstruation) occurs. Boys become more muscular, the voice deepens, and the genitals begin to increase in size. The first attraction, either heterosexual or homosexual, may occur during this stage, and the child may begin to masturbate more frequently, but privately. For information on the Tanner stages of sexual development in boys and girls, see Chapter 19.

Many school-age children are curious about sex, reproduction, and sex roles, and they may ask explicit questions. Parents and nurses should answer with facts and follow up with age-appropriate printed material. By age 10, parents should begin teaching children basic information about approaching body changes, menstruation, sexual intercourse, and reproduction.

Adolescents

Adolescence is a time of heightened sexual interest and activity. There are two reasons for this: (1) the hormonal changes accompanying puberty and (2) the culture's emphasis on sex. As might be expected, masturbation is common. It is a safe and comforting sexual activity that has neither interpersonal nor disease risks. However, some adolescents may encounter parental, cultural, or religious disapproval of masturbation.

Sexual exploration usually begins with kissing, moves on to fondling, and culminates in genital contact. This progression may occur over a period of years, or there may be an early initiation of oral, vaginal, or anal intercourse. Although about 75% of adolescents are sexually active by their late teen years, the teen pregnancy rate is slowly dropping (Alan Guttmacher Institute, 2002). However, the increasing incidence of oral sex in early adolescence is a troubling phenomenon. Many teens argue that this behavior allows them to maintain their virginity and incorrectly assume that it carries no health risks.

Sexuality education in the home and school dispels myths and prepares teens for adult roles. To make informed choices as they move toward adulthood, adolescents need information about body changes, interpersonal relationships, **contraception** (birth control), and preventing STIs. To review physical changes of adolescence, see Chapters 9 and 19.

Young Adults

Not so many years ago it was generally assumed that young adults would remain virgins until marriage, when the husband and wife could become sexually active and start a family. Today, marriage is often delayed, and young adults engage more openly in premarital sex. Many young adults practice **serial monogamy,** in which the partners are mutually faithful but make no lifelong commitment. When the relationship ends, each partner usually enters another monogamous relationship.

During early adulthood, people define their sexual identity and resolve issues related to their sexual orientation. As a part of sexual maturity, they develop an intimate relationship in which there is both communication and respect. Many people find a life partner during this period and make long-term plans, which often include parenting. However, some adults continue to struggle with their sexual identity, sexual orientation, or ability to form or commit to intimate relationships.

Young adults often wonder whether their sexual behaviors and responses are normal (e.g., "How often do most people have intercourse?" "Do other women have an orgasm every time they have sex?"). Many still need information about birth control, prevention of STIs, and relationship and communication issues.

Middle Adults

Many middle adults experience life changes that may enhance their physical and emotional intimacy. The children have left the home, college and weddings are

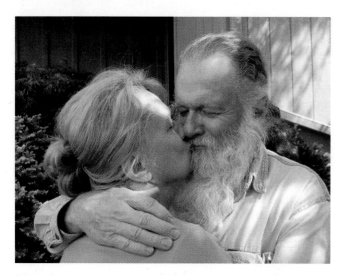

FIGURE 32–6 **Healthy older adults maintain sexual intimacy.**

paid for, careers are settled or winding down, and concerns about pregnancy are gone. However, this may also be a time when physical changes and chronic diseases emerge to affect sexual patterns.

Women transition through **menopause** (cessation of menstruation), a process that varies widely. Some are relieved that the prospect of childbearing has ended; others may mourn the loss of the ability to give birth. Normal physiological changes that result from decreased levels of estrogen and progesterone include decreased vaginal secretions and vaginal wall thinning. These changes may result in painful intercourse and decrease a woman's desire for sexual activity. Some women also experience hot flashes, sleep disturbances, and mood changes.

Men, as a result of the aging process or diseases (e.g., type II diabetes or hypertension), may experience erectile difficulty. They may perceive this problem as a threat to their masculinity, and their self-image may suffer. Men also experience a decrease in the sex hormone testosterone. Sexual desire and the ability to achieve and maintain erection may decrease gradually, but many men remain fertile into old age.

It is important to recognize that middle adults may have sexual concerns that should be addressed. This may be difficult for young nurses, because patients of this age may remind them of their parents. It can be a challenge to view them as individuals who engage in and enjoy sexual relations.

Aging Adults

Healthy adults have sexual intercourse in their 60s and 70s and may continue, with less frequency, into their 80s. Men may need more time and more direct genital stimulation to achieve erection. It may take longer to ejaculate, and the orgasmic contractions

may be less intense. When penetration is not possible (e.g., because of male erectile dysfunction), many couples find satisfaction with alternate forms of sexual stimulation and expression.

Women remain capable of orgasm and may even "rediscover" sexual desire after menopause. Water-soluble lubricants counteract vaginal dryness and enhance pleasurable sensations during sexual activity.

Loss of health or of a partner are the main reasons for decreased sexual activity in the aging population. Other difficulties are a lack of privacy (e.g., for those who live in a nursing home), discomfort associated with arthritis, and activity intolerance (e.g., from heart disease). Nevertheless, research from both *Modern Maturity* and the National Council on Aging has found that older adults generally have more romantic encounters and view their sexual relations as at least as satisfying or more satisfying than in their youth (Jacoby, 1999; Dunn & Culter, 2000).

You can help aging clients to understand that sexual feelings do not necessarily disappear with age; and sexual expression need not stop (Figure 32–6). Suggest alternatives to intercourse when illness or disability interfere. For example, sexual expression may include hugging, caressing, oral sex, and mutual manual stimulation. In addition, you may suggest ways to adapt coital positions to accommodate body changes, for example, when a partner is obese or has joint immobility.

KnowledgeCheck 32–4

- Why is it important to consider sexuality throughout the life cycle?
- What are the two major contributing factors to adolescents' heightened sexual interest and activity?
- What aspects of human sexuality are associated with young and middle adulthood?
- What challenges to sexuality may be found in the aging adult?

 Go to Chapter 32, **Knowledge Check Response Sheet and Answers,** on the Electronic Study Guide.

What Factors Affect Sexuality?

Culture, religion, lifestyle, sexual knowledge, and physical health all influence our attitudes toward sexuality, sexual behaviors, and intimate relationships. This knowledge can help you to provide nonjudgmental, holistic care to people who have a wide range of values, lifestyles, and states of well-being.

Culture

Culture influences our ideas about gender role, gender identity, marriage, sexual expression, and social responsibilities. However, it is not unusual for people

| toward evidence-based practice |

There is great concern regarding high-risk sexual behaviors in adolescent and young adult women. Education is vital to decrease the transmission of sexually transmitted infections. Questions remain as to what approach or which variables are most effective in promoting abstinence or "safer sex" behaviors.

Haglund, K. A. P. (2002). *A life history study of sexually abstinent, adolescent, African-American females*. Unpublished Doctoral Dissertation, University of Wisconsin, Milwaukee.

Researchers collected life histories of 14 sexually abstinent African American females between the ages of 15 and 18 through two 60-minute semistructured interviews. The study revealed that the subjects lacked accurate knowledge regarding reproductive anatomy and physiology, had a personal sense of maturity, avoided situations that would put them at risk, were at ease with being different, aspired to become mature woman like their role models (mother and maternal grandmother), possessed faith in God, and demonstrated futuristic thinking. The researcher concluded that nurses could assist adolescents with their sexuality choices as they provided information regarding human sexuality and reproduction.

Hulton, L. J. (2001). The application of the Transtheoretical Model of Change to adolescent sexual decision-making. *Issues in Comprehensive Pediatric Nursing, 24*(2), 95–115.

This study of 694 students in the seventh grade revealed that the virgins followed a highly predictable pattern of sexual decision making that resulted in a decision to remain abstinent. Knowledge of this process can enable nurses to be aware of the differences in adolescent decision making and allow for appropriate intervention strategies.

Langille, D. B. (2002, Summer). Factors associated with sexual intercourse before age 15 among female adolescents in Nova Scotia. *Canadian Journal of Human Sexuality, 11*(2), 91–99.

A study of 1132 female students aged 15–20 explored the factors that were associated with participation in sexual intercourse. Girls who had sexual intercourse prior to age 15 were less likely to live with both parents, have more educated parents, to have fathers employed full time, have higher school grades, and attend church regularly. Researchers concluded that an understanding of these factors can help educators and other service providers to identify and respond to the needs of young women.

1. Based on the above studies, which variables would you determine to be the best predictors of abstinence or "safer sex" behaviors?

2. What nursing interventions may be most effective in maintaining abstinence and decreasing high-risk sexual behaviors in this population?

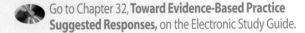 Go to Chapter 32, **Toward Evidence-Based Practice Suggested Responses,** on the Electronic Study Guide.

---

to be ethnocentric—that is, to see their own culture and sexual behaviors as the norm for all. Because the United States is a multicultural country, beliefs and practices related to human sexuality vary widely. But compared to other regions of the world, sexuality in the United States has often been described as repressed. Consider the following examples of cultural influence.

- Victorian-era legacies have influenced many European Americans, some of whom consider sex to be "not nice."
- African Americans are influenced by the dominant Anglo-Saxon culture as well as by their African heritage, history in America, and current economic and social situation. Marriage rates for African Americans are lower than for other ethnic groups in part because of an unequal gender ratio (84 males per 100 females), as well as economic issues that have led to decreased employment for black men (Hyde & DeLamater, 2003).
- Many Latinos have strong ties to the Roman Catholic Church and a tradition of rigidly defined gender roles. The norm is for the man to be given more freedom as a child, but he is expected to be a virile, responsible provider for his family as an adult. In contrast, the female is typically raised to be more passive and obedient throughout her life.
- Asian Americans tend to be the most sexually conservative of the major U.S. cultural groups.

Culture determines what is acceptable and what is not. In some societies, **polygamy** (marriage to more than one partner) may be acceptable. Another culture

may permit or prohibit sexual play among children. Many cultures have special rites of passage at puberty, such as the Jewish bar mitzvah for boys and bat mitzvah for girls, or the Native American vision quest.

Generally, you should honor cultural practices unless they are harmful. An example of a harmful practice is **female circumcision** (female genital mutilation), which is illegal in most countries but is still performed among certain tribes. In this procedure, the labia majora, labia minora, and clitoris are excised, and/or the vagina is sutured closed **(infibulation).** Infibulation may be done to ensure that the girl remains a virgin, whereas clitoral excision is meant to reduce sexual desire and ensure that the woman remains faithful to her husband. In addition to its psychosocial consequences, the procedure carries a high risk of infection and can cause the development of scar tissue that makes vaginal birth impossible. In 1980, the World Health Organization and the United Nations Children's Fund recommended the abolishment of female circumcision, and in 1996, the U.S. Congress passed a law making female circumcision on girls under 18 a federal offense (Brady, 1998).

Religion

Religion also has a powerful influence on sexuality. Religious restrictions against premarital sex, birth control, homosexuality, abortion, extramarital relationships, and masturbation are common. Some religions have rules about body coverings, modesty, and the gender of healthcare providers. Even education about the structure and function of the human body is governed by some religions. The "sexual revolution" that began in the 1960s has led to permissive sexual values in the wider North American society. When these values conflict with a person's traditional religious values, anxiety and sexual dysfunction may result. To review the influence of religion on health, see Chapter 14.

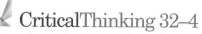 CriticalThinking 32–4

How have religion and culture influenced your views on sexuality?

Lifestyle

Life experiences encompass our interactions with others and the environment. Family, socioeconomic status, employment factors, and interpersonal relationships shape our lifestyle, although they do not fully determine it. Consider the following examples:

- Having a beloved brother reveal to you that he is gay might alter your perception of homosexuality. Similarly, being raised by a lesbian couple might affect your view of gender roles.

- Growing up in a low-income neighborhood in which prostitution is a visible and accepted part of the environment might influence your views on what is acceptable sexual behavior.

- Dedication to a high-stress job or the demands of raising young children might leave you too exhausted to desire sex with your spouse, whereas retirement might bring time to develop your range of intimate expression.

- Being in an abusive relationship would affect how you feel about yourself and might cause you to avoid intimacy in the future.

Lessons learned through day-to-day experience create powerful impressions on our views and often modify cultural and religious influences.

Sexual Knowledge

Although sexuality and family life are part of the curriculum in many public schools, you cannot assume that young adults have adequate sexual knowledge. Community values play a large role in determining how sexuality is viewed and taught. Thus, even if a state mandates sex education, a particular school may limit discussion on reproduction, sexually transmitted infections, birth control, intimacy, exploitive relationships, domestic abuse, and/or rape, believing that these topics are best addressed by the family or church. In addition, many children are home-schooled or taught in private or religious schools that do not allocate any class time to sex education. Even in schools with a comprehensive curriculum, parents have the right to exclude their child from sex education classes.

Do not let your clients' age, level of education, or life experiences lead you to make assumptions about their knowledge of sexuality. For example:

- A married person may not be sexually active.

- A woman with several children may not know what is involved in a pelvic exam or how conception occurs.

- A highly educated person may be woefully uninformed regarding his body structure and function.

It is difficult for most people to admit to a professional that they lack knowledge. Therefore, you must assess each client's knowledge and understanding of sexual terms. At times you may need to use the vernacular or "street" terminology to be understood. You can then introduce correct terminology.

KnowledgeCheck 32–5

- What sexual knowledge would you expect an adult male with children to have?
- What sexual knowledge would you expect a nursing student to have?

 Go to Chapter 32, **Knowledge Check Response Sheet and Answers,** on the Electronic Study Guide.

Health and Illness

Sexuality involves body, mind, and spirit; so, it is not surprising that health status affects sexuality. For example, healthful nutrition and physical exercise are commonly reported to increase satisfaction in sexual relationships, whereas overweight and inactivity can undermine one's own feelings of attractiveness or one's attraction for one's partner. The importance of sexuality is readily apparent in the clinical setting. For example, the clients in the "Meet Your Patients" scenarios all expressed concerns related to their sexuality.

Physical Illness

Diseases, injuries, and medical treatments may demand lifestyle changes in multiple areas, including sexual functioning.

- *Heart disease or respiratory disease* may cause people to restrict sexual activity because of fatigue, dyspnea, or fear of harming the heart.
- *Diabetes mellitus* leads to neurological changes that may cause male erectile dysfunction; women may experience vaginal dryness and loss of orgasmic ability. In addition, vaginal yeast infections are common with diabetes, causing itching and painful intercourse.
- *Cancer* may be accompanied by body image changes, fatigue, treatments that create nausea, and fear of death—all of which lead to decreased desire for sexual activity.
- *Spinal cord injury* may make it impossible for the person to feel physical stimulation. Depending on the level of the injury, the person may or may not experience psychogenic or reflexogenic genital arousal. Some men may be able to achieve erection and ejaculation and are fertile; others may have no genital response.
- *Surgeries,* in addition to causing pain in the early preoperative period, may harm a person's body image. At the least, surgery leaves a physical scar. At worst, it removes a body part or creates other disfigurement. When the surgery involves body parts important to sexual functioning (e.g., a breast, a testicle), the effect is even more likely to be negative. Because some people feel ugly after such procedures and worry about their partner's reactions to their appearance, they may avoid having sex. Two very common surgeries are hysterectomy and prostatectomy:

    Hysterectomy (surgical removal of a uterus) may enhance the sexual experience if it relieves pain and bleeding that were present before surgery. In contrast, some women report difficulty becoming aroused or having less intense orgasm after hysterectomy. These problems may be related to trauma to nerves in the pelvic area, to the absence of uterine contractions during orgasm, or to anxiety because so much of the woman's gender identity had been tied to childbearing.

    Prostatectomy (removal of the prostate gland, usually to treat prostate cancer) may be accompanied by erectile and other sexual dysfunction.

If a person becomes disabled while in a marriage or other committed relationship, the strain can threaten the partnership. In contrast, a person who is single or has a life-long disability may experience difficulty establishing an intimate relationship because of physical limitations, social isolation, or discrimination. Even when people lose interest in sexual intercourse, a need for intimacy still exists. Communication about sexual needs and desires may be difficult for couples, but as a nurse, you can support and facilitate it. Rehabilitation programs ideally offer holistic services and facilitate discussion regarding sexuality and relationship issues.

Psychiatric Disorders

Psychiatric disorders can lead to interpersonal disruptions and difficulty with sexual expression.

- A depressed person experiences significant loss of interest in activities that previously brought pleasure. Thus it is common for people with depression to avoid engaging in interpersonal activities, including sex.
- Conversely, a person with hypomania or mania may be preoccupied with pleasurable activities and increased sexual activity, as well as verbalization and acting out. Both extremes are disruptive to a relationship.
- For a person with psychosis, interpersonal relationships and sexual patterns are disrupted by lack of contact with reality or frank delusions.

Counseling for the couple is important when symptoms are controlled. During times of acute illness, support for the partner is vital.

Medications and Other Drugs

Many medications used to treat health problems affect sexuality. Gabriel Thomas ("Meet Your Patients") clearly illustrates the concern some clients have about commonly prescribed medications. Table 32–1 lists a number of medications and their effects on sexual function.

Until recently, the effects of medications on sexual functioning were almost always experienced as unwanted side effects. Today, however, there are medications that alter sexual function in a positive manner. These include sidenafil citrate (Viagra), vardenafil (Levitra), and tadalafil (Cialis). These nitric oxide–releasing medications treat erectile dysfunction

TABLE 32-1 Effects of Drugs on Sexual Function

Medication	Possible Effect
Alcohol	In limited quantities, alcohol may enhance desire and function. However, heavy or chronic use may lead to decreased libido, orgasmic dysfunction, and erectile dysfunction.
Antianxiety agents	Decreased libido, delayed ejaculation.
Anticonvulsants	Decreased libido, prolonged painful erections, difficulty achieving orgasm.
Antidepressants	Decreased libido, difficulty achieving orgasm. Bupropion (Wellbutrin) and trazodone (Desyrel) are least likely to cause sexual side effects.
Antihistamines	Decreased libido, decreased vaginal lubrication.
Antihypertensives	Decreased libido, erectile dysfunction, delayed ejaculation. Calcium channel blockers are least likely to cause sexual difficulties.
Chemotherapy	Fatigue, decreased libido.
Opioids	Decreased libido, erectile dysfunction.
Stimulants (cocaine, methamphetamines)	Initially stimulants cause increased intensity of the sexual encounter; however, with continued use, sexual dysfunction develops.

(ED) that is caused by poor blood flow to the penis (Silverman, 2002). They are frequently given to patients who have diabetes mellitus or who are taking beta-adrenergic blocking agents (medications used to treat high blood pressure and cardiac problems).

KnowledgeCheck 32–6

- Identify four factors associated with physical illness that may affect sexuality or sexual functioning.
- What determines our sexual attitudes?

 Go to Chapter 32, **Knowledge Check Response Sheet and Answers,** on the Electronic Study Guide.

SEXUAL HEALTH

The World Health Organization defines **sexual health** as a state of physical, emotional, mental, and social well-being related to sexuality; it is not merely the absence of disease, dysfunction, or infirmity. Sexual health requires a positive and respectful approach to sexuality and sexual relationships, as well as the openness and opportunity to have pleasurable and safe sexual experiences, free of coercion, discrimination, and violence. For sexual health to be attained and maintained, the sexual rights of all persons must be respected, protected, and fulfilled (WHO, 2002). To promote sexual health effectively, you will need theoretical knowledge about sexual responses, modes of sexual expression, and problems affecting sexuality.

 CriticalThinking 32–5

Examine your own beliefs about sexuality. Identify areas of concern you have regarding sexuality. How do you think this will affect your ability to assist patients with sexual health concerns?

What Is the Sexual Response Cycle?

The **sexual response cycle** is the sequence of physiological events that occur when a person becomes sexually aroused. Based on research conducted in the 1950s, William Masters and Virginia Johnson identified a four-stage sexual response: excitement, plateau, orgasm, and resolution (Figure 32–7). A growing body

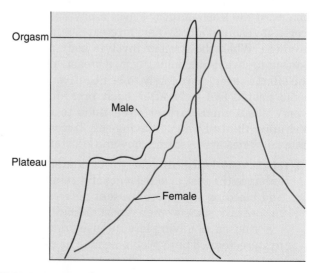

FIGURE 32–7 **The sexual response cycle.**

BOX 32-1 Normal Physiological Changes in Sexual Response That Occur with Aging

Sexual Response Stage	Changes in Women	Changes in Men
Desire	Decreased libido	Decreased libido
Excitement and plateau	Delayed nipple erection Reduced labial separation and swelling Reduced vaginal expansion Reduced lubrication Decreased elevation of the uterus Reduced muscle tension Reduced vaginal tone (in those who have had multiple vaginal deliveries); results in less stimulation during intercourse	Delayed nipple erection Delayed and less-firm erection Longer excitement stage Decreased preejaculatory emissions Reduced muscle tension Reduced lifting of the scrotum and testes Shorter phase of impending orgasm May require more direct stimulation to achieve and maintain an erection
Orgasm	Reduced spread of sexual flush	Shorter ejaculation time Fewer ejaculatory contractions Reduced volume of ejaculate
Resolution	No cervical dilation	More rapid loss of erection Longer refractory period Nipple erection lasts longer after orgasm

Sources: Stanley, M., et al., (2005). *Gerontological nursing: Promoting successful aging with older adults.* Philadelphia: F. A. Davis Company; Kennedy-Malone, L., Fletcher, K., & Plank, L. (2004). *Management guidelines for nurse practitioners working with older adults.* Philadelphia: F. A. Davis Company; Running, A., & Berndt, A. (2003). *Management guidelines for nurse practitioners working in family practice.* Philadelphia: F. A. Davis Company; EngenderHealth. (2004). Sexual response and sexual practices: Normal changes in response with aging. *Sexuality and Sexual Health: An Online MiniCourse.* Retrieved September 2, 2004, from http://www.engenderhealth .org/res/onc/sexuality/response/ miw/pg5.html/

of research has called into question this four-stage model. One suggested alteration of the original Masters and Johnson model is to add a stage of desire, which in some people precedes and in some people follows, excitement (Basson, 2001).

Although it is most intense in the genitals, sexual response is a total body response, involving many physiological changes (e.g., increased heart rate, flushing). The emotional and mental aspects of sexual activity are equally important to the person's satisfaction. The body has many **erogenous zones** (areas that cause sexual arousal when stimulated): the genitals, the skin, lips, ears, breasts, buttocks, and thighs. Box 32–1 shows normal physiological changes in sexual response that occur with aging.

Desire

Desire is a stage of varying length characterized by an interest in sexual intimacy. Desire occurs in the mind and is communicated either verbally or through body language. This communication may be subtle and easily misread. In different cultures, behaviors meant to communicate desire may vary along gender lines. **Libido** is an individual's typical level of desire. In many people, desire is readily aroused by erotic stimuli, such as sights, sounds, and fantasies. However, recent research indicates that a majority of women and a minority of men do not experience desire until after they have become aroused; in these people, physical excitement prompts the desire for sex (Basson, 2001).

Although desire depends on both psychic stimulation and local sexual stimulation, it does increase in proportion to the level of the sex hormones (e.g., a man with low testosterone is not as interested in sex). For women, desire reaches a peak each month near the time of ovulation, when estrogen levels are high.

What is considered "sexual" or "attractive" can vary greatly, because societal, cultural, and personal values influence the range of stimuli that provoke sexual desire. Desire may last only moments or be ongoing for years. Transient sexual thoughts are fleeting moments of desire. Unrequited love is an example of desire that lasts for years.

Excitement

Excitement is the body's physical response to desire. During excitement the following bodily changes occur: Heart rate, blood pressure, and respiratory rate increase; muscles tense *(myotonia);* nipples become erect; and genital and pelvic blood supply increases *(vasocongestion)*. In women, vasocongestion leads to vaginal lubrication, swelling of the breasts, rise of the uterus, and swelling of the labia and clitoris. In men, erection begins as the penis increases in length and diameter. The testes rise closer to the body, and the scrotum thickens.

Excitement may lead to further sexual activity, but this is not inevitable. For both sexes, the person may lose and regain initial physical excitement many times without progressing to the next stage. Excitement may be communicated verbally or through body language.

Plateau

If stimulation continues, the person reaches the **plateau** phase. Plateau is associated with continued increases in pulse, respiratory rate, blood pressure, and muscle tension. Some people flush around the face, neck, and chest in this phase. In women, the areolae become larger, the clitoris retracts into the clitoral hood, Bartholin's glands lubricate, and the lower vagina swells and narrows. With a male partner, the vagina tightens around the man's penis, increasing his sexual stimulation. In men, the ridge of the glans penis becomes more prominent, pre-ejaculate (2 or 3 drops of fluid) is emitted, and the testes rise closer to the body. The person may achieve, lose, and regain the plateau phase several times without experiencing orgasm.

Orgasm

Orgasm occurs at the peak of the plateau phase. At the moment of orgasm, the sexual tension that has been building is released. The heart rate, respiratory rate, and blood pressure reach their peak, and there is loss of voluntary muscle tone.

- *In women,* spinal cord reflexes cause powerful rhythmic contractions of the vagina, uterus, anus, and pelvic floor muscles; feelings of warmth spread through the pelvic area. The cervical canal dilates, allowing easy transport of the sperm to the uterus. Orgasm may last for a few seconds or up to nearly a minute.

- *In men,* spinal cord reflexes cause the urethra, anus, and pelvic floor muscles to contract. Thrusting movements of the pelvis and penis occur, followed by **ejaculation** (the expelling of semen through the urethra). For men, orgasm usually lasts no more than 30 seconds.

The intensity of orgasm varies among individuals and in each individual from one sexual experience to another. Orgasm may involve intense spasm and loss of awareness, or it may be signaled by as little as a sigh or subtle relaxation.

Resolution

Resolution is the period of time following orgasm. The muscles relax, and the body returns to its pre-excitement state. Immediately following orgasm, men experience a **refractory period,** during which they cannot achieve an erection. The duration of this period varies among individuals and increases with age. Women experience no refractory period—they can either enter the resolution stage or return to the excitement or plateau stage immediately following orgasm.

KnowledgeCheck 32–7

Identify the phase described.

- This phase is reached if there is ongoing stimulation. This stage may be achieved, lost, and regained several times without the occurrence of orgasm.
- This stage occurs in the mind and may be communicated between potential sexual partners either verbally or through body language.
- This phase is associated with the release of sexual tension.

 Go to Chapter 32, **Knowledge Check Response Sheet and Answers,** on the Electronic Study Guide.

 CriticalThinking 32–6

Critique the theory of Masters and Johnson, as represented in the preceding discussion of the sexual response cycle. How would you respond to the statement that the theory does not adequately address variation among individuals and even within an individual's sexual response?

What Are Some Forms of Sexual Expression?

People express their sexuality and gain sexual satisfaction in many different ways. There is a range of behaviors that are socially acceptable and therefore considered "normal" by most people in our society. These are discussed in the next few sections. Keep in mind that people vary in what they consider to be "normal," as well as in their modes of sexual expression.

Developing Intimate Relationships

Developing intimate relationships involves a willingness to take risks and offer trust. Intimacy involves openness, mutual respect, caring, commitment, protection, honesty, and devotion. Although we often think of intimate relationships as sexual, they are not necessarily so. Furthermore, in our society, many sexual relationships occur without intimacy.

Fantasies and Erotic Dreams

It is fair to say that all men and women have sexual fantasies. They may be related to past experiences, dreams, desires, or stories heard, seen, or read. Sexual fantasies serve to increase self-esteem and sexual arousal and serve as an outlet to explore sexual desires. Fantasies may occur without sexual activity, during masturbation, or during intercourse. People in long-term monogamous relationships may use fantasy to bring variety and excitement into a routine sexual encounter. Erotic dreams are also common, among both men and women. Nocturnal orgasm may or may not occur.

Masturbation

Masturbation is self-stimulation of the genitals. Although there are many techniques, men typically hold and stroke the shaft of the penis, and women typically stimulate the clitoris manually. Young children touch their genitals as a part of body exploration, but they quickly learn either that touching certain areas is not acceptable or that it should be done in private. Adolescents, particularly males, may masturbate frequently. Adults may masturbate for sexual release when a partner is not available or for variety in a partnered relationship. Sex therapists often recommend masturbation as a means to resolve orgasm difficulties in women and ejaculatory problems in men.

Religious and social taboos discouraging masturbation are plentiful. Many people mistakenly believe that masturbation is harmful, causing acne, warts, blindness, or insanity. Although most people masturbate, most do not talk about it openly in our society. For example, in 1994, U.S. Surgeon General Joycelyn Elder was removed from her position for advocating masturbation and suggesting, at an AIDS conference, that it should perhaps be taught as a method of safe sex (Frankel, 1994).

Shared Touching

An alternative to sexual intercourse may be mutual masturbation, or shared touching. This is particularly appealing to individuals who seek to maintain virginity, wish to decrease the risk of sexually transmitted infection, or have mobility or other physical problems that make intercourse difficult. Mutual masturbation is recognized as a form of safer sex because body fluids are not likely to be exchanged. This behavior can be satisfying because it allows for a significant level of sexual intimacy and allows participants to experience orgasm.

Sexual Intercourse

Sexual intercourse and **coitus** are terms used to describe penile penetration of the vagina. People use a variety of positions for intercourse: one partner supine (woman on top or man on top), side-lying, standing, sitting, and rear entry, for example. With the penis in the vagina, the man thrusts his hips to move the penis back and forth. The woman may make similar hip-thrusting movements, continuing until orgasm is achieved. For some women, manual stimulation of the clitoris is also necessary to achieve orgasm. Partners usually do not reach orgasm at the same time, despite the romantic preoccupation with this phenomenon.

Unprotected coitus may lead to conception, so the couple should use some method of contraception if they want to avoid pregnancy. Because it involves exchange of body fluids, sexual intercourse may also lead to the transmission of infections. Using a lubricated latex condom decreases this risk.

Oral-Genital Stimulation

Both heterosexual and homosexual couples practice oral-genital stimulation (oral sex). Couples in committed relationships may engage in it for sexual variety or as foreplay. Others may engage in oral sex because it provides intimacy yet cannot result in pregnancy, and many believe that it does not affect their virginity status. For the latter reasons, oral sex is becoming much more prevalent among adolescents. Oral-genital contact may, however, lead to sexually transmitted infections (STIs).

When a woman is the recipient of oral stimulation to her genitals, the practice is called **cunnilingus. Fellatio** is stimulation of the male genitals by a partner's mouth. Although swallowing semen is not a health issue, it may be a matter of personal preference whether the recipient ejaculates in his partner's mouth. If the couple is not in a long-term monogamous relationship, dental dams, plastic wrap, or latex condoms should be used to prevent the transmission of STIs.

Anal Stimulation or Anal Intercourse

Both homosexual and heterosexual couples engage in oral anal stimulation (called **anilingus**). A sex toy

(dildo or vibrator), or the partner's tongue and mouth may be used to stimulate the anus. **Anal intercourse** (also termed *sodomy*) is the insertion of the penis into the partner's rectum. When a couple engages in anal intercourse, lubrication is essential to lessen the chance of minute tears to the rectal mucosa or damage to the anal sphincter. Unless the couple is in a long-term monogamous relationship, they should use a lubricated latex condom to lessen the chance of STIs. The condom must be changed prior to vaginal penetration to avoid the transfer of *Escherichia coli* bacteria from the rectum to the vagina. Couples should follow the same precaution when using sex toys.

Celibacy

Celibacy is a state in which an individual refrains from sexual activity. Traditionally, a celibate is a person who remains unmarried, usually for religious reasons, and sublimates sexual desire through prayer, meditation, and service. However, some people choose to remain celibate out of fear of intimate relationships. Childhood sexual trauma, for example, may lead an adult to choose celibacy. Some people are celibate because a developmental or physical disability limits their opportunities for meeting prospective partners, their privacy, or their ability to communicate or act on their desires. Some celibate people simply have a low libido and prefer to focus their energies elsewhere. Married couples may be happily celibate and very content with their situation, whereas people who are celibate following the loss of a relationship, whether through separation, divorce, or death, often feel a considerable void.

Alternative Forms of Sexual Expression

The *Diagnostic and Statistical Manual of Mental Disorders* (American Psychiatric Association, 2000) describes eight categories of sexual deviation or **paraphilias:** exhibitionism, fetishism, frotteurism, pedophilia, sexual masochism, sexual sadism, transvestic fetishism, and voyeurism. Whereas some people experience guilt, shame, and depression about their paraphilia, others are distressed only by the societal disapproval, restrictions, and possible criminal charges associated with their mode of expression. For more information about paraphilias,

 Go to Chapter 32, **Supplemental Materials: Alternative Forms of Sexual Expression,** on the Electronic Study Guide.

KnowledgeCheck 32–8
- What are aspects of an intimate relationship?
- Identify solitary types of sexual expression and those that may be conducted with a partner.

 Go to Chapter 32, **Knowledge Check Response Sheet and Answers,** on the Electronic Study Guide.

What Problems Affect Sexuality?

Sexual well-being is a complex mesh of physical, emotional, cognitive, social, and spiritual components. Therefore, it is not surprising that many people experience challenges to their sexual health. Difficulties can arise in loving, healthy relationships as well as in dysfunctional couplings. Sexual dysfunction may be temporary and situational, or it may be long-standing.

Sexually Transmitted Infections

A **sexually transmitted infection (STI)** is one that is almost always spread through direct sexual contact. STIs are not transmitted by casual contact, such as touching, coughing, shaking hands, or sharing a glass with someone. They are spread by direct contact with a sore or with body fluids, such as semen, vaginal secretions, or blood that contains pathogens. An STI may be caused by bacteria, viruses, fungi, or parasites.

STIs are among the most common infectious diseases in the United States today. More than 20 different STIs have been identified, and they affect millions of men and women each year. In the United States in 2000, an estimated 18.9 million new cases were reported to the Centers for Disease Control and Prevention (CDC, 2001). Nearly two-thirds of all STIs occur in people younger than 25 years. However, at least one in ten newly diagnosed cases of HIV occurs in a person older than 50 years.

Many STIs have few or no symptoms, allowing a person to be infected and transmit the infection without knowing it. For example, up to 90% of women infected with gonorrhea or chlamydia have no symptoms. To find out whether a patient has an STI, you must obtain a culture, that is, a swab of secretions from the genitals. In a man, the swab is put into the urethral opening. In a woman, the swab is obtained from secretions near the cervix. A culture of the throat or rectum is obtained if the person has had oral or anal sex.

Many STIs can be treated fairly easily with antibiotics; however, if left untreated, they may cause serious problems. In women, the pathogens can travel up through the uterus into the fallopian tubes and cause pelvic inflammatory disease (PID). Unchecked PID may cause sterility. One STI, human papillomavirus infection (HPV), causes genital warts and cervical and other genital cancers.

The best ways to prevent STIs are to be celibate or participate only in a committed, mutually monogamous sexual relationship with someone who has never had an STI and has never shared needles. Risk for an STI increases if a person has unprotected sex or has more than one sex partner. The more sexual partners, the greater the risk. Other risk factors include alcohol and drug use, sexual activity at an early age, intercourse with a new partner, prior history of an

STI, failure to utilize latex barriers with sexual contact, genital piercings, intercourse between men, intercourse with someone who has recently been in prison, sexual assault, sexual abuse, and failure to comply with prescribed treatment for an STI (Davidson, 2004).

To read about a number of STIs, their symptoms, treatment, and effect on sexual functioning, fertility, and childbearing,

 Go to Chapter 32, **Tables, Boxes, Figures: ESG Table 32–1,** on the Electronic Study Guide.

Dysmenorrhea

Dysmenorrhea is painful menstruation caused by strong uterine contractions that cause ischemia of the uterus. Most common among adolescents, the patient may experience cramping, lower abdominal pain, back and upper thigh pain, headache, vomiting, and diarrhea. Treatments include analgesics such as aspirin and other nonsteroidal anti-inflammatory drugs (NSAIDS), for example, ibuprofen (Advil), bedrest, and application of heat to the back and abdomen.

Premenstrual Syndrome

Premenstrual syndrome (PMS) is characterized by physical and emotional changes occurring 3 to 14 days prior to the onset of the woman's menstrual period. Estimates are that 50 to 90% of women experience PMS. Physical symptoms include headaches, constipation, breast tenderness, and weight gain associated with bloating, abdominal swelling, or swelling of the hands and feet. Some women feel as though they are on an emotional roller coaster, with periods of depression, anxiety, irritability, tension, and an inability to concentrate. Some women have difficulty maintaining social interactions at work or school because of severe emotional symptoms. Client teaching for PMS is discussed later in this chapter.

KnowledgeCheck 32–9

- Identify three methods to decrease the transmission of STIs.
- What are physical and emotional symptoms of premenstrual syndrome (PMS)?

 Go to Chapter 32, **Knowledge Check Response Sheet and Answers,** on the Electronic Study Guide.

Negative Intimate Relationships

Many couples are happy, and their relationship becomes even more satisfying as they mature. However, some intimate relationships are not satisfying, even though they do not involve physical or emotional abuse. These are sometimes described as loveless marriages or marriages of convenience. Couples may continue loveless marriages for financial gain, social status, for "the sake of the children," or because of cultural or religious restrictions regarding divorce.

The most negative relationships involve *domestic violence* (also called *intimate partner violence*), which may include physical and/or emotional intimidation and assault, and/or rape. Although either gender partner may be a victim of domestic violence, most often a man is the perpetrator. The anger, domination, and physical violence of the partner leads to fear, intimidation, and submission in the victim. Often victims come to believe that they deserve the abuse and thus may hesitate to admit the cause of their injuries, even in the hospital setting. Many abused women are either emotionally or financially dependent on their partner and believe they have no options except to stay in the relationship.

Sexual Harassment

Sexual harassment occurs when a person in power makes unwelcome sexual advances that implicitly or explicitly relate to the victim's employment, academic status, or success. "Advances" can take the form of sexual comments or behaviors (such as touching). Because of the power imbalance, the victim may keep silent and suffer physically and psychologically.

Sexual harassment may take two forms: (1) In *quid pro quo* cases, the employer makes the employee feel that she must engage in unwelcome sexual advances to maintain employment; (2) In *hostile environment* cases, the sexual advances are more subtle, but persistent, and create an intimidating environment.

Rape

Although rape is actually a crime of violence rather than of sex, we discuss it here because it often involves the sexual organs and usually has negative effects on the victim's sexuality. **Rape** is nonconsensual vaginal, anal, or oral penetration. It occurs through force, by the threat of bodily harm, or when the victim is incapable of giving consent. Victims of rape range from infants to older adults and may be either gender, although female adolescents and young women are the most frequent victims. In 69% of cases, the assailant is known to the victim (Rennison & Rand, 2003). Younger children are most likely to be sexually assaulted by an acquaintance or relative. All 50 states now agree that rape within a marriage is a crime.

Gang rape occurs when more than one person sexually assaults a victim. Group rape perpetrators are usually young men, and drugs and alcohol are frequently involved. **Statutory rape** is sexual activity between an adult and a person under the "age of consent" (this ranges from 14 to 18 years of age, depending on state regulations). This charge may be filed

even when the sex is consensual. **Date rape** is rape by an acquaintance when the assault occurs during an agreed-on social encounter. Although date rape is not a lesser violation, our society tends to blame the woman when date rape occurs.

Unfortunately, many women fail to report incidents of rape. An assault that involves significant physical injury is most likely to become known to the authorities because the victim requires medical attention. Reasons for not reporting rape include fear of the assailant, knowledge of the low conviction rate for rapists, the wish to avoid a trial, shame and embarrassment, past sexual history, wanting to "move on," and self-blame. If you follow accounts of rape charges and trials in the media, you can easily understand how victims may conclude that reporting a rape does not ensure that justice will be served. In addition to psychological and physiological trauma, the rape victim is at risk for STIs and pregnancy. Referral to a local sexual assault support group is critical. A *sexual assault nurse examiner (SANE)* is a registered nurse who has received special training in the immediate care of sexual assault victims.

Sexual Response Cycle Disorders

A variety of disorders may occur throughout the sexual response cycle. These disorders affect desire, arousal, excitement, and orgasm.

Low Libido

A significant decrease in or absence of both sexual fantasies and sexual activity characterizes decreased sexual desire, or **low libido (hypoactive sexual desire).** Low libido may affect both men and women. It can be transient or long term. The person may experience low libido only with one particular partner, or the lack of desire can extend to all sexual activity. Persons with low libido may reluctantly engage in sexual encounters or avoid all sexual contact. However, once sexual activity has been initiated, the person is usually able to achieve orgasm.

Factors contributing to hypoactive sexual desire include sexual trauma, a negative attitude toward sex, negative relationships, and biological factors, including hormone deficiencies and side effects of various medications. Hypoactive sexual desire, in both men and women, may respond positively to testosterone administration.

Arousal Disorders

Disorders of arousal may affect men and women. In a woman, it manifests as minimal or absent pelvic congestion and vaginal lubrication even though desire may be present. Hormonal changes, the aging process, tampons, and medications, including antihistamines,

also cause vaginal dryness. Vaginal dryness may result in **dyspareunia,** or painful intercourse, which further decreases sexual desire. A water-based lubricant or saliva is helpful in resolving vaginal dryness. Other significant causes of female dyspareunia include vaginal or urinary tract infections, pelvic inflammatory disease, and endometriosis.

A rare disorder affecting desire and arousal is vaginismus. **Vaginismus** is characterized by intense involuntary contractions of the perineal muscles, which close the vaginal opening and prevent penile penetration. Vaginismus may be associated with negative attitudes toward sex or a history of sexual abuse or trauma. Physiological disorders may also be the cause.

Sexual arousal disorders in men manifest as **erectile dysfunction (ED),** also called *impotence*. Men with ED have persistent or recurring inability either to achieve or to maintain an erection sufficient for satisfactory sexual performance. Although ED may result from a psychological problem, more frequently it is the result of a medical situation or a medication. Physical causes are best treated with medications that produce engorgement of the penis. As already mentioned, older men need more stimulation and more time to achieve an erection; this is not considered ED.

Dyspareunia in men most commonly results from urinary tract infection or **phimosis,** a condition in which the foreskin of the penis is too tight. **Balanitis,** inflammation of the penis, is another cause of dyspareunia in men.

Orgasmic Disorders

Orgasmic disorder is a delay in or absence of orgasm after a normal sexual excitement phase. Once a woman has had orgasms, it is uncommon for her to lose that ability unless there has been a sexual trauma, poor sexual communication, a conflicted sexual relationship, a mood disorder, a medical condition, or direct physiological effects from a drug. Orgasmic disorder is more prevalent in younger women who have not had adequate sexual experience to learn how to reach orgasm. It is not unusual for a woman to require manual clitoral stimulation to reach orgasm; not all women can achieve orgasm through intercourse alone.

Men, too, can experience orgasmic disorders. Some cannot achieve orgasm during intercourse but are able to reach orgasm through masturbation or manual or oral stimulation by their partner.

In **premature ejaculation,** the male reaches orgasm and ejaculates before, at the time of, or shortly after penetration. The disappointment of both partners may lead to issues with self-esteem, sexual avoidance, and ED. There are sexual techniques as well as medications that help to delay ejaculation.

Retrograde ejaculation occurs when the semen empties into the bladder instead of being ejaculated through the urethra. Normally this cannot occur because the internal bladder sphincter closes in the orgasmic phase. However, some medications, prostate surgery, and spinal cord injuries may lead to retrograde ejaculation, with resulting sterility.

KnowledgeCheck 32–10

- Identify three forms of sexual victimization.
- In which phases of the sexual response cycle can sexual dysfunction occur?

 Go to Chapter 32, **Knowledge Check Response Sheet and Answers,** on the Electronic Study Guide.

Practical Knowledge
knowing how

Although you understand the importance of comprehensive client assessment, you may find it difficult to gather information related to sexuality. Students, and some nurses, may be embarrassed, or may be concerned that the client will be embarrassed, to talk about sexual matters. These matters are personal and private, and they can threaten a person's self-esteem. But including sexuality as a routine part of your nursing assessment reinforces the concept that sexuality is an integral part of life. It also provides an opportunity for much-needed patient teaching. Many patients will not raise the topic of sexuality, so if you do not mention it, you cannot meet patient needs.

| Assessment |

The extent to which you will assess a client's sexual health status varies. For example, for a woman with a suspected STI, you would perform a comprehensive health assessment in addition to a focused sexual health assessment. Similarly, clients with illnesses that affect their sexual functioning should receive a full assessment. Jocelyn Carter ("Meet Your Patients") is an example. Recall that chronic illness has a profound effect on sexual functioning. Frank Thanee and Gabriel Thomas ("Meet Your Patients") have chronic health problems that have created concerns related to their sexuality. A focused sexual health assessment is needed in the following situations:

- Pregnancy, infertility workup, request for birth control
- Menstrual cycle irregularities or problems
- Annual health visit
- Unusual discharge from or change in genital organs

- Urination problems
- As part of a comprehensive physical examination
- A known sexual problem (e.g., dyspareunia)
- Illness that may affect sexual function (e.g., arthritis)

Sexual History

Most healthcare facilities use a standard nursing assessment form. Some address sexuality in a comprehensive manner, but most have only a few superficial questions or nothing at all. You will need to be sensitive to your client's verbal and nonverbal cues to identify and explore relevant areas that are not on the form. For topics to include in a sexual history and for suggestions for questions to ask,

 Go to Chapter 32, **Assessment Guidelines and Tools,** in Volume 2.

Tips for Taking a Sexual History

When you are asking personal questions, be sure to provide privacy. It is not usually enough merely to pull the curtains around the bed. At some point, you will probably want to talk with both partners, because the client and partner are a unit. Nevertheless, you should be aware that a patient may prefer to be alone when you take a sexual history. It is one thing to discuss blood pressure in the presence of family, but quite another to discuss sexual health issues, which may threaten the very core of a relationship. For example, a wife is not likely to discuss domestic violence with her abusing husband at her side. An 18-year-old man will probably not admit to having sex with another man when his father is present. An adolescent daughter may not want to discuss her STI in front of her mother.

For other suggestions,

 Go to Chapter 32, **Technique 32–1: Taking a Sexual History,** in Volume 2.

Physical Examination

Sexual health assessment includes a physical examination focused on the reproductive system. For detailed instructions about performing these examinations,

 Go to Chapter 19, **Procedure 19–17: Assessing the Male Genitourinary System,** and **Procedure 19–18: Assessing the Female Genitourinary System,** in Volume 2.

If there is reason to suspect that a client has a STI, you should obtain cultures of any discharge or lesions. Other laboratory tests may be ordered, as well.

KnowledgeCheck 32–11

What techniques can you use to increase comfort and communication during a sexual history assessment?

 Go to Chapter 32, **Knowledge Check Response Sheet and Answers,** on the Electronic Study Guide.

 CriticalThinking 32–7

Review the three case scenarios in the "Meet Your Patients" discussion. Consider the following questions:

- Would you be comfortable caring for and responding to each of these clients?
- What topics, if any, that have been raised by these clients would be difficult for you to handle?
- How would you answer each of the client's questions?

| Nursing Diagnosis |

NANDA has two nursing diagnoses for describing sexual problems. Use a diagnosis of:

- *Ineffective Sexuality Patterns* when the patient expresses concerns about his own sexuality. Examples of such concerns might include conflict about sexual orientation, fear of acquiring an STI, lack of knowledge about how to adapt sexual techniques to altered body function, lack of privacy, not having a partner, or impaired relationship with the partner.

- *Sexual Dysfunction* when there is an actual change in sexual function that the patient views as unsatisfying, unrewarding, or inadequate. This includes sexual response cycle disorders, such as low libido, arousal disorders, orgasmic disorders, vaginismus, premature ejaculation, and erectile dysfunction.

There is much overlap between these two NANDA diagnoses; however, Sexual Dysfunction is the more specific diagnosis for physiological problems. Thus, it is best to use Sexual Dysfunction when the patient has one or more of the following defining characteristics:

- Changes in achieving sexual satisfaction
- Change of interest in self or others
- Inability to achieve sexual satisfaction
- Verbalization of a sexual problem
- Actual or perceived limitations imposed by disease or therapy
- Changes in ability to fulfill perceived sex role
- Change in relationship with significant other
- Values conflicts

If these defining characteristics do not seem to "fit" the patient, then use the more general diagnosis, Ineffective Sexuality Patterns (concern about one's sexuality). The only defining characteristic needed to make

that diagnosis is that the patient reports difficulties, limitations, or changes in sexual behaviors or activities.

Jocelyn Carter ("Meet Your Patients"), for example, is not actually experiencing problems with sexual satisfaction or performance. She is expressing a broader concern about her sexuality—about her future desirability as a sex partner. Therefore, the better diagnosis for her is Ineffective Sexuality Patterns. The same is true for Gabriel Thomas, who is expressing fear that he may have sexual problems in the future. You could diagnose Sexual Dysfunction for Frank Thanee because he is experiencing a values conflict. He is expressing concerns, not about his sexual orientation, but about how it will affect his parents.

Etiologies of Sexuality Diagnoses

Several other nursing diagnoses may be the cause of sexuality problems. The following are the more common ones:

- *Activity Intolerance* and *Fatigue* may result from cardiac or respiratory disease, cancer, immune dysfunction, chronic pain, and morbid obesity. People with such conditions must alter their lifestyle, including sexual activity, to conserve energy. Lack of energy may decrease the person's interest in sex, or it may require a change in the mode of sexual expression.

- *Impaired Physical Mobility* (e.g., as occurs with arthritis, spinal cord injuries, or cerebral palsy) may affect a person's ability to interact, meet potential partners, and perform sexually (e.g., assume certain positions, make certain movements).

- *Fear* that sexual activity may be dangerous can inhibit desire and the ability to perform. This may occur, for example, after heart surgery. This diagnosis may also apply to the client's partner. A partner may be afraid that sexual activity will hurt the client after surgery, or if the partner is pregnant.

- *Chronic pain* may directly affect interpersonal relationships, interest in sex, or comfort during sexual intimacy. It may cause fatigue, indirectly affecting sexuality.

- *Chronic Low Self-Esteem* may result from chronic health problems and their consequences (e.g., loss of employment, inability to perform parenting roles). Sexual expression may also become a challenge, yet the intimacy and reassurance that accompanies sexual encounters can be vital to self-esteem and a sense of wholeness.

- *Self-Care Deficits.* For clients who need assistance with activities of daily living (ADLs), family or caretakers often find it difficult to accept and facilitate sexual relationships. When a person with a physical disability lives in a residential facility, lack of

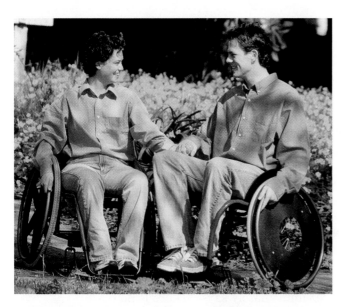

FIGURE 32–8 Sexual expression may be a challenge, yet the intimacy and reassurance that accompanies sexual encounters can be vital to self-esteem and a sense of wholeness.

opportunity and privacy may interfere with sexual expression (Figure 32–8).

- *Delayed Development.* Relationship challenges also exist for people who are developmentally disabled. Those with very low cognitive functioning are unable to seek out or understand sexual relationships. Unfortunately, this makes them vulnerable to sexual abuse. At a higher level of functioning, adolescents and adults have, as would be expected, a physical desire for sexual activity and often an accompanying desire for a loving, intimate relationship. Sex education is vital for these individuals to help them understand body structure and function, relationship issues, and ways to avoid exploitation and abuse.

Sexuality Problems as Etiologies of Other Diagnoses

Sexuality problems can be the etiology of other nursing diagnoses, for example:

- *Disturbed Body Image* related to change in appearance secondary to orchiectomy (removal of a testicle)
- *Pain (during coitus)* related to inadequate vaginal lubrication secondary to aging
- *Fear* related to sexual abuse by father
- *Rape Trauma Syndrome* (Note that you do not need an etiology for this nursing diagnosis. It is self-explanatory, as are most syndrome diagnoses.)

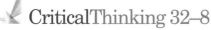 CriticalThinking 32–8

Give a specific example (patient situation) for each of the defining characteristics of Sexual Dysfunction given in the preceding section.

Planning Outcomes/Evaluation

For *NOC standardized outcomes* associated with Ineffective Sexuality Patterns and Sexual Dysfunction,

 Go to Chapter 32, **Standardized Language, Examples of NOC Outcomes for Sexuality Problems,** in Volume 2.

Individualized client outcomes and goals, as always, depend on the nursing diagnosis you identify. For either Sexual Dysfunction or Ineffective Sexuality Patterns, you might write the following desired outcomes:

- Expresses comfort with sexual orientation.
- Describes plans for resolving values conflicts about extramarital sex (e.g., will talk to his minister).
- Describes techniques for preventing STIs.
- Reports using a condom for all sexual activities involving exchange of body fluids.

The following are examples of outcomes that apply to Sexual Dysfunction:

- Communicates sexual needs and preferences to partner.
- Maintains penile erection through orgasm.
- Describes ways to adapt positions for intercourse to accommodate painful knee joints.

Planning Interventions/Implementation

For *NIC standardized interventions* and selected nursing activities for sexuality,

 Go to Chapter 32, **Standardized Language, Examples of NIC Interventions and Nursing Activities for Sexuality,** in Volume 2.

Specific nursing activities for sexuality problems depend on the etiology of the problem and on the goals selected. Broadly speaking, nursing interventions center around teaching about sexual health and self-care, counseling for altered sexual functioning, and dealing with inappropriate sexual behavior. Those interventions are discussed in the following sections.

Teaching About Sexual Health

Before you begin teaching, take the time to get to know your client and find out what she already knows about sexuality. Rapport and trust are essential to encourage clients to speak openly with you about sensitive or embarrassing topics. The time you spend putting the client at ease is well spent. If the client is comfortable, she is more likely to retain what you teach and to feel comfortable asking questions. Offer to include the partner in the discussion if the client wishes.

Text continues on page 788.

Nursing Care Plan

Client Data

Emilio Juarez is a 50-year-old Latino man recovering from an acute myocardial infarction (MI; heart attack). He has no history of diabetes or hypertension. Mr. Juarez owns his own computer consulting company and is active in the community (he is current president of the Chamber of Commerce). He is in a private room on the telemetry floor.

After dinner, Mr. Juarez's nurse sits down to teach Mr. Juarez and his wife, Luz, about the medications he will be taking. She also begins to talk to them about a cardiac rehabilitation program. Mr. Juarez asks, "What do you mean by 'activity restriction'? Do I have to stop doing all the things I did before?" The nurse asks, "What things are you thinking about?" Mr. Juarez hesitates, then says, "Oh, like working in the yard, going up the stairs, and, you know, personal things." Mrs. Juarez immediately says, "There is no need to talk about that now. The most important thing is for my Emilio to feel better and get home—there is plenty of time for other things later." The nurse tells the couple that many couples are anxious about resuming sexual activity after a heart attack and says, "I'd like to give you some information about that and answer any questions you might have."

Nursing Diagnosis

Ineffective Sexuality Patterns related to lack of knowledge about post-MI sexual activity and reluctance to ask questions, as evidenced by Mrs. Juarez's comment, "There is no need to talk about that now."

NOC Outcomes

Sexual Identity (1207)
Sexual Functioning (0119)
Body Image (1200)

Individualized Goals/Expected Outcomes

By discharge, Mr. Juarez will:
1. Be able to identify two resources he can use to learn more about sexual activity after myocardial infarction.
2. Commit to attending the cardiac rehabilitation classes offered at the hospital.

During and by the end of the cardiac rehabilitation program, Mr. Juarez will:
1. Identify stressors in his life related to sexual activity.
2. Report a desire to resume sexual activity to pre-MI levels.
3. Resume previous sexual activity.

NIC Interventions/Activities	Rationale
NIC Interventions Sexual counseling #5248 Body image enhancement #5220 Anxiety reduction #5820 **Nursing Activities** 1. Initiate discussions about sexual activity after MI, beginning with general, nonthreatening statements.	Clients and significant others are often too embarrassed to ask about sexual matters. The client's perception of his sexuality impacts personal and social behavior outside the bedroom (Steinke, 2002; Steinke & Patterson-Midgley, 1996).
2. Allow Mr. Juarez to control the discussion of sexual matters.	This shows respect for the client's privacy and his sexual being. Controlling what issues are discussed and when enhances self-esteem (Steinke, 2000).
3. Listen carefully to Mr. Juarez's expression of concerns, jokes, and nonverbal communication.	Men who are uncomfortable starting a discussion about sexual matters may send signals by making jokes, avoiding eye contact with female staff, and being "rowdy" with other men in a class situation (Steinke, 2000).
4. Seek consultation from other members of the health team as needed.	When nurses are uncomfortable talking about sexual matters and do not initiate the conversation, the client may think sexual activity is prohibited after MI. If the nurse is personally uncomfortable discussing these matters, it is imperative to consult with other members of the team who can meet the client's needs (Steinke, 2000; Steinke & Patterson-Midgley, 1996).
5. Include Mrs. Juarez in counseling as much as possible, with Mr. Juarez's consent.	Marriage and close interpersonal relationships allow each member to support the other and alleviate negative effects of stress. The client's ability to adapt physically and emotionally after MI depends on the spouse's ability to cope with situational stressors (Beach et al., 1992).

➤

Nursing Care Plan *(continued)*

Nursing Interventions/Activities	Rationale
6. Be clear about exploring Mr. and Mrs. Juarez's specific concerns, and correct any misinformation.	Anxiety about sexual activity after MI often arises from misconceptions. The incidence of sexual dysfunction after MI is estimated at 50 to 75% of all clients (Friedman, 2000). Regular exercise, such as in a cardiac rehab program, reduces the risk of MI from sexual activity (Muller, 2000; DeBusk et al., 2000). Sexual intercourse does not lead to exaggerated heart rate or blood pressure responses (Jackson, 2000). The period of maximum risk (which is still very low) is within 2 weeks of the MI (DeBusk et al., 2000).
7. Discuss the danger of using drugs for erectile dysfunction together with nitrates.	A profound and potentially dangerous drop in BP can occur when erectile dysfunction medication is used in the presence of oral, topical, or sublingual nitrates (Jackson, 2000).

Evaluation

After Mrs. Juarez left for the evening, the nurse returned to bring Mr. Juarez a medication. He said, "Thanks for bringing that up and for leaving the booklet. I love my wife, and I was worried. I sure didn't want to have another heart attack. She was embarrassed to let on that it is important to her, but we will be sure to make use of the rehab program." The nurse followed up later by giving the Juarezes a videotape that discusses sexual issues, which they can take home and watch in privacy and comfort when they are ready to do so.

References for Interventions

Beach, E. K., Maloney, B. H., Plocica, A. R., Sherry, S. E., Weaver, M., Luthringer, L., et al. (1992). The spouse: A factor in recovery after acute myocardial infarction. *Heart & Lung, 21*(1), 30–38.

DeBusk, R., Drory, Y., Goldstein, I., Jackson, G., Kaul, S., Kimmel, S. E., et al. (2000). Management of sexual dysfunction in patients with cardiovascular disease: Recommendations of the Princeton consensus panel. *American Journal of Cardiology, 86*(2), 175–181.

Friedman, S. (2000). Cardiac disease, anxiety and sexual functioning. *American Journal of Cardiology, 86 (Supplement)* (2A), 46F–50F.

Jackson, G. (2000). Sexual intercourse and stable angina pectoris. *American Journal of Cardiology, 86 (Supplement)* (2A), 35F–37F.

Muller, J. E. (2000). Triggering of cardiac events by sexual activity: Findings from a case-crossover analysis. *American Journal of Cardiology, 86 (Supplement)* (2A), 14F–18F.

Steinke, E. E. (2000). Sexual counseling after myocardial infarction. *American Journal of Nursing, 100*(12), 38–43.

Steinke, E. E. (2002). A videotape intervention for sexual counseling after myocardial infarction. *Heart & Lung, 31*(5), 348–354.

Steinke, E. E., & Patterson-Midgley, P. (1996). Sexual counseling of MI patients: Nurses' comfort, responsibility, and practice. *Dimensions of Critical Care Nursing, 15*(4), 216–223.

Care Map

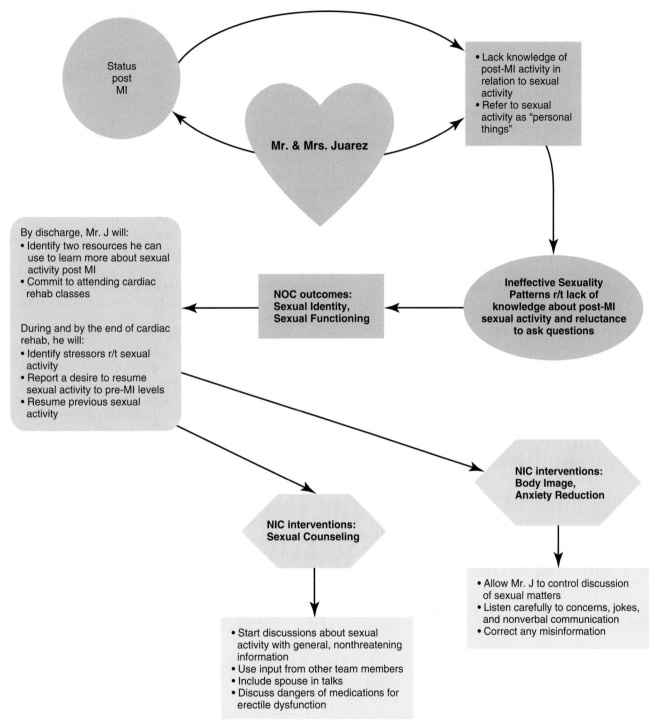

Status post MI

Mr. & Mrs. Juarez

- Lack knowledge of post-MI activity in relation to sexual activity
- Refer to sexual activity as "personal things"

Ineffective Sexuality Patterns r/t lack of knowledge about post-MI sexual activity and reluctance to ask questions

NOC outcomes: Sexual Identity, Sexual Functioning

By discharge, Mr. J will:
- Identify two resources he can use to learn more about sexual activity post MI
- Commit to attending cardiac rehab classes

During and by the end of cardiac rehab, he will:
- Identify stressors r/t sexual activity
- Report a desire to resume sexual activity to pre-MI levels
- Resume previous sexual activity

NIC interventions: Sexual Counseling

NIC interventions: Body Image, Anxiety Reduction

- Start discussions about sexual activity with general, nonthreatening information
- Use input from other team members
- Include spouse in talks
- Discuss dangers of medications for erectile dysfunction

- Allow Mr. J to control discussion of sexual matters
- Listen carefully to concerns, jokes, and nonverbal communication
- Correct any misinformation

Key:
- Data
- Nursing diagnosis
- NOC outcomes
- Other outcomes
- NIC interventions
- Nursing actions

As part of teaching focused on sexuality, you should discuss prevention of STIs with all clients and discuss contraception with clients who are heterosexual or bisexual. Other common topics are presented in the next sections.

Body Function and Reproduction

A person's age, experience, and educational level do not ensure knowledge of sexual functioning. Before you begin any teaching, explore your client's knowledge base by asking open-ended questions such as "What questions do you have about sex?"

Visual aids (e.g., a diagram of reproductive system anatomy) are helpful (see Chapter 24). For example, for pregnant clients you could use a pictorial guide illustrating fetal development. Most agencies provide handouts and brochures so that clients can review information at home.

As part of your general discussion on sexuality and body function, you may wish to discuss common myths and misconceptions about sex. Below are several statements about sex—all false—that provide a good starting point for discussion.

- You can't get pregnant the first time you have sex.
- You can tell the size of a man's penis by the size of his feet.
- You always have symptoms if you have an STI.
- You can tell from looking at someone if they have an STI. They will be dirty looking.
- People over 60 don't have sex.
- A vaginal orgasm is better than a clitoral orgasm.
- If the relationship is good, the man and woman will achieve simultaneous orgasm.
- It is not healthful to have intercourse during menstruation.
- The only normal position for intercourse is face to face. Anything else is deviant or at least "not nice."
- Only "dirty" people have STIs. You will not get an STI if your partner has good hygiene habits.
- If a person does not have an orgasm, they do not really love their partner.

Douching

Teach women that douching is unnecessary and is associated with significant risks. It can wash away the lactobacilli that clean the vagina and protect it from infection. Women who douche are at increased risk for some STIs and for pelvic inflammatory disease. Furthermore, douching is essentially useless as a method of contraception. Some women douche because they notice an odor. Reassure them that this is normal during certain times of their menstrual cycle. If the odor

doesn't disappear after washing, they should see their healthcare provider (Iannacchione, 2004).

Menstruation

Many women require information about self-care to dispel myths about menstruation. For example, it is not dangerous to engage in sexual activity during menstruation. The bloody fluid is from the uterus, not the vagina, so intercourse will not harm the vagina. Actually, some women enjoy sex more during menstruation because the increased vascularity in the pelvic region increases their pleasurable sensations, and orgasm may relieve their menstrual cramps. Some men, too, enjoy the warm, wet sensations. If the flow is very heavy, the woman can place a towel under her buttocks to protect the bed linens. Some women use a diaphragm to keep the flow from entering the vagina during sexual activity.

To prevent odor, the woman should use good perineal hygiene, bathe or shower every day, and change pads or tampons frequently. Advise women to follow the manufacturer's directions for reducing the risk for toxic shock syndrome. Deodorized pads and tampons are not very effective and can cause irritation to the vulva and vagina.

For mild cramping occurring before or during menses, aspirin and other nonsteroidal antiinflammatory drugs, such as ibuprofen (Motrin) are effective and can be taken unless contraindicated for other reasons. These drugs inhibit uterine contractions as well as having analgesic properties. A heating pad or warm bath may be comforting; lying supine also keeps the abdomen warm.

Premenstrual Syndrome

For women with PMS, you may suggest a variety of nonpharmacological treatments: eating small, frequent meals; reducing sugar, caffeine, alcohol, and salt in the diet; taking vitamin and mineral supplements; and exercising. Pharmaceutical studies have demonstrated the effectiveness of selective serotonin reuptake-inhibiting drugs (SSRIs) such as fluoxetine (Prozac) and sertraline (Zoloft) in managing symptoms (Dimmock, Wyatt, Jones, & O'Brien, 2000; Steiner, 2000).

Menopause

Traditionally, many physicians prescribed hormone replacement therapy (HRT) usually consisting of synthetic estrogens and progestin to relieve symptoms of menopause. However, recent research suggests that there is increased risk of vascular events (e.g., thrombophlebitis) and dementia with long-term use of HRT. Counsel women to discuss the risks and benefits of

HRT with their primary care provider, and inform them that there are some natural remedies that may provide symptom relief. Refer to the accompanying Complementary and Alternative Modalities (CAM) box.

Self-Examination

Breast self-examination and testicular self-examination are vital aspects of sexual health. Although there has recently been controversy about whether to advise routine breast self-examination, there seems to be little harm in encouraging your clients to routinely perform these assessments until more conclusive evidence is discovered. For more information and for details about the assessments, see Chapters 19 and 41.

Preventing Sexually Transmitted Infections

Preventing the spread of STIs is a worldwide health concern, and education is a key component. The only absolutely safe sex is total avoidance of sexual activity with a partner. However, most adults do not choose abstinence. The next safest sex occurs within a long-term, mutually monogamous relationship. Other safer sex practices involve the consistent, correct use of a condom and limiting the number of sexual partners. The Self-Care box on page 790 provides information on the use of male and female condoms. You should teach your clients the proper use of condoms and encourage them to discuss sexual feelings, activity, and safety with their partners. If people are not comfortable talking about birth control, STIs, and safer sex with a potential partner, they need to consider whether it is wise to begin a sexual relationship. Planned Parenthood (2004) advocates the following behaviors for safer sex:

- Be honest about current sexual practices and sexual history, as well as sexual health concerns.
- Avoid the exchange of body fluids, including semen, blood, and vaginal secretions, by correctly and consistently using latex barriers.
- Avoid contact with genital sores or growths.
- Have routine checkups for infection.
- Consult a healthcare provider for diagnosis and treatment of symptoms such as abnormal discharge from the vagina, penis, or rectum; a burning sensation with urination; sores in the genital area; or painful intercourse.
- Accept responsibility for your actions.

Also advise clients to choose a healthcare provider with whom they are comfortable while discussing these issues and to keep themselves healthy by speaking frankly and openly about their sexual health concerns. Assure them that testing, examination, and treatment for STIs are always confidential.

CAM for Menopause Symptoms

complementary and alternative modalities (CAM)

Help, including hormone therapy, is available for menopause symptoms. In addition to finding a primary care provider with whom to discuss their symptoms, advise women to:

- Eat a balanced diet, low in fat and rich in calcium.
- Use supplemental vitamins, if necessary.
- Take supplemental calcium and magnesium.
- Exercise daily.
- Avoid smoking.
- Limit alcohol and caffeine.
- Drink plenty of water to counteract the drying effect of low estrogen levels.
- Use soy products (e.g., soy milk, tofu, and soy flour), which are rich in *phytoestrogens* that are converted during digestion to very weak estrogens.
- Try the herbal remedies red clover and black cohosh.
- Use natural progesterone cream, which is made from a yam root. Women usually apply a small amount of the cream for 12 days out of each month.

Contraception

For clients who are heterosexual or bisexual, your sexual health teaching may include methods for preventing unwanted pregnancies. Several fertility control and family planning strategies are available, each with advantages and disadvantages. For information on several fertility control methods,

 Go to Chapter 32, **Tables, Fertility Control Methods,** in Volume 2.

Counseling for Sexual Problems

The PLISSIT model was developed as a guideline for sex therapy (Annon, 1974). Basic nursing education does not prepare you to provide sex therapy. However, the first three PLISSIT steps have been successfully adapted to address sexual knowledge deficits, which you are qualified to treat. The acronym, PLISSIT, represents the following:

P-permission. Permission means that you communicate an open, accepting attitude so that the client

Teaching Your Patient to Use a Condom

Using Male Condoms

The male condom is a sheath that covers the penis during sexual activity.

- Put the condom on before the penis touches the vagina, mouth, or anus.
- Inspect the package to ensure that the condom has not been damaged.
- Open the package without tearing the condom.
- Squeeze out the air at the tip of the condom, and unroll it over the erect penis, leaving some space at the tip to collect the ejaculate.
- After sex, to avoid breaking the condom, hold the condom at the rim as the penis is withdrawn.
- Use a new condom if you want to have sex again.

Using Female Condoms

The female condom is a plastic pouch that fits inside the vagina so that all vaginal tissue is protected from contact with the penis. The condom is inserted with the inner ring placed high in the vagina near the cervix and the outer ring on the labia.

- Insert the condom before the penis touches the vagina.
- Inspect the package to ensure that the condom has not been damaged.
- Open the package without tearing the condom.
- Put the inner ring and pouch inside the vagina.
- Push the inner ring as far into the vagina as it will go.
- Ensure that the outer ring stays outside the vagina.
- If needed, add lubricant to the inside of the condom.
- After sex, gently pull out the condom and discard.

Do

- Use latex condoms unless you or your partner are allergic to latex, or use polyurethane condoms.
- Treat condoms gently, and keep them out of the sun.
- Use only water-based lubricants to reduce friction and prevent tearing.
- Check the expiration date of the condom and packaging. Old condoms may be brittle and more likely to break.

Don't

- Don't store condoms in your wallet for a long period of time.
- Don't use fingernails or teeth to open the condom wrapper; doing so can tear the condom.
- Don't reuse a condom.
- Don't use lotions or oils with condoms; these may cause breakage.

---

feels free to ask questions and express concerns and feelings and to engage in sexual behaviors with a consenting partner. For example, you might state, "Many women experience decreased vaginal lubrication after menopause. Have you noticed anything like this?"

LI-limited information. Supplying limited information may include teaching about normal sexual functioning, expected changes in sexual functioning, medication side effects, and medical and surgical impacts on sexuality. For example, you might say, "Some women experience decreased vaginal lubrication because of decreased levels of certain hormones."

SS-specific suggestions. You might make specific suggestions for self-care, as presented in this chapter. For example: "You might consider using a water-soluble lubricant."

IT-intensive therapy. If these interventions do not relieve the client's concerns, you should refer the client to someone with specialized knowledge of sexual health. For example: "You might consider discussing this with your gynecologist."

Dealing with Inappropriate Sexual Behavior

Nursing involves intimate contact. We see people disrobed, touch their bodies, and discuss private topics. In most cases, patients recognize this as professional behavior associated with providing health care. Occasionally they may respond inappropriately. For example, a client may make sexually suggestive comments, request sexually related care that is not required (e.g., ask you to bathe his genitalia when he can do it adequately himself), disrobe or expose body parts that are not involved in the care delivered, or touch or grab you as you provide care. The following are the most common reasons for sexually inappropriate behaviors:

- Confusion
- Neurological disorders, especially those involving the frontal lobe
- Psychiatric problems resulting in poor impulse control
- Misinterpretation of nursing care

- Need to have power or control over others, especially when the client feels powerless in other aspects of his life

- Worries about sexual functioning

- Unrealistic view of nursing based on sexual stereotypes

If you believe a client is demonstrating inappropriate sexual behaviors, immediately tell the client that his behavior is inappropriate. Do not express anger, but use clear statements, such as, "I do not like your comments. They are inappropriate. Please stop." Next, let the client know what behavior you expect. Be direct with your comments. If the client is exposing himself, let him know what you expect him to wear ("I expect you to keep your pajama bottoms on)." If the client is attempting to touch you, tell him, "Do not touch me." Refocus the client's attention to the care you are delivering ("Hold still now, while I tape your IV"). If you are extremely uncomfortable or the client persists in his comments or actions, leave the room and report the incident to your instructor or the nurse assigned to the client. Your instructor may need to change your assignment. You may also wish to consider discussing the situation with the client while another person is in the room.

Sexual harassment is a unique form of inappropriate sexual behavior (refer to "Sexual Harassment" in the "Theoretical Knowledge" section). If you believe you are being sexually harassed, you should confront your harasser and clearly state your concerns. If you feel unable to confront your harasser (for example, if the harasser is a teacher or supervisor), keep a written record of the events, and report your concerns to the worksite or school official in charge of personnel. By law, all worksites and educational environments must have a written procedure for handling cases of sexual harassment. It will tell you how to file a grievance, what forms you need to use, to whom the incident is reported, and what the procedure is for hearing and resolution. For further information, see Chapter 45.

PUTTING IT ALL TOGETHER

Consider the three patients discussed in the "Meet Your Patients" scenario. Each situation illustrates how important sexual identity is to the sense of self.

- Jocelyn Carter is having a breast removed secondary to cancer. However, her question focuses not on the threat from cancer, but on how this surgery will affect her relationship with her husband.

- Gabriel Thomas has extremely high blood pressure, yet he is concerned that medications will impair his sexual abilities.

- Frank Thanee is recovering from open heart surgery but is focused on explaining to his visiting family his long-term relationship with a man.

The full-spectrum nursing model can help you to find the best approach when dealing with sexual health. We have used the three patients in "Meet Your Patients" to illustrate how this works.

- *Self-knowledge.* To help patients identify and resolve sexual health concerns, you will need to examine your own beliefs and values. The self-knowledge gained from examining your own views on sexuality will help you to be open to your patients' sexual concerns. What are your beliefs about sex and sexuality? Are you uncomfortable around people whose sexual orientation is different from yours? Imagine how you would feel if Frank Thanee asked you for help.

- *Theoretical knowledge.* You will need theoretical knowledge about sexuality, the effect of health concerns on sexual function and expression, and treatment of sexual health problems. Many myths and taboos surround the subject of sexuality, so it is important that you remain objective and current regarding these topics. A sound knowledge base enables you to teach and respond sensitively to all your clients. What knowledge do you already have that would enable you to address Gabriel Thomas's concerns? What knowledge do you still need?

- *Practical knowledge.* When dealing with sexuality, communication skills are essential practical knowledge. Your verbal and nonverbal skills demonstrate to patients your comfort with sensitive topics. Consider the situation of Jocelyn Carter. Suppose you responded to Jocelyn's question by telling her, "That's the least of your worries." How do you think she would feel? Now consider what might happen if you responded, "You must be worried about your sexual relationship. Tell me a little more about what you're feeling."

- *Critical thinking and the nursing process.* Consider Gabriel Thomas. Mr. Thomas has a markedly elevated blood pressure but is concerned about the effects of medications on his sexual function. To help him, you will need to assess his knowledge and concerns, critically examine his issues in light of what is known about hypertension and its treatment, and use the nursing process to develop a plan of care that is acceptable to him. When working with patients with sexual health concerns, tailor your approach to each individual's needs, just as you do in all areas of health.

 Go to Chapter 32, **Resources for Caregivers and Health Professionals,** on the Electronic Study Guide.

 Suggested Readings: Go to Chapter 32, **Reading More About Sexual Health,** on the Electronic Study Guide.

 Bibliography: Go to Volume 2, Bibliography.

33 Sleep & Rest

CHAPTER

Learning Outcomes

After completing this chapter, you should be able to:

* Explain why rest and sleep are important.

* Describe the functions and physiology of sleep.

* Explain circadian rhythms and how they relate to sleep.

* Identify factors that influence rest and sleep.

* Describe nursing implications for age-related differences in the sleep cycle.

* Identify at least five common sleep disorders.

* Perform a comprehensive sleep assessment using appropriate interview questions, a sleep diary, and a sleep history.

* Formulate nursing diagnoses that identify sleep problems that may be treated through specific nursing interventions.

* Plan, implement, and evaluate nursing care related to specific nursing diagnoses addressing sleep problems.

Your Patient

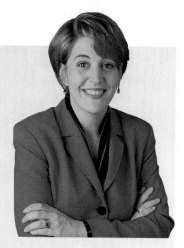

You are a nurse working on a surgical unit. Today you are meeting with Anne for preoperative teaching. She is scheduled for a complete hysterectomy, bilateral salpingo-oophorectomy, and cystocele and rectocele repair next Monday. She has a secondary diagnosis of fibromyalgia, a painful muscle disorder.

Anne is a 49-year-old married woman with three children. She works full time and manages the family with her husband, Evan. She says, "I'm a little nervous about the surgery, but I know I need it. But I haven't been sleeping well because of thinking about it." Anne tells you that she has actually had trouble sleeping for the last 20 years. "I take an Ambien pill, 10 mg, every night to help me sleep. Will I be able to get that in the hospital? I really can't sleep at all without it," explains Anne.

As you continue the interview, Anne explains that she suffered from physical and emotional abuse as a young woman and has had sleep problems ever since. She has been to counseling, but that did not improve her sleep. Recently her sleep has been even more troublesome. Aside from her upcoming surgery, she has been coping with the recent death of her father. After meeting with Anne, you realize that sleep-promoting measures will be an important part of her nursing care while she is in the hospital.

What clues in Anne's situation would cause you to suspect that she will have difficulty sleeping while in the hospital? What characteristics of the hospital environment might interfere with Anne's sleep? You may not have enough theoretical knowledge and experience to feel confident about your answers to these questions, but use your present knowledge base and your life experiences to think about them.

Theoretical Knowledge
knowing why

Have you felt tired after waking up from a night's sleep? Have you ever been tired, but not sleepy, and, after relaxing a while, felt your normal energy return? How do you think sleep and rest are different? How are they alike?

Rest is a condition in which the body is inactive or engaging in mild activity, after which the person feels refreshed. A person at rest is calm, at ease, relaxed, and free of anxiety and stress (Figure 33–1). People rest by doing things that they find calming and relaxing, for example reading, listening to music, watching television, doing needlework, praying or meditating, gardening, baking, playing golf, walking, and camping.

Sleep is a cyclically occurring state of decreased motor activity and perception (Germann & Stanfield, 2002) (Figure 33–2). Body functions slow, and metabolism falls by 20 to 30%, so the body conserves energy. Sleep is characterized by altered consciousness: a sleeping person is unaware of the environment and responds selectively to external stimuli. For example,

an alarm clock, bright light, or other "meaningful" stimuli usually will awaken a sleeper, but everyday background noises and soft light will not.

Although necessary and beneficial, rest without sleep is inadequate. At rest, the body is disturbed by

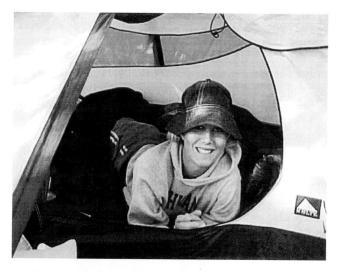

FIGURE 33–1 Girl resting.

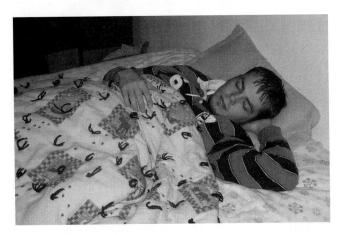

FIGURE 33–2   Boy sleeping.

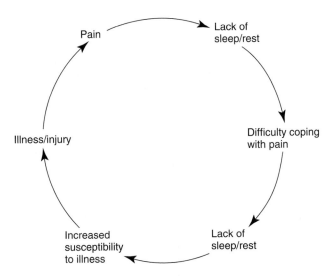

FIGURE 33–3   Relationship between sleep/rest and illness. Lack of sleep and rest increases our susceptibility to illness, and the pain of illness and injury increases our susceptibility to disturbed sleep.

all exterior stimuli, whereas in sleep it is screened from them by altered consciousness. Thus, as we discuss next, sleep restores the body; rest alone cannot do this.

WHY DO WE NEED TO SLEEP?

We spend more time sleeping than engaging in any other single activity: about 8 hours a day, or 2688 hours a year—nearly one-third of our lives! So why is sleep so important? Before you try to answer, think back to the last time you had a poor night's sleep. Remember the mental fogginess, the physical fatigue, the feeling of slight nausea? Missing even one night of sleep can reduce mental performance, and long periods of sleep deprivation can result in stress-related illnesses and injuries (e.g., from an automobile accident). The reason is that sleep and rest are essential for physical, mental, and spiritual well-being.

Theorists do not agree on all of the functions of sleep, but studies have shown that adequate sleep restores energy. Despite the fact that some regions of the brain are more active during sleep than when we are awake, our total energy output is reduced while we sleep, giving the body time for restoration and repair. Research also indicates that sleep strengthens the immune system: Animals deprived of sleep are more vulnerable to infection (Germann & Stanfield, 2002). Sleep may also improve learning and adaptation, giving the individual a chance to mentally repeat and rehearse facts and situations before they are encountered in wakeful life. Some evidence suggests that sleep and dreaming may facilitate the storage of long-term memory (Germann & Stanfield, 2002), perhaps by assisting the brain in reorganizing and storing information. Sleep also appears to reduce stress and anxiety, improving our ability to cope and concentrate on activities of daily living. For further discussion of sleep theories,

 Go to Chapter 33, **Supplemental Materials: Theories of Sleep,** on the Electronic Study Guide.

Sleep/rest and illness are interrelated (Figure 33–3). Illness and injury increase the need to sleep and at the same time make it difficult to sleep. In turn, lack of sleep increases the susceptibility to illness by compromising the immune system. People who are ill or injured need more sleep than usual to restore energy needed for tissue repair and healing. However, they often have difficulty resting because of pain and other symptoms of their illness.

Because sleep enhances wellness and speeds recovery from illness, promoting sleep is an important independent nursing intervention. In this chapter, you'll learn how to recognize signs of sleep disturbance, as well as factors that interfere with patients' sleep, and specific measures to facilitate sleep for each client.

KnowledgeCheck 33–1

- Compare and contrast sleep and rest. How are they different? Alike?
- Why is promoting sleep an important nursing intervention?

 Go to Chapter 33, **Knowledge Check Response Sheet and Answers,** on the Electronic Study Guide.

CriticalThinking 33–1

 What effect do you think surgery will have on Anne's sleep ("Meet Your Patient")? Why?

HOW MUCH SLEEP DO WE NEED?

Sleep needs vary widely among individuals. Even though the accepted standard has been 8 hours per night for adults, there is really no "correct" amount or pattern of sleep that maintains well-being in all people.

In spite of individual variations, however, different sleep patterns are characteristic of different age groups.

Infants have an overall greater total sleep time than any other age group. Newborns sleep as much as 16 to 20 hours a day, in periods ranging from one to several hours. Sleep time gradually decreases over the next few months, but throughout the first year of life, a minimum of 14 hours of sleep per day is recommended (Tuller, 2004). Most infants sleep several hours during one overnight period, with a morning and afternoon nap each day.

After the first year of life, sleep duration gradually decreases (Table 33–1). In most adults, sleep of 7 to 8 hours is fully restorative; however, there are wide individual variations. In some cultures, total sleep time is divided into an overnight sleep period and a midafternoon nap.

Older adults spend significantly less time sleeping but need more rest than younger adults. Usually older adults rest or nap during the day, go to bed early, and get up early. They take longer falling asleep, and their arousal periods during sleep are longer and more frequent. Frequent waking is commonly due to physical discomfort, anxiety, and nocturia (Polan & Taylor, 2003). If the sleep is interrupted, the person will need to sleep longer to feel restored. If the older adult does not increase the total time in bed, she may experience fatigue, irritability, and impaired cognition.

CriticalThinking 33–2

- How much sleep might Anne (Meet Your Patient) need in a normal night?
- How will a good night of sleep benefit Anne while she is in the hospital?
- If you were preparing for an important test, would it be better to stay up all night studying, or should you try to get a good night of sleep?
- How many hours of sleep do *you* need to feel rested and function well the next day? Compare notes with family members, friends, and classmates. Do they all need the same amount of sleep as you?

PHYSIOLOGY OF SLEEP

Our environment plays a role in the physiology of our sleep, so we begin with an exploration of circadian rhythms, by which the body maintains synchronicity with the natural world.

How Do Circadian Rhythms Influence Sleep?

Biorhythms are "biological clocks" that are controlled within the body and synchronized with environmental factors (e.g., gravity, electromagnetic forces, light, and darkness). Biorhythms influence many

TABLE 33–1 Average Sleep Requirements	
Age Group	**Hours per Day**
Newborns (birth to 4 weeks)	16–20
Infants (4 weeks to 1 year)	14–16
Toddlers (1–3 years)	12–14
Preschoolers (3–6 years)	11–13
Middle and late childhood (6–12 years)	10–11
Adolescents (12–18 years)	8–9
Young adults (18–40 years)	7–8
Middle-age adults (40–65 years)	7
Older adults (65 years and older)	5–7

physical and mental functions. For example, body temperature is typically lowest when the person wakes up in the morning, and female menstruation follows an approximately 28-day cycle, like the lunar cycle on which our calendar months are based.

A **circadian rhythm** is a biorhythm based on the day-night pattern in a 24-hour cycle. The term comes from the Latin words *circa,* meaning "about" and *dies,* meaning "day"—once a day. A person's circadian rhythm is regulated by a cluster of cells in the hypothalamus of the brain stem that respond to changing levels of light. Circadian rhythm affects our overall level of functioning; most people have a higher energy level in the daytime and less energy at night. However, some people are more alert and active in the morning, whereas others function at a higher level in the afternoon or evening.

Do you find yourself feeling sleepy at about the same time each night? Do you often awaken before the alarm clock goes off? If so, that's because the timing of sleep and waking is also influenced by your circadian biorhythm. Sleep quality is best when the time at which you go to sleep and wake up is in synchrony with your circadian rhythm. For this reason, people who work evening and night shifts (e.g., healthcare workers, police officers, and so on) can suffer significant sleep deprivation until their bodies adjust to the new pattern. Changing time zones can also disrupt sleep-wake cycles and can thus be troublesome for people who travel frequently on business. Hospitalization can also interfere with a patient's circadian rhythm. Noises, lights, waking the patient for assessments or medications, absence of normal bedtime rituals, absence or presence of family members, recent losses, or fear of the unknown may hinder the patient's ability to sleep at his usual time.

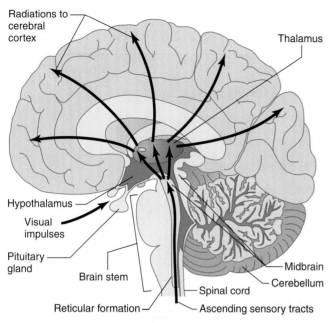

FIGURE 33–4 **The reticular activating system, consisting of the reticular formation and certain areas in the cerebral cortex, works to regulate sleep and wakefulness.**

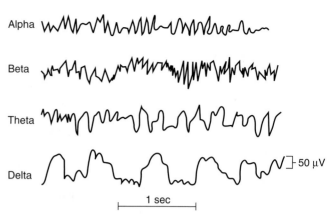

FIGURE 33–5 **Four different types of brain waves.**

![CriticalThinking 33–3]

CriticalThinking 33–3

What may upset Anne's circadian rhythm?

How Is Sleep Regulated?

What makes us fall asleep? What happens in the brain during sleep? The mechanisms of sleep are complex and poorly understood, but we know that sleep is controlled by centers in the lower part of the brain, which produce sleep by actively inhibiting wakefulness. As just noted, a major factor in regulating sleep is the amount of light received through the eyes. The increasing light of a dawning sky signals the hypothalamus (Figure 33–4) to induce gradual arousal from sleep. Another collection of nerve cell bodies within the brain stem, called the **reticular formation,** is responsible for maintaining wakefulness. The reticular formation is activated by stimuli from the cerebral cortex. Together, these reticular and cortical neurons are called the **reticular activating system (RAS).** Neurotransmitters associated with excitatory and inhibitory sleep mechanisms include catecholamines, acetylcholine, serotonin, histamine, and prostaglandins. L-tryptophan and adenosine promote feelings of sleepiness.

An **electroencephalogram (EEG)** is a machine that is used to record the electrical activity of the neurons in the brain. Electrical impulses are transmitted from the brain to the machine through electrodes attached to the scalp. These impulses create wave patterns commonly known as *brain waves.* Any of four different types of brain waves may be recorded (Figure 33–5):

- *Alpha waves* are high-frequency, medium-amplitude, irregular waves.
- *Beta waves* are high-frequency, low-amplitude, irregular waves.
- *Theta waves* are high-amplitude waves that are common in children but rare in adults.
- *Delta waves* are low-frequency, high-amplitude, regular waves common in deep sleep.

The EEG of a waking person differs greatly from that of a sleeping person. In general, the greater the brain activity, the more rapid the brain waves on the EEG. While the person is awake, brain waves are very rapid, irregular, and low in amplitude, mostly alpha and beta waves. Many neurons are firing at different intervals, at different times, and with different strengths. When a person is relaxed (e.g., sitting on the couch watching TV without any mental arousal), the EEG records mostly alpha activity. During sleep, alpha waves disappear. They are replaced by slower, higher amplitude delta waves.

What Are the Stages of Sleep?

There are two distinct types of sleep:

1. **NREM** (non–rapid eye movement) sleep is produced by withdrawal of neurotransmitters from the reticular formation and inhibition of arousal mechanisms in the cerebral cortex.
2. In **REM** (rapid eye movement) sleep, the brain is highly active with rapid, low-amplitude waves similar to those that occur when a person is awake and alert. REM sleep is primarily initiated by the reticular formation.

Five stages of sleep (four NREM stages and the REM stage) have been identified, based on brain activity and other physiological characteristics. See Table 33–2 for characteristics of each stage of sleep.

TABLE 33-2 Characteristics of Stages of Sleep

Stage	Typical Duration	Characteristics
I	5–10 minutes	• Transition between wakefulness and sleep • Light sleep; can be awakened easily • Relaxed but aware of surroundings • Groggy, heavy lidded • Regular, deep breathing; eyelids open and close slowly • Accounts for about 5% of total sleep • Dreams usually not remembered
II	10–15 minutes	• Light sleep • Easily roused • Temperature, heart rate, and blood pressure decrease slightly • Accounts for about 50% of total sleep
III	5–15 minutes	• Deep sleep • Difficult to rouse • Parasympathetic nervous system predominates: temperature, pulse, respirations, and blood pressure slow even more • Skeletal muscles very relaxed • Snoring may occur • Accounts for about 8% of total sleep
IV	20–50 minutes	• The deepest sleep • Difficult to awaken • Body, mind, and muscles very relaxed • Parasympathetic nervous system still predominates; heart rate and respirations are slow and regular; temperature and BP are low • If roused, may be confused • Accounts for about 11% of total sleep
REM (V)	5–30 minutes (usually at least 20–30)	• Paradoxical sleep • Less restful than NREM sleep • Eyes move rapidly • Small muscles twitch • Metabolism, temperature, pulse, and BP increase • Pulse may be rapid and irregular • Apnea may occur • Gastric secretions increase • Large muscle activity and deep-tendon reflexes are depressed • Dreaming occurs • If awakened, will react normally • Accounts for about 25% of total sleep

NREM Sleep Stages

NREM sleep is also called *slow-wave sleep (SWS)* because it is characterized by the presence of delta waves. NREM is divided into four stages, each deeper than the one preceding it. The parasympathetic branch of the autonomic nervous system becomes progressively more dominant during each stage of NREM sleep, so the metabolic rate and all vital signs progressively decrease.

• **Stage I** is a light sleep from which the sleeper can easily be awakened. The person is relaxed; breath-

ing is regular and deep; the eyelids slowly open and close, and the eyes roll from side to side. The person feels groggy, the eyelids feel heavy, and suddenly without notice the person falls asleep. Within 5 to 10 minutes, sleep progresses to stage II. Stage I accounts for about 5% of our total sleep during the night. Brain activity consists of alpha waves, with occasional low-frequency theta waves (McCance & Heuther, 2002).

• **Stage II** is also light sleep. Brain activity slows. The eyes are still, and body processes begin to slow down

34 CHAPTER

Skin Integrity

& Wound Healing

Learning Outcomes

After completing this chapter, you should be able to:

* Discuss the factors that affect skin integrity.

* Identify wounds based on accepted classification schemes.

* Describe the three phases of wound healing.

* Distinguish primary intention healing, secondary intention healing, and tertiary intention healing.

* Describe three types of wound drainage.

* Review the major complications of wound healing.

* Explain the factors involved in the development of pressure ulcers.

* Use the Braden and Norton scales to assess risk for pressure ulcers.

* Assess and categorize pressure ulcers based on the pressure ulcer staging system.

* Provide nursing care that limits the risk of pressure ulcer development.

* Accurately chart assessment of a wound.

* Demonstrate appropriate technique for irrigating a wound.

* Describe care of a wound with a drain.

* Differentiate the four forms of wound debridement.

* Discuss the RYB color code system for wound management.

* Discuss when and how to use gauze dressings, transparent films, hydrocolloids, hydrogels, and absorbent dressings.

* Describe guidelines to follow when applying heat or cold therapy.

* Demonstrate bandage and binder application.

MEET Your Patient

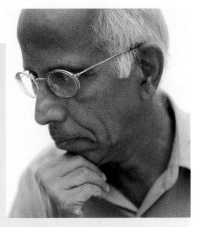

William Harmon is a 78-year-old man who fell 3 days ago. His fall resulted in a fractured left hip. He was admitted to the hospital and underwent an open reduction and internal fixation (ORIF) of the left hip. Today is his second postoperative day.

Mr. Harmon's weight on admission was 140 lb (63.64 kg). His height is 73 inches. His family reports that he has been steadily losing weight. He expresses little interest in eating and says he has been depressed since his wife died last year.

While performing your assessment of Mr. Harmon, you notice that a large dressing covers the left hip incision. You loosen the dressing and see that the staples are intact at the incision site and that there is a minimal amount of serosanguineous drainage on the bandage. As you turn him in bed, you see a 10 cm by 6 cm reddened area on his coccyx. William now has two wounds, an intentional surgical wound and a pressure ulcer that has resulted from his impaired mobility. How will you care for each of these wounds? What factors contributed to each of the wounds, and how will you promote healing?

Theoretical Knowledge
knowing why

The integumentary system consists of the skin, hair, nails, sweat glands, and the subcutaneous tissue below the skin. The skin is the largest organ of the body. The major functions of the skin include protection of the internal organs, unique identification of an individual, thermoregulation, metabolism of nutrients and metabolic waste products, and sensation.

FACTORS AFFECTING SKIN INTEGRITY

It is important first to understand the structure of the skin (Figure 34–1). The **epidermis** is the outer portion of the skin. The epidermis is made up of four or five layers, of which the most important are the inner and outer layers. The outermost layer of the epidermis, the **stratum corneum,** is composed of numerous thicknesses of dead cells. Functioning as a barrier, it restricts water loss and prevents fluids, pathogens, and chemicals from entering the body. The innermost layer of the epidermis, the **stratum germinativum,** continually produces new cells, pushing the older cells toward the skin surface. Keratinocytes, melanocytes, and Langerhan cells are located in the epidermal layer. The **keratinocytes** are protein-containing cells that give the skin strength and elasticity. Deeper in the epidermis are **melanocytes,** which produce **melanin,** a pigment that gives skin its color and provides protection from ultraviolet light. **Langerhans cells** are mobile. Their function is to phagocytize (engulf) foreign material and trigger an immune response.

The **dermis** lies below the epidermis and above the subcutaneous tissue. It is made of irregular fibrous connective tissue that provides strength and elasticity to the skin and is generously supplied with blood vessels. Within the dermis are sweat glands, sebaceous glands, ceruminous glands, hair and nail follicles, sensory receptors, elastin, and collagen.

The **subcutaneous layer** is composed primarily of connective and adipose tissue. It provides insulation, protection, and a reserve of calories in the event of severe malnutrition. This layer varies in thickness in different body sites. Sex hormones, genetics, age, and nutrition also influence the distribution of subcutaneous tissue.

For optimal function, all layers of the skin must be intact. Breaks in the skin increase the risk of infection, for example, and may lead to significant harm. Surgery and injuries may result in a loss of skin integrity. Several factors affect the ability to maintain intact skin and heal a break in the skin.

Factors that influence the ability to maintain intact skin and heal wounds include: age, mobility, nutrition, hydration, diminished sensation, impaired circulation, medications, moisture on the skin, fever, contamination, and lifestyle.

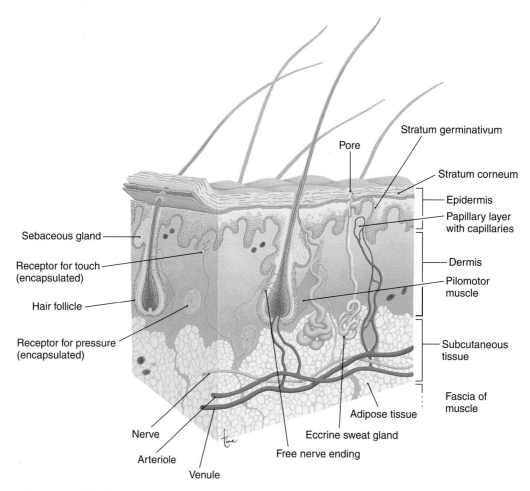

FIGURE 34–1   **The structure of the skin.**

Age-Related Variations

Age affects the condition and structure of the skin. Infants, for example, are born with varying amounts of *vernix caseosa,* a creamy substance that protects their skin. Infants' skin is thinner and more permeable than that of adults, qualities that predispose infants to skin breakdown (e.g., diaper rash). The subcutaneous layer and sweat glands are not fully developed. As a result, thermoregulation is inadequate, and the infant must be swaddled to maintain body heat.

The skin of infants and young children feels smooth because it has not been exposed to the environment. As children are exposed to sun and other elements, skin texture becomes coarser. Sex hormones released during puberty increase sebaceous and sweat gland activity, which leads to perspiration and sometimes acne. In women, high estrogen levels may contribute to the softening of connective tissue and cause striae and darkening of the skin, particularly on the face, areolae, nipples, vulva, and umbilicus.

As adults age, the activity of the sebaceous and sweat glands diminishes, resulting in drier skin. Along with loss of lean body mass, the subcutaneous tissue layer thins, giving the individual a sharp angular appearance. Excess weight can offset this change of appearance, though. The strong bond between the epidermal and dermal layer decreases as the dermal layer loses elasticity as a result of changes in its collagen fibers. These changes make the skin prone to breakdown and prolong wound-healing time. Regeneration of healthy skin takes twice as long in an 80-year-old than in a 30-year-old. Additionally, many older adults have chronic diseases that interfere with healing. Diabetes, for instance, predisposes to infection, and liver dysfunction interferes with synthesis of blood clotting factors.

Impaired Mobility

A healthy person moves and shifts position unconsciously when he senses pressure or discomfort. However, many people are unable to move independently. For them, immobility causes an increase in pressure and may lead to skin breakdown. Impaired mobility is caused by conditions that require complete bedrest or that seriously limit activity. Examples are paralysis, extreme fatigue, high-risk pregnancy, sedation, altered levels of conciousness, casts, traction, and altered sensory perception.

KnowledgeCheck 34–1

- Identify the major functions of the skin.
- What is the function of the stratum corneum, the outermost layer of the skin?
- What is the function of the subcutaneous layer?
- What effect does aging have on skin?
- What effect does immobility have on skin?

 Go to Chapter 34, **Knowledge Check Response Sheet and Answers,** on the Electronic Study Guide.

Nutrition and Hydration

Skin condition reflects overall nutritional status, while at the same time, nutritional intake affects the skin. Adequate intake of protein, cholesterol, calories, fluid, vitamin C, and minerals is essential to maintaining skin integrity. *Protein* is necessary to maintain the skin, repair minor defects, and preserve intravascular volume. As protein levels decline from excess loss or inadequate intake, minor defects cannot be repaired, fluid leaks from the vascular compartment of dependent areas, and edema (excess fluid in the tissues) develops. Edema decreases skin elasticity and interferes with the diffusion of oxygen to the cells. Therefore, the skin becomes prone to breakdown.

Abnormally low *cholesterol* levels predispose patients to skin breakdown and inhibit wound healing. Patients on low-fat tube feedings may experience deficiencies in cholesterol, fatty acids, and linoleic acid. Together, these fats aid in providing fuel for wound healing and maintain a waterproof barrier in the stratum corneum (Stone, Wyman, Salisbury, & Chenitz, 1999).

If *calorie intake* is inadequate, the body uses proteins for energy; they are then unavailable for building and maintenance functions (see Chapter 26). When undernutrition is prolonged, the person experiences weight loss, loss of subcutaneous tissue, and muscle atrophy. As a result, padding between the skin and the bones decreases, predisposing to pressure ulcers.

Ascorbic acid (vitamin C) is involved in the formation and maintenance of collagen, so a deficiency can delay wound healing. *Zinc* and *copper* are also involved in collagen formation, and deficiencies of either may impair healing.

Hydration is an essential element of skin turgor. Poor skin turgor may occur as a result of dehydration, whereas swelling may result from overhydration. For further discussion on fluid requirements, see Chapter 36.

Diminished Sensation

Clients with peripheral vascular disease, spinal cord injury, diabetes, cerebrovascular accident, trauma, or fractures often have diminished tactile sense, and they are therefore more prone to skin breakdown. If you've ever touched a hot surface and quickly pulled back your hand, you know the importance of tactile sensation. A client with diminished sensation may be unable to sense the hot surface and would experience a burn. For such a client, a cut or wound in an area with limited sensation may go unnoticed and therefore untreated. The client with diminished sensation is also unable to feel pressure in an affected area. As a result, he may not shift position to relieve pressure over bony prominences or be aware that shoes or clothing are constricting.

Impaired Circulation

The vascular system brings oxygen-rich blood to the tissues and removes metabolic waste products. Any form of circulatory impairment adversely affects tissue metabolism. Impaired arterial circulation restricts activity, produces pain, and leads to muscle atrophy and development of thin tissue that is prone to ischemia and necrosis. Impaired venous circulation results in engorged tissues with high levels of metabolic waste products that are prone to edema, ulceration, and breakdown. Both forms of circulatory impairment delay wound healing. In fact, circulatory impairment is one of the main causes of chronic wounds.

Medications

Side effects and idiosyncratic reactions to medications can affect skin integrity and wound healing. Any medication that causes pruritus (itching), dermatoses (rashes), photosensitivity, alopecia, or pigmentation changes can result in changes that impair skin integrity or delay healing. The following are examples:

- Blood pressure medications decrease the amount of pressure required to occlude blood flow to an area, creating a risk for ischemia.
- Anti-inflammatory medications, such as over-the-counter NSAIDs (e.g., ibuprofen [Motrin]) and steroids (e.g., prednisone [Deltasone]) inhibit wound healing.
- Anticoagulants (e.g., heparin, warfarin [Coumadin]) can lead to extravasation of blood into subcutaneous tissue. As a result, even minimal pressure or injury can cause a hematoma.
- Chemotherapeutic agents delay wound healing because of their cellular toxicity.
- Certain antibiotics, psychotherapeutic drugs, and chemotherapy agents for cancer increase sensitivity to sunlight, increasing the risk for sunburn.
- Several herbal products, such as those containing lavender and tea tree oil, cleanse the skin but also have a drying effect.

Moisture on the Skin

Exposure to moisture leads to **maceration** (softening of the skin) and increases the likelihood of skin breakdown. Incontinence and fever are the most common sources of moisture. Bowel incontinence is particularly

troublesome because feces contain digestive enzymes and microorganisms that can readily lead to **excoriation** (denuding) of superficial skin layers, placing such a patient at risk for skin breakdown and infection.

Fever

Fever is a risk factor for skin breakdown for several reasons. First, it leads to sweating, which can cause maceration. Second, it increases the metabolic rate, thereby raising the tissue demand for oxygen. An increased demand for oxygen is difficult to meet if there is any circulatory impairment or tissue compression secondary to pressure. Finally, fever is a sign of infection. An infection triggers an immune response, which uses calories and nutrients, making them unavailable for wound healing.

Contamination or Infection

Contamination of a wound refers to the presence of microorganisms in the wound. A wound is said to be **colonized** if the microorganisms are creating no harm. In contrast, an **infection** implies that the microorganisms are causing harm by releasing toxins, invading body tissues, or increasing the metabolic demand of the tissue. Infection of the skin makes it more vulnerable to breakdown and impedes healing of open wounds.

Lifestyle

Some lifestyle habits affect skin integrity:

- *Tanning* exposes the skin to ultraviolet radiation, thereby increasing the risk for skin cancer.
- *Frequent bathing and use of soap* removes skin oils and may lead to drying, which jeopardizes the skin's barrier function.
- *Regular exercise* improves circulation, which is necessary for maintaining skin integrity and wound healing.
- *A nutritious diet* helps maintain skin integrity, as already discussed.
- *Smoking* limits the oxygen supply to the tissues, making skin more prone to breakdown and delaying wound healing.
- *Body piercings and tattoos* present a risk for infection and scarring. Complications, which occur in about 20% of piercings, include local infections, sepsis, endocarditis, hepatitis, and toxic shock syndrome. Intraoral and perioral piercings can result in gingivitis, damage to teeth and gums, and choking. Advise patients to become informed about the procedure and about aftercare and to find reputable, professional piercers.

 Go to **www.safepiercing.org**

KnowledgeCheck 34–2

- Identify the factors that affect skin integrity.
- What nutritional components are essential to maintain skin?

Go to Chapter 34, **Knowledge Check Response Sheet and Answers,** on the Electronic Study Guide.

CriticalThinking 34–1

- Review the case of William Harmon ("Meet Your Patient"). What risks, if any, does William have for skin breakdown or delayed healing? What additional information do you need to know to fully evaluate his risk?
- What risks do you have for impaired skin integrity? What actions can you take to protect your skin?

WOUNDS

Wounds are a disruption in the normal integrity of the skin. Wounds may be intentional, such as a surgical wound, or unintentional, such as a cut or a pressure ulcer. As a nurse, you will be responsible for monitoring skin integrity and providing wound care.

Types of Wounds

Wounds are classified according to length of time the wound has existed, as well as the condition of the wound (e.g., contamination, severity).

- *Skin integrity.* The simplest wound classification system is based on the integrity of the skin. If there are no breaks in the skin, the wound is described as **closed.** *Contusions* (bruises) or tissue swelling from fractures are common closed wounds. A wound is considered **open** if there is a break in the skin or mucous membranes. Open wounds include abrasions, lacerations, puncture wounds, and surgical incisions. A compound fracture may also lead to an open wound caused by the projection of bone through the skin. Several open and closed wounds are described in Table 34–1.
- *Length of time for healing.* The length of time for wound healing varies according to the skin integrity and the factors (discussed in the previous section) affecting it. **Acute wounds** are expected to be of short duration. Wounds that exceed the anticipated length of recovery are classified as **chronic wounds.** Chronic wounds include pressure, arterial, venous, and diabetic ulcers. These wounds are frequently colonized with bacteria, and healing is slow because of the underlying disease process. A chronic wound may linger for months or years. Table 34–2 provides further information about chronic wounds.
- *Level of contamination.* **Clean wounds** are uninfected wounds with minimal inflammation. They

TABLE 34-1 Types of Wounds (Based on Condition of Tissues)

Type	Description
Abrasion	A scrape of the superficial layers of the skin; usually unintentional but may be performed intentionally for cosmetic purposes to smooth skin surfaces.
Abscess	A localized collection of pus due to invasion from a pyogenic bacterium or other pathogen; must be opened and drained to heal.
Contusion	A closed wound caused by blunt trauma. May be referred to as a bruise or ecchymotic area.
Crushing	A wound caused by force leading to compression or disruption of tissues. Often associated with fracture. Usually there is minimal or no break in the skin.
Incision	An open, intentional wound caused by a sharp instrument.
Laceration	The skin or mucous membranes are torn open, resulting in a wound with jagged margins.
Penetrating	An open wound in which the agent causing the wound lodges in body tissue.
Puncture	An open wound caused by a sharp object. Often there is collapse of tissue around the entry point, making this wound prone to infection.
Tunnel	A wound with an entrance and exit site.

TABLE 34-2 Chronic Wounds

Type	Etiology	Characteristics
Pressure ulcers	Caused by pressure resulting in tissue ischemia and injury.	Appearance depends on the stage. Tends to be located over bony prominences.
Arterial ulcers	Caused by inadequate circulation of oxygenated blood to the tissue.	Surrounding skin appears shiny, thin, and dry and is cool to touch. Often there is loss of hair in the surrounding area. Area has delayed capillary refill time, and patients may complain of pain that worsens with increased activity. Most common in lower extremities but can occur anywhere.
Venous stasis ulcers	Caused by venous pooling, resulting in edema and blood stagnation.	Surrounding skin is reddened or brown. Skin temperature and peripheral pulses are normal. Wounds are usually shallow, with irregular wound margins. The wound bed often contains exudate. Patients usually have minimal pain. Most common below the knee.
Diabetic ulcers	May develop as a result of vascular changes associated with diabetes or impaired sensation secondary to neuropathy.	Surrounding skin appears shiny, thin, and dry and is cool to touch. Often there is loss of hair in the surrounding area.

may be open or closed and do not involve the gastrointestinal, respiratory, or genitourinary tracts (these systems frequently harbor bacteria). There is very little risk of infection for a clean wound. **Clean-contaminated wounds** are surgical incisions that enter the gastrointestinal, respiratory, or genitourinary tracts. There is an increased risk of infection for these wounds, but there is no obvious infection. **Contaminated wounds** include open, traumatic wounds or surgical incisions in which a major break in asepsis occurred. The risk of infection is high for these wounds. **Infected wounds** are wounds with evidence of infection, such as purulent drainage or necrotic tissue. Wounds are considered infected when bacteria counts in the wound tissues are above 100,000 organisms per gram of tissue. A wound is considered to be **colonized** if microorganisms are present but are creating no harm.

- *Depth of the wound.* **Superficial wounds** involve only the epidermal layer of the skin. The injury is usually the result of friction, shearing, or burning. **Partial-thickness wounds** extend through the epidermis into the dermis. **Full-thickness wounds** extend into the subcutaneous tissue and beyond (Sussmen & Bates-Jensen, 2001). The descriptor **penetrating** is sometimes added to indicate that the wound involves internal organs. Wound depth is a major determinant of healing time: The deeper the wound, the longer the healing time.

KnowledgeCheck 34–3

- Explain the difference between an acute and a chronic wound.
- Describe the wound categorization system based on contamination.
- How does wound depth affect healing?

 Go to Chapter 34, **Knowledge Check Response Sheet and Answers,** on the Electronic Study Guide.

Wound Healing Process

All wounds heal through a physiological process in which epithelial, endothelial, and inflammatory cells, platelets, and fibroblasts migrate into the wound to bring about tissue repair and regeneration. The process is essentially the same regardless of the type of injury or the type of tissues involved. Wounds may heal by regeneration or by primary, secondary, or tertiary intention.

- *Regenerative/epithelial* healing takes place when a wound affects only the epidermis. No scar forms, and the new (regenerated) epithelial cells form new skin that cannot be distinguished from the intact skin.
- *Primary (first) intention* healing takes place when a wound involves minimal tissue loss and has edges

that are well approximated (closed) (Figure 34–2A). Little scarring is expected. A clean surgical incision heals by this method.

- *Secondary (second) intention* healing occurs when a wound (1) involves extensive tissue loss, which prevents wound edges from approximating, or (2) should not be closed (e.g., because it is infected). Because the wound is left open, it heals from the inner layer to the surface by filling in with beefy red **granulation tissue** (a form of connective tissue with an abundant blood supply) (Figure 34–2B). Epithelial tissue may appear in the wound as small pink or pearl-like areas. Do not mistake this as a sign of infection.

Wounds that heal by secondary intention heal more slowly, are more prone to infection, and develop more scar tissue. Pressure ulcers (discussed later) and infected wounds are examples.

- *Tertiary (third) intention* healing, also called *delayed primary closure,* occurs when two surfaces of granulation tissue are brought together (Figure 34–2C). This technique may be used when the wound is clean-contaminated or contaminated. Initially the wound is allowed to heal by secondary intention. When there is no evidence of edema, infection, or foreign matter, the wound edges are closed by bringing together the granulating tissue and suturing the surface. These wounds require strict aseptic technique during all dressing changes because they are prone to infection. Tertiary intention healing creates less scarring than does secondary, but more than primary intention healing.

Wound healing occurs in three stages: inflammatory, proliferative, and maturation (Figure 34–3). We discuss these stages next.

The Inflammatory Phase—Cleansing

The inflammatory phase is a cleansing phase. It lasts from 1 to 5 days and consists of two major processes: hemostasis and inflammation.

- *Hemostasis.* At the time of injury, tissue and capillaries are destroyed, causing blood and plasma to leak into the wound. Area vessels constrict to limit blood loss. Platelets are called to the site and aggregate (clump together) to slow bleeding. At the same time, the clotting mechanism is activated to form a blood clot.
- *Inflammation.* The inflammatory reaction is characterized by edema, erythema, pain, temperature elevation, and migration of white blood cells into the wound tissues. Within 24 hours, macrophages begin engulfing bacteria (**phagocytosis**) and clearing debris. In conjunction with plasma proteins and fibrin, they form a scab at the surface of the wound, which seals the wound and helps prevent microbial invasion.

(a) Primary intention

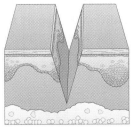 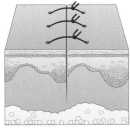 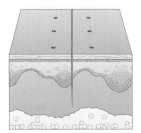

Clean wound   Sutured early   Results in hairline scar

(b) Secondary intention

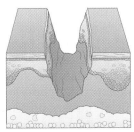 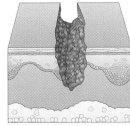 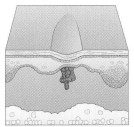

Wound gaping and irregular   Granulation occurring   Epithelium fills in scar

(c) Tertiary intention

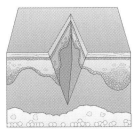 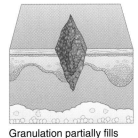 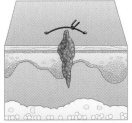

Wound not sutured   Granulation partially fills in wound   Granulating tissue sutured together

FIGURE 34–2 *A,* In a wound with minimal tissue loss, the edges may be sutured together, resulting in rapid healing and minimal scarring. *B,* A wound that heals by secondary intention heals from the inner layer to the surface. Healing takes longer, and there is scarring. *C,* A wound that heals by tertiary intention is initially healed by secondary intention and later sutured.

The Proliferative Phase—Granulation

The proliferative (also called *regeneration*) phase occurs from days 5 to 21. Cells develop to fill the wound defect and resurface the skin. **Fibroblasts** (connective tissue cells) migrate to the wound where they form **collagen,** a protein substance that adds strength to the healing wound. New blood and lymph vessels sprout from the existing capillaries at the edge of the wound. The result is the formation of granulation tissue, a beefy red tissue that bleeds readily and is easily damaged. As the clot or scab is dissolved, epithelial cells begin to grow into the wound from surrounding healthy tissue and seal over the wound (**epithelialization**).

The Maturation Phase—Epithelialization

The *maturation phase* is the final phase of the healing process. It begins in the second or third week and continues until the wound is completely healed. Collagen fibers that have been laid in the wound bed during the proliferative phase are remodeled into an organized structure (e.g., scar tissue), increasing the tensile strength of the wound. Epithelialization continues. A wound that has healed by primary intention leaves little scarring. Even so, a scar is only 80% as strong as the original tissue.

KnowledgeCheck 34–4

Identify the type of wound healing (primary, secondary, or tertiary intention):

• A wound that heals from inner layer to the surface
• A wound with approximated edges
• A wound that heals by approximating two surfaces of granulation tissue
• A wound that is sutured and has minimal or no tissue loss

 Go to Chapter 34, **Knowledge Check Response Sheet and Answers,** on the Electronic Study Guide.

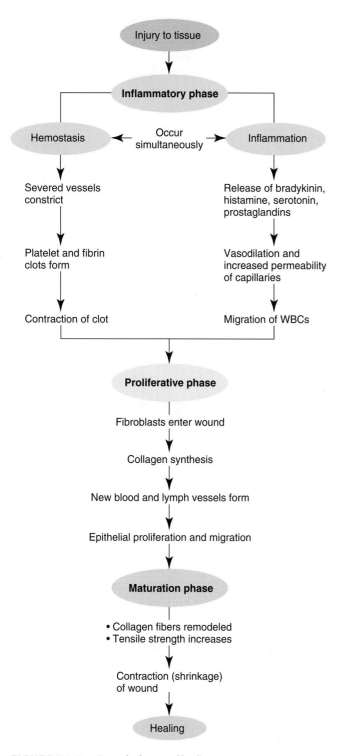

FIGURE 34–3   Stages in the wound healing process.

Wound Closures

Wounds that heal by primary and tertiary intention may be closed in a number of ways. Adhesive strips, sutures, staples, surgical glue, vacuum-assisted closure, and compression are the current choices.

• *Adhesive strips (Steri-Strips)* are used to close superficial low-tension wounds, such as skin tears or lacerations, or to close the skin on a wound that has been closed subcutaneously. They may also be used to give additional support to a wound after sutures or staples have been removed. Adhesive strips are often kept in place until they begin to separate from the skin on their own. For instructions on applying Steri-Strips,

 Go to Chapter 34, **Technique 34–1: Placing Steri-Strips,** in Volume 2.

• *Sutures* ("stitches") are the traditional wound closures. Several types of suture materials are available. *Absorbent* sutures are used deep in the tissues, for example, to close an organ or **anastomose** (connect) tissue. Because they are made of material that will gradually dissolve, there is no need to remove absorbent sutures. *Nonabsorbent* sutures are placed in superficial tissues and require removal, often by a nurse. Suturing leads to small puncture wounds along the track of the laceration or incision. For instructions on removing sutures and staples,

Go to Chapter 34, **Technique 34–2: Removing Sutures and Staples,** in Volume 2.

• *Surgical staples* are made of lightweight titanium. They provide a fast, easy way to close an incision.
• *Surgical glue* is a relatively new method for wound closure. It is safe for use in clean, low-tension wounds. It is an ideal wound closure method for skin tears.
• *In vacuum-assisted wound closure,* a piece of foam in the wound is attached by a tube to a negative-pressure pump to remove wound drainage, provide subatmospheric pressure to improve healing, create a clean and moist environment, and form a barrier to bacterial infection. The vacuum device is computerized and can be programmed for continuous or intermittent negative pressure.
• *Compression stockings* are used with venous stasis ulcers of the lower extremities. They apply continuous pressure to the veins, which facilitates venous return and allows the ulcers to heal.

Collaborative Wound Treatments

Collaborative treatments are necessary for wounds that will not heal despite aggressive care. Such treatments include the following:

• *Surgical options* such as extensive debridement, skin grafts, secondary closure of the wound, and flap techniques (partially detached tissue placed over a wound) are used on complicated wounds.

- *Hyperbaric oxygen therapy (HBOT)* is the administration of 100% oxygen under pressure to a wound site. HBOT increases oxygen concentration in the tissue, stimulates the growth of new blood vessels, and enhances white blood cell (WBC) action.
- *Platelet-derived growth factor* augments the inflammatory phase of wound healing and accelerates collagen formation in the wound.

Types of Wound Drainage

Drainage is the flow of fluids from a wound or cavity. It is often referred to as **exudate**—fluid that oozes as a result of inflammation. Exudate may take several forms.

- **Serous exudate** consists of *serum,* the straw-colored fluid that separates out of blood when a clot is formed. It is watery in consistency and contains very little cellular matter. You can expect this type of drainage from a clean wound.
- **Sanguineous exudate** is bloody drainage. It indicates damage to capillaries. Fresh bleeding produces bright red drainage, whereas older, dried blood is a dark, red-brown color. You will often see sanguineous exudate with deep wounds or wounds in highly vascular areas. **Serosanguineous** drainage, a combination of bloody and serous drainage, is most commonly seen in new wounds.
- **Purulent exudate** is thick, often malodorous, drainage that is seen in infected wounds. It contains pus, a protein-rich fluid filled with WBCs, bacteria, and cellular debris. It is commonly caused by infection from a **pyogenic** (pus-forming) bacteria, such as streptococci or staphylococci. Normally, pus is yellow in color, although it may take on a blue-green color if the bacterium *Pseudomonas aeruginosa* is present.
- **Purosanguineous exudate** is pus that is red-tinged. It indicates that small vessels in the wound area have ruptured.

Complications of Wound Healing

Recall that wounds heal by moving through the phases of inflammation, proliferation, and maturation. At times this process is interrupted by complications. The most common complications are discussed below.

Hemorrhage

Whenever a capillary network is interrupted or a blood vessel is severed, bleeding occurs. **Hemostasis** (cessation of bleeding) usually occurs within minutes of the injury. Hemostasis is delayed, however, when large vessels are injured, a clotting disorder exists, or the client is on anticoagulant therapy. If bleeding begins again after initial hemostasis, something is probably wrong. Possible causes include a slipped suture, erosion of a blood vessel, a dislodged clot, or infection. Bleeding may be internal or external. The risk of hemorrhage is greatest in the first 24 to 48 hours following surgery or injury.

- *Internal bleeding* causes swelling of the affected body part, pain, and changes in vital signs (i.e., decreased blood pressure, elevated pulse). A **hematoma,** a red-blue collection of blood under the skin, forms as a result of internal bleeding. The amount of blood in a hematoma varies. A large hematoma causes pressure on surrounding tissues. If the hematoma is located near a major artery or vein, it may impede blood flow.
- *External hemorrhage* is easier to recognize. You will see bloody drainage on the dressings and in the wound drainage devices. When there is a brisk hemorrhage, blood often pools underneath the client as the dressings become saturated. To be sure that you recognize the full extent of the bleeding, remember to look underneath the patient.

Infection

Microorganisms can be introduced to a wound during an injury, during surgery, or after surgery. Suspect infection if a wound fails to heal. Localized swelling, redness, heat, pain, fever (temperatures higher than 38°C, or 100.4°F), foul-smelling or purulent drainage, or a change in the color of the drainage may also indicate infection. The symptoms are likely to occur in a contaminated or traumatic wound within 2 to 3 days. In a clean surgical wound, you will usually not see signs and symptoms of an infection until the 4th or 5th postoperative day.

Dehiscence

Rupture (separation) of one or more layers of a wound is called **dehiscence** (Figure 34–4). Wound dehiscence is most likely to occur in the inflammatory phase of healing, before large amounts of collagen have been deposited in the wound to strengthen it. The most common causes of dehiscence are poor nutritional status, inadequate closure of the muscles, or wound infection. Obese clients are also more likely to experience dehiscence because fatty tissue does not heal readily and the patient's mass increases the strain on the suture line.

Dehiscence is usually associated with abdominal wounds. Patients often report feeling a pop or tear, especially with sudden straining from coughing, vomiting, or changing positions in bed. Usually there is an immediate increase in serosanguineous drainage.

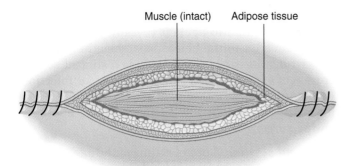

FIGURE 34–4 **Dehiscence is separation of one or more layers of a wound. It is most common in the inflammatory phase of healing.**

Nursing interventions include applying a binder and modifying activity to prevent evisceration.

Evisceration

Evisceration is total separation of the layers of a wound in which internal viscera protrude through the incision (Figure 34–5). This is a rare complication and is a surgical emergency. Immediately cover the wound with sterile towels or dressings soaked in sterile saline solution to prevent the organs from drying out and becoming contaminated with environmental bacteria. Have the patient stay in bed with knees bent to minimize strain on the incision. Notify the surgeon and ready the patient for a surgical procedure (see Chapter 37).

Fistulas

A **fistula** is an abnormal passage connecting two body cavities or a cavity and the skin. Fistulas often result from infection. An abscess forms, which breaks down surrounding tissue and creates the abnormal passageway. Chronic drainage from the fistula may lead to skin breakdown and delayed wound healing. The most common sites where fistulas form are the gastrointestinal and genitourinary tracts. Figure 34–6 illustrates a fistula between the rectum and vagina.

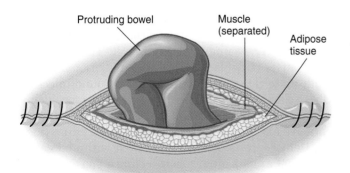

FIGURE 34–5 **Evisceration is total separation of the layers of a wound with internal viscera protruding through the incision.**

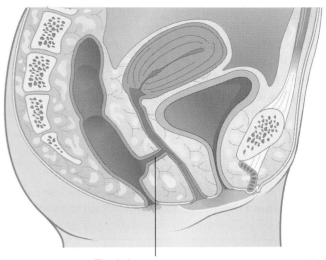

Fistula between rectum and vagina (enterovaginal)

FIGURE 34–6 **A fistula is an abnormal passage connecting two body cavities or a cavity and the skin. Fistulas are most common in the gastrointestinal and genitourinary tracts.**

KnowledgeCheck 34–5

- Describe four types of wound closures.
- Identify five types of wound complications.
- Describe three signs of internal hemorrhage.
- Differentiate between dehiscence and evisceration.

Go to Chapter 34, **Knowledge Check Response Sheet and Answers,** on the Electronic Study Guide.

CriticalThinking 34–2

Recall the case of Mr. Harmon ("Meet Your Patient"). What form of wound healing (primary, secondary, or tertiary) is he undergoing? How long would you expect it to take before his wounds heal?

PRESSURE ULCERS

A pressure ulcer is a type of chronic wound. We discuss it separately because vigilant nursing care can prevent pressure ulcers. In the event they do form, nursing plays a major role in their treatment. It is estimated that 1 million people in the United States have pressure ulcers: about 15% of hospital patients, 10% of home care patients, and 20% of long-term care patients (Cuddigan, Berlowitz, & Ayello, 2001; "Nutritional Support in Wound Care," 2004; Smith, 1995). Treatment is estimated to cost between $5 and 8.5 billion annually.

Pressure Ulcer Development

Pressure ulcers (also called *decubitus ulcers, pressure sores,* and *bedsores*) are caused by unrelieved

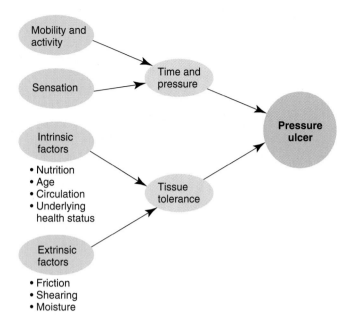

FIGURE 34–7 Several factors contribute to the development of pressure ulcers.

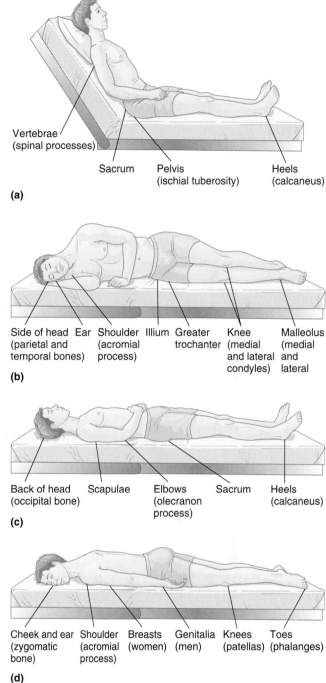

FIGURE 34–8 Most commonly, pressure ulcers develop over the bony prominences. (Adapted from AHRQ Clinical Practice Guidelines.)

pressure that compromises blood flow to an area, resulting in *ischemia* (inadequate blood supply) in the underlying tissue. The key variables in ischemia are time and pressure. Small amounts of pressure over an extended period of time or a large amount of pressure for a short period of time results in tissue ischemia.

Although time and pressure are the key variables, several other factors predict the likelihood of pressure ulcer formation (Figure 34–7). Some factors are intrinsic and some are extrinsic. **Intrinsic factors** alter skin characteristics or oxygen delivery capabilities, decreasing the amount of force required to create a pressure ulcer. Examples include immobility and impaired sensation, as occur with spinal cord injuries, stroke, or coma; malnourishment; aging; low arteriolar pressure; and fever. Review the previous section, "Factors Affecting Skin Integrity," for further discussion of intrinsic factors. **Extrinsic factors** include friction, shearing, and exposure to moisture.

- *Friction* damages the outer protective epidermal layer, decreasing the amount of pressure needed to develop skin lesions (Graff, Bryant, & Beinlich, 2000).

- *Shearing* occurs when the epidermal layer slides over the dermis, causing damage to the vascular bed. It most commonly occurs when the head of the bed is elevated and the patient slides downward, causing shear to develop in the sacral area. When shearing occurs, the amount of pressure needed to occlude circulation is cut in half.

- *Moisture,* especially in the form of urine or feces, macerates the skin and also decreases the amount of pressure required to produce ulceration.

The most common sites where pressure ulcers develop are over the bony prominences. Skin is compressed between the bone and the hard surface of the bed or chair, reducing blood flow to the area. When the patient is supine, these pressure points are the occiput, scapulae, elbows, sacrum, and heels. Figure 34–8 illustrates the pressure points in the supine, lateral, prone, and sitting positions.

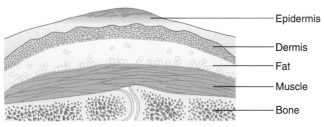

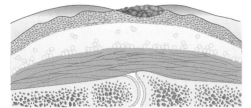

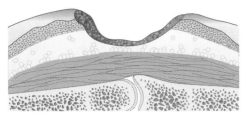

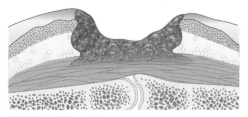

(a) Stage I

(b) Stage II

(c) Stage III

(d) Stage IV

FIGURE 34–9 *A,* Stage I pressure ulcer. *B,* Stage II pressure ulcer. *C,* Stage III pressure ulcer. *D,* Stage IV pressure ulcer.

Staging of Pressure Ulcers

Pressure ulcers are classified by the degree of tissue involvement. The following standardized staging system, developed by the Agency for Healthcare Research Quality (AHRQ) and the National Pressure Ulcer Advisory Panel (NPUAP), is used to describe pressure ulcers.

- *A stage I pressure ulcer* (Figure 34–9A) is as an area of nonblanchable erythema of intact skin. It appears as redness in lightly pigmented individuals. In clients with dark skin, the area may have red, blue, or purple hues. The discoloration remains for more than 30 minutes after the pressure is relieved. The surrounding skin may be warmer or cooler. With the initial injury, skin temperature rises, but later it cools as continued pressure interferes with circulation. Tissue consistency is firm at first and

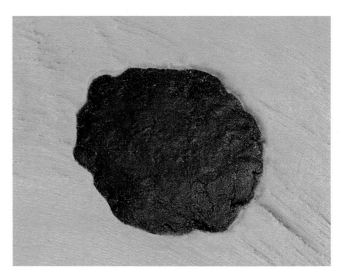

FIGURE 34–10   Ulcers that are covered with an eschar cannot be staged.

later becomes soft and boggy. The patient may feel pain and itching.

- *A stage II pressure ulcer* involves partial-thickness skin loss of the epidermis, dermis, or both. The skin is no longer intact and may appear as an abrasion, blister, or shallow crater (Figure 34–9B).
- *A stage III pressure ulcer* (Figure 34–9C) is characterized by full-thickness skin loss involving damage or necrosis of subcutaneous tissue, which may extend down to, but not through, the underlying fascia. The ulcer appears as a deep crater. **Undermining** (deeper-level damage under boggy superficial layers) of adjacent tissue may be present.
- *A stage IV pressure ulcer* (Figure 34–9D) involves full-thickness skin loss with extensive destruction, tissue necrosis, or damage to muscle, bone, or support structures. Undermining and **sinus tracts** (blind tracts underneath the epidermis) are common.

An **eschar** (Figure 34–10) is a black, leathery covering comprised of *necrotic tissue* (dead cells) and plasma proteins. An eschar forms when a wound cannot close by epithelialization (e.g., because the surface is too large). An ulcer covered by an eschar cannot be classified using this staging method because it is impossible to determine the depth. The eschar must be removed to stage the wound.

Reverse staging does not occur as an ulcer heals. The healing process cannot cause a stage IV pressure ulcer to become a stage III. Pressure ulcers become progressively more shallow by filling with granulation tissue, but lost muscle, subcutaneous fat, and dermis are not replaced. Therefore, reverse staging does not accurately characterize what is physiologically occurring in the ulcer. Instead, pressure ulcers maintain their original staging classification throughout the healing process, but they are described by the modifier *healing* (e.g., "stage IV ulcer: healing").

<table>
<tr><td colspan="2">

BOX 34-1 **History Questions for Skin and Wound Assessment**

- What is your typical activity level?
- Tell me about your usual diet.
- How much liquid do you drink each day?
- Do you have any areas of numbness and tingling?
- Have you had any recent changes in your skin?
- Do you have any sores or open areas? If so, how long have you had the wound?
- Have you ever had difficulty healing a wound?
- What kinds of healthcare problems have you been experiencing?
- What medications—prescribed, herbal, or over-the-counter—are you taking?
- What is your typical hygiene routine?
- Do you smoke?
- How much time do you spend outdoors?
- Do you have diabetes? If so, how often do you check your feet? How often do you see a podiatrist?

</td></tr>
</table>

KnowledgeCheck 34–6

- What stage pressure ulcer does Mr. Harmon ("Meet Your Patient") have?
- What factors have contributed to its development?

 Go to Chapter 34, **Knowledge Check Response Sheet and Answers,** on the Electronic Study Guide.

 CriticalThinking 34–3

Based on your knowledge of the factors that have contributed to Mr. Harmon's pressure ulcer development, what actions may lead to healing of the pressure ulcer? *Note:* To answer this question, you do not need to know about wound care (e.g., irrigation) for a pressure ulcer.

Practical Knowledge
knowing how

As a nurse, you will care for many patients who have wounds or who are at risk for skin breakdown. In the remainder of the chapter, we will discuss how to maintain skin integrity, prevent pressure ulcers, and treat wounds.

| Assessment |

You should perform a focused assessment of the skin, including risk factors for skin breakdown, for all patients who are in inpatient facilities or who have known risk factors for impaired skin integrity. Existing wounds require additional assessment. A thorough skin assessment includes a nursing history, physical examination, and diagnostic testing.

Nursing History

To assess wound healing ability and the risk for skin breakdown, you will need to gather data on factors that affect skin integrity (discussed previously): age, mobility, nutrition, hydration, sensation, circulation, medications, moisture, lifestyle, underlying health and disease status, and the presence of microorganisms. Box 34–1 provides questions you can ask to assess these factors.

Risk Assessment Measures

Many facilities use comprehensive risk assessment tools to evaluate the patient's risk for skin problems. Patients may have multiple risk factors, and such assessment tools enable you to evaluate the cumulative risk. Among the most commonly used tools are the Braden and Norton scales.

The *Braden scale* is used to identify persons at risk for developing pressure ulcers. Research has shown it to be reliable and valid in several settings (Armstong, Bortz, & Halter, 2001; Bergstrom, Braden, Kemp, Champagne, & Ruby, 1998). The Braden scale (Figure 34–11) evaluates six major risk factors. The final score reflects the patient's risk; the lower the score, the more likely the patient will develop a pressure ulcer. A score of 18 or less for hospitalized patients indicates risk (Bergstrom, Braden, et al., 1998). You should use this scale to assess the patient on admission to the facility and again in 48 to 72 hours. Studies have shown the second score to be more predictive, probably related to increased awareness of the patient's status.

The *Norton scale* (Figure 34–12) assesses risk based on the patient's physical condition, mental state, activity, mobility, and incontinence. A low score indicates a high risk. Some have suggested that the Norton scale should be modified by adding categories for skin appearance, medication, and nutrition.

 CriticalThinking 34–4

Review the Braden and Norton scales. Apply these risk assessment scales to Mr. Harmon ("Meet Your Patient").

- What additional information, if any, do you need to complete these assessments?
- Which scale do you find most useful?

BRADEN SCALE FOR PREDICTING PRESSURE SORE RISK

Patient's Name _____ Evaluator's Name _____ Date of Assessment _____

	1	2	3	4
SENSORY PERCEPTION ability to respond meaningfully to pressure-related discomfort	**1. Completely Limited** Unresponsive (does not moan, flinch, or grasp) to painful stimuli, due to diminished level of consciousness or sedation. OR limited ability to feel pain over most of body.	**2. Very Limited** Responds only to painful stimuli. Cannot communicate discomfort except by moaning or restlessness. OR has a sensory impairment which limits the ability to feel pain or discomfort over 1/2 of body.	**3. Slightly Limited** Responds to verbal commands, but cannot always communicate discomfort or the need to be turned. OR has some sensory impairment which limits ability to feel pain or discomfort in 1 or 2 extremities.	**4. No Impairment** Responds to verbal commands. Has no sensory deficit which would limit ability to feel or voice pain or discomfort.
MOISTURE degree to which skin is exposed to moisture	**1. Constantly Moist** Skin is kept moist almost constantly by perspiration, urine, etc. Dampness is detected every time patient is moved or turned.	**2. Very Moist** Skin is often, but not always moist. Linen must be changed at least once a shift.	**3. Occasionally Moist:** Skin is occasionally moist, requiring an extra linen change approximately once a day.	**4. Rarely Moist** Skin is usually dry, linen only requires changing at routine intervals.
ACTIVITY degree of physical activity	**1. Bedfast** Confined to bed.	**2. Chairfast** Ability to walk severely limited or non-existent. Cannot bear own weight and/or must be assisted into chair or wheelchair.	**3. Walks Occasionally** Walks occasionally during day, but for very short distances, with or without assistance. Spends majority of each shift in bed or chair.	**4. Walks Frequently** Walks outside room at least twice a day and inside room at least once every two hours during waking hours.
MOBILITY ability to change and control body position	**1. Completely Immobile** Does not make even slight changes in body or extremity position without assistance.	**2. Very Limited** Makes occasional slight changes in body or extremity position but unable to make frequent or significant changes independently.	**3. Slightly Limited** Makes frequent though slight changes in body or extremity position independently.	**4. No Limitation** Makes major and frequent changes in position without assistance.
NUTRITION usual food intake pattern	**1. Very Poor** Never eats a complete meal. Rarely eats more than 1/2 of any food offered. Eats 2 servings or less of protein (meat or dairy products) per day. Takes fluids poorly. Does not take a liquid dietary supplement OR is NPO and/or maintained on clear liquids or IVs for more than 5 days.	**2. Probably Inadequate** Rarely eats a complete meal and generally eats only about 1/2 of any food offered. Protein intake includes only 3 servings of meat or dairy products per day. Occasionally will take a dietary supplement. OR receives less than optimum amount of liquid diet or tube feeding.	**3. Adequate** Eats over half of most meals. Eats a total of 4 servings of protein (meat, dairy products) per day. Occasionally will refuse a meal, but will usually take a supplement when offered OR is on a tube feeding or TPN regimen which probably meets most of nutritional needs.	**4. Excellent** Eats most of every meal. Never refuses a meal. Usually eats a total of 4 or more servings of meat and dairy products. Occasionally eats between meals. Does not require supplementation.
FRICTION & SHEAR	**1. Problem** Requires moderate to maximum assistance in moving. Complete lifting without sliding against sheets is impossible. Frequently slides down in bed or chair, requiring frequent repositioning with maximum assistance. Spasticity, contractures or agitation leads to almost constant friction.	**2. Potential Problem** Moves feebly or requires minimum assistance. During a move skin probably slides to some extent against sheets, chair, restraints or other devices. Maintains relatively good position in chair or bed most of the time but occasionally slides down.	**3. No Apparent Problem** Moves in bed and in chair independently and has sufficient muscle strength to lift up completely during move. Maintains good position in bed or chair.	

Total Score _____

FIGURE 34–11 The Braden scale for predicting pressure sore risk. *Source:* U.S. Department of Health and Human Services. (1992). Clinical practice guideline. Pressure ulcers in adults: Prediction and prevention. PPPPUA Publication No.92-0047. Rockville, MD: Public Health Service, pp. 16–17. Copyright © Barbara Braden and Nancy Bergstrom, 1988. Reprinted with permission.

<table>
<tr><td colspan="7" align="center">**Norton Scale for Assessing Risk of Pressure Ulcers**</td></tr>
<tr><td></td><td>Physical Condition</td><td>Mental Condition</td><td>Activity</td><td>Mobility</td><td>Incontinent</td><td></td></tr>
<tr><td></td><td>Good 4
Fair 3
Poor 2
Very bad 1</td><td>Alert 4
Apathetic 3
Confused 2
Stupor 1</td><td>Ambulant 4
Walk/help 3
Chair-bound 2
Bed 1</td><td>Full 4
Slightly limited 3
Very limited 2
Immobile 1</td><td>Not 4
Occasional 3
Usually/urine 2
Doubly 1</td><td>Total Score</td></tr>
<tr><td>Name/Date</td><td></td><td></td><td></td><td></td><td></td><td></td></tr>
<tr><td></td><td></td><td></td><td></td><td></td><td></td><td></td></tr>
<tr><td></td><td></td><td></td><td></td><td></td><td></td><td></td></tr>
<tr><td></td><td></td><td></td><td></td><td></td><td></td><td></td></tr>
<tr><td colspan="7">The Norton Scale uses five criteria to assess patients' risk for pressure ulcers. Scores of 14 or less indicate liability to ulcers; scores of <12 indicate very high risk.</td></tr>
<tr><td colspan="7">Norton, D., McLaren, R. & Exton-Smith, A. N. (1975). *An investigation of geriatric nursing problems in hospitals.* Edinburgh, UK: Churchill Livingstone. Used with permission.</td></tr>
</table>

FIGURE 34–12 **Norton scale for assessing risk of pressure ulcers.** *Source:* Norton, D., McLaren, R., & Exton-Smith, A. N. (1975). *An investigation of geriatric nursing problems in hospitals.* Edinburgh, UK: Churchill Livingstone. Used with permission.

Physical Examination

Physical assessment of skin integrity focuses on the following areas:

- *Inspecting the skin.* Inspect all areas of the body routinely. Evaluate the skin for color, integrity, temperature, texture, turgor, mobility, moisture, lesions, and hair distribution. See Chapter 19 for more details on skin assessment.

- *Assessing mobility and activity level.* As you know, activity level and mobility affect skin integrity. Assess the musculoskeletal system, as described in Chapter 19. See Chapter 31 for additional information on activity and mobility.

Assessing Wounds

All wounds require a focused assessment. Assessment frequency depends on the condition of the wound, the work setting, the patient's overall condition and underlying disease process, the type of wound, and the type of treatment used for the wound. If you are providing wound care, you will assess the wound with every treatment. Assessment parameters include the following:

- *Location.* Describe the location of the wound in anatomic terms. For example, you would describe an incision from cardiac surgery as a midsternal incision extending from the manubrium to the xiphoid process. An accurate description of the location is important because location influences the rate of healing. Wounds in highly vascular regions, such as the scalp or hands, heal more rapidly than wounds in less vascular regions, such as the abdomen or heel. Location also affects movement. Wounds that can be readily stabilized heal more rapidly than those in areas that are affected by the constant stress of movement (Goldberg & Tomaselli, 2002).

- *Size.* Measure the length and width of the wound in centimeters. Many clinicians recommend photo documentation, with the wound's dimensions indicated on the photo. This is especially useful if the wound has an irregular border. To measure wound depth, gently insert a sterile cotton-tip applicator into the deepest part of the wound. Measure the applicator from skin level to the tip. If you are evaluating a pressure ulcer, your staging of the wound will also provide information on its depth.

- *Appearance.* Your description of the appearance of the wound should be very detailed. You must describe:
  1. *The type of wound (open or closed).* If the wound is sutured, examine the closure. Are the wound edges approximated? Is there tension on any aspect of the wound? Are the stitches intact?
  2. *The color of the wound.* Redness and inflammation for the first 2 to 3 days is normal, but erythema or swelling beyond that time may indicate infection.
  3. *Condition of the wound bed (in an open wound).* A beefy red, moist appearance is evidence of healing. A pale color or dry texture indicates a delay in healing. Necrotic tissue is devitalized tissue, which becomes slough or eschar. **Slough** is usually soft, stringy, and pale yellow or gray. Eschar is thick, hard, and black or brown. Removal of slough or eschar is essential for a wound to heal. If there is a tunnel or sinus tract in the wound bed, inspect and probe for depth and characteristics. Look for openings in the

deep areas of the wound. Document the position and depth of any tunneling. Assess the wound edges. Look for undermining, the loss of tissue underneath surface structures.

- *The skin surrounding the wound.* Skin discoloration may indicate a hematoma or additional injury to the surrounding tissue. Look for maceration, undermining, crepitus, blistering, or erythema. Maceration is caused by excessive moisture and appears as pale, wrinkled skin, which may flake and peel. Undermining will produce a boggy feel around the wound. **Crepitus** is gas trapped under the skin. If you palpate the surrounding skin and feel a crackling sensation, this is crepitus. Crepitus may be due to air leaking from the lung in a chest wound or may indicate the presence of gas-producing bacteria. Look for erythema, swelling, or other signs of irritation; these signs indicate that the surrounding tissue is in jeopardy. Examine the edges of the wound for epithelial tissue and contraction.

- *Drainage.* Determine whether exudate is present. If so, describe the color, consistency, amount, and odor. When it is important to assess the exact quantity of wound drainage, you may be asked to weigh dressings before they are applied and again when they have been removed. The change in weight reflects the amount of drainage that they have absorbed. If a drain is present, simply measure the amount of fluid in the collection container. Drainage amounts vary according to the type of wound. Odor may indicate fistula formation or bacterial contamination. For example, if a patient has an abdominal wound that was odorless but begins to smell of bile or feces, you should carefully assess for presence of a fistula.

- *Patient responses.* Ask your patients about pain or discomfort related to the wound or wound care. You will need to develop a pain management plan if the patient is uncomfortable. Always take seriously the patient's complaint of pain, especially if there is a sudden increase. Pain is often an early symptom of infection. In the immunocompromised patient, pain may be the only symptom of infection (Branom, 2002).

For a wound assessment summary,

Go to Chapter 34, **Assessment Guidelines and Tools, Wound Assessment,** in Volume 2.

Assessing Untreated Wounds

For an untreated wound, make the same assessments as for a treated wound. Also, make additional assessments that allow you to determine the immediate treatment needed. For example, assess for bleeding. If bleeding is profuse, apply direct pressure to the site. If bleeding continues after you apply pressure for 5 minutes or if blood is spurting from the wound, call the physician immediately. Severe pain, numbness, or loss of movement below the wound also requires immediate, comprehensive evaluation. For a description of the assessment process for an untreated wound,

Go to Chapter 34, **Assessment Guidelines and Tools, Assessing an Untreated Wound,** in Volume 2.

Also determine whether the patient needs a tetanus immunization. Tetanus-prone wounds include compound fractures, gunshot wounds, crush injuries, burns, punctures, foreign object injuries, wounds contaminated with soil, and wounds neglected for more than 24 hours.

An immunization should be given if:

- The last immunization was 10 years ago or longer.
- The wound is contaminated with dirt or debris, and the most recent tetanus immunization was given more than 5 years ago.
- It is uncertain when the patient last received an immunization.

Assessing Pressure Ulcers

When ischemia first occurs, the skin over the area is pale and cool. When you relieve the pressure (e.g., by turning the patient), vasodilation occurs, and extra blood rushes to the area to compensate for the ischemic period. The area flushes bright red (**reactive hyperemia**). If the redness does not disappear quickly, tissue damage has occurred. The redness should last about half as long as the duration of the ischemia. For example, if the tissue was compressed for an hour, reactive hyperemia should not last more than about 30 minutes.

In addition to the wound assessments just described, the AHRQ and NPUAP recommend use of the *PUSH tool* (Figure 34–13) to evaluate pressure ulcers (National Pressure Ulcer Advisory Panel, 2002). The tool provides a comprehensive means of reporting the progression of a pressure ulcer. Surface area, exudate, and type of wound tissue are scored and totaled. As the ulcer heals, the total score falls.

Laboratory Data

You should integrate laboratory data with your history and physical assessment findings. The most common laboratory assessments performed on clients with wounds or risk for skin breakdown are leukocyte count, serum protein levels, coagulation studies, and wound cultures.

Go to Chapter 34, **Diagnostic Testing: Tests for Assessing Wounds,** in Volume 2.

PUSH Tool - Version 3.0

Patient Name:_____   Patient ID#:_____

Ulcer Location: _____   Date:_____

DIRECTIONS:
Observe and measure the pressure ulcer. Categorize the ulcer with respect to surface area, exudate, and type of wound tissue. Record a sub-score for each of these ulcer characteristics. Add the sub-scores to obtain the total score. A comparison of total scores measured over time provides an indication of the improvement or deterioration in pressure ulcer healing.

Length x Width	0	1	2	3	4	5	Subscore
	0 cm^2	$<0.3 \text{ cm}^2$	$0.3 - 0.6 \text{ cm}^2$	$0.7 - 1.0 \text{ cm}^2$	$1.1 - 2.0 \text{ cm}^2$	$2.1 - 3.0 \text{ cm}^2$	
		6	7	8	9	10	
		$3.1 - 4.0 \text{ cm}^2$	$4.1 - 8.0 \text{ cm}^2$	$8.1 - 12.0 \text{ cm}^2$	$12.1 - 24.0 \text{ cm}^2$	$> 24 \text{ cm}^2$	
Exudate Amount	0	1	2	3			Subscore
	None	Light	Moderate	Heavy			
Tissue Type	0	1	2	3	4		Subscore
	Closed	Epithelial Tissue	Granulation Tissue	Slough	Necrotic Tissue		
							Total Score

Length x Width: Measure the greatest length (head to toe) and the greatest width (side to side) using a centimeter ruler. Multiply these two measurements (length • width) to obtain an estimate of surface area in square centimeters (cm^2). **Caveat:** Do not guess! Always use a centimeter ruler and always use the same method each time the ulcer is measured.

Exudate Amount: Estimate the amount of exudate (drainage) present after removal of the dressing and before applying any topical agent to the ulcer. Estimate the exudate (drainage) as none, light, moderate, or heavy.

Tissue Type: This refers to the types of tissue that are present in the wound (ulcer) bed. Score as a "4" if there is any necrotic tissue present. Score as a "3" if there is any amount of slough present and necrotic tissue is absent. Score as a "2" if the wound is clean and contains granulation tissue. A superficial wound that is reepithelializing is scored as a "1". When the wound is closed, score as a "0".

> **4 - Necrotic Tissue (Eschar):** black, brown, or tan tissue that adheres firmly to the wound bed or ulcer edges and may be either firmer or softer than surrounding skin.
> **3 - Slough:** yellow or white tissue that adheres to the ulcer bed in strings or thick clumps, or is mucinous.
> **2 - Granulation Tissue:** pink or beefy red tissue with a shiny, moist, granular appearance.
> **1 - Epithelial Tissue:** for superficial ulcers, new pink or shiny tissue (skin) that grows in from the edges or as islands on the ulcer surface.
> **0 - Closed/Resurfaced:** the wound is completely covered with epithelium (new skin).

Note: Refer to the NPUAP Website (www.npuap.org) for further information regarding development and use of the PUSH Tool.

Version 3.0: 9/15/98
© National Pressure Ulcer Advisory Panel

FIGURE 34–13   **The PUSH tool for evaluation of pressure ulcers.** *Source:* National Pressure Ulcer Advisory Panel. (2002). Retrieved August 8, 2004, from *http://www.npuap.org/pushins.htm*

PRESSURE ULCER HEALING CHART
(use a separate page for each pressure ulcer)

Patient Name:_____   Patient ID#:_____

Ulcer Location: _____   Date:_____

Directions: Observe and measure pressure ulcers at regular intervals using the PUSH Tool. Date and record PUSH Sub-scale and Total Scores on the Pressure Ulcer Healing Record below.

	PRESSURE ULCER HEALING RECORD															
DATE																
Length x Width																
Exudate Amount																
Tissue Type																
Total Score																

Graph the PUSH Total Score on the Pressure Ulcer Healing Graph below.

PUSH Total Score	PRESSURE ULCER HEALING GRAPH															
17																
16																
15																
14																
13																
12																
11																
10																
9																
8																
7																
6																
5																
4																
3																
2																
1																
Healed 0																
DATE:																

Version 3.0: 9/15/98
© National Pressure Ulcer Advisory Panel

FIGURE 34–13   **The PUSH tool for evaluation of pressure ulcers** *(continued).*

Wound cultures may be ordered to determine the types of bacteria present in the wound. Cultures may be obtained by swab, aspiration, or tissue biopsy.

- *Swabbing* the wound is a common, noninvasive method to obtain a culture. However, this method has limited merit. A positive culture may not indicate an infection, because chronic wounds are colonized with bacteria. Although the value of a swab culture is limited, it may be ordered, particularly if there has been a sudden change in the nature of the drainage.

 Go to Chapter 34, **Procedure 34–1: Obtaining a Wound Culture by Swab,** in Volume 2.

Also see the Critical Aspects box below.

- *Needle aspiration* of a wound is the preferred method for a culture obtained by nursing staff. It should be used to assess chronic wounds with clinical indications of infection, such as erythema, edema, foul odor, or drainage.

 Go to Chapter 34, **Procedure 34–2: Obtaining a Needle Aspiration Culture from a Wound,** in Volume 2.

Also see the Critical Aspects box.

- *Tissue biopsy* is the most accurate method for culturing a chronic wound or pressure ulcer. However,

this procedure is invasive, requires specially trained providers, and consequently is expensive. There is also a risk of sepsis from the biopsy (Branom, 2002). Wounds are not considered infected unless the bacteria count exceeds 100,000 organisms per gram of tissue. However, the presence of beta hemolytic streptococci, in any number, is considered an infection.

Knowledge Check 34–7

- What should be included in a wound assessment?
- What is the preferred method of wound culture that may be performed by a registered nurse?
- Identify three types of laboratory data that may be associated with a delay in wound healing.

 Go to Chapter 34, **Knowledge Check Response Sheet and Answers,** on the Electronic Study Guide.

What Assessments Can I Delegate?

Initial assessment of a wound, as well as ongoing evaluation of a wound that requires treatment, must be done by the licensed nurse. You may delegate to unlicensed assistive personnel (UAP) inspection of the skin for evidence of skin breakdown. Instruct the UAP to notify you of redness, tissue warmth, or drainage. You may also delegate turning and position changes to the UAP. Turning and movement prevent tissue damage from ischemia, thereby preventing pressure ulcers.

---

critical aspects of procedures 34–1 through 34–7

 For steps to follow in *all* procedures, refer to the inside back cover of Volume 2.

Procedure 34–1: Obtaining a Wound Culture by Swab

- Position the patient for easy access to the wound and in a manner that will allow the irrigation solution to flow freely from the wound with the assistance of gravity.

- Don protective equipment: gown, face shield, and clean gloves.

- Remove the soiled dressing, and dispose of gloves and dressing.

- Wearing clean gloves, fill a 35 mL syringe, with attached 19-gauge angiocath, with 0.9% (normal) saline solution.

- Holding the angiocath tip 2 cm from the wound bed, gently irrigate the wound (superior to inferior).

- Press the culture swab against an area of red granulating tissue, and rotate.

- Reinsert the swab into the culturette tube, label the tube, and transport it to the lab.

Procedure 34–2: Obtaining a Needle Aspiration Culture from a Wound

- Administer pain medication 30 minutes prior to the procedure, if necessary.

- Cleanse the wound with saline-moistened gauze, wiping from the center of the wound toward the edge.

- Draw up 1 mL of 0.9% (normal) saline for injection into a 22-gauge needle attached to a 3 mL syringe.

- Insert the needle 1 to 2 mm into the wound bed, and inject 1 mL of normal saline.

- Aspirate 1 mL of fluid from the wound bed.

- Express the fluid into the culture tube.

- Label the culture tube, and transport it to the lab.

- Apply a clean dressing to the wound as ordered.

Procedure 34–3: Performing a Sterile Wound Irrigation

- Administer pain medication 30 minutes prior to the procedure, if necessary.

- Position the patient for easy access to the wound and in a manner that will allow the irrigation solution to flow freely from the wound with the assistance of gravity.

- Don protective equipment: gown, face shield, and clean gloves.

- Remove the soiled dressing, and dispose of gloves.

- Set up a sterile field with a sterile irrigation kit or a 35 mL syringe and a 19-gauge angiocath, dressing supplies, and irrigation solution.

- Wearing sterile gloves, fill either the syringe and angiocath or the piston-tip syringe with irrigation solution.

- Holding the syringe 2 cm from the wound bed, gently irrigate the wound with a back-and-forth motion, moving from the superior aspect to the inferior aspect.

- Dry the tissue surrounding the wound with sterile gauze.

- Apply a new dressing as ordered.

- Dispose of used equipment and soiled dressings in a biohazard container.

- Reposition the patient.

Procedure 34–4: Removing and Applying Dry Dressings

- Administer pain medication 30 minutes prior to the procedure, if necessary.

- Place the patient in a comfortable position that provides easy access to the wound.

- Wearing clean gloves, remove the soiled dressing and discard it in a biohazard receptacle.

- Cleanse the wound with saline-moistened gauze.

- Assess the wound for location, appearance, odor, and drainage.

- Apply a dry dressing.

- Secure the dressing with tape.

Procedure 34–5: Removing and Applying Wet-to-Damp Dressings

- Assess for pain, and medicate 30 minutes prior to procedure, if necessary.

- Place the patient in a comfortable position that provides easy access to the wound.

- Wearing clean gloves, remove the soiled dressing and discard it in a biohazard receptacle.

- Cleanse the wound with saline-moistened gauze.

- Assess the wound for location, appearance, odor, and drainage.

- Apply a single layer of moist, fine-mesh gauze to the wound. Be sure to place gauze in all depressions of the wound.

- Apply a secondary moist layer over the first layer. Repeat this process until the wound is filled with moistened sterile gauze.

- Cover the moistened gauze with a surgipad.

- Secure the dressing with tape or Montgomery straps.

Procedure 34–6: Applying a Transparent Film Dressing

- Place the patient in a comfortable position that provides easy access to the wound.

- Remove the soiled dressing, if necessary.

- Cleanse the surrounding skin and wound.

- Assess the condition of the wound.

- Apply the transparent film dressing to the wound by removing the center backing and holding the dressing firmly by the edges.

- Remove the edge liners.

Procedure 34–7: Applying a Hydrocolloid Dressing

- Place the patient in a comfortable position.

- Remove the soiled dressing, if necessary.

- Cleanse the wound, if necessary.

- Assess the wound, or other area where hydrocolloid dressing will be applied, for size, location, appearance, exudate, odor, and signs and symptoms of infection.

- Shave the area around the wound if necessary.

- Apply the hydrocolloid dressing.

| Diagnosis |

The following nursing diagnoses are appropriate for patients who are at risk for skin breakdown or for patients who have wounds.

- *Risk for Impaired Skin Integrity* is appropriate for patients who have one or more risk factors for skin breakdown (e.g., immobility, incontinence, extremes of age, impaired circulation, impaired sensation, undernutrition, emaciation). NANDA International (2005) recommends that you use a risk assessment tool (e.g., Norton or Braden Scale) to identify these patients.

- *Impaired Skin Integrity* is appropriate for patients who have experienced damage to the epidermis or dermis, for example, patients who have superficial wounds or stage I or II pressure ulcers.

- *Impaired Tissue Integrity* is appropriate for patients with wounds that extend into the subcutaneous tissue, muscle, or bone. Use this diagnosis for patients with deep wounds or stage III or IV pressure ulcers.

- *Risk for Impaired Tissue Integrity* is appropriate for clients with impaired skin integrity who are at risk for delayed healing. For example, Mr. Harmon ("Meet Your Patient") has a stage I pressure ulcer but is at risk for further progression of the ulcer because of his age, nutritional state, and the presence of another wound. Note that this is not a NANDA diagnosis; however, it is useful in the situation described.

Skin problems and wounds can be the etiology for other nursing diagnoses, for example:

- *Risk for Infection* is an appropriate diagnosis if the patient has a traumatic wound or is immunosuppressed, undernourished, or immobile.

- *Pain* is a diagnosis that may be used for patients who are experiencing discomfort from the wound or from the treatments required to heal the wound.

- *Body Image Disturbance* should be used if the patient is experiencing distress about the wound. Consider this diagnosis even if the patient is expected to make a complete recovery. Some patients experience extreme distress about wounds. You will certainly want to consider this diagnosis if the patient experiences an injury that is expected to result in disfigurement.

| Planning Outcomes/Evaluation |

For associated NOC standardized outcomes for skin and tissue integrity diagnoses,

 Go to Chapter 34, **Standardized Language, Selected Standardized Outcomes and Interventions for Skin and Wound Diagnoses,** in Volume 2.

Individualized goals/outcome statements should address the need to maintain intact skin or heal the wound. For patients who have a diagnosis of Risk for Impaired Skin Integrity, you might write a goal such as the following:

> Maintains intact skin throughout treatment, as evidenced by good skin turgor with no erythema, edema, or breaks in the skin.

For patients who have a wound (actual Impaired Skin Integrity or Impaired Tissue Integrity), you might write a goal such as the following:

> Wound will heal by May 1, as evidenced by a progressive decrease in the size of the wound, a decrease in drainage from the wound, improvement in the condition of the surrounding skin, and no evidence of infection (erythema, purulent drainage, or odor).

Healthy People 2010 (U. S. Department of Health and Human Services, 2000) has set a public health objective to reduce the prevalence of pressure ulcers in nursing homes by 50%. The document cites an incidence of 16 per 1,000 residents in 1997 but acknowledges that it is difficult to determine the exact number of people who have pressure ulcers (pp. 1-32 and 1-33).

| Planning Interventions/Implementation |

For NIC standardized interventions for skin and tissue integrity problems,

 Go to Chapter 34, **Standardized Language, Selected Standardized Outcomes and Interventions for Skin and Wound Diagnoses,** in Volume 2.

Specific nursing activities directed at maintaining skin integrity or healing wounds focus on preventing and treating pressure ulcers, providing wound care, and applying heat and cold therapies. In the next section we will discuss these nursing therapeutic measures.

Preventing Pressure Ulcers

Pressure ulcers are extremely difficult and time-consuming to treat. As a result, prevention is the most important nursing intervention. Prevention involves reducing risk factors by providing skin care, nutrition, positioning, therapeutic mattresses and cushions, and patient/family teaching.

Providing Skin Care

Skin care begins with regular inspection of the skin—at least daily for patients at risk—and usually every 8 to 12 hours for institutionalized patients. You must have adequate light to detect subtle, early skin changes. Be sure to check pressure points for erythema, tenderness, or edema. Instruct family members and caregivers in the importance of early detection of skin problems.

Bathing techniques and soaps can contribute to skin breakdown, so meticulous care is necessary to

BOX 34–2   Scheduled Position Changes

0600–0800	Right lateral
0800–0830	Fowler's position for breakfast
0830–1030	Left lateral
1030–1230	Left Sims'
1230–1300	Fowler's position for lunch
1300–1500	Supine
1500–1700	Right lateral
1700–1800	Right Sims'
1800–1900	Up in chair for dinner and visitors
1900–2100	Left lateral
2100–2300	Left Sims'
2300–0100	Supine
0100–0300	Right lateral
0300–0500	Left lateral
0500–0600	Left Sims'

keep the skin clean and intact. If the patient is diaphoretic (sweaty), he may need frequent bathing. Use warm water; hot water will increase skin dryness. Gently bathe fragile skin using a minimum of force and friction. Use a mild cleansing soap, and be sure to rinse thoroughly and gently pat the skin dry. Use soap only as needed, not routinely. Soaps are drying to the skin because they remove oils from the skin and may interfere with the ability of the skin to hold water. If the patient's skin is dry, apply a moisturizing lotion. Lightly apply the lotion, and do not massage over bony prominences.

Keep the linen soft, clean, dry, and free from wrinkles by changing it frequently. Provide skin care regularly. Prevent maceration and secondary infection by providing skin care after each incidence of incontinence.

Providing Nutrition

Nutrition is vital to skin integrity. Patients with rapid weight loss, high metabolic demands, limited intake, or decreased serum albumin are particularly at risk for pressure ulcer development.

Carefully review the diet ordered for at-risk patients, and assess what the patient is eating. The diet may need to be modified for the patient to consume adequate calories and protein. Protein requirements may be as high as 2 grams per kilogram of body weight in the malnourished individual with a wound. High-protein supplements may be necessary.

Consider the consistency of the diet as well. A soft diet that is easy to chew may be helpful for a patient who is frail or is missing teeth. Tube feeding or parenteral nutrition may be ordered to supplement oral intake if the patient is unable to consume adequate quantities of calories and protein. Often a dietary referral is helpful.

Frequent Positioning

Pressure ulcers develop from unrelieved pressure. Most patients who are at risk for pressure ulcers have mobility problems. As a result, you must provide frequent position changes. This is one of the most important interventions for preventing pressure ulcers.

AHRQ guidelines and NPUAP recommendations support repositioning the patient at least every 2 hours. Use the "rule of 30" to guide the positioning of the patient: Elevate the head of the bed 30° or less, and when the patient is on her side, position the patient at a 30° angle to avoid direct pressure on the trochanter. If the head of the bed is elevated more than 30°, limit the time in this position to minimize pressure and shear. Generally, a patient can be placed in the following positions: supine, right lateral, right Sims', left lateral, left Sims', prone, and Fowler's.

The prone position has limited use because many patients are unable to assume this position as a result of mobility or respiratory problems. You can include Fowler's position in the positioning schedule, but use it only for short periods of time because it creates high pressure and shear forces.

Box 34–2 is an example of a turning schedule. It is helpful to place a schedule at the bedside so that all caregivers can participate in the prevention strategy.

Therapeutic Mattresses and Cushions

Use pillows, blankets, or foam wedges as needed to help position a patient. These devices expand the weight-bearing area by molding to the body. Numerous support surfaces have been developed for use in preventing and treating pressure ulcers. Examples include chair pads, mattress overlays, mattress replacements, and specialty beds.

A *mattress overlay* is placed over a standard mattress. It may be made of foam or gel or may be air filled. The most commonly used overlays are egg crate mattresses (Figure 34–14) and alternating air overlays. *Mattress replacements* replace the standard

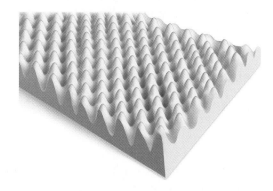

FIGURE 34–14   An egg crate mattress is a static mattress overlay used to reduce pressure.

TABLE 34-3 The Red-Yellow-Black (RYB) Color Code System of Wound Care

Wound Color	Type of Tissue	Nursing Goal	Nursing and Collaborative Activities
Red	Granulation tissue	Protect the wound.	Keep the wound moist and covered.
Yellow	Moist, devitalized tissue (slough)	Cleanse the wound.	Wound irrigation and dressings. May consider debridement.
Black	Eschar	Debride the wound.	Sharp, mechanical, enzymatic, or autolytic debridement.

mattress with an alternative surface that reduces pressure. They may be constructed of foam, air, gel, or water. *Specialized beds* are complete bed units composed of air, water, or gel. These beds are often used for clients with stage III and IV ulcers. Figure 34–15 is a decision-making tree developed by AHRQ to guide selection of appropriate support surfaces.

Patient and Family Teaching

Teaching the at-risk patient and family about pressure ulcer prevention is a key prevention strategy. Include the following topics in your teaching:

- Characteristics of healthy skin
- Appearance of skin that has experienced unrelieved pressure
- Skin care and hygiene
- Protection of the skin
- Importance of adequate nutrition
- Techniques for turning and positioning
- Importance of frequent position changes
- Use of pillows and pressure-reducing devices
- Skin changes that should be reported to health professionals

KnowledgeCheck 34–8

- Identify the major interventions for preventing pressure ulcers.
- What nursing diagnosis is most appropriate for a patient at risk for pressure ulcer development?

 Go to Chapter 34, **Knowledge Check Response Sheet and Answers,** on the Electronic Study Guide.

Providing Wound Care

Nursing care of a patient with a wound incorporates all of the strategies for preventing pressure ulcers, as well as wound treatment strategies. Treatment depends on the nature of the wound. In 1988, the Universal Classification of Wounds by Color system was introduced in the United States by Marion Merrell Dow, Inc. This system, also known as the Red-Yellow-Black (RYB) Color Code (Table 34–3), classifies wounds based on surface appearance and provides guidance for treating wounds.

- *Red wounds* may range from pink to beefy red, based on the amount of granulation tissue in the wound bed. A red wound is ideal because redness is an indication of healing. A clean, moist environment protects the granulating tissue. To protect a red (healing) wound, gently cleanse the wound, and apply a dressing that keeps it moist and clean. The dressing should protect the wound from friction or other disruption of the healing tissue.

- *Yellow wounds* may range from pale beige to shades of green and brown. This color is a result of moist devitalized tissue. These wounds produce a significant amount of drainage, usually purulent. To treat a yellow wound, cleanse the wound to remove the slough. Cleansing may include wound irrigation, wet-to-damp dressings, and absorptive dressings. Collaborative treatment frequently includes application of topical antibiotics and debridement (removal of devitalized tissue).

- *Black wounds* range in color from brown to black. The shiny leathery covering, eschar, indicates the presence of dried necrotic tissue. Necrotic tissue is an excellent medium for bacterial growth. Therefore, treatment of a black wound requires debridement of the necrotic tissue. The exception is the presence of an eschar at the heel. AHRQ does not recommend debridement of this site.

Cleansing Wounds

Wounds are cleansed to remove exudate, slough, foreign materials, and microorganisms. Historically, antiseptic solutions such as Dakin's, acetic acid, hydrogen peroxide, povidone-iodine, and alcohol were used to cleanse wounds. However, research has demonstrated that these antiseptic solutions damage granulating tissue and should not be used. Currently, cleansing agents

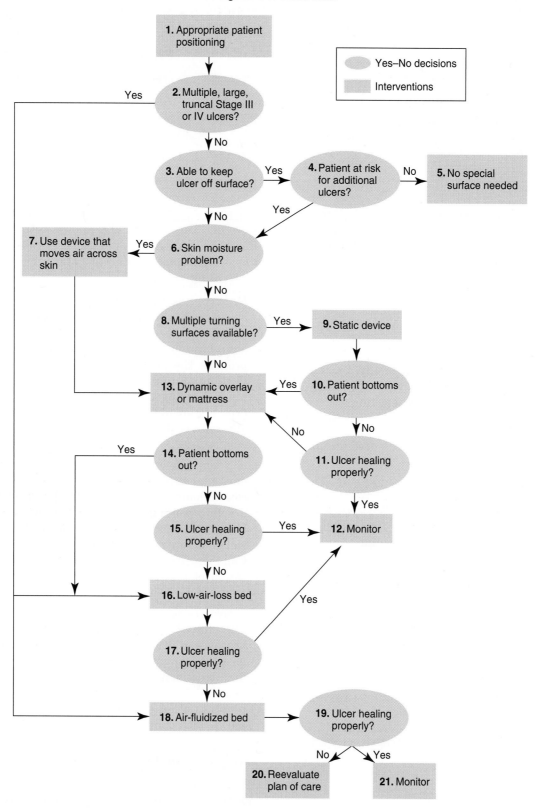

Management of tissue loads

FIGURE 34–15 **A decision-making tree to guide selection of appropriate support surfaces.**

Source: Agency for Healthcare Quality and Research. (1994). *Clinical practice guidelines: Pressure ulcer treatment.* Rockville, MD: Author.

include saline, dilute antimicrobial solutions, and commercially prepared wound cleansers. Liquid or foam skin cleansers may be used to cleanse periwound skin or incontinence effluent. They are not for use in wounds.

To cleanse a wound, gently pat the surface with gauze soaked with saline or other prescribed wound cleanser. If there is granulation tissue, be careful not to disrupt it. Wound irrigation is a gentle technique. As you know from Table 34–3, though, some wounds do require vigorous cleansing. Hydrotherapy is an example of an aggressive cleansing method and is a form of debridement.

Irrigating Wounds

Nurses commonly use irrigation (**lavage**) to cleanse wounds gently by flushing. To remove debris from a wound, you must introduce the irrigation solution with a mild amount of force. Ideal irrigation pressures range from 4 pounds per square inch (psi) to 15 psi. Pressures below 4 psi may not be adequate. Pressures above 15 psi increase the risk of driving bacteria into the tissues as well as causing mechanical damage. A 35 mL syringe attached to a 19-gauge angiocath will deliver the solution at approximately 8 psi (Branom, 2002; Campton-Johnston & Wilson, 2001).

Some agencies use a piston syringe for irrigation. Do not use a bulb syringe; it increases the risk of aspirating the drainage. Commercial irrigation systems are also available. Closely evaluate the amount of pressure they deliver before you use these devices.

There is a risk of splattering with this technique, so you must use gowns, masks, and goggles. Sterile technique is used for acute surgical wounds, wounds that have recently undergone sharp debridement, or when ordered by the physician. The majority of wound irrigation uses clean technique. The Critical Aspects box on p. 830 provides a summary of the procedure. For the complete steps,

 Go to Chapter 34, **Procedure 34–3: Performing a Sterile Wound Irrigation,** in Volume 2.

Caring for Wounds with Drainage Devices

A variety of drains may be inserted into wounds to allow fluid and exudate to exit. Drainage prevents excessive pressure building up in the tissues. Drains are usually placed during a surgical procedure. Some drains are sutured into place, whereas others are simply placed into the cavity.

Types of Drains

A *Penrose drain* is a flexible latex tube that is placed in the wound bed but usually not sutured into place. A clip or pin may be attached to keep it from slipping further into the wound. You may be asked to advance

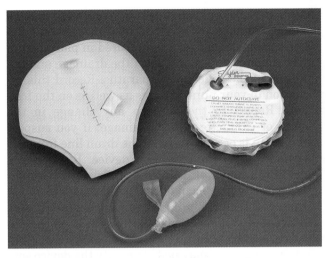

FIGURE 34–16 *Left,* Penrose drain. *Center,* Jackson-Pratt device. *Right,* Hemovac drainage system.

the drain by gradually removing it from the wound bed. For example, the surgeon may order "Advance the Penrose drain 6 mm ($\frac{1}{4}$ inch) per day." Each day you pull the drain out of the wound 6 mm ($\frac{1}{4}$ inch) until the drain is finally removed. For guidelines,

 Go to Chapter 34, **Technique 34–3: Shortening a Drain,** in Volume 2.

Some drains are attached to a collection device. Examples include *Hemovac, Jackson-Pratt,* and *Davol drains* (Figure 34–16). The surgeon may order a device to be "placed to suction." This means that you will compress the device to create suction and facilitate removal of drainage. For guidelines,

 Go to Chapter 34, **Technique 34–4: Emptying a Closed-Wound Drainage System,** in Volume 2.

If a specific pressure is to be applied, some drains can be connected to wall suction. The physician's orders will specify the amount of suction. For example, a surgeon may order: "Place Hemovac to 20 mm Hg suction at all times."

Nursing Activities for Maintaining Drains

You are responsible for monitoring wound drains. The surgeon will describe the number and type of drains present. Describe drain placement according to the position on the clock face. Consider the patient's head to be at the 12 o'clock position (e.g., "Penrose drain at 3 o'clock"). Some patients have more than one drainage device in a wound. Label the drains numerically with a marker or by placing tape on the collection apparatus so that each caregiver provides consistent care.

CHAPTER 35 Oxygenation

Learning Outcomes

After completing this chapter, you should be able to:

✳ Describe the structure and function of the respiratory and cardiovascular systems.

✳ Identify individual, environmental, and pathological factors that influence oxygenation.

✳ Assess oxygenation, breathing, circulation, and gas exchange.

✳ Interpret diagnostic testing related to oxygenation, breathing, circulation, and gas exchange.

✳ Develop nursing diagnoses related to oxygenation, breathing, circulation, and gas exchange.

✳ Plan outcomes and care for maintaining and improving oxygenation.

✳ Safely and correctly perform common nursing procedures related to oxygenation, breathing, perfusion, and gas exchange.

✳ Evaluate adequacy of oxygenation, breathing, perfusion, and gas exchange, and modify nursing activities appropriately based on outcomes.

Your Patients

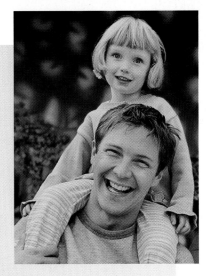

You are scheduled for a clinical placement in a pulmonary clinic. Your assignment is to (1) measure vital signs and perform a basic assessment related to breathing and oxygenation, (2) perform common therapeutic interventions related to breathing and oxygenation, (3) identify desired outcomes and evaluate achievement of those outcomes, and (4) plan for follow-up and home care needs. In the course of your clinical day, you care for the following clients:

• Mary is a 4-year-old girl with a history of asthma. Her mother, Ms Green, has brought her in for an "asthma attack." Mary is sitting in her mother's lap and breathing rapidly through an open mouth. She has a cough that sounds congested and wheezy. The physician has already ordered a nebulized treatment containing albuterol (Proventil) and ipratropium bromide (Atrovent).

• Mr. Chu is a 68-year-old man complaining of cough, sore throat, fatigue, and weakness. His blood pressure (BP) is 166/82 mm Hg, pulse is 90 bpm, respirations are 26 per minute, and temperature is 100.4°F (38°C).

• William is a 19-year-old man who has had a sudden onset of right-sided chest pain and shortness of breath. His chest x-ray film revealed a right pneumothorax, and he is currently receiving 35% oxygen by face mask while waiting for an ambulance to transport him to the hospital for further evaluation.

• Ms Saunders is a 45-year-old homemaker. She says she has been extremely tired, easily becomes short of breath, and is unable to complete her chores without frequent rest breaks. She is pale and seems tired. Her vital signs are as follows: BP, 136/78 mm Hg; pulse, 86 bpm; respirations 24 per minute and unlabored; temperature 98.4° F (36.7°C); and pulse oximetry 98% on room air. She is now waiting for her lab results, which include a complete blood count (CBC).

Each of these patients is experiencing a respiratory problem. In this chapter we will describe a variety of assessment techniques and interventions to support breathing, oxygenation, circulation, and gas exchange for patients such as these.

Theoretical Knowledge
knowing why

Respiratory function is a complex phenomenon involving the musculoskeletal, neurological, respiratory, and cardiovascular systems. The musculoskeletal and neurological systems regulate the movement of air into and out of the lungs. The cardiovascular system transports oxygen and carbon dioxide, which are exchanged in the lungs.

THE PULMONARY SYSTEM

This section describes the structures and functions of the pulmonary system and explains how breathing is controlled. The pulmonary system has two major components: the *airway* and the *lungs*.

What Are the Structures of the Airway?

The airway consists of the nasal passages, mouth, pharynx, larynx, trachea, bronchi, and bronchioles (Figure 35–1). Air flows through these structures into and out of the lungs. In addition, the airway structures moisten, warm, and filter inhaled air. This is accomplished in four ways:

• A moist mucous membrane lining adds water to inhaled air.

• Blood flowing through the vessels of airway walls transfers body heat to the inhaled air.

• Specialized cells in the lining of the airways secrete sticky mucus to trap foreign particles.

• **Cilia,** tiny hairlike projections from the walls of the airways, move rhythmically to sweep trapped debris up and out of the airway.

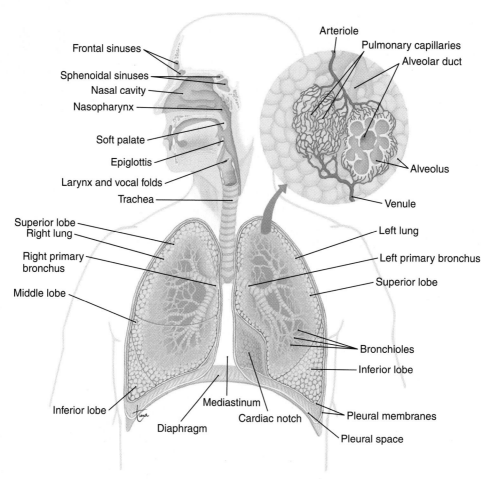

FIGURE 35-1 An anterior view of the respiratory system. The upper airway starts at the nose and continues to the level of the larynx. The lower airway, located below the larynx, is considered sterile. The lungs are soft, spongy organs that are composed of millions of alveoli, the gas exchange units of the pulmonary system.

The larynx divides the airway into two sections. The **upper airway,** located above the larynx, includes the nasal passages, mouth, and pharynx. The **lower airway,** located below the larynx, includes the trachea, bronchi, and bronchioles. The lower airway is considered sterile.

Normally we inhale air through the nose. The *nasal passages* contain coarse hairs that filter air and vascular mucous membranes that warm and moisten the air. When nasal passages are blocked or we need increased airflow, we use mouth breathing. The mouth, however, is not efficient at warming and moistening inhaled air and has no filtering capacity. Thus the mouth quickly becomes dry as inhaled air robs it of moisture. In addition, air inhaled through the mouth is not as warm, moist, or cleared of debris as is air inhaled through the nose.

The *pharynx* (throat) contains lymphoid tissue (called *tonsils*) on both sides. The pharynx contains the openings to the esophagus and trachea. The *trachea* lies just in front of the esophagus; thus, the openings to both lie next to each other in the pharynx. The

epiglottis, a small flap of tissue superior to the larynx, closes off the trachea during swallowing so that food and fluid do not enter the lower airway. The epiglottis opens during breathing to allow air to move through the airway.

The *larynx* is the narrowest portion of the upper airway, so it is a common site for airway obstruction. It is composed of cartilage and muscles. Spasm of these muscles (**laryngospasm**) can close off the entire lower airway and create a respiratory emergency.

The trachea and bronchial tree make up the lower airway. The trachea is supported by horseshoe-shaped rings of cartilage that keep it from collapsing during inhalation. The trachea lies just under the skin of the anterior neck, making it accessible for creation of an emergency surgical airway opening.

The trachea divides to form the right and left mainstem bronchi. The *left mainstem bronchus* is narrower, longer, and leaves the trachea at a sharper, more horizontal angle than the right. The *right mainstem bronchus* is shorter and fatter than the left and leaves the trachea at a more vertical angle. Thus, it is

more susceptible to aspiration of foreign bodies, food, and fluid than the left.

As with the trachea, there are cartilage rings supporting the mainstem bronchi. However, as the airways branch and become smaller, the cartilage support becomes progressively thinner until it disappears in the smaller bronchioles. The walls of the bronchi and bronchioles contain layers of criss-crossing smooth muscles. Spasm of these muscles (**broncho-spasm**) narrows the airway and obstructs airflow.

What Are the Structures of the Lungs?

The chest cavity is a closed compartment sealed with neck muscles at the top, ribs and intercostal muscles all around, and the large diaphragm muscle at the bottom. The *lungs* are soft, spongy, cone-shaped organs that lie on each side of the chest cavity, separated by the **mediastinum,** which contains the heart and great vessels. The right lung is composed of three lobes; the left lung has two lobes. The upper portion of each lung, the *apex,* extends upward above the clavicle. The lower portion of each lung, the *base,* rests on the diaphragm. Knowing the location of lung tissue beneath the chest wall helps you to perform a complete and accurate assessment of the lungs.

The lungs are composed of millions of alveoli. The **alveoli** are tiny air sacs with thin walls surrounded by a fine network of capillaries. Gases easily pass back and forth between the alveoli and capillaries. It is in the *alveolar-capillary membrane* that inhaled air in the lungs comes in contact with the blood of the pulmonary circulation.

Alveoli are composed of two types of cells (Figure 35–2). *Type I alveolar cells* are the gas exchange cells. *Type II alveolar cells* are not involved in gas exchange; they produce **surfactant,** a lipoprotein that lowers the surface tension within alveoli and prevents their walls from adhering together. The moist, membranous inner walls of the alveoli tend to draw together because of the high surface tension inside the alveoli. Therefore, adequate surfactant levels are key to allowing the alveoli to inflate during breathing.

The **pleura** is a thin, double-layered membrane. One layer lines the inside of the chest cavity, and the other covers the outside of the lungs. Between the two layers is the **pleural space,** a thin film of fluid that allows the two layers to remain in contact but glide over each other during breathing movements. Although the pleural membranes glide over each other, they also cling to each other because the negative pressure inside the pleural space creates a mild suction. This suction effect is important because the outside of the lungs must be in constant contact with the inside of the chest cavity for normal function to occur. As long as the pleural space is intact with negative

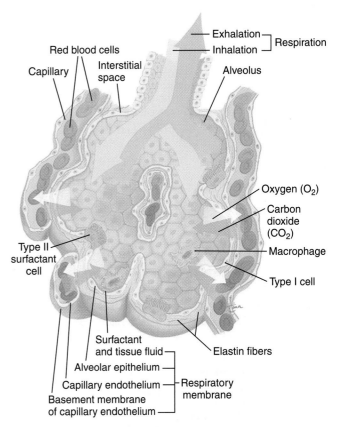

FIGURE 35–2 **Alveolar structure showing type I and type II cells. Type I alveolar cells are the gas exchange cells. Type II alveolar cells produce surfactant, a lipoprotein that decreases the surface tension within alveoli.**

pressure and only a thin film of fluid inside, the lungs expand and contract as the chest expands and contracts. If the pleural space fills with air or fluid, or the chest cavity is opened, the lungs will no longer be in contact with the inside of the chest wall, altering lung expansion and pulmonary function.

KnowledgeCheck 35–1

- What happens to inhaled air in the airways? How does this occur?
- What portion of the upper airway is most prone to airway obstruction? Why?
- Which lung is more susceptible to aspiration? Why?
- What does surfactant do for alveoli?

 Go to Chapter 35, **Knowledge Check Response Sheet and Answers,** on the Electronic Study Guide.

CriticalThinking 35–1

You are assigned to care for a patient who has a medical condition with which you are not familiar. You look it up and find that the condition causes a dramatic loss of surfactant. Based on your knowledge of the function of surfactant, what problems is this patient at high risk for developing?

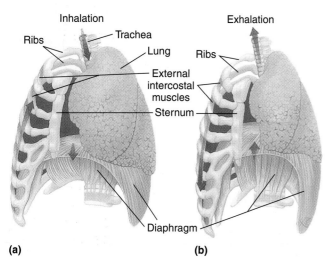

(a)   **(b)**

FIGURE 35–3   During inhalation, the diaphragm contracts, pulling the chest cavity and lung bases downward; the intercostal muscles pull the rib cage up and outward. In exhalation, the diaphragm relaxes, the lung bases move upward, and the ribs and intercostal muscles move down and in, resulting in lung compression.

What Are the Functions of the Pulmonary System?

Two major processes occur in the pulmonary system: ventilation and respiration. **Ventilation** is the movement of air into and out of the lungs through the act of breathing. **Respiration** refers to the exchange of gases (oxygen and carbon dioxide) in the lungs.

The term **oxygenation** refers to how well cells, tissues, and organs are supplied with oxygen. At the alveolar-capillary membrane, oxygen diffuses into the blood cells. If blood is not adequately oxygenated at the alveolar-capillary membrane, **hypoxemia** (low blood-oxygen levels) exists. Getting oxygen into the blood as it flows through the lungs is only the first step in oxygenation. In the second step, blood is transported to the tissues so that oxygen is available for their use. This is the job of the cardiovascular system. **Perfusion** refers to the circulation of blood to all body regions. **Hypoxia** refers to inadequate oxygen levels in the tissues and organs.

Pulmonary Ventilation

Pulmonary ventilation (breathing) is the movement of air into and out of the lungs. Oxygenation of the blood, and ultimately of organs and tissues, depends on adequate ventilation. Poor ventilation results in insufficient amounts of oxygen available in the lungs for diffusion into the blood. Ventilation is accomplished through cycles of inhalation and exhalation.

- **Inhalation** is caused by expansion of the chest cavity and lungs, which creates negative pressure inside the lungs; this causes air to be drawn in through the nose or mouth and airways. The **diaphragm** is the major muscle of breathing. When it contracts with

each inhalation, the chest cavity is pulled downward. The lung bases descend with the chest cavity. *Intercostal muscles,* the small muscles around the ribs, also contract on inhalation and pull the ribs outward, slightly expanding the chest cavity and lungs. Recall that the pleural membrane covering the lungs adheres to the pleural membrane lining the chest cavity. Lung expansion creates negative pressure and draws air in through the only opening to the outside, the trachea. See Figure 35–3A.

- **Exhalation** occurs when the diaphragm and intercostal muscles relax, allowing the chest and lungs to return to their normal resting size (Figure 35–3B). The reduction in size causes the pressure inside the chest and lungs to rise above atmospheric pressure, so air flows out of the lungs. Exhalation requires no energy or effort.

The rate and depth of respirations affect ventilation. **Hyperventilation** occurs when a person's rate and depth of breathing increase enough to move a large amount of air through the lungs. Mild hyperventilation can occur in response to hypoxemia; ventilation increases to draw additional air (and oxygen) into the lungs. However, as ventilation increases, carbon dioxide levels fall. More severe hyperventilation is usually caused by drugs, central nervous system abnormalities, high altitude, heat, exercise, panic, fear, or anxiety. **Hypoventilation** occurs when a decreased rate or depth of breathing moves only a small amount of air into and out of the lungs. Hypoventilation predisposes to the development of hypoxemia because less air (carrying oxygen) reaches the alveoli. The concern is that hypoxemia will lead to hypoxia.

The adequacy of ventilation is also affected by lung compliance, lung elasticity, and airway resistance:

- **Lung compliance** refers to the ease of lung inflation. Normally the lungs inflate easily because of their stretchy elastin fibers, low water content, and low alveolar surface tension. Conditions that cause elastin fibers to be replaced with scar tissue (collagen), increased lung water (edema), or loss of surfactant all reduce lung compliance.

- **Elastic recoil** refers to the tendency of the elastin fibers to return to their original position away from the chest wall after being stretched. Alveoli that have been overstretched, as with emphysema, lose their elastic recoil over time. This loss of elasticity allows the lungs to inflate easily but inhibits deflation, leaving stale air trapped in the alveoli.

- **Airway resistance** is the resistance to airflow within the airways. The larger the diameter of the airway, the more easily air moves through it. Normally, airway resistance is very low, so it takes little effort to move large volumes of air into and out of the lungs. However, even small decreases in airway diameter (as

Lung Volumes and Capacities

Title	Definition	Significance
Tidal volume (V_T)	The amount of air moved into and out of the lungs with each normal breath. Normally around 500 mL.	In a healthy state, V_T increases when oxygen demand increases. Diseases that restrict lung inflation, create muscular weakness, or paralyze the diaphragm limit the ability of the body to increase tidal volume. When such disorders become severe, V_T will fall too low to support even resting oxygen demands.
Inspiratory reserve volume (IRV)	The maximum amount of air that can be inhaled above and beyond the normal tidal volume. Ranges from 2000 to 3000 mL.	IRV determines how much the tidal volume can increase when oxygen demands increase.
Expiratory reserve volume (ERV)	The maximum extra amount of air that can be forcefully exhaled after the end of a normal tidal expiration. Ranges from 1000 to 1500 mL.	Some diseases (e.g., emphysema) cause collapse of alveoli and airways, which traps extra air in the lungs. This "trapped" air cannot be exhaled and lowers ERV.
Residual volume (RV)	The amount of air remaining in the lungs after the most forceful exhalation. Ranges from 1000 to 1500 mL	Diseases that reduce ERV lead to an increase in RV. As more air is trapped in the lungs and cannot be exhaled even with forceful attempts (ERV), it becomes part of the residual volume that is never completely exhaled.
Inspiratory capacity (IC)	The combination of the tidal volume and inspiratory reserve volume (V_T + IRV). Ranges from 2500 to 3500 mL.	This is the amount of air that can be inhaled with maximum effort. It reflects the capacity one has to inhale deeply.
Functional residual capacity (FRC)	The combination of expiratory reserve volume and residual volume (ERV + RV). Ranges from 2000 to 3000 mL. Exhalation of additional air requires effort to force more air out.	This is the amount of air that stays in the lungs at the end of a normal passive quiet exhalation. Disorders that cause air trapping increase the FRC.
Vital capacity (VC)	The combination of inspiratory reserve volume and expiratory reserve volume (IRV + ERV). Ranges from 3000 to 4500 mL	This is the maximum amount of air that can be forcefully exhaled after filling the lungs to their maximum level with the deepest possible inspiratory effort.

might occur with secretions in the airway or mild bronchospasm) markedly increase airway resistance.

The process of ventilation can be studied clinically through **spirometry,** a measure of air that moves into and out of the lungs. To describe the events of pulmonary ventilation, the air in the lungs is divided into four volumes and four capacities. Normal lung volumes and capacities vary with body size, age, and exercise. Volumes and capacities are higher in men, in large people, and in athletes. The accompanying Diagnostic Testing box summarizes this information. The

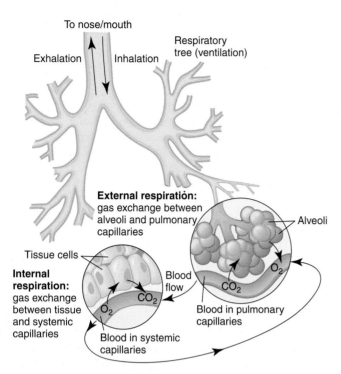

FIGURE 35–4 External respiration occurs at the alveolar-capillary membrane. Internal respiration occurs at the tissue-capillary membrane.

norms presented are based on averages for a young adult man.

KnowledgeCheck 35–2

- What is the difference between ventilation and respiration?
- Describe oxygenation and perfusion.
- Describe how the diaphragm, accessory muscles, and pressure changes within the lungs create inhalation and exhalation.
- How does hypoventilation affect risk for hypoxemia and hypoxia?
- Does poor peripheral perfusion increase risk for hypoxemia?

 Go to Chapter 35, **Knowledge Check Response Sheet and Answers,** on the Electronic Study Guide.

 ## CriticalThinking 35–2

Ms Saunders ("Meet Your Patient") has adequate blood oxygen levels based on a pulse oximeter reading of 98%. Can you conclude that organ and tissue oxygenation is adequate? Explain your thinking.

Respiration (Gas Exchange)

Respiration refers to gas exchange, that is, the oxygenation of blood and elimination of carbon dioxide in the lungs. Although the plural form *respirations* is used to mean "breaths" in an assessment of vital signs, this is a misnomer: you cannot measure gas exchange by counting breaths per minute. Later in this chapter we will discuss diagnostic tests that do measure gas exchange.

Gas exchange occurs at two equally essential levels: (1) at the alveolar-capillary membrane in the lungs (external), and (2) at the capillary-cellular membrane in body tissues (internal). See Figure 35–4.

External Respiration: Alveolar-Capillary Gas Exchange

External respiration occurs in the lungs at the alveolar-capillary membrane. In the alveoli, oxygen (O_2) diffuses across the alveolar-capillary membrane into the blood of the pulmonary capillaries; carbon dioxide (CO_2) diffuses into the alveoli to be exhaled. Several important principles govern this gas exchange:

- **Diffusion** is the tendency of molecules of a substance to move from a region of high concentration to one of lower concentration. Therefore, the higher the O_2 pressure in the alveoli, the faster oxygen will diffuse into the blood.
- Oxygen and CO_2 diffuse more rapidly through a thin membrane. Conditions that thicken the membrane itself or that create a greater distance for gases to travel (e.g., through fluid or secretions) slow the rate of gas diffusion through the membrane.
- Loss of functional lung due to secretions, lung collapse, or bronchospasm reduces the total surface area available for gas exchange.
- Carbon dioxide is much more soluble in water than O_2. It thus diffuses 20 times more rapidly across the membrane than oxygen, and it will continue to diffuse across an abnormal capillary membrane long after O_2 diffusion has slowed dramatically.

Internal Respiration: Capillary-Tissue Gas Exchange

Internal respiration occurs in body organs and tissues. Oxygen diffuses from the blood through the capillary-cellular membrane into the cell, where it is used for metabolism. From the cells, CO_2, a waste product of cell metabolism, diffuses through the capillary-cellular membrane into the blood, from where it is transported to the lungs and exhaled. Tissue oxygenation requires both adequate external respiration and adequate peripheral circulation. Limitations in either function may lead to tissue hypoxia. In addition, if tissue cells are using more oxygen for metabolism than normal (e.g., during a high fever), hypoxia will occur unless more oxygen is made available to the tissues.

How Is Breathing Controlled?

The respiratory centers in the brain stem drive breathing based on feedback from chemoreceptors and lung receptors. *Chemoreceptors* located in the medulla of the brainstem, the carotid arteries, and the aorta detect changes in blood pH, O_2 levels, and CO_2 levels, and they send messages back to the central respiratory center in the brain stem. In response, the respiratory center

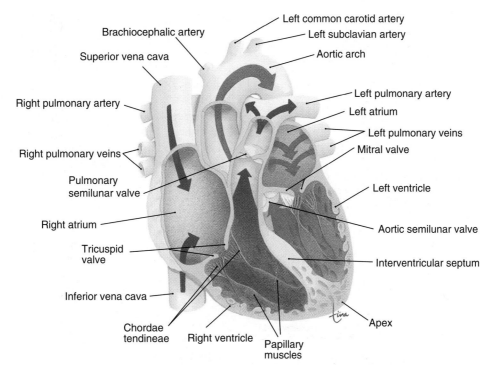

FIGURE 35–5 The heart is a four-chamber muscular organ. Thin-walled atria receive blood into the heart; thick-walled ventricles pump blood out of the heart. Valves between chambers in the heart allow blood to flow easily from one chamber to another and prevent backflow of blood.

increases or decreases ventilation to maintain normal blood levels of pH, O_2 (pO_2), and CO_2 (pCO_2). Normally the blood CO_2 level provides the primary stimulus to breathe. High CO_2 levels stimulate breathing to eliminate the excess CO_2. A secondary, though important, drive to breathe is hypoxemia. Low blood O_2 levels stimulate breathing to get more oxygen into the lungs.

In addition, *lung receptors,* located in the lung and chest wall, are sensitive to breathing patterns, lung expansion, lung compliance, airway resistance, and respiratory irritants. The respiratory center uses feedback from the lung receptors to adjust ventilation. For example, if the lung receptors sense respiratory irritants such as dust, cold air, or tobacco smoke, the respiratory center triggers airway constriction and a more rapid, shallow pattern of breathing.

Voluntary control from the *motor cortex* can override the involuntary respiratory centers, but only temporarily. Voluntary control of breathing allows a person to integrate activities such as talking, singing, swallowing, whistling, and blowing with breathing.

KnowledgeCheck 35–3

- Which gas (oxygen or carbon dioxide) is more diffusible through capillary membranes?
- The level of which gas (oxygen or carbon dioxide) is the primary stimulant for breathing?

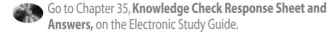

Go to Chapter 35, **Knowledge Check Response Sheet and Answers,** on the Electronic Study Guide.

THE CARDIOVASCULAR SYSTEM

This section discusses the structures, functions, and regulation of the cardiovascular system.

What Are the Structures of the Cardiovascular System?

The structures of the cardiovascular system are the heart and the blood vessels.

The Heart

The heart is a four-chambered muscular organ encased in the **pericardium** (a sac of connective tissue) located inside the chest cavity. The two thin-walled **atria** receive blood into the heart, and the two thick-walled **ventricles** pump blood out of the heart. Valves between the heart chambers open widely to allow blood to flow easily and without turbulence from one chamber to another, and the valves close tightly to prevent backflow of blood. The **base,** or broadest side of the heart, which houses the atria, faces upward. The **apex,** or tip of the heart, which houses the ventricles, faces downward (Figure 35–5).

A strong, efficient heartbeat keeps blood flowing through the vascular system. Deoxygenated blood from organs and tissues flows through the venous system into the right side of the heart and then into the pulmonary circulation. At the alveolar-capillary membrane,

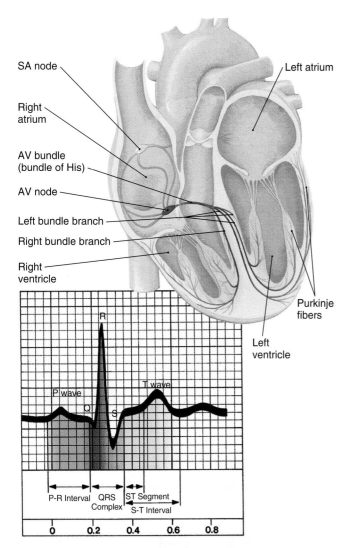

FIGURE 35–6 **The SA node initiates an electrical impulse that is conducted through the intra-atrial pathways to all parts of the atrial muscle and to the AV node. These electrical impulses travel through the AV node to the bundle of His (AV bundle). From the bundle of His, the electrical impulses are conducted very rapidly through the bundle branches and Purkinje fibers that are spread throughout the ventricular muscles. The electrocardiogram is one of normal heartbeat.**

external gas exchange occurs. The newly oxygenated blood then flows from the lungs into the left side of the heart and out into the arterial circulation.

The **cardiac cycle** is the sequence of mechanical events that occurs during a single heartbeat. Very simply, it is the simultaneous contraction of the two atria, followed a fraction of a second later by the simultaneous contraction of the ventricles. The electrical activity of the myocardium regulates the cardiac cycle (Figure 35–6).

The heart contains specialized areas of nerve tissue that initiate electrical impulses. The **sinoatrial (SA) node** (which acts as the pacemaker) in the right atrium initiates an impulse that triggers each heart-

beat. The impulse travels rapidly down the atrial conduction system so that both atria contract as a unit. There is a slight delay at the **atrio-ventricular (AV) node.** From the AV node, impulses pass into the left and right bundles of His and into the Purkinje fibers. In this way, myocardial fibers are electrically stimulated almost simultaneously to create a unified cardiac muscle contraction strong enough to pump blood out of a heart chamber. If there are defects in this electrical system, impulses travel more slowly through the heart and some areas contract before others. This can lead to ineffective heart pumping and decreased cardiac output.

Normally, the SA node is in charge and initiates a rate of 60 to 100 beats per minute, depending upon the body's oxygen needs. If the SA node fails, the AV node can take over as the pacemaker, but it generally triggers a slower heart rate. If both the SA and AV nodes fail, the conduction fibers can initiate impulses. Ventricular conduction generates a very slow rate, usually less than 40 beats per minute; however, this can be life-saving if no other node or fiber is initiating an impulse.

Systemic and Pulmonary Blood Vessels

The vascular system is composed of three types of vessels: arteries, veins, and capillaries. All vessels are lined with a smooth endothelial layer that promotes nonturbulent blood flow and prevents platelets from sticking to the sides of the walls and beginning a clot.

Arteries have thick, elastic walls that allow them to stretch during cardiac contraction (**systole**) and to recoil when the heart relaxes (**diastole**). The walls of **arterioles** (smaller branches of arteries) are primarily smooth muscle. Under control by the sympathetic nervous system, the arterioles constrict or dilate to vary the amount of blood flowing into capillaries and help maintain blood pressure.

Arterioles branch into smaller and smaller vessels until they become **capillaries,** microscopic vessels. Because they are only one cell thick, they facilitate the exchange of gases, nutrients, and wastes between the tissue cells and the blood. Billions of capillaries provide blood flow to every cell in the body. For illustrations of the systemic arteries and veins,

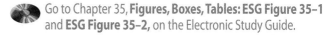

Go to Chapter 35, **Figures, Boxes, Tables: ESG Figure 35–1** and **ESG Figure 35–2,** on the Electronic Study Guide.

Capillaries connect the arterial and venous systems and carry blood from arterioles to venules; the venous system returns the deoxygenated blood to the heart. **Veins** and **venules** have thin, muscular, but inelastic walls that collapse easily. These walls contract or relax in response to feedback from the sympathetic nervous system: When blood volume is low, the

veins contract to provide a smaller space for the low volume of blood; when blood volume is high, veins relax and enlarge to accommodate the large volume of blood. You can think of the venous system as a holding tank for variations in blood volume.

The Coronary Arteries

The heart has its own blood supply through the coronary arteries (Figure 35–7). The coronary sinus (not shown), located just above the aortic valve, fills with blood during diastole. From the coronary sinus, blood flows into the two main coronary arteries, which branch into several sections to supply the heart muscle with blood. The coronary arteries are the only arteries in the body that fill during diastole.

KnowledgeCheck 35–4

- Trace the path of normal electrical impulses in the heart.
- How do the walls of arteries, veins, and capillaries differ?
- What is the importance of diastole to perfusion of the heart?

 Go to Chapter 35, **Knowledge Check Response Sheet and Answers,** on the Electronic Study Guide.

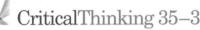 CriticalThinking 35–3

Your patient has a condition that has caused the mitral valve to become stiff with only a narrow opening for blood flow. What type of problems related to oxygenation would you anticipate in this patient?

How Are Oxygen and Carbon Dioxide Transported?

The cardiovascular system circulates oxygenated blood to organs and tissues and returns deoxygenated blood to the heart. Maintaining this blood flow requires adequate cardiac output, adequate circulation, and effective regulation of cardiovascular function. A full 97% of blood oxygen is bound to hemoglobin, the iron-containing protein in red blood cells; only 3% is in a dissolved state. At the tissue level, O_2 leaves the hemoglobin, becomes dissolved in the blood, and passes through the capillary membrane. Only the dissolved form of O_2 can pass through capillary membranes. Hemoglobin thereby serves as a reservoir for oxygen until it is needed in the dissolved state.

Carbon dioxide is a waste product of normal aerobic tissue metabolism. Carbon dioxide can be carried in the blood in three ways: about 7% of CO_2 is dissolved in plasma, 23% attaches to hemoglobin, and 70% is converted into bicarbonate ions. However, CO_2 diffuses through cellular- and alveolar-capillary membranes only in its dissolved state. The CO_2 bound to hemoglobin eventually detaches and becomes dissolved in the plasma for diffusion into the alveoli. The

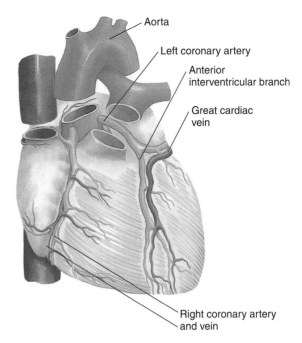

FIGURE 35–7   **Coronary vessels in anterior view. The pulmonary artery has been cut to show the left coronary artery emerging from the ascending aorta.**

bicarbonate ions in the plasma are converted back to CO_2, which becomes dissolved, diffuses into the alveoli, and is exhaled.

How Is Cardiovascular Function Regulated?

Cardiovascular function is regulated by the autonomic nervous system (ANS) and by control centers in the brain stem.

Autonomic Nervous System

The autonomic nervous system regulates cardiovascular function through its influence on heart rate, cardiac muscle contractility, and vascular tone.

- *The heart.* Through branches at the thoracic level of the spinal cord, *sympathetic fibers* stimulate the heart to beat faster and contract more strongly. *Parasympathetic fibers* innervate the heart through the vagus nerve. Parasympathetic stimulation results in a slowed heart rate, but it does not influence myocardial contractility.

- *The vascular system.* All blood vessels are innervated by *sympathetic fibers* that maintain them in a constant baseline state of partial contraction (tone). Vascular tone maintains blood pressure and blood flow even when a person is resting or asleep. Sympathetic stimulation above and beyond this baseline varies in response to body needs. Increased sympathetic stimulation causes constriction of some vessels

(e.g., skin, gastrointestinal tract, and kidneys) and dilatation of other vessels (skeletal muscle). This serves to shunt blood flow to the skeletal muscles for a fight-or-flight response. The *parasympathetic nervous system* has no significant control over blood vessels.

For a brief overview of the nervous system,

 Go to Chapter 35, **Supplemental Materials: The Nervous System,** on the Electronic Study Guide.

For more complete information, consult an anatomy and physiology text.

Brain Stem Centers

The brain stem centers integrate feedback from baroreceptors and chemoreceptors in the body to regulate cardiac function and blood pressure. The *vasomotor center* controls sympathetic stimulation of the heart and vascular system. The *cardioinhibitory center* controls parasympathetic slowing of the heart rate.

Baroreceptors located in the walls of the heart and blood vessels are sensitive to pressure changes. The aortic arch and carotid artery baroreceptors are particularly important in the regulation of heart rate and vascular tone. When baroreceptors sense even a small drop in pressure, they send messages to the brain stem centers to stimulate the sympathetic nervous system to increase heart rate and induce vasoconstriction. This mechanism allows us to change positions and maintain blood pressure.

Chemoreceptors located in the aortic arch and the carotid arteries are sensitive to changes in blood pH, oxygen levels, and carbon dioxide levels. Their main function is to regulate ventilation, but they also send information to the vasomotor center in response to lack of oxygen. The vasomotor center responds by activating sympathetic stimulation.

KnowledgeCheck 35–5
- How are oxygen and carbon dioxide transported in the blood?
- How is the cardiovascular system regulated?

 Go to Chapter 35, **Knowledge Check Response Sheet and Answers,** on the Electronic Study Guide.

 ## CriticalThinking 35–4

The second person you meet at the pulmonary clinic is Mary, a 4-year-old girl with a history of asthma ("Meet Your Patient"). She is receiving a nebulized treatment containing Proventil (albuterol) and Atrovent (ipratropium bromide). These medications stimulate the sympathetic nervous system.

- What cardiovascular side effects can you anticipate?
- How might these side effects affect oxygenation?
- What do you need to know about the patient's history to safely administer the drugs?

WHAT FACTORS INFLUENCE OXYGENATION?

Factors that influence oxygenation include developmental stage, the environment, individual and lifestyle factors, medications, and pathophysiological states.

Developmental Stage

Normal development influences lung, heart, and circulatory function, all of which affect oxygenation. Developmental factors have less effect on function in young and middle adults than in older adults.

Infants

Premature infants (fewer than 33 weeks gestation) are born before the alveolar surfactant system is fully developed. Therefore, they are at high risk for respiratory distress syndrome (RDS), also called hyaline membrane disease. RDS is characterized by widespread **atelectasis** (collapse of alveoli). The premature infant also has immature pulmonary circulation. Together with hypoventilation, this leads to hypercarbia (high CO_2 blood levels) and hypoxemia.

Even infants born at term are at risk for oxygenation problems, for example, infection and airway obstruction. Newborns have diminished ability to produce mucus, so their inhaled air is dryer and they have less protection against infection. Because their lower airway structures are located very close to each other, an infectious agent can spread rapidly. The infant's airways are quite small and therefore are easily obstructed by edema, mucus, or a foreign body. By 6 months of age, infants can grasp small objects and put them in their mouth. This new skill, combined with small airway diameter, puts the infant at risk for choking on small objects.

Toddlers

As the toddler's respiratory and immune systems mature, his risk for frequent and serious infections diminishes. However, the incidence of upper respiratory infections (URI) remains high because (1) the tonsils and adenoids are relatively large, predisposing to tonsillitis; and (2) many children are exposed to new infectious agents in preschool and day care. Most children recover from URIs without difficulty.

Although growing, toddlers' airways are still relatively short and small and may be easily obstructed. Toddlers often put objects in their mouths as part of exploring their environment. Thus they are at risk for transmitting infections through toys and other objects, as well as for airway obstruction from aspiration of small objects (e.g., candy, buttons, coins, peanuts, grapes, and so on). In addition, toddlers are at high risk

for drowning in very small amounts of water around the home (e.g., in a bucket of water or toilet bowl).

Preschool and School-Age Children

Preschool and school-age children have developed mature body systems that can adapt to moderate stress and change, including the lungs, heart, and circulatory systems. They have bouts of tonsillitis or URIs, which usually resolve without difficulty. Unfortunately, children as young as school age sometimes begin social habits, such as cigarette smoking, that can have long-term adverse effects on oxygenation. Young people often begin smoking for social reasons (e.g., peer pressure, advertising), but nicotine addiction perpetuates the habit.

Adolescents

In adolescence, the lungs, heart, and blood components develop adult characteristics. The average adolescent is developmentally at little risk for lung, heart, or circulatory disorders. They are, however, developing behaviors and habits that can create risk throughout life. By 12th grade in the United States, 62% of students have tried cigarettes, with one-fourth reporting that they smoke at least one cigarette per day (Wong, Perry, & Hockenberry, 2002). The U.S. incidence of childhood obesity is also rising, causing some adolescents to exhibit signs of cardiovascular disease at an early age. Sedentary lifestyle and a diet high in calories, fat, and sugar are thought to be major causes.

Young and Middle Adults

The unhealthful diets of adolescence often continue into adulthood as people become "too busy" to prepare and eat nourishing foods, or simply prefer the taste of high-fat, high-sugar foods. A sedentary lifestyle, lack of aerobic exercise, and smoking also contribute to cardiovascular and lung disorders in this group.

Older Adults

In general, the number of cells and the efficiency of the organs decline in a subtle and progressive way as a person ages. Keep in mind, though, that endurance training and regular exercise minimize the rate of these changes. In fact, an older person who is physically conditioned by regular exercise may have better lung, heart, and circulatory function than a younger adult who is not well conditioned (Eliopoulos, 2001). Older adults tend to experience:

- *Reduced lung expansion and less alveolar inflation,* especially in the bases of the lungs. This is because (1) costal cartilage begins to calcify, reducing chest wall movement during breathing; (2) the lungs have less recoil ability; and (3) the alveoli lose elasticity.

- *Difficulty expelling mucus or foreign material* due to a less effective cough reflex and fewer cilia in the airways.

- *Diminished ability to increase ventilation* when oxygenation demands increase (e.g., with exercise). The reason is that exhalation becomes less efficient, causing progressive air-trapping.

- *Declining immune response,* especially cell-mediated immunity, T-cell activity, and the inflammatory response.

All of these changes put older adults at risk for respiratory infections. Upper respiratory infections that would be mild and short-lived in a younger person may quickly lead to pneumonia in the older adult. In addition, chemoreceptors that control breathing respond more slowly to increased O_2 demand or rising levels of CO_2.

Cardiac efficiency gradually declines as the heart muscle loses contractile strength and heart valves become thicker and more rigid. The peripheral vessels become less elastic, which creates more resistance to ejection of blood from the heart. As a result of these changes, the heart becomes less able to respond to increased oxygen demands, and it needs longer recovery times after responding. For example, in response to exercise, an older adult's heart rate does not increase as much as a younger person's, but it will remain elevated longer. Thus, older adults have lower exercise tolerance and need more rest after exercise.

Environment

Environmental factors, such as stress, allergic reactions, altitude, and temperature, affect oxygenation. These factors are discussed below.

Stress

The stress response stimulates:

- *Release of catecholamines* from the sympathetic nervous system. This results in increased heart rate and contractility, vasoconstriction, and increased tendency of blood to clot.

- *Suppression of the immune and inflammatory responses,* which decreases resistance to infection.

- *Release of cortisol* from the adrenal cortex, which results in altered glucose, fat, and protein metabolism.

Sustained stimulation of the sympathetic nervous system can lead to cardiovascular disease. In addition, a chronically suppressed immune and inflammatory response increases the risk for all infections, including respiratory. For additional information on the effects of stress, see Chapter 25.

Allergic Reactions

An **allergy** is a hypersensitivity, or over-response, to an antigen. Pulmonary allergens include such things as dust, dust mites, cockroach particles, pollen, molds, newsprint, tobacco smoke, animal dander, and sometimes foods. Inflammatory substances released during an allergic response (e.g., histamine, protease) cause the following cardiovascular events:

- Dilation of blood vessels in areas affected (which increases blood flow to the areas)
- Attraction of eosinophils and neutrophils to the reaction site
- Damage of local tissues by protease
- Increased permeability of capillaries, with resulting fluid leak into tissues
- Contraction of local (e.g., vascular) smooth muscle cells.

Hay fever is an allergic reaction affecting the eyes, nose, and/or sinuses and causing the release of *histamine,* which is largely responsible for accumulation of nasal fluid and swollen nasal membranes. Antihistamines are effective in combating hay fever. **Asthma** is an allergic reaction occurring in the bronchioles of the lungs, causing release of *slow reacting substance of anaphylaxis,* which causes lower airway edema and spasms, making breathing difficult and ineffective. Because histamine is not a major factor in causing the asthmatic reaction, antihistamines have little effect in the treatment of asthma.

Air Quality

Air pollution triggers respiratory problems (e.g., lung cancer, carbon monoxide poisoning) that interfere with oxygenation. Even healthy people may experience headache, coughing, and other symptoms when exposed to air pollution. People with existing respiratory disease may become unable to function. Some sources of air pollution are natural (e.g., forest fires), but the most common and damaging sources result from human activities (e.g., automobile exhaust emissions). Indoor air pollutants include carbon monoxide, nitrogen oxides, radon, and suspended particles (dust, mold spores, soot, ash, aerosols, tobacco smoke, and asbestos). Pollutants are most harmful to infants and toddlers, older adults, and people with heart or lung disease. For more information about air quality,

 Go to Chapter 35, **Supplemental Materials: Air Quality Affects Oxygenation,** on the Electronic Study Guide.

Altitude

Atmospheric pressure falls from 760 mm Hg at sea level to 523 mm Hg at 10,000 feet. Oxygen pressure falls proportionally, leading to decreased oxygen diffusion from alveoli into capillaries. Low oxygen levels at high altitudes can cause hypoxemia and hypoxia. If a person is suddenly exposed to low oxygen levels, arterial chemoreceptors stimulate ventilation, making more oxygen available in the alveoli and at the tissue level. Over the long term, people who live at high altitudes undergo physiological changes that facilitate oxygenation. Changes include increased:

- Ventilation
- Production of red blood cells (RBCs)
- Lung volume and pulmonary vasculature (resulting in increased surface area for alveolar-capillary gas exchange)
- Vascularity of body tissues
- Ability of tissue cells to use oxygen even when atmospheric oxygen pressure is low (Guyton & Hall, 2000).

Heat and Cold

Heat generally causes vasodilatation, which increases cardiac output and oxygenation. However, heat also increases metabolism. As a result, people are naturally more sedentary in hot weather.

Cold slows cell metabolism (reducing O_2 demand), causes vasoconstriction, and slows the heart rate. Artificial hypothermia is used in surgery quite successfully. As another example, victims of cold-water near-drowning have been revived after long periods of time, in part because of the reduced O_2 demands associated with hypothermia. Of course, prolonged exposure to cold causes frostbite, loss of hypothalamic temperature regulation, and death (Guyton & Hall, 2000).

Lifestyle

Lifestyle factors that affect oxygenation include pregnancy, occupational exposure to hazards, nutrition, obesity, exercise, smoking, and substance abuse.

Pregnancy

During pregnancy, oxygen demand increases dramatically. To compensate, the mother's blood volume increases by 30%. The woman requires additional iron to produce this blood as well as to meet fetal requirements. Failure to meet these iron demands can result in maternal anemia, reducing tissue oxygenation of the mother.

Maternal metabolism increases by approximately 15% during the last half of pregnancy, increasing the demand for O_2. Simultaneously, the enlarging uterus pushes upward against the diaphragm, limiting its downward movement. In response, the maternal respiratory rate increases in order to increase *minute*

ventilation (amount of air moved into and out of the lungs in 1 minute) (Guyton & Hall, 2000).

Occupational Hazards

Occupational hazards may affect oxygenation by irritating airways, causing cardiovascular disease, interfering with blood cell function, or causing cancer. Toxic agents may be categorized as follows:

- *Chemicals and their fumes* irritate the sensitive membranous lining of the lungs and airways and may lead to lung cancer or leukemia. Even common household cleaners can emit toxic fumes.
- *Products of combustion* (e.g., carbon monoxide) are known causes of lung cancer and chronic lung disease.
- *Organisms,* such as fungi and mold, may lead to infections and precipitate asthma.
- *Fine particles (e.g., coal dust and asbestos)* suspended in the air can be inhaled into the smallest airways, causing irritation and toxic reactions, including cancer.
- *Radiation* is a known cause of leukemia.

Nutrition

The body needs an appropriate balance of proteins, carbohydrates, fats, and other nutrients for proper immune function, resistance to disease and infection, normal cellular function and tissue repair, and maintenance of a healthy weight. A diet high in saturated fat predisposes to the development of atherosclerosis, coronary artery disease, and hypertension, all of which can negatively affect circulation and oxygenation. Vitamins, minerals (especially iron), and protein are important to prevent anemia, which reduces blood-oxygen carrying capacity. Poor nutrition, especially in those with pulmonary disorders, can lead to loss of ventilatory muscle strength, making breathing more difficult.

Obesity

Obesity is BMI above 30. Obesity causes multiple health problems, many of which affect the lungs, heart, and circulation.

- *Respiratory infections.* Large abdominal fat stores press upward on the diaphragm, preventing full chest expansion, leading to hypoventilation and dyspnea on exertion. The risk for respiratory infection then increases because lower lung lobes are poorly ventilated and secretions are not removed effectively.
- *Sleep apnea.* When the person lies down, chest expansion is limited even more. Excess neck girth and fat stores in the upper airway often lead to obstructive

sleep apnea, a condition characterized by daytime sleepiness, loud snoring, and periods of apnea lasting 10 to 120 seconds (Porth, 2002).

- *Cardiovascular effects.* Obesity also increases the risk of developing atherosclerosis and hypertension. Excess fat stores in and around the heart itself reduce its effectiveness as a pump. At the same time, the workload of the heart is increased by the need to perfuse the excess body tissues.

Exercise

Exercise increases metabolic demands. The body responds by increasing the heart rate and the rate and depth of breathing. Like skeletal muscles, the heart muscle is strengthened with regular aerobic exercise. As the heart becomes stronger, it becomes a more efficient pump. As a result, resting heart rate is slower because a higher heart rate is not required to maintain cardiac output. Lack of exercise has the opposite effect. A sedentary lifestyle reduces the efficiency of the heart and the capacity to increase ventilation in response to exercise.

Smoking

Tobacco smoke contains tiny particles of tar and approximately 200 known toxic chemicals. *Mainstream smoke* (inhaled directly from the cigarette) and *sidestream smoke* (released from the burning tip of a cigarette into the air) are harmful to everyone in the environment, especially children, older adults, and people with allergies or lung disorders. Sidestream smoke has actually been found to have higher concentrations of harmful compounds than mainstream smoke, thus posing a significant health risk to nonsmokers (American Lung Association, 2002b).

Tobacco smoke constricts bronchioles, increases fluid secretion into the airways, causes inflammation and swelling of the bronchial lining, and paralyzes cilia. These effects lead to reduced airflow and increased production of secretions not easily removed from the airways. Lung inflammation stimulates the release of enzymes that break down elastin and other alveolar wall components. Continued smoking leads to chronic bronchitis, obstruction of bronchioles and alveolar walls, and emphysema. Cigarette smoking is estimated to be the cause of over 80% of cases of lung cancer. The incidence of cancer rises as the number of cigarettes smoked and the length of time smoking increases (American Lung Association, 2002b).

Once a person stops smoking, the body begins to repair the damage. In the first few days, the person will cough more as the cilia begin to clear the airways. Then the coughing subsides, and breathing becomes easier. Even long-time smokers can benefit from smoking cessation. Box 35–1 highlights some of the benefits of

BOX 35-1   Health Effects of Smoking Cessation

- Blood pressure and heart rate decrease.
- Circulation to the extremities improves within 2 hours.
- Carbon dioxide levels in the blood begin to drop within 4 hours.
- Oxygen levels in the blood begin to improve within 8 hours.
- Digestion improves.
- Coughing, congestion, and shortness of breath decrease.
- Overall energy increases.
- Lungs increase ability to clean themselves, thereby reducing the risk of infection.
- Risk of heart attack decreases and returns to that of a nonsmoker in 1 year.
- Risk of lung and other cancers, stroke, and chronic obstructive lung disease decreases.

smoking cessation. The accompanying Self-Care box provides suggestions for helping patients stop smoking.

Substance Abuse

Abused substances include over-the-counter and prescription medications, commonly available commercial products, and illegal substances. Excess use or overdose of respiratory depressants such as opioids, sedatives, antianxiety agents, and hypnotics can cause death due to hypoventilation, apnea, and respiratory failure. Commonly available products such as alcohol, caffeine, glue, aerosols, and other inhalants also have abuse potential and can be lethal. Large amounts of alcohol depress respiratory, cardiac, and vasomotor centers of the brain. Chronic alcohol abuse causes fatty infiltration of the heart muscle, thrombi in the coronary arteries, heart enlargement, and dysrhythmias, all of which can ultimately lead to heart failure (Mulvihill, Zelman, Holdaway, Tompary, & Turchaney, 2001). Illicit drugs, including stimulants (e.g., amphetamines, cocaine), hallucinogens (e.g., LSD, PCP), and marijuana also have adverse effects on the respiratory and cardiovascular systems.

KnowledgeCheck 35–6

- What are the major risks to oxygenation related to developmental factors?
- What environmental and lifestyle factors that influence ventilation and circulation can be avoided or minimized?

 Go to Chapter 35, **Knowledge Check Response Sheet and Answers,** on the Electronic Study Guide.

self-care   Smoking Cessation Tips

- Identify several personal reasons to quit smoking, such as: "I'll live longer and be able to spend more time with my children and grandchildren," or "My father died of lung cancer. He really suffered. I have no desire to experience that."
- Make a list of things you enjoy doing. Choose one of these items as a reward for not smoking.
- Before smoking, ask yourself, "What can I do instead of smoking this cigarette?"
- Identify friends who do not smoke, and plan to spend time with them.
- Have carrot sticks, celery, gum, or sunflower seeds available to chew instead of smoking a cigarette.
- Learn several relaxation techniques, such as meditation or visualization, to help you through the stress of quitting.
- Use positive affirmations daily. "I can successfully quit smoking. I am no longer a smoker."
- Tell several supportive people of your plan to quit. Ask them to help you be successful.
- Plan a time to quit. Choose a time that will not require many additional demands on you.
- Talk with friends and co-workers who have successfully quit smoking.
- Tell your healthcare providers that you would like to quit smoking.
- Save the money you would have spent on cigarettes. Treat yourself to an activity or event with the money you have saved.

 CriticalThinking 35–5

Review the "Meet Your Patients" scenario at the beginning of this chapter.

- Which patient(s) may be experiencing developmental, environmental, or lifestyle-related problems with oxygenation?
- Identify any additional information you need to know to answer this question.

Medications

Many drugs can interfere with oxygenation by depressing respirations or cardiovascular function. For a more complete discussion,

 Go to Chapter 35, **Supplemental Materials: Medications That Can Interfere with Oxygenation** and **Medications Used to Improve Oxygenation,** on the Electronic Study Guide.

Respiratory Effects

Respiratory depressants generally act by depressing central nervous system control of breathing or by weakening the muscles of breathing. They include general anesthetics, opioids (e.g., morphine), antianxiety drugs (e.g., diazepam [Valium]), sedative-hypnotics (e.g., barbiturates), neuromuscular blocking agents, and magnesium sulfate.

Drugs that block beta-2 adrenergic receptors have little effect on healthy lungs but can lead to serious bronchiole constriction in people with asthma.

Cardiovascular Effects

Cardiovascular depressants are used therapeutically to slow the heart rate or reduce the force of myocardial contraction. This may lead to a drop in cardiac output and impair tissue oxygenation. The following are the most commonly used cardiovascular depressants:

- *Beta-adrenergic blocking agents* (e.g., bisoprolol fumarate [Zebeta]) are used therapeutically to reduce the work load of the heart, to control abnormal heart rhythms (dysrhythmias), and to control hypertension. Drugs that block beta-1 receptors slow the heart rate and decrease the strength of myocardial contraction.
- *Calcium channel blocking agents* (e.g., nifedipine [Procardia]) block the flow of calcium into cells of the heart and vessels. They decrease blood pressure and the strength of myocardial contraction, slow the heart rate, and dilate the arteries and arterioles.

CriticalThinking 35–6

You are caring for a 60-year-old patient immediately following a surgical procedure under general anesthesia. He has a history of chronic asthma. The physician has written an order for a medication that is a nonselective beta-blocking agent. What actions should you take? Explain your thinking. (*Note:* To answer this question, you will need to review the complete discussion of medications affecting cardiovascular function on the Electronic Study Guide.)

Pathophysiological Conditions

Alterations in oxygen and carbon dioxide levels at the alveolar-capillary membrane or the tissue level may be life threatening. The following are common alterations:

- *Hypoxemia.* Recall that hypoxemia means low arterial blood oxygen levels. It is caused by poor oxygen diffusion into the blood across the alveolar-capillary membrane (ineffective external respiration) due to lung or pulmonary circulation disorders. Hypoventilation predisposes to the development of hypoxemia and may lead to hypoxia. However, even if the blood is adequately oxygenated, you cannot conclude that adequate oxygen will reach organs and tissues. You must also assess how well blood is circulating to specific tissues and how well the tissues are receiving and using the oxygen. Assessment techniques for this purpose are discussed later in this chapter.
- *Hypoxia.* Recall that hypoxia means poor oxygenation of organs and tissues. It may be due to hypoxemia or circulatory disorders. To determine adequacy of tissue oxygenation, you must assess both circulation and tissue/organ function. Poor peripheral circulation is characterized by weak or absent pulses; pale, ashen, or cyanotic skin and mucous membranes; and cool skin temperature. You can indirectly assess tissue oxygenation by determining whether organs are functioning normally. For example, hypoxic central nervous system tissue causes abnormal brain functioning (e.g., altered level of consciousness), whereas hypoxic renal tissue causes abnormal kidney functioning (e.g., poor urine output), and hypoxic limb tissue results in abnormal muscle functioning (e.g., muscle weakness and pain with exercise).
- *Hypercarbia.* **Hypercarbia (hypercapnia)** refers to an excess of dissolved CO_2 in the blood due to hypoventilation. Hypoventilation is caused by abnormalities affecting the lungs or chest cavity or by neuromuscular abnormalities that interfere with normal breathing. Hypercarbia can occur suddenly, as in acute airway obstruction or drug overdose, or chronically, as in chronic lung disease. Very high blood levels of CO_2 have an anesthetic effect on the nervous system and can lead to somnolence progressing to coma and death, a syndrome known as *carbon dioxide narcosis*.
- *Hypocarbia.* **Hypocarbia (hypocapnia)** is a low level of dissolved CO_2 in the blood due to hyperventilation. In most cases (except high altitude), blood O_2 levels remain normal. Severe hypocarbia stimulates the nervous system, leading to muscle twitching or spasm (especially in the hands and feet) and numbness and tingling in the face and lips.

Alterations in gas exchange are caused by a number of disorders that affect the structure, function, and regulation of the pulmonary and cardiovascular. The next few sections highlight these disorders. For a more complete discussion of these pathological conditions,

 Go to Chapter 35, **Supplemental Materials: Pathophysiological Conditions That Influence Gas Exchange,** on the Electronic Study Guide.

KnowledgeCheck 35–7

- How do you assess for adequate tissue oxygenation?
- How are hyperventilation and hypoventilation related to carbon dioxide levels?
- What are the effects of carbon dioxide levels on the nervous system?

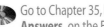 Go to Chapter 35, **Knowledge Check Response Sheet and Answers,** on the Electronic Study Guide.

CriticalThinking 35–7

You are assessing a very anxious young man who looks scared and is complaining of trouble breathing. His respiratory rate is 32 and deep. He states his fingers and hands are numb.

- What is the most likely cause?
- What blood levels would help you clarify what is going on?

Pulmonary System Abnormalities

A variety of pulmonary abnormalities can lead to alterations in gas exchange. Here we briefly discuss the major causes.

- *Structural abnormalities.* Structural abnormalities include anything that restricts or limits the free movement of the chest wall (e.g., fractured ribs, kyphosis), interruptions in the chest cavity that inhibit inflation of the lungs (e.g., pneumothorax), or a collection of fluid (blood, lymph, pus) in the pleural space that inhibits lung expansion.

- *Airway inflammation and obstruction.* Allergic reactions (e.g., asthma) or irritation from smoke or other irritants may cause airway inflammation. Obstruction may be mechanical, as with a foreign object or bolus of food, or due to spasm (e.g., laryngospasm). Swollen tonsils and a swollen epiglottis may also cause obstruction.

- *Infections.* Respiratory infections (e.g., influenza, common colds) are among the most common causes of short-term disability in the United States. Lower respiratory tract infections (acute bronchitis, pneumonia, and tuberculosis) occur more often in children, older adults, and people with impaired immunity or lung function.

- *Alveolar-capillary membrane disorders.* These disorders are characterized by a change in the consistency of the lung tissue, especially at the alveolar level. The alveoli become stiff and difficult to ventilate, and gas exchange is impaired. Pulmonary edema, acute respiratory distress syndrome (ARDS), and pulmonary fibrosis are examples.

- *Atelectasis.* **Atelectasis** is alveolar collapse. Anything that reduces ventilation (e.g., tumor, obstructed airway) can cause atelectasis.

Pulmonary Circulation Abnormalities

For gas exchange to occur in the alveoli, there must be adequate blood flow through the pulmonary circulation. The most common causes of impaired pulmonary circulation are pulmonary embolus and pulmonary hypertension. A **pulmonary embolus** is obstruction of pulmonary arterial circulation by a foreign substance (e.g., a blood clot, air, or fat).

Pulmonary hypertension is elevated pressure within the pulmonary arterial system. Normally this is a low-pressure system with thin-walled, compliant vessels. High pressure in the pulmonary circulation increases the workload of the heart. Over time, this causes right-sided heart failure, with a reduced amount of blood pumped into the pulmonary circulation.

Neuromuscular Abnormalities

Neuromuscular abnormalities can affect gas exchange by interfering with the regulation of breathing or limiting movement of the muscles involved with breathing. Any condition that alters CNS function can interfere with the regulation of breathing. Trauma, stroke, and medications are the most common causes. Neuromuscular disorders that affect the nerves involved in breathing can also depress respiratory function. Guillain-Barré syndrome, amyotrophic lateral sclerosis, and myasthenia gravis are examples.

Cardiovascular Abnormalities

Cardiovascular abnormalities interfere with the flow of oxygenated blood to organs and tissues. Major abnormalities are as follows:

- **Heart failure** occurs when the heart becomes an inefficient pump and is unable to meet the body's demands. Blood is oxygenated when it passes through the lungs, but it is not well circulated to the organs and tissues. Impaired circulation leads to systemic and pulmonary edema, which further impairs gas exchange.

- **Cardiomyopathy** is a heart muscle disorder that results in heart enlargement and impaired cardiac contractility.

- **Cardiac ischemia** occurs when oxygen requirements of the heart are unmet. Prolonged ischemia leads to myocardial infarction (MI) as parts of the heart *necrose* (die) from inadequate oxygen. **Angina pectoris** is transient chest pain due to myocardial ischemia. The tissue becomes injured but does not necrose.

- **Dysrhythmias** (alterations in heart rate or rhythm) can lower cardiac output and decrease tissue oxygenation.

- **Heart valve abnormalities** create turbulent flow, leading to a decrease in cardiac output and compromised tissue oxygenation. Often there is an audible murmur. The valves most commonly affected are the mitral and aortic valves.

Peripheral Vascular Abnormalities

Disorders of peripheral blood vessels impair blood flow to and from organs and tissues. Arterial abnormalities disrupt flow of oxygenated blood to tissues. When arterial blood flow is compromised, signs and

symptoms include pallor, pain, weak or absent pulses, poor capillary refill, cool skin, and tissue dysfunction. Venous abnormalities disrupt blood return to the heart. When venous blood flow is compromised, signs and symptoms include edema, brown skin discoloration, and tissue dysfunction (e.g., stasis ulcers).

Oxygen Transport Abnormalities

Even if the heart is functioning well and arterial blood flow is intact, tissues can become hypoxic if the blood is unable to carry adequate amounts of oxygen. The most common causes are anemia and carbon monoxide poisoning. **Anemia** is an abnormally low level of red blood cells, hemoglobin, or both. **Carbon monoxide** is a colorless, odorless gas that is produced by the combustion of flammable materials and fuels. When inhaled, carbon monoxide binds tightly to hemoglobin at the oxygen receptor sites, making it impossible for hemoglobin to carry oxygen.

Metabolism Extremes and Oxygen Demand

In the assessment of oxygenation, metabolic rate and organ oxygen demand must be considered. Hypermetabolic states (e.g., severe burns, sepsis) increase oxygen demands. If the cardiovascular system cannot keep up with the increased oxygen demands, tissue hypoxia will result. Hypometabolic states (e.g., hypothermia) reduce oxygen demands. Victims of hypothermia can sometimes be resuscitated after long periods of time without brain injury because of the brain's low oxygen requirements in the hypometabolic state.

KnowledgeCheck 35–8

- Identify seven types of conditions that affect ventilation and oxygenation. How are they similar? How are they different?
- What types of injuries are most likely to be associated with oxygenation problems?

 Go to Chapter 35, **Knowledge Check Response Sheet and Answers,** on the Electronic Study Guide.

CriticalThinking 35–8

You are the nursing supervisor on the night shift in a small community hospital. You are responsible for monitoring bed status. At the beginning of the shift, you have only one critical care bed available. During your shift, you receive calls for assistance on the following patients:

- Patient A has burns on her face, scalp, and chest and is coughing up sputum with black streaks.
- Patient B has pneumonia but has suddenly become confused.
- Patient C is short of breath and complaining that he can't breathe. His skin is cool and moist, and he is coughing up clear sputum with small bubbles in it.

Which patient would you admit to the critical care bed? Why?

Practical Knowledge
knowing how

Nursing care for patients with oxygenation concerns is directed at assessing for and maximizing the effectiveness of ventilation and gas exchange. In this part of the chapter, we discuss these nursing activities.

| Assessment |

Assessment of oxygenation status includes a history and examination that gathers information relevant to lung, heart, and circulatory function. The order in which you gather information and the priorities of assessment vary with the patient's condition and the purpose of the assessment. For example, for someone in obvious respiratory distress, the immediate assessment focus includes asking simple questions about current symptoms while performing a quick examination to determine adequacy of breathing, circulation, and oxygenation. In contrast, the assessment for risk of respiratory disease in a healthy individual might include more extensive questions about occupation, smoking habits, and living environment; a medical history; and an extensive physical examination.

Assessing Risk for Impaired Oxygenation

A health history related to oxygenation includes questions about the presence of risk factors that affect lung, heart, and vascular function. Topics to assess include the following:

- Demographic data
- Health history
- Respiratory history
- Cardiovascular history
- Environmental history
- Lifestyle

For a detailed list of interview questions for each of these topics,

 Go to Chapter 35, **Assessment Guidelines and Tools, Questions to Assess Risk for Impaired Oxygenation,** in Volume 2.

Physical Examination

Assessment of heart, vessel, and lung function includes inspection, palpation, percussion, and auscultation. Use inspection to observe respiratory patterns, signs of respiratory distress, chest structures and movement, skin and mucous membrane color, presence or absence of edema, sputum characteristics, and

overall general appearance. Palpate pulses, skin temperature, heart pulsations through the chest wall, and areas of tenderness. Perform percussion over the lung fields to screen for areas of consolidation or excess air pockets in the lungs. Auscultate breath sounds, heart sounds, and vascular sounds. For a step-by-step discussion of how to assess the heart, lungs, and vascular system,

 Go to Chapter 19, **Procedure 19–12: Assessing the Chest and Lungs,** and **Procedure 19–13: Assessing the Heart and Vascular System,** in Volume 2.

Patients experiencing shortness of breath or difficulty breathing become very anxious. Your assessment must be done quickly. When a patient complains, "I can't breathe," you should be concerned with three questions:

1. How well is the patient ventilating right now?
2. How well are the blood and tissues being oxygenated?
3. What immediate intervention is required?

To answer the first two questions, look for signs of respiratory distress, auscultate breath sounds, and assess for signs of adequate organ and tissue oxygenation. The answers to these questions will determine the type of intervention required. Below we examine a variety of focused physical assessments.

Breathing Patterns

Assess for normal and altered breathing patterns. They include the following: eupnea, tachypnea, bradypnea, apnea, Kussmaul's breathing, Biot's breathing, and Cheyne-Stokes respirations. These patterns are defined in Table 17–2. Also,

 Go to Chapter 35, **Technique 35–1: Assessing Respiratory Patterns,** in Volume 2.

Recall that pain alters the rate and depth of respirations. Often patients in pain breathe shallowly and are at risk for atelectasis. Regularly assess all patients for pain. Once you have medicated the patient, reassess breath sounds, and encourage the patient to cough and breathe deeply.

Cough

Everyone coughs from time to time to remove small amounts of mucus and debris from the airways. Coughing is a normal protective response to known respiratory irritants (e.g., cigarette smoke, irritating fumes, dust particles) or when food or fluid accidentally gets into the airways. A cough becomes significant

---

BOX 35-2 Significance of Sputum Appearance and Odor

Color/appearance	Significance
White or clear	Usually present in viral infections (e.g., common cold, viral bronchitis), often requiring only supportive care.
Yellow or green	A sign of infection.
Black	Caused by coal dust, smoke, or soot inhalation.
Rust colored	Associated with pneumococcal pneumonia, tuberculosis, and possibly the presence of blood.
Hempotysis	The coughing up of blood or bloody sputum. It may range from small streaks of blood to large amounts of frank blood.
Pink and frothy	Associated with pulmonary edema.

Foul-smelling sputum usually indicates bacterial infection (e.g., pneumonia, lung abscess).

---

if it persists, is recurring, or is productive. A persistent or recurring cough may indicate ongoing or recurring airway irritation. Advise patients to obtain medical evaluation for a cough that lasts more than 3 weeks and cannot be explained.

- *Assess for signs and symptoms associated with a cough.* This helps determine its cause. A cough associated with nasal congestion, sneezing, or watery eyes or nose discharge is most likely due to allergies and may be successfully treated with over-the-counter remedies. A cough occurring with fever, chest congestion, noisy breath sounds, and sputum production is more likely to be due to an upper respiratory tract infection, which may require antibiotics. A cough associated with dyspnea, chest tightness, and wheezing may be due to an airway obstruction disorder such as asthma, which requires corticosteroids and bronchodilating medications.

- *Assess sputum appearance, color, and odor.* A cough is described as **productive** if it raises sputum (mucus and debris) up from the airways. Sputum appearance and odor provide valuable clues about the cause and significance of a cough (see Box 35–2).

- *Assess sputum amount.* The amount of sputum can vary from a teaspoon to pints. In general, sputum production increases with the severity of the underlying condition. However, limited sputum production does not always indicate a minor problem, because

excess mucus and debris may be trapped in the airways and the patient unable to raise it. Nursing measures discussed later in the chapter are aimed at helping loosen and mobilize pulmonary secretions.

- *Assess sputum timing.* Sputum production ranges from constant to once per day. Tobacco smokers often have a "morning cough," which helps clear their airways of mucus and debris accumulated overnight. They may not realize that this is a result of long-term lung irritation and damage and is not a normal occurrence for everyone. In contrast, someone with an upper respiratory tract infection is more likely to produce sputum throughout the day.

- *Obtain sputum samples.* Laboratory examination of sputum is a valuable diagnostic tool. Sputum samples are examined microscopically and cultured in the lab to identify organisms and test for sensitivity to different anti-infective agents. You may be responsible for collecting sputum specimens. For a summary of this procedure, see the Critical Aspects box. For the complete steps,

 Go to Chapter 35, **Procedure 35–1: Collecting a Sputum Specimen,** in Volume 2.

Respiratory Effort

A healthy person breathes effortlessly. A patient experiencing shortness of breath or dyspnea requires a thorough assessment. However, you must take care not to increase his respiratory effort. Use closed questions the patient can answer with yes, no, or only a few words. Ask whether the shortness of breath began suddenly or gradually, how severe it is right now, and whether it is getting better or worse. At the same time, observe for the signs of increased respiratory effort discussed below. Note that these signs are most easy visible in infants and small children.

- **Nasal flaring** is the visible enlargement of the nostrils with inhalation. It helps reduce resistance to airflow in the nose and keep the nasal passages open to take in more air.

- Head bobbing (i.e., the neck flexes and the head bobs forward with each inhalation) is a sign of difficulty inhaling air.

- **Retractions** are the visible "sinking in" of intercostal, supraclavicular, and subcostal tissue, caused by excessive negative pressures generated in the chest to try to increase the depth of inhalation.

- Use of accessory muscles during inspiration. The patient may use the intercostals, abdominal muscles, and muscles of the neck and shoulders when there is an increased demand for oxygen or problems with ventilation.

- Grunting reflects involuntary muscle contraction during expiration to help keep alveoli open and enhance gas exchange.

- Body positioning to facilitate respirations. The patient usually finds upright posture the most comfortable. In the upright position, gravity pulls the abdominal organs down and allows the diaphragm more room to contract. Most patients with dyspnea cannot tolerate lying down. **Orthopnea** is the term used to describe difficulty breathing when lying down. Ask how the patient usually sleeps. Some patients may report sleeping in a recliner or chair.

- Ask about **paroxysmal nocturnal dyspnea (PND),** sudden awakening due to shortness of breath that begins during sleep. The patient feels panic and extreme dyspnea and must sit upright to ease breathing.

- Observe for **conversational dyspnea,** the inability to speak complete sentences without stopping to breathe. The more frequently the patient pauses when speaking, the more severe the dyspnea.

- Listen for the sounds of respiratory distress. **Stridor** is a high-pitched, harsh, crowing, inspiratory sound caused by partial obstruction of the larynx or trachea. You can hear it without a stethoscope. Common causes are croup, acute epiglottis, vocal cord edema, and lodged foreign bodies. Partial airway obstruction can easily become complete airway obstruction. Therefore the patient with stridor needs immediate care.

  Wheezing is a musical sound produced by air passing through partially obstructed small airways. It is often heard in patients with asthma and lung congestion. Diminished or absent breath sounds in a patient experiencing dyspnea are signs of worsening ventilation and oxygenation. Oxygen therapy and measures to restore adequate ventilation may be required. These therapies are discussed in the interventions section of this chapter.

KnowledgeCheck 35–9

- What areas should you include in a nursing history for a patient with oxygenation concerns who is undergoing a comprehensive assessment?
- When is a cough significant? What aspects of a cough should be assessed?
- Identify at least five signs that you may observe in a patient experiencing dyspnea.
- A patient has a respiratory rate of 30 that is rhythmic and moderate in depth. What term would you use to describe this breathing pattern?

 Go to Chapter 35, **Knowledge Check Response Sheet and Answers,** on the Electronic Study Guide.

critical aspects of procedures 35–1 through 35–12

 For steps to follow in *all* procedures, refer to the inside back cover of Volume 2.

Procedure 35–1A: Obtaining an Expectorated Specimen

- Position the patient in high or semi-Fowler's position.

- Caution the patient not to touch the inside of the sterile container or lid.

- Instruct the patient to breathe deeply for three or four breaths, then expectorate the specimen with a deep cough.

- Label the specimen container with the name of the patient, the test, and the collection date and time.

- Place the specimen in a plastic bag labeled with a biohazard label. Follow agency policy.

- Send the specimen to the laboratory immediately. If specimen transport is delayed, consult the lab; refrigeration may be required.

Procedure 35–1B: Obtaining a Specimen by Suction

- Position the patient in high or semi-Fowler's position.

- Don protective eyewear.

- Attach the suction tubing to the male adapter of the inline sputum specimen container.

- Don sterile gloves.

- Attach the sterile suction catheter to the rubber tubing on the inline sputum specimen container.

- Lubricate the suction catheter with sterile saline solution.

- Insert the tip of the suction catheter gently through the nasopharynx, endotracheal tube, or tracheostomy tube. Advance the tip into the trachea (see Procedure 35–6 or Procedure 35–7).

- When the patient begins coughing, apply suction for 5 to 10 seconds to collect the specimen.

- If an adequate specimen (5 to 10 mL) is not obtained, allow the patient to rest for 1 minute, and then repeat the procedure. Administer oxygen to the patient at this time, if indicated.

- When an adequate specimen is collected, discontinue suction, and gently remove the suction catheter.

- Label the specimen container with the name of the patient, the test, and the collection date and time.

- Place the specimen in a plastic bag labeled with a biohazard label. Follow agency policy.

- Send the specimen to the laboratory immediately. If specimen transport is delayed, consult the lab; refrigeration may be required.

Procedure 35–2: Monitoring Pulse Oximetry (Arterial Oxygen Saturation)

- Choose a sensor that is appropriate for the patient's age, size, and weight and for the desired location.

- Attach the probe sensor to the site. Make sure that the photodetector and light-emitting diodes on the probe sensor face each other.

- Connect the sensor probe to the oximeter, and turn it on.

- Read the SaO_2 measurement on the digital display when it reaches a constant value, usually in 10 to 30 seconds.

- Set and turn on the alarm limits for SaO_2 and pulse rate, according to the manufacturer's instructions, patient condition, and agency policy if continuous monitoring is necessary.

- Remove the probe sensor, and turn off the oximeter.

Procedure 35–3: Applying and Caring for a Patient with a Cardiac Monitor

- Expose the patient's chest, and identify electrode sites based on the monitoring system and the patient's anatomy.

- With an alcohol pad, clean the areas where electrodes will be placed, and allow them to dry.

- Gently rub the placement sites with a washcloth or gauze pad until the skin reddens slightly.

- Remove the electrode backing, and make sure the gel is moist.

- Apply the electrodes to the sites by pressing firmly.

- Check the patient's ECG tracing on the monitor. If necessary, adjust the gain on the monitor to increase the waveform size.

- Set the upper and lower heart rate alarm limits according to agency policy, and turn them on.

- Obtain a rhythm strip by pressing the "record" button.

Procedure 35–4: Performing Percussion, Vibration, and Postural Drainage

- Help the patient assume the appropriate position based on the lung field that requires drainage.

- Keep the patient in the desired position for 10 to 15 minutes.

- Using cupped hands, perform percussion over the affected lung area for 1 to 3 minutes while the patient is in the desired drainage position.

- Next, perform vibration.

Procedure 35–4: *(continued)*

- Assist the patient to sit up. Have him cough at the end of a deep inspiration to clear the airways of secretions.

- Repeat postural drainage, percussion, and vibration for each lung field that requires treatment. The entire treatment should not exceed 60 minutes.

- Provide mouth care.

Procedure 35–5: Administering Oxygen by Cannula, Face Mask, or Face Tent

- Attach the flow meter to the wall oxygen source.

- Assemble and apply the oxygen equipment according to the device prescribed (nasal cannula, face mask, or face tent).

- Turn on the oxygen using the flow meter, and adjust it according to the prescribed flow rate.

- Make sure that the oxygen equipment is set up correctly and functioning properly before you leave the patient's bedside.

Procedure 35–6: Performing Tracheostomy Care

- No formal recommendation can be made about wearing sterile rather than clean gloves when performing endotracheal care according to the Centers for Disease Control (Tablan, Anderson, Besser, Bridges, and Hajjeh, 2004).

- Position the patient in semi-Fowler's position.

- Suction the tracheostomy (see Procedure 35–9).

- Place the tracheostomy care equipment on the overbed table, and prepare the equipment, using sterile or modified sterile technique, depending on agency policy.

- Remove the oxygen source, if the patient is receiving supplemental oxygen.

- Remove the inner cannula with your nondominant hand, and dispose of it (if it is a disposable cannula) or clean it (if it is a reusable cannula).

- Attach the oxygen source to the outer cannula, if possible.

- Clean the stoma under the faceplate with the cotton-tipped applicators saturated with hydrogen peroxide or half-strength hydrogen peroxide.

- Clean the top surface of the faceplate and the skin around it with the gauze pads saturated with hydrogen peroxide or half-strength hydrogen peroxide.

- Clean areas using the cotton-tipped applicators and gauze pads saturated with normal saline solution.

- Dry the skin around the faceplate and stoma with dry sterile gauze.

- Remove soiled tracheostomy stablizers.

- Have the patient flex his neck, and apply new tracheostomy stabilizers.

- Insert a precut, sterile tracheostomy dressing under the faceplate and new tracheostomy stabilizers.

Procedure 35–7: Performing Oropharyngeal and Nasopharygeal Suctioning

- Position the patient in semi-Fowler's position, with the face turned toward you for oropharyngeal suctioning or the neck hyperextended for nasopharyngeal suctioning.

- Turn on the suction and adjust the pressure regulator according to agency policy (typically 100 to 120 mm Hg for adults, 95 to 110 mm Hg for children, and 50 to 95 mm Hg for infants).

- Prepare the suction equipment. If you are using the nasal approach, open the water-soluble lubricant.

- Pick up the suction catheter with your dominant hand, and attach it to the connection tubing.

- Approximate the depth the suction catheter should be inserted.

- Remove the oxygen delivery device.

- If the patient's oxygen saturation is less than 94%, or if he is in any distress, you may need to administer supplemental oxygen before, during, and after suctioning (see Procedure 35–5).

- Lubricate and insert the suction catheter into the mouth or naris.

- Gently advance the catheter the premeasured distance into the pharynx.

- Place a finger over the suction control port of the catheter to engage the suction.

- Apply suction while you withdraw the catheter, using a continuous rotating motion.

- After you withdraw the catheter, clear it by placing the tip into the container of sterile saline and applying suction.

- Lubricate the catheter, and repeat suctioning as needed, allowing 20-second intervals between suctioning.

- Dispose of equipment in a biohazard receptacle.

Procedure 35–8: Performing Orotracheal and Nasotracheal Suctioning

- Position the patient in semi-Fowler's position.

- Turn on the wall suction or portable suction machine, and adjust the pressure regulator according to agency policy (typically 100 to 120 mm Hg for adults, 95 to 110 mm Hg for children, and 50 to 95 mm Hg for infants).

- Prepare the suction equipment. If you are using the nasal approach, open the water-soluble lubricant.

- Don sterile glove(s).

▶

Procedure 35–8: *(continued)*

- Pick up the suction catheter with your dominant hand, and attach it to the connection tubing.

- Approximate the depth the suction catheter should be inserted.

- Insert the catheter in the nose or mouth, and advance it to the pharynx.

- Advance the catheter from the pharynx to the trachea by passing the catheter when the patient inhales.

- Place a finger over the suction control port of the catheter.

- Apply suction while you withdraw the catheter, using a continuous rotating motion. Apply suction for no longer than 10 seconds.

- After you withdraw the catheter, clear it by placing the tip of the catheter into the container of sterile saline and applying suction.

- Lubricate the catheter, and repeat suctioning as needed, allowing intervals of at least 30 seconds between suctioning.

- Replace the oxygen source.

- Coil the suction catheter in your dominant hand. Pull the sterile glove off over the coiled catheter. Discard the glove containing the catheter in a receptacle designated by your agency.

- Dispose of equipment, and make sure new suction supplies are readily available for future suctioning.

- Provide mouth care.

Procedure 35–9: Performing Tracheostomy or Endotracheal Suctioning

- Use sterile, modified sterile, or clean technique, according to agency policy and patient status.

- Position the patient in semi-Fowler's position, unless contraindicated.

- Turn on the wall suction or portable suction machine, and adjust the pressure regulator (typically 100 to 120 mm Hg for adults, 95 to 110 mm Hg for children, and 50 to 95 mm Hg for infants).

- Pick up the suction catheter with your dominant hand, and attach it to the connection tubing. (Consider your dominant hand sterile and your nondominant hand unsterile.)

- Hyperoxygenate the patient according to agency policy and patient need by using the resuscitation bag or the 100% button on the ventilator.

- Insert the suction catheter gently, with suction off, into the endotracheal tube or tracheostomy tube.

- Advance the suction catheter, gently aiming downward and being careful not to force the catheter. Advance the catheter until you meet resistance.

- Apply suction while you withdraw the catheter. Make sure to apply suction for no longer than 10 seconds.

- Repeat suctioning as needed, allowing intervals of at least 30 seconds between suctioning. Make sure to hyperoxygentate the patient between each pass.

- Replace the oxygen source, if you removed the patient from the source during suctioning.

- Provide mouth care.

- Reposition the patient to provide comfort and prevent pressure ulcers.

Procedure 35–9A: Performing Tracheostomy or Endotracheal Suctioning Using Inline Closed Suction Equipment

- Prepare the equipment. You need to perform these steps only once per day:
  - (a) Open the inline suction catheter, using sterile technique.
  - (b) Remove the adapter on the ventilator tubing.
  - (c) Attach the inline suction catheter equipment to the ventilator tubing.
  - (d) Reconnect the adapter on the ventilator tubing.
  - (e) Attach the other end of the inline suction catheter to the connection tubing placed to suction.

- Position the patient in semi-Fowler's position, unless contraindicated.

- Turn on the wall suction or portable suction machine, and adjust the pressure regulator (typically 100 to 120 mm Hg for adults, 95 to 110 mm Hg for children, and 50 to 95 mm Hg for infants).

- Hyperoxygenate the patient according to agency policy.

- Don clean procedure gloves.

- If a lock is present on the suction control port, unlock it.

- Gently insert the suction catheter into the airway by maneuvering the catheter within the sterile sleeve.

- Advance the suction catheter into the airway, being careful not to force the catheter. Advance the catheter until you meet resistance.

- Apply suction while withdrawing the catheter. Make sure to apply suction for no longer than 10 seconds.

- Withdraw the inline suction catheter completely into the sleeve. The indicator line on the catheter should appear through the sleeve.

- Attach the prefilled, 10 mL container of normal saline solution to the saline port located on the inline equipment. Squeeze the 10 mL container of normal saline solution while applying suction. Lock the suction regulator port.

Procedure 35–10: Caring for a Patient on a Mechanical Ventilator

- Prepare the resuscitation bag; keep it at the bedside.

- The respiratory therapy department is responsible for setting up mechanical ventilation in most agencies. If you must assume the responsibility, refer to the manufacturer's instructions.

- Verify ventilator settings with the physician's order.

- Check the ventilator alarm limits. Make sure they are set appropriately.

- Attach the ventilator tubing to the endotracheal tube or tracheostomy tube.

- Prepare the suctioning equipment.

- Check the ventilator tubing frequently for condensation. Drain the condensate into a collection device, or briefly disconnect the patient from the ventilator and empty the tubing into a waste receptacle, according to agency policy. Never drain the condensate into the humidifier.

- Provide the patient with an alternative form of communication, such as a letter board or white board.

- Check ventilator settings regularly.

- Give sedatives or antianxiety drugs as needed; request an order if necessary. Try to determine the cause of anxiety.

- Reposition the patient regularly, being careful not to pull on the ventilator tubing.

- Provide frequent oral care. Moisten the lips with a cool, damp cloth and water-based lubricant.

- Ensure that the call light is always within reach, and answer call light and ventilator alarms promptly.

Procedure 35–11: Caring for the Patient with Chest Tubes (Disposable Water Seal System)

- Obtain and prepare the prescribed drainage system.

- Position the patient according to the indicated insertion site.

- As soon as the chest tube is inserted, attach it to the drainage system using a connector.

- Using sterile technique, wrap petroleum gauze around the chest tube insertion site, and dress the site with two precut sterile drain dressings covered by a large drainage dressing (ABD).

- Secure the dressing in place with 2-inch silk tape, making sure to cover the dressing completely.

- Using the spiral taping technique, wrap 1-inch silk tape around the connections. Wrap from top to bottom and bottom to top.

- If suction is prescribed, attach the suction tubing to the suction source. Alternatively, if suction is not prescribed, leave the suction vent on the drainage system open.

- Prepare the patient for a portable chest x-ray exam.

- Keep emergency supplies at the bedside in the event of tube dislodgement or system failure.

- Maintain the chest tube and drainage system by preventing kinks, ensuring patency of the air vent, and keeping the system below the level of the chest tube.

Procedure 35–12: Performing Cardiopulmonary Resuscitation, One- and Two-Person

- Establish whether the patient is unresponsive. (Shake the patient and shout, "Are you OK?")

- Activate the emergency response system immediately if the patient is an adult. If you are alone and the patient is an infant or child, perform CPR for 1 minute, and then activate the emergency response system.

- Carefully place the patient on a hard surface. Logroll the patient if you suspect a cervical spine injury. If the patient is in a hospital bed, place a CPR board under the patient's back.

- Properly position yourself.

- A—Airway. Open the patient's airway. Use either the head-tilt–chin-lift maneuver or the jaw-thrust maneuver.

- B—Breathing. Check for breathing. (Place your ear over the patient's mouth and nose. Look, listen, and feel for breathing for no longer than 10 seconds.) If the patient is breathing, continue to hold the airway open. If the patient is not breathing, administer two slow breaths.

- C—Circulation. Check for signs of circulation. Use the carotid pulse in adults and children, and the brachial or femoral pulse in infants. Assess for a pulse for 5 to 10 seconds. Also check for other signs of circulation, such as movement.

- If signs of circulation are absent, correctly position your hands and begin chest compressions.

- Continue CPR for four cycles, then reassess pulse.

- Stop CPR if the patient responds, regains an adequate pulse, and begins to breathe; if you are too exhausted to continue; or if signs of death are obvious.

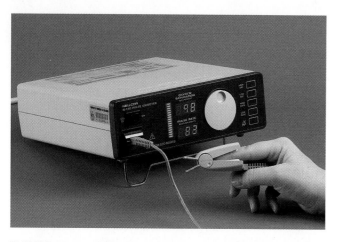

FIGURE 35–8   Pulse oximetry is a noninvasive estimate of arterial blood oxygen saturation (Sao_2). It uses a light-emitting diode (LED) probe to measure light absorption by hemoglobin in the circulating red blood cells.

 CriticalThinking 35–9

Review the patients presented in the "Meet Your Patients" scenario.

- Which patients are experiencing respiratory distress? Identify the signs of distress in these patients.
- Which patients require a comprehensive assessment, and which patients will need a rapid assessment and immediate treatment because of the severity of their symptoms?

Pulse Oximetry

Pulse oximetry is a noninvasive estimate of arterial blood oxygen saturation (Sao_2). **Sao_2** reflects the percentage of hemoglobin molecules carrying oxygen. The normal value is 95 to 100%. Values below 94% are considered abnormal in healthy people and should be investigated to determine the cause. Pulse oximetry works by measuring light absorption by hemoglobin in the circulating red blood cells. Because well-oxygenated hemoglobin and deoxygenated hemoglobin absorb light differently, the oximeter is able to detect this difference and calculate the percentage of oxygenated hemoglobin.

Pulse oximetry is simple to perform, provides a rapid reading, and can be used intermittently or continuously (Figure 35–8). A probe is placed on a part of the body where capillary blood flow is near the surface (e.g., a nail bed, earlobe, nose, or forehead). Be aware that factors such as movement and acrylic fingernails can interfere with the accuracy of the readings. The preceding Critical Aspects box explains the use of pulse oximetry. For the complete procedure,

 Go to Chapter 35, **Procedure 35–2: Monitoring Pulse Oximetry (Arterial Oxygen Saturation)**, in Volume 2.

Also,

 Go to Chapter 35, **Technique 35–2: Tips for Obtaining Accurate Pulse Oximetry Readings**, in Volume 2.

 CriticalThinking 35–10

You hear a pulse oximeter alarm sound in a nearby patient room and find it reading 75%.

- What observations should you make?
- What action should you take?

Diagnostic Testing

Diagnostic testing helps clinicians identify the causes of impaired oxygenation and monitor patient responses to treatment.

 Go to Chapter 35, **Diagnostic Testing: Tests Related to Oxygenation**, in Volume 2.

We discuss several of these tests in the next sections. For additional information on interpreting arterial blood gases, see Chapter 36.

Skin Testing

Skin testing is widely used to detect exposure and antibody formation to the tubercle bacillus. A positive skin test is defined as an area of induration (hardness) at the test site. The size of the induration that indicates a positive result depends on risk factors. Patients with positive tuberculosis (TB) skin tests must undergo further testing (chest x-ray study and sputum cultures) to determine whether they have merely been exposed to disease or whether they have active disease.

 Go to Chapter 35, **Diagnostic Testing: Reading a Tuberculin Skin Result**, in Volume 2.

Allergy testing also uses skin testing to identify antigens that may cause hypersensitivity reactions in susceptible individuals. Testing is performed by scratching antigen samples onto the skin. The area is then observed for allergic skin reactions. Skin testing is performed in facilities with resuscitation equipment and personnel trained in its use, because life-threatening airway obstruction sometimes occurs in response to the allergens.

Arterial Blood Gases

Arterial blood gas (ABG) analysis measures the levels of oxygen and carbon dioxide in arterial blood.

As the name suggests, an artery (usually the brachial, radial, or femoral) is used to obtain the blood sample. Arteries are located deep under the surface of the skin adjacent to nerves, making needle insertion painful. The blood sample may be obtained by arterial puncture or by withdrawal from an arterial line. Nurses in critical care units routinely draw ABGs and monitor patients with invasive arterial monitoring; however, you may care for patients on medical-surgical units, or even outpatients, who will undergo periodic ABG evaluation. ABG analysis measures pH, partial pressure of oxygen (PO_2), partial pressure of carbon dioxide (PCO_2), saturation of oxygen (SaO_2), and bicarbonate (HCO_3) level. Here, we discuss only PO_2 and PCO_2. For full discussion of arterial blood gas values, see Chapter 36.

Measuring Arterial Blood Oxygen

The **PO_2 (partial pressure of oxygen)** is the amount of oxygen available to combine with hemoglobin to form *oxyhemoglobin,* the form in which oxygen is transported through the body. At sea level, the normal range is 80 to 100 mm Hg. After tissues have extracted oxygen from arterial blood and the blood enters the veins to return to the heart, the venous blood PO_2 has fallen to around 40 mm Hg. The SaO_2 (saturation of oxygen) reflects oxygen that is bound to hemoglobin. The SaO_2, along with the PO_2 and hemoglobin level, indicates the degree to which the tissues are receiving oxygen. Small changes in SaO_2 are associated with large changes in PO_2.

 Go to Chapter 35, **Diagnostic Testing: Arterial Blood Gas Values: Evaluating Adequacy of Oxygenation,** in Volume 2.

To fully interpret PO_2 and SaO_2 values, you need to know the percentage of oxygen in the air the patient is inhaling. This is known as the **fraction of inspired oxygen, or FIO_2.** At sea level, atmospheric air (commonly known as *room air*) is 21% oxygen (FIO_2 = 21%). The norms quoted for PO_2 and SaO_2 are based on an FIO_2 of 21%. If a healthy patient receives 100% oxygen for a few minutes, the arterial PO_2 would rise to 500 to 600 mm Hg, and the SaO_2 would remain at 100%. The reason is that the hemoglobin can be "filled" with oxygen only to 100% capacity. When gas exchange is impaired as a result of disease or injury, PO_2 and SaO_2 levels begin to fall. However, they can be kept at normal levels if supplemental oxygen is given.

Measuring Arterial Blood Carbon Dioxide

The **partial pressure of carbon dioxide (PCO_2)** is a measure of the CO_2 dissolved in the blood. Normal arterial PCO_2 is 35 to 45 mm Hg. Carbon dioxide readily diffuses across the alveolar-capillary membrane even in the face of obstacles such as alveolar fluid or thickened membranes. As a result, PCO_2 levels remain normal until a severe disorder interferes with all gas exchange. Once in the alveoli, the amount of carbon dioxide exhaled from the lungs is directly influenced by how well air is moving into and out of the lungs (ventilation).

• *Hypocarbia.* Recall that when a person hyperventilates, he exhales large amounts of CO_2, causing arterial PCO_2 values to fall. Hyperventilation brings more oxygen into the lungs, so unless it is triggered by hypoxemia, oxygen levels (PO_2) usually remain normal.

• *Hypercarbia.* Conversely, in hypoventilation less CO_2 diffuses into the alveoli for exhalation, leaving more CO_2 in the arterial blood; this causes PCO_2 values to rise. High PCO_2 levels have an anesthetic effect on the nervous system and can be toxic. Hypoventilation severe enough to cause hypercarbia is usually associated with hypoxemia because inadequate amounts of oxygen are inhaled.

KnowledgeCheck 35–10

- What does a pulse oximetry reading tell you?
- What is the relationship between arterial PO_2 and SaO_2 levels?
- Identify normal PO_2, SaO_2, and PCO_2 levels.
- What effect does ventilation have on arterial PCO_2?
- How is PCO_2 related to oxygenation?

 Go to Chapter 35, **Knowledge Check Response Sheet and Answers,** on the Electronic Study Guide.

CriticalThinking 35–11

You are caring for two patients, both of whom have a PO_2 of 95 mm Hg and SaO_2 of 99%. Do they have similar lung function? Explain your answer.

Peak Flow Monitoring

Peak expiratory flow rate (PEFR) measures the amount of air that can be exhaled with forcible effort. Patients with asthma use PEFR monitoring to detect subtle changes in their condition often before symptoms occur. A peak flow meter is used to monitor these changes (Figure 35–9). Peak flow is expressed in liters per minute. Patients with asthma are often asked to measure their peak flow daily and with the onset of any symptoms. Treatment protocols describe the use and frequency of medications based on individualized peak flow rates. The Home Care box on page 870 describes self-monitoring with a peak flow meter.

Cardiac Monitoring

Cardiac monitoring is the continuous monitoring of the **electrocardiogram (ECG),** a rendering of the electrical activity of the heart. Electrodes placed on the skin of the chest display a wave-form on a monitor screen or printout. The ECG illustrates electrical activity, but

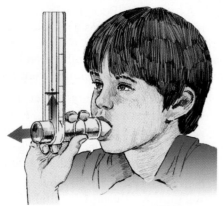

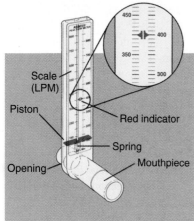

FIGURE 35–9 **A patient with asthma using a peak flow meter to monitor peak expiratory flow rate (PEFR).**

not mechanical activity. In other words, the ECG reflects what the nerves are telling the heart muscle to do, but NOT what the heart muscle is actually doing in response. The purposes of cardiac monitoring are to:

- Identify the patient's baseline rhythm and rate.
- Recognize significant changes in the baseline rhythm and rate.
- Recognize lethal dysrhythmias that require immediate intervention.

The ECG reading illustrates the complete cardiac cycle. Each part of the ECG complex has been given a letter to identify it: **P, Q, R, S** and **T** (Figure 35–6).

- The **P wave** represents the firing of the SA node and conduction of the impulse through the atria. In the healthy heart, this leads to atrial contraction.
- The **QRS complex** represents *ventricular depolarization* and leads to ventricular contraction.
- The **T wave** represents the return of the ventricles to an electrical resting state so they can be stimulated again (*ventricular repolarization*). The atria also repolarize, but they do so during the time of

Home Use of a Peak Flow Meter

People with asthma are often asked to monitor their peak flow readings at home and to compare their current readings to their baseline "personal best."

- Teach patients that to get an accurate reading, they need to take a deep breath and forcefully exhale.

- Teach patients to take a series of three readings and record the highest reading.

- Teach patients to maintain or adjust their medication use according to their highest reading. They should follow the color-coded treatment protocols prescribed by their physician. These are individualized for each patient. Notice that these correspond to the color-coded markers on their peak flow meter.

> *Green: Baseline peak flow—***Peak flow is within 85% of personal best baseline.**

Treatment protocol calls for routine medication use.

> *Yellow: 15 to 50% reduction in peak flow—***This reading signals the onset of airway changes.**

Treatment protocols usually specify an increase in the dosage of maintenance medications, use of rescue therapies (e.g., fast-acting bronchodilators), or a call to the healthcare provider. These measures are designed to reverse acute exacerbations before they become severe.

> *Red: Severe reduction in peak flow—***This reading signals a reduction of more than 50% of personal best baseline.**

Treatment protocols usually specify immediate treatment with rescue medications and to seek emergency treatment if symptoms do not improve.

ventricular depolarization; thus, they are obscured by the QRS complex and cannot be seen on the ECG complex.

Dysrhythmias are abnormal heart rhythms. Dysrhythmias can be broadly categorized as *tachydysrhythmias* (rates greater than 100 beats per minute), *bradydysrhythmias* (rates less than 60 beats per minute), or *ectopy* (extra beats). Within each category, dysrhythmias can be further classified by their site of origin, which includes *supraventricular* (above the ventricles), *junctional* (within the AV node), or *ventricular* (in the ventricles). All dysrhythmias have the potential to decrease cardiac output, resulting in

hypotension and tissue hypoxia. Skill in identifying cardiac rhythms (both normal and abnormal) requires study and experience and is beyond the scope of this chapter. However, the Critical Aspects box highlights activities involved with the care of a patient on a cardiac monitor. For the complete procedure,

VOL 2 Go to Chapter 35, **Procedure 35–3: Applying and Caring for a Patient with a Cardiac Monitor,** in Volume 2.

Twelve-Lead Electrocardiogram

Continuous monitoring, which uses electrodes attached to the chest, detects a single view of the heart. In contrast, a standard 12-lead electrocardiogram can provide 12 views of the electrical activity of the heart, like a camera that takes pictures from various angles. Electrodes are placed on each of the four limbs, and six electrodes are placed on the chest (Figure 35–10). The 12-lead ECG analyzes the electrical activity between various lead combinations. If a portion of the heart muscle is damaged, the lead(s) capturing the activity in the damaged area will illustrate this damage as an altered complex. A small section of the view from each lead is printed on one sheet of paper so that all 12 views can be compared (Figure 35–11). If you work in cardiovascular nursing, you will develop skill in 12-lead ECG interpretation.

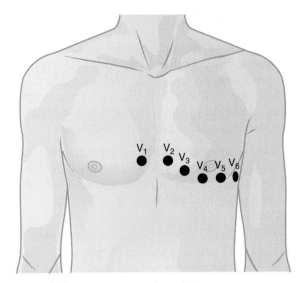

FIGURE 35–10   Chest lead placements for a 12-lead ECG.

KnowledgeCheck 35–11

- What does the P wave, QRS complex, and T wave of an ECG complex represent?
- How is a 12-lead ECG different from continuous cardiac monitoring?

Go to Chapter 35, **Knowledge Check Response Sheet and Answers,** on the Electronic Study Guide.

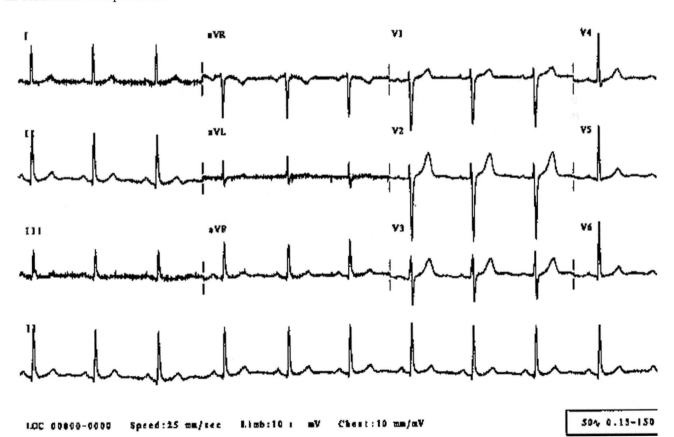

LOC 00000-0000   Speed:25 mm/sec   Limb:10 mV   Chest:10 mm/mV   50~ 0.15-150

FIGURE 35–11   A normal 12-lead ECG tracing.

| Nursing Diagnosis |

Alterations in oxygenation can be nursing diagnoses, etiologies of other problems, or merely symptoms of other problems. In analyzing the assessment data, you must determine which. For example, suppose a patient is breathing shallowly and slowly. The nursing diagnosis might be one of the following:

- *Ineffective Breathing Pattern (hypoventilation)* related to pain secondary to rib fractures. In this case, you would provide pain relief; the desired outcome is that the patient will have effective (normal) ventilation.

- *Ineffective Tissue Perfusion (Cerebral)* related to Ineffective Breathing Pattern (hypoventilation), as manifested by slurred speech and drowsiness. In this case, you would address the etiology by administering oxygen; the desired outcome would be effective cerebral perfusion, evidenced by normal speech and alertness.

- *Ineffective Tissue Perfusion (Cerebral)* related to edema from head trauma, as manifested by Ineffective Breathing Pattern (hypoventilation). In this situation, you would, of course, support ventilation until the problem subsides. However, the primary interventions would be directed toward the edema and head trauma. Once these etiologies were corrected, the hypoventilation would disappear. The goal would be effective cerebral perfusion, evidenced by normal breathing pattern.

Problems of Ventilation and Gas Exchange

Five NANDA diagnoses directly describe problems with ventilation and gas exchange. Use these diagnoses when they are the central problem and you intend to use interventions to eliminate the cause of the problem. For further discussion of these diagnoses,

 Go to Chapter 35, **Standardized Language, Nursing Diagnoses Associated with Impaired Ventilation and Gas Exchange,** in Volume 2.

- *Ineffective Airway Clearance* is the inability to maintain a clear airway. The main mechanism for keeping airways open is a strong cough that moves secretions into the throat to be expectorated or swallowed.

- *Ineffective Breathing Pattern* is used to describe inadequate ventilation, such as hypoventilation, hyperventilation, tachypnea, or bradypnea.

- *Impaired Gas Exchange* is the appropriate diagnosis if the patient is adequately ventilating but diffusion across the alveolar-capillary membrane is impaired. The NANDA definition specifies "excess or deficit in oxygenation and/or CO_2 elimination at the alveolar-capillary membrane" (NANDA International, 2005, p. 82). Although ABG analysis is the most accurate way to detect Impaired Gas Exchange, you will be called on to assess adequacy of gas exchange without having this information available.

- *Impaired Spontaneous Ventilation* describes a condition in which a patient, as a result of decreased energy reserves, is unable to maintain breathing adequate to support life. This situation requires collaborative emergency intervention, including resuscitation and mechanical ventilation.

- *Dysfunctional Ventilatory Weaning Response* represents a specific situation in which a patient who is being mechanically ventilated cannot adjust to lower levels of ventilator support, prolonging the ventilatory weaning process. Etiologies may be psychological (e.g., anxiety), situational (e.g., low nurse-to-patient ratio), or physiological (e.g., uncontrolled pain).

Problems of Circulation

Several nursing diagnoses address impaired circulation and tissue or organ hypoxia. They are briefly discussed below. For additional information,

 Go to Chapter 35, **Standardized Language, Nursing Diagnoses Associated with Impaired Circulation,** in Volume 2.

- *Decreased Cardiac Output* is the appropriate diagnosis when the heart is unable to pump adequate amounts of blood to meet the metabolic demands of the body. Definitive interventions for this problem are collaborative.

- *Ineffective Tissue Perfusion (Renal, Cerebral, Cardiopulmonary, Gastrointestinal, or Peripheral)* is appropriate for a patient experiencing poor perfusion to an organ or tissue, specifically, for a patient experiencing organ dysfunction rather than the overall effects of poor circulation that is evident with decreased cardiac output.

Impaired Oxygenation as Etiology

The following are examples of problems that are caused by impaired oxygenation:

- Activity Intolerance due to dyspnea or imbalance between oxygen supply and demand

- Risk for Activity Intolerance related to decreased oxygen-carrying capacity of the blood secondary to anemia

- Acute Pain related to chest trauma or chest wall pain

- Anxiety related to shortness of breath
- Disturbed Sleep Pattern due to dyspnea, orthopnea, or agitation from respiratory medications
- Fatigue related to impaired gas exchange
- Fear related to frequent episodes of dyspnea
- Ineffective Coping related to hospitalization for oxygenation impairment
- Ineffective Health Maintenance related to tobacco use
- Chronic Low Self-Esteem or Situational Low Self-Esteem related to impaired role performance secondary to chronic or acute respiratory illness
- Risk for Aspiration related to decreased level of consciousness, medications, or swallowing difficulties
- Risk for Infection related to chronic lung disease, tracheal intubation, or impaired cough
- Social Isolation related to inability to attend usual activities because of frequent respiratory illness

| Planning Outcomes/Evaluation |

Associated NOC standardized outcomes and evaluation criteria related to oxygenation are included in the Cardiopulmonary class of NOC Domain II: Physiologic Health. NOC outcomes that are appropriate for patients with oxygenation problems include the following: Blood Loss Severity, Cardiac Pump Effectiveness, Circulation Status, Mechanical Ventilation Weaning Response: Adult, Respiratory Status: Airway Patency, Respiratory Status: Gas Exchange, Respiratory Status: Ventilation, Tissue Perfusion (Abdominal Organs, Cardiac, Peripheral, Pulmonary), and Vital Signs.

Individualized goals/outcome statements depend on the nursing diagnosis you identify. For diagnoses related to gas exchange or circulation, the following are examples of goals you might write:

- Expectorates secretions effectively.
- No dyspnea or shortness of breath.
- Symmetrical chest expansion.
- Lungs clear; no adventitious sounds present.
- Respiratory rate and rhythm within normal limits for patient.
- Heart rate in expected range.
- Brisk capillary refill.
- Normal skin color (no pallor or cyanosis).

| Planning Interventions/Implementation |

Associated NIC standardized interventions related to oxygenation are found in NIC Domain 2: Physiological Interventions: Complex. They are further subdivided into the subcategories Respiratory Management and Tissue Perfusion Management. Respiratory Management interventions focus on maintaining a patent airway and promoting gas exchange. Tissue Perfusion Management focuses on optimizing circulation. For examples of NOC outcomes and NIC interventions for selected oxygenation nursing diagnoses,

 Go to Chapter 35, **Standardized Language, Examples of NOC Outcomes and NIC Interventions Linked to Oxygenation Diagnoses,** in Volume 2.

These provide a general care planning guide. Depending on individual patient needs, other NOC outcomes or NIC interventions may also be appropriate.

Specific nursing interventions for patients with oxygenation problems address ventilation, gas exchange, and circulation. These interventions are discussed below.

Promoting Optimal Respiratory Function

Deep, regular breathing promotes ventilation and optimizes gas exchange. Other interventions to promote optimal function include disease screening and prevention, positioning, incentive spirometry, and preventing aspiration.

Perform Immunizations and Screening

Measures to prevent or minimize the impact of disease on respiratory function include immunizations for influenza and pneumonia and screening for tuberculosis.

Influenza immunizations are developed annually to closely match the major known strains of the virus that have evolved. An immunization given to a healthy young adult is 70 to 80% effective. Though less effective in preventing the disease in older adults, immunization decreases the severity and complications of the disease by 50 to 60% and the incidence of death by 80% (Allender & Spradley, 2001). Adults aged 65 years and older, people with respiratory diseases or suppressed immune systems, residents in congregate living conditions (e.g., mental and correctional facilities), and healthcare workers are encouraged to receive influenza immunization annually. The federal government has set a goal that 90% of these risk groups will be vaccinated annually against influenza by 2010 (U.S. Department of Health and Human Services, 2000).

Pneumonia is a leading cause of infectious death in the United States, with a mortality rate of approximately 50% in people over age 65. Therefore, people who are most susceptible should be immunized against pneumonia annually. This includes people over age 65 and those who have chronic disease, compromised immune system, or conditions involving the lower respiratory tract. The immunization is not effective for children under age 2 years and is not routinely administered to healthy people between 2 and

65 years of age. In this healthy population, measures to prevent the spread of respiratory infections are the most effective means of preventing pneumonia (Allender & Spradley, 2001).

The recommendation for annual pneumonia immunizations is somewhat controversial. Historically this vaccine was thought to convey lifetime immunity, but recent data illustrate that this may not be so. As a result, the vaccine is recommended every year for high-risk groups. In light of the current controversy, look for updates on this recommendation (Lackner, Hamilton, Hill, Davy, & Guay, 2003).

Tuberculosis screening (skin testing) is recommended annually for low-income populations, residents in congregate living conditions, immigrants from countries with a high prevalence of TB, and healthcare workers. For it to be effective, you must administer the antigen intradermally, not subcutaneously. Read the test site 48 to 72 hours after administration. For interpreting test results,

 Go to Chapter 35, **Diagnostic Testing: Reading a Tuberculin Skin Test Result,** in Volume 2.

Prevent Upper Respiratory Infections

Teach clients measures for preventing upper respiratory infections (URIs). Many URIs, including the common cold, are caused by viruses and are not cured by antibiotics. Although URIs are usually self-limiting, they may lead to other respiratory diseases and seriously compromised oxygenation in children, older adults, and people who have other illnesses. For teaching tips, see the box Self-Care: Teaching Patients to Prevent URIs, in Chapter 41.

Position for Maximum Ventilation

Position affects ventilation. An upright or elevated position pulls abdominal organs down, allowing maximum diaphragm excursion and lung expansion.

- If the patient is short of breath, provide an overbed table so the patient can lean forward on it.
- When the patient is lying on her side, provide pillows to support the upper arm.
- Assist with frequent position changes to keep all areas of lungs well ventilated, and ambulate as often as possible without creating fatigue.

Teach and Assist with Incentive Spirometry

Incentive spirometers are designed to encourage patients to take deep breaths by reaching a goal-directed volume of air. Incentive spirometry is usually reserved for patients at risk for developing atelectasis or pneumonia, such as patients who have had abdominal,

chest, or pelvic surgery, patients on prolonged bedrest, or patients with a history of respiratory problems. Incentive spirometers offer various visual cues (such as elevation of a ball or piston) to show patients whether they are inhaling deeply enough. You can delegate incentive spirometry coaching to LPNs and qualified unlicensed assistive personnel (UAPs). However, as the RN, you are responsible for ensuring that incentive spirometry is carried out correctly, and at required frequencies, for evaluating patient responses, airway clearance, and ventilation. See Figure 37–7 and the box Self-Care: Teaching Your Patient About Incentive Spirometery, in Chapter 37.

Take Aspiration Precautions

Aspiration is a risk for patients with a decreased level of consciousness, diminished gag or cough reflex, or difficulty with swallowing. You should keep a suction setup available for routine and emergency use. Preventing aspiration requires you to have practical knowledge about positioning, enteral and oral feedings, and administering medications. For guidelines to use with at-risk patients,

 Go to Chapter 35, **Technique 35–3: Guidelines for Preventing Aspiration,** in Volume 2.

Many of the guidelines involve basic care and can be delegated to qualified LPNs and UAPs. You are responsible for monitoring for aspiration. Record in the nurse's notes any preventive measures taken.

KnowledgeCheck 35–12

Identify at least three nursing interventions to promote optimal respiratory function in a hospitalized patient with chronic lung disease.

 Go to Chapter 35, **Knowledge Check Response Sheet and Answers,** on the Electronic Study Guide.

CriticalThinking 35–12

- Review the "Meet Your Patients" scenario. For which of these patients should you recommend annual flu or pneumonia immunizations? Why?
- A 24-year-old nursing student has no previous hospitalizations or known chronic health problems, takes no medications, and has no current respiratory symptoms. On routine purified protein derivative, or PPD, testing (tuberulin skin testing), the student has an area of induration measuring 5 mm. How would you interpret these results?

Mobilizing Secretions

Coughing promotes deep inhalation and forceful expulsion of secretions. Interventions that help enhance

coughing and mobilize secretions include deep breathing, coughing exercises, and hydration.

Teach Deep Breathing and Coughing

Deep breathing promotes ventilation and gas exchange. Coughing after deep breathing mobilizes secretions, which keeps airways and alevoli open and provides greater surface area for gas exchange. For information about teaching patients to deep-breathe,

 Go to Chapter 35, **Procedure 37–1: Collecting a Sputum Specimen,** in Volume 2.

Alter this procedure for patients with chronic lung disease. Have the patient exhale through pursed lips and cough throughout expiration in several short bursts to avoid high expiratory pressures, which collapse diseased airways.

Maintain Hydration

The following activities are important to keep pulmonary secretions thin and mobile:

- *Maintain systemic hydration.* Encourage oral fluid intake as much as possible. Supplement oral intake by intravenous fluid administration if the patient cannot ingest adequate amounts of fluid.

- *Humidify inhaled air.* You can accomplish this with humidification devices or nebulizers. A **nebulizer** is a device that turns liquids into an aerosol mist that can be inhaled directly into the lungs. Nebulizers are often used to deliver medications to the lungs, but they can also be used to deliver moisture to the airways and lungs. See "Administering Respiratory Inhalations" in Chapter 23, and Figure 23–19. Also,

 Go to Chapter 35, **Technique 35–4: Oxygen Therapy Safety Precautions,** in Volume 2.

Humidifiers are also used to keep secretions thin and mobile. A **humidifier** is a device that delivers small water droplets from a reservoir. Small humidifiers filled with sterile distilled water are attached to oxygen delivery systems to moisten the dry oxygen.

Perform Chest Physiotherapy

Chest physiotherapy moves secretions to the large, central airways for expectoration or suctioning. It involves postural drainage, chest percussion, and chest vibration. These procedures are briefly discussed below and in the Critical Aspects box. For detailed discussion,

 Go to Chapter 35, **Procedure 35–4: Performing Percussion, Vibration, and Postural Drainage,** in Volume 2.

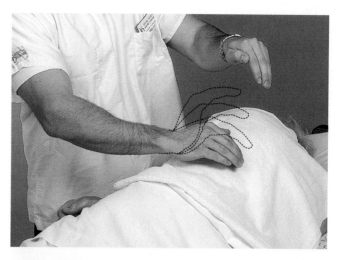

FIGURE 35–12   Chest percussion is the rhythmic clapping of the chest wall using cupped hands.

- *Postural drainage* is the use of positioning to promote drainage from the lungs. Check chest x-ray results to see what segments of the lungs are affected. With this information, you can plan your treatment. Postural drainage uses gravity to drain the lungs; therefore, you will place the affected area in an uppermost position so that secretions will drain down toward the large, central airways. For example, if the patient has pneumonia of the right lower lobe, you would place her on her left side and elevate the foot of the bed. This position allows the right lower lobe to drain.

- *Chest percussion and chest vibration* are used in conjunction with postural drainage. Have the patient assume the desired position for 10 to 15 minutes. Then percuss and vibrate to loosen and mobilize the secretions. **Chest percussion** is the rhythmic clapping of the chest wall using cupped hands (Figure 35–12). **Chest vibration** is the vibration of the chest wall with the palms of the hands (Figure 35–13). Vibration is a gentle procedure, so you can use it in frail patients

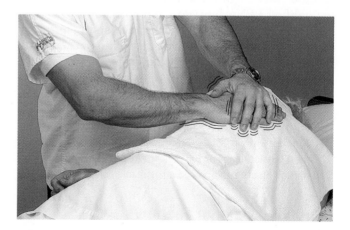

FIGURE 35–13   Chest vibration is the vibration of the chest wall with the palms of the hands.

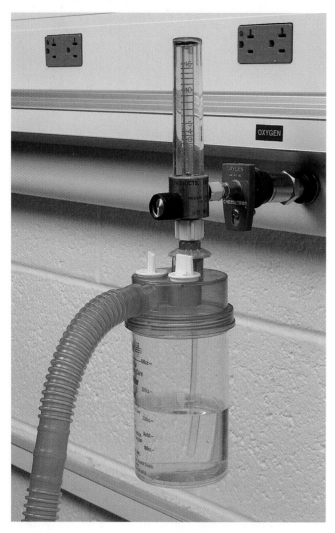

FIGURE 35–14 Healthcare facilities usually have oxygen available through wall outlets connected to a large central tank of oxygen.

who cannot tolerate percussion. If one is available, you may wish to use a vibrating machine instead of the palms of your hands.

You can delegate chest physiotherapy techniques to qualified LPNs, but you are responsible for assessing and monitoring airway clearance and respiratory status. In many institutions, respiratory therapists routinely perform chest physiotherapy.

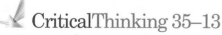 CriticalThinking 35–13

Your patient has pneumonia in the right lower lobe. She is mildly dyspneic with any activity. Strategize how you would perform chest physiotherapy on this patient. What activities would you consider to make this procedure more tolerable for the patient?

Supplying Oxygen Therapy

Oxygen is a medication and requires a physician order for dosage and route. Often agencies have protocols with

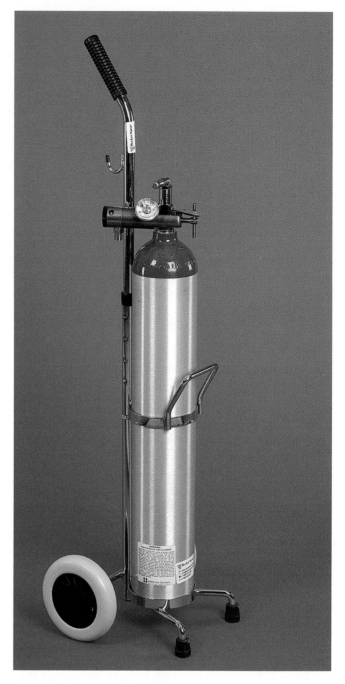

FIGURE 35–15 Portable oxygen tanks come in a variety of sizes.

standing orders for oxygen administration in an emergency. Oxygen is supplied in several different ways.

- *Wall outlets* connected to a large central tank of oxygen are usually provided in healthcare facilities (Figure 35–14).
- *Compressed O₂ in portable tanks* may also be available (Figure 35–15).
- *Liquid oxygen units* are often used for home oxygen therapy (Figure 35–16).
- *Oxygen concentrator.* An oxygen concentrator removes nitrogen from room air and concentrates O_2.

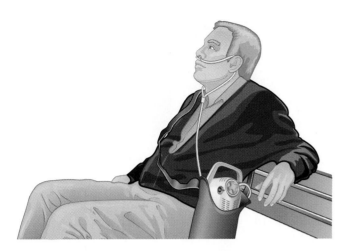

FIGURE 35–16 Liquid oxygen units are small and portable. They are ideal for home use.

It requires a battery pack or electrical outlet for power. Oxygen concentrators can deliver flow up to 4 liters per minute (L/min) to create an F_{IO_2} of approximately 36%. Concentrations are higher at lower flow rates (e.g., an F_{IO_2} of 95% at 1 L/min). These devices eliminate the need for buying oxygen cylinders, relieving clients' anxiety about running out of oxygen. However, they are expensive, noisy, and not portable; moreover, the client must still have backup oxygen in case of a power failure.

An oxygen flow meter must be connected to the oxygen source to control the flow rate of oxygen from its source to the patient. Flow meters are set in liters per minute.

Various devices (e.g., mask, cannula) are used to deliver oxygen to a patient. They differ in the amount of oxygen they can deliver and the degree to which they enclose the patient. The Critical Aspects box summarizes how to set up and apply oxygen therapy. For the complete procedure,

 Go to Chapter 35, **Procedure 35–5: Administering Oxygen by Cannula, Face Mask, or Face Tent,** in Volume 2.

Because oxygen is a medication, its administration is a nursing responsibility. UAPs may assist in maintaining oxygen use (e.g., adjusting the face mask), but you are responsible for monitoring the patient's response to therapy.

Transtracheal Oxygen Delivery

A **tracheostomy** is a direct surgical opening into the trachea through the neck. Inhaled air bypasses the upper airway, which normally warms and moistens air before it reaches the lower airway. Oxygen may be delivered through the tracheostomy via a collar or an adapter. A **transtracheal catheter** is a catheter

placed into the tracheostomy to deliver O_2 directly into the trachea. Because oxygen cannot be humidified through this device, it is rarely used.

Oxygen Hazards

The following risks are associated with oxygen therapy:

- *Oxygen toxicity can develop* when O_2 concentrations of more than 50% are administered for longer than 48 to 72 hours. Prolonged use of high O_2 concentrations reduces surfactant production, which leads to alveolar collapse and reduced lung elasticity.
- *Oxygen supports combustion,* although it does not burn. High concentrations of oxygen will turn a small spark or fire into a large fire. Fire prevention precautions must be used near oxygen delivery systems.

 Go to Chapter 35, **Technique 35-4: Oxygen Therapy Safety Precautions,** in Volume 2.

- *Oxygen tanks contain oxygen under pressure.* If the tank ruptures or falls, compressed oxygen spews from the tank and turns it into an unguided missile. Oxygen tanks have been known to shoot through walls when ruptured. They must be handled carefully, and secured well, to prevent this hazard.

KnowledgeCheck 35–13

- Why is oxygen humidified?
- Which oxygen delivery method is appropriate for the following patients?

    A patient ordered to receive 2 L/min of oxygen

    A patient who complains of being claustrophobic and requires low-flow humidified oxygen

    A patient with chronic obstructive pulmonary disease (COPD) with an order for oxygen at an F_{IO_2} of 24%

    A patient who wants to avoid intubation but requires an F_{IO_2} of 100%

 Go to Chapter 35, **Knowledge Check Response Sheet and Answers,** on the Electronic Study Guide.

Using Artificial Airways

Artificial airways provide an open airway for patients who have or who are at risk for airway obstruction. The most common artificial airways are discussed in the following sections.

Pharyngeal Airways

Pharyngeal airways provide an open air passage by holding the tongue away from the back of the pharynx. When they are properly placed, air can flow around and through them, and suction catheters can be passed through them.

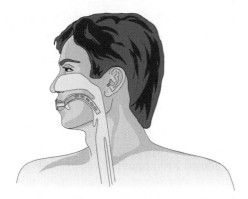

FIGURE 35–17 Oropharyngeal airway in place.

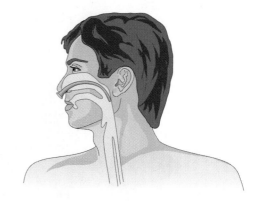

FIGURE 35–18 A nasopharyngeal airway in proper position.

Oropharyngeal airways (Figure 35–17) should be used only in unconscious patients because they are likely to trigger gagging, vomiting, or laryngospasm if airway reflexes are intact. They are C-shaped plastic devices available in infant, pediatric, and adult sizes. To select the appropriate size, hold the airway next to the patient's face. The length of the airway should extend from the front of the teeth to the end of the jawline. If it is *too short,* it will not keep the tongue pulled forward; if it is *too long,* it may push the epiglottis against the laryngeal opening and completely obstruct the airway.

 VOL 2 Go to Chapter 35, **Technique 35-5: Inserting an Oropharyngeal Airway,** in Volume 2.

Nasopharyngeal airways (Figure 35–18) are flexible rubber tubes that are inserted through a nostril into the pharynx. Patients who are semiconscious can tolerate nasal airways because they do not stimulate the gag reflex. They are available in a variety of pediatric and adult sizes. Generally, the larger the internal diameter, the longer the tube. To select the appropriate size, hold the airway next to the patient's face. The length of the airway should extend from the nares to the end of the jawline.

VOL 2 Go to Chapter 35, **Technique 35-6: Inserting a Nasopharyngeal Airway,** in Volume 2.

Endotracheal Airways

Patients who are unable to breathe because of airway obstruction or respiratory failure require airway insertion directly into the trachea. **Endotracheal airways** are pliable tubes inserted into the trachea through the mouth *(orotracheal tube),* nose *(nasotracheal tube),* or an opening directly into the trachea *(tracheostomy tube).* Because they bypass the upper airway, inhaled air is drawn directly into the lower airway without humidification, filtering, or warming. For this reason, devices that warm and humidify inhaled air

are used with endotracheal airways. Figure 35–19*A* illustrates the parts of an endotracheal airway. Figure 35–19*B* shows the placement of an orotracheal tube.

Managing endotracheal and tracheostomy tubes generally requires the expertise of a respiratory therapist or an RN, but you can delegate this activity to specially trained and skilled LPNs, especially in critical care areas. In acute care settings, you should not delegate this activity to unlicensed assistive personnel. However, doing so may be acceptable in long-term

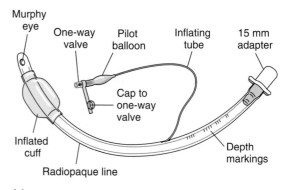

Murphy eye

One-way valve

Pilot balloon

Inflating tube

15 mm adapter

Cap to one-way valve

Inflated cuff

Radiopaque line

Depth markings

(a)

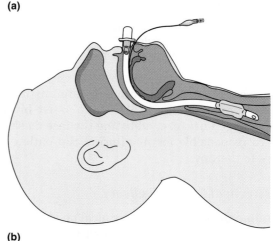

(b)

FIGURE 35–19 *A,* An endotracheal tube. *B,* Placement of an orotracheal tube.

care situations for patients who have healed, permanent tracheostomies. Once the ostomy is well healed, the airway will not collapse if the tracheostomy tube is dislodged; therefore, the UAP, or even the patient, can reinsert it if necessary. Many patients with permanent tracheostomies perform self-care at home.

Nursing responsibilities related to endotracheal airways are to assist in their insertion, maintain stabilization, and provide routine suctioning and management. Insertion of endotracheal airways is within the scope of practice of certain specially trained nurses (e.g., nurse anesthetist). As an RN, you will assist with insertion by gathering equipment and preparing the patient.

On most units, you will find intubation equipment in the resuscitation cart. You will need a laryngoscope, endotracheal tubes of various sizes, water-soluble lubricant, a syringe to inflate the cuff, and tape to secure the tube in place. If a tracheostomy is performed, a surgical tray will be needed to create the direct opening into the trachea.

Intubation is often a hurried procedure, performed in response to a decline in the patient's respiratory function. Remain calm, and explain to the patient that the airway will enable him to breathe effectively. Once the airway is in place, listen to breath sounds to establish that both lungs are ventilated. Reassess breath sounds periodically. After the airway is inserted, record the type and size, as well as the patient's response to the insertion.

 Go to Chapter 35, **Technique 35–7: Caring for Patients with Endotracheal Airways,** in Volume 2.

The Critical Aspects box also summarizes care specifically for patients with a tracheostomy. For the complete procedure,

 Go to Chapter 35, **Procedure 35–6: Performing Tracheostomy Care,** in Volume 2.

KnowledgeCheck 35–14

- In what circumstances would you use an oropharyngeal airway? A nasopharyngeal airway?
- What facts should you record if a patient is intubated?
- Describe seven interventions associated with caring for a patient with an endotracheal tube.

 Go to Chapter 35, **Knowledge Check Response Sheet and Answers,** on the Electronic Study Guide.

Suctioning Airways

Airways are suctioned to remove secretions and maintain patency. Signs that indicate the need for suctioning include gurgling sounds during respiration, restlessness, labored respirations, decreased oxygen

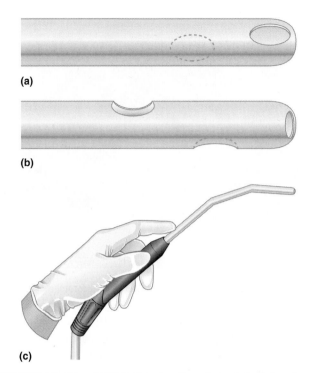

FIGURE 35–20 *A,* Whistle-tipped suction catheter. *B,* Open-tipped suction catheter. *C,* Yankauer (oral) suction tube.

saturation (SaO_2), increased heart and respiratory rates, and adventitious breath sounds on auscultation. Although suctioning the airways helps remove secretions, it also removes air from the airways; thus, each time suction is applied, the patient's O_2 levels diminish. As a result, suctioning must be done quickly and is often accompanied by supplemental oxygen. Suctioning can also irritate mucous membranes if done too frequently.

Suction catheters may be open tipped or "whistle-tipped" (Figure 35–20*A* and *B*). Most suction catheters have a port on the side, over which you place your thumb to control the suction. A Yankauer tube (Figure 35–20*C*) is a rigid device for suctioning the oral cavity.

Airway suctioning is usually performed by RNs and LPNs, but not by unlicensed assistive personnel. UAPs may use a Yankauer tube to suction the oral cavity as part of maintaining hygiene and preventing aspiration of oral secretions.

Oropharyngeal and Nasopharyngeal Suctioning

Pharyngeal suctioning is performed to prevent oral and nasal secretions from entering the lower airway when the patient is too weak to cough up secretions. The patient's condition determines whether you suction the pharynx through the mouth or nose. Most patients find oropharyngeal suctioning more comfortable than the nasal approach. However, if the patient is unable to cooperate and automatically bites down

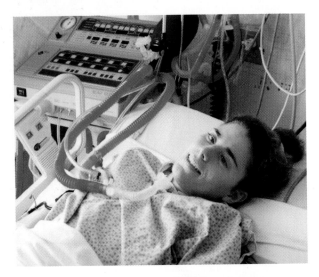

FIGURE 35–21 A patient on a ventilator via tracheosotomy.

when anything is placed in his mouth, use a nasal approach. To suction the pharynx you must first estimate the distance to which you will advance the catheter. Suctioning the pharynx triggers a cough, which helps loosen and mobilize secretions. Use a gentle approach and do not force the catheter to advance. The Critical Aspects box summarizes this procedure. For the complete steps,

 Go to Chapter 35, **Procedure 35–7: Performing Oropharyngeal and Nasopharyngeal Suctioning,** in Volume 2.

If an oropharyngeal or nasopharyngeal airway is in place, follow the same procedure, but insert the suction catheter through the nasal airway or alongside the oral airway.

Orotracheal and Nasotracheal Suctioning

In tracheal suctioning, a catheter is passed beyond the pharynx into the trachea to remove secretions from the lower airways. The trachea may be suctioned through the mouth, nose, or an endotracheal airway. When suctioning through the nose or mouth, insert the catheter into the pharynx, and advance it into the trachea during inspiration. This prevents the catheter from entering the esophagus and causing the patient to gag or vomit. When the suction catheter enters the trachea, it will stimulate coughing. The Critical Aspects box provides highlights of this procedure. For the complete steps,

 Go to Chapter 35, **Procedure 35–8: Performing Orotracheal and Nasotracheal Suctioning,** in Volume 2.

An endotracheal or tracheostomy tube provides a direct path into the trachea. To suction, insert the catheter through the artificial airway into the trachea. You do not have to insert the catheter as far into a tracheostomy tube, because you are bypassing the long up-

per airway. Before suctioning, make sure the airway is secured so it is not dislodged by the coughing or suctioning. At present the issue of whether to use sterile, modified sterile, or clean technique is unresolved according to the Centers for Disease Control (Tablan, Anderson, Besser, Bridges, and Hajjeh, 2004). The Critical Aspects further describes this procedure. For the complete steps,

 Go to Chapter 35, **Procedure 35–9: Performing Tracheostomy or Endotracheal Suctioning,** in Volume 2.

KnowledgeCheck 35–15

- Describe the difference between pharyngeal and tracheal suctioning.
- How can you ensure that the suction catheter enters the trachea and not the esophagus?

 Go to Chapter 35, **Knowledge Check Response Sheet and Answers,** on the Electronic Study Guide.

Caring for a Patient on a Mechanical Ventilator

A **mechanical ventilator** is a machine that assists a patient to breathe. Usually the patient is intubated before he is placed on the ventilator. An endotracheal tube or a tracheosotomy tube is connected by oxygen tubing to the ventilator.

Negative pressure ventilators consist of shells that fit around the chest. Negative pressure generated inside the shell pulls the chest outward and forces the patient to inhale air, similar to normal breathing. These ventilators are rarely used for acutely ill patients, but they are occasionally used for chronic conditions, for example, in patients with muscle weakness from neuromuscular disease.

Positive pressure ventilators, the most widely used type, require the patient to have an artificial airway (Figure 35–21). Positive pressure ventilation carries risks, including *barotrauma* (injury to the airways due to pressure changes) and drop in cardiac output as the positive pressure in the chest decreases venous return to the heart.

To care for a patient on a mechanical ventilator, you need a thorough understanding of the ventilator, its settings, and how to troubleshoot problems. To work with patients receiving mechanical ventilation, you will need to familiarize yourself with the types of machines in use. In the event of a malfunction, if the repair is not readily obvious, manually ventilate the patient with an Ambu bag (resuscitation bag) while a colleague troubleshoots the problem. The Critical Aspects box describes care of the patient on a mechanical ventilator, including ventilator terminology you will hear used. For the complete procedure,

 Go to Chapter 35, **Procedure 35–10: Caring for a Patient on a Mechanical Ventilator,** in Volume 2.

Patients receiving mechanical ventilation are usually cared for by RNs. In critical care settings, specially trained LPNs may provide care, but the RN is responsible for ensuring that procedures are implemented safely and effectively and for providing ongoing assessment of the patient's ventilatory and oxygenation status. Mechanical ventilation may be a short- or long-term therapy. Patients requiring long-term ventilation are often cared for at home or in specialized long-term care units. As a result, LPNs and family members provide care.

Caring for a Patient Requiring Chest Tubes

Recall that normally there is negative pressure in the pleural space and only a thin layer of fluid between the membranes. Accumulation of fluid in the pleural space interferes with lung expansion, ventilation, and gas exchange. Air in the pleural space creates positive pressure, causing lung tissue to collapse. Chest tubes remove air or fluid from the pleural space to make room for the lungs to fully expand. A chest-drainage system is composed of a chest tube inserted into the pleural space and a drainage collection system.

To understand how a chest-drainage system works, think of the chest tube as an extension of the pleural space. To provide negative pressure within the chest tube, the open end of the tube is placed under water. With each exhalation, air is expelled through the chest tube into the water, but no air is drawn in during inhalation. Once all air is expelled, negative pressure has been reestablished in the chest tube and in the pleural space. Once the lung tissue is reexpanded, the chest tube can be safely removed. Four types of chest drainage systems are available.

A *one-bottle system* is the most basic chest drainage system. It consists of a chest tube connected to one water-sealed drainage bottle (Figure 35–22*A*). The single bottle is both collector and water seal. This system cannot handle large volumes of fluid or air drainage. As fluid drains from the chest tube, it mixes with the water in the bottle and raises the water level, making it harder for the patient to exhale. The following are key points for managing a one-bottle system:

- Keep the intake tube below the fluid level in the drainage bottle to prevent drawing air into the pleural space with inhalation.

- Maintain the tubing about 2 cm below the water level. As tubing length below the water increases, more effort is required to exhale.

- Take precautions to see that the bottle is not accidentally tipped over, uncovering the long vent tube and allowing air to enter the pleural space.

A *two-bottle system* has one bottle that connects directly with the chest tube and serves as a collection

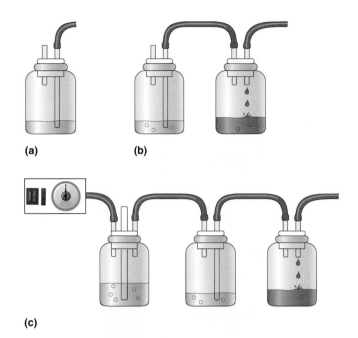

FIGURE 35–22 **Chest drainage systems.** *A,* A one-bottle system. *B,* A two-bottle system. *C,* A three-bottle system.

bottle. The second bottle serves as the water-seal bottle (Figure 35–22*B*); it maintains negative pressure. Because no water is mixed with chest drainage, the amount of drainage can be measured more accurately. The two-bottle system can handle large amounts of fluid drainage, but its design can still contribute to labored breathing.

In the *three-bottle system,* a third bottle is connected to the water-seal bottle and placed to suction (Figure 35–22*C*). This creates controlled negative pressure within the system. The suction control bottle has three vent tubes: one connected to suction, one connected to the water seal bottle, and a long middle tube with one end open to air at the top and the other end submerged in sterile water inside the bottle. Suction pressure is expressed in centimeters of water; the length of the long tube that is submerged in water is usually 15 to 20 cm for adults.

The depth of submersion determines the maximum suction possible within the system. Adjusting the suction regulator does not increase the amount of suction. Instead, it simply draws more air in from the atmosphere and causes more bubbling within the bottle. This is a safety feature that prevents excessive negative pressure from being created in the system. For proper functioning, adjust the suction regulator to create gentle bubbling in the suction control bottle.

Disposable chest drainage systems have all the advantages of a three-bottle system but are compact and lightweight. Each chamber of the disposable system represents one of the bottles in the three-bottle system (Figure 35–23). This system is the most commonly used system. The Critical Aspects box summarizes

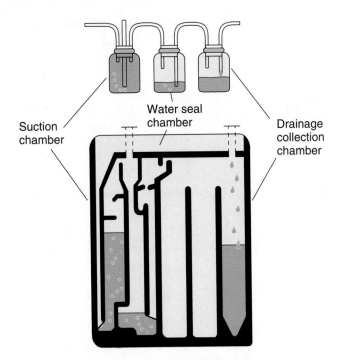

Suction chamber

Water seal chamber

Drainage collection chamber

FIGURE 35–23 **A disposable chest drainage system.**

how to care for patients with a disposable chest drainage system. For the complete procedure,

Go to Chapter 35, **Procedure 35–11: Caring for a Patient with Chest Tubes (Disposable Water Seal System),** in Volume 2.

Care of a patient with a chest drainage system involves four broad nursing interventions: (1) monitor breathing, gas exchange, and chest drainage; (2) maintain an intact, properly functioning drainage system; (3) promote lung reexpansion; and (4) prevent complications or intervene promptly if complications occur.

Monitor Breathing, Gas Exchange, and Drainage

When caring for patients requiring chest tubes, perform the following actions:

- Frequently assess breathing patterns, breathing effort, and breath sounds.
- Assess mental status, heart rate and rhythm, and pulse oximetry readings. These reflect adequacy of oxygenation.
- Monitor character, color, and amount of chest drainage. Drainage is usually greatest when the chest tube is initially inserted and decreases as the lung reexpands. Immediately report sudden or large increases in drainage or new onset of bright red blood, along with an assessment of the patient's condition at that time.

Maintain Drainage System

In addition, maintain the drainage system by performing the following actions:

- Regularly inspect and ensure that tubing and connections are air-tight, free of kinking or occlusion, and maintained at consistent negative pressure levels.
- Tape connections to prevent air leaks.
- Make sure that the chest dressing around the tube insertion site is occlusive. Usually, petroleum gauze is wrapped around the insertion site to ensure occlusion.
- Monitor drainage. Blood or purulent matter can occlude the tubing.
- Do not "milk" or strip the tubing; doing so can create excess negative pressure.

Promote Lung Reexpansion

To promote lung reexpansion, encourage the patient to be as active as his condition permits and to cough and perform deep-breathing exercises regularly. Chest drainage systems are bulky, but with disposable systems, patients can still get out of bed and ambulate. Most patients will need assistance from one or two staff members to protect and monitor the system and the patient.

Prevent Complications or Intervene

A *tension pneumothorax* is a life-threatening complication of chest drainage. It occurs when positive pressure builds up in the pleural space and pushes the lungs, great vessels, and heart toward the other side of the chest. If a patient with a chest drainage system becomes acutely short of breath, immediately check for occlusion of the system. Relieve the occlusion to prevent pressure buildup.

Recollapse of the lung can occur because of loss of negative pressure within the system. This is commonly caused by air leaks, disconnections, or breaks or cracks of the bottles or chambers. If any of these occur, immediately place the disconnected end nearest the patient into a bottle of sterile water or saline to a depth of 2 cm to serve as an emergency water-seal until a new system can be connected.

Do not clamp the chest tube; doing so can rapidly lead to a tension pneumothorax. Chest tubes should be clamped only for changing the drainage system. Limit the clamp time, and monitor the patient's respiratory status constantly until the clamp is removed.

You can delegate routine care of a patient with chest tubes to LPNs and qualified UAPs, but responsibility to monitor the chest drainage system and patient status remains with the RN.

| toward evidence-based practice |

Ramsay, J., & Hoffmann, A. (2004). Smoking cessation and relapse prevention among undergraduate students: A pilot demonstration project. *Journal of American College Health, 53*(1), 11–18.

This pilot study explored the feasibility of training peers to lead cessation and relapse-prevention programs for undergraduates. Among participants there was a quit rate of 88.2%, suggesting that peers were effective facilitators. Relapse-prevention interventions included six monthly group programs and individual meetings. Each session provided education and training in stress management, nutrition and exercise habits, managing environmental smoking triggers, and coping in social situations. After participating in the relapse-prevention programs, 63.3% of the initial quitters remained smoke free, another indication that peers were effective facilitators.

Lipkus, I. M., McBride, C. M., Pollak, K. I., Schwartz-Bloom, R. D., Tilson, E., & Bloom, P. N. (2004). A randomized trial comparing the effects of self-help materials and proactive telephone counseling on teen smoking cessation. *Health Psychology, 23*(4), 397–406.

This study tested the efficacy of self-help materials with or without telephone counseling to increase cessation among teen smokers. Teen smokers (N = 402) recruited from 11 shopping malls and 1 amusement park in the southeastern United States were randomized to one of two groups: these who were given written self-help material plus video, and those who were given written self-help material, video, and telephone counseling. Cessation rates for the self-help and self-help with counseling were 11% and 16%, respectively (p = 0.25), at the end of 4 months; and 19% and 21%, respectively (p = 0.8), at the end of 8 months. Results suggest that telephone counseling offers a slight advantage over purely independent cessation.

Use the information provided above as you answer the following questions:

1. What is the incidence of smoking at your school?

2. Would either of the approaches discussed above be effective in helping to curb smoking at the school you attend?

3. What is the feasibility of your nursing program's sponsoring a smoking cessation program that includes peer facilitators and telephone follow-up at your school or the local high school?

 Go to Chapter 35, **Toward Evidence-Based Practice Suggested Responses,** on the Electronic Study Guide.

KnowledgeCheck 35–16
- What is the purpose of mechanical ventilation?
- Why is a chest tube inserted?
- What is the advantage of a three-bottle system (compared to a one-bottle or two-bottle system)?
- How does a disposable chest drainage system compare to the bottle drainage system?

 Go to Chapter 35, **Knowledge Check Response Sheet and Answers,** on the Electronic Study Guide.

Promoting Circulation

Adequate circulation ensures that oxygenated blood reaches tissues and organs and venous blood returns to the heart. Two important nursing interventions are to promote venous return and prevent clot formation.

Promote Venous Return

Measures that promote venous return increase the flow of blood back to the vena cava and the right side of the heart.

- Elevate the patient's legs above the level of the heart. This promotes venous return from the feet and legs. However, flexion of the hips, legs, and knees constricts the veins and slows venous blood flow. If one is available, have the patient sit in a recliner that elevates the legs rather than sitting upright in a chair with legs elevated on a stool.

- Encourage and support early and frequent ambulation.

- Teach patients to avoid sitting with the legs crossed; this interferes with blood flow.

- Encourage or provide range-of-motion (ROM) exercises, which increase venous blood flow through rhythmic massaging of the veins by the active muscles (see Chapter 31).

- Apply compression devices. *Antiembolism stockings (TED hose)* are elastic stockings that compress superficial leg veins and promote venous return. *Sequential compression devices (SCD),* also called *pneumatic compression devices,* are cuffs that surround the legs and alternately inflate and deflate to promote venous return to the heart. Antiembolism stockings and SCD are frequently used in perioperative patients to promote venous return and prevent clot formation. See Chapter 37 for further discussion

and instructions on how to apply these stockings and appropriate follow-up care.

 Go to Chapter 37, **Procedure 37–2: Applying Antiembolism Stockings,** in Volume 2.

Prevent Clot Formation

A **thrombus** is a stationary clot adhering to the wall of a vessel. An **embolus** is a clot that travels in the bloodstream. Clots can form following injury to vessels, or in response to hypercoaguability. Of course, all the strategies to promote venous return also help prevent clot formation.

- Turn patients frequently; teach patients to change positions frequently. This prevents vessel injury from prolonged pressure in one position.

- Use scrupulous sterile technique when inserting or handling intravenous lines. This prevents infection that can damage the vessel lumens.

- Be sure intravenous medications are adequately diluted. This prevents chemical irritation of veins during IV medication therapy. Promote adequate hydration (i.e., monitor intake and output, assess hydration, manage fluid intake, teach patients to drink plenty of fluids). Unless contraindicated, adult fluid intake should be approximately 2000 mL per day to keep urine output around 1500 mL per day (Kidd & Wagner, 2001). Adequate hydration keeps respiratory secretions thin but also keeps the blood from becoming viscous ("thick"); viscous blood clots more readily.

- Promote smoking cessation. Nicotine increases the risk for thrombus formation because of its constricting effects on vessel walls.

- Patients at particularly high risk for thrombus formation may receive anticoagulant therapy to help prevent abnormal clot formation.

Administering Medications

Medications used to treat disorders that affect oxygenation include oral and inhaled respiratory medications, cardiovascular medications, antianxiety agents, and analgesics.

Respiratory Medications

Respiratory medications promote ventilation and oxygenation by their effects on the respiratory system. The major types of respiratory medicines include bronchodilators, corticosteroids, cough preparations, decongestants, antihistamines, and mucolytics.

- *Bronchodilators* relax the smooth muscles lining the airways. They can be administered as oral or inhaled medicines. The main types of bronchodilators are beta-2 adrenergic agonists, anticholinergics, and methylzanthines.

- *Respiratory anti-inflammatory agents* combat inflammation in the airways. They are important in treating and controlling respiratory conditions characterized by hypersensitive airways and airway inflammation (e.g., asthma). The major categories include corticosteroids, cromolyn, and leukotriene modifiers.

- *Cough preparations* include antitussives (cough suppressants) to reduce the frequency of an involuntary, hacking, nonproductive cough and expectorants, which help make coughing more productive. These agents are often found mixed together in one preparation to achieve both desirable effects with one medication. The goal is to reduce the frequency of dry, unproductive coughing while making voluntary coughing more productive.

- *Nasal decongestants* relieve stuffy, blocked nasal passages by constricting local blood vessels through stimulation of alpha-1 adrenergic nerve receptors in the vessels. Although the desired effect is on the nasal mucosa, these medications can have systemic adrenergic effects causing elevated blood pressure, tachycardia, and palpitations, especially in those with a history of cardiovascular conditions.

- *Antihistamines* are drugs that prevent the effects of histamine release. They are used to treat upper respiratory and nasal allergy symptoms and include such drugs as diphenhydramine (Benadryl), chlorpheniramine (Chlor-Trimeton), brompheniramine (Dimetane), loratadine (Claritin), fexofenadine (Allegra), and cetirizine (Zyrtec).

- *Mucolytic agents* react directly with mucus to reduce viscosity and make secretions easier to remove from the airways. Concentrated saline and acetylcysteine (Mucomist), both of which are administered by inhalation, are available. Aceytylcysteine can trigger bronchospasm and smells like rotten eggs. Therefore, its use is limited. Saline is well tolerated and is frequently instilled into artificial airways to liquefy secretions.

Cardiovascular Medications

Cardiovascular drugs are used to enhance cardiac output, thus providing increased blood flow and oxygenation to organs and tissues. They include vasodilators, beta-adrenergic blocking agents, diuretics, and positive inotropes.

- *Vasodilators* cause vessel dilatation, which eases the work of the heart. Drugs that dilate arterioles decrease the resistance against which the heart pumps (afterload). Drugs that dilate veins decrease venous

return to the heart (preload). Vasodilators can cause hypotension, especially when the person rises from a sitting or lying position. Patients should be warned of this effect. You will need to monitor the patient's blood pressure and observe for symptoms of hypotension. Vasodilating agents include angiotensin-converting enzyme (ACE) inhibitors, angiotensin II receptor blockers, and nitrates.

- *Beta-adrenegic agents* block stimulation of beta receptors, which are located primarily in the heart, lungs, and blood vessels. Beta-1 selective agents are used to treat angina, acute myocardial infarction, and congestive heart failure. They decrease heart rate, slow conduction through the AV node, and decrease myocardial oxygen demand by reducing myocardial contractility.

- *Diuretics* increase removal of sodium and water from the body by increasing urine output. Diuretics reduce the volume of circulating blood and prevent accumulation of fluid in the pulmonary circulation.

- *Positive inotropes* increase cardiac contractility. They are used therapeutically to make the heart a more effective pump. The goal is to improve pumping effectiveness without creating excess heart work and oxygen demand. The two main classes of positive inotropes are cardiac glycosides and phosphodiesterase inhibitors.

Performing Cardiopulmonary Resuscitation

All of the previously discussed nursing interventions are designed to promote circulation, ventilation, and gas exchange. However, the patient's condition can rapidly deteriorate. You must be prepared to perform *cardiopulmonary resuscitation (CPR)* in the event that your patient experiences a respiratory, cardiac, or cardiopulmonary arrest. **Cardiac arrest** is the cessation of heart function. Signs of cardiac arrest are pale, cool, grayish skin; absence of femoral or carotid pulses; apnea; and pupil dilation. In the event of cardiac arrest, you have only 4 to 6 minutes before the brain is damaged by lack of oxygen. **Respiratory (pulmonary) arrest** is cessation of breathing. It can be caused by a blocked airway or occur following a cardiac arrest; it may be sudden or preceded by increasingly labored breathing.

CPR procedures are regularly updated as new knowledge is gained. The American Heart Association provides training sessions for health professionals to become certified in CPR. This is a prerequisite for employment and clinical practice. The Critical Aspects box summarizes key steps in performing CPR. For the complete procedure,

 Go to Chapter 35, **Procedure 35–12: Performing Cardiopulmonary Resuscitation, One- and Two-Person,** in Volume 2.

All agencies have procedures (called a "Code Blue" in many agencies) for announcing cardiac or respiratory arrest, and there are usually emergency buttons in the patient rooms in acute care facilities. Pressing the button summons a code team, trained in CPR. However, you will probably need to begin CPR before they arrive. Before beginning CPR, you are responsible for knowing whether your patient has an advance directive stating that he does not want CPR.

KnowledgeCheck 35–17

- Identify three strategies that prevent clot formation.
- How do inhaled bronchodilators affect oxygenation?
- What is the most commonly used mucolytic agent?
- How do diuretics affect oxygenation?

 Go to Chapter 35, **Knowledge Check Response Sheet and Answers,** on the Electronic Study Guide.

 Go to Chapter 35, **Resources for Caregivers and Health Professionals,** on the Electronic Study Guide.

 Suggested Readings: Go to Chapter 35, **Reading More About Oxygenation,** on the Electronic Study Guide.

 Bibliography: Go to Volume 2, Bibliography.

36 Fluids, Electrolytes, & Acid-Base Balance

Learning Outcomes

After completing this chapter, you should be able to:

* Identify the fluid compartments within the body.

* Describe the location and function of the major electrolytes of the body.

* Differentiate between active and passive transport, osmosis, diffusion, and filtration.

* Describe the body mechanisms for maintaining fluid and electrolyte balance.

* Summarize the major fluid and electrolyte balance disorders.

* Describe respiratory and metabolic acidosis and alkalosis.

* Describe compensatory mechanisms for acid-base imbalances.

* Provide nursing interventions for clients with fluid, electrolyte, and acid-base imbalances.

Your Patients

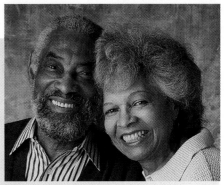

Your instructor has assigned you to care for Jackson LaGuardia, a 60-year-old man with end-stage renal disease. You have arrived at the hospital to review his chart so that you can provide care the following day. When you arrive on the unit, the charge nurse informs you that Mr. LaGuardia is still in the emergency department (ED). You go to the ED to review his chart and gather data.

In the ED, you introduce yourself and explain your purpose. The charge nurse tells you that five members of the LaGuardia family have all come to the ED complaining of nausea, vomiting, and diarrhea related to severe gastroenteritis, a viral intestinal disorder. The family members include the following:

8-month-old Jason, grandson of Jackson
26-year-old Susanna, Jackson's daughter and Jason's mother

60-year-old Jackson
58-year-old Gemma, Jackson's wife
82-year-old Martha, Jackson's mother

Jason, Jackson, and Martha are being admitted to the hospital. However, Susanna and Gemma have been asked to follow up tomorrow in the urgent care clinic. As you prepare for your clinical day, you think, "If they all have the same disorder, why are only three family members being admitted? What makes these patients different?" In this chapter we will follow the LaGuardias and answer these questions.

Theoretical Knowledge
knowing why

In a healthy state, the fluid and chemical state of our bodies is in balance. However, illness can disturb this balance and threaten our existence. In this chapter we examine how fluid, electrolyte, and acid-base balance are maintained, as well as what happens when there are disturbances in each of these areas.

BODY FLUIDS

Body fluid is primarily water with various dissolved substances. Gases, such as carbon dioxide and oxygen, readily dissolve in body fluids. In fact, it is through body fluids that they are transported in the body. Solid substances, called **solutes,** also dissolve in body fluids. Many solutes are **electrolytes**—substances (e.g., sodium, potassium) that develop an electrical charge when dissolved in water. Other solutes are nonelectrolytes. **Nonelectrolytes** (e.g., glucose, urea) do not conduct electricity. Body fluids perform several important functions:

- Maintaining blood volume
- Regulating body temperature
- Transporting material to and from cells
- Serving as an aqueous medium for cellular metabolism
- Assisting with digestion of food
- Serving as a medium for excreting waste

Fluid makes up about 60% of an average adult's body weight. However, total body water content varies with the number of fat cells, age, and sex. Women have less body fluid than men because they have proportionately more body fat. An obese person has less fluid than a person of lean build. Body water progressively decreases with age. Table 36–1 demonstrates the distribution of fluid based on age and gender.

What Are the Body Fluids Compartments?

Most body fluid is contained within two compartments. **Intracellular fluid (ICF)** is contained within the cells. Essential for cell function and metabolism, it accounts for approximately 40% of body weight. **Extracellular fluid (ECF)** is outside the cells. ECF carries water, electrolytes, nutrients, and oxygen to the cells and removes the waste products of cell

TABLE 36-1	Total Body Fluid in Relation to Sex and Age	
Age	**Total Body Fluid (Percentage of Body Weight)**	
Full-term newborn	70–80%	
1 year old	64%	
Young adult	Men: 60% Women: 50–55%	
Middle adult	Men: 55% Women: 45–50%	
Older adult	Men: 50% Women: 45%	

metabolism. ECF accounts for 20% of body weight. ECF is of three types:

- *Interstitial fluid* lies in the spaces between the body cells. Excess fluid within the interstitial space is called edema.
- *Intravascular fluid* is the plasma within the blood. Its main function is to transport blood cells.
- *Transcellular fluid* includes specialized fluids, such as cerebrospinal, pleural, peritoneal, and synovial fluid; and digestive juices.

Figure 36–1 illustrates the distribution of body fluids. In times of illness, fluid may move into an area that makes it physiologically unavailable, such as the

peritoneal space (a condition called ascites), the pericardial space (a condition called pericardial effusion), or the vesicles produced by a burn wound. This phenomenon is known as **third spacing** because fluid is literally trapped in a third compartment.

What Electrolytes Are Present in Body Fluids?

In addition to water, body fluid is composed of oxygen, carbon dioxide, dissolved nutrients, metabolic waste products, and electrolytes. Electrolytes that carry a positive charge are called **cations.** They include sodium (Na^+), potassium (K^+), calcium (Ca^{2+}) and magnesium (Mg^{2+}). Electrolytes that carry a negative charge are called **anions.** Examples are chloride (Cl^-), bicarbonate (HCO_3^-), phosphate (HPO_4^{2-}), and sulfate (SO_4^{2-}). Electrolytes are measured in milliequivalents per liter of water (mEq/L) or milligrams per 100 mL (mg/100mL or mg/dL). Note that 1 dL, or deciliter, equals 100 mL. *Milliequivalent* is a measure of chemical combining power, whereas *milligram* is a weight measure.

The composition of body fluids varies between compartments:

- In the ICF, the major cations are potassium and magnesium. The major anions are phosphate and sulfate. Other electrolytes are present, but to a lesser degree.
- In the ECF, the major electrolytes are sodium, chloride, and bicarbonate. Albumin is also present in the ECF, mostly in the intravascular fluid. Gastric and intestinal secretions (transcellular fluids) also contain electrolytes.
- Severe electrolyte imbalances can occur if electrolytes move into a compartment they do not normally occupy or if they are lost from the body through perspiration, wounds, injury, or illness.

KnowledgeCheck 36–1
- Define *solute, electrolyte, intracellular fluid, extracellular fluid, cation,* and *anion.*
- Identify the major electrolytes in the ICF and ECF.

Go to Chapter 36, **Knowledge Check Response Sheet and Answers,** on the Electronic Study Guide.

CriticalThinking 36–1
- Based on the information presented in the "Meet Your Patients" scenario, rank the members of the LaGuardia family based on total body water content.
- Does this information help you understand which family members were admitted to the hospital?

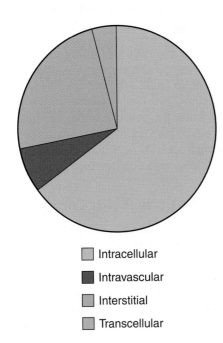

☐ Intracellular

☐ Intravascular

☐ Interstitial

☐ Transcellular

FIGURE 36–1   Normal distribution of body fluids.

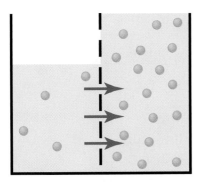

FIGURE 36–2 Osmosis is the movement of water across a membrane from a less concentrated solution to a more concentrated solution.

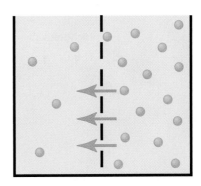

FIGURE 36–3 Diffusion is the movement of molecules of a solute through a cell membrane from an area of higher concentration to an area of lower concentration.

How Do Fluids and Electrolytes Move in the Body?

The selectively permeable membranes of cells and capillaries separate ICF and ECF. Fluid and electrolytes move across these membranes by passive and active mechanisms. In **active transport,** movement of fluid and solutes requires energy. **Passive transport** requires no energy. The three passive transport systems are osmosis, diffusion, and filtration.

Osmosis

Osmosis involves movement of water (or other pure solute) across a membrane from an area of a less concentrated solution to an area of more concentrated solution. Water moves across the membrane to dilute the higher concentration of solutes (Figure 36–2). As you may recall, a solute is a substance dissolved in body fluid. Solutes may be crystalloids or colloids. **Crytalloids** are solutes that readily dissolve. **Colloids** are larger molecules that do not dissolve readily.

The concentration of solutes in body fluid is called **osmolality. Osmols** refers to the number of particles of solute per kilogram of water and is expressed as milliosmoles per kilogram (mOsm/kg). Sodium is the greatest determinant of serum osmolality, and potassium is the greatest determinant of intracellular osmolality. Glucose and urea also contribute to osmolality in the ICF and ECF.

Another term for osmolality is **tonicity.** A fluid that is of the same osmolality as blood is called **isotonic.** An isotonic solution is often given by IV infusion if blood volume is low. Because the solution is the same concentration as blood, the fluid will remain in the vascular space, and no osmosis will occur. A **hypotonic solution** is of lower osmolality than blood. When a hypotonic solution is infused, water moves by osmosis from the vascular system into the cells. A **hypertonic solution** contains a higher concentration of solutes than blood. When a hypertonic solution is given to a patient, water moves by osmosis from the cells into the ECF.

Diffusion

Diffusion is a passive process by which molecules of a solute move through a cell membrane from an area of higher concentration to an area of lower concentration. Movement occurs (Figure 36–3) until the concentrations are equivalent on both sides of the membrane. For an example of diffusion, pour yourself a cup of coffee. Now add cream to the coffee. Initially, the cream is concentrated in the area where you have poured it. However, within a short period of time the cream is evenly dispersed throughout the coffee. If you stir the coffee, the cream mixes evenly more quickly. Fluids within the human body work on a similar principle; movement of the body speeds the diffusion of molecules.

The rate of diffusion varies according to the size of the molecules, the concentration of the solution, and the temperature of the solution. Small molecules move more rapidly than larger molecules. Large discrepancies in concentration require a longer period of time to reach equilibration. Higher temperatures cause molecules to move faster, so that diffusion occurs more rapidly.

Filtration

Filtration is the movement of both water and smaller particles from an area of high pressure to low pressure (Figure 36–4). **Hydrostatic pressure** is the force created by fluid within a closed system; it is responsible for normal circulation of blood. In other words, blood flows from the high-pressure arterial system to the lower pressure capillaries and veins. As fluid (plasma) moves through the capillary membrane, only solutes of a certain size can flow with it. For example, the membrane pores of Bowman's capsule in the kidneys are very small, and only albumin, the smallest of the proteins, can be filtered through the membrane. By contrast, the membrane pores of liver cells are extremely large, so that a variety of solutes can pass through and be metabolized.

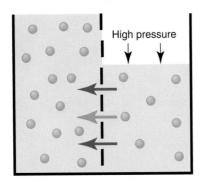

FIGURE 36–4 Filtration is the movement of water and smaller particles from an area of high pressure to an area of low pressure.

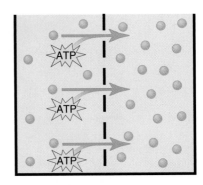

FIGURE 36–5 Active transport is the movement of electrolytes against a concentration gradient. For the movement to occur, active transport requires energy expenditure.

Osmotic pressure is the power of a solution to draw water. A highly concentrated solution (with many molecules in solution) draws water and has a high osmotic pressure. The plasma proteins in the blood exert osmotic, or colloidal, pressure to help maintain fluid in the vascular space. However, when hydrostatic pressure exceeds osmotic pressure, fluid leaves the vessels. This difference, known as the **filtration pressure,** represents the net pressures that move fluid and solutes.

Active Transport

Active transport occurs when molecules (e.g., electrolytes) move across cell membranes from an area of low concentration to an area of high concentration. Active transport requires energy expenditure for the movement to occur against a concentration gradient (Figure 36–5). Adenosine triphosphate (ATP) is released from the cell to enable certain substances to acquire the energy needed to pass through the cell membrane. For example, sodium concentration is greater in ECF; therefore, sodium tends to enter by diffusion into the intracellular compartment. This tendency is offset by the sodium-potassium pump, which is located on the cell membrane. In the presence of ATP, the sodium-potassium pump actively moves sodium from the cell into the ECF. Active transport is vital for maintaining the unique composition of both the extracellular and intracellular compartments.

Table 36–2 summarizes the processes of fluid and electrolyte movement.

KnowledgeCheck 36–2

Identify the appropriate mechanism: osmosis, diffusion, filtration, or active transport:

* Molecules move across a membrane to equalize concentration.
* Fluid moves across a membrane to equalize concentration.
* Molecules move against a concentration gradient.
* Molecules move to equalize pressure.

Go to Chapter 36, **Knowledge Check Response Sheet and Answers,** on the Electronic Study Guide.

How Does the Body Regulate Fluids?

A balance between fluid intake and output is essential to maintain homeostasis. Excesses or deficits of intake or output can lead to severe disorders.

Fluid Intake

You have undoubtedly been told to drink eight to ten glasses of water per day. Did you ever wonder where

TABLE 36-2   Processes of Fluid and Electrolyte Movement

Process	What Moves	From Area Of	To Area Of
Diffusion	Molecules (solute)	High concentration	Low concentration
Active transport	Molecules (solute)	Low concentration	High concentration
Osmosis	Water	Low concentration	High concentration
Filtration	Water and small particles	High pressure	Low pressure

that recommendation came from or why that volume is important? Eight to ten 8-ounce glasses of water provide 1920 to 2400 mL of fluid. The Institute of Medicine (IOM) (2004), however, has recommended a total fluid intake of 2700 mL per day for women and 3700 mL per day for men. This is higher than the previous recommendation of 2500 mL per day for the average adult engaged in moderate activity in moderate temperature, which you may have learned in a biology class. The IOM states that we should obtain 80% of our intake from drinking fluids and the remaining 20% from food and cellular metabolism of foods. Prolonged exercise and heat exposure increase the requirements. The IOM did not set an upper limit on fluid intake (IOM, 2004).

Habit and culture influence fluid consumption. However, thirst is the major regulator of fluid intake. Changes in plasma osmolality signal the thirst center in the hypothalamus, which leads to the urge to drink. Situations that increase plasma osmolality (and promote thirst) include excessive fluid loss, excessive sodium intake, and decreased fluid intake. Situations that inhibit the thirst mechanism include a high intake of fluids, fluid retention, excessive IV infusion of hypotonic solutions, and low sodium intake.

Fluid Output

Fluid loss occurs throughout the day, creating a constant need to replenish fluid. In a healthy state, fluid losses are equivalent to fluid intake. The following are sources of fluid loss:

- *Urine* (1500 mL per day). Urine accounts for the greatest amount of fluid loss. Urine output varies according to intake and activity but should remain at least 30 to 50 mL per hour. The volume of urine increases as intake increases, and it decreases to compensate for other fluid losses (e.g., vomiting and excessive perspiration).

- *Skin* (650 to 900 mL per day). Sensible (perceived) fluid loss through the skin occurs through perspiration, at 300 to 500 mL per day. Perspiration varies based on temperature, skeletal muscle activity, and metabolic activity. Fever, exercise, and some disease processes increase metabolic activity and heat production, leading to increased fluid loss. Insensible water loss (loss that we do not perceive) occurs by diffusion through the skin; it accounts for 350 to 400 mL per day. Insensible loss increases with open wounds, burns, or other breaks in the protective layer of the skin.

- *Lungs* (350 to 400 mL per day). Insensible loss also occurs through the lungs as water is exhaled with the breath. An increase in respiratory rate increases the amount of fluid lost.

- *Feces* (100 to 200 mL per day). Soft stools contain more water than hard stool. As stool frequency increases, water loss also increases.

Hormonal Regulation

The kidneys are the principal regulator of fluid and electrolyte balance. The following hormones are involved:

- *Antidiuretic hormone*. Pressure sensors in the vascular system stimulate or inhibit the release of **antidiuretic hormone (ADH)** from the pituitary gland. ADH causes the kidneys to retain fluid. If fluid volume within the vascular system is low, fluid pressures within the system decrease, and more ADH is released. If fluid volume (and therefore pressure) increases, less ADH is released, and the kidneys eliminate more fluid. ADH is also produced in response to a rise in serum osmolality, fever, pain, stress, and some opioids.

- *Renin-angiotensin system*. When extracellular (i.e., intravascular) fluid volume is decreased, receptors in the glomeruli respond to the decreased perfusion of the kidneys by releasing renin. **Renin** is an enzyme responsible for the chain of reactions that converts angiotensinogen to angiotensin II. **Angiotensin II** acts on the nephrons to retain sodium and water and directs the adrenal cortex to release aldosterone.

- *Aldosterone*. **Aldosterone** promotes the reabsorption of sodium and the excretion of potassium in the distal tubules of the kidneys. Sodium reabsorption results in passive reabsorption of water, thereby increasing plasma volume and improving kidney perfusion. When fluid excess is present, renin is not released, and this process stops.

- *Other hormones*. (1) Thyroid hormone affects fluid volume by influencing cardiac regulation. An increase in thyroid hormone causes an increase in cardiac output thereby increasing glomerular filtration rate and urine output. A decrease has the opposite effect. (2) Atrial natriuretic factor (ANF) is released from the atrium of the heart when the atrial walls are stretched because of fluid excess. ANF promotes sodium and water excretion from the kidneys and inhibits thirst.

 CriticalThinking 36–2

Apply the information on fluid balance to the LaGuardia family ("Meet Your Patients"). What have you learned that helps you explain why some family members require hospitalization? What additional information do you need to be able to predict each person's fluid balance?

How Does the Body Regulate Electrolytes?

To maintain health, the body must balance electrolyte losses and intake. For example, potassium lost through diarrhea and vomiting must be replaced by dietary potassium or potassium supplements. Table 36–3 provides information about the function, regulation, and

TABLE 36-3   Major Electrolytes

Electrolyte	Function	Regulation	Sources
Sodium (Na⁺) $Sodium\ (Na^+)$ • Major cation in the ECF • Normal serum level = 135–145 mEq/L	• Regulates fluid volume • Helps maintain blood volume • Interacts with calcium to maintain muscle contraction • Stimulates conduction of nerve impulses	• Moves by active transport across cell membranes • Regulated by aldosterone and ADH levels • Reabsorbed and excreted through the kidneys • Minimal loss through perspiration and feces • Low levels may be caused by excess water intake	Table salt, soy sauce, cured pork, cheese, milk, processed foods, canned products, and foods preserved with salt
Potassium (K⁺) $Potassium\ (K^+)$ • Major cation in the ICF • Normal serum level = 3.5–5 mEq/L	• Maintains ICF osmolality • Regulates conduction of cardiac rhythm • Transmits electrical impulses in multiple body systems • Assists with acid-base balance	• Regulated by aldosterone • Excreted and conserved through the kidneys • Lost through vomiting and diarrhea • Loss triggered by many diuretics	Common food sources include bananas, oranges, apricots, figs, dates, carrots, potatoes, tomatoes, spinach, dairy products, and meats
Calcium (Ca²⁺) $Calcium\ (Ca^{2+})$ • Most abundant electrolyte in the body • Normal serum level = 8.5–10.5 mg/dL	• Promotes transmission of nerve impulses • Regulates muscle contractions • Maintains cardiac automaticity • Essential factor in the formation of blood clots • Catalyst for many cellular activities	• Combines with phosphorus to form the mineral salts of the teeth and bones • Calcium and phosphorous levels inversely proportional • Parathyroid hormone (PTH) stimulates release of calcium from bones and reabsorption from kidneys and intestines • Calcitonin (from the thyroid) blocks bone breakdown and lowers calcium levels • Absorption stimulated by vitamin D	• See Table 36–4 for average daily requirements • Common food sources include milk, milk products, dark green leafy vegetables, and salmon
Magnesium (Mg²⁺) $Magnesium\ (Mg^{2+})$ • Present in skeleton and ICF; second most abundant cation in ICF • Normal serum level = 1.3–2.1 mEq/L	• Involved in protein and carbohydrate metabolism • Necessary for protein and DNA synthesis within the cell • Maintains normal intracellular levels of potassium • Involved in electrical activity in nerve and muscle membranes • May have a role in regulating blood pressure and may influence the release and activity of insulin (IOM, 2004).	• Ingested in the diet and absorbed through the small intestine • Excreted by kidneys • Loss may be triggered by diuretics, poorly controlled diabetes mellitus, and excess alcohol intake	• Average daily requirement is 18–30 mEq • Found in most foods, but high levels are present in green vegetables, cereal grains, and nuts

TABLE 36–3 *(continued)*

Electrolyte	Function	Regulation	Sources
Chloride (Cl⁻)	• Works with Na⁺ to maintain osmotic pressure between fluid compartments	• Reabsorbed and excreted through the kidneys along with sodium	Found in foods high in sodium
• Major anion in the ECF	• Essential for production of HCl for gastric secretions	• Regulated by aldosterone and ADH levels	
• Normal serum level = 95–105 mEq/L	• Functions as buffer in oxygen–carbon dioxide exchange in RBCs	• Deficits lead to potassium deficits; potassium deficits lead to chloride deficits	
	• Assists with acid-base balance		
Phosphate (PO₄⁻)	• Serves as a catalyst for many intracellular activities	• Combines with calcium to form the mineral salts of the teeth and bones	Foods high in phosphate are meat, fish, poultry, milk products, carbonated beverages, and legumes
• Major anion in the ICF	• Promotes muscle and nerve action	• Calcium and phosphorous levels inversely proportional	
• Normal serum level = 1.7–2.6 mEq/L	• Assists with acid-base balance	• Regulated by PTH; has inverse response to calcium	
	• Important for cell division and transmission of hereditary traits		
Bicarbonate (HCO₃⁻)	• Maintains acid-base balance by functioning as the primary buffer in the body	• Excreted and reabsorbed by the kidneys	• Readily available in body as a result of metabolism
• Major buffer in the body		• Lost through diarrhea, diuretics, renal insufficiency	• Present in acid neutralizers (e.g., sodium bicarbonate)
• In ECF and ICF		• Excess possible if person ingests quantities of acid neutralizers	
• Normal serum level = 22–26 mEq/L			

food sources of major electrolytes in the body. The body has various mechanisms for regulating electrolyte balance, which are discussed later in this chapter. Maintenance of normal serum levels also depends on dietary intake, discussed in the remainder of this section.

Sodium (Na⁺)

Sodium is the major cation in the ECF. Its primary function is to regulate fluid volume. When sodium is reabsorbed in the kidney, water and potassium are also reabsorbed, thereby maintaining ECF volume. According to the 2004 Dietary References Intake report (IOM, 2004), a healthy adult between the ages of 19 and 50 should consume 1.5 grams of sodium and 2.3 grams of chloride each day—or 3.8 grams of salt—to replace daily losses and maintain serum blood levels. Intake should not exceed 5.8 grams per day. However, among persons 31 to 50 years of age, more than 95% of American men,

90% of Canadian men, 75% of American women, and 50% of Canadian women regularly consume salt in excess of 5.8 g/day. Older adults, African Americans, and people with chronic diseases including hypertension, diabetes, and kidney disease are especially sensitive to the blood pressure raising effects of salt. As a result, they are advised to limit salt to 2.0 g/day (IOM, 2004).

Potassium (K⁺)

Potassium is the major cation of the ICF; only 2% of body potassium is found in the extracellular fluid. Potassium is a key electrolyte in cellular metabolism. The 2004 Dietary References Intake report (IOM, 2004) recommends that adults consume at least 4.7 grams of potassium per day. However, most American and Canadian women aged 31 to 50 years old consume less than half of the recommended amount of potassium, and intake is only moderately higher for men. Moderate potassium deficiency is associated with increased

TABLE 36-4 Recommended Calcium Intake

Age	Optimal Calcium Intake
Birth to 6 months	400 mg/day
6–12 months	600 mg/day
1–5 years	800 mg/day
6–10 years	800–1200 mg/day
Adolescents and young adults (11–24 years)	1200–1500 mg/day
Women between 25 and 50 years	1000 mg/day
Pregnant or lactating women	1200–1500 mg/day
Postmenopausal women and men over 65	1500 mg/day

Source: National Institutes of Health (NIH). (1994). NIH Consensus Development Conference: Statement on Optimal Calcium Intake. Washington, D.C.: Author.

blood pressure, increased salt sensitivity, increased risk of kidney stones, and increased risk of bone turnover. Because of its effect on blood pressure, low intake of dietary potassium is associated with increased risk of stroke.

The DRIs do not specify an upper limit of potassium intake because there is no evidence of problems associated with higher potassium intake (IOM, 2004). In a healthy person, a high potassium intake does not result in a high serum potassium (hyperkalemia), because the kidneys efficiently eliminate excess dietary potassium.

Calcium (Ca²⁺)

Calcium is responsible for bone health and neuromuscular and cardiac function. It is also an essential factor in blood clotting. Approximately 99% of body calcium is located in the bones and teeth. The remaining 1% circulates in the blood and affects system functions. Because calcium is so vital for cardiac and muscle function, serum levels are tightly regulated. As serum levels drop, calcium leaches from the bones into the blood to compensate. If dietary intake is insufficient, bone loss occurs; prolonged deficiencies lead to osteoporosis.

An estimated 44 million American men and women aged 50 and older have osteoporosis (U.S. Department of Health and Human Services, 2004). That number is expected to escalate as the population ages, because most Americans do not include the recommended amount of calcium in their diets. Most calcium should be obtained from naturally calcium-rich foods, such as dairy products. Calcium-fortified foods and calcium supplements can be used as a secondary source (U.S. Department of Health and Human Services, 2004). For recommended calcium intake by age group, see Table 36–4 ([NIH], 1994).

Magnesium (Mg²⁺)

Magnesium is a mineral used in more than 300 biochemical reactions in the body. Like calcium, only about 1% of magnesium is found in the blood. The remaining 99% is divided between the ICF and bone (in combination with calcium and phosphorus). Although magnesium deficiency is rare, you may find low levels in individuals who have a high alcohol intake. Some malabsorption disorders may also cause magnesium depletion.

Chloride (Cl⁻)

Chloride is the most abundant anion in the extracellular fluid. It is usually bound with other ions, especially sodium or potassium (e.g., as sodium chloride, or salt). A healthy adult between the ages of 19 and 50 should consume 2.3 grams of chloride each day along with 1.5 grams of sodium to replace daily losses and maintain serum blood levels (IOM, 2004).

Phosphate (PO₄⁻)

Phosphate is the most abundant intracellular anion. Phosphate in the ECF is known as **phosphorus.** Most phosphate is bound with calcium in teeth and bones. Phosphate and calcium exist in an inverse relationship; as one increases, the other one decreases. As a result, high blood phosphorus levels decrease the movement of calcium from the bones.

Bicarbonate (HCO₃⁻)

Bicarbonate is present in both ICF and ECF. The kidneys regulate extracellular bicarbonate levels. When serum levels rise, the kidneys excrete excess bicarbonate. If serum levels are low, the kidneys conserve bicarbonate. Bicarbonate is not consumed in the diet but is produced by the body to meet current needs.

KnowledgeCheck 36–3

- Identify the major functions of sodium, potassium, calcium, magnesium, chloride, phosphate, and bicarbonate.
- What are the major concerns associated with sodium and potassium intake?
- Identify at least five potassium-rich foods.
- Identify the ideal calcium intakes for each member of the LaGuardia family ("Meet Your Patients").

 Go to Chapter 36, **Knowledge Check Response Sheet and Answers,** on the Electronic Study Guide.

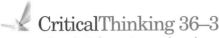

CriticalThinking 36–3

Based on the information you have learned about the major electrolytes of the body, which electrolytes are most likely to be out of balance in members of the LaGuardia family? Explain your answer.

How Is Acid-Base Balance Regulated?

Acids and bases are formed in the body as part of normal metabolic processes. An **acid** is any compound that contains hydrogen ions (H^+) that can be released. For this reason, acids are referred to as cation donors. A common strong acid is hydrochloric acid (HCl), which is present in gastric secretions. A **base or alkali** is a compound that combines with (accepts) hydrogen ions in solution. Therefore, bases are referred to as cation acceptors. A strong base has a tendency to bind hydrogen ions, whereas a weak base binds only a small portion of the available hydrogen ions.

The amount of acid or base present in a solution is measured as **pH.** The pH is reported on a scale of 1 to 14: 1 to 6.9 is acidic, 7 is neutral, and 7.1 to 14 is basic, or alkaline. Arterial blood and tissue fluid normally have a pH of 7.35 to 7.45; therefore, they are slightly alkaline. The stronger an acid, the lower the pH. In contrast, a strong base has a high pH. The pH is a logarithmic scale. For example, a pH of 4 is ten times more acidic than a pH of 5. A serum pH below 7.30 or above 7.52 alters enzymatic activity and creates myocardial irritability. A serum pH above 7.8 or below 6.9 is usually fatal. Three complex mechanisms maintain acid-base balance: (1) buffers, (2) respiratory control of carbon dioxide, and (3) renal regulation of bicarbonate (HCO_3^-).

Buffers

Buffer systems prevent wide swings in pH. A buffer system consists of a weak acid and a weak base. Buffer molecules keep strong acids or bases from altering the pH either by absorbing or releasing free hydrogen ions.

- *Carbonic acid–sodium bicarbonate system.* Carbonic acid (H_2CO_3) and sodium bicarbonate ($NaHCO_3^-$) buffer almost 90% of metabolic processes in the ECF. Blood and tissue fluid depend on this buffer system to maintain a relatively constant pH. During normal metabolism, blood and tissue fluids tend to become acidic; therefore, more sodium bicarbonate is required than carbonic acid. The usual ratio of $NaHCO_3^-$ to H_2CO_3 is 20:1. As long as this ratio is maintained, the pH remains within its normal range. If bicarbonate is depleted while neutralizing a strong acid, the pH may drop below 7.35, resulting in a condition called **acidosis.** If a strong base is added to extracellular fluid and depletes carbonic acid, the pH may rise above 7.45, resulting in a condition called **alkalosis.**

- *Phosphate system.* The phosphate system helps regulate acid-base balance in intracellular fluids. The phosphate system works in the same way as the bicarbonate system but converts alkaline sodium phosphate (Na_2HPO_4) to acid sodium phosphate (NaH_2PO_4).

- *Protein system.* Plasma proteins and the globin portion of hemoglobin (in red blood cells) contain chemical groups that can either combine with or liberate hydrogen ions. This system helps buffer intracellular fluid and plasma to maintain pH balance.

Respiratory Mechanisms

The lungs, which control the body's carbonic acid supply, are the second line of defense to restore normal pH. When the serum pH is too acidic (pH is low), the lungs remove carbon dioxide through rapid, deep breathing. This reduces the amount of carbon dioxide available to make carbonic acid. If the serum pH is too alkaline (pH is high), the lungs try to conserve carbon dioxide through shallow respirations. This system works with the carbonic acid–sodium bicarbonate buffer system to maintain the 20:1 ratio of base to acid.

Renal Mechanisms

The last line of defense is the kidneys, which regulate the concentration of plasma bicarbonate. They can neutralize more acid or base than either the respiratory system or the chemical buffers. If the serum pH is too acidic, the kidneys conserve additional bicarbonate to neutralize the acid. If the serum pH is too alkaline, the kidneys excrete additional bicarbonate to lower the amount of base and thereby decrease the pH. The kidneys also buffer pH by forming acids and ammonium (a base).

Although the renal system is very effective at altering pH, it is slow. It may take up to 3 days to return the pH to normal limits. This process is known as *compensation.* The pH returns to normal, but the carbon dioxide or bicarbonate level is abnormal. Over time, or when the original problem is corrected, these levels also return to normal.

KnowledgeCheck 36–4

- Briefly describe the three mechanisms used to maintain pH.
- Rank order the acid-base balance mechanisms from the most rapidly acting to the most slowly acting.

 Go to Chapter 36, **Knowledge Check Response Sheet and Answers,** on the Electronic Study Guide.

FLUID, ELECTROLYTE, AND ACID-BASE IMBALANCES

Illness or disease may lead to imbalances of fluid, electrolytes, or pH. These are discussed in the next sections. The "Practical Knowledge" section, later in the chapter, presents interventions to correct these imbalances.

Fluid Imbalances

Fluid imbalances involve a deficit or excess in fluid volume or an alteration in distribution among the fluid compartments.

Fluid Volume Deficit

Fluid volume deficit (hypovolemia) occurs when there is a proportional loss of water and electrolytes from the ECF. You will also hear the term *dehydration*. However, **dehydration** implies the loss of water only, so the two terms are not interchangeable. Hypovolemia may result from insufficient intake of isotonic fluid; bleeding; excessive loss through urine, skin, insensible losses, or the gastrointestinal tract; or loss of fluid into a third space.

The first symptom of hypovolemia is thirst. If the patient is able to recognize thirst and respond by drinking liquid, no further treatment may be required. If fluid is not available or the patient is unable to drink, hypovolemia progresses. As fluid volume decreases, the heart pumps the remaining blood faster but not as powerfully, resulting in a rapid, weak pulse and a low blood pressure. Water is pulled from the interstitial spaces and the ICF into the vascular system, resulting in dry skin and mucous membranes, decreased skin turgor, and decreased urine output. Patients complain of muscle weakness, fatigue, and feeling warm. Temperature increases because the body is less able to cool itself through perspiration. In an older adult, temperature will rise but may not be elevated above normal body temperature.

Weight is a sensitive measure of fluid loss. A sudden 5% loss of body weight is considered clinically significant. When loss approaches 8%, fluid loss is severe. A sudden loss of 15% of body weight due to fluid loss is usually fatal. The patient with fluid volume deficit usually has an elevated blood urea nitrogen (BUN) level and elevated hematocrit. Both values increase because there is less water in proportion to the solid substances being measured. Specific gravity of the urine increases as the kidneys attempt to conserve water, resulting in more concentrated urine.

You can help prevent fluid volume deficit by identifying patients who have the highest risk for developing this condition. High-risk patients include older adults, infants, children, and any patients with conditions associated with fluid loss (e.g., vomiting, fever). Encourage patients to drink adequate fluids to maintain fluid balance. If the patient is unable to take enough fluid by mouth, you may need to administer parenteral fluids.

Fluid Volume Excess

Fluid volume excess (hypervolemia) involves excessive retention of sodium and water in the ECF. *Overhydration* is not a synonym for hypervolemia, because overhydration means excess water in the ECF but does not denote electrolyte changes. Fluid volume excess results from excessive salt intake, disease affecting kidney or liver function, or poor pumping action of the heart. The retained sodium increases osmotic pressure in the ECF. This pressure pulls fluid from the cells into the ECF.

The vital sign changes in a patient with hypervolemia are the opposite of those in a patient with hypovolemia. The blood pressure is elevated, pulse is bounding, and respirations are increased and shallow. The neck veins may become distended. Along with increased intravascular volume, excess ECF may accumulate in the tissues, especially in dependent areas, as edema. The skin is pale and cool. Urine output becomes dilute, and volume increases. The patient rapidly gains weight. In severe fluid overload, the patient develops moist crackles in the lungs, dyspnea, and ascites (excess peritoneal fluid). Hemodilution causes BUN, hematocrit, and the specific gravity of the urine to decrease.

You can help prevent fluid overload by monitoring intake and output and observing patients for signs and symptoms of fluid overload. Electronic infusion pumps control the rate of infusion of intravenous fluid, thereby limiting the risk for patients receiving IV therapy.

KnowledgeCheck 36–5

- Define *fluid volume deficit* and *fluid volume excess*.
- Identify the signs and symptoms of fluid volume deficit and fluid volume excess.
- Describe dehydration and overhydration.

 Go to Chapter 36, **Knowledge Check Response Sheet and Answers,** on the Electronic Study Guide.

Electrolyte Imbalances

All the electrolytes may become imbalanced. Table 36–5 discusses the common causes, signs and symptoms, and treatment of sodium, potassium, calcium, magnesium, and phosphate imbalances. Disorders affecting chloride ions occur in conjunction with sodium disorders. As sodium levels rise, chloride levels also rise. Decreases also occur simultaneously. Manifestations and treatments are identical to the treatments used for sodium imbalances. Because of the role of bicarbonate as a buffer, bicarbonate levels rise and fall to maintain pH. Further discussion of abnormal bicarbonate levels is included in the "Acid-Base Imbalances" section, which follows.

We can apply the information in Table 36–5 to the LaGuardia family ("Meet Your Patients"). Jackson LaGuardia has end-stage renal disease (ESRD), or renal failure. As a result, he is at risk for imbalances in all of his electrolytes. Now he is experiencing nausea, vomiting, and diarrhea. This will further alter the imbalance of potassium and sodium. Due to his complex imbalances, he is a candidate for admission to the hospital. He will need careful rehydration and monitoring of his electrolytes. The remaining family members are likely to be experiencing sodium, potassium, and fluid deficits.

TABLE
36-5 Electrolyte Imbalances

Disorder	Common Causes	Signs and Symptoms	Treatment
Hyponatremia $Na^+ < 135$ mEq/L	Diuretics GI fluid loss Adrenal insufficiency Excessive intake of hypotonic solutions, such as water or D_5W IV fluids Syndrome of inappropriate ADH	Anorexia, nausea, and vomiting Weakness Lethargy Confusion Muscle cramps or twitching Seizures	Monitor I & O Monitor sodium level Increase oral sodium intake Administer IV saline infusion, if severe
Hypernatremia $Na^+ > 145$ mEq/L	Excessive sodium intake Water deprivation Increased water loss through profuse sweating, heat stroke, or diabetes insipidus Administration of hypertonic tube feeding	Thirst Elevated temperature Dry mouth and sticky mucous membranes If severe: • Hallucinations • Irritability • Lethargy • Seizures	Monitor I & O Monitor sodium level Monitor vital signs and level of consciousness Restrict sodium in the diet Beware of hidden sodium in foods and medications Increase water intake Administer IV solutions that do not contain sodium
Hypokalemia $K^+ < 3.5$ mEq/L	Diuretics GI fluid loss through vomiting, gastric suction, or diarrhea Steroid administration Hyperaldosteronism Anorexia or bulimia	Fatigue Anorexia, nausea, and vomiting Muscle weakness Decreased GI motility Dysrhythmias Paresthesia Flat T wave on ECG Increased sensitivity to digitalis	Monitor potassium level If client is taking digoxin, monitor pulse and observe for toxicity Encourage foods rich in potassium Administer potassium supplements (*Note:* IV supplements must be well diluted and administered slowly)
Hyperkalemia $K^+ > 5.0$ mEq/L	Renal failure Potassium-sparing diuretics Hypoaldosteronism High potassium intake coupled with renal insufficiency Acidosis Major trauma Hemolyzed serum sample produces pseudohyperkalemia	Muscle weakness Dysrhythmias Flaccid paralysis Intestinal colic Tall T waves on ECG	Monitor potassium level Caution about potassium-rich food intake in patients with elevated creatinine levels Cautiously administer IV potassium supplements If severe, monitor ECG; prepare to administer a cation exchange resin and glucose and insulin Renal dialysis may be required
Hypocalcemia $Ca^{2+} < 8.5$ mg/dL	Hypoparathyroidism Malabsorption Pancreatitis Alkalosis Vitamin D deficiency	Diarrhea Numbness and tingling of extremities Muscle cramps Tetany Convulsions Laryngeal spasms Cardiac irritability Positive Trousseau's and Chvostek's signs	Monitor serum calcium Encourage increased calcium intake Administer calcium supplements If severe, monitor patency of airway, institute seizure and safety precautions, and administer parenteral calcium

Go to Chapter 36, **Technique 36–1: Assessing for Trousseau's and Chvostek's Signs,** in Volume 2.

VOL 2

Daily Weights

Monitoring daily change in weight is an accurate method of assessing fluid status. Weight changes over time are usually related to diet and exercise levels. In contrast, short-term changes usually indicate changes in fluid status. Each kilogram (2.2 lb) of weight is equivalent to 1 liter (1000 mL) of fluid. Thus, a sudden drop in weight of 5 pounds in a client with diarrhea is equivalent to a fluid loss of almost 2300 mL.

To accurately monitor fluid status by weight, you must use the same balanced scale each day. Weigh the client at the same time of day, making sure that the client is wearing the same amount of clothing. Clients undergoing hemodialysis (blood cleansing through an artificial kidney) are usually weighed before and after dialysis treatments. Many lose 3 to 4 kg over the course of several hours of dialysis. As a result, hypotension, tachycardia, and feelings of lightheadedness are common after a dialysis treatment.

Weight monitoring is a valuable tool for assessing fluid status when it is impractical or impossible to measure intake and output. For example, it is impossible to know how much fluid a breast-fed infant receives with each feeding. If the infant is feeding well but experiencing diarrhea, weight monitoring will help the parents and pediatrician assess fluid status. Incontinence, draining wounds, and limited resources may also make it difficult to monitor intake and output. Weight monitoring is a practical solution that may be initiated as a nursing order.

Fluid Intake and Output

Intake and output (I&O) are monitored to assess fluid status. I&O are usually tallied at the end of each shift, as well as for each 24-hour period. In intensive care units, I&O are measured hourly. To monitor, measure all fluids the client consumes or excretes. Although this sounds simple, it may be difficult to quantify all losses. For example, if the client passes a large soft stool, how much fluid is contained within that stool? That question cannot be answered without chemical analysis. As a result, I&O are correlated with daily weights to determine fluid status.

Most healthcare facilities have standardized I&O forms. I&O may be recorded on a separate form or be part of a flowsheet.

 Go to Chapter 16, **Forms: Intake and Output Record,** in Volume 2.

 Go to Chapter 16, **Forms: Nursing Assessment Flow Sheet,** in Volume 2.

Explain to the client, family members, and all caregivers that I&O are being monitored. Posting a sign at the bedside or on the door to the room is a helpful reminder. When possible, have the client assist you with monitoring.

Include the following items as fluid intake: oral fluids, semiliquid foods, ice chips, parenteral fluids, enteral feedings, and irrigations instilled and not withdrawn immediately. Fluid output includes the following items: urine output, gastrointestinal fluid loss (e.g., emesis), feces, and drainage (e.g., from suction devices or wounds).

KnowledgeCheck 36–7

- Identify ten physical assessment components that can be used to monitor fluid, electrolyte, and acid-base balance.
- What aspects should be evaluated in a nursing history focused on fluid, electrolyte, and acid-base balance?

 Go to Chapter 36, **Knowledge Check Response Sheet and Answers,** on the Electronic Study Guide.

CriticalThinking 36–5

What vital sign changes would you expect to find when assessing Jackson LaGuardia ("Meet Your Patients")?

Laboratory Studies

Several laboratory tests are performed to evaluate fluid, electrolyte, and acid-base status.

- *Serum electrolytes.* Venous blood samples are taken to measure sodium, potassium, chloride, and bicarbonate levels. In many labs, electrolyte panels also include blood urea nitrogen (BUN), creatinine, and glucose. BUN and creatinine are sensitive measures of fluid status and kidney function.

- *Serum osmolality* is a measure of the solute concentration of the blood. It is expressed as milliosmoles per kilogram (mOsm/kg). Sodium is the greatest determinant of serum osmolality. Glucose and urea also contribute to serum osmolality. Serum osmolality may be directly measured with venous blood or estimated by doubling the serum sodium level. A rise in serum osmolality indicates fluid volume deficit; a decrease indicates fluid volume excess. Changes in serum osmolality usually indicate alterations in sodium levels.

- *Urine osmolality* measures the solute concentration of urine. The body excretes nitrogenous wastes as well as electrolytes. As a result, urine osmolality is substantially higher than serum levels. Fluid volume deficit increases urine osmolality; fluid volume excess decreases urine osmolality.

- A *complete blood count (CBC)* is a measure of red blood cells (RBCs), white blood cells (WBCs), and platelets. Included in the CBC is the hematocrit, a measure of the percentage of RBCs in whole blood.

As fluid levels decrease, the percentage of blood made up by cells increases, and the hematocrit rises. As fluid levels increase, the hematocrit falls.

- *Urinalysis* is a routine screening test. It includes a measure of urine pH and specific gravity. Urine pH normally ranges from 4.6 to 8.0.

    pH. Urine becomes more acidic in respiratory or metabolic acidosis, starvation, or fluid volume deficit. An alkaline urine is associated with an alkaline state in the blood.

    Specific gravity. Specific gravity rises and falls in opposition to fluid status. A low specific gravity occurs when fluid is plentiful. When fluid levels decrease, urine becomes more concentrated, and specific gravity increases.

- *ABGs.* Interpretation of ABGs was discussed earlier in this chapter. For a list of these values, along with other lab studies discussed above,

 Go to Chapter 36, **Diagnostic Testing: Assessing Fluid, Electrolyte, and Acid-Base Balance,** in Volume 2.

Nursing Diagnosis

Nursing diagnoses directly related to fluid, electrolyte, and acid-base balance include the following:

- *Deficient Fluid Volume. Etiologies* include decreased fluid intake, fluid restrictions, inability to obtain or swallow fluids, abnormal fluid losses (e.g., through vomiting, diarrhea, or blood loss), increased need for fluids due to fever, extreme heat, or increased metabolic demands. *Defining characteristics* include dry mucous membranes, scant urine output, increased urine concentration, elevated hematocrit, thirst, weakness, weight loss, decreased skin and tongue turgor, decreased blood pressure, and elevated temperature, pulse, and respirations.

- *Excess Fluid Volume. Etiologies* include excessive fluid intake, limited fluid output (e.g., due to renal failure or low cardiac output), or excess sodium intake. *Defining characteristics* include decreased hemoglobin and hematocrit, decreased urine specific gravity, oliguria, restlessness, anxiety, weight gain, edema, venous distention, increased blood pressure, bounding pulse volume, rales and crackles on auscultation, and rapid respirations.

- *Risk for Deficient Fluid Volume* is a potential diagnosis appropriate for a client experiencing vascular, cellular, or intracellular dehydration (recall that this is a loss of total water volume). *Risk factors* include use of diuretic medications, loss of fluid through tubes (e.g., gastric suction), extremes of age, problems affecting access to or swallowing of fluids, and hypermetabolic state.

- *Risk for Imbalanced Fluid Volume* is a potential diagnosis appropriate for a client at risk for increase or decrease of fluids or for rapid fluid shifts in the intravascular, intracellular, or interstitial space. NANDA (2005) has established only one *risk factor:* impending major invasive procedures.

- *Impaired Gas Exchange* is an appropriate diagnosis for a client with a disorder affecting gas exchange at the alveolar-capillary membrane (see Chapter 35). Impaired Gas Exchange limits the effectiveness of the carbonic acid–bicarbonate buffer system and alters serum pH.

Fluid, electrolyte, and acid-base imbalances may be etiologies of other nursing diagnoses. Below are several examples:

- Activity Intolerance related to excess fluid and electrolyte loss through diarrhea
- Impaired Oral Mucous Membrane related to Deficient Fluid Volume
- Impaired Skin Integrity related to dehydration
- Decreased Cardiac Output related to hypovolemia

Planning Outcomes/Evaluation

The overall goal for a client experiencing an imbalance of fluid, electrolytes, or acid-base is to restore balance.

NOC standardized outcomes for describing fluid and electrolyte status include the following: Electrolyte & Acid/Base Balance, Fluid Balance, Fluid Overload Severity, and Hydration. For selected indicators for these outcomes,

 Go to Chapter 36, **Standardized Language, Selected Nursing Diagnoses, Outcomes, and Interventions for Fluid and Electrolyte Problems,** in Volume 2.

Individualized goals/outcome statements you might write for a client include the following examples:

- Maintains fluid balance, as evidenced by balanced 24-hr intake and output; good skin turgor; eyeballs firm; blood pressure within normal limits; and no adventitious breath sounds.
- Electrolyte balance restored, as evidenced by alertness and cognitive orientation.
- Drinks at least 2500 mL in 24 hours.
- Urine specific gravity within normal limits.

Planning Interventions/Implementation

NIC standardized interventions related to fluid, electrolyte, and acid-base balance include Acid-Base

Teaching Patients to Prevent Fluid and Electrolyte Imbalances

Teach clients to:

- Drink at least eight to ten 8-ounce glasses of water per day.
- Use thirst as a guide to fluid intake.
- Limit consumption of fluids high in salt, sugar, caffeine, or alcohol.
- Drink water before, during, and after strenuous exercise.
- Avoid routine use of laxatives, antacids, weight-loss products, or enemas. All of these products may cause imbalances.
- Weigh yourself daily if fluid balance is critical or if you are experiencing excessive loss.
- Contact a health professional if there is a sudden change of weight, decreased urine output, swelling in dependent areas, shortness of breath, or dizziness.

- Contact a healthcare provider if you experience prolonged vomiting, diarrhea, or inability to tolerate liquids or food.
- Eat a well-balanced diet, including dairy products rich in calcium.

In addition:

- Teach the client about usual fluid needs and circumstances that increase fluid needs, such as high environmental temperature, fever, GI fluid loss, or draining wounds. Base your teaching on the client's current intake and the changes required to meet fluid goals.
- Identify medications or conditions that place the client at risk for imbalances. For example, if the client is receiving a potassium-wasting diuretic, she will need to increase potassium intake, either by taking a supplement or by altering the diet.

Management, Electrolyte Management, and Fluid Management. For a listing of other interventions,

Go to Chapter 36, **Standardized Language, Selected Nursing Diagnoses, Outcomes, and Interventions for Fluid and Electrolyte Problems,** in Volume 2.

Individualized interventions are aimed at correcting the underlying disorder that led to imbalance. Your care will focus on preventing imbalances, modifying oral intake, providing parenteral fluids, and transfusing blood products, all of which are discussed below.

Preventing Fluid and Electrolyte Imbalances

Preventing imbalances is preferable to treating imbalances. Use the data you obtained from your assessment to plan how to help your client avoid imbalances. Common strategies are listed in the accompanying Self-Care box.

Dietary Changes

To promote fluid and electrolyte balance, most people need to limit their sodium intake and increase their dietary potassium and calcium. As previously discussed, most North Americans consume more sodium than they should and not enough potassium and calcium. Teach clients to eat foods rich in potassium and calcium every day and to avoid sodium-rich foods (see Chapter 26). For example, instruct clients to read food labels, particularly when trying to limit sodium intake.

Oral Electrolyte Supplements

Many clients are unable to correct electrolyte disturbances with dietary changes alone. This is especially true for clients who have food intolerances, who rely on prepared meals, or who live in group settings. Such clients may need oral supplements to meet their requirements. Potassium and calcium are among the most common supplements. Most adults consume less calcium per day than the recommended amount, so supplementation is advisable. Calcium supplements come in many forms, including tablet, liquid, and chewable form. Potassium supplements are available in pill and liquid form. Many have an unpleasant taste. The following are suggested nursing activities:

- Encourage clients to take potassium supplements with juice to mask the taste.
- Teach clients to take supplements regularly to maintain electrolyte balance.
- Remind clients that supplements are medications and should be viewed as part of the treatment plan.
- If the client's medications are altered, review the continued need for supplements.
- Caution clients that salt substitutes contain potassium. If the client has been advised to use salt substitutes, review the need for potassium supplements.
- Encourage clients who take calcium supplements to consume at least 2500 mL of fluid per day to avoid constipation and reduce the risk of kidney stone formation.

KnowledgeCheck 36–8

- Identify laboratory tests that monitor fluid, electrolyte, and acid-base balance.
- Give at least five strategies to prevent fluid and electrolyte imbalance.

 Go to Chapter 36, **Knowledge Check Response Sheet and Answers,** on the Electronic Study Guide.

Modifying Oral Fluid Intake

Clients experiencing fluid imbalances may need to restrict or increase their daily oral intake to correct the underlying disorder.

Facilitating Fluid Intake

Clients with actual or potential fluid volume deficit may need to increase their fluid intake. Whenever possible, clients should take fluids by mouth. You may provide enteral replacement through a nasogastric or feeding tube if the client can tolerate fluids in the gastrointestinal tract but is unable to meet his needs independently. Parenteral fluid replacement is used only when enteral replacement cannot meet the client's fluid needs.

To successfully increase fluid intake, you must establish the desired amount of fluid intake for the client. The target amount reflects the client's current fluid balance and underlying condition. For example, if a client is dehydrated, an order might read: "Force fluids: 2500 mL oral fluids per 24 hours." From this order you can develop a plan to increase fluids. Typically people drink more fluid during the day and early evening, when they are more likely to be active. A large volume of fluid late in the evening may interrupt sleep because it may prompt the need to urinate. Therefore, you should distribute fluids to reflect the time of day, for example:

7:00 A.M. to 3:00 P.M.—1200 mL
3:00 P.M. to 11:00 P.M.—900 mL
11:00 P.M. to 7:00 A.M.—300 mL

Strategies to increase fluid intake include the following:

- Offer a variety of fluids throughout the day. Vary hot and cold liquids, and offer a choice of juices and other drinks.
- Each time you are at the bedside, remind the patient to drink.
- Break daily goals into hourly increments. For example, in the 8 hours between 7:00 A.M. and 3:00 P.M. (see the preceding example), have the patient drink 150 mL of fluid every hour. Give him a written schedule.
- Provide a glass with milliliter markings on it so that the patient will know how much he is drinking.

- Always have fluid readily available to the client. For example, keep a pitcher of water at the bedside.
- When possible, have the client and family members participate in tracking fluid intake.

Facilitating Fluid Restriction

Patients may be placed on fluid restriction for a variety of reasons (e.g., cardiovascular, liver, or renal impairment). Inform patients and caregivers of the reason for the restriction, as well as the amount of fluid allowed. If you do not educate the patient and family, they may not restrict fluids adequately.

Typically, fluid volume is divided into amounts allotted per shift. However, fluid restrictions usually include *all* forms of intake. For example, an order might read: "Limit total fluid intake to 1500 mL per 24 hours." If the patient is receiving IV antibiotics four times per day, you must include that volume as a part of the total fluids. If 75 mL is infused with each administration, total IV fluids equal 300 mL. So, the oral intake must be limited to 1200 mL per day. This amount may be distributed as 700 mL on the day shift, 400 mL on the evening shift, and 100 mL at night. Strategies to restrict fluid intake include the following:

- Do not offer liquids with meals, because food may quench thirst. Reserve liquids for between meals.
- Limit intake of dry, salty, or spicy foods; these foods increase thirst.
- Offer ice chips to help quench thirst.
- Provide frequent oral hygiene.
- Keep liquids away from the bedside.
- Provide diversional activities for the patient.

Parenteral Replacement of Fluids and Electrolytes

When fluid loss is severe or the client cannot tolerate oral or tube feedings, fluid volume is replaced parenterally. Intravenous therapy is the administration of fluids, electrolytes, medications, or nutrients by the venous route. Intravenous fluids are used to:

1. Expand intravascular volume.
2. Correct an underlying imbalance in fluids or electrolytes.
3. Compensate for an ongoing problem that is affecting either fluid or electrolytes.

For instance, Martha LaGuardia ("Meet Your Patients") is being treated in the emergency department (ED) for gastroenteritis. She is experiencing fluid loss from vomiting and diarrhea, complicated by her use of a diuretic. IV therapy will allow her to receive fluid to expand her intravascular volume and to maintain her hydration until the vomiting and diarrhea subside. It

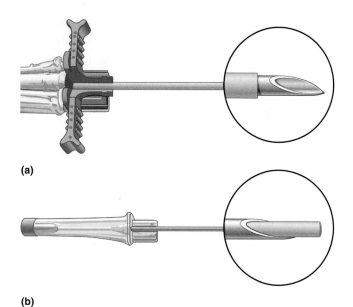

(a)

(b)

FIGURE 36–7   Typical IV access devices. A, An over–the–needle catheter. B, An inside-the-needle catheter.

will also provide electrolyte replacement based on her laboratory studies. Mrs. LaGuardia will remain on IV fluids until she can meet her fluid and electrolyte needs orally. All of the members of the LaGuardia family are experiencing fluid losses and would benefit from increasing their fluid intake. When fluid balance is fragile, or when the client cannot tolerate oral fluids, replacement may be supervised in an inpatient setting.

Types of Solutions

As we explained earlier, solutions are classified according to how they compare to the osmolality of blood serum. Intravenous fluids are these classified as isotonic, hypotonic, and hypertonic solutions. The osmolality of isotonic fluids is similar to that of blood serum.

- *Isotonic fluids.* When infused, isotonic solutions remain inside the intravascular compartment. As a result, they are useful for clients with hypotension or hypovolemia. Clients at risk for fluid volume excess due to congestive heart failure (CHF) must be closely monitored when they receive isotonic fluid replacement, because they may easily develop fluid overload. Examples of isotonic fluids are lactated Ringer's solution and 0.9% saline.

- *Hypotonic solutions.* Examples include 5% dextrose (D_5W) and 0.45% saline (½NS). The osmolality of a hypotonic solution is less than that of serum. When infused, these solutions pull body water from the intravascular compartment into the interstitial fluid compartment. As the interstitial fluid is diluted, its osmolarity decreases, drawing water into the adjacent cells. Hypotonic fluid is used for hyperglycemic

conditions, such as diabetic ketoacidosis, in which high serum glucose draws fluid out of the cells and into the vascular and interstitial compartments. Hypotonic fluids must be administered carefully to prevent a sudden fluid shift from the intravascular space to the cells.

- *Hypertonic fluids.* Examples include volume expanders, such as dextran and serum albumin. The osmolality of hypertonic fluids is higher than that of serum. When administered, they pull fluids and electrolytes from the intracellular and interstitial compartments into the intravascular compartment. Hypertonic fluids can help stabilize blood pressure, increase urine output, and reduce edema. Volume expanders are used to increase blood volume following severe loss of blood or plasma, such as in major burns or hemorrhage.

Vascular Access Devices

Intravenous therapy requires placement of a vascular access device. You will choose the type of device on the basis of the client's condition, type of fluid that will be infused, and the anticipated length of treatment.

Peripheral Access Devices

IV catheters (and needles) are sized by their diameter, which is called the **gauge.** The smaller the diameter, the larger the gauge. Therefore, the greater the diameter, the more rapidly fluid can be delivered. Several types of catheters are used to access peripheral veins, including the following:

- *Over-the-needle catheters* (Figure 36–7A). These are also called angiocaths. A polyurethane or Teflon catheter is threaded over a metal stylet (needle). You pierce the skin and vein with the stylet, advance the catheter into the vein, and remove the metal. In most cases, the plastic catheter is less than 7.5 cm (3 inches) in length. This type of access device is ideal for brief therapy. However, you cannot give highly irritating or hyperosmolar solutions through this type of catheter because it may cause severe damage to the vein. Ordinarily, the site is rotated every 72 to 96 hours (CDC, 2002).

- *Inside-the-needle catheters* (Figure 36–7B). This catheter is similar to the over-the-needle catheter; however, the polyurethane or Teflon catheter lies inside the metal needle. After you advance the catheter into the vein, you withdraw the needle.

- The *butterfly needle,* also called a scalp vein needle or wing-tipped catheter, is a short, beveled metal needle with flexible plastic flaps attached to the shaft (Figure 36–8). You can pinch the flaps and hold them tightly together to facilitate insertion. After insertion, flatten them out and tape them against the

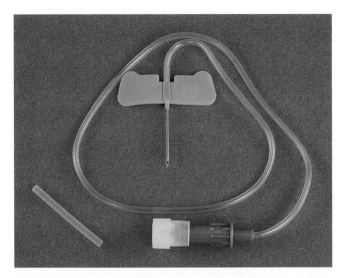

FIGURE 36-8 The butterfly, or scalp vein, needle is commonly used for intermittent or short-term therapy for children and infants.

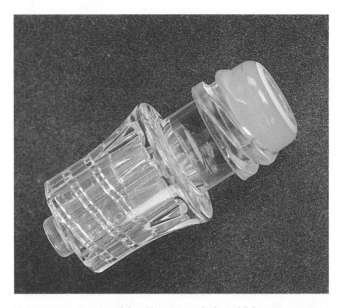

FIGURE 36-9 A peripheral intravenous lock establishes a venous route as a precautionary measure for clients whose condition may change rapidly or who may require intermittent infusion therapy.

skin to prevent dislodgement during the infusion process. These needles are commonly used for intermittent or short-term therapy for children and infants. Because the inflexible metal needle remains in the vein, a butterfly needle is more likely to infiltrate (damage the vein and allow fluid to leak into the interstitial spaces) than a plastic catheter.

- A *midline peripheral catheter* is a peripherally inserted flexible IV catheter, typically inserted into the antecubital fossa and then advanced into the larger vessels of the upper arm for greater hemodilution. It is 15 cm (6 inches) long, so it can be used for a longer period of time than a shorter angiocath. A midline peripheral catheter may remain in place for as long as 49 days, although the median length of use is 7 days (CDC, 2002). A midline catheter is still considered a peripheral line, so you cannot administer highly osmolar and irritating solutions through it.

In response to the Needlestick Safety and Prevention Act passed by Congress in 2000, the Centers for Disease Control and Prevention (CDC) and the Occupational Safety and Health Administration (OSHA) require the use of "needleless" systems. Therefore, you will usually have available access devices with safety features to prevent accidental "sticks." But if you find you must use an older, nonsafety device, do not attempt to recap the stylet after removing it from the vein.

Peripheral Intravenous Lock

A peripheral intravenous lock (also called a heparin lock or a saline lock) establishes a venous route as a precautionary measure for clients whose condition may change rapidly or who may require intermittent infusion therapy. Insert a peripheral IV catheter or butterfly wing-tipped catheter into a vein, and cap the hub with a lock port (Figure 36–9). Maintain the patency of the lock by injecting normal saline or a dilute heparin solution, depending on agency policy.

Central Venous Access Devices

A **central venous access device (CVAD)** is an intravenous line inserted into a major vein; typically, the subclavian or internal jugular vein is used. A catheter is advanced from the insertion site into the superior vena cava. A central line offers several advantages: (1) It can accommodate highly irritating and hyperosmolar solutions because the blood and solution mix rapidly at the infusion site; (2) central veins are accessible even if the patient is experiencing severe fluid depletion; and (3) central lines may also be used to monitor central venous pressure. CVADs require radiographic confirmation of placement. The following are types of CVADs:

- *Peripherally inserted central catheters (PICC lines)* are long, soft, flexible catheters inserted through a vein in the arm and threaded into a central vessel (Figure 36–10). A physician or specially trained registered nurse performs the insertion. Prolonged IV antibiotic therapy, parenteral nutrition, and chemotherapy are the most common uses for a PICC line. Nursing interventions for patients with PICC lines include providing sterile dressing changes per protocol and observing the site for complications, such as cellulitis or infection. A PICC line is intended for long-term use and does not need to be replaced unless the site appears infected or the catheter is no longer patent.

- *Nontunneled central venous catheters* are inserted through the skin into the jugular, subclavian, and,

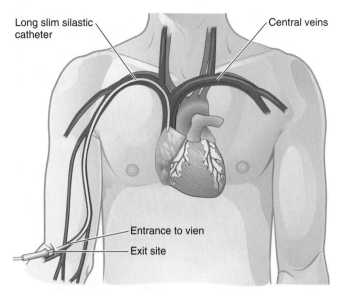

FIGURE 36–10 reference labels: Long slim silastic catheter, Central veins, Entrance to vien, Exit site

FIGURE 36–10 A PICC line is a long, soft, flexible catheter inserted through a vein in the arm and threaded into a central vessel.

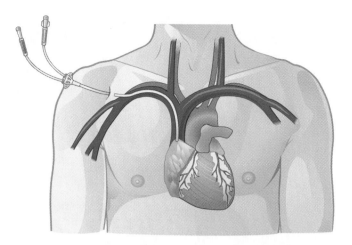

FIGURE 36–11 Nontunneled central venous catheters are inserted into the jugular, subclavian, and occasionally, femoral veins.

occasionally, femoral veins, and they are sutured in place. Often these are referred to as double-, triple-, or quadruple-lumen catheters, depending on the number of ports in the line (Figure 36–11). These CVADs are intended for shorter use (3 to 10 days) than a PICC line and offer the advantage of allowing multiple fluids to infuse simultaneously. Because they are frequently inserted in the chest, insertion poses a risk of pneumothorax.

- *Tunneled central venous catheters* are intended for long-term use. The catheter is inserted through a 7.5- to 15-cm (3- to 6-inch) subcutaneous tunnel in the chest wall and then into the jugular or subclavian vein (Figure 36–12). The catheter is sutured in place, but the sutures are removed after 1 or 2 weeks because the tunneling provides additional support to the catheter at the skin insertion site.

- *Implanted ports* are devices made of a radiopaque silicone catheter and a plastic or stainless steel injection port with a self-sealing silicone-rubber septum. The catheter enters the internal jugular vein in the neck, and it may be tunneled or untunneled to a completely implanted subcutaneous reservoir (port) in the upper chest (Figure 36–13). Only specially trained nurses are allowed to access an implanted port because of the risk of infiltration into the tissue if the needle placement is not correct.

KnowledgeCheck 36–9
- What is the purpose of intravenous fluids?
- Describe the types and functions of three IV solutions.
- Under what conditions would a central venous access device be preferable to a peripheral device?

Go to Chapter 36, **Knowledge Check Response Sheet and Answers,** on the Electronic Study Guide.

 CriticalThinking 36–6
What type of venous access device would you expect Martha LaGuardia ("Meet Your Patients") to receive in the hospital? Why?

Starting an Intravenous Infusion

To start an IV infusion, you will need to gather equipment and supplies, set up the solution and administration set, select a venipuncture site, and perform venipuncture.

Obtain Equipment and Supplies

You will need both venipuncture supplies and IV infusion equipment. Usually this consists of an IV catheter,

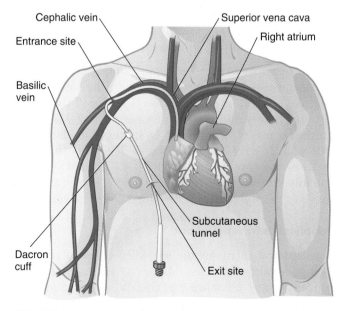

FIGURE 36–12 reference labels: Cephalic vein, Superior vena cava, Entrance site, Right atrium, Basilic vein, Subcutaneous tunnel, Dacron cuff, Exit site

FIGURE 36–12 A tunneled central venous catheter is inserted through subcutaneous tissue in the chest wall into the jugular or subclavian vein.

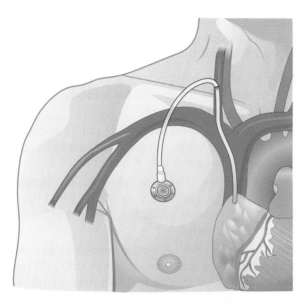

FIGURE 36–13 An implanted port is a CVAD that enters the internal jugular vein in the neck but is tunneled to a completely implanted subcutaneous reservoir (port) in the upper chest.

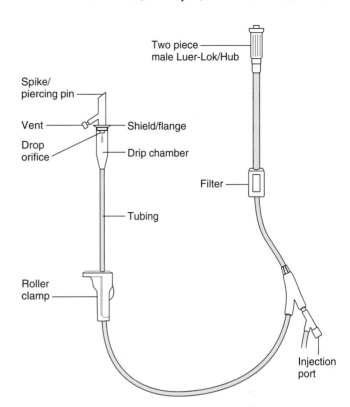

FIGURE 36–14 A basic administration set, or infusion kit.

a prepackaged administration set, extension tubing, and the IV solution. Intravenous supplies are sterile, prepackaged, and disposable. They vary based on manufacturer, so familiarize yourself with what is available in your facility.

- *IV catheter.* When selecting the access device, consider the type of fluid and the speed at which you are to infuse it. Traditionally, for most IV fluids, nurses use a 20- to 24-gauge catheter. For most peripheral infusions (with rates of 50 to 175 mL per hour), a 24-gauge thin-walled catheter or a 22-gauge non-thin-walled catheter is sufficient and will deliver over 1400 mL/hr if needed (Macklin, 2003). However, you will need a larger size for rapid infusions, to infuse viscous fluids, or for surgical or trauma patients. Select the smallest diameter and the shortest length catheter that will accommodate the prescribed therapy (Intravenous Nursing Society, 2000, p. 44).

- *Administration set (infusion kit).* The administration set connects the fluid container to the catheter you insert in the patient. An administration set consists of a plastic insertion spike, a drip chamber, tubing with a regulating (roller) clamp, a rubber injection port, and a catheter adapter (hub) (Figure 36–14). Both ends of the infusion set (over the spike and the catheter adapter) are sterile. Remove the protective caps just before use. Insert the spike into the port of the IV solution container; the adapter (hub) at the other end of the tubing fits into the IV catheter in the patient's vein.

  The drip chamber is calibrated to allow a predictable amount of fluid to be delivered in each drop. A macrodrip delivers 10 to 20 drops per milliliter of solution; a microdrip delivers 60 drops per milliliter. The drop factor is indicated on the package and

varies with the manufacturer. Select a microdrip or a macrodrip administration set based on the client's fluid needs. For very slow infusion rates or for children, use a microdrip. A roller clamp on the tubing controls the rate of flow.

- *Extension tubing and filters.* The end of the IV tubing contains a needle adapter that attaches to the inserted sterile IV catheter. You may use extension tubing to lengthen the primary tubing or to provide additional Y-injection ports for administration of other IV solutions or medications.

  Occasionally, an intravenous filter will be used on the tubing. Some administration sets have built-in filters. Usually the filter is placed at the end of the tubing. Filters remove particulate matter from the solution. They are used for additives or medications that have a tendency to clump and also to filter microorganisms. Filters come in a variety of sizes; the finer the filter, the greater the degree of solution filtration. Many facilities do not use IV filters because of cost, but studies have shown that IV filters reduce the rate of phlebitis and bacteremia by as much as 40% (Intravenous Nursing Society, 2000).

- *Injection port.* Use the injection port to administer a secondary IV fluid or medication (see Chapter 23).

- *Solutions.* Inspect the IV solution to be certain that it contains the desired fluid, the fluid is clear, the bag is intact, and the solution has not expired. IV solutions are available in glass or plastic containers. Glass containers were the first IV systems available,

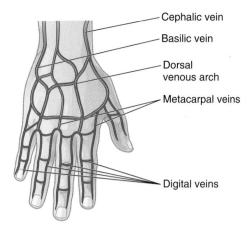

(a) Superficial veins of the hand

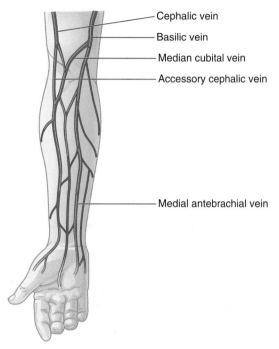

(b) Superficial veins of the forearm

FIGURE 36–15   *A,* Superficial veins of the hand. *B,* Superficial veins of the forearm.

but today about 90% of all IV fluids are packaged in plastic (Phillips, 2005). Fluids for continuous infusions are packed in 1-liter or 500-mL bags. Smaller solution bags (50 mL, 100 mL, and 250 mL) are used for intermittent infusions, such as antibiotics or other medications. Plastic containers collapse as fluid infuses, so you can use a nonvented administration set. Glass bottles do not collapse and therefore require a vented administration set. Set up the solution and administration set prior to performing the venipuncture.

Select a Peripheral Intravenous Site

To select a venipuncture site when initiating IV therapy, consider the client's age, condition of his veins,

presence of disease or previous surgery, anticipated duration of the infusion, the type of solution used, and the speed at which the infusion is to run.

- *Age.* For adults, you will usually use veins in the hand or arm (Figure 36–15); for infants, veins in the scalp or dorsum of the foot.
- *Type of solution.* For hypertonic solutions, viscous solutions, or irritating medications, use a large vein to cause the least amount of trauma.
- *Speed of infusion.* The faster the rate, the larger the vein (and the larger the IV catheter) you will need. Use the largest vein available, keeping other selection criteria in mind.
- *Duration of infusion.* Keep in mind that peripheral IV catheter sites are changed every 72 to 96 hours. Initiate the infusion with the vein most distal to the heart, and move toward the heart on subsequent insertions. If you start an IV below an already used site (i.e., to change the site or after a failed attempt at insertion), fluid may leak from the old site.
- *Presence of disease or previous surgery.* Avoid areas with scarring or with impaired circulation or neurological status (for example, the affected arm following a mastectomy; an area with signs of infection, previous infiltration or thrombosis; an arm with an arteriovenous fistula [shunt for dialysis]; or the affected side after cerebrovascular accident [stroke]).

Also consider the following:

- If possible, select a vein on the patient's nondominant hand or arm. This preserves functional ability.
- Look for a vein that has a firm, round appearance with a relatively straight pathway. Do not use a red, hot, or hard vein.
- Avoid areas where the vein crosses over joints. If you must use such an area, you will need to splint the joint.
- Avoid veins that are highly visible; they tend to roll.
- The cephalic vein is one of the best veins to use because it is relatively large, and the forearm provides a natural splint.
- The dorsal veins of the hand are easy to access and are splinted by the metacarpals, but these veins are often quite small and fragile.
- Avoid the antecubital veins if possible. If the patient flexes her arm, the IV catheter may become displaced; so you would probably need to splint her elbow. Furthermore, if a PICC line is needed at a later time, you will still have the antecubital veins available for it.
- Do not use veins in the legs and feet unless there is no other option. Peripheral circulation may not be adequate in the lower limbs, so there is increased danger of thrombus formation.

Perform Venipuncture

If you have difficulty locating a suitable vein, gently tap on the vein with the pads of two or three fingers to dilate them. If the vein is still difficult to find, cover the arm with a warm moist compress to stimulate vasodilatation. If, after a meticulous search, no veins can be found, release the tourniquet and move it up higher on the same extremity, or move to the other arm if not contraindicated.

Enter the skin at a 20 to 30° angle in the direction of the vein. Use a quick, smooth motion to pierce the skin. After piercing the skin, reduce the angle of the IV needle until it is almost parallel with the skin. If the vein appears to roll, apply counter tension against the skin just above and below the entry site, using your nondominant hand. Pull the skin in the opposite direction the needle will be advancing. Do not press too hard; doing so will compress blood flow in the vein and cause it to collapse.

If you are not successful, release the tourniquet, and place gauze over the skin puncture site. Make a second attempt above the initial site or in the opposite extremity. Although it is rare, you may inadvertently enter an artery. You'll recognize this because bright red blood is quickly seen in the IV tubing. If this occurs, remove the catheter and apply direct pressure for at least 5 minutes. For a summary of key points in starting a peripheral IV line, see the accompanying Critical Aspects box for Procedures 36–1 through 36–7. For the complete procedure,

 Go to Chapter 36, **Procedure 36–1: Initiating a Peripheral Intravenous Infusion,** in Volume 2.

Regulating and Maintaining an Intravenous Infusion

You are responsible for maintaining the correct rate of flow and for monitoring the client's response to the infusion. Many factors can influence the rate of flow of an IV solution:

- *The height of the solution container in relation to the insertion site.* The greater the distance, the faster the flow. Check the flow rate each time the client or IV solution is repositioned to ensure that the flow rate is correct.
- *Client position.* Pressure on the IV site decreases flow. If an IV is infusing in the right arm and the patient is positioned on his right side, the pressure on the right arm will be greater than if the client were positioned supine or on the left.
- *Blood pressure.* As blood pressure rises, more force is required to infuse into the vein.
- *The internal diameter of the IV catheter.* The smaller the diameter (the higher the gauge), the more you

must open the roller clamp to achieve the flow rate desired.

- *Condition of the catheter and tubing.* If the catheter is dislodged from the vein, flow may stop entirely or continue at a slowed rate. A knot or kink at any point in the tubing will slow flow.

Intravenous fluids can flow by gravity or be regulated by an electronic infusion control device.

Gravity Flow

When gravity flow is used, adjust the rate with the roller clamp on the tubing. Check the infusion rate hourly. If the fluid is running too slowly, adjust the flow rate, but do not attempt to catch up by administering extra fluid rapidly. If the fluid is running too fast, slow the rate, and assess the client for signs of fluid volume excess. If the client is ambulatory, attach the fluid container to a pole with wheels. Instruct the client to keep the solution container above the infusion site and to avoid pulling on the tubing or the infusion site. The Critical Aspects box summarizes how to regulate an IV by gravity flow. For the complete procedure,

 Go to Chapter 36, **Procedure 36–2: Regulating the IV Flow Rate,** Volume 2.

Volume-Control Set

A volume-control set (e.g., Buretrol, Soluset, Volutrol) is another method for regulating an IV infusion (see Figure 23–44 in Chapter 23). You will drain fluid from the larger IV solution container into the volume-control container. Typically, the volume placed in the volume-control container is equal to the prescribed hourly infusion rate. The rate is regulated in the same way as other administration sets (the drip factor is usually 60 gtts per mL); however, the maximum amount of fluid that can enter a patient is limited to the volume in the volume-control set. Use this type of equipment when the client is at risk for fluid volume excess and for infants and children, who require close supervision of fluid intake. An advantage of this system is that medications can be added to the volume-control set and diluted with IV fluid for intermittent administration.

Infusion Pump

If you are using an electronic infusion-control device (pump), the machine will maintain the infusion rate after you program it. Most infusion pumps sound an alarm when the fluid bag is almost empty, when air is in the line, or when there is resistance to flow. Infusion control devices save time and prevent accidental delivery of large amounts of fluid. They do not, however, excuse you from regularly monitoring the flow rate and assessing the needle insertion site.

VOL 2 For steps to follow in *all* procedures, refer to inside of back cover of Volume 2.

critical aspects of procedures 36–1 through 36–7

Procedure 36–1: Initiating a Peripheral Intravenous Infusion

- Prepare the intravenous solution and administration set.
- Locate a vein for placing the IV catheter. Select the most distal vein on the hand or arm initially.
- Clip excessive hair at the site with scissors.
- Don procedure gloves.
- Apply the tourniquet, and cleanse the site. Allow the antiseptic to dry on the skin.
- Using your nondominant hand, stabilize the vein, making sure not to contaminate the insertion site.
- Inform the patient that you are about to insert the catheter.
- Open the catheter. Grasp it with the thumb and forefinger of your dominant hand, making sure that the bevel is up.
- Holding the catheter at a 20 to 30° angle, pierce the skin.
- Lower the catheter so that it is parallel to the skin and insert the catheter.
- Watch for a flashback of blood; then disengage the stylet, and advance the catheter.
- While holding the catheter in place with one hand, release the tourniquet with your other hand.
- Quickly connect the tubing adapter to the IV catheter, using aseptic technique.
- Open the roller clamp, and allow the IV fluid to flush the catheter, and then adjust the flow rate according to the physician's order.
- Cover the insertion site with a sterile, semipermeable, transparent dressing.
- Loop and tape the administration tubing, and the connection between the catheter and tubing, and the looped section of the tubing.
- Label the dressing with the date and time of insertion, catheter size, and your initials.
- If the insertion site is located near a joint, place an arm board under the joint, and secure it with tape.

Procedure 36–2: Regulating the IV Flow Rate

- Check the solution to make sure that you have the proper IV fluid with the prescribed additives.
- Verify the prescribed infusion rate.
- Calculate the drip rate.
- Apply a time tape to the IV solution container. Mark the time the infusion was started.
- Open the roller clamp so that IV fluid begins to flow.
- Using a watch, count the number of drops entering the drip chamber in 1 minute.
- Adjust the roller clamp, increasing or decreasing the flow until you achieve the prescribed drip rate.
- Monitor the infusion rate 15 minutes after you begin the infusion; then monitor the rate hourly.

Procedure 36–3: Setting Up and Using IV Pumps

- Calculate the infusion rate.
- Attach the IV pump to the IV pole, and plug it into the nearest electrical outlet.
- Take the administration set from the package, label the tubing with the date and time, and close the clamp on the administration set.
- Remove the protective covers, and spike the port of the solution container with the administration set. Hang the IV solution container on the IV pole.
- If a filter is required, attach it to the end of the administration set.
- Compress the drip chamber of the administration set, and allow it to fill halfway.
- Place the electronic eye on the drip chamber between the fluid level and the origin of the drip. (If there is no electronic eye, consult the manufacturer's instructions for setup.)
- Prime the administration set with fluid by opening the roller clamp and allowing the fluid to flow slowly through the tubing. Close the clamp.
- Inspect the tubing for the presence of air. If air bubbles remain in the tubing, flick the tubing with a fingernail to mobilize the bubbles.
- Turn on the IV pump, and load the administration tubing into the pump according to the manufacturer's instructions.
- Program the pump with the prescribed infusion rate (hourly rate) and the volume to be infused (usually the total amount in the IV bag). Again, follow the manufacturer's instructions—each type pump is different.

Procedure 36–3: (continued)

- Apply procedure gloves, and connect the administration set adapter to the IV catheter. Take care not to contaminate the adapter hub, the IV catheter, or the insertion site.

- Unclamp the administration set tubing, and press the start button on the IV pump.

- Make sure that the alarms are turned on and audible.

- Check the pump hourly to make sure that the correct volume is infusing.

- At the end of your shift (or at the time specified by your healthcare facility), clear the pump of the volume infused, and record the volume on the patient's I & O form.

Procedure 36–4: Changing IV Solutions, Tubing, and Dressings

Procedure 36–4A: Changing the IV Solution

- Prepare and label your next container of IV solution 1 hour before the present infusion is scheduled to finish.

- Close the roller clamp on the infusing (empty) administration set.

- Wearing procedure gloves, remove the old IV solution container from the IV pole. Remove the spike from the bag, keeping the spike sterile.

- Spike the new IV solution bag.

- Hang the new IV solution container on the IV pole, and inspect the tubing for air.

- Open the roller clamp, and adjust the drip rate.

- Adhere the time tape to the new IV solution container. Mark the times.

Procedure 36–4B: Changing the IV Solution and Tubing

- Prepare the new IV solution and tubing.

- Wearing procedure gloves, carefully remove the tape securing the connection between the catheter and tubing.

- Close the roller clamp on the administration set.

- Remove the protective cover from the distal end of the new administration set.

- Stabilize the IV catheter with your nondominant hand while applying pressure over the vein just above the insertion site.

- Quickly, but gently, disengage the old tubing from the IV catheter, and insert the new tubing into the IV catheter. Use a hemostat ("mosquito" clamp) to hold the catheter hub if the old tubing does not come loose easily.

- Open the roller clamp, and adjust the drip rate.

- Resecure the IV catheter and tubing connection.

Procedure 36–4C: Changing the IV Dressing

- Wearing procedure gloves, stabilize the catheter with your nondominant hand, and carefully remove the dressing.

- Inspect the insertion site. Using a circular motion, cleanse the insertion site with an antiseptic swab containing 2% tincture of iodine, alcohol, or chlorhexidine.

- Allow the antiseptic to dry on the skin.

- Cover the insertion site with a sterile semipermeable transparent dressing.

- Loop and tape the administration tubing, and the connection between the catheter and tubing.

- Label the dressing with the date and time of insertion, catheter size, and your initials.

Procedure 36–5: Converting a Primary Line to a Heparin or Saline Lock

- Assist the client to a comfortable position.

- Place a linen-saver pad under the extremity with the IV catheter.

- Don procedure gloves.

- Remove the IV lock from the package, and flush the adapter with saline or dilute heparin, according to unit policy.

- Carefully remove the IV dressing and the tape that is securing the tubing.

- Close the roller clamp on the administration set.

- With your nondominant hand, apply pressure over the vein just above the insertion site.

- Disengage the old tubing from the IV catheter. Grasp the catheter hub with a hemostat ("mosquito" clamp) if the tubing does not disengage readily.

- Quickly insert the lock adapter into the IV catheter.

- Flush the lock adapter again.

- Apply a sterile transparent semipermeable dressing.

- Discard the used supplies.

Procedure 36–6: Discontinuing an IV Line

- Assist the client to a comfortable position.

- Place a linen-saver pad under the extremity that contains the IV catheter.

Procedure 36–6: *(continued)*

- Apply procedure gloves, and close the roller clamp on the administration set.

- Carefully remove the IV dressing and the tape that is securing the tubing.

- Apply a sterile 2 × 2 gauze pad above the IV insertion site and gently remove the catheter, directing it straight along the vein. Do not press on the gauze pad while removing the catheter.

- Apply firm pressure with the gauze pad over the insertion site. Hold pressure for 2 to 3 minutes; hold longer if bleeding persists.

- Remove the soiled 2 × 2 gauze pad and replace it with a new sterile 2 × 2 gauze pad. Secure it with a piece of 1-inch tape.

- Dispose of the IV catheter, IV supplies, and gloves in the appropriate containers.

Procedure 36–7: Administering a Blood Transfusion

- Verify that informed consent has been obtained.

- Verify the physician's order, noting the indication, rate of infusion, and any pretransfusion or post-transfusion medication orders. Administer any pretransfusion medications as prescribed.

- Obtain a blood administration set and IV container of normal saline solution.

- Obtain the blood product from the blood bank according to your institution's policy.

- Recheck the physician's order.

- With another qualified staff member (as deemed by your institution), verify the patient and blood product identification.

- Remove the blood administration set from the package, and label the tubing with the date and time. Then, close the clamps on the administration set.

- Spike the port of the normal saline solution container, and hang the IV solution.

- Compress the drip chamber of the administration, set and prime the tubing with the saline solution.

- Invert the blood filter on the administration set, and prime it with normal saline solution.

- Gently invert the blood product container several times.

- Spike the blood product container through the port, and hang the blood on the IV pole.

- Slowly open the roller clamp closest to the blood product.

- Obtain a set of vital signs.

- Attach the distal end of the administration set to the IV catheter.

- Measure vital signs in 5 minutes, 15 minutes, then 30 minutes, then hourly.

- When the blood has transfused, flush the line with normal saline solution.

- Disconnect the tubing from the IV catheter, and dispose of the blood product container and tubing per agency policy.

- If a second unit of blood is to be transfused, the same administration set may be used.

- Administer any post-transfusion medications ordered.

Procedure Variation: Managing a Transfusion Reaction

- Stop the transfusion immediately. Do not flush the tubing with the normal saline solution.

- Disconnect the administration set from the IV catheter. Obtain vital signs, and auscultate heart and breath sounds.

- Maintain patency of the IV catheter by hanging a new infusion of normal saline solution.

- Notify the physician.

- Place the administration set and blood product container, with the blood bank form attached, inside a biohazard bag. Send the bag to the blood bank immediately.

- Obtain blood (in the extremity opposite the transfusion site) and urine specimens according to your institution's policy.

- Continue to monitor vital signs frequently.

- Administer medications, as prescribed.

The Critical Aspects box describes how to regulate an IV using an infusion control device. For the complete procedure,

 Go to Chapter 36, **Procedure 36–3: Setting Up and Using IV Pumps,** in Volume 2.

KnowledgeCheck 36–10

- What factors should you consider when selecting an insertion site for a peripheral IV line?
- What are the preferred locations for peripheral IV lines?
- Describe the most common components used for infusing IV fluid.
- Identify three ways to regulate the flow rate of IV fluid.

 Go to Chapter 36, **Knowledge Check Response Sheet and Answers,** on the Electronic Study Guide.

Calculating Flow Rates

As you already know, intravenous administration sets are sized as microdrips or macrodrips. Microdrips deliver fluid at a rate of 60 drops per mL. Macrodrips deliver fluid at a rate of 10 to 20 drops per mL (depending on the manufacturer). To begin, you need to know the ordered infusion rate and the flow rate of the administration set in drops per minute. First multiply the number of mL to be infused in 60 minutes (hourly rate) by the drop factor in drops per milliliter to obtain the total drops per hour. Then divide by 60 to get the drip rate in drops per minute. For example, an hourly rate of 100 mL multiplied by 15 drops per milliliter and divided by 60 equals the drip rate. Therefore, the drip rate equals 25 drops per minute. Use this formula to calculate flow:

$$\frac{\text{Hourly rate in mL} \times \text{drop factor (drops/mL)}}{60 \text{ minutes}} = \text{drip rate}$$

Using the preceding example:

$$\frac{100 \text{ (mL per hour)} \times 15 \text{ (gtts/mL)}}{60 \text{ minutes}} = 25 \text{ gtts per minute}$$

Managing Multiple Lines

If the client is receiving multiple IV solutions, you must label all lines. For example, a client requiring the simultaneous infusion of IV fluid and antibiotics, blood products, and TPN requires three separate lines because none of these products should be mixed. To monitor the lines, clearly identify each line. Use RA for right arm, LA for left arm, and so on. Also, designate a number for each site (e.g., RA#1, RA#2, LA#1), because there may be more than one line in each extremity. If the lines are in separate arms, giving each one a number may seem unnecessary; however, over the course of therapy some lines may need to be discontinued and others started. If the client has a multiport central line, be sure that each port has its own designation.

Complications of Intravenous Therapy

Inserting an IV catheter breaks the body's first line of defense (the skin) and provides a portal of entry for microorganisms. In addition, trauma roughens the vein wall and predisposes the person to platelet clumping and thrombus formation. Minimize this effect by swiftly piercing the skin and anchoring the catheter and tubing to reduce tissue trauma. Complications at the IV site include infiltration, extravasation, infection, thrombus, and thrombophlebitis. Systemic complications occur less frequently than local complications but may be life-threatening. They include fluid volume excess, sepsis, and embolus. Table 36–8 describes potential complications of IV therapy.

Changing Intravenous Solutions, Tubing, and Dressings

The infusion rate dictates how often you need to change the IV solution. You should hang a new container of fluid when the previous container is nearly empty but fluid still remains at the appropriate level in the drip chamber. A liter of IV fluid infusing at 125 mL/hr must be changed every 8 hours, whereas a liter infused at 50 mL/hr will hang for 20 hours. Regardless of rate, do not leave an intravenous solution hanging for more than 24 hours because the likelihood of contamination increases with time. For instructions on changing a solution container, see the Critical Aspects box, and

 Go to Chapter 36, **Procedure 36–4: Changing IV Solutions, Tubing, and Dressings,** Volume 2.

Administration sets for continuous peripheral and central infusions are usually changed every 72 hours (every 24 hours for total parenteral nutrition). Because most peripheral catheters are changed every 72 to 96 hours (CDC, 2002), changing the administration set frequently coincides with inserting a new intravenous catheter. As a rule, if you start an IV at a new site, use a new administration set. Reusing a set from a previous site increases the risk of contamination. Procedure 36–4B explains how to change the administration tubing and solution.

CVADs usually remain in place for lengthy periods of time. The dressing at the site must be changed periodically. In the acute care setting, you will usually change the dressing every 72 hours. However, in home care, the dressing may be left in place for 1 week. You will probably dress both central and peripheral lines with transparent, semipermeable dressings. These dressings allow direct visualization of the site between dressing changes, permit evaporation of moisture, and provide a secure anchor for the catheter. At times, you may still see tape securing a catheter at the insertion site. This trend has diminished though because of the risk of contamination at the site (Intravenous Nursing

TABLE 36-8 Complications of Intravenous Therapy

Local Complications

Complication	Causes	Signs and Symptoms	Nursing Response
Hematoma—a localized mass of blood outside the blood vessel	Nicking the vein during an unsuccessful insertion, discontinuing an IV line without holding pressure over the site, or applying a tourniquet too tightly above a previously attempted venipucture site.	Ecchymosis, swelling, discomfort	Be gentle with venipuncture technique. Apply pressure when discontinuing an IV.
Infiltration—the seepage of nonvesicant solution or medication into surrounding tissues	IV catheter becomes dislodged or the tip penetrates the vessel wall.	Slowed or stopped flow Swelling, tenderness, pallor, hardness and coolness at the site The patient may report a burning sensation in the area.	Stop the infusion immediately. Restart the IV infusion in a different vein, higher in the extremity or in another extremity. Elevate the affected arm on a pillow to promote absorption of excess fluid.
Extravasation—infiltration of a vesicant substance into the tissues (A vesicant is a solution that causes the formation of blisters and subsequent tissue sloughing and necrosis)	IV catheter becomes dislodged, or the tip penetrates the vessel wall.	Slowed or stopped flow Pain, burning, and swelling at IV site, blanching and coolness of the surrounding skin Blistering is a late sign.	Treatment depends on the severity of the infiltration. Stop the IV infusion immediately. Administer an antidote, if one is available. (Antidotes alter the pH, alter DNA binding, neutralize the drug, or dilute the extravasated drug.) Apply cold compresses, and elevate the extremity.
Phlebitis—inflammation of the vein	May be due to mechanical irritation, infusion of solutions that are irritating to the vessel, or sepsis. Dextrose solutions, potassium chloride, antibiotics, and vitamin C are associated with a higher risk of phlebitis.	Redness, pain, and warmth at the site, local swelling, palpable cord along the vein, sluggish infusion rate, and elevated temperature	Discontinue the IV infusion. Initially, apply cold compresses to the site. Thereafter, use warm compresses. Consult the primary care provider if there is streaking or erythema along the vein or a palpable cord. Prevention measures: • Use the smallest catheter practical (usually 22-gauge or 24-gauge thin-walled catheter). • Use polyurethane catheters instead of Teflon. • Stabilize and secure the catheter to minimize movement in the vein. • Rotate the site at least every 96 hours.

TABLE 36–8 (continued)

Local Complications

Complication	Causes	Signs and Symptoms	Nursing Response
Thrombosis—clot formation at the insertion site	Trauma to the vessel, compression of the line by client movement, or a low flow rate.	Slowed or stopped infusion, localized warmth at the site, inability to restart flow of IV	Discontinue the IV infusion, and restart in a new location. Apply cold compresses to the site if the site is warm and tender. Assess for circulatory impairment.
Thrombophlebitis—thrombosis and inflammation	Use of veins in the legs for infusion, use of a hypertonic or highly acidic solution. Can be a result of untreated phlebitis.	Sluggish flow rate, edema, tender and cordlike veins, warmth and erythema at site	Discontinue the IV infusion, and restart in the opposite extremity, using all new equipment. Apply warm, moist compresses. Consult the primary care provider.
Local infection—microbial contamination of the cannula or IV site	Using poor technique when inserting the catheter, leaving the catheter in place for longer than 72 hours, or direct contamination.	Redness, swelling, exudate, elevated temperature	Remove the IV line. Apply a sterile dressing over the site. Administer antibiotics, if necessary.

Systemic Complications

Complication	Causes	Signs and Symptoms	Nursing Response
Septicemia—the presence of microorganisms or their toxic products in the circulatory system	A break in aseptic technique, or contaminated IV solution.	Fluctuating fever, chills, tachycardia, confusion, hypotension, altered mental status, elevated WBC count	Discontinue the IV infusion immediately. Consult the primary care provider. Treatment often involves antibiotics, fluids, and medications to support vital signs.
Fluid overload	Infusing excessive amounts of IV fluids or administering fluid too rapidly.	Weight gain, edema, hypertension, shortness of breath, crackles, distended neck veins	Slow the IV flow rate. Place the client in high-Fowler's position. Monitor vital signs. Administer oxygen, if needed. If severe, diuretics may be ordered.
Air embolus—a rare complication involving the introduction of air into the vascular system	Loose connections, adding a new IV bag to a line that has run dry without clearing the line of air; air in tubing cassette of infusion pump.	Palpitations, chest pain, lightheadedness, dyspnea, cough, hypotension, tachycardia, sudden change in mental status	Call for help. Place client in Trendelenburg's position on the left side. Administer oxygen. Have emergency equipment available.
Catheter embolus—a piece of catheter breaks off and travels through the vascular system	Reinserting a catheter used in an unsuccessful insertion; removing and reinserting a stylet, causing shearing of the catheter; placing the catheter in a joint flexion.	Sharp, sudden pain at IV site, jagged catheter end on removal, cyanosis, chest pain, tachycardia, hypotension	Apply a tourniquet above the site. Notify the physician and radiologist. Start a new IV line. Prepare the patient for radiographic examination.

Source: Phillips, L. D. (2005). *Manual of IV Therapeutics* (4th ed.). Philadelphia: F. A. Davis Company.

| toward evidence-based practice |

Niesen, K. M., Harris, D. Y., Parkin, L. S., & Henn, L. T. (2003). The effects of heparin versus normal saline for maintenance of peripheral intravenous locks in pregnant women. *Journal of Obstetrics, Gynecology, & Neonatal Nursing, 32*(4), 503–508.

Researchers in a large academic medical center in the Midwest compared the efficacy of two available preparations (1 mL heparin, 10 units/mL; and 1 mL normal saline) to maintain patency in peripheral intravenous locks during pregnancy. A convenience sample of 73 hospitalized pregnant women who were between 24 and 42 weeks' gestation were randomly assigned to receive either heparin flushes or normal saline flushes for IV lock maintenance. IV locks were flushed after each medication administration, or at least every 24 hours, with the assigned blinded flush solution. Intermittent IV lock sites were also evaluated every 12 hours for the development of phlebitis. Data revealed no statistically significant differences in IV lock patency nor in phlebitis between heparin or normal saline flushes.

1. Based on this study, if your unit had been using heparin flushes, would you recommend using only saline flushes on your unit? Why or why not? (To answer this question, identify at least three limiting factors in this study. Look up any terms you do not know.)

 Go to Chapter 36, **Toward Evidence-Based Practice Suggested Responses,** on the Electronic Study Guide.

Society, 2000). Procedure 36–4C discusses how to change the IV dressing.

Converting to a Peripheral Intravenous Lock

Some clients require only intermittent infusion of medications or venous access for emergencies. They do not need the fluids provided by a constant infusion of solution. A peripheral intravenous lock is used for this purpose. The terms *peripheral lock, heparin lock, saline lock,* or *PRN adapter* are used interchangeably. A peripheral infusion can be easily converted to a peripheral lock when no further infusion is required.

To create a peripheral lock, attach the sterile injection cap of the PRN adapter to the IV catheter. Some IV locks also contain a short segment of tubing. Each time you give a medication through the lock, you will need to flush the lock before and after you administer the medication. Consult your agency policy regarding the type of solution to use (saline or a dilute heparin solution). Converting an IV line to an IV lock is described in the Critical Aspects box. For complete instructions,

 Go to Chapter 36, **Procedure 36–5: Converting a Primary Line to a Heparin or Saline Lock,** Volume 2.

Discontinuing an Intravenous Line

Discontinue the IV line when IV fluids or medications are no longer needed or if the integrity of the line is in question. Inspect the catheter to ensure that it is intact when you remove the line. The Critical Aspects box summarizes removal of an IV catheter. For the complete procedure,

 Go to Chapter 36, **Procedure 36–6: Discontinuing an IV Line,** in Volume 2.

KnowledgeCheck 36–11

- The order reads, "5% dextrose in water/ 0.45% saline solution with 20 mEq KCl; infuse 1 liter in 5 hours." Calculate the hourly rate and the drip rate using (1) a macrodrip administration set with 15 drops/mL and (2) a microdrip set.
- Describe the difference between infiltration and extravasation as a complication of IV therapy.
- In general, how often are administration sets changed on peripheral IV lines? When TPN is infused?

 Go to Chapter 36, **Knowledge Check Response Sheet and Answers,** on the Electronic Study Guide.

Replacement of Blood and Blood Products

Intravenous fluids can replace fluid volume, but they do not restore oxygen-carrying capacity or replace clotting factors. Blood products are infused when the patient has experienced significant blood loss, diminished oxygen-carrying capacity, or a deficiency in one of the blood components. The American Association of Blood Banks (AABB) estimates that 8 million volunteers donate blood each year, for a total of 15 million units of whole blood and red blood cells (AABB, 2004). Each unit of donated blood is separated into multiple components, such as red blood cells, plasma, platelets, and clotting factors. Thus, one unit of donated blood may be used in the care of four clients. Unfortunately, fewer than 5% of eligible persons donate blood each year. To be eligible to donate blood, a person must be in good health, at least 17 years of age (although some states permit younger people, with parental consent, to donate) and weigh at least 110 pounds. In addition, each potential donor is screened for a variety of disorders, such as hepatitis, HIV, and Creutzfeldt-Jakob disease (the human form of mad cow disease).

TABLE 36-9 Blood Transfusions

Blood Group	Antigens	Antibodies	Can Give Blood To	Can Receive Blood From
AB	A and B	None	AB	AB, A, B, and O
A	A	B	A and AB	A and O
B	B	A	B and AB	B and O
O	None	A and B	AB, A, B, and O	O

Blood Groups

Human blood is classified into four main groups based on the presence or absence of certain antigens and antibodies. The antigens are located on the surface of the red blood cells, and the antibodies are in the plasma. You inherit the blood group you belong to from your parents. The four main blood groups are A, B, AB, and O.

If you belong to blood group A, you have A antigens on the surface of your RBCs, and B antibodies in your plasma. The opposite is true for persons with blood group B. Blood group AB has both antigens on the surface of the red blood cells and no antibodies at all in the plasma. In contrast, blood group O has neither A or B antigens on the surface of the red blood cells but both A and B antibodies in the blood plasma (Table 36–9). Patients must be transfused only with blood that is compatible with their own blood group.

An additional antigen, known as Rh factor, is also important with blood typing. If the antigen is present, you are referred to as Rh+. If it is absent, you are Rh−. Thus, you can belong to one of the following eight groups:

A Rh+	B Rh+	AB Rh+	O Rh+
A Rh−	B Rh−	AB Rh−	O Rh−

Blood Typing and Crossmatching

Once blood is donated, several tests are performed on the sample. First the sample is tested for ABO group (blood type) and Rh type (positive or negative), as well as for any unexpected red blood cell antibodies that may cause problems in a recipient. Screening tests assess for evidence of donor infection with hepatitis B and C viruses, HIV, human T-lymphotropic viruses, and syphilis. More recently, screening for West Nile virus has been added. Screening determines whether the blood is acceptable for transfusion. If all disease screens are negative, the blood is placed in the pool of available products.

When a potential donor is identified, additional testing, known as crossmatching, is performed. **Crossmatching** identifies possible minor antigens that will affect the compatibility of the donor blood in the recipient. RBCs from the donor blood are mixed with plasma from the potential recipient. A reagent is added, and the sample is observed for clumping or agglutination. If

no clumping is observed, the risk of transfusion reaction is low, and it is considered safe to transfuse the sample of blood. Table 36–9 summarizes blood group matching. As you can see, people with blood group O are considered universal donors, whereas people with blood group AB are considered universal recipients. In regard to Rh factor, people who are Rh+ may receive blood with or without Rh factor. However, people who are Rh− may only receive Rh− blood.

When possible, autologous (self-donated) units of blood are given instead of blood from a donor. This negates the risk of a mismatch or exposure to undetected disease. Autologous blood is usually collected as a preoperative donation for possible transfusion during elective surgery. Autologous donation is most often done with orthopedic, cardiac, and vascular surgery. Autologous blood accounted for 4.7% of all donated blood in 1999 (AABB, 2004). The process of donating autologous blood stimulates the bone marrow to produce new blood cells. Given adequate time for recovery, the collected cells may be wholly or partially replaced prior to surgery.

Blood Products

Several blood products are available for transfusion:

- *Whole blood* contains red blood cells, white blood cells, and platelets suspended in plasma.

- *Red blood cells* are prepared from whole blood by removing the plasma. RBCs can raise the client's hematocrit and hemoglobin levels while minimizing an increase in volume. RBCs are available for transfusion as packed RBCs (PRBC).

- *Plasma* is the liquid portion of the blood. It is 90% water and constitutes about 55% of blood volume. Plasma may be transfused whole or may be separated into specific products, such as albumin, clotting factor concentrates, and immune globulins.

- *Platelets* help the clotting process by sticking to the lining of blood vessels. Units of platelets are prepared by using a centrifuge to separate the platelet-rich plasma from the donated unit of whole blood. The platelet-rich plasma is then centrifuged again to concentrate the platelets further. Platelets are used

TABLE 36-10 Transfusion Reactions

Type of Reaction	Signs and Symptoms	Nursing Responsibilities
Allergic—allergy to blood being transfused	Flushing, itching, wheezing, urticaria (hives); anaphylaxis, if severe	Stop the transfusion. Replace with a saline infusion. Notify the physician immediately. Administer prescribed antihistamine.
Bacterial—contamination of the blood	Fever, chills, vomiting, diarrhea, hypertension	Stop the transfusion. Replace with a saline infusion. Notify the physician. Administer antibiotics as ordered. Treat symptoms.
Febrile—temperature elevation due to sensitivity to WBCs, plasma proteins, or platelets	Fever, chills, warm, flushed skin, aches	Stop the transfusion. Replace with a saline infusion. Notify the physician. Treat symptoms.
Hemolytic reactions—destruction of RBCs as a result of infusing incompatible blood; occurs in 1 in 600,000 transfusions	Fever, chills, dyspnea, chest pain, tachycardia, hypotension; can be fatal	Stop the transfusion immediately. Replace with a saline infusion. Notify the physician immediately. Send the remaining blood, including tubing and filter; a sample of venous blood; and the first voided urine to the lab for analysis. Treat shock.
Circulatory overload—administering too great a volume or too rapidly	Persistent cough, crackles, hypertension, distended neck veins	Slow or stop the transfusion. Monitor vital signs. Place the client upright. Notify the physician.

to treat clients who have a shortage of platelets or have abnormal platelet function.

- *White blood cells,* specifically granulocytes, can be collected by centrifugation of whole blood. They are transfused within 24 hours after collection and are used for infections that are unresponsive to antibiotic therapy. The effectiveness of white blood cell transfusion is still being investigated.

- *Plasma derivatives* are concentrates of specific plasma proteins that are prepared from many units of plasma. Plasma derivatives include a variety of clotting factors, immune globulins, and albumin.

Initiating a Transfusion

Before beginning a transfusion, verify the written order for the blood product, and perform a set of vital signs. If the patient's temperature is elevated, inform the primary care provider before hanging the transfusion. Most patients experience a minor elevation in temperature after a transfusion is given. A preexisting

elevated temperature may exacerbate this response. As a result, the physician may order premedication.

Inspect the IV site before hanging the transfusion. Make sure that it is patent. When infusing blood products, generally you will use an 18-gauge catheter. You can use a 20-gauge catheter if necessary. In fact, the *Technical Manual of the American Association of Blood Banks* (1996) says that a 22-gauge thin-wall catheter can be used without difficulty and without damage to the red blood cells (Macklin, 2003). The Critical Aspects box describes the procedure for initiating and monitoring a blood transfusion. For the complete procedure,

 Go to Chapter 36, **Procedure 36-7: Administering a Blood Transfusion,** in Volume 2.

Transfusion Reactions

Even though you use scrupulous technique, transfusion reactions can and do occur. Five types of reaction are possible: allergic, bacterial, febrile, or hemolytic reactions, and circulatory overload. Table 36-10

describes each of these transfusion reactions. To help prevent transfusion reactions, be extremely careful in identifying the patient and the blood, start the transfusion slowly, and remain with the patient for the first 5 to 15 minutes of the transfusion.

KnowledgeCheck 36–12

- Identify eight potential blood types.
- Describe the types of blood products that are available for transfusion.
- Identify and describe types of transfusion reactions.

 Go to Chapter 36, **Knowledge Check Response Sheet and Answers,** on the Electronic Study Guide.

 Go to Chapter 36, **Resources for Caregivers and Health Professionals,** on the Electronic Study Guide.

 Suggested Readings: Go to Chapter 36, **Reading More About Fluids, Electrolytes, and Acid-Base Balance,** on the Electronic Study Guide.

 Bibliography: Go to Volume 2, Bibliography.

37 Perioperative Nursing

CHAPTER

Learning Outcomes

After completing this chapter, you should be able to:

＊ Name and differentiate the three phases of the perioperative period.

＊ Describe the ways in which surgeries can be classified.

＊ Discuss factors that affect the degree of risk of surgery.

＊ Identify nursing actions associated with the preoperative phase, including physical preparations for surgery.

＊ Overview preoperative teaching.

＊ Describe the nurse's responsibilities with regard to surgical consent forms.

＊ Compare and contrast the roles of the circulating and scrub nurse.

＊ Compare and contrast general anesthesia, local anesthesia, regional anesthesia, and conscious sedation.

＊ Discuss common nursing interventions during the intraoperative phase, including skin preparation, positioning for surgery, and intraoperative safety measures.

＊ Describe nursing assessments appropriate for surgical clients on admission to the nursing unit.

＊ Identify potential postoperative complications.

＊ Provide nursing care to prevent postoperative complications, including application of sequential compression devices and use of incentive spirometry.

＊ Use nursing diagnoses appropriately to describe a patient's unique needs during the preoperative, intraoperative, and postoperative periods.

Your Patient

Nishad Singh is a 68-year-old man who came to the emergency department (ED) with sudden onset of rectal bleeding. He tells the ED nurse, "I've been real tired and dragging for several months. This morning I felt a little worse than usual. When I went to the bathroom, there was a lot of blood. I've never had that before, and it scared me. I've had to go to the bathroom a couple times this morning, and it's all blood." The ED nurse collects the following data:

> BP: 138/88 mm Hg
> Pulse: 104 bpm and regular
> Respiratory rate: 20 breaths per minute
> Temperature: 36.7°C (98.0°F)
> Oxygen saturation: 98%

The ED nurse assesses that Mr. Singh is mildly anxious. His breath sounds are clear, but his abdomen is tender in the left lower quadrant (LLQ). The nurse draws blood to be sent to the lab. While they are waiting for the lab results, Mr. Singh tells the nurse, "My stomach is cramping down low, and I need to go to the bathroom." She provides him with a bed pan. He passes approximately 200 mL of bright red blood with a small amount of fecal material. He becomes sweaty and lightheaded after the BM. The nurse rechecks his vital signs and notes that his BP is now 120/76 mm Hg and that his pulse is up to 120 beats per minute. The nurse shows the ED physician the bloody bowel movement and updates him on the change in vital signs.

When the ED physician examines Mr. Singh, he tells Mr. Singh that he will be admitted to the hospital for further evaluation of the bleeding.

You are the nurse assigned to care for Mr. Singh on the medical-surgical unit. Mr. Singh is sent from the ED directly to radiology for a CT scan of his abdomen. The scan reveals a tumor in the sigmoid colon. Since leaving the ED, Mr. Singh has had three more bloody bowel movements. His blood pressure is 100/72 mm Hg, and his pulse rate is up to 134 bpm. The physician orders a bolus of 1000 mL of lactated Ringer's solution and a unit of packed red blood cells as soon as it is available. Mr. Singh is scheduled for colon resection surgery, which will occur as soon as the surgical team can be assembled and the room prepared.

In this chapter we will discuss how to prepare a client for surgery and the activities that occur before, during, and after surgery. We will follow Mr. Singh through the stages of perioperative care.

Perioperative nursing involves the care of clients before, during, and after surgery. Historically, perioperative nursing practice was called "operating room nursing" and was limited to transferring patients into and out of operating rooms and handing instruments to surgeons during surgical procedures. Now nurses are active in all phases of the operative experience.

The Association of periOperative Registered Nurses (the AORN) is one of the most highly organized and powerful specialty organizations within the profession of nursing. The *AORN Standards, Recommended Practices, and Guidelines* (Lobb, 2003) inform perioperative nursing practice.

PREOPERATIVE CARE

The **preoperative phase** begins with the client's decision to have surgery and ends when the client enters the operating room.

Theoretical Knowledge
knowing why

Nursing care during the preoperative phase focuses on identifying existing health concerns, planning for intraoperative and postoperative needs, and providing preoperative teaching for the patient and family. Preoperative nursing care is delivered in a variety of settings. More than 70% of surgeries in the United States are performed in outpatient settings, such as endoscopy suites, physicians' offices, and ambulatory surgery centers (Johnson, Holm, & Godshall, 2000). The length of the preoperative period and the extent of the patient teaching depend on the type of surgery to be done and the patient's overall health status.

How Can Surgeries Be Classified?

Surgeries can be classified by body system, purpose, level of urgency, and degree of seriousness. The classifications often overlap. Knowing the type of surgery helps you identify the patient's perioperative needs and plan patient care.

By Body System

The body system classification is useful for determining the risk of infection postoperatively. Surgical incisions that enter the gastrointestinal, respiratory, or genitourinary tracts have a higher risk for infection than does surgery of other body systems. However, if an organ ruptures or surgery is required to repair a penetrating injury, the risk of infection is very high regardless of the body system involved. Mr. Singh ("Meet Your Patient") will have surgery of the gastrointestinal system.

By Purpose

The following purposes are used to describe surgery. See whether you can identify the purpose that describes Mr. Singh's ("Meet Your Patient") surgery.

- **Ablative surgery** involves removal of a diseased body part. For example, a cholecystectomy removes a diseased gallbladder.
- **Diagnostic surgery** is undertaken to confirm or negate a diagnosis. Examples include a biopsy, a fine-needle aspiration, or invasive testing, such as a cardiac catherization.
- **Palliative surgery** is done to alleviate discomfort or other disease symptoms without producing a cure. Examples include nerve root destruction for chronic pain or *tumor debulking* (removal of a portion of a mass when complete excision is not possible).
- **Reconstructive surgery** is performed to restore function. A rotator cuff repair and repair of a torn ligament are examples.
- **Cosmetic surgery** is done to improve appearance. A face-lift is an example.
- **Transplant surgery** replaces a malfunctioning body part, tissue, or organ. Joint replacements and organ replacement procedures are included in this category. A related procedure, in which an organ or tissue is harvested from someone pronounced brain dead for transplantation into another person, is called **procurement** surgery.

By Degree of Urgency

Emergency surgery requires transport to the operating suite as soon as possible to preserve the patient's life or function. The surgical team is summoned and preparations are made rapidly. Internal hemorrhage, rupture of an organ, and trauma are common causes of emergency surgery. **Urgent surgery** is scheduled within 24 to 48 hours to alleviate symptoms, repair a body part, or restore function. Removal of a cancerous breast and internal fixation of a fracture are examples. **Elective surgery** is performed when surgery is the recommended course of action, but the condition is not time-sensitive. The client may delay surgery to gather information, consider options, or organize care for the family. Examples include repair of a torn ligament, removal of rectal polyps, or a rhinoplasty (repair of the nose). How would you describe the degree of urgency for Mr. Singh's surgery?

By Degree of Risk

There is an old adage that "the only minor surgery is someone else's surgery." This statement reflects the anxiety that often accompanies surgery. Nevertheless, surgery is defined as major or minor based on the degree of seriousness or risk associated with the procedure.

- **Major surgery** is associated with a high degree of risk. For example, it may be associated with the potential for significant blood loss, involve vital organs, be a prolonged or complicated procedure, or have significant potential for postoperative complications. Some examples of major procedures are CABG (coronary artery bypass graft), organ transplantation, nephrectomy (removal of a kidney), and colon resection.
- **Minor surgery**, often performed on an outpatient basis, involves little risk and usually has few complications. Examples include arthroscopy, breast biopsy, and inguinal hernia repair.

The degree of risk varies with the condition of the client, as well as with the type of surgery.

What Factors Affect Surgical Risk?

The patient's age, general health, and personal habits can contribute to increased risk during any surgical procedure.

- *Age.* The very young and very old are at greatest risk during surgical procedures. Infants have limited ability to regulate temperature and have immature immune, cardiovascular, liver, and renal systems. Because an infant's blood volume is small, even minor blood losses may represent a substantial portion of the total blood volume. In addition, infants are unable to comprehend what is happening and may have difficulty calming. Toddlers understand simple explanations but may fear separation from parents or caregivers. Be sure to include parents and caregivers in your plan of care.

TABLE 37-1 Wound Type and Potential for Infection

Wound Potential for Infection	Wound Characteristics	Examples of Surgery Associated with the Wound
Clean wounds	• Uninfected; minimal inflammation; little risk of infection • Surgery does not involve the gastrointestinal, respiratory, or genitourinary tract	Face lift, cataract surgery, joint replacement, breast biopsy, tonsillectomy
Clean-contaminated wounds	Not infected, but carry increased risk for infection	Surgical incisions that enter the gastrointestinal, respiratory, or genitourinary tracts
Contaminated wounds	Not infected, but risk for infection is high	Surgery to repair trauma to open wounds, such as compound fractures; surgery in which a major break in surgical asepsis occurred
Infected wounds	There is evidence of infection, such as, purulent drainage, necrotic tissue or bacterial counts above 100,000 organisms per gram of tissue	A postoperative surgical incision of any type that has evidence of infection

Older adults are at increased risk because they have less physiological reserve and often have comorbid conditions (other illness not related to the surgery). Many of the physiological changes of aging predispose older adults to increased risk. Among these changes are decreased kidney function, decreased bone and lean body mass, increased peripheral vascular resistance, decreased cardiac output, decreased cough reflex, and increased time required for healing wounds.

• *Type of wound.* Both preexisting wounds (e.g., from trauma) and the wounds (incisions) created by the surgical procedure can pose a risk for infection. See Table 37–1. Risk to the patient increases along with the risk for or presence of infection. Which type of wound will Mr. Singh have immediately after surgery?

• *Preexisting conditions.* The ideal surgical candidate is a healthy young adult who takes no medications. Unfortunately, many surgical clients have underlying acute or chronic disorders that increase surgical risk. Chronic health problems of particular concern are cardiovascular disease, coagulation disorders, respiratory illness, renal disease, diabetes, liver disease, neurological disorders, and nutritional disorders. Acute health concerns that increase surgical risk include infections, such as upper respiratory tract infections. Box 37–1 provides additional information on preexisting conditions.

• *Mental status.* Patients with altered cognition, from either physical or mental illness, may be unable to comprehend preoperative instructions or give informed consent for surgical procedures. They may also require medications (e.g., antipsychotic agents) that interact with anesthetics and analgesics given in the perioperative period. Surgery may aggravate preexisting dementia, confusion, and disorientation.

• *Medications.* Both prescribed and over-the-counter medications may increase surgical risk. For example, many herbs can cause potassium loss and increase the risk for cardiac dysrhythmias, and patients who self-prescribe high doses of vitamin E may be at increased risk for bleeding. See Box 37–2.

• *Personal habits.* Habits such as smoking or abusing alcohol or other substances can increase surgical risk. Smoking affects pulmonary function; long-term alcohol use contributes to liver disease, predisposing the patient to bleeding. Alcohol and drugs interact with anesthetic agents and medications to create adverse effects. Also, habitual substance abusers may have a cross-tolerance to anesthetic and analgesic agents, causing them to need higher than normal doses.

• *Allergies.* Patients may be allergic to medications, tape, latex, and solutions used in surgery. Reactions range from unpleasant to life-threatening.

KnowledgeCheck 37–1

• Define *preoperative phase.*
• What are the four ways surgery can be classified?
• What factors affect surgical risk?

 Go to Chapter 37, **Knowledge Check Response Sheet and Answers**, on the Electronic Study Guide.

BOX 37-1 Preexisting Conditions That Increase Surgical Risk

Chronic Conditions

- *Cardiovascular diseases,* such as hypertension, congestive heart failure, and myocardial infarction affect the ability of the heart to work as an efficient pump. If these disorders are well controlled (e.g., with blood pressure medications or cardiotonic medications), risk is limited.

- *Coagulation disorders* delay clotting and increase blood loss, placing the patient at risk for hemorrhage and hypovolemic shock. In contrast, a hypercoagulation state increases the risk of stroke, embolism, or intravascular clotting.

- *Chronic respiratory disorders,* such as emphysema, asthma, or bronchitis, decrease pulmonary function, increase the risk of respiratory infection, and may be exacerbated (made worse) by general anesthesia.

- *Renal disease* affects the patient's ability to excrete many medications, including anesthetic agents. It also affects the ability to regulate fluid and electrolytes.

- *Diabetes mellitus* delays wound healing and increases the risk of infection and cardiovascular disorders associated with diabetes.

- *Liver disease* affects the body's ability to metabolize amino acids, carbohydrates, and fat; to manufacture prothrombin for clotting; and to detoxify medications. Therefore, the patient is at increased risk for poor wound healing, hemorrhage, and toxic reactions to anesthetics and medications.

- *Neurological disorders,* such as paralysis or spinal cord injury, increase the risk for vasomotor instability and thus create the potential for wide swings in blood pressure. In addition, patients with seizure disorders are more likely to have a seizure in the perioperative period.

- *Nutritional disorders* can affect surgical outcomes. Patients who are malnourished or obese are at risk for delayed wound healing, infection, and fatigue. Obese clients are also more prone to cardiovascular disorders and impaired pulmonary function.

Acute Conditions

- *Upper respiratory tract infections* are associated with increased risk of postoperative pneumonia, especially if the patient receives a general anesthetic.

- *Acute infections* tax the patient's energy and physiological reserves, increasing the risk for various postoperative complications.

BOX 37-2 Medications That Increase Surgical Risk

Antibiotics	May potentiate the action of anesthetic agents
Anticoagulants	Increase risk for bleeding
Antidysrhythmics	May impair cardiac function during anesthesia
Antihypertensives	Increase the risk for hypotension during surgery; may interact with anesthetic agents to cause bradycardia and impaired circulation
Aspirin	Increases risk for bleeding
Corticosteroids	Delay wound healing and increase risk for infection
Diuretics	Alter fluid and electrolyte balance (especially potassium balance)
Opioids	Increase risk of respiratory depression
NSAIDs	Inhibit platelet aggregation, increasing the risk for bleeding
Tranquilizers	Increase risk of respiratory depression

CriticalThinking 37-1

How would you evaluate Mr. Singh's ("Meet Your Patient") surgical risk? What additional information do you need to answer this question?

Practical Knowledge
knowing how

The nursing focus in the preoperative phase is to prepare the patient for surgery. You will use the nursing process to identify any unique nursing diagnoses a patient might have. However, many, if not most, perioperative nursing interventions are routine, preventive measures that you will use for *all* surgical patients.

Perioperative Nursing Data Set (PNDS)

In the late 1980s, the AORN began to develop the Perioperative Nursing Data Set (PNDS), a standardized vocabulary specifically designed to describe the care of perioperative clients. The PNDS is derived from the Perioperative Patient-Focused Model (Figure 37–1), which consists of four domains: the health system, behavioral responses, physiological responses, and

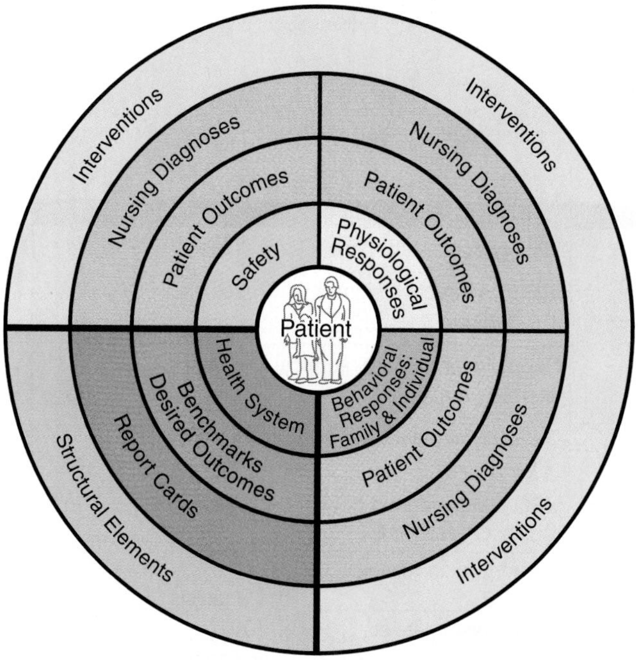

FIGURE 37–1 Association of periOperative Registered Nurses Perioperative Patient-Focused Model. *Source:* Reprinted with permission from AORN, *Perioperative Nursing Data Set,* 2nd ed. Copyright 2002 © AORN, Inc., 2170 Parker Rd, Suite 300, Denver, CO 80231.

safety. The perioperative nurse intervenes within the context of the healthcare system to assist the client to achieve physiological, behavioral, and safety outcomes throughout the perioperative experience.

The PNDS is the first nursing language developed by a specialty organization that has been recognized by the American Nurses Association. The PNDS consists of 74 nursing diagnoses, 133 nursing interventions, and 28 nurse-sensitive patient outcomes appropriate for use in any surgical setting. For additional information on the PNDS,

Go to the **AORN web site at www.aorn.org.**

In this chapter, we will continue to use the NANDA, NOC, and NIC standardized languages because you have already been introduced to them in previous chapters.

| Assessment |

To prevent omission of important information, many facilities have developed a preoperative checklist. Figure 37–2 is an example of a preoperative checklist developed by the AORN. Although the forms may vary at each institution, the areas for assessment are the same. Those areas are discussed below.

Nursing History

It is essential to determine whether the client is physiologically, cognitively, and psychologically prepared for the intraoperative and postoperative phases of surgery. Collect assessment data from the client, significant others, medical records, and other members of the healthcare team. Include the following topics in your preoperative assessment:

- Health history
- Physical status
- Allergies
- Medications
- Mental status
- Knowledge and understanding of the surgery and anesthesia
- Cultural and spiritual factors
- Access to social resources
- Coping strategies
- Use of alcohol and drugs

For further discussion about preoperative assessment

VOL 2 Go to Chapter 37, **Assessment Guidelines and Tools, Preoperative Assessment,** in Volume 2.

Additional assessments may be needed if the client is undergoing outpatient surgery or has a planned short stay after surgery. The accompanying Home Care box discusses the preoperative assessment for a client who will be discharged to home after surgery.

home care

Preoperative Assessment for the Surgical Client Who Will Be Discharged to Home

The type of surgery, the client's condition, and the support system determine whether it is safe to discharge a client to home after surgery. Your assessment for home care should focus on these questions:

- What kind of care will be needed?
- Is the client able to take care of himself? If not, who is available to assist with care?
- Does the caregiver have the necessary skills to provide care?
- If not, can these skills be taught before the client is discharged?
- What features in the home environment will facilitate the client's progress? What features will inhibit progress? For example, can the client get to the bathroom? Can the client negotiate the stairs in the house?
- How will the client be followed after discharge? That is, how soon should he visit his physician? Will he receive home nursing care?

AORN *SAMPLE* Preoperative Assessment Form
(Facility Name and Address)

NOTE: *This record is a sample only. Clinical records should be customized to incorporate data fields that represent the setting, facility, procedure, and patient. Reproductions and variations are encouraged, provided credit is given to AORN.*

Date:_____

Addressograph

(Patient Information: name, age, gender, medical record number, date)

Structural Data:

Admitted via:
- ☐ Ambulatory   ☐ Wheelchair   ☐ Stretcher
- ☐ Other assistive devices:_____

Admitted from:
- ☐ Home   ☐ Transferring hospital
- ☐ Acute rehab facility   ☐ Extended/skilled care facility

Date of preoperative assessment:_____

Planned procedure:_____

Language(s) spoken: ☐ English ☐ Spanish ☐ Other:_____

☐ Patient's records, belongings, valuables secured (I115)
- Belonging inventory: ☐ Watch   ☐ Jewelry
- ☐ Contacts/glasses   ☐ Dentures/partial(s)   ☐ Hearing aid

Identity confirmed (I26):   ☐ Yes   ☐ No

Advance directive signed: ☐ Yes   ☐ No
 Location:_____

Operative procedure, surgical site, and laterality verified (I143):   ☐ Yes   ☐ No

Consent for planned procedures verified (I124):
   ☐ Yes   ☐ No

NPO status verified (I138):   ☐ Yes   ☐ No
 Since: (date/time)_____

Preadmission testing
- ☐ CBC_____   ☐ Urinalysis_____
- ☐ Potassium level_____   ☐ EKG_____
- ☐ CXR_____   ☐ Pregnancy test:_____
- ☐ Type and cross   # of units:_____

Nursing Data Elements:

General health status: (check when present)
- ☐ Diabetes   ☐ Cancer   ☐ Obesity   ☐ Pregnancy
- ☐ Hematologic disorders (anemia, sickle cell disease or conditions)

☐ Vital signs:
- Temperature:_____   Pulse:_____   BP:_____
- Respirations:_____   Height:_____   Weight:_____

☐ Allergies verified (note type of reaction) (I123)
- Latex allergy: ☐ Yes   ☐ No
- Medications: ☐ Yes:_____   ☐ No
  - _____
  - _____
- Food: ☐ Yes:_____   ☐ No
  - _____

☐ Daily medications (prescription, OTC, vitamins, alternative medication, herbal remedies, chemotherapy):
- _____
- _____
- _____
- Medications taken day of surgery:_____

☐ Alcohol/Drug social use:_____

☐ **Neurologic assessment:** ☐ Alert and oriented
- ☐ Speech intact   ☐ Follows simple commands
- ☐ Risk of falls   ☐ History of seizures
- LOC: ☐ Alert/oriented   ☐ Drowsy   ☐ Sedated
- ☐ Asleep   ☐ Unresponsive   ☐ Disoriented
- ☐ Other:_____

☐ **Sensory assessment:**
- ☐ No limitations   ☐ Hearing impairment   ☐ Visual impairment

☐ **Cardiovascular assessment:**
- ☐ Pacemaker   ☐ Implanted defibrillator
- ☐ Chest pain
- ☐ Peripheral edema: Location:_____
- ☐ DVT/PE risk:
  - ☐ None ☐ Low ☐ Med ☐ High
  - _____
  - _____

☐ **Respiratory assessment:**
- ☐ Tracheotomy
- ☐ Intubated
- ☐ Chest tube
- Respirations: ☐ Regular   ☐ Labored
- Smoking history ☐ Yes   ☐ No
  - Packs/day:_____ Years smoked:_____
  - Quit date:_____
- ☐ Cough   ☐ Cold symptoms
- ☐ Current or recent respiratory infection
- ☐ Preexisting respiratory problems (specify):
  - _____
  - _____

☐ **Musculoskeletal assessment:**
- ☐ No limitations
- ☐ Paralysis
- ☐ Traction
- ☐ Limited ROM
- ☐ Amputation:_____
- ☐ Prosthesis:_____

FIGURE 37–2   Example of a preoperative checklist. *Source:* Reprinted with permission from AORN *Perioperative Patient-Focused Model.* Copyright 2002 © AORN, Inc., 2170 Parker Rd, Suite 300, Denver, CO 80231.

Nursing Data Elements (continued):

☐ **Skin assessment:**
    ☐ Cool   ☐ Warm   ☐ Intact
    ☐ Dry   ☐ Moist
    ☐ Body jewelry removed
    ☐ Makeup removed
    ☐ Tattoos: _____
    ☐ Rash:_____
    ☐ Bruises: _____
    ☐ Wounds: _____
    ☐ Ostomy:_____
    ☐ Catheter/Drain: _____
    ☐ Venous access device: _____

☐ **Gastrointestinal assessment:**
    Last bowel movement (date/time):_____
    Usual diet: _____
    _____

    Recent unexplained weight loss
    ☐ Yes: Amount:_____ Time frame:_____
    ☐ No
    Problems chewing or swallowing
    ☐ Yes   ☐ No
    Special needs:
    ☐ Chewing   ☐ Swallowing
    ☐ Appetite   ☐ Diet preferences

☐ **Genitourinary/Gynecology assessment:**
    ☐ Voided on call to OR
       Time:_____ Amount:_____
    ☐ Urinary catheter: Amount in bag:_____
    ☐ Urinary incontinence

☐ **Psychosocial assessment:**
    ☐ Calm/relaxed ☐ Anxious ☐ Talkative
    ☐ Crying   ☐ Restless ☐ Withdrawn
    ☐ Other:_____
    ☐ Concerns regarding surgery or hospitalization:
    _____

    ☐ Religious/cultural concerns/requests:
    _____

    ☐ Receives help from:
       ☐ Children ☐ Support person
       ☐ Other (specify):
    _____

    ☐ Patient cares for:
       ☐ Children: Ages:_____
       ☐ Self   ☐ Spouse
       ☐ Other (specify):
    _____

☐ Determine level of knowledge (I135):
    ☐ Barriers to learning:_____
    ☐ Motivation to learn
       ☐ excellent   ☐ average   ☐ limited

☐ Abuse screening
    Have you ever felt threatened verbally,
    emotionally, or physically in any of your
    relationships?
    ☐ Yes   ☐ No
    Have you been hit, slapped, kicked, or other-
    wise physically hurt by an intimate partner?
    ☐ Yes   ☐ No
    Are you afraid of your partner or anyone you
    live with?
    ☐ Yes   ☐ No
    If yes, describe and make appropriate referral

☐ **Pain assessment**
    ☐ Instructed on use of pain scale
    ☐ Pain assessment (0-10): _____
       Location: _____

☐ **Discharge planning**
    Will require assistance after discharge
    ☐ Yes   ☐ No
    Discharge plan:
    ☐ Home
    ☐ Home nursing service
    ☐ Short-term care facility
    ☐ Extended care facility
    ☐ Other:_____

    Individual who will escort patient home:
    Name: _____
    Phone number: _____
    Relationship: _____

Comments:
_____
_____
_____
_____
_____

Preoperative nursing diagnoses
☐ Anxiety/fear (X4)
☐ Therapeutic regimen management ineffective (X33)
☐ Deficient knowledge (X30)
☐ Risk for injury (X29)
☐ Pain (X38)
☐ Other:_____

RN Signature:
X

Comments:

Physical Assessment

If you identify risk factors from the nursing history, focus on these aspects during your brief head-to-toe physical assessment. For example, if the patient states she had a cough last week, perform a focused assessment of the ear, nose, throat, and lungs to determine how the cough may affect the patient's risk. If the patient has chest congestion, as evidenced by rhonchi and productive cough, communicate these findings to the surgeon and the anesthesia team; if a general anesthetic is planned, it may be necessary to delay the surgery. For additional details on physical assessment, see Chapter 19.

Diagnostic Testing

Preoperative screening tests are usually ordered before surgical procedures. The type of testing depends on the patient's age, health history, and facility policies. For example, most institutions require a complete blood count and urinalysis prior to surgery, as well as an ECG for patients over age 50. Patients with chronic health problems may require additional testing.

 Go to Chapter 37, **Diagnostic Testing: Common Preoperative Screening Tests,** in Volume 2.

KnowledgeCheck 37–2

- Identify the information that you should gather in the preoperative nursing history.
- What type of physical assessment is performed as part of the preoperative assessment?
- What laboratory tests are most commonly ordered before surgery?

 Go to Chapter 37, **Knowledge Check Response Sheet and Answers,** on the Electronic Study Guide.

CriticalThinking 37–2

- What factors will affect your preoperative assessment of Mr. Singh ("Meet Your Patient")?
- Describe how you might perform the assessment as well as provide physical care. What modifications, if any, should you make in his assessment?

| Nursing Diagnosis |

As you learned in Chapter 4, nursing diagnoses describe the individualized needs of patients. However, preoperative patients all have a common set of needs, regardless of their individual differences and regardless of the type of surgery they are to have. For example, all patients need diagnostic tests, physical preparation for surgery, and preoperative teaching.

Nursing diagnoses for the preoperative client evolve from your assessment. You should identify a nursing diagnosis only if the patient has the defining characteristics for it. Identify "risk" diagnoses only if the patient has an underlying condition that places him at higher risk than the average surgical patient. For example, all preoperative patients need preoperative teaching, so it makes no sense to write a nursing diagnosis of Deficient Knowledge for every patient. Agency protocols or critical pathways will almost certainly mandate teaching. As another example, almost all surgical patients have at least mild anxiety, and many of your routine actions will help to relieve anxiety, so there is no need to write a diagnosis of Anxiety. Do not put any nursing diagnosis on the care plan unless you plan to address it with something other than the routine preoperative interventions.

The following NANDA nursing diagnoses may be useful for some preoperative clients:

- *Anticipatory Grieving* is useful for patients who will be losing body function or a body part (e.g., a limb, a uterus) as a result of the surgery. Use this diagnosis only if the patient shows symptoms such as denial, anger, withdrawal, and so on. This diagnosis may be difficult to identify in the brief preoperative encounter.
- *Anxiety* may be mild, moderate, severe, or at panic level. In the preoperative client, anxiety may be related to the current change in health status or due to concerns about loved ones because the client will be unable to provide care. Make this diagnosis only if the client has symptoms such as restlessness, trembling, and other defining characteristics.
- *Fear* is a common reaction to surgery. Fear may be related to the unknown outcome of the surgery, to the diagnosis after a diagnostic procedure, and to the fear of pain during and after surgery. Many of your routine interventions help to address Fear.
- *Ineffective airway clearance* may be used for clients who have a preexisting health problem, such as bronchitis or emphysema.
- *Disturbed Sleep Pattern* often results from anxiety about the upcoming surgery.
- *Ineffective Coping* may be appropriate for a client with extreme anxiety and concerns about the outcomes of the surgery.
- *Latex Allergy Response* is appropriate for clients who have a known allergy to latex.
- *Risk for Latex Allergy Response* is appropriate for clients who have had multiple surgeries or urinary catheterizations, are in professions with daily exposure to latex, have a history of asthma, or are allergic to bananas, avocados, kiwi, chestnuts, or poinsettia plants.

• *Deficient Knowledge.* As previously mentioned, all clients need preoperative teaching, a routine intervention; so, you do not need a Deficient Knowledge diagnosis. If you believe the client may not learn, or that the information is too complex to remember, then identify the problem likely to result from the Deficient Knowledge. For example:

Ineffective Management of Therapeutic Regimen related to Deficient Knowledge of postoperative medications and office visits

Risk for Infection related to Deficient Knowledge of wound care and asepsis.

 CriticalThinking 37–3

Which, if any, of the preceding nursing diagnoses would be most appropriate for Mr. Singh ("Meet Your Patient")? Explain your reasoning.

| Planning Outcomes/Evaluation |

The overall nursing goal in the preoperative phase is to prepare the patient adequately for surgery and to deliver him to the operating suite in the best condition possible. Outcomes that provide evidence of achieving this goal are that the patient:

• Is well-informed about his surgery.
• Provides informed consent.
• Knows what to expect postoperatively.
• Has a minimum of anxiety.

These goals are appropriate for nearly all preoperative patients.

Associated NOC outcomes for the preoperative nursing client depend, of course, on the nursing diagnoses you identify. For outcomes and goals using NOC terminology for the diagnoses Anxiety, Fear, Deficient Knowledge, and Disturbed Sleep Pattern, as well as *individualized goals/outcome statements* you might write for those diagnoses,

 Go to Chapter 37, **Standardized Language, Selected Standardized Nursing Diagnoses, Outcomes, and Interventions for Preoperative Patients,** in Volume 2.

| Planning Interventions/Implementation |

For *NIC standardized interventions* designed to achieve the expected outcomes and resolve or alleviate the identified nursing diagnoses of Anxiety, Fear, Deficient Knowledge, and Disturbed Sleep Pattern,

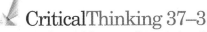 Go to Chapter 37, **Standardized Language, Selected Standardized Nursing Diagnoses, Outcomes, and Interventions for Preoperative Patients,** in Volume 2.

Many preoperative nursing activities are routine interventions to be used for *all* preoperative patients, regardless of their nursing diagnoses. NIC has a special Perioperative Care domain (category) for such interventions. The following are the NIC interventions in the Perioperative Care domain (category):

• *Preoperative Coordination:* Facilitating preadmission diagnostic testing and preparation of the surgical patient. (Activity example: Notify physician of abnormal diagnostic test results.)

• *Surgical Preparation:* Providing care to a patient immediately prior to surgery and verifying required procedures/tests and documentation in the clinical record. (Activity example: Complete preoperative checklist.)

• *Teaching: Preoperative:* Assisting a patient to understand and mentally prepare for surgery and the postoperative recovery period. (Activity example: Correct unrealistic expectations of the surgery, as appropriate.)

The following sections explain in more detail how to carry out routine interventions such as obtaining informed consent for the surgery, providing preoperative teaching, and preparing the client physically.

Confirm That Surgical Consent Has Been Obtained

Before a surgical procedure is performed, the law requires the surgeon to obtain the patient's informed consent. Consent is nearly always obtained by having the patient sign a form provided by the healthcare agency. Once signed and witnessed, the surgical consent form is part of the client's record and accompanies the client to the operating room.

The signed consent form verifies that the surgeon and patient have communicated adequately about the surgery (Dale, Rothrock, & McEwen, 2003). Informed consent helps protect patients from having a surgery they do not understand or want, and the signed document protects the healthcare agency and workers from later claims that the patient did not consent to have the procedure. Also see Chapters 44 and 45 regarding informed consent.

Informed consent means that the physician presented information about the surgery and that the patient understood it and was not coerced (pressured) to consent. The patient must be alert, rational, mentally competent, and not sedated when he signs; and the information must be given to him in a language and vocabulary that he can understand. If a patient is not capable of giving informed consent (e.g., is unconscious or has dementia) or if the client is a minor

child, in most states a family member, conservator, or legal guardian may give consent for the procedure.

The surgical consent form includes the following information:

- The type of surgery being performed
- The name and qualifications of the person performing the surgery (e.g., Jason Esmar, MD)
- A statement that the risks and benefits of surgery, as well as alternative options, have been explained to the client
- A statement that the client has the right to refuse surgery or withdraw consent at any time

The surgeon is responsible for (1) giving the patient the necessary information, and (2) determining the patient's competence to make an informed decision about the surgery. You are responsible for verifying that the surgical consent form is signed and witnessed. Often you will obtain the signature and document on the preoperative checklist that you have done so. As a patient advocate, you should first verify with the patient that the physician has explained the procedure and answered all his questions. If the patient has further questions or if you have any questions about the patient's competence, notify the surgeon, and delay sending the patient to surgery. Be sure to document these conversations, and document in the nurse's notes that the surgeon was notified of any additional questions or concerns.

KnowledgeCheck 37–3

- Who is responsible for obtaining informed consent for the surgical procedure?
- What are the nursing responsibilities related to informed consent?

 Go to Chapter 37, **Knowledge Check Response Sheet and Answers,** on the Electronic Study Guide.

Provide Preoperative Teaching

Preoperative teaching prepares the patient for the surgical experience, allays fears, and decreases the risks of postoperative complications. See Chapter 24 as needed to review patient teaching. The content of the teaching plan should focus on:

- Explaining what will happen before, during, and after surgery, and how the patient can participate in the care.
- Discussing common feelings and concerns that patients have about surgery. This helps the patient feel supported and less anxious.

What to Teach

The type of surgery influences the content of your teaching. For example, if the patient is scheduled for an outpatient knee arthroscopy (visualization of the joint)

under spinal anesthesia, the teaching plan needs to describe the procedure and the anticipated discharge of the patient within hours after surgery. This is different from the teaching for a patient who will have cardiac surgery and spend a number of days in the hospital. Box 37–3 describes content to discuss with all preoperative patients. The Critical Aspects box summarizes preoperative teaching of coughing, deep-breathing, moving in bed, and leg exercises. For the complete steps,

 Go to Chapter 37, **Procedure 37–1: Teaching a Patient to Cough, Deep-Breathe, Move in Bed, and Perform Leg Exercises,** in Volume 2.

How to Teach

You can use written instructions, video presentations, phone contact, or face-to-face discussion to provide preoperative teaching. Teach in a language the patient understands and at a level that is easily understood. Obtain an interpreter for translation if the patient speaks a language that you do not speak. When possible, avoid using family members as translators (see Chapter 13).

Include family members in the teaching as much as possible, and provide written materials to reinforce your instruction. If the patient is a child, be sure to include the parents or caregivers in the teaching and assessments. To facilitate the child's understanding, use dolls or age-appropriate toys, simple language (e.g., "Lie on your tummy, please"), and play (e.g., have the child give medicine to her doll with an empty syringe or listen to its "heart" with your stethoscope).

When to Teach

Patients undergoing emergency surgery usually require extensive physical care preoperatively. You may need to give IV fluids, transfuse blood, treat for pain, and administer many medications, as in the case of Mr. Singh ("Meet Your Patient"). Because of the urgency of some surgery, you may have limited time for preoperative teaching. However, you should always teach the patient as much as possible to prepare him for the surgical experience.

For elective surgery, patients usually have a scheduled preoperative assessment about a week before the surgery. The session may include preoperative testing, an appointment with the anesthesia staff, signing the consent form, and planned preoperative teaching.

Prepare the Patient Physically for Surgery

Physical preparation of the client for surgery involves the following nursing concerns:

- *Nutritional status.* Anxiety and anesthesia reduce gastrointestinal motility. To decrease the risk of

BOX 37-3 Preoperative Teaching

What to Expect Before Surgery

- Explain the planned preoperative testing—lab tests, x-ray studies, ECG, and so on.

- Discuss skin preparation, including preoperative wash with an antibacterial product.

- Discuss ordered preoperative medications.

- Outline activities that will occur prior to surgery, such as insertion of an IV line, placement of a urinary catheter, or cardiac monitoring.

- Review the preoperative restriction of fluid and food. Usually the client is to be NPO for at least 8 hours prior to the planned start of surgery. If the client Is having surgery on the GI tract, an additional bowel prep may be ordered (e.g., a low-residue diet beginning 1 week prior to surgery, and a liquid diet for the 48 hours preceding surgery). Clients having GI surgery also may have enemas prior to surgery.

- Explain the need to remove jewelry, makeup, hearing aids, glasses, contact lenses, and any removable dental prostheses prior to being transported to the operating suite.

- Tell the client that a member of the anesthesia team will speak with him about the proposed anesthesia before surgery.

- Give the client and family a tentative schedule for the operative day, including the time to arrive at the hospital or surgery center.

- Teach the client the importance of deep breathing and coughing, especially after general anesthesia. Demonstrate how to splint the incision to facilitate deep breathing and coughing.

- Teach the client how to move into and out of bed after surgery.

- Teach the importance of leg exercises to minimize the risk of thrombus formation. If decreased activity or prolonged bedrest is anticipated, explain the use of anitembolism stockings or sequential compression devices.

- Explain to the client and family where relatives may wait during surgery.

What to Expect in the Operative Suite

- Discuss the preoperative holding area and activities that may occur there.

- Describe the operating room and the activities that the client may anticipate prior to the surgery.

- Explain that the anesthesiologist or nurse anesthetist will monitor the client throughout the entire surgery and is responsible for keeping him comfortable with medications throughout the procedure.

- Describe the types of people who may be present in the operative suite. This is particularly important if the client is not receiving a general anesthetic.

What to Expect After Surgery

- Explain that the client will initially be cared for in the postanesthesia care unit. After a period of observation, he will be transferred to the surgical unit. Note that some clients may be transferred directly to the critical care unit after surgery. If this is expected, tell the client and family about this preoperatively.

- Family may visit after the client has been admitted and assessed on the surgical unit.

- Tell the client what to expect in terms of dressings, equipment, and monitoring devices.

- Describe the types of assessments that will be performed.

- Explain that pain medication will be given to keep the client comfortable. If he experiences pain, he should tell the nursing staff.

- Discuss the usual progression 3f recovery, including activity level, coughing, deep breathing, leg exercises, and dietary intake.

- Discuss the anticipated length of stay.

Note: If the client is to be discharged the day of surgery, inform her in advance about what to wear to the facility, and explain that she must arrange for a responsible adult to drive her home.

---

nausea and vomiting, clients usually fast, taking no food or liquids for 8 hours prior to surgery. Stress to patients and family the importance of fasting to avoid the danger of aspiration.

- *Skin preparation.* Depending on the surgery and facility, clients may be asked to shower or scrub the surgical site with an antibacterial solution (e.g., Phisohex or Betadine) the evening before surgery and the morning of the surgery. Hair removal and final skin preparation are performed in the operating room immediately before surgery.

- *Bowel preparation.* Historically, clients received enemas prior to all surgeries. Now, however, enemas are used only for surgical procedures of the colon. To empty the colon of feces, clients are asked to consume a low-residue diet for several days before surgery and are given a regimen of medications and/or enemas to clear the bowel. Stress the importance of adhering to the regimen to limit the risk of contaminating the operative site with feces.

- *Urinary elimination.* Indwelling catheters are not routinely inserted for surgery. However, catheterization

For steps to follow in *all* procedures, refer to the inside back cover of Volume 2.

critical aspects of procedures 37–1 through 37–3

Procedure 37–1: Teaching a Patient to Cough and Deep Breathe, Move in Bed, Perform Leg Exercises

- Assess the patient's readiness to learn.

- Ensure that the patient is clear about the difference between coughing and merely clearing the throat.

- Demonstrate how to splint a potential chest or abdominal incision.

- Make sure the patient flexes her knees prior to turning on her side in bed.

- Support the patient who is unable to maintain a side-lying position with pillows.

- Teach the patient to alternately flex and extend the knees.

- Teach the patient to alternately dorsiflex and plantar flex the foot.

- Teach the patient to rotate her ankles in a complete circle.

Procedure 37–2: Applying Antiembolism Stockings

- Measure the patient's leg to ensure that you select stockings of the correct size.

- Inspect the legs and feet for edema, abrasions, lesions, open areas, and circulatory changes.

- Elevate the patient's legs for at least 15 minutes prior to applying stockings.

- Turn the stocking inside out to the level of the heel.

- Insert patient's foot into stocking. Gradually unroll and pull the remaining portion of the stocking up and over the leg.

  Keep knee-high stockings 2.5 to 5 cm (1 to 2 inches) below the joint.

  Do not apply thigh-high stockings if the thigh circumference is greater than 100 cm (25 inches).

- Make sure the stocking is free of wrinkles and is not rolled at the top or bunched.

Procedure 37–3: Applying Sequential Compression Devices

- Determine whether elastic stockings are to be used concurrently with the sequential device. If so, apply them (see Procedure 37–2).

- Place the regulating pump for the sequential compression in a location that will ensure patient safety.

- Place the patient in a supine position.

- If you are using SCD and PAS brand thigh-high compression sleeves, measure the thigh.

- Place the lower extremity on the open sleeve, ensuring that the compression chambers are located over the correct anatomical structure (e.g., knee opening is at the level of the joint)

- Leave 1 to 2 fingerbreadths between the sleeve and the extremity.

- Set the regulating pump to the correct pressure, as ordered.

- Instruct the patient to call for assistance in disconnecting the tubing from the sleeve.

---

may be ordered if it is important to keep the bladder empty during surgery or if fluid status is being carefully monitored. If a catheter is not ordered, have the client void before receiving preoperative medications. The patient could fall if he gets out of bed to use the bathroom after being sedated or given opioids for pain.

- *Preoperative medications.* The anesthesia team may order preoperative medications to relax the patient, reduce respiratory secretions, or reduce the risk of vomiting and aspiration. Table 37–2 discusses types of medications used. If the surgery time is known, the medication is ordered at a prearranged time (e.g., at 0915). If the surgery time is likely to vary, the medication may be ordered to give "on call." You will give the on-call medication when the operating suite staff notify you it is time to do so.

- *Routine medications.* Many routine medications are held (not administered) on the day of surgery. For example, an insulin-dependent diabetic may be instructed to hold her morning injection or administer half of the normal dose. The patient needs less insulin because her NPO status will keep her blood sugar lower than usual. The anesthesiologist will monitor the blood sugar in the operating room and give additional insulin if needed. Patients may also be instructed to stop routine medications several days prior to surgery. For example, a client receiving warfarin for anticoagulation may be instructed to stop the medication 7 days prior to surgery.

- *Prostheses.* Before being transported to the operating suite, the patient must remove all artificial body parts, such as dentures, artificial limbs, or contact

TABLE 37-2 Preoperative Medications

Type of Medication	Use	Examples
Anticholinergics (e.g., phenothiazines)	Reduce oral and pulmonary secretions, prevent laryngospasms, prevent bradycardia	atropine (Atropisol), chlorpromazine (Thorazine), scopolamine (Hyoscine), glycopyrrolate (Robinul)
Anxiolytics (e.g., benzodiazepines)	Control anxiety, calming	alprazolam (Xanax), clonazepam (Klonipin), diazepam (Valium), lorazepam (Ativan), midazolam (Versed)
Antihistamines	Provide sedation and antiemetic effects	hydroxyzine (Vistaril), diphenhydramine (Benadryl)
Barbiturates	Provide sedation without significant cardiopulmonary depression	secobarbital (Seconal), pentobarbital (Nembutal)
H_2 receptor antagonists	Reduce gastric acidity	cimetidine (Tagamet), ranitidine (Zantac)
Hypnotics	Provide sedation and increase the duration of sleep	temazepam (Restoril)
Neuroleptics	Provide sedative, antiemetic, and anticonvulsant effects	droperidol (Inapsine), Innovar (fentanyl and droperidol)
Opioid analgesics	Provide pain relief and sedation; induce anesthesia	fentanyl (Sublimaze), meperidine (Demerol), morphine (Duramorph)

lenses. Wigs, eyeglasses, makeup, and jewelry must also be removed.

- *Antiembolism stockings.* **Antiembolism stockings** are elastic stockings that compress the veins of the legs and increase venous return to the heart (Figure 37–3). They may be applied preoperatively to prevent venous pooling during surgery and decrease the risk of thrombus formation. Stockings may extend from foot to knee, or foot to thigh. Some have an opening at the toes that allows you to assess circulation in the feet.

The Critical Aspects box summarizes the application of antiembolism stockings. For the complete steps,

VOL 2 Go to Chapter 37, **Procedure 37–2: Applying Antiembolism Stockings,** in Volume 2.

As a part of their National Patient Safety Goals, implemented in 2003, the Joint Commission on Accreditation of Healthcare Organizations (JCAHO) includes a focus on eliminating patient misidentification and wrong-site surgery. JCAHO suggests the following safety measures ("JCAHO Sets," 2002):

- Use a preoperative checklist to confirm that appropriate documents are available.
- Mark the surgical site before surgery, and involve the patient in the marking process.

KnowledgeCheck 37–4

- Identify topics that should be discussed in preoperative teaching.
- Describe the typical physical preparation of a client undergoing surgery.

 Go to Chapter 37, **Knowledge Check Response Sheet and Answers,** on the Electronic Study Guide.

CriticalThinking 37–4

- What aspects of preoperative teaching should you stress when caring for Mr. Singh ("Meet Your Patient")?
- A bowel preparation is typically part of preoperative preparation for a client having colon surgery. Do you think this will be part of Mr. Singh's physical preparation? Why or why not?

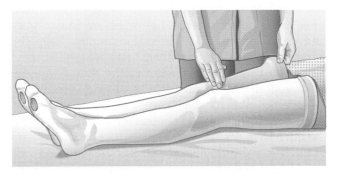

FIGURE 37–3 Antiembolism stockings compress the veins of the legs and increase venous return to the heart.

| toward evidence-based practice |

Gilmartin, J. (2004). Day surgery: Patients' perceptions of a nurse-led preadmission clinic. *Journal of Clinical Nursing, 13*(2), 243–250.

Thirty patients undergoing same-day surgery in a large teaching hospital in the north of England were interviewed about their experience of the preoperative preparation and assessment. The surgery unit consisted of a preassessment unit, a seated preoperative area, three ORs, a six-bed PACU, a 24-bed second-stage recovery area, and a separate recovery area where patients are seated. The patients were undergoing a variety of surgical procedures, including general surgery, gynecology, and urology procedures.

Patients felt they needed comprehensive information about procedures, health education, and an opportunity to ask questions. A few patients pointed to deficits in information that left them feeling anxious. Others noted that delays in surgical start times or unexpected cancellation of surgery threw them into states of disequilibrium.

Bernier, M. J., Sanares, D. C., Owen, S. V., & Newhouse, P. L. (2003). Preoperative teaching received and valued in a day surgery setting. *AORN Journal, 77*(3), 563–572, 575–578, 581–582.

Using a convenience sample of 116 patients, this study examined the congruence between the preoperative teaching delivered by perioperative nurses and the information desired by day-surgery patients. Five dimensions of preoperative information were explored: situational/procedural information, sensation/discomfort information, patient role information, psychosocial support, and skills training. Researchers found a high congruence between information offered and information received. Patients from higher income levels favored situational/procedural information, and women preferred psychosocial support information.

---

1. How would these studies influence your preoperative teaching?

2. These studies focused on clients scheduled for outpatient surgery. How might the studies affect preoperative care for inpatients scheduled for surgery?

 Go to Chapter 37, **Toward Evidence-Based Practice Suggested Responses,** on the Electronic Study Guide.

Transfer to the Operative Suite

Once you have completed your preoperative care, the client is ready for transport to the OR. The completed preoperative checklist and the patient's chart must accompany the patient. Lock up valuables according to agency policy, or have the patient's family keep them. Occasionally, especially if the patient has a significant sensory deficit, the patient can wear his hearing aid or glasses to the OR. You will need to make advance arrangements with the operating suite staff or anesthesia team for this to occur. Often children are permitted to bring a favorite toy with them to the OR to provide comfort. Children may fear being separated from their parents. Arrange for parents to spend time with the child immediately before the surgery and as soon as possible after the surgery. Keep the parents informed, and let them know what to expect.

If you transfer the patient to the operating room (OR) from a nursing unit in the hospital, you should prepare the room for the patient's return after surgery. Put clean linens on the bed, including pads to protect the linen from drainage. Fold the linens back to the end of the bed, raise the bed to stretcher height, and lock the wheels. Move furniture and equipment so that the stretcher can be placed directly against the bed. You will need equipment for measuring vital signs, an IV pole, an emesis basin, tissues, a clean gown, washcloth, towel, and extra pillows for positioning the patient. You may also need to set up suction and oxygen equipment, depending on the type of surgery the patient is having.

 Go to Chapter 37, **Technique 37–1: Preparing a Room for a Patient's Return from Surgery**, in Volume 2.

INTRAOPERATIVE CARE

The **intraoperative phase** begins when the patient enters the operating suite and ends when she is admitted to the postanesthesia care unit.

Theoretical Knowledge
knowing why

To provide intraoperative care, you will need theoretical knowledge of the roles of the various members of the intraoperative team and of the different types of anesthesia that are used.

Operative Personnel

The personnel who attend the client during the surgical procedure are called the *intraoperative team*. The

team is divided into members who must use sterile technique and those who use clean technique (see Chapter 20 to review medical and surgical asepsis, as needed). During the intraoperative phase, registered nurses can function as the scrub nurse, circulating nurse, or registered nurse first assistant. Each of these roles contributes to the safe care of surgical clients.

Sterile Team

Members of the sterile team include the surgeon, surgical assistant, and scrub person. Before beginning the surgery, they perform a surgical scrub of the hands and arms, dry with sterile towels, and don sterile gowns and gloves. (To review these procedures, see Chapter 20.)

The **scrub nurse** is a member of the sterile intraoperative team. He can be an RN, LVN, or a surgical technician. The scrub nurse sets up the sterile field, prepares the surgical instruments, assists with the sterile draping of the patient, anticipates and responds to the surgeon's needs, and maintains the integrity of the sterile field. The **registered nurse first assistant (RNFA)** is an RN with additional education and training in surgical technique and is also part of the sterile team. The RNFA serves as an assistant to the surgeon, a role that has historically been filled by physicians. The RNFA works with the surgeon to perform the surgical procedure. The RNFA is employed by the surgeon or the hospital.

Sterile team members are the only persons allowed to enter the sterile field. The sterile field encompasses the client and the area immediately surrounding the client. Creation of the sterile field proceeds as follows:

- The scrub person performs a surgical prep, using Betadine scrub and Betadine paint, to cleanse the operative site.
- The area surrounding the operative site is then covered with sterile drapes so that only the operative area is exposed.
- Sterile draping is placed over the remainder of the client's body.
- In most cases a vertical drape is suspended at neck level so the client's head and airway are accessible to the anesthesiologist or nurse anesthetist (who is not sterile). For neurosurgery, even the head is draped, and the anesthesiologist or nurse anesthetist sits to the side of the head.

 Go to Chapter 37, **Technique 37–2: Creating an Operative Field,** in Volume 2.

Clean Team

Team members who abide by clean technique (medical asepsis) include the anesthesiologist or nurse anes-

thetist, the circulating RN, biomedical technicians, and radiology technicians. These personnel never enter the sterile field, but instead function around and beyond it.

A physician **anesthesiologist** or a **nurse anesthetist (CRNA)** may administer anesthesia. Their role is to continuously monitor and evaluate the client's responses to the anesthetic agent and the surgical procedure. In 2003, CRNAs administered 65% of all anesthetics in the United States (American Association of Nurse Anesthetists [AANA], 2004).

The **circulating nurse** is a registered nurse who applies the nursing process to coordinate all activities in the operating room. She is a strong client advocate who continuously monitors the client and the sterile field. The circulating nurse maintains a safe, comfortable environment, communicates with appropriate personnel outside the operating room, manages care of the intraoperative client, and responds to emergencies. An important aspect of the circulating nurse's role is to attend to the patient during the induction of anesthesia. In some cases, the circulating nurse administers sedation to the client.

KnowledgeCheck 37–5

- Identify the intraoperative nursing roles that are part of the sterile intraoperative team and those that are part of the clean intraoperative team.
- Which nursing roles are always held by a registered nurse?

 Go to Chapter 37, **Knowledge Check Response Sheet and Answers,** on the Electronic Study Guide.

Types of Anesthesia

During surgery, anesthesia is used to obtain analgesia (control of pain), muscle relaxation, and amnesia (memory loss). Anesthesia is classified as general, conscious sedation, or regional.

General Anesthesia

General anesthesia produces rapid unconsciousness and loss of sensation. The anesthesiologist or nurse anesthetist administers inhaled and intravenous medications that depress the patient's central nervous system (CNS) and relax the musculature. Muscle relaxants, paralyzing agents, narcotics, barbiturates, and inhaled gases are some of the agents used during general anesthesia.

Advantages of general anesthesia are that:

- The patient is unconscious, so she experiences no anxiety that might affect cardiac and respiratory functioning.
- The muscles are relaxed, so the client remains completely motionless during the surgical procedure.
- Anesthesia can be adjusted to accommodate the length of the procedure and the patient's age and

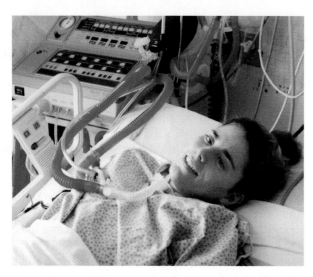

FIGURE 37–4   Clients who receive general anesthesia may require mechanical ventilation for respiratory support during surgery. Some clients require ongoing mechanical ventilation.

physical condition. For example, an older adult may require less anesthetic than anticipated; if so, the anesthetist can decrease the dosage without interrupting the procedure. Also, if complications occur, the anesthesia can be continued for longer than originally planned.

Disadvantages of general anesthesia are that:

- The respiratory and circulatory muscles are depressed, so mechanical ventilation is often needed while the patient is under the effects of the anesthetic agent(s) (Figure 37–4). These effects predispose the patient to pneumonia and thrombophlebitis in the postoperative period.
- General anesthesia creates a risk for death, heart attack, stroke, and malignant hyperthermia. **Malignant hyperthermia** is a rare, often fatal, metabolic condition that occurs during the use of muscle relaxants and inhalation anesthesia. Metabolism increases in the skeletal muscles, and they become rigid. The temperature rises rapidly. Predisposition to this condition is inherited.

Frequent minor complaints after general anesthesia include sore throat (from intubation), nausea and vomiting (from relaxation of gastrointestinal smooth muscle), headache, uncontrollable shivering, and confusion.

Conscious Sedation

Conscious sedation is an alternative form of anesthesia that provides intravenous sedation and analgesia without producing unconsciousness. The patient is aware of his surroundings and can talk with the surgical team during the procedure. During conscious sedation, the client may feel sleepy but can be easily aroused by touch or speech. Nevertheless, blood pressure, heart rate, respiratory rate, and oxygen saturation are monitored, and the patient usually receives oxygen via nasal cannula during the procedure. Because of the amnesic effect of many of the medications, the patient may not recall aspects of the procedure afterwards. Advantages are that (1) pain and anxiety are adequately controlled without the risks of general anesthesia, and (2) recovery is rapid. Conscious sedation is used for procedures such as bronchoscopy and cosmetic surgery.

Regional Anesthesia

Regional anesthesia prevents pain in the area of the procedure by interrupting nerve impulses to and from the area. The client remains alert but is numb in the involved area. Regional anesthesia may be administered by infiltration of the surgical site and surrounding tissue with local anesthetics, such as lidocaine (Xylocaine) or bupivacaine (Marcaine). These medications may also be injected into and around specific nerves (nerve block) to depress the sensory, motor, and/or sympathetic impulses of a limited area of the body.

Regional anesthesia is low in cost, is simple to administer, and requires a minimal recovery period. It is especially suitable for minor, ambulatory procedures. However, many patients are apprehensive about being able to see and hear the procedure. Regional anesthesia may not be practical if the client is highly anxious or if adequate pain control cannot be achieved. Techniques for achieving regional anesthesia include the following.

Local Anesthesia

Local anesthesia produces loss of pain sensation at the desired site (e.g., a wound to be sutured, a growth on the skin). Local anesthesia is typically used for minor procedures. However, after finishing a major surgery, the surgeon may infiltrate the operative area with local anesthetics to provide postoperative pain relief. Local anesthetics may be applied topically or injected. A **topical anesthetic** is applied directly to the skin and mucous membranes. Lidocaine (Xylocaine) and benzocaine (Orajel, T-caine) are commonly used because they are rapidly absorbed and rapid-acting.

Nerve Block

A **nerve block** is the injection of an anesthetic into and around a nerve or group of nerves (e.g., the facial nerve, the brachial plexus). A **Bier (intravenous) block** is a nerve block technique in which the anesthetist places a tourniquet on an arm or leg, and then injects a local anesthetic agent intravenously below the level of the tourniquet. The tourniquet is maintained at a pressure that limits venous return but continues to allow arterial circulation. The patient feels no pain

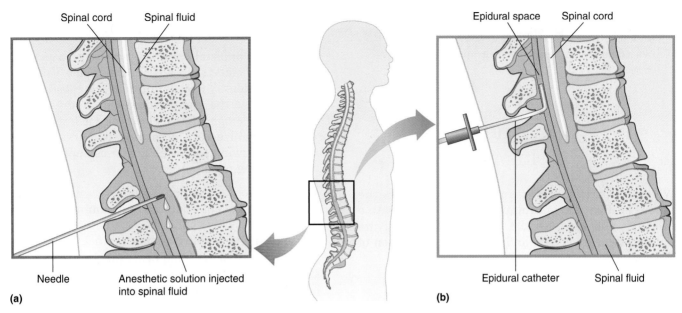

Spinal cord   Spinal fluid

Needle   Anesthetic solution injected
into spinal fluid

(a)

Epidural space   Spinal cord

Epidural catheter   Spinal fluid

(b)

FIGURE 37–5   *A,* Spinal anesthesia is the injection of a local anesthetic into the subarachnoid space to block sensation and movement. *B,* Continuous epidural anesthesia can be used to provide postoperative analgesia.

in the extremity as long as the tourniquet is in place. Advantages of the Bier block are its rapid onset and recovery time. Also, the tourniquet decreases bleeding during the surgical procedure and prevents systemic absorption of the local anesthetic. However, when the procedure is finished, the tourniquet is deflated, and there is potential for systemic absorption of the anesthetic. To prevent tissue damage, the tourniquet must not be left in place for more than 2 hours.

Spinal Anesthesia

Spinal anesthesia is the injection of an anesthetic into the cerebrospinal fluid (CSF) in the subarachnoid space (Figure 37–5*A*). This injection blocks sensation and movement below the level of the injection. Spinal anesthesia is often used for surgical procedures in the lower abdomen, pelvis, and lower extremities. This technique allows the patient to remain conscious during the procedure and usually does not depress respirations.

Side effects of spinal anesthesia include hypotension, nausea, vomiting, urinary retention, or a headache from leakage of CSF. A headache after spinal anesthesia must be closely monitored and may require additional treatment by the anesthesia staff.

Occasionally a higher level of spinal anesthesia is achieved than intended—that is, the medication may migrate upward in the spinal cord. This can depress respirations and cardiac rate. Placing the patient in Fowler's position may prevent respiratory paralysis.

The blood pressure may also decrease suddenly due to pervasive vasodilatation—the anesthesia blocks the sympathetic vasomotor nerves, which normally maintain muscle tone in peripheral blood vessels.

Patients with these complications often require ventilation and support of blood pressure during surgery, so they must be carefully monitored during surgery and in the recovery period.

Epidural Anesthesia

Epidural anesthesia requires insertion of a thin catheter into the epidural space (Figure 37–5*B*). Anesthetic agents are infused through the catheter to produce loss of sensation. Epidural anesthesia can be used as a surgical anesthetic and to provide postoperative analgesia. Advantages and disadvantages of epidural anesthesia are similar to those of spinal anesthesia. Epidural anesthesia is safer than spinal anesthesia because the anesthetic does not enter the subarachnoid space and the depth of anesthesia is not as great. However, drugs intended for epidural administration are of a higher concentration than those for spinal administration; so if the medication is inadvertently injected too deeply (into the subarachnoid space), hypotension and respiratory paralysis occur, and mechanical ventilation is necessary.

Epidural anesthesia is ideal for obstetrics procedures (e.g., cesarean birth or pain control with vaginal birth) because the mother is awake to bond with the newborn, and her mobility is not limited for long.

KnowledgeCheck 37–6

- What is the purpose of anesthesia?
- Under what type(s) of anesthesia does the client remain conscious?

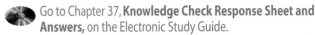
Go to Chapter 37, **Knowledge Check Response Sheet and Answers,** on the Electronic Study Guide.

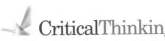

Critical Thinking 37–5

What form of anesthesia is Mr. Singh most likely to receive? Why?

Practical Knowledge
knowing how

When the patient arrives in the surgical suite, the nurse verifies the information on the preoperative checklist and assesses the patient. After that, the nursing focus is on safe and successful completion of the surgery.

| Assessment |

The circulating nurse greets the client in the preoperative holding area and performs a brief assessment. The nurse begins by verifying that the surgical consent has been signed and witnessed and that the preoperative checklist is complete. The nurse then assesses the client's anxiety level and physical condition. The next steps are to measure the vital signs, examine the surgical site, and inspect IV lines, drainage tubes, and catheters. Often the circulating nurse or the anesthetist starts an IV line in the holding area if there is not already one present. A preoperative medication may be given in the holding area. For common interview questions in the intraoperative phase,

Go to Chapter 37, **Assessment Guidelines and Tools, Intraoperative Care Questionnaire,** in Volume 2.

| Nursing Diagnosis |

The circulating nurse uses the information from the assessment to develop relevant nursing diagnoses. As in the preoperative phase, most intraoperative nursing care consists of standard activities to be used for all patients. Most intraoperative patients, regardless of the surgery, have the following potential complications (collaborative problems):

- Potential Complications of surgery:
  Hypothermia
  Fluid and electrolyte imbalance
  Excessive bleeding or hemorrhage
  Musculoskeletal injury secondary to positioning
- Potential Complications of anesthesia:
  Aspiration
  Vasomotor instability (and resultant hypotension and diminished peripheral perfusion)

Respiratory depression
Cardiovascular compromise

Except in unusual circumstances (e.g., a patient in poor nutritional status, a very old patient), you may not need to identify specific nursing diagnoses for a patient because the standardized care addresses all the potential complications. However, for nurses who prefer to organize care according to nursing diagnoses, the following potential diagnoses apply to most patients having major surgery:

- *Risk for Imbalanced Body Temperature* related to exposure in cool environment and administration of cool IV fluids. This applies especially to very young, very old, and very thin patients.
- *Risk for Aspiration* related to depressed respirations and reflexes. For patients who have weak muscles for coughing or a poor gag reflex, this diagnosis is especially relevant.
- *Risk for Imbalanced Fluid Volume* related to NPO status and blood loss from surgery. Some patients are at higher than normal risk, for example, patients with renal or cardiac problems.
- *Risk for Perioperative Positioning Injury* related to patient factors such as edema, emaciation, obesity, and sensory perceptual disturbances secondary to anesthesia.

Use the following nursing diagnoses only if the patient has the necessary defining characteristics or risk factors. Do not use them for all patients.

- *Risk for Latex Allergy Response* related to multiple exposures (e.g., multiple surgeries, catheterizations) or history of related allergies
  Latex Allergy Response (needs no etiology)

| Planning Outcomes/Evaluation |

The overarching goals in the intraoperative phase are that the patient will:

- Be free from injury.
- Remain physiologically stable.
- Experience optimal surgical outcomes.

For *associated NOC standardized outcomes* for intraoperative patients, along with examples of goals created with NOC indicators and scales,

Go to Chapter 37, **Standardized Language, Selected Standardized Nursing Diagnoses, Outcomes, and Interventions for Intraoperative Patients,** in Volume 2.

Notice that the goals are appropriate for nearly all surgical patients.

Individualized goals/outcome statements are formulated from the patient's nursing diagnoses. The following are examples:

• Maintains body temperature within normal range.

• Has clear lung sounds and patent airway.

• Has urine output of at least 30 mL/hr.

• Will have no skin, tissue, or neuromuscular injury as a result of positioning.

| Planning Interventions/Implementation |

Intraoperative care focuses on maintaining a safe environment and assisting the intraoperative team to provide appropriate care for the client. The nurse anesthetist manages the interventions for most of the patient's potential problems, for example, fluid volume status, airway protection, and vital signs monitoring.

NIC standardized interventions for the intraoperative period come from the domain of Perioperative Care. They include interventions for all intraoperative patients, regardless of their individual nursing diagnoses. One intervention, Anesthesia Administration, must be performed by an anesthesiologist or nurse anesthetist. The RN assists in implementing a number of interventions:

• Anesthesia Administration

• Autotransfusion

• Infection Control: Intraoperative

• Positioning: Intraoperative

• Surgical Assistance

• Surgical Precautions

• Temperature Regulation: Intraoperative

For *NIC standardized interventions* for specific intraoperative nursing diagnoses,

 Go to Chapter 37, **Standardized Language, Selected Standardized Nursing Diagnoses, Outcomes, and Interventions for Intraoperative Patients,** in Volume 2.

Notice, however, that most of the interventions apply to all surgical patients and are subsumed by the preceding Perioperative Care interventions.

The following sections explain in more detail how to carry out "routine" interventions, such as providing skin preparation, positioning, and carrying out intraoperative safety measures. Note that "routine" in this context means that the activities are planned and performed for all patients. Nursing interventions are *never* routine in the general sense; they must always be performed with thought and skill.

Skin Preparation

Surgical skin preparation reduces the risk of postoperative wound infection by reducing the microbial count at the operative site. Skin preparation typically begins in the preoperative phase, when the client cleanses the skin with an antimicrobial solution the evening before and the morning of surgery. The intraoperative nurse provides additional skin preparation. If you are the intraoperative nurse, you will do the following:

• *Assess the skin.* Assess skin for signs of infection, rash, or other forms of skin irritation. Document the condition of the skin on the intraoperative record.

• *Remove hair from the site only if necessary.* Historically, the surgical site was routinely shaved. Now, however, you will remove hair only if it is abundant in the area of the surgery or if the surgeon specifies a preference for hair removal. Hair removal increases the risk of abrasions or nicks in the skin, which can provide a portal of entry for bacteria. As a rule, remove hair in the preoperative holding area immediately before surgery to reduce the time for bacterial growth. Use clippers to trim hair because they are less likely than a razor to cause skin irritation.

• *Cleanse the surgical site.* In the operative suite, skin preparation precedes draping of the client. Cleanse the surgical site and a generous area of surrounding skin with povidone-iodine (Betadine) scrub; then paint it with Betadine solution. If the client has an allergy to iodine, use an alternative preparation solution.

Positioning

Five variables determine the position of the patient in the OR: the surgical site, access to the patient's airway, the need to monitor vital signs, comfort, and safety. A position that is ideal for accessing the surgical site may not be used if any of the other factors are compromised. If the patient has preexisting injuries or discomfort, this information is also factored into the decision about how to position.

The patient is usually positioned after anesthesia has begun. Use straps, wedges, pillows, and surgical table attachments to maintain the position during the surgery. To prevent shearing, lift, do not slide, the patient into position. In many cases, the surgical team assists with positioning.

The circulating nurse is responsible for preventing positioning injuries. Surgical patients often spend 3 to 4 hours, or even longer, in the same position. This places them at risk for pressure ulcer formation. Some anesthetic agents decrease tissue perfusion, thereby increasing the patient's risk for sustaining positioning injuries. Padding the bony prominences is one measure to protect the client during surgery. For

nursing interventions to address the NANDA diagnosis Risk for Perioperative Positioning Injury,

 VOL 2 Go to Chapter 37, **Standardized Language, Selected Standardized Nursing Diagnoses, Outcomes, and Interventions for Intraoperative Patients,** in Volume 2.

Intraoperative Safety Measures

As a part of their National Patient Safety Goals, implemented in 2003, the Joint Commission on Accreditation of Healthcare Organizations suggests that just before starting any surgical or invasive procedure, you conduct a final verification process to confirm the correct patient, procedure, and site. ("JCAHO Sets," 2002).

The circulating nurse is responsible for a variety of other measures that protect the patient in the intraoperative phase. These measures are briefly explained here.

- Assist the scrub nurse to prepare and maintain the sterile field. The circulating nurse gathers surgical supplies and equipment for use during surgery. She then works with the scrub nurse to transfer the supplies to the sterile field.

- Provide supplies and materials during surgery. During surgery, if additional supplies are needed, the circulating nurse gathers the supplies and opens them onto the sterile field. Supplies may include dressings, surgical equipment, medications, irrigating solutions, or sutures.

- Monitor intake and output of the client. Together with the anesthetist, the circulating nurse monitors the fluid infused, as well as urine output, drainage, and blood loss.

- Handle specimens. Often the surgeon will obtain a sample of tissue that must be analyzed during the operative procedure. The circulating nurse receives the specimen, coordinates with the pathologist to review the sample, and reports the pathology findings to the surgeon. The circulator also handles specimens that will be sent for evaluation after the surgery is complete.

- Perform sponge, sharps, and instrument counts. The circulating nurse and the scrub nurse count the material that is added to the sterile field. As the surgery comes to an end, a repeat count is performed to ensure that no instruments, sponges, or sharps are left inside the client.

- Document care and the client's response to care on the surgical record.

KnowledgeCheck 37–7

- For what activities is the circulating nurse responsible in the OR?
- Describe six intraoperative safety measures performed by the circulating nurse.

 Go to Chapter 37, **Knowledge Check Response Sheet and Answers,** on the Electronic Study Guide.

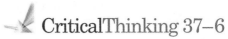 CriticalThinking 37–6

What special concerns, if any, may affect Mr. Singh ("Meet Your Patient") during the intraoperative phase of care?

POSTOPERATIVE CARE

The postoperative phase begins when the client enters the postanesthesia care unit and ends when the client has healed from the surgical procedure. This phase consists of two parts: recovery from anesthesia and recovery from surgery.

Theoretical Knowledge
knowing why

When the surgical procedure is complete, members of the surgical team prepare the patient for transfer to the postanesthesia care unit (PACU), also called the recovery room. The PACU is located near the OR. In the immediate postoperative phase, the patient is at high risk for respiratory and cardiovascular compromise. As a precaution, the circulating nurse and the anesthesiologist accompany the patient during transport to the PACU.

Recovery from Anesthesia

The first postoperative phase is often known as the *postanesthesia phase* or the *immediate postoperative phase*. This phase begins when the client is transferred from the operating table to a bed (or gurney) for transport to the PACU. The anesthetist and the circulating nurse attend to the client's needs during the transfer to the PACU and are responsible for giving a comprehensive report to the PACU nurse.

The PACU is typically an open unit that allows nurses to observe patients easily. PACU nurses have specialized education and experience in caring for postoperative clients. Normally, nurses working in the PACU have experience in critical care. The PACU nurse receives a comprehensive report from the anesthesia provider and circulating RN. Box 37–4 outlines the content of that report.

Recovery from Surgery

The second phase of postoperative care begins when the patient is discharged from the PACU and admitted to the surgical nursing unit. The patient is transported to the surgical unit only after he has recovered from anesthesia and his condition is stable. The goal of this phase is to facilitate healing and prevent postoperative complications.

37-4 Information Contained in the Report from the OR

- Procedure performed
- Type of anesthesia
- Medications administered in the OR
- Duration of the procedure and anesthesia
- Postoperative vital signs
- Pulse oximetry values
- Allergies
- Lab values
- Estimated blood loss
- Fluid intake and output
- Preoperative mobility status, skin integrity, and sensory perception abilities
- Surgical complications
- Presence of tubes, drains, catheters
- Existing IV lines
- Postoperative orders

Practical Knowledge
knowing how

In the next sections we discuss nursing care associated with both phases of postoperative care.

Nursing Care in the Postanesthesia Care Unit

The PACU nurse performs a quick, focused initial assessment of the surgical patient in the presence of the anesthesia provider and circulating RN. After that, she assesses the patient every 5 to 15 minutes. The American Society of Perianesthesia Nurses (ASPAN) has identified the following essential elements of the initial assessment of the postoperative patient (Zeckuhr, 1999):

- Integration of preoperative, intraoperative, and transfer data.
- Airway assessment. Assess airway patency, presence of artificial airway, mechanical ventilator settings, and oxygen saturation. Many patients arrive in the PACU with an artificial airway or endotracheal tube in place. For most, the PACU nurse will remove the airway or tube once she determines that the patient is able to maintain his own airway.
- Vital signs, including respiratory rate, respiratory competence, and breath sounds; cuff or arterial blood pressure; temperature and type of measurement used; pulse (apical and peripheral); and oxygen saturation

- Level of consciousness
- Central venous pressure (CVP), arterial BP, pulmonary wedge pressure, and intracranial pressure (as indicated)
- Patient position. An unconscious client is usually positioned on his side to help maintain an open airway and decrease the likelihood of aspirating mucus or saliva. Ensure optimal chest expansion by elevating the superior arm on a pillow.
- Skin color and condition
- Safety needs (e.g., siderails raised)
- Neurovascular assessment, such as peripheral pulses and sensation at extremities, as indicated
- Condition of dressing(s)
- Condition of suture line(s), if visible
- Type, patency, security of drainage tubes, catheters
- Amount and type of drainage (dressings, tubes, catheters)
- Muscular response and muscle strength
- Pupil response
- Fluid therapy, location of sites, condition of IV sites, and types and rates of solution(s) and/or blood products infusing
- Level of comfort

The only postoperative intervention from NIC's Perioperative Care category is Postanesthesia Care. Postanesthesia Care encompasses the preceding assessments and adds measures such as providing for safety and administering oxygen. For *NIC interventions* for other postoperative nursing diagnoses,

Go to Chapter 37, **Standardized Language, Selected Standardized Nursing Diagnoses, Outcomes, and Interventions for Postoperative Patients,** in Volume 2.

The client remains in the PACU until he has recovered from the effects of anesthesia. See Box 37–5 for signs of recovery from anesthesia.

Postoperative Nursing Care on the Surgical Unit

The assigned nurse admits the patient to the surgical unit. If the patient is transported by gurney, assist him to the bed. As soon as the patient has arrived, perform an assessment, and listen to a summary report from the PACU nurse.

| Assessment |

The initial postoperative assessment is identical to the assessment performed by the PACU nurse (see above). However, the patient has undergone a period

BOX 37–5 Evidence of Recovery from Anesthesia

- The patient is conscious and easily reoriented. Often patients will drift off to sleep between arousals; however, they easily reorient and are generally aware of circumstances and surroundings.
- The patient is able to maintain a patent airway independently and to deep-breathe, cough, and expectorate secretions.
- Vital signs are stable and within an acceptable range. The blood pressure may be markedly different from the immediate preoperative measures, because BP is often elevated preoperatively because of anxiety. BP may also be elevated postoperatively because of pain or because routine BP medicines were held. The patient may require medication to control pain or BP before he can be discharged from the PACU.
- The patient is able to move all extremities that he could move preoperatively. The patient regains movement and sensation once spinal or epidural anesthesia has worn off.
- The patient is urinating at least 30 mL/hr and is in relative fluid balance. Consider blood loss, urine output, gastric drainage, and emesis when calculating fluid balance.
- Dressings are dry and intact, or wound drainage is considered appropriate for the procedure. The client should have no overt signs of excessive blood or fluid loss before he is transferred to the surgical unit.

of stabilization since surgery, so the frequency of assessment can be less than in the PACU, where the patient was assessed every 5 to 15 minutes. Agency protocols vary, but a common pattern is to assess the patient:

- On arrival to the nursing unit
- Every 15 minutes for the first hour
- Every 30 minutes for the next 2 hours
- Every hour for the next 4 hours
- Then every 4 hours

You may increase the frequency of assessments if the patient's condition changes.

KnowledgeCheck 37–8

- What are the two parts of the postoperative phase of care?
- How often is a patient typically assessed after surgery?
- What assessments are made?

 Go to Chapter 37, **Knowledge Check Response Sheet and Answers**, on the Electronic Study Guide.

| Nursing Diagnosis |

If healing proceeds normally and no complications develop, most postoperative patients have a common set of collaborative problems (Table 37–3), regardless of the type of surgery they underwent. Except in special situations (e.g., patients with comorbid conditions such as diabetes or asthma), you will not need to write potential ("risk for") nursing diagnoses. Write potential nursing diagnoses only if a patient has a higher risk for the problem than the average surgical patient. For example, you might use:

- *Risk for Ineffective Peripheral Tissue Perfusion* for patients who have a history of peripheral arterial disease or cardiac insufficiency.
- *Risk for Deficient Fluid Volume* for patients who have lost a large amount of blood in surgery or who are dehydrated on admission.
- *Risk for Ineffective Breathing Pattern* for patients with weak accessory muscles for breathing, with a decreased level of consciousness, or with a respiratory condition such as emphysema.
- *Risk for Infection* for patients who have compromised immune status or who may not be capable of managing their own wound care at home.

Of course, you will use a nursing diagnosis whenever a problem becomes actual instead of merely potential. Nursing diagnoses will vary based on the surgical procedure and the client situation. One common postoperative nursing diagnosis is Delayed Surgical Recovery, which is appropriate when the patient requires more days to recover than the anticipated length of stay for the surgery. There is no need for a Deficient Knowledge diagnosis because patient teaching is a routine intervention for all postoperative patients. For the most frequently used diagnoses,

 Go to Chapter 37, **Standardized Language, Selected Standardized Nursing Diagnoses, Outcomes, and Interventions for Postoperative Patients,** in Volume 2.

| Planning Outcomes/Evaluation |

A comprehensive plan of care for common postoperative nursing diagnoses includes NOC standardized outcomes as well as individualized goals. Because of shortened hospital stays, the postoperative period now extends well past the patient's discharge from the hospital. Often, especially for those who have had major procedures, a home health nurse continues to follow the patient at home to facilitate a smoother

Complication	Description	Clinical Signs	Interventions for Prevention and Early Detection
		Respiratory System	
Aspiration pneumonia	Airway inflammation caused by gastric secretions (especially hydrochloric acid from the stomach) inhaled into lungs because of absent gag reflex secondary to anesthesia.	Cough, fever, elevated WBC, decreased or absent breath sounds, decreased oxygen saturation (SaO_2), tachypnea, dyspnea, blood-tinged sputum.	*Preoperative:* Emphasize the importance of NPO for at least 8 hours prior to surgery. *Postoperative:* Continue NPO until intestinal motility returns; carefully monitor the patient and position on the side when sedated.
Atelectasis	Collapse of alveoli due to hypoventilation, mucus plugs blocking airways, narcotic analgesics, immobility.	Decreased or absent breath sounds, decreased oxygen saturation (SaO_2), fever, tachypnea, dyspnea, tachycardia, diaphoresis, pleural pain.	• Encourage deep breathing, coughing, moving in bed, ambulation, use of incentive spirometry. • See interventions for NIC category Respiratory Monitoring. • Monitor rate, rhythm, depth, and effort of respirations. • Note chest movement, symmetry, accessory muscle use, retractions. • Listen for noisy respirations. • Note location of trachea. • Determine need for suctioning by listening for crackles and rhonchi over major airways. • Suction, as needed. Auscultate lung sounds after suctioning, and other respiratory treatments to determine effectiveness. • Monitor for increased restlessness, anxiety. • Monitor ability to cough effectively.
Pneumonia	Inflammation of the alveoli due to infection with bacteria, viruses, toxins, or irritants. Caused by hypoventilation secondary to anesthesia and narcotic analgesics, and by poor cough effort as a result of aging or weakness.	Productive cough with blood-tinged or purulent sputum, fever, elevated WBC, decreased or absent breath sounds, decreased SaO_2, chest pain, tachypnea, dyspnea.	Encourage and assist with deep breathing, coughing, moving in bed, ambulation, use of incentive spirometry. Teach how to splint incision to control pain when moving.
Pulmonary embolism	A clot that occludes blood flow to a portion of the lungs; usually a result of clot formation in the lower extremities, which breaks loose and migrates to the lungs. May also be due to venous injuries, hypercoagulable state, use of high-dose estrogen, preexisting circulatory disorders.	Sudden onset of dyspnea, shortness of breath, chest pain, hypotension, tachycardia, decreased SaO_2, cyanosis.	Encourage and assist with leg exercises, ambulation, antiembolism stockings, and sequential compression devices.

➤

TABLE 37-3 Potential Postoperative Complications (Collaborative Problems) *(continued)*

Complication	Description	Clinical Signs	Interventions for Prevention and Early Detection
		Cardiovascular System	
Thrombophlebitis	Blood clot and inflammation of the vein, usually in the legs. Results from increasesd coagulability and venous stasis due to immobility during and after surgery.	*Superficial:* Vein is red, hard, and hot to touch. *Deep:* Limb is pale and edematous; aching, cramping in limb; Homans' sign (pain in calf when foot is dorsiflexed).	Promote leg exercises, ambulation, antiembolism stockings, sequential compression devices, hydration.
Embolus	Movement of a thrombus or foreign body from its original location. In the venous system, often results in pulmonary embolus. Movement in the arterial system will result in symptoms in the area affected—often results in cerebrovascular accident (CVA), myocardial infarction (MI), or loss of circulation to an area.	See pulmonary embolus. For arterial emboli, symptoms depend on the location.	Prevent thrombophlebitis. If thrombophlebitis occurs, position and immobilize the limb. Do not massage calves.
Hemorrhage	Bleeding may be internal or external. May be caused by slipped ligature, uncontrolled bleeder, or infection.	*If external:* dressings saturated with bright red blood; increased output in drains or chest tubes. *If internal:* increased pain, increasing abdominal girth, ecchymosis or swelling around incision, tachycardia, hypotension.	Frequently monitor vital signs, dressings, and wound drainage.
Hypovolemia	Decreased blood volume; may be due to blood loss during and after surgery, dehydration, or excess loss through vomiting, diarrhea, or drains.	Hypotension, tacycardia, decreased urine output, fatigue, thirst.	• Carefully monitor vital signs and I & O. • Monitor skin color, temperature, and moistness. • Monitor for central and peripheral cyanosis. • Identify possible causes of changes in vital signs. • Insert urinary catheter, if appropriate. • Monitor hydration status (moist mucous membranes). • Administer IV therapy as prescribed. • Promote oral intake when tolerated. • Prepare to administer blood or blood products, as ordered.
		Gastrointestinal System	
Nausea and vomiting	Stomach upset or vomiting related to pain, anxiety, anesthesia, medications, or oral intake before peristalsis returns.		• Have patient remain NPO until return of bowel sounds. • Advance diet slowly. • Treat pain.

TABLE 37–3 *(continued)*

Complication	Description	Clinical Signs	Interventions for Prevention and Early Detection
Gastrointestinal System			
Abdominal distention (tympanites)	Excess gas within the intestines; may be due to a slow return of peristalsis or from handling of the intestines during surgery.	Abdominal discomfort, bloating, hypoactive or absent bowel sounds.	• Encourage and assist to move in bed and ambulate. • Have patient remain NPO until return of bowel sounds and avoid drinking with a straw. • Provide fluids at room temperature.
Constipation	A decrease in the frequency of bowel movements, resulting in the passage of hard stool. Usually related to use of opioids, immobility, inadequate fluid intake, or low-fiber diet.		Encourage and assist to move in bed, ambulate, and increase fluid and fiber intake after bowel sounds return.
Ileus	Loss of the forward flow of intestinal contents due to decreased peristalsis secondary to anesthesia, handling of the intestines during surgery, electrolyte imbalances, infection, or ischemic bowel.	Abdominal pain, distention, absent bowel sounds, vomiting.	Independent preventive measures are minimal. Observe for symptoms; notify surgeon.
Genitourinary System			
Renal failure	Decreased or absent urine output due to hypovolemia, shock, or toxic reaction to medications.	Urine output < 30 mL/hr; Rising BUN and creatinine levels.	Carefully monitor I & O and lab values.
Urinary retention	Accumulation of urine in the bladder; may result from diminished muscle tone as a result of anesthesia and anticholinergic medications, handling of tissues during surgery, or inflammation in the pelvic region.	Bladder distention, suprapubic pain, diminished urine output or output less than fluid intake, inability to void or small frequent voidings, hypertension, restlessness.	• Provide privacy and adequate time to urinate. • May need catherization.
Urinary tract infection	Infection in the urinary tract related to catherization, stagnant urine in the bladder secondary to immobility or anticholinergic medications, or instrumentation of the urinary tract.	Urinary frequency, suprapubic discomfort, burning on urination, cloudy urine.	• Carefully monitor I & O. • Maintain aseptic technique with catherization and perineal care. • Provide adequate IV and oral fluids.
Surgical Incision			
Dehiscence	Separation of one or more layers of the wound due to poor nutritional status, obesity or other strain on suture line, inadequate closure of the muscles, or wound infection.	A pop or tear sensation, especially with sudden straining from coughing, vomiting, or changing positions in bed. Usually there is an immediate increase in serosanguinous drainage when dehiscence occurs.	• Provide adequate nutrition. • Use binders to support the incision. • Have client avoid strain. • Monitor for infection.

TABLE 37-3   Potential Postoperative Complications (Collaborative Problems)
(continued)

Complication	Description	Clinical Signs	Interventions for Prevention and Early Detection
		Surgical Incision	
Evisceration	Protrusion of organs or tissues through the separated incision. For causes, see dehiscence.	Visible protrusion of organs through incision.	Same as for dehiscence.
Wound infection	Inflammation or drainage from a wound due to growth of microorganisms secondary to poor aseptic technique.	Localized swelling, redness, heat, pain, fever (>38°C), foul-smelling drainage, or a change in the color of the drainage.	• Maintain aseptic technique with surgical dressing changes. • See interventions for NIC category Infection Protection. • Monitor for systemic and localized signs and symptoms of infection. • Assess vulnerability to infection. • Limit the number of visitors, as appropriate. • Inspect incision and drain areas for redness and extreme warmth. • Inspect surgical dressings for drainage and odor. • Obtain cultures as needed. • Encourage sufficient nuitritional and fluid intake. • Monitor vital signs, especially temperature. • Teach client about signs of infection.

transition through the postoperative process. For *NOC standardized outcomes and individualized goals,*

Go to Chapter 37, **Standardized Language, Selected Standardized Nursing Diagnoses, Outcomes, and Interventions for Postoperative Patients,** in Volume 2.

| Planning Interventions/Implementation |

Most postoperative interventions focus on prevention and early detection of potential complications (collaborative problems). Many such interventions are done as a part of the preoperative teaching. Others are described in Table 37–3. These are routines that are followed for all postoperative patients, regardless of type of surgery. For *NIC interventions* for postoperative nursing diagnoses,

Go to Chapter 37, **Standardized Language, Selected Standardized Nursing Diagnoses, Outcomes, and Interventions for Postoperative Patients,** in Volume 2.

Specific nursing activities should be designed to relieve identified nursing diagnoses. In the next sections, we discuss the content of routine postoperative teaching and the use of sequential compression devices.

Postoperative Teaching

Teaching is especially important postoperatively because most patients must perform quite a bit of self-care. Postoperative teaching should reinforce content taught preoperatively. In addition, you should teach the patient about the following:

• Postoperative treatment regimen (e.g., dressing changes, exercises), including rationale for the treatments

• Self-management of the treatment regimen

• Expected results and effects of the surgery

• The prescribed diet, and how to select foods on the diet

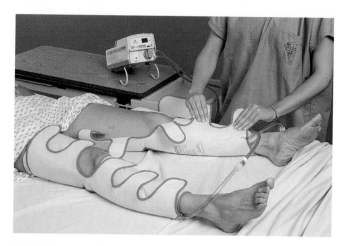

FIGURE 37–6 Sequential compression devices (SCDs) may be ordered for clients at high risk for thrombophlebitis.

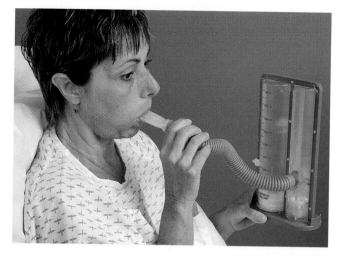

FIGURE 37–7 Incentive spirometry facilitates lung expansion and coughing to clear mucus from airways.

- Prescribed activity
- Signs and symptoms of complications that require the patient to notify the surgeon or primary care provider
- Return office or clinic visits
- Lifestyle changes that may be needed
- Community resources available (e.g., Reach for Recovery)

To use time efficiently, try to do some teaching each time you are at the bedside for other care. Be sure the patient is comfortable but alert. Do not attempt teaching when the patient is in pain, needs to void, or is drowsy from opioid analgesics.

Sequential Compression Device (SCD)

In addition to previously discussed postoperative exercises, clients at high risk for thrombophlebitis may have a sequential compression device (SCD) ordered. The SCD is a plastic sleeve with chambers that is wrapped around the client's legs. Connecting tubes extend from the sleeve and are attached to an air pump (Figure 37–6). The sleeve may extend from ankles to knees or up to the top of the thighs. The SCD provides sequential pressure to the chambers of the plastic sleeve. Starting at the ankle, the first chamber is inflated. When the second chamber inflates, the first chamber deflates. This process continues up to

the top of the sleeve and then resumes again at the base by the ankle. SCDs apply brief pressure to each segment of the leg. The pressure compresses the veins and promotes venous return to the heart. The Critical Aspects box summarizes application of sequential compression devices. For the complete steps,

VOL 2 | Go to Chapter 37, **Procedure 37-3: Applying Sequential Compression Devices,** in Volume 2.

Incentive Spirometry

Incentive spirometry may be ordered for patients who are at high risk for atelectasis and pneumonia. Incentive spirometry facilitates deep breathing, increases lung volume, and promotes coughing to clear mucus from the respiratory tree. The equipment (Figure 37–7) varies in appearance, but all devices include a gauge to monitor the patient's progress visibly.

Incentive spirometry is especially useful if the client has a history of lung problems or smoking or will experience a prolonged period of inactivity. If you know that the client will be using an incentive spirometer postoperatively, include its use in your preoperative teaching. If it is ordered postoperatively, explain to the client that this is a method to monitor his deep breathing. Refer to the accompanying Self-Care box for patient teaching.

self-care

Teaching Your Patient About Incentive Spirometry

- Explain to the patient that the machine will enable him to monitor the depth of his breathing.

- Clients with abdominal or chest incisions may require pain medication to use the incentive spirometer.

- Assist the patient to an upright position in the bed or chair.

- Instruct the patient to do the following:

  1. Breathe out normally.
  2. Place the mouthpiece in the mouth, and create a seal.
  3. Breathe in slowly and as deeply as possible through the mouthpiece. Monitor the depth of inspiration by viewing the gauge. (Establish goals for the client so that progress can be monitored.)
  4. Hold breath as long as possible, at least to a slow count of 3.
  5. Remove the mouthpiece from the mouth, and exhale.
  6. Rest for a few seconds
  7. Repeat this process 10 times every hour while awake, if possible.
  8. After each set of 10 deep breaths, cough to be sure lungs are clear. Support any incision when coughing by placing a pillow firmly against it.

KnowledgeCheck 37–9

- Identify six potential postoperative complications.
- Why are sequential compression devices used?

 Go to Chapter 37, **Knowledge Check Response Sheet and Answers,** on the Electronic Study Guide.

 Go to Chapter 37, **Resources for Caregivers and Health Professionals,** on the Electronic Study Guide.

 Suggested Readings: Go to Chapter 34, **Reading More About Perioperative Nursing,** on the Electronic Study Guide.

 Bibliography: Go to Volume 2, Bibliography.

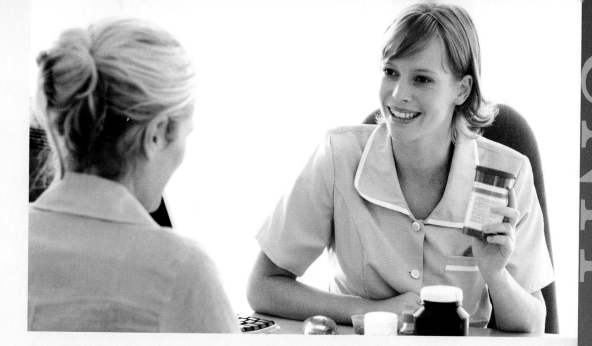

Nursing Functions

38 CHAPTER

Leading
& Managing

Learning Outcomes

After completing this chapter, you should be able to:

* Distinguish leadership, followership, and management.

* Discuss the qualities and behaviors that contribute to effective leadership and followership.

* Discuss the qualities and behaviors that contribute to effective management.

* Define *power* and *empowerment*.

* Describe several ways in which nurses can be empowered.

* Discuss the qualities of preceptors and mentors.

* Describe the change process.

* Identify methods of dealing with change.

* Describe the major concepts of conflict and conflict resolution.

* Describe the major concepts of safe and effective delegation.

* Set short- and long-term personal and career goals.

* Organize patient care to make effective use of time.

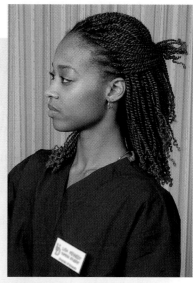

MEET Your Peer

Mary is a student in a nursing program. She considers herself a "pretty good test-taker" and has a GPA of 3.4. She received her first test grade in the Nursing Fundamentals class, and it was a C. Mary is sure that she will never pass this course and that her dream of becoming a nurse will vanish. On discussing the test with her classmates, she realized that there are several other disappointed students who have been used to making As and Bs on exams. The nursing exams seem different, because they do not just ask students to recall memorized material, but also apply what they have learned. Mary decides to get the group together and plan some strategies for study groups. She asks the instructor whether she will meet with them and go over their plan to make sure they are on the "right track." Mary has exhibited some leadership qualities.

Theoretical Knowledge
knowing why

In this chapter we define *leadership, management, followership,* and the relationships among them. We discuss the challenges to nurses today as they lead and manage others. Those challenges also involve the concepts of power and empowerment.

WHAT IS LEADERSHIP?

You may be thinking, "I just started in my nursing program. How can you expect me to be a leader now?" As a student, you do need time to learn how registered nurses function in a work environment. However, you can begin to assume some leadership skills as a new student. The essence of leadership is the ability to influence other people. Effective **leaders** enable people to move "in the same direction, toward the same destination, at the same speed, not because they have been forced to, but because they want to" (Lansdale, 2002, p. 63). A leader has three primary tasks:

1. Help people develop a sense of direction and purpose.
2. Build the group's commitment to its goals.
3. Face the numerous challenges that arise on a daily basis (Drath, 2001).

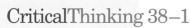

CriticalThinking 38–1

Think of a goal your class might have. Obviously, each student wants to develop the skills necessary to provide excellent patient care and learn the theory content to pass the course and continue in the program. What other goals might you have, as a group? As a leader, how might you help the group meet their goals?

Leadership Theories

How does a person become a leader? What type of leader is most effective? Although much research has been done on these questions, no theory has yet emerged as the clear answer. The reason may be that different situations require different qualities and behaviors. In nursing, for example, some situations require quick thinking and fast action. Others require time to reflect on the best solution to a complicated problem. Let's look now at some of the best-known leadership theories and the leader qualities and behaviors that have been identified as effective (Pavitt, 1999; Tappen, 2001).

Trait Theories

Have you ever heard someone say, "Leaders are born, not made"? That implies that some of us are natural leaders, but others of us are not. Many of the early research studies on leadership were done in an attempt to identify the qualities, or **traits,** that distinguish a leader from a nonleader. The traits most often identified are intelligence and initiative. Other qualities that were found to be associated with leadership are excellent interpersonal skills, high self-esteem, creativity, willingness to take risks, and ability to tolerate the consequences of taking risks (White & Lippitt, 1960). Leadership may come more easily to some than to others, but everyone can be a leader, at least in certain areas, if she develops the necessary knowledge and skills.

Behavioral Theories

The trait theories were concerned with what a leader *is;* the behavior theories are concerned with what the leader *does.* One of the most influential of these behavioral theories is concerned with leadership style. Three styles have been identified (White & Lippett, 1960):

- **Authoritarian** leadership (also called *autocratic, directive, controlling*). The authoritarian leader gives orders, makes decisions for the group as a whole, and bears most of the responsibility for the outcomes. For example, when a decision needs to be made, an authoritarian leader would say, "I've given this a great deal of thought and decided that this is the way we're going to solve our problem." Although authoritarian leadership is an efficient way to run things, it usually stifles creativity and may inhibit motivation. Authoritarian leadership may be either punitive or kind and compassionate.
- **Democratic** leadership (also called *participative*). In contrast to the authoritarian leader, the democratic leader shares the planning, decision making, and responsibility for outcomes with other members of the group. Although this is often a less efficient way to run things, it is more flexible and more likely to foster motivation and creativity. A democratic leader tends to provide guidance rather than control.
- **Laissez-faire** leadership (also called *permissive, nondirective*). The laissez-faire ("let it alone") leader does very little planning or decision making and does not encourage others to participate, either. In fact, laissez-faire leadership is really a lack of leadership. For example, when a decision needs to be made, a laissez-faire leader may postpone making the decision or never make the decision at all. In most instances, the leader leaves people feeling confused and frustrated because there is no goal, no guidance, and no direction. Some very mature individuals thrive under laissez-faire leadership because they need little guidance. However, most people do not work effectively under this kind of leadership.

Pavitt summed up the difference between these three styles nicely: A democratic leader tries to move the group toward its goals, an autocratic leader tries to move the group toward the leader's goals, and a laissez-faire leader makes no attempt to move the group (Pavitt, 1999, pp. 330ff).

KnowledgeCheck 38–1

Identify the three common styles of leadership in the behavioral theories of leadership.

 Go to Chapter 38, **Knowledge Check Response Sheet and Answers,** on the Electronic Study Guide.

Task-Relationship Theories

Another important distinction in leadership style is the one between a *task* focus and a *relationship* focus (Blake, Mouton, & Tapper, 1981). Some leaders emphasize the tasks (e.g., keeping the nursing station neat, getting charting done) and fail to realize that interpersonal relationships (e.g., attitude of physicians toward nursing staff, treating housekeeping staff with respect) have considerable impact on employee morale and productivity. Others focus on the interpersonal aspects and ignore the quality of the job being done as long as people get along with each other. The most effective leader is able to balance the two, attending to both the task and the relationship aspects of working together.

Situational Theories

We know now that people and leadership situations are far more complex than the early theories recognized. Furthermore, situations may change rapidly, requiring even more complex theory to explain people's responses (Bennis, Spreitzer, & Cummings, 2001). In recognition of this, less simplistic theories have evolved to replace the trait and behavioral theories.

Adaptability is the key to the situational approach (McNichol, 2000). Instead of assuming that one particular approach works in all situations, situational theories recognize the complexity of work situations and encourage the leader to consider a number of factors when deciding what action to take. Every situation is different. A change that is welcomed by one group may be strongly resisted by another group. The type of leadership approach is one factor that may affect people's responses to change. The type of organization is another important situational factor. Situational theories emphasize the importance of understanding all of the factors that affect a particular group of people in a particular environment and of varying the type of leadership to meet the needs of the situation.

Transformational Theories

Although the situational theories were an improvement over earlier theories in recognizing how complex the process of influencing others really is, they were still missing something. They did not address meaning, inspiration, and vision (Tappen, 2001), which are the distinguishing features of transformational leadership theory.

According to transformational theory, people need a sense of mission that goes beyond good interpersonal relationships or the appropriate reward for a job well done (Bass & Avolio, 1993). This is especially true in nursing. Caring for people, sick or well, is the goal

of our profession. Most of us chose nursing to do something for the good of humankind; this is our vision. One goal of nursing leadership should be to guide us toward achieving that vision.

Transformational leaders can communicate their vision in a way that is so meaningful and exciting that it inspires commitment in the people with whom they work (Trofino, 1995). If successful, the goals of the leader and staff will "become fused, creating unity, wholeness, and a collective purpose" (Barker, 1992, p. 42). The qualities and behaviors associated with transformational leadership are included in Table 38–1.

 CriticalThinking 38–2

Observe a nurse in one of the healthcare agencies where you are doing a clinical rotation. What leadership qualities and behaviors do you see the nurse exhibiting? How do these behaviors help in planning nursing care?

WHAT IS MANAGEMENT?

Whereas leaders may or may not have official appointments to the position, managers are usually officially appointed to a position that has power and authority to enforce decisions. A **manager** is an employee of an organization who has the power, authority, and responsibility for planning, organizing, coordinating, and directing the work of others.

Management Theories

Although there are many management theories, it is most important to be familiar with the two major, but opposing, schools of thought in management: (1) scientific management and (2) the human relations approach to management. As you will see, one emphasizes the task aspects of managing people, and the other emphasizes the relationship aspects.

Scientific Management

Almost 100 years ago, Frederick Taylor argued that most jobs could be done more efficiently if they were thoroughly analyzed (Lee, 1980; Locke, 1982). Given a properly designed task and sufficient incentive to get the work done, workers would be more productive. For example, Taylor encouraged paying people "by the piece," that is, by the number of "widgets" made (in health care, the equivalent would be, for example, by the number of clients bathed or monitored), rather than by the number of hours worked. This encourages workers to get the most work done in the least amount of time, Taylor said. The work itself was also analyzed to improve efficiency.

Which do you think would take the least amount of time and manpower: bringing patients to the radiology

TABLE 38-1	Qualities and Behaviors Associated with Transformational Leadership

Qualities of Effective Leaders	Behaviors of Effective Leaders
Integrity	Think critically
Courage	Solve problems
Initiative	Respect others
Energy	Listen to others
Optimism	Communicate skillfully
Persistence	
Balance	
Self-awareness	

department or bringing a portable x-ray machine to the bedside? What about physical therapy: taking patients to the PT department or having the therapist come to the patient's room? In health care, there has been a lot of discussion about these kinds of questions. This kind of thinking is the basis for the emphasis on eliminating excess staff and increasing the productivity of remaining employees.

Human Relations-Oriented Management

McGregor's (1960) theory X and theory Y are good examples of the difference between scientific management and human relations-oriented management.

- **Theory X,** says McGregor, reflects a common attitude among managers that most people really do not want to work very hard and that the manager's job is to make sure that they do work hard. According to theory X, a manager needs to employ strict rules, constant supervision, and the threat of punishment (reprimands, withheld raises, and threats of job loss) to create industrious, conscientious workers.

- **Theory Y,** which McGregor prefers, is the opposite viewpoint. Theory Y managers believe that work itself can be motivating and that people will work hard if their managers provide a supportive atmosphere. A theory Y manager emphasizes guidance rather than control, development rather than close supervision, and reward rather than punishment.

A human relations-oriented (theory Y) nurse manager is concerned with keeping staff morale as high as possible, assuming that satisfied, motivated

staff will do the best work. Employees' attitudes, opinions, hopes, and fears are important to this type of leader. Such a manager would spend considerable effort to work out conflicts and promote mutual understanding among the staff to provide an atmosphere in which people can do their best work.

Qualities of an Effective Manager

The effective nurse manager possesses a combination of qualities: leadership, clinical expertise, and business sense. None of these alone is enough; it is the combination that prepares a person for the complex task of managing a group or team of healthcare providers. Let's look at each of these briefly:

- *Leadership.* All of the "people skills" of the leader are essential to the effective manager. They are the core skills the nurse needs to function as a manager.
- *Clinical expertise.* If a nurse manager is to help others develop their skills and evaluate how well they have done so, she needs a certain amount of clinical expertise. It is not necessary (or even possible) to know everything every other professional on the team knows, but it is important to be able to assess the effectiveness of their work in terms of patient outcomes.
- *Business sense.* Nurse managers also need to be concerned with the "bottom line," that is, with the cost of providing the care that is given, especially in comparison with the benefit received from that care. In other words, nurse managers need to be able to analyze how much time is spent to provide a given amount of client care, how effective that client care has been, and how much will be paid to the institution for the care delivered.

These are complex tasks that require knowledge of budgeting, staffing, and measurement of patient outcomes, much of which is beyond the scope of this textbook. There is some controversy over the amount of clinical expertise versus business sense that is needed to be an effective nurse manager. Some argue that a person can be a "generic" manager—that the job of managing people is the same, no matter what tasks they perform. Others argue that the manager must understand the tasks better than anyone else in the work group. Our position is that both are needed, along with excellent leadership skills.

You are probably saying to yourself, " I don't want to be a manager. I just want to take care of patients." However, as a registered nurse, you will manage groups of patients, and you will be responsible for supervising nursing assistants, licensed practical nurses, and other ancillary staff. Even as a staff nurse, you will be a manager of care.

Activities of an Effective Manager

Mintzberg (1989) divides the manager's activities into three categories: interpersonal, decisional, and informational.

- *Interpersonal skills* are important to both leaders and managers. In fact, one might say that interpersonal skills are important to everyone! From the beginning of your career in nursing school, you will have many opportunities to develop positive working relationships with other disciplines, departments, and units within the organization. Can you see how Mary ("Meet Your Peer") would need interpersonal skills to accomplish her goals?
- *Decisional skills.* From the very beginning of your career, you will be expected to develop critical-thinking skills and an ability to prioritize and make decisions for your clients. Even as a student, you will need to know what information to report to your instructor and when to provide it. What decisions did Mary ("Meet Your Peer") make?
- *Informational responsibilities.* Side by side with decisional responsibilities are the informational responsibilities of a manager. The nurse must be able to relay information to other staff members and monitor the activities and decisions the staff have made with that information. What are some kinds of information Mary would need to communicate to the students interested in forming a study group?

KnowledgeCheck 38–2

- How is transformational leadership different from the other theories of leadership?
- Define *manager*.
- In McGregor's management theory, which is more like scientific management: theory X or theory Y?

 Go to Chapter 38, **Knowledge Check Response Sheet and Answers,** on the Electronic Study Guide.

GETTING READY TO BECOME A LEADER AND MANAGER

You may still be asking yourself, "What does all this leadership and management stuff have to do with me?" Besides learning the role of the registered nurse, you should begin at this point to look at the skills employers think you need to be ready to work for them. Along with passing the NCLEX examination, employers cite the skills listed in Box 38–1 as desirable in job candidates (Shingleton, 1994).

Many of these skills have been identified in our discussion of leading and managing. It is not too early to begin to develop your abilities in these areas. These skills not only will assist you as you go through your

BOX 38-1 Desirable Job Candidate Skills

- Ability to assume responsibility
- Computer knowledge
- Critical-thinking and analytical skills
- Interpersonal skills
- Leadership abilities
- Motivation, initiative, and flexibility
- Oral and written communication skills
- Organizational skills
- Problem-solving and decision-making abilities
- Proficiency in field of study or technical competence
- Self-discipline
- Teamwork ability
- Willingness to work hard

nursing program, but also will make the adjustment to the RN role much easier.

One of the first steps in identifying what skills you need to develop and what skills you already possess is to do a brief SWOT analysis. A SWOT (strengths, weaknesses, opportunities, threats) analysis plan, borrowed from the corporate world, can guide you through an analysis of your own internal strengths and weaknesses and reveal external opportunities and threats that may help or hinder your leadership and management skills (Ellis, 1999). Your SWOT analysis may include the factors listed as examples in Table 38–2 (Pratt, 1994), but certainly you will have others.

CriticalThinking 38–3

Stop and think! Take some time to personalize the SWOT analysis in Table 38–2. What weaknesses do you need to minimize, or which strengths do you need to develop as you begin to develop your leadership and management skills?

Mentors and Preceptors

There are two aspects to consider as you get ready to become a leader and manager. The first part, discussed above, consists of developing self. The second part is really a combination of developing self and developing others: preceptorship and mentorship. A **mentor** is someone more experienced who provides career development assistance, such as coaching, sponsoring advancement, providing challenging assignments, protecting protégés from adversity, and promoting positive visibility. Mentors provide guidance to the new student or graduate as he continues in the profession. Mentors can also fulfill psychosocial roles, such as personal support, friendship, acceptance, role modeling, and counseling.

Many organizations have preceptors for the new employee. A **preceptor** is someone with more experience who provides practical teaching and guidance for a student or new employee. As a student, you may be assigned an RN preceptor in your clinical rotations. You may work side by side with a preceptor to provide patient care now and as a new graduate. In many instances, the preceptor will become your mentor. However, the mentor role is much more encompassing than the preceptor role. The mentor relationship is a voluntary one and is built on mutual respect and development of the mentee. Box 38–2 identifies responsibilities of the mentor and mentee in this relationship.

TABLE 38-2 SWOT Analysis Plan—Examples

Strengths	Weaknesses	Opportunities	Threats
Relevant work experience	Poor communication and people skills	Nursing shortage	Competition from other students and other nursing programs
Advanced education	Inflexibility	Availability of mentors and preceptors	Lack of time
Good communication and people skills	Lack of interest in self-learning	Variety of experiences in clinical rotations	
Computer skills	Difficulty adapting to change	Many leadership and management books and self-learning programs available	

BOX 38-2 Mentor and Mentee Responsibilites

Mentor Responsibilites

- Demonstrate excellent communication and listening skills.
- Be sensitive to the needs of nurses, patients, and the workplace.
- Encourage excellence in others.
- Share and provide counsel.
- Exhibit good decision-making skills.
- Demonstrate an understanding of power and politics.
- Demonstrate trustworthiness.

Mentee Responsibilities

- Demonstrate eagerness to learn.
- Participate actively in the relationship by keeping all appointments and commitments.
- Seek feedback, and use it to modify behaviors.
- Demonstrate flexibility and an ability to change.
- Be open in the relationship with the mentor.
- Demonstrate an ability to move toward independence.
- Evaluate choices and outcomes.

Sources: Scheetz, L. J. (2000). *Nursing faculty secrets.* Philadelphia: Hanley & Belfus; Simonetti, J., & Ariss, S. (1999). *Business Horizons,* *42*(6), 56–73.

You should look for a mentor in the nursing program right now. A student who has already completed several semesters and appears to be a leader is a good choice. Perhaps this is a project for your student nurses association: pairing up mentors and mentees. You may also be assigned a student preceptor while you are in the program. Although this student may or may not become your mentor, you will need to have leadership and management skills to work side by side effectively.

Will you assume the role of preceptor or mentor while you are still in school? We hope your response is yes. As you progress in the program, remember the feelings of uncertainly and anxiety that you probably now have, and volunteer to mentor another new student. Through the mentoring process, you can continue to develop yourself as a leader. Mentoring and preceptoring are part of your professional responsibilities, as the ANA Standard of Nursing Practice 10 (2004) states:

> *Collegiality. The registered nurse interacts with and contributes to the professional development of peers and colleagues.*

How Will This Change As I Grow in My Nursing Career?

As you begin your nursing clinical experiences, your nursing instructor will supervise most of your decisions. As you continue to develop your knowledge and skills, you will begin working more as a member of the team. You will be expected to prioritize patient care, work with a variety of team members and families, and provide care for groups of clients. You may go to community agencies and network with community groups. To be successful in your continued role development as an RN, you must work on perfecting the skills discussed in this chapter.

KnowledgeCheck 38–3

- Identify four skills that employers cite as desirable in job candidates.
- Identify three responsibilities of a mentor and three responsibilities of a mentee.

 Go to Chapter 38, **Knowledge Check Response Sheet and Answers,** on the Electronic Study Guide.

 CriticalThinking 38–4

Think about how you are working with your peers at this time. What mentor responsibilities are you exhibiting? Is there someone who is already mentoring you? If so, what qualities does this person exhibit?

WHAT IS FOLLOWERSHIP?

Leadership and followership are two separate concepts, two separate roles that are complementary, not competitive. There would be no leaders without followers, and there can be no followers without leaders. No one person can have the best strategy, have the clearest vision, or identify the most effective approaches to solve problems. All participants need to be recognized as full partners in the organizational venture. If we define **followers** as individuals who take another as a role model and who act in accordance with, imitate, support, and advocate the ideas and opinions of another (Grossman & Valiga, 2000), then we can define **followership** as the act of being an effective follower.

An organization is a community of many leaders and many followers, frequently changing places depending on the particular activity that is occurring. To participate fully and provide significant feedback,

BOX 38-3 Developing Effective Follower Skills

- Continue your formal and informal education.
- Get involved in your nursing program and later in your profession—be a steward, not a spectator!
- Take initiative and action without being told to. Be creative.
- Be committed to something other than your own career development—find passion in life.
- Set high values, and hold on to them.
- Seek mentors, or accept an offer of mentorship if it is made.
- Be reflective.
- Develop a sense of humor.
- Develop positive relationships with colleagues, rely on each other, and be responsible to each other.
- Develop a wide array of skills, including communication, assertiveness, clinical practice, decision-making, and writing skills.
- Seek feedback on your own performance.
- Independently think up and champion new ideas.
- Feel free to criticize, but do not just complain and walk away.
- Be proactive. Advocate and be a catalyst for change.
- Remain fully accountable for your actions.
- Share information rather than hoard it.
- Be willing to stand up, stand out, risk rejection, and play devil's advocate.
- Present your position in a forthright and respectful manner.
- Give credit when credit is due.
- Follow through on your commitments.
- Try to solve difficult problems rather than expecting the leader to do it all.
- Figure out the steps that are needed for the group to meet its goals, and be part of those steps.
- Stand up and support your leader, but do not expect perfection from him or her.
- Be comfortable with uncertainty and ambiguity.
- Discover or create opportunities to fulfill and maximize your value to the organization. Take time to understand the "big picture."
- Develop self-confidence.
- When appropriate, challenge established beliefs so that all subjects are open to discussion.
- Seek wise counsel.
- Set personal goals, and take responsibility to meet them (Grossman & Valiga, 2000).
- Do not give in to peer pressure.
- Learn about leadership, but recognize that that it is OK to be a follower.

followers need to demonstrate a number of important qualities and behaviors (Grossman & Valiga, 2000):

- Function independently; be a self-starter
- Think critically about ideas that are proposed
- Challenge ideas of the leader
- Give honest feedback and constructive criticism; suggest alternative courses of action
- Be actively involved
- Invest time and energy to arrive at the best possible solution for the group
- Think and act as a team; be cooperative and collaborative
- Draw on and complement each other's and the leader's specialties, strengths, and areas of expertise
- Work on behalf of the organization and the mutually agreed on vision and goals
- Know their own strengths and what their unique contributions to the effort can be
- Seek information so they have the larger picture
- Know when and how to assume the role of the leader when necessary
- Have a positive sense of self-worth and a "can do" attitude
- Be innovative and creative
- Be attentive to what is happening around them
- Be responsible and hold up their end of the bargain

Blindly following some leader without question or taking a passive role in one's work, one's community, or one's professional organization will do little to advance the profession, promote individual growth, or achieve quality patient care. How can you develop your skills as an effective follower? The suggestions in Box 38–3 are only some of many to consider. What else can you add to this list?

WHAT ARE THE CHALLENGES TO BEING AN EFFECTIVE LEADER AND MANAGER?

Individual challenges to being an effective leader and manager center around your ability to develop the skills necessary to assume these roles. Challenges also occur in the healthcare environment. These challenges include the economic climate of healthcare and the nursing labor market.

Economic Climate of Health Care

One of the attractive features of nursing as a career is the wide variety of settings in which nurses can work. From rural migrant health clinics to organ transplant units, nurses' skills are needed wherever there are concerns about people's health. Relationships with clients may extend for months or years, as they do in school health or in nursing homes, or they may be brief and never repeated, as often happens in hospitals, clinics, and emergency departments.

For many years, decisions about care were based primarily on providing the best quality care, whatever the cost. More recently, however, healthcare providers are pressured to seek methods of care delivery that achieve quality outcomes at lower cost. This economic perspective is rooted in three fundamental observations:

• *Resources are scarce.* The scarcity of resources means that three decisions must be made:
  1. How much do we spend on healthcare services, and what do those services consist of?
  2. How will those healthcare services be produced?
  3. How should, or can, we distribute health care? In other words, how are services apportioned within the population? For example, it is hard to believe that the healthcare needs of more than 40 million uninsured individuals in America are not being met because these people cannot afford to pay insurance premiums.

• *Resources have alternative uses.* Because resources are limited, a choice to spend resources in one area eliminates the allocation of those same resources for another use. If we wish to build more nursing homes, for example, we must be willing to accept fewer hospitals or less housing, education, or other uses of those same resources.

• *Individuals want different things or have different preferences.* Some people choose alternative treatment modalities, such as acupuncture, herbal therapy, or massage therapy, rather than traditional health care. The assumption exists that preferences for products and services can be influenced—hence, the extensive marketing of healthcare services.

Nursing Labor Market

Registered nurses make up 77% of the nurse workforce in the U.S., with almost 60% employed in hospitals (Spratley, Johnson, Sochalski, Fritz, & Spencer, 2000). The nationwide unemployment rate for RNs is only 1%, but job vacancy rates in hospitals range from 13 to 20% (First Consulting Group for the American Hospital Association, 2001). A serious nursing shortage is here and will continue until 2020. The demand for nurses is expected to increase even more dramatically as the baby boomers reach their 60s, 70s, and beyond. From now until 2030, the population aged 65 and older will double.

As in the past, cost control and demand for nursing services will most likely involve changing nurse staffing patterns, the model of care, or professional nursing practice (Ritter-Teitel, 2002). All of these changes will affect you, the RN. Regardless of the changes, the shortage of RNs will demand that the RN lead and manage personnel delivering patient care while maintaining fiscal responsibility. Health care is big business. Nurses must juggle the needs of their patients with the needs of the organization (Nelson, 2002). How can we do that?

 CriticalThinking 38–5

Identify changes in your community that will affect you as you embark upon your nursing career? What will you do to prepare for these changes?

WHAT ARE POWER AND EMPOWERMENT?

The leadership and management techniques discussed so far will help you to achieve your goals; however, there are times when these attempts to influence others are overwhelmed by other forces or individuals. Where does this power come from? Who has it? Who does not?

Although people at the top of the organization have most of the *authority* in the organization, they do not have all of the *power*. In fact, the people at the bottom of the hierarchy also have some power. **Power** is the ability to influence other people despite resistance from them. In other words, one person or group can impose its will on another person or group (Haslan, 2001). Power may be actual or potential, intended or unintended. It may also be used for good or for evil, for serious purposes or for selfish ones.

Sources of Power

There are many sources of power. Many of them are readily available to nurses, but some of them are not (Barraclough & Stewart, 1992).

• *Authority:* The power granted to an individual or a group by virtue of position (within the organizational hierarchy, for example).

• *Reward:* The promise of money, goods, services, recognition, or other benefits.

• *Expertise:* The special knowledge an individual is believed to possess. As Sir Francis Bacon said long ago, "Knowledge is power" (Bacon, 1597, quoted in Fitton, 1997, p. 150).

• *Coercion:* The threat of pain or of harm, which may be physical, economic, or psychological.

Let's look at various groups of people in a health-care organization in terms of the types of power that may be available to them.

Managers are able to reward people with salary increases, promotions, and recognition. They can also use coercion—cause economic or psychological pain for the people who work for them, particularly through their authority to evaluate and fire people.

Patients at first appear to be relatively powerless in a healthcare organization. However, if patients refused to use the services of a particular organization, that organization would eventually cease to exist. Patients reward healthcare workers by praising them to their supervisors. They can also cause discomfort by complaining about them.

Nurses have expertise power, as well as authority over licensed practical nurses, UAPs, and other personnel by virtue of their position in the hierarchy. They are critical to the operation of most healthcare organizations and could cause considerable trouble if they refused to work, another source of power (coercion).

Assistants and technicians may appear to be relatively powerless because of their low position in the hierarchy. Imagine, however, how the work of the organization (e.g., hospital, nursing home) would grind to a halt if all the nursing aides failed to appear one morning. Therefore, they have both expertise and coercive power.

Fralic (2000, p. 340) offers a good example of the power of information, or expertise, that nurses have:

> *Florence Nightingale showed very graphically in the 1800s that wherever her nurses were, far fewer died, and wherever they were not, far more died. Think of the power of that information. Immediately people were saying, "What would you like, Miss Nightingale? Would you like more money? Would you like a school of nursing? What else can we do for you?" She had solid data, she knew how to collect it, and she knew how to interpret and distribute it in terms of things that people valued.*

KnowledgeCheck 38–4

What are the sources of power available to nurses?

 Go to Chapter 38, **Knowledge Check Response Sheet and Answers,** on the Electronic Study Guide.

Sources of Empowerment

How can nurses, either individually or collectively, maximize their power and increase their feelings of empowerment? To answer this question, you should first distinguish between the concepts of power and empowerment. Recall that power is the ability to influence other people despite resistance from them. **Empowerment** is a psychological state, a feeling of competence,

control, and entitlement that a person experiences. Given these definitions, it is possible to be powerful and yet not feel empowered. Power refers to action, and empowerment refers to feelings. Both are of interest to nursing leaders and managers. Feeling empowered includes the following (Spreitzer & Quinn, 2001):

- *Self-determination:* Feeling free to decide how to do your work.
- *Meaning:* Caring about your work, enjoying it, and taking it seriously.
- *Competence:* Confidence in your ability to do your work well.
- *Impact:* Feeling that people listen to your ideas, that you can make a difference.

Nurses, like most people, want to have some power and to feel empowered. They want to be heard, to be recognized, to be valued, and to be respected. They do not want to feel unimportant or insignificant to society or to the organization in which they work. You can become empowered by enhancing and sharing expertise.

Enhancing Expertise

Most healthcare professionals, including nurses, are empowered to some degree by their own professional knowledge and competence. Following are some ways in which you can enhance your competence, thereby increasing your own sense of empowerment:

- Actively participate in interdisciplinary team conferences and patient-centered conferences on your unit.
- Attend continuing education offerings to enhance your expertise.
- Attend local, regional, and national conferences sponsored by nursing organizations.
- Read journals and books in your specialty area.
- Participate in nursing research projects related to your clinical area.
- Discuss with colleagues in nursing and other disciplines how to handle a difficult clinical situation.
- Observe the practice of experienced nurses.
- Return to school to earn additional degrees in nursing.

Although you have just begun your nursing career, it is not too early to begin thinking of ways to become empowered.

Sharing Expertise

The second part of the effort to become empowered is to share with others the knowledge and experience you have. This means not only using your knowledge to improve your own practice, but also communicating what you have learned to other students and, later, to your colleagues in nursing. It also means letting your

instructors and supervisors know that you have enhanced your professional competence. You can share your knowledge with your clients, empowering them as well. In the future, you may even reach the point at which you have learned more about a particular subject than most nurses have and want to write about it for publication.

Practical Knowledge
knowing how

As a leader or manager, you will need to get people to work together to make things happen. To do so, you will need to communicate effectively, delegate, deal with conflict and change, and manage your time appropriately.

COMMUNICATING

Communication is the core of leadership. Leadership arises through relationships with other people, and leaders use communication to engage and support these relationships (Mulholland, 1991). One model of communication views it as a circular process that is affected by many factors. Communication in this model has both content and a relationship context. This means the activity is continuous, mutually interdependent, and influenced by the behaviors of each communicator. You need to use active listening (see Chapter 18) to pick up all levels of meaning in a communication. Surface listening, or inattention, often causes a misinterpretation of the message. A person's attitude also influences what he hears and how he interprets the message. To manage client care effectively, it is important to keep the lines of communication open on all levels.

As a professional nurse, you will need to communicate client information to other members of the nursing team, to families, and to the individual client. Promoting trust and sincerity enhances communication among team members. Congruence (agreement) between your words and your deeds promotes trust. If team members feel that you are trustworthy and sincere, they will be more likely to ask questions and seek clarification when they are uncertain of something.

DELEGATING

An important aspect of leadership and management is learning how to delegate. You can apply the nursing process to delegating to safely provide patient care (Hansten & Washburn, 1998).

- *Assess and diagnose.* Before deciding who should care for a particular client, you must assess each client's particular needs.
- *Plan goals and interventions.* Set client-specific goals, and identify what interventions are required to achieve these goals. Mentally identify which staff member is best suited for the task or activities. Thinking this through before delegating helps prevent problems later.
- *Implement.* Next, determine which personnel have the knowledge and skill to care for the client, and assign the tasks to the appropriate person.
- *Evaluate.* You must still oversee care and determine whether client care needs have been met. Be sure to allow time for feedback during the day. This enables all personnel to see how they are doing and what they still need to do.

The National Council of the State Boards of Nursing (1995) developed a concept called the "Five Rights of Delegation." You will find this in Chapter 7.

Often, a manager must first determine the mix of personnel (RN, LVN, or UAP) required to deliver care on a unit before being able to delegate tasks to individuals. By looking at the needs of each client, you can make an educated decision about which staff members have the appropriate education and skill to deliver safe, quality care.

What If I Lack the Experience to Delegate?

The added responsibility of delegation often causes discomfort for new graduates. You may be used to providing total patient care for one or more clients but lack the experience of organizing care for groups of clients with other team members. To decrease this discomfort, you need to observe how more experienced nurses delegate to others. Working with a preceptor will also give you experience in delegation. The American Nurses Association (2002) has issued a Position Statement on Unlicensed Assistive Personnel. Box 38–4 lists the direct and indirect client care that may be performed by UAPs.

What Are the Concerns About Delegating?

Today's healthcare environment requires nurses to delegate. Many nurses voice concerns about the personal risk regarding their licensure if they delegate inappropriately. The courts have usually ruled that nurses are not liable for the negligence of other workers, provided that the nurse delegated appropriately. Delegation is within the scope of nursing practice (Parkman, 1996).

Nurses have expressed concern over the effects of delegation on the quality of client care. When you delegate, you control the delegation. You decide to whom

BOX 38-4 Care that May Be Performed by Unlicensed Assistive Personnel

Direct Client Care Activities

- Assisting with feeding and drinking
- Assisting with ambulation
- Assisting with grooming
- Assisting with toileting
- Assisting with dressing
- Assisting with socializing

Indirect Client Care Activities

- Providing a clean environment
- Providing a safe environment
- Providing companion care
- Providing transport for noncritical clients
- Assisting with stocking nursing units
- Providing messenger and delivery services

Source: American Nurses Association. (2002). *Position statements: Registered nurse utilization of unlicensed assistive personnel.* Washington, D.C.: Author.

you will delegate the task. Remember that there are levels of acceptable performance and that not every task needs to be done perfectly.

KnowledgeCheck 38–5

Explain the relationship of delegation and the nursing process.

 Go to Chapter 38, **Knowledge Check Response Sheet and Answers,** on the Electronic Study Guide.

MANAGING CHANGE

Change is a naturally occurring phenomenon, a part of everyone's life. Every day, we have new experiences, meet new people, and learn something new. We grow up, leave home, graduate from college, and begin a new career, perhaps a new family as well. Some of these changes are milestones in our lives, ones we have prepared for and anticipated for some time. Others are entirely unexpected—sometimes welcome and sometimes not. Many are exciting, leading us to new opportunities and challenges. When change occurs too rapidly or demands too much of us, though, it can make us very uncomfortable (Bilchik, 2002).

The Comfort Zone

Let's assume that your daily routine was basically stable before you started nursing school. You took care of the kids or worked during the day and took a class or two each term. You knew what to expect and how to deal with whatever problems arose in the course of a day. In other words, you were operating within your "comfort zone" (Farrell & Broude, 1987; Lapp, 2002). A change of any magnitude is likely to move you out of this comfort zone into discomfort. Now you are most likely attending a full-time nursing program and juggling changes in finances, child-care arrangements,

and planning options. This first stage in the change process is called *unfreezing*. You are moving out of your comfort zone.

Resistance to Change

People resist change for a variety of reasons. For example, you may find that that you can manage the change in class schedule, but that the child-care arrangements are more difficult. Resistance to change comes from three major sources: technical concerns, psychosocial needs, and threats to a person's position and power (Araujo Group, n.d.). For a student, technical concerns may involve issues related to transportation to school or work, getting children to school, or managing household responsibilities.

Recall Maslow's (1970) hierarchy of needs, discussed in Chapters 3, 9, and 11. Maslow observed that the more basic needs (e.g., physiological and safety needs) must be at least partially met before a person is motivated to seek fulfillment of the higher-order needs. Change can make it more difficult for a person to meet any or all of these physiological and psychosocial needs. Status, power, and influence, once gained within families and organizations, are hard to give up. You may be totally in charge in the family and in the office, yet be a novice in the nursing program.

Recognizing Resistance

It is easy to recognize resistance to a change when it is expressed directly. When a person says to you, "That's not a very good idea," "I am going to quit if I can't get better grades," or "There's no way I'm going to do that," there is no doubt that you are encountering resistance. When resistance is less direct, however, you may have difficulty recognizing it unless you know what to look for.

Resistance may be active or passive (Heller, 1998). **Active resistance** can take the form of attacks or outright refusals to comply, such as the statements in the previous paragraph, writing "killer" memos that destroy the idea or the person who suggested it, quoting existing rules that make the change difficult or impossible to implement, or organizing resistance to the change (encouraging others to resist). **Passive approaches** entail avoidance: canceling appointments to discuss implementing the change, being "too busy" to make the change, agreeing to the change but doing nothing to effect the change, and simply ignoring the entire process as much as possible.

Lowering Resistance

You can use various approaches to lower people's resistance to change. Strategies fall into four categories: disseminating information, refuting currently held beliefs, providing psychological safety, and commanding (Tappen, Weiss, & Whitehead, 2004).

CriticalThinking 38–6

Recall one change that you have experienced that was put into effect by a command (or a new rule, policy, or law).

- What effects did this change have on your life (e.g., work, school, home)?
- How did the command make you feel?
- What would have made this change easier for you?

Obviously, the quickest way to implement change, if you have the authority to do so, is to issue a command. Issuing a command is not necessarily the best strategy, but it is sometimes necessary when the change must be made quickly. The other strategies are:

- *Disseminating information.* Much resistance is simply the result of misunderstandings about a proposed change. Information about the change can be shared on a one-to-one basis, in group meetings, or through written materials distributed by print or electronic means. As a student, it is important that any changes in the program are communicated to you on a timely basis. You should also communicate any changes in your plans to the appropriate people, such as other students, your nurse team leader, or your instructor. As a student nurse or staff member, you should treat client resistance to change in the same manner. The more information that you give the client, the more likely she will be to cooperate with the change.

- *Refuting currently held beliefs.* Leaders often can take action that provides a catalyst for change (Lichiello & Madden, 1996). For example, simply providing evidence that what people are doing or believing is inadequate, incorrect, or inefficient can

increase their willingness to change. For example, patients may enter the hospitals with horror stories from friends and family but may then find that there was no basis for the stories. For example, how have your ideas about the nursing program changed since you first began? What happened, or what information did you receive, that caused you to change your beliefs?

- *Providing psychological safety.* When a proposed change threatens basic human needs in some way, reducing that threat can lower resistance. This leaves people feeling more comfortable about the change. Although each situation poses different kinds of threats and requires different actions to reduce these threats, Box 38–5 identifies common strategies that help increase psychological safety and reduce resistance to change.

Implementing the Change

Now, finally, you are ready to make the change that has been so carefully planned. In addition to employing strategies to lower resistance, increase motivation, and help people work well together, consider the following factors related to change. Ask yourself:

- What is the magnitude of this change? Is this a major change that affects almost everything people do, or is it a minor one with little impact on what people do every day?

- What is the complexity of this change? Is this a difficult change to make? Does it require much new knowledge or skill, or both? How long will it take for people to acquire the necessary knowledge and skill?

- What is the pace of the change? How urgent is this change? Can it be done gradually, or must it be implemented all at once?

- What is the current stress level of the people involved in this change? Is this the only change that is taking place, or is it just one of many changes taking place? How stressful are these changes? How can I help people keep their stress levels within tolerable bounds?

As indicated earlier, some discomfort is likely to occur with almost any change, but it is important to keep it within tolerable limits. You need sufficient pressure to get people to pay attention to the change process, but not so much that they are overstressed by it. In other words, you want to raise the heat enough to get them moving, but not so high that they boil over (Heifetz & Linsky, 2002).

Integrating the Change

Integrating the change is the last step. After the change has been made, it is important to make sure

Common Strategies to Increase Psychological Safety and Reduce Resistance to Change

BOX 38-5

- Point out similarities between old and new procedures.
- Suggest ways in which the change can provide new opportunities and challenges.
- Allow time for learning and practice of any new procedures, if possible, before a change is implemented.
- Recognize the competence and skill of the people involved.
- Ensure involvement of as many people as possible in both the design of the change and the implementation.
- Express approval of people's concern for providing the best care possible.

- Express your appreciation for each individual's and group's contributions in general and to the proposed change.
- Provide a climate of trust and acceptance in which mistakes can be made without negative consequences for individuals.
- If possible, provide assurance that no one will lose his or her position because of the change.
- Provide opportunities for people to express their feelings and ask questions about the proposed change.

that everyone has moved into a new "comfort zone." Ask yourself:

- Is the change well integrated into everyday operations?
- Are people comfortable with it now?
- Is it well accepted? If not, why not? What can be done to increase acceptance?
- Is there any residual resistance that could still undermine full integration of the change? If there is, how can this resistance be overcome?

As Kotter noted, change "sticks" when, instead of being the new way to do something, it has become "the way we always do things around here" (1999, p. 18).

Change is an inevitable part of living and working. Your leadership can influence how people respond to change, the amount of stress it causes, and the amount of resistance it provokes. Handled well, most changes can become opportunities for professional growth and development rather than just additional stressors for students, nurses, and their clients.

CONFLICT

Why do conflicts occur? Nursing education and working in health care bring together people of different ages, genders, income levels, statuses, ethnic groups, educational levels, lifestyles, and professions for the purpose of restoring or maintaining people's health. Differences of opinion over how to best accomplish goals are a normal part of working with people of various skill levels and backgrounds. Each of us brings different experiences, beliefs, values, and habits to interactions with others. These differences are a natural part of our being unique individuals and members of different segments of our society. Various pressures and demands in the classroom, clinical setting, and workplace also generate problems and conflicts among

people. Any or all of these can interfere with our ability to work together.

Conflicts Occur at All Levels

Conflicts can occur at any level and involve any number of people, including your boss, subordinates, peers, or patients (Sanon-Rollins, 2000). On the *individual level,* they can occur between two people working together on a classroom or clinical project, between two people in different departments, or even between a staff member and a client or family member. On the *group level,* conflict can occur between two or more teams, departments, or professional groups (e.g., nurses and social workers may conflict over who is responsible for discharge planning). On the *organizational level,* conflicts can occur between two or more hospitals, health agencies, or community organizations.

"Win-Win" Resolutions

Some people think about problems and conflicts in the same way as they think about a football game or tennis match: Someone has to win, and someone has to lose. There are some problems with this comparison to sports competition:

- Our aim is to work together more effectively, not to defeat the other party.
- The people who lose are likely to feel bad about losing. As a result, they may spend their time and energy preparing to win the next round, rather than on their work.
- A tie (neither side wins or loses) may be just a stalemate; no one has won or lost, but the problem is also still there.

So the answer to the question, "Win, lose, or draw?" is, "None of the above." Instead, a win-win result, in

which both sides gain some benefit, is the best resolution (Haslan, 2001). Following are two erroneous beliefs that can be serious barriers to achieving a mutually beneficial (win-win) resolution of a conflict:

1. *Fixed-pie myth.* Many people think of what can be "won" or gained in a negotiation as a fixed amount, even with a win-win outcome: "I get half, and you get half." The problem is that if I get three-quarters or all of what I wanted, then you will only get one-quarter or less of what you wanted. This is the "fixed pie" myth of conflict resolution (Thompson & Fox, 2001).
2. *Devaluation reaction.* In another erroneous assumption, the devaluation reaction, the person thinks, "If what we've agreed to is good for them, then it has to be bad for us."

Conflict Resolution

When differences and disagreements first arise, problem solving may be sufficient. If the situation has already developed into a full-blown conflict, however, negotiation, either informal or formal, of a settlement may be necessary.

Step 1: Identify the problem. Sometimes, it is easy to identify the real issue or problem. At other times, however, some discussion and exploration of the issues are necessary before the real problem emerges. "It would be nice," say Browne and Kelley, "if what other people were really saying was always obvious, if all their essential thoughts were clearly labeled for us . . . and if all knowledgeable people agreed about answers to important questions" (1994, p. 5). Of course, this is not what usually happens. People are often vague about what their real concern is; sometimes they are genuinely uncertain about what the real problem is. Emotional involvement may further cloud the issue. All of this needs to be sorted out so that the problem is clearly identified and a solution can be sought.

Step 2: Generate possible solutions. Here creativity is especially important. As a leader, begin the process of trying to find new, creative solutions. It is natural for people to try to repeat something that worked well for them in the past, but solutions that were previously successful may not work in the future. Instead, encourage people to spend some time searching for innovative solutions (Smialek, 2001).

Step 3: Evaluate suggested solutions. An open-minded, objective evaluation of each suggestion is needed, but you may find that this is not always easy to accomplish. When a group engages in problem solving, it is sometimes difficult to separate the suggestion from its source. For example, on a team, the status of the person who made the suggestion may influence whether the suggestion is judged to be useful. Judge the suggestion on its merits, not its source.

Step 4: Choose the best solution. Choose the solution that is most likely to work—one that will give you the best results with the fewest negative effects. A combination of suggestions is often the best solution.

Step 5: Implement the solution chosen. The true test of any solution is how well it actually works. Once a solution has been implemented, it is important to give it time to work. Impatience may lead you to abandon a good solution prematurely.

Step 6: Evaluate—Is the problem resolved? Not every problem is resolved successfully on the first attempt. If the problem has not been resolved, you need to resume the process with even greater attention to identifying the real problem and how it can be successfully resolved.

Informal Negotiation

If the conflict is not resolved by your chosen solution, you may have to move on to the next step—informal negotiation. The following steps may prove useful.

1. Ask yourself:
   - What am I trying to achieve?
   - What is the environment in which I am operating?
   - What problems am I likely to encounter?
   - What does the other side want?
2. Set the stage.
3. Conduct the negotiation.
   - Set the ground rules.
   - Clarify the problem.
   - Make your opening move.
4. Continue with offers and counteroffers.
5. Agree on the resolution of the conflict.

Conflict is inevitable within any large or diverse group of people who are trying to work together over an extended period of time. However, it does not have to be destructive, and it does not even have to be a negative experience if everyone involved handles it skillfully. In fact, conflict can stimulate people to learn more about each other and how to work together in more effective ways. Resolution of a conflict, when it is done well, can lead to improved relationships, more creative methods of problem solving, and higher productivity.

TIME MANAGEMENT

Many of the personal management and organizational skills related to the workplace focus on time management and scheduling. Although new nurses may have the required job skills, many lack personal management skills, specifically time management. You might be able to handle conflict and change, delegate appropriately, and be a strong leader among your peers, your faculty, and staff. But if you can't organize and manage your time, you will never gain your full potential.

Many nurses "punch a time clock" that records the minute they enter and leave work, and management considers very few excuses for being late acceptable. Timesheets and schedules are part of most healthcare workers' lives. We are expected to follow precisely set schedules and meet deadlines for virtually everything we do, from distributing medications to getting reports done on time. Many agencies analyze vast quantities of computer-generated data to determine the amount of time spent on various activities. It is no wonder some of us seem obsessed with time. Consider how you can use the following suggestions to improve your time management.

Setting Your Own Goals

It is difficult to decide how to spend your time, because there are so many things that need time. A good first step is to get an overview of the situation. Then ask yourself, "What are my goals?" Goals help clarify what you want and give you energy, direction, and focus. Once you know where you want to go, set priorities. This is not an easy task. Keep in mind Alice's conversation with the Cheshire Cat in Lewis Carroll's *Alice's Adventures in Wonderland* (1865/1965)?

> *"Would you tell me please, which way I ought to go from here?" asked Alice.*
> *"That depends a good deal on where you want to go to," said the Cat.*
> *"I don't care where," said Alice.*
> *"Then it doesn't matter which way you go," said the Cat.*

How can you get somewhere if you do not know where you want to go? It is important to explore your personal and career goals. This can help you make decisions about the future. You can apply these concepts to daily activities as well as to career decisions. Ask yourself questions about what you want to accomplish over a particular time period.

To help organize your time, you need to set both short- and long-term goals. *Short-term goals* are goals that you wish to accomplish within the near future. Setting up your day in an organized fashion is a short-term goal, and so is scheduling a time to study. *Long-term goals* are goals you wish to complete over a long period of time. Advanced education and career goals are examples. A good question to ask yourself is, "What do I see myself doing 5 years from now?" Every choice you make requires a different allocation of time (Moshovitz, 1993).

Organizing Your Work

Many healthcare professionals are linear, fast-tempo, achievement-oriented people. However, working at a fast pace is not necessarily the same as accomplishing a great deal. You can spend much energy in rushing around and stirring things up while actually achieving very little.

To "manage" time, you need to handle time with a measure of skill. Therefore, time management includes efficiently meeting client care needs during a nursing shift (Navuluri, 2001). Organizing your work can eliminate extra steps or serious delays in completing your work. It can also reduce the amount of time you spend doing things that are neither productive nor satisfying. As you begin your nursing program, you may care for only one to two clients. However, as you develop time management skills, you will be able to handle a workload of seven or eight inpatients. The following are some suggestions:

- *Work on the most difficult tasks when you have the most energy.* This decreases frustration later in the day, when you may be more tired and less efficient. Also consider your energy levels when beginning a big task. Start when levels are high and not at, say, 4:00 in the afternoon, if that is when you find yourself winding down (Baldwin, 2002). For example, if you are a "morning person," plan your demanding work in the morning. If you get energy spurts later in the morning or early afternoon, plan to work on larger or heavier tasks at that time.

  Of course, this choice is not always within your control. Many nursing tasks are based on a schedule. If the wound care is due at 1:00 P.M., you must carry out the task then, even if you would prefer to eat lunch and rest. Analyze your work to determine which tasks are fixed and what you can manipulate to match your energy.

- *Create a personal time inventory.* To begin managing your time, you need to develop a clearer understanding of how you use your time. A personal time inventory helps you estimate how much time you spend in typical activities. Keeping the inventory for a week gives a fairly accurate estimate of how you spend your time. The inventory also helps identify "time wasters" (Gahar, 2000).

- *To avoid time wasters, take control.* It is important to prevent endless activities and other people controlling you. Every day, set priorities to help you meet your goals. Learn when to say no. Learn to say, "I would really like to help you; can it wait until I finish this?"

| **toward evidence-based practice** |

Upenieks, V. (2002). What constitutes successful nurse leadership? *Journal of Nursing Administration, 32* (12), 622–632.

Healthcare organizations have come to realize that strong nursing leaders are the key to retention and recruitment of nurses. These organizations are seeking answers to what constitutes successful nursing leadership in today's healthcare environment. A sample population of 16 nurse leaders from four acute care hospitals were interviewed. A set interview form was used so that all nursing leaders were asked the same questions.

Eighty-eight percent of the nurse leaders interviewed confirmed that access to information, opportunity, and resources in the work environment produced a climate for leadership effectiveness. These empowering structures created a supportive and productive climate, enhancing the success of the nurse leader. The study participants also perceived that a nurse leader who has informal and formal power and the opportunity to grow from new challenges can empower clinical staff by sharing power and opportunity.

1. What was the method used to collect the data? Was it written or oral?

2. Describe an environment that helps a leader to be effective, according to this study. Then give an example of each of the factors mentioned.

3. According to this study, how can nurse leaders empower clinical staff?

 Go to Chapter 38, **Toward Evidence-Based Practice Suggested Responses,** on the Electronic Study Guide.

- *Make a daily worksheet.* Providing yourself with reminders of various tasks and when they need to be done can help you organize your day. Without some type of schedule, you are more likely to drift through a day or bounce from one activity to another in a disorganized fashion. The danger in using schedules, however, is that the more they divide the day into discrete segments, the more they fragment the work and discourage a holistic approach. Use the schedule as an organizational tool, but focus on your clients.

- *Learn to delegate.* See previous discussions about delegation.

- *Streamline your work.* Many tasks cannot be eliminated or delegated, but they can be done more efficiently. Here are three wise sayings in time management:

  1. "Work smarter, not harder." This should appeal to nurses facing increasing demands on time. See Box 38–6.

  2. "Never handle a piece of paper more than once." This philosophy can be used to handle patient care, as well as office work and school work. Handle an issue now rather than putting it off until later.

  3. "A stitch in time saves nine." Preventive action saves time in the long run.

Summary

Time can be your best friend or your worst enemy. It is important to identify how you feel about time and to assess your own time management skills. Nursing requires that you perform numerous activities within what often seems to be a very short period of time, so learn how to make the most of your day. Finally, remember that you should set aside 8 hours for sleep and several more for personal or leisure ("time off") time. Use Table 38–3 to help you to review the necessary components of time management.

BOX 38-6 **Work Smarter, Not Harder**

- Gather materials, such as bed linens, for all of your clients at one time. As you go to each room, leave the linen so that it will be there when you need it.

- While giving a bed bath or providing other personal care, perform some of the aspects of the physical assessment, such as taking vital signs, skin assessment, and parts of the neurological and musculoskeletal assessment.

- If a client does not "look right," do not ignore your instincts. The client is probably having a problem.

- Prevention is always a good idea. If you are not sure about a treatment or medication, ask before you proceed. It is usually less time-consuming to prevent a problem than it is to resolve one.

- When you set aside time to do a specific task that has a high priority, stick to your schedule and complete it.

- Do not allow interruptions while you are completing paperwork. Focus on the task at hand.

TABLE 38-3 Components of Time Management

Action	Examples
Prioritize	List tasks in order of importance. Remember that some tasks must be done at specific times, whereas others can be done at any time. Emergencies take precedence. Identify events you control and events others control. Use critical-thinking skills to assign priorities.
Question • Effectiveness • Efficiency • Efficacy	 • Did the task produce the desired outcome? • How can I accomplish the plan with the least expenditure of time? • Is there a way to break this down into simpler tasks? • Do I have the skill and ability to obtain the desired effect?
Recheck	Mentally and physically recheck an unfinished or delegated task.
Practice self-reliance	Identify tasks that are within your control and those that are not. Use critical-thinking skills and adaptability to revise priorities. "Go with the flow."
Treat	Treat yourself to a break when you can. Treat yourself to time off. Treat yourself to an educational experience: Commit yourself to excellence. Treat others with courtesy and respect.

KnowledgeCheck 38–6

- Name and define two erroneous beliefs that can be barriers to achieving a win-win conflict resolution.
- List the steps of conflict resolution.
- List several suggestions for organizing your work.
- State one "wise saying" to guide you in streamlining your work.

 Go to Chapter 38, **Knowledge Check Response Sheet and Answers,** on the Electronic Study Guide.

PUTTING IT ALL TOGETHER

Begin now to look at your strengths and weaknesses. Work on improving the weaknesses and maximizing your strengths. Focus on the concepts of leadership as you work with your classmates, your instructors, and the clinical facilities. Recognize that conflict and change are a normal part of life, and become proactive as issues arise. Observe how "real" nurses delegate and manage their time. Take what is useful, and learn from their examples. Watch for opportunities to be mentored, and make time to mentor others. Above all, remember that you may be the most important person in the life of your client during the time you are with him or her—a very big responsibility, but one you will meet with honor and courage.

 Go to Chapter 38, **Resources for Caregivers and Health Professionals,** on the Electronic Study Guide.

 Suggested Readings: Go to Chapter 38, **Reading More About Leading and Managing,** on the Electronic Study Guide.

 Bibliography: Go to Volume 2, Bibliography.

Portions of this chapter were taken from R. M. Tappen, S. A. Weiss, & D. K. Whitehead (2004), *Essentials of nursing leadership and management* (3rd ed.). Philadelphia: F. A. Davis Company. Used with permission.

39 Nursing Informatics

Learning Outcomes

After completing this chapter, you should be able to:

* Define informatics and its three components.

* Explain how computers work.

* List types of connectivity.

* Describe several forms of electronic communication.

* Describe the importance of computers in evidence-based nursing practice.

* Discuss the benefits of the electronic health record.

* Explain the relationship between computers and standardized nursing languages.

* Identify at least two ways that automation decreases error in health care.

* Defend the assertion that computerized medical records are more private than paper records.

* Explain how computers can reduce some of the barriers to evidence-based practice.

* Identify at least four online sources of nursing research.

* Describe the process of literature database searching.

* Outline a process for evaluating evidence and determining a solution.

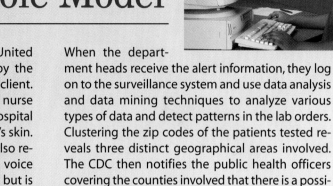

MEET Your Nurse Role Model

In a small rural clinic in the midwestern United States, the nurse practitioner is puzzled by the raised, oozing pustules on her 23-year-old client. Using a camera linked to a web system, the nurse transmits to a dermatologist in a research hospital 60 miles away pictures of the young woman's skin. As the dermatologist views the images, he also reviews the symptoms with the woman via voice transmittal. The physician suspects smallpox but is stunned because smallpox was eradicated many years ago. He orders lab tests to confirm his diagnosis. The order for the test is logged into the automated laboratory system at the hospital, which is linked to the nationwide surveillance database.

At the Centers for Disease Control and Prevention (CDC), the home of the nationwide centralized database, red alerts appear. They signify that there has been an unusual number of laboratory tests for smallpox. The data technician monitoring the system uses a videophone to notify the director of the CDC of the alert. The director stores the videophone conversation and picture so he can forward it to several department heads, including the departments of bioterrorism and epidemiology.

When the department heads receive the alert information, they log on to the surveillance system and use data analysis and data mining techniques to analyze various types of data and detect patterns in the lab orders. Clustering the zip codes of the patients tested reveals three distinct geographical areas involved. The CDC then notifies the public health officers covering the counties involved that there is a possible smallpox outbreak.

The county health officers view the gathered data, using the Internet to access the National Electronic Disease Surveillance System (NEDSS) at the CDC. Using wireless technology to communicate with personal digital assistants (PDAs), they notify the physicians who ordered the tests. The message alerts them to a possible outbreak and directs them to a web site containing the latest research evidence for diagnosing and treating smallpox. The public health department then uses an automated **algorithm,** or automated set of rules, to determine whether to begin mass vaccination, to alert the media, and to disseminate information to other counties.

CriticalThinking 39–1

Reflect on this scenario. Identify how information was managed and processed.

- What mechanisms for gathering and disseminating information were used?
- How did automation assist decision making?
- How was evidence used in decision making?
- Why is informatics important to biodefense?

Theoretical Knowledge
knowing why

The opening scenario is an example of how healthcare professionals encounter and use vast amounts of information to make decisions in practice. This chapter will give you an overview of how this works.

WHAT IS NURSING INFORMATICS?

Whether you become a staff nurse, an administrator, a researcher, primary health care provider, or an educator, you will need current, accurate, and "best available" information to do your job well. The good news is that plenty of information is available. MEDLINE, the premier medical literature database at the National Institutes of Health, currently houses 11.7 million citations and is growing at the rate of more than 400,000 new entries per year (Masys, 2002). If a conscientious nurse read two articles every evening, by the end of the year she would be 550 years behind in keeping up with the literature. The bad news (if you want to call it that) is that we are drowning in information while still lacking in knowledge. Do you ever feel that way as a student?

It is not possible to keep all the necessary information in your head. No one can. We need critical thinking and tools to manage the information to make

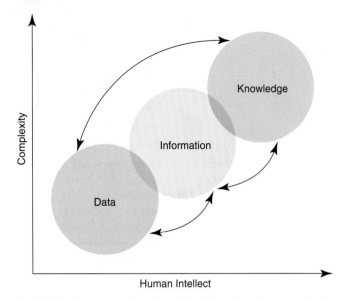

FIGURE 39–1 **Transformation of data to knowledge.** *Source:* Reprinted with permission from the American Nurses Association, *Scope and standards of nursing informatics practice (2001)*, American Nurses Publishing, ANA, Washington, DC.

it useful to us. If it is not possible to learn and retain all the information, then you must know how to find, process, and manage it to arrive at the best decisions for your practice. In essence, this is the definition of **informatics:** the managing and processing of information necessary to make decisions. **Nursing informatics** is informatics applied to nursing practice, education, and research. The first conceptual framework for informatics envisioned the elements ("stuff") of informatics as *data, information,* and *knowledge* (Graves & Corcoran, 1989). Full-spectrum nurses interact with all three of these elements in daily practice, so you need to understand how they interrelate.

Data

Data are "discrete entities that are described objectively without interpretation" (American Nurses Association [ANA], 2001). In other words, data are raw, unprocessed numbers, symbols, or words that have no meaning by themselves. For example, what does 101 mean? It could indicate the movie title *101 Dalmatians,* a piece of programming language, or someone's body temperature, pulse rate, weight, or age. Without a context, data are meaningless.

In nursing, we speak of data as those primary facts and observations acquired in the course of providing services, such as the numerical value of a blood pressure measurement or factual data such as, "Father died of prostate cancer." Notice that even this data has no meaning until the nurse interprets it: The meaning of "Father died of prostate cancer" changes if the client is a healthy 24-year-old female versus a 54-year-old male experiencing bleeding from the bowel.

Information

Information consists of groupings of data processed into a meaningful, structured form (ANA, 2001). If you combine 101 from the previous example with a degree symbol, you know that the number represents a temperature. If other data—gender (female), age (23), and 3 days of decreasing temperatures—are grouped together, information is formed. You now know that this young woman had a high fever but appears to be getting better.

Data:	101, female, 23, three
Grouped data:	101 degrees Fahrenheit, female gender, age 23, 3 days of decreasing temperatures
Information:	Woman with high fever appears to be getting better

In the opening scenario, what information did the CDC receive that triggered an alert?

Knowledge

In the "Meet Your Nurse Role Model" scenario, what *information* did the CDC use to create knowledge of the counties involved? Take a minute to write your answer.

The answer to the question is that the CDC received information on the number of lab tests performed for smallpox. Grouping this with other information (e.g., the normal number of lab tests performed) and existing knowledge (i.e., about smallpox and about bioterrorism), the CDC personnel created *knowledge* of the potential for a smallpox epidemic and perhaps even an attack of bioterrorism.

Knowledge is formed when data are grouped, creating meaningful information and relationships, which are then added to other structured information (ANA, 2001). The knowledge can either be previously known or new. In the preceding scenario of the 23-year-old female with the temperature of 101°F, we can add information about pathophysiology, pharmacokinetics (how medications work), patient history, and physical assessment, providing the knowledge to make an informed decision about the patient's current condition and further treatment.

Figure 39–1 depicts the transformation of data into knowledge. As we have come to realize that the gathering of data and information to make decisions is neverending, the model has evolved to depict overlapping circles and both forward and backward movement.

Wisdom

Nelson and Joos (1989) added *wisdom* to the Graves and Corcoran model. **Wisdom** is defined as the *appropriate use* of knowledge in managing or solving human problems. As we discussed in Chapter 1, wisdom develops as

an outcome of your clinical experience, theoretical knowledge, critical thinking, and intuition—as you progress from novice to expert in the practice of full-spectrum nursing.

KnowledgeCheck 39–1

- What is the difference between knowledge and wisdom?
- Define the following: *data, information, knowledge.*
- Give an example of each: data, information, knowledge.

 Go to Chapter 39, **Knowledge Check Response Sheet and Answers,** on the Electronic Study Guide.

UNDERSTANDING COMPUTERS AND CONNECTIVITY

Before you can appreciate the tremendous benefits of automation for nursing practice, you need to understand some fundamentals of computers and connectivity.

How Do Computers Work?

Computers are so embedded in our daily lives that we are hardly aware of their existence. In addition to the common personal computer and laptop, computers function in personal digital assistants (PDAs), robots, video games, and most electronic devices from TVs to telephones. A **computer** is an electronic device with four main functions: input, process, output, and storage. Collectively, these operations are known as **information processing** (or *data processing*). The power of a computer is twofold:

1. The speed, accuracy, and reliability with which it operates
2. The enormous amounts of data it is capable of storing and keeping readily available for processing

Computer operations require electronic circuits. These circuits are embedded on small *microchips* or, using *nanotechnology,* on even smaller atoms. Figure 39–2 is a picture of a microchip containing the electronic circuits that perform the operations of a computer. In the future, developers predict that nanotechnology will create nanorobots the size of molecules that will attack cancer cells and viruses to make them harmless. Nanorobots could be programmed to do cellular-level surgery without leaving the scars of conventional surgery (Bonsor, 2002).

If you are a sophisticated computer user, you probably already know how hardware, storage media, and software enable a computer to function (Figure 39–3). If you cannot answer the following questions,

 Go to Chapter 39, **Supplemental Materials: How Does a Computer Work?** and **Tables, Boxes, Figures: ESG Figure 39–1,** on the Electronic Study Guide.

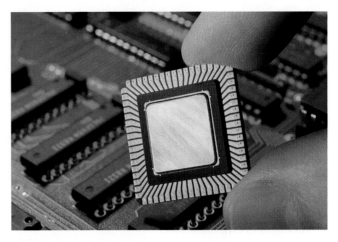

FIGURE 39–2 A microchip that performs the operations of a computer is as small as the end of a finger.

Pretest: Computers

1. List and describe three kinds of computer storage media.
2. Name and describe two computer input devices (hardware).
3. Name and describe two computer output devices (hardware).
4. What is the central processing unit in a computer?
5. What is the difference between ROM and RAM memory?
6. Explain the difference between an operating system and application software.
7. Name three different kinds of application software (e.g., spreadsheet).
8. Define *bit, byte, kilobyte, megabyte,* and *gigabyte.*
9. What is the term *megahertz* used to describe?

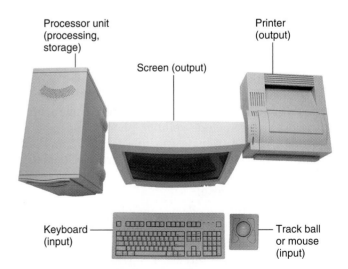

FIGURE 39–3 Basic microcomputer hardware: screen (output), processor unit (processing, storage), keyboard (input), mouse (input), and printer (output).

10. Match the following applications with the types of activities (administration, clinical, or education) with which they may be associated. Some applications may be associated with multiple activities. Explain your thinking.

Applications	*Types of activity*
Word processing	Administration
Databases	Clinical
Spreadsheets	Education
E-mail	
Computer-assisted instruction (CAI)	
Graphics programs	
Clinical documentation	

If you want to check your answers,

 Go to Chapter 39, **Pretest Answer Key,** on the Electronic Study Guide.

If you were able to answer most of the pretest questions, proceed to the next section.

What Are Some Different Types of Connectivity?

Communication in health care must be efficient, fast, and reliable. **Connectivity** is a term referring to the ways in which computers and other hardware communicate and share information. For example, several computers can print to one printer, files can be shared, and individuals can communicate using e-mail or Listservs. Connecting technology has many forms.

- *Wired.* In a "wired" environment, all of the devices are connected by a physical wiring system of cables. For example, if you have a home computer, it is probably cabled to a keyboard and a printer. What examples of wired connectivity can you find in the opening scenario?

- *Wireless. Wireless* is a term used to describe telecommunications in which electromagnetic waves (rather than some form of wire) carry the signal over part or the entire communication path. Some common wireless examples include cellular phones and pagers, cordless mouse, remote controls for TV and VCR, baby monitors, satellite television, and personal digital assistants (PDAs) such as those mentioned in the opening scenario.

- *Modem.* The term *modem* stands for "modulator/demodulator." It changes computer codes into pulses or signals that can travel over telephone lines (e.g., to connect to the Internet). The transmission speed for modems can be as high as 56 kbps. A home computer or a laptop is often connected to the telephone with either an internal or an external modem.

- *Cable.* Cable modems connect computers to the Internet with the same technology as cable television. Cable modems are typically faster than regular telephone modems, but when many subscribers are online, using the same cable, speed is not as fast. Because the service is "always available," you don't need to dial in or wait for call setup.

- *Digital subscriber line (DSL).* This technology is another high-speed connection to the Internet. It exploits unused frequencies on copper telephone lines to transmit data at multi-megabit speeds. Voice and high-speed data can be sent simultaneously over the same line. Like cable connectivity, the service is always available and needs no dialup. DSL is not shared in the same manner as cable, so you always have the same speed, no matter how many people are online. However, DSL speed is limited by the distance from a switching station. The farther away from a station you are, the slower your access speed.

- *Internet.* The Internet is an international network linking millions of computers via cable, phone lines, or wireless technology. Tens of millions of people use it every day. It operates on a backbone system without a true central host computer. Technically, *Internet* and *World Wide Web* are not interchangeable terms. The Web is a child of the Internet, whose ease of use has made it much more popular than the original, text-based Internet. The Web allows for use of photographs, sound, and moving pictures to create visually exciting and interactive web sites.

  How was the Internet used in the small rural clinic in the opening scenario? Besides the nurse, who else used the Internet, and how?

What Are Some Forms of Electronic Communication?

Electronic communication can be very simple, such as "plain old telephone service" (POTS) or very complex, such as telehealth. Electronic forms of communication use all the different forms of connectivity.

Telephone

Telephone service is so pervasive, economical, and simple to use, that we may not even think of it as "technology." But it is the backbone of any organization's communication system. Telephony is *synchronous* (real-time) and supports the subtle verbal cues needed to understand the speaker's meaning. Because it is so commonplace, people often take telephony for granted and do not look for new ways to use it. However, innovative use of the telephone can make significant improvements to the delivery of care. For example, follow-up calls can be made after same-day surgery

Use of Informatics in Home Care

A telephony documentation application has been developed for home health aides. On arriving at a patient's home, the aide uses the patient's phone to dial in to a central number and keys in her identification. The time of the call, telephone number from which it came, and identification of the worker are automatically recorded. At the end of the visit, the aide again calls from the patient's phone. Again, the location, time, and identification of the caller are recorded. Using the telephone key pad, the aide then keys in codes indicating the tasks accomplished. She never has to physically write a documentation record; it is accomplished using the telephone. This reduces the amount of time the aide must spend in recording care, improves accuracy, and prevents lost documentation.

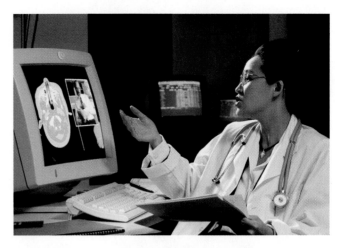

FIGURE 39–4 Videoconferencing permits face-to-face interaction without requiring the participants to travel to a central location.

rather than requiring a return visit. See the Home Care box for a home health example.

Undoubtedly the biggest change in voice telephony in recent years is the expanded use of mobile phones. Mobile communication reduces the effort required to locate people to speak to them. The combination of mobile telephony and paging systems can reduce the time clinicians spend answering pagers or responding to telephone messages. Increasingly, nurses in both home care and acute care are carrying cellular phones rather than taking the time to find a wired telephone. They are instantly available for communication.

Videoconferencing

Videoconferencing allows face-to-face interactions when participants are geographically separated (Figure 39–4). This medium is also synchronous (real-time) and allows participants to see the nonverbal cues and gestures of other participants. The addition of video to voice technology adds cost and complexity to the communication process. However, the increased cost of communication may be offset by the reduced cost for travel (e.g., to a meeting, workshop, seminar, or national conference).

Facsimile (Fax)

Facsimile, or fax, was one of the first technologies to use telephone lines for data transmission. It is sometimes called *telecopying*. When you feed a printed document into the sending machine, an optical scanner digitizes the text and images and transmits the digital data via telephone lines. The receiving machine reconverts the digital message and prints a paper copy of the document. Faxing works well if the recipient wants only to read the document. The recipient cannot manipulate or alter the message.

Electronic Mail

One of the earliest, and still most popular, methods of electronic communication is the use of electronic mail, or e-mail. It is useful because of its speed of transfer and almost universal accessibility. People typically use e-mail to send short textual messages between computer users across a computer network. You can create documents in other applications (e.g., word processing documents, photographs, spreadsheets) and "attach" them to send with the e-mail message. Popular e-mail applications include Netscape's Messenger, Eudora, and Microsoft's Outlook Express. Nurses and other healthcare providers can use e-mail to interact with patients, consult with colleagues, and communicate with insurance industry representatives, pharmacies, and hospitals.

Be aware that privacy is not assured with electronic mail. For example, it is entirely legal for employers to read incoming and outgoing employee messages when they are sent on company equipment. In addition, once a message has been sent, you have no control over who may actually read it or to whom it might be forwarded. For more information about e-mail security,

 Go to Chapter 39, **Supplemental Materials: E-mail Security,** on the Electronic Study Guide.

Listserv

Mailing lists are an extension of e-mail use. The most common mailing list application is called a **Listserv** (standing for *list server*). The names and

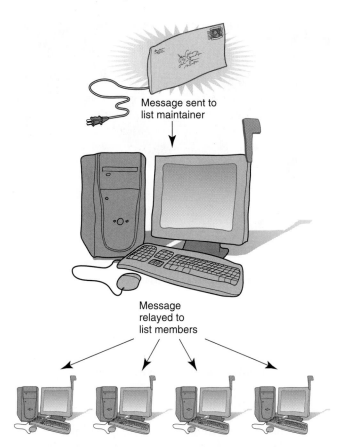

FIGURE 39–5 A message sent to the Listserv server is relayed to all list members.

BOX 39–1 Listservs for Nurses

Go to the **American Nursing Informatics Association** web site at **www.ania.org**

The following are some web sites that will help you find a professional Listserv in your area of interest.

- **American Nurses Association: www.ana.org/listserv/**
- **Nurse-Beat Connections: www.nurse-beat.com/ links/listserves.htm**
- **NurseNet listing of nursing discussion forums: http://ualberta.ca.~jrnorris/nursenet/nurlists.html**
- **NMAP listing of mailing lists: http://nmap.ac.uk**

To join a Listserv:

1. Address your e-mail request to the list management address, for example:
   LISTSERV@UVVM.UVIC.CA
2. Leave the subject line blank.
3. In the body of the email type: subscribe nameoflistserv yourfirstname yourlastname
   For example: subscribe nrsinged Sarah Moffett
4. You should receive an email welcoming you to the Listserv and giving a set of instructions about interacting with the Listserv. Print and save the instructions for future reference.

addresses of the people on the mailing list, called **subscribers,** are stored by the Listserv on a single server. A single address is then designated for the group to use. When a message is sent to that address, it is delivered to the Listserv server, which then distributes the message via e-mail to all subscribers (Figure 39–5).

Virtually all subspecialties and special interest groups in health care have a Listserv. Interested professionals subscribe to the list and receive mailings from others on the list. If you use a Listserv, be aware that any message you send through the mailing list goes to *everyone* on the mailing list. So be careful when you hit the "Reply" command!

Listservs are a powerful communication tool. Communication is global and almost instantaneous. Ideas and protocols can be shared, questions asked and answered, and surveys taken. Everyone on the list has equal opportunity to share in the discussion. See Box 39–1 for the addresses of some listservs that might be of interest to you.

Telehealth

Telehealth is the use of telecommunication to send healthcare information between patients and professionals at different locations (Figure 39–6). It improves access to health care by providing long-distance

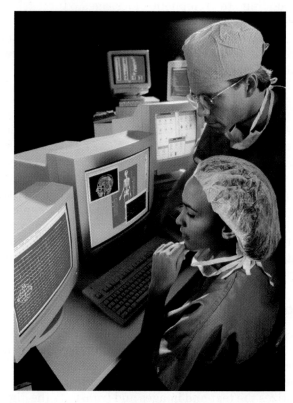

FIGURE 39–6 Telehealth helps to solve time and distance problems in healthcare.

BOX 39-2 Use of Computer Information Systems in Nursing

Nursing Practice	Nursing Education	Nursing Administration	Nursing Research
Literature access and retrieval (e.g., for evidence-based practice)	Literature access and retrieval	Quality assurance and utilization review	Literature review
Care planning	Computer-assisted instruction (CAI) programs	Employee records (e.g., to track licenses, immunizations)	Data collection
Client records (e.g., documenting, order entry, retrieving lab results)	Classroom technology	Staffing patterns, hiring	Data analysis (both qualitative and quantitative)
Telenursing (e.g., in home health)	Distance learning	Buildings and facilities management	Research dissemination
Case management	Testing and grading	Finance and budgets	Applying for grants
Documenting medications	Student records	Accreditation reviews (e.g., monitoring quality indicators for JCAHO)	
Transcribing orders	Development of electronic and learning communities using the World Wide Web		
Reordering medications			
Identifying drug interactions			
Warning practitioners about drug incompatibilities			

clinical health care, patient and professional education, and health administration. The U.S. Department of Defense is a pioneer in telehealth and continues to explore new avenues of use, including providing healthcare services to soldiers in combat and dependent families in outlying posts. The following are other examples of the use of telehealth:

- When the consultation of a specialist is required in a rural healthcare site, telecommunications equipment at both the rural site and the specialist's site can connect the patient to the specialist in a minimum amount of time without requiring the patient to travel. The specialist can see and talk to the client, as well as view his records, x-ray films, lab results, and so on. Refer back to the "Meet Your Nurse Role Model" scenario. How did the nurse make use of telehealth?

- A more common use of telehealth is the use of home health monitoring devices. These devices allow the healthcare professional to monitor vital sign status and other indicators without physically entering a home or requiring a patient to make a clinic trip. This allows for more frequent monitoring of patients.

Despite barriers, such as cost and issues surrounding licensing and reimbursement, telehealth applications will continue to expand in the future. For information about barriers that slow the growth of telehealth,

 Go to Chapter 39, **Supplemental Materials: Barriers to Telehealth,** on the Electronic Study Guide.

CriticalThinking 39-2

- As a patient, would you prefer a telehealth or a face-to-face consultation? Why?
- Now imagine that you are an accident victim brought to a rural clinic staffed only with paraprofessionals. Does your answer change? If so, why?

THE ROLE OF INFORMATICS IN NURSING PRACTICE

You have been introduced to several ways in which computer information systems are used in nursing care. In this section, we describe the role of informatics and standardized nursing languages in promoting evidence-based practice, maintaining health records, decreasing medical error, and protecting patient privacy and confidentiality. Box 39–2 summarizes the use of computers in practice, education, administration, and research.

Why Are Computers Important for Evidence-Based Practice?

The ever-increasing volume of knowledge changes the way decisions are made in health care. The *traditional model of healthcare decision making* relies on each practitioner's personal experience and judgment. But health care is now so complex that problems routinely exceed the clinical decision-making capacity and reliability of individual practitioners. The *new*

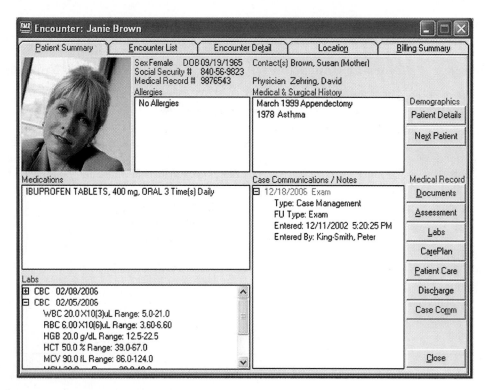

FIGURE 39–7 **Computer screen from an electronic health record.** *Source:* Courtesy of Per Se Technologies, Atlanta, GA. Used with permission.

model of decision making is evidence-based practice. As we discussed in Chapter 8, evidence-based practice uses a knowledge base of accumulated "best evidence" that can change quickly and continuously. To find the current *best* evidence, you must be able to locate the evidence, evaluate its quality and relevance to the problem, and apply the solution. Because of the large volume of information that you must process and manage, you will undoubtedly use computers to help you locate the evidence on which to base your practice.

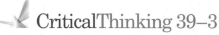

CriticalThinking 39–3

Analyze the "Meet Your Nurse Role Model" scenario. What example of evidence-based practice do you find in it?

What Are the Benefits of an Electronic Health Record?

The *electronic health record (EHR)* is also commonly known as the *electronic medical record, computerized medical record,* and *computer-based patient record.* EHR software allows clinicians to create, store, edit, and retrieve patient charts on a computer. Figure 39–7 is an example of a computer screen using EHR software. Notice the "tab" for "Encounter List," which you would click to get information about this patient's previous visits to the hospital or clinic. Notice, too, that there is a tab for "Billing Summary" so that the record includes business-related as well as clinical information.

A successful EHR project allows an organization to replace its paper charts and care plans with electronic records. Other benefits of the EHR include the following:

- *Improved access to patient data.* Improved data access can increase efficiency, productivity, and continuity of care. A paperless health record stores all patient information in one location, rather than in bits and pieces in many different files and locations. A person's complete health information is available at the touch of a button.

- *Privacy.* Access to sensitive patient information can be limited only to individuals with proper authorization, and each retrieval of data can be logged electronically—a vast improvement over the folders and charts that can pass through many hands without a record of who examines them.

- *Accessibility.* Have you ever needed to write your nurses' notes before leaving the clinical setting, only to discover that the chart was in the x-ray department with the patient? Or that the physician was making rounds with it in her hands? In contrast, any number of people in different locations can access a computerized record—and all at the same time. A physician can view lab results from his office while a nurse views them in the hospital and a lab technician adds more data. In addition, computers allow for point-of-care access to patient information. A variety of hardware supports this need, from stationary bedside terminals,

wireless laptops mounted on mobile carts, and hand-held devices such as PDAs (Figure 39–8).

• *Research and public health benefits.* Many healthcare leaders find themselves overwhelmed with data but lack the information they need to make informed decisions. Computerized records place data in repositories (storage areas) so that the information can be sorted and collated to create the information and knowledge necessary to aid decision-making research. For example, state health departments can access population-based medical information to track communicable diseases, possibly preventing epidemics. Health researchers and analysts can also take advantage of aggregate health information to find out, for example, which treatment is most effective for a disease, thus improving patient outcomes over time.

Some EHR systems are designed for planning as well as for documenting care. Other applications are designed to support efficient patient care workflow. Studies (e.g., Ammenwerth, Mansmann, Iller, & Eichstadter, 2003) demonstrate that nurses who understand the nursing process and are familiar with computers are more accepting of automated documentation. As younger people who have grown up with technology enter the workforce, the nursing profession's comfort level with computers is increasing.

Although most organizations understand the advantages of an EHR, up-front costs and the change in organizational culture that must occur with automation are major deterrents to implementation.

KnowledgeCheck 39–2

- What is the difference between application software and operating system software?
- What is the difference between modem and cable connectivity?
- How is a Listserv different from regular e-mail?

 Go to Chapter 39, **Knowledge Check Response Sheet and Answers,** on the Electronic Study Guide

Why Are Standardized Nursing Languages Needed for EHRs?

Suppose you wanted to find out how many patients on your hospital unit had a nursing diagnosis of Impaired Skin Integrity during the past year. If the hospital uses paper medical records, how could you find out? If the records are on computer, would that make a difference?

You probably said something like: Pull all the charts, and look at the nurses' notes. Or maybe, search for the words *Impaired Skin Integrity* in the computerized records. That's a beginning. But think about this: Nurses use a variety of terms to describe the same data. For example, in some charts you would find the term *skin breakdown;* in others, *a reddened area, bedsore,* or a *stage III pressure ulcer.* Would you count all of these as Impaired Skin Integrity? What if the nurses

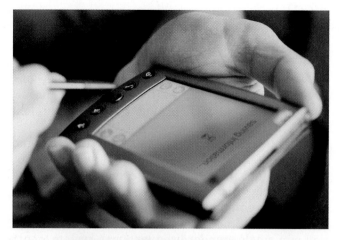

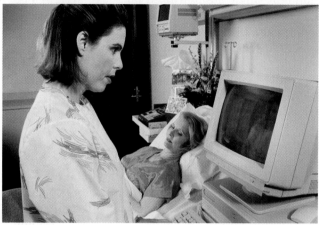

FIGURE 39–8 Point-of-access computing. *A,* Hand-held computer. *B,* Bedside terminal.

used some terms you didn't think to search for? Do you see how the lack of a uniform way to describe patient problems can hamper efforts to create and retrieve nursing data from automated documentation systems?

Nurses do not describe clinical interventions uniformly, either. Inconsistent language and meaning make it impossible to compare and research nursing contributions to patient care (Beyea, 2000). Use of standardized nursing languages helps to ensure that nursing contributions are an integral component of any electronic health record. Understanding those nursing contributions through research and teaching will help to further define the scope of nursing practice and make visible the contributions of nursing in healthcare.

The first use of standardized nursing language began in the 1970s, with the NANDA classification of nursing diagnoses. Since then, several initiatives to develop standardized languages for nursing practice have arisen. By 2003, the American Nurses Association Committee for Nursing Practice Information Infrastructure had recognized 13 standardized languages.

 Go to Chapter 39, **Standardized Language, American Nurses Association Recognized Languages for Nursing,** in Volume 2.

Each of these languages makes a unique contribution to knowledge development in nursing. At this time, it appears that no single language has captured nursing practice in its entirety. Each language is currently in the process of revision and further development. This is, of course, true of *all* languages, including English and Spanish and other national languages.

This text primarily uses the NANDA, NIC, and NOC classifications for describing patient problems, outcomes, and interventions (see Chapters 4, 5, and 6). Other classifications, such as the Omaha system and CCC, are intended for specific settings (i.e., community health and home health, respectively). Adoption of a single standardized language system would enhance communication among nurses, with other healthcare professionals, and with the public. Because this does not appear likely, however, nurses are working to "map" terms from each system to their equivalents in other systems (e.g., Impaired Skin Integrity in NANDA might map to Integument in the Omaha system).

How Does Automation Decrease Error in Healthcare?

As health care becomes more complex, the opportunities for error increase exponentially. Misdiagnosing, overlooking an allergy, or erroneously transcribing a medication order can carry serious consequences. A hospital stay can be prolonged or death can result from a seemingly simple mistake. Medical error is the 8th leading cause of death in the United States. As many as 44,000 to 98,000 people die annually in the United States as a result of medical error, more than from motor vehicle accidents, breast cancer, or AIDS (Institute of Medicine [IOM], 2000, p. 1). In addition to the anxiety and suffering caused, the IOM report estimates that medical error costs $8.5 to $14.5 billion per year in the United States (p. 2). The most common errors are drug complications (19%), wound infections (14%), and technical complications (13%) (IOM, 2000, p. 30).

The *American Journal of Nursing* (*AJN* Reports, 2003) recently cited an expert in medication safety whose study revealed that 19% of nurses' medication doses were incorrect. Errors included giving at the wrong time, omitting doses, giving the wrong dose, and giving without authorization. Seven percent of the errors were clinically significant (p. 25). For a more extensive discussion on the use of automation to decrease medication errors,

 Go to Chapter 39, **Supplemental Materials: How Does Automation Decrease Error in Healthcare?,** on the Electronic Study Guide.

In health care, building a safer system means designing processes of care to ensure that patients are protected from accidental injury. Automation provides a secure way for providers to quickly and efficiently communicate with each other regarding a patient's allergies, medications, or current health status, so that an emerging situation does not become deadly. A computerized record can be quickly accessed, updated, and forwarded simultaneously to all members of the healthcare team. For example, many different departments (e.g., x-ray department, nursing, pharmacy) need to know about a patient's allergies. Rather than continually asking the patient to recite his allergies, the computer can record the information one time and send it to every department that needs it. Computers help decrease errors in other ways, as well:

1. *Computerized physician order entry* helps prevent errors in reading and transcribing orders.
2. *Bar-coding medications at the unit-dose level* helps to prevent nurses from selecting an incorrect medication.
3. *Use of smart technologies (e.g., infusion devices) at the point of care* helps to ensure that the correct dose is delivered to the patient.

 CriticalThinking 39–4
- How does automation contribute to or decrease errors in health care?

How Can I Use Electronic Health Records Ethically?

No information is more sensitive than medical records. Patients confide in nurses and physicians, trusting that their information will remain private. Only one person at a time can view a paper record, and that person and the record must be in the same geographical location. With an automated record, many people can view the information at the same time, and they can be in many different geographical locations. Still, in some ways the automated record is more secure than the paper record. Almost anyone who wears a white coat and has a stethoscope around her neck can view the paper record. There is no record to show who has looked at the information. In contrast, several measures protect the confidentiality of the electronic health record:

- *Passwords* for all users are probably the most obvious protection. In most institutions, passwords are tied to the responsibilities of the job designation. For example, the business office does not have access to clinical information, and nurses do not have access to data about the patient's bill-paying arrangement.

- *Audit trails.* Organizations are required to have software that tracks each person who accesses information. This is called an audit trail. Anything a person adds to or changes in the record is recorded automatically on the audit trail and can be investigated.
- *HIPAA regulations.* As of April 2003, most health plans and care providers are required to comply with the Department of Health and Human Services (HHS) Privacy Rule (also referred to as "the HIPAA regulations"), which was mandated in response to the Health Insurance Portability and Accountability Act (HIPAA) of 1996. This is the first comprehensive federal protection for the privacy of individually identifiable health information. Some of the requirements are that health plans and providers must (1) obtain consent before disclosing health information used for treatment or payment options; and (2) limit disclosure of information to the minimum necessary to accomplish intended purposes. These rules apply to all forms of communication: electronic, written and oral. For full information,

Go to the **U.S. Department of Health and Human Services** web site at www.hhs.gov/ocr/hipaa/

Although it is important to protect the privacy of healthcare records from outside observers, professionals who have password access but are not assigned to the patient to provide care make most breaches of confidentiality. Strong personal integrity and adherence to nursing and other codes of ethics are necessary to protect patient privacy within healthcare organizations.

KnowledgeCheck 39–3

- List at least three ways in which computers can help reduce healthcare errors.
- Discuss at least three measures to protect the confidentiality of patients' electronic health records.

Go to Chapter 39, **Knowledge Check Response Sheet and Answers,** on the Electronic Study Guide.

Practical Knowledge
knowing how

Professional standards require accountable practitioners to keep up to date with research and new knowledge. For example, ANA Professional Performance Standard 3, Criteria 2 and 3, state that the nurse should demonstrate a commitment to lifelong learning and seek experiences that reflect current practice to maintain skills and competence (ANA, 2004). You can accomplish this by knowing how to search literature databases efficiently and use web resources discriminately.

USING INFORMATICS TO SUPPORT EVIDENCE-BASED PRACTICE

As you have learned in previous chapters, evidence-based practice involves (1) identifying a clinical problem, (2) searching the literature, (3) evaluating evidence, and (4) deciding on the intervention (Stevens, 2001). It is not enough to find one journal article in support of an intervention. Managing and processing information are essential for these tasks. Nurses require the most current, best-quality information for making decisions in their practice. In hospital settings, nurses need information mainly on medical/surgical topics, clinical nursing issues, and drug therapy (Bradshaw & Dale, 1999). But how do nurses use automated systems to access that information? See Box 39–3 for a profile of an information-literate person.

How Do Computers Reduce Barriers to Evidence-Based Practice?

Most nurses are action oriented, preferring to learn by looking, listening, and talking. It may seem easier to seek information from colleagues, rely on past experience, draw on knowledge of pathophysiology, and read whatever references are closest at hand. However, in the clinical setting, the closest references may not contain the most current information or the best possible evidence. Computers at the worksite help overcome this barrier to evidence-based practice by providing fast, easy access to current practice information from around the world. For example, when traditional methods have failed, you could quickly use a computer to look up the latest, tested interventions for a patient who is incontinent of urine.

One barrier to evidence-based nursing practice is the rigid schedule of many nurses, which prevents them from using libraries. Because the Internet is available 24 hours a day, you can access libraries and other information sources on your own schedule.

Even though most professionals believe that searching literature in the workplace benefits care, some supervisors and managers fail to facilitate or reward the practice, focusing instead on immediate patient care tasks (e.g., "Are the assessments all done and charted?"). Employers need to provide systems to access current literature and databases at the point of care, as well as giving nurses time and encouragement to use them. Literature use should be considered an intrinsic part of practice and rewarded as such. In a time-limited work environment, accessibility to current information sources is critical. As a professional, you should urge employers to provide quick access to evidence on which to base your practice decisions.

BOX 39-3 Profile of an Information-Literate Person

An information literate person *accesses* information:

- Recognizes the need for information
- Recognizes that accurate and complete information is the basis for intelligent decision making
- Formulates questions based on information needs
- Identifies potential sources of information
- Develops successful search strategies
- Accesses print and technology-based sources of information
- Is a competent reader

An information literate person *evaluates* information:

- Establishes authority
- Determines accuracy and relevance
- Distinguishes opinion from factual knowledge
- Rejects inaccurate and misleading information
- Creates new information to replace inaccurate or missing information as needed

An information literate person *uses* information:

- Organizes information for practical application
- Integrates new information into an existing body of knowledge
- Applies information in critical thinking and problem solving

Other characteristics:

- A resourceful and independent learner
- Confident in his or her ability to solve problems
- Able to function independently and work equally well in groups
- Creative and able to adapt to change

Source: Krumsieg, K., & Baehr, M. (2000). *Foundations of learning* (3rd ed.). Corvallis, OR: Pacific Crest.

How Do I Use Computers to Search the Literature?

Lack of literature-searching skills is another reason why many nurses fail to capitalize on the automated information available to them to enrich their practice. There are several steps to conducting an automated search of the literature.

A critical first step is to identify the need for information. When you clearly understand the need for information and how it will be used, it is easier and more efficient to search, locate, evaluate, retrieve, organize, and manage the resources required to answer your question. The next step is to formulate a precise definition of the problem. This is usually in the form of a question, for example, "What are the leading causes of falls in older adults?" This question guides your search for information. After formulating a question, you can then conduct a search of the most recent literature and most relevant studies.

CriticalThinking 39–5

Before reading the next section, see whether you can puzzle out the answers to the following two questions. Consult with your classmates and instructors, if necessary, after finishing the chapter.

- Why must a question be formed before initiating the search?
- The suggested question in the preceding section was "What are the leading causes of falls in older adults?" Why can't you use a general topic such as "falls" for your search topic?

Online Sources of Nursing Research

You must evaluate the *type* of literature you need to answer the question. For instance, a research report provides better support for an intervention than does an opinion article. Although some information is classic and timeless, it is usually best to find the most current studies.

- *Textbooks,* although good for general information, are not the most current source of information. The information in a textbook is generally 3 to 5 years old the day the book is published.
- *Printed journal articles* are more current, but the information may still be 6 months to 2 years old by the time the article is published. Journals come in varying degrees of academic rigor. You must discriminate among scholarly, general interest, and popular periodical literature.
- *Scholarly journals* generally have a sober, serious look. They usually contain many graphs and charts, but few glossy pages or pictures. A scholar or researcher in the field writes the articles, carefully footnoting and citing references. Articles submitted to scholarly journals are reviewed by a group of experts to determine if they are suitable for publication. This process is known as **peer review.** The main purpose of a scholarly journal is to report on original research to make the information available to others. Examples of scholarly journals include: *Journal of Nursing Scholarship, Journal of Nursing Administration, Nursing Research, Nurse Educator,* and *International Journal of Nursing Terminologies and Classifications.*

| toward evidence-based practice |

Low, D. K. & Belcher, J. V. R. (2002). Reporting medication errors through computerized medication administration. *CIN: Computers, Informatics, Nursing, 20*(5), 178–183.

This study compared the incidence of medication errors 12 months before the implementation of a bar code medication administration system to 12 months after implementation. The study revealed an 18% increase in errors.

1. At first glance, what seems to be the obvious conclusion you can draw about the bar code system?

2. On the basis of this report, you might jump to a conclusion that the bar code system was not a good idea. Before drawing that conclusion, though, what questions do you need to ask about what might have been going on in this institution (or on this unit) that might have made it *appear* there was more error when that really was not the case?

3. What other things, besides the bar code system, can cause medication errors?

4. How might an automation system make it appear there was nurse error when no error actually occurred?

This last question is difficult, so you are not expected to figure it out on your own. The answer follows:

Although automation is unfailingly consistent, if the correct rules are not programmed into the system, an error may be reported that is not usually considered an error. For instance, the window of opportunity for proper administration of a medication is usually one half-hour either before or after the assigned time. However, for many medications, such as vitamins and stool softeners, the window of opportunity can be widened without harming the patient or affecting the efficiency of the drug. If this variation is not accounted for in the programming, giving a vitamin 1 hour after the assigned time will show as an error when, in fact, it was not.

You must carefully analyze the results of automating procedures before jumping to any conclusions about practice. What may appear to be an increased incidence of medication errors may actually reveal that medication errors were previously underreported and that some variation in administration is acceptable and not actually an error.

 Go to Chapter 39, **Toward Evidence-Based Practice Suggested Responses,** on the Electronic Study Guide.

- *General interest periodicals* are usually quite attractive. Articles are heavily illustrated, commonly with photographs. News and general interest periodicals sometimes cite sources, but not always. Articles may be written by a member of the editorial staff, a scholar, or a freelance writer and are often peer reviewed. The language is geared to any educated audience. A specialty is not assumed. Some examples of general interest nursing periodicals include the *American Journal of Nursing, RN,* and *Nursing* [*current year*].

- *Popular periodicals* are usually slick and attractive in appearance. They include many graphics and photographs. These publications rarely, if ever, cite sources. Information in such journals is often second- or third-hand, and the original source is sometimes obscure. Articles are usually very short, lack depth, and are written in simple language and designed to meet a minimal education level. The main purpose is to promote a product or viewpoint. Examples include *Parents, Readers Digest,* and *Modern Healthcare.*

- *The World Wide Web* contains the most current information, including some well-respected nursing

journals (e.g., *American Journal of Nursing, NurseWeek, Online Journal of Issues in Nursing* and *Nursing Standard Online*). A new discovery can be published on the Web for the entire world to see on the day of discovery.

Literature Databases

Literature databases are a powerful tool for finding information. Literature databases are catalogues of articles, usually sorted by discipline. Databases exist for engineering, education, law, medicine, nursing, and other disciplines. These databases often overlap—what is found in one database can also be found in another. For example, MEDLINE is the largest medical database and lists internationally published articles from journals covering all areas of biomedicine. The Cumulative Index for Nursing and Allied Health Literature (CINAHL) is a smaller database covering nursing, allied health, biomedical, and consumer health journal articles. Most of the articles in CINAHL are also listed in MEDLINE. If, however, you are looking for a nursing-focused article, it is more efficient to use CINAHL because the search is already narrowed to nursing and allied health.

BOX 39-4 Example of a Database Entry

Author(s):	Lacey, MD
Title:	The experience of using decisional support aids by patients with breast cancer
Source:	*Oncology Nursing Forum 2002* Nov–Dec: 29(10): 1491-7 (19 ref)
Standard No:	ISSN: 0190-535X Serial Identifier: 006740000 NLM Unique Identifier: 7809033
Language:	English
Descriptor:	Cancer Patients Breast Neoplasms Decision Making, Patient
Document Type:	Journal article; research; tables/charts
Database:	CINAHL

The search results may also contain an abstract of the article, and in some instances, the full-text article is available either for a fee or at no charge.

People are understandably confused by the distinction between materials found on the free public Web and those on the "private" Web, because the Web is used as a delivery method for both. Whereas the *public Web* is easy to use, its search engines retrieve a large number of irrelevant pages, and many scholarly publications are not available on the public web. In contrast, on the *private Web,* electronic indexes provided by organizations and universities give students access to more reliable and accurate information, including scholarly articles that have undergone a peer review process. The private Web is a collection of subscribed services purchased by the provider. Individuals can also subscribe on a yearly basis to journal indexes.

Each entry in a database contains an article citation, subject headings describing the article, and a text summary of the article called an *abstract.* Other information about the article may also be included, such as the name of the author(s), the name of the institution at which the research was done, and the language in which the article was published (Box 39–4). Many full-text journal articles are available online, some free and some for a fee. Table 39–1 includes descriptions of some commonly used databases in health care. Do not limit your search to a single database. You will find valuable information in the databases of

TABLE 39-1 Selected Databases

Database	Description
CINAHL (Cumulative Index for Nursing and Allied Health Literature)	Covers nearly 1175 nursing, allied health, biomedical, and consumer health journals, publications of the American Nursing Association, and the National League for Nursing. Coverage with abstracts is from January 1986 to the present. Coverage with indexing from 1982 to the present. Updated monthly.
Cochrane Library	A regularly updated collection of evidence-based medicine databases, including systematic reviews, reviews of effectiveness, and a controlled trials register. This is a source of reliable evidence about the effects of health care.
Health and Wellness Resource Center	Provides integrated access to medical, health, and wellness information from reference sources, magazines and journal articles, pamphlets, and some Web resources. Quick Start links include a medical encyclopedia, dictionary, drug and herb finder, health organization directory, health assessment links, health news, and a few select medical Web sites.
MEDLINE	Produced by the U.S. National Library of Medicine, MEDLINE is one of the major sources for biomedical literature. Coverage includes every subject in the broad field of biomedicine, indexing articles from over 9075 international journals published in the United States and 70 other countries.
PsycINFO 1887	Covers worldwide literature in psychology and related disciplines, such as psychiatry, sociology, anthropology, education, linguistics, and pharmacology. Journal articles, technical reports, and dissertations are included. Coverage is from 1887 to the present. Updated weekly.

other disciplines (e.g., psychology, education, business, law, and engineering).

How Do I Evaluate Evidence and Determine a Solution?

Evaluating the evidence may be as simple as reading a research study and applying the results to your current situation. For example, in the search for information about falls in older adults, you may find research to indicate a number of safety measures that can be easily implemented to create a safer environment for your patients. However, evaluating evidence can also be very complicated, requiring an understanding of statistics and research methodologies. Just because one research study indicates that sugar causes cancer does not mean that the study was valid or reliable; therefore, you must not base conclusions on the results of only one study. Experience and further study about research will increase your ability to evaluate your findings in the literature.

CAUTION! Although an article you find on the Web may be quite current, it is not necessarily accurate, valid, or reliable. Many sites are created by individuals with questionable credentials or by companies attempting to sell their product or service. Such sites may not provide the best information to support your research; even worse, their information may be incomplete, inaccurate, biased, or unreliable. See Box 39–5 for suggestions on evaluating materials you obtain from a website. For ethical principles to guide health information web sites,

 Go to **Chapter 39, ESG Box 39–1,** on the Electronic Study Guide.

BOX 39–5 How to Evaluate a Health Information Web Site

Remember, anyone can publish anything on the Web. The information you obtain may have been created by an expert, but most World Wide Web sites are authored by nonexperts. They may contain fact or opinion. Do not believe everything you read on the Web! Use the following questions to guide your evaluation.

Evaluate For	Questions to Ask
Authority	1. Who is the author? What are his credentials and qualifications to speak on this topic? Are the sources of information stated? Don't confuse the author with the webmaster. 2. Check the URL domain (e.g., *www.nih.gov*). What institution published the document? The Web address provides clues to this: .com—a company .mil—the U.S. military .edu—a school or university .net—a network of computers .gov—the U.S. government .org—a nonprofit organization The domain symbols ~ or % or a name (e.g., jsmith), "users" or "members" indicate a personal web page. 3. Who is the sponsor? The name right after "www" will provide a clue (e.g., see "nih"), but the full name (e.g., National Institutes of Health) should be on the page. 4. Can you contact the author for clarification or more information?
Currency	1. When was it produced? For some topics, you need current information. 2. When was it updated? Note that the fact that the Web page was "updated" may not mean that the information was updated at the same time. It may simply mean that the physical file was changed in some way (e.g., a misspelled word corrected) 3. Are the links up to date? Check the links to see whether they work.
Purpose	1. Why was the page put on the Web? Remember that many sites are for the purpose of selling a product or an idea. Other purposes may be to entertain, to give facts, to share humor, or to provide a forum for ideas and opinions. 2. Look for words like "about our company," "mission," "philosophy," "who am I," and so on. 3. Who are the intended users of the page? Students, experts, patients? 4. Are there advertisements on the page? This may be a clue.
Availability	1. Can you view or download the information without a special browser or special software? 2. Are there fees for viewing the full content?

➤

BOX 39-5 How to Evaluate a Health Information Web Site *(continued)*

Evaluate For	Questions to Ask
Content quality (accuracy, objectivity, coverage)	1. Are the sources documented with footnotes or links? Are they scholarly links or information sources? 2. Is the information provided by the site, or is it reproduced from another source? 3. Are there links to the original sources (if they are online)? Or a reason for not providing a link? Do they work? 4. Look for bias (e.g., political or ideological), especially when you agree with it! Are there links to opposing views if it is an opinion page? 5. *Is the information reliable and error-free?* Is there someone who verifies or checks the information? 6. *How in-depth* is the material? 7. *What does the page offer* that you can't find elsewhere? 8. *Look up the page* in a directory that evaluates its contents. For example: *www.ipl.org* *www.sitegrade.com* (SiteGrade) *www.ciolek.com/WWWVLPages/QltyPages/QltyLinks.html* (WWW Virtual Library Maintainers: Criteria Used to Select Links for Resources' Catalogues)
Usability	1. Is it easy to read and navigate? 2. Are HELP screens available? 3. Is there a search engine on the site? 4. Is it frequently offline or slow to load?

 CriticalThinking 39–6

Why is the Web an unreliable source of accurate information?

 Go to Chapter 39, **Resources for Caregivers and Health Professionals,** on the Electronic Study Guide.

 Suggested Readings: Go to Chapter 39, **Reading More About Nursing Informatics,** on the Electronic Study Guide.

 Bibliography: Go to Volume 2, Bibliography.

Holistic Healing

Learning Outcomes

After completing this chapter, you should be able to:

* Explain holism and holistic care.

* Compare and contrast complementary, alternative, integrative, and allopathic health care.

* Explain how the placebo response relates to holistic care.

* Discuss the trends in use of complementary and alternative modalities (CAM).

* Differentiate the five types of CAM.

* Discuss the most commonly used CAM therapies.

* Identify ways to integrate CAM into nursing care.

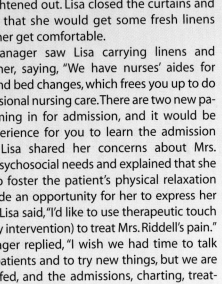

Your Patient

MEET

Lisa Jackson is a new graduate RN at her first nursing job on a surgical unit of the local community hospital. When Lisa entered the room to assess Mrs. Riddell, a surgical patient, she found her lying in bed, crying softly. Mrs. Riddell sobbed, "I don't think I can handle this. All the pain. I feel terrible. I'm so worried about cancer. I don't have any sick time left at work; how am I going to manage?" Lisa put her hand gently on the patient's arm and said, "It sounds like you're going through a lot right now. It must be very difficult for you." Mrs. Riddell reached for Lisa's hand and began sobbing, "I'm so afraid."

Just then Joy Lensen, the manager of the surgical unit, walked into the room, speaking quickly as she entered, "Lisa, you forgot to turn the call light off. Oh, Mrs. Riddell, you seem upset. Are you in pain?" Mrs. Riddell struggled to speak through her tears and nodded her head yes. "On a scale of 1 to 10, how strong is the pain?" Ms Lensen asked. "About a 5," the patient replied. Looking at Lisa, the manager said, "Ms Jackson will check when you can have your next dose of pain medication."

On the way to the nurses' station, Lisa explained to her manager that Mrs. Riddell was worried and frightened about her diagnosis. "First things first, Lisa, get the patient's pain under control," replied the manager. Lisa wanted to spend a few moments with the patient, giving her time to express her feelings and concerns. She realized that pain relief was important but that Mrs. Riddell's pain was complicated by her anxious feelings. However, Lisa was new on the unit and decided to follow the manager's orders to address the physical pain, hoping to continue her dialogue with the patient when she returned with the analgesic.

When Lisa returned with the medication, Mrs. Riddell refused it. She was still weepy and distressed and complained that she really just needed to have her bed straightened out. Lisa closed the curtains and explained that she would get some fresh linens and help her get comfortable.

The manager saw Lisa carrying linens and stopped her, saying, "We have nurses' aides for cleanup and bed changes, which frees you up to do the professional nursing care. There are two new patients coming in for admission, and it would be good experience for you to learn the admission process." Lisa shared her concerns about Mrs. Riddell's psychosocial needs and explained that she wanted to foster the patient's physical relaxation and provide an opportunity for her to express her concerns. Lisa said, "I'd like to use therapeutic touch (an energy intervention) to treat Mrs. Riddell's pain." The manager replied, "I wish we had time to talk more to patients and to try new things, but we are short-staffed, and the admissions, charting, treatments, dressing changes, IVs, medications, and phone calls will never be done by the end of shift if we don't do first things first. I'm sorry to disillusion you, but welcome to the real world of nursing."

Lisa and Mrs. Riddell are experiencing some problems common to contemporary health care: inadequate staff, time, and resources for the care we know our patients deserve. Today many patients and nurses feel caught in a model of sick care that emphasizes disease and professional emotional neutrality.

Theoretical Knowledge
knowing why

Holistic healing and nontraditional health care are a growing trend. Some say this interest is a direct result of dissatisfaction with the impersonal nature of traditional health care. In this chapter, we will explore holistic care and the use of complementary and alternative modalities (CAM).

HOLISM

The concept of **holism** focuses on the relationships among all living things. Holism was the dominant philosophy throughout early history, but it fell out of

favor in the 17th century, when René Descartes and other influential philosophers of the time introduced the notion that the mind and body are split. Descartes' thinking strongly influenced the emerging discipline of medicine and is largely responsible for Western medicine's separate treatment of physical and mental health. However, in 1926, South African statesman Jan Christian Smuts reinvigorated the belief in holism by declaring that living entities are more than the sum of their parts.

Biomedical and holistic perspectives consider health and disease from different perspectives. Consider the case of a person with bacterial pneumonia. Conventional biomedical treatment uses antibiotics to kill the bacteria, an antipyretic to suppress fever and other uncomfortable symptoms, an expectorant to liquefy secretions, increased fluids, and rest. Treatment is successful when the pathology (i.e., infection) and symptoms (e.g., fever) are gone. Conventional medicine is often referred to as **allopathy,** a term used to indicate medical practice focused on counteracting symptoms.

A holistic approach expands the therapeutic encounter to include methods of enhancing the person's resistance to the illness, including rest, fluids, nutritional counseling, reduction of aggravating behaviors, and stress management. Holism emphasizes the need to change lifestyle behaviors that trigger vulnerability to illness. Holistic treatment is complete when the person has healed into an optimal state of wellness (as defined by the individual), has developed an understanding of why the illness occurred, and has adopted lifestyle changes.

What Is Holistic Health Care?

The public's current interest in holistic healing is the result of a culmination of forces, including the focus of Western medicine on illness, in spite of many people's desire to promote health, avoid illness, and use treatments with fewer side effects. Because many people are interested in holistic care, you need to have theoretical knowledge of holistic practices, be aware of the effects of holistic treatments, and help patients achieve holistic care.

Holistic health care is founded on the following beliefs:

- Each person is unique.
- Each person is a whole in constant interaction with the environment. The body, mind, and spirit must come together to achieve harmony and healing.
- Disease is a result of multiple contributing factors rather than one cause.
- Factors essential to health are social support, health practices, family illness patterns, personality traits, culture, child-rearing practices, and relatedness to nature.
- All healing is self-healing.
- Hope, faith, and the will to live are important to maintaining health and recovering from illness.
- The patient's expectation that the treatment will be effective is part of the self-healing process. A positive state of mind is necessary to bring harmony to the body.
- Each person is interconnected to others, nature, and to the world.
- Health is achieved when there is balance, integration, and harmony in life.
- Healthcare resources are better used when they focus on health promotion and disease prevention.
- Illness is an opportunity for growth and has meaning within the context of the life experience.
- Illness occurs when there is a shift in an individual's balance.

A **modality** is a technique or method of treating a disorder, for example, therapeutic touch and antibiotics. *Holistic health care* is a term often used interchangeably with *complementary health care* and *alternative health care,* but they do not have the same meaning. A **complementary** modality is one that is used together with traditional medical care. An **alternative** modality is one that is used instead of traditional medical care. Complementary and alternative modalities (CAM) encompass a wide range of philosophies, approaches, and therapies that the conventional healthcare system does not commonly use, accept, understand, study, or make available. Although a number of CAM treatments are holistic, many are narrowly focused.

Until recently there was limited scientific evidence regarding the effectiveness of CAM therapies in Western society. The creation of the National Center for Complementary and Alternative Medicine (NCCAM), a division of the National Institutes of Health, has stimulated research in this area. As a result, the list of what is considered CAM is continually changing, and therapies that are proven to be safe and effective are incorporated into conventional health care while new modalities emerge.

Integrative health care, a term coined by physician Andrew Weil, refers to coordinated care that encompasses all treatments and health practices a patient uses. To provide integrative care requires a practitioner who is knowledgeable about interactive effects of conventional and CAM treatments and able to coordinate all the care modalities. The practitioner must establish trust so that the patient will disclose CAM use and must communicate with other health providers for referral and coordination of care. Integrative health care is holistic because it considers all aspects of the patient's care.

KnowledgeCheck 40–1

- Compare and contrast alternative, complementary, and integrative modalities.
- What is the relationship between allopathy and holistic health care?

 Go to Chapter 40, **Knowledge Check Response Sheet and Answers,** on the Electronic Study Guide.

CriticalThinking 40–1

- Review the "Meet Your Patient" scenario. What kind of care is Mrs. Riddell receiving: allopathic, complementary, alternative, or integrative? Would you be comfortable offering CAM therapies to Mrs. Riddell?
- As a holistic healer, should Lisa administer pain medications to Mrs. Riddell if she agrees to take them? Why or why not?

The Placebo Response

The **placebo response,** the client's expectation that a treatment will be effective, is a basic underlying principle of holistic care. The placebo response is an expression of mind-body unity. The stronger a person's belief in treatment efficacy, the stronger the placebo effect. It's opposite, the **nocebo effect,** is a demonstration of the power of the mind to create bodily distress. For example, expecting that a treatment will be painful tends to increase treatment discomfort. These responses illustrate the powerful influence of the mind on states of health and disease.

In holistic care, treatment outcomes are enhanced if the practitioner and the patient believe that the treatment will be effective and if the practitioner establishes an empathetic and supportive relationship with the patient.

The ideal relationship is mutual and based on equality, with the patient assuming an active role in the treatment plan. The practitioner acts as a role model and negotiates care that incorporates a number of healing modalities. Practitioners teach patients to strengthen their intent to heal by focusing their minds to influence the course of illness and recovery. Techniques such as visual imagery, affirmations, and relaxation techniques enhance treatment outcomes because the mind and body function as a unit. Holistic healers believe that all healing is self-healing, and the placebo response demonstrates this natural phenomenon.

Spirituality and Holism

To fully understand the experience of health and illness, you must include the spiritual dimension. Spirituality is the vital process of discovering meaning, purpose, fulfillment, and value in life. As such, it has tremendous influence on health and an individual's ability to heal

(see Chapter 14). According to Levine (1984), absence of spirituality creates a sense of disconnection from one's true source, a loss of meaning to one's life, and a state of *dis-ease*. A holistic perspective incorporates the realities of the human condition—disease, disability, misfortune, aging, pain, and death—into the life experience. Illness and disease are viewed as opportunities for transformation and growth.

Holism is not a set of self-improvement strategies. A holistic context fosters maturation through illness, disability, deformity, and even death. Holism helps to answer some vital questions: Who am I? How do I choose to live? And what is the value of my life?

CriticalThinking 40–2

Holistic health care relies on the placebo effect. However, traditional therapy discourages the use of placebos for pain control (ethicists hold that placebos are deceptive and do not respect patient autonomy). Traditional researchers attempt to factor out the placebo effect when conducting clinical research trials. React to these two belief systems. Which belief is most congruent with your view of health care? How do you think these divergent views might affect research on CAM?

Who Is a Holistic Patient?

In May 2004, NCCAM and the National Center for Health Statistics (NCHS) released findings on Americans' use of CAM. The results came from a 2002 survey completed by 31,044 adults aged 18 years or older. The study found that 36% of adults used some form of CAM over the previous 12 months. When megavitamin therapy and prayer for health reasons are included in the definition of CAM, that number rises to 62%.

Data revealed that women, people with higher educational levels, and people who have been hospitalized in the past year are more likely to use CAM. The U.S. public spent an estimated $36 to $47 billion on CAM therapies in 1997. Approximately half of these costs were paid out-of-pocket. These fees were more than out-of-pocket expenses for all hospitalizations in 1997 and about half of all out-of-pocket physician services expenses (NCCAM, 2004).

In a nationwide study of what motivates people to use CAM, Astin (1998) discovered that most people who use CAM do so because they find it more in harmony with their own values, beliefs, and philosophical orientation toward health and life. Cassidy (1994) identified characteristics of persons likely to benefit from holistic care:

- Have a high need for affiliation and relational style of health care
- Wish to alleviate symptoms gently or with fewer side effects
- Will not take "hopeless" for an answer

- Wish to prevent disease or enhance wellness
- Interpret the body-person as being more than just physical and want to address energetic, psychosocial, and spiritual needs
- Are concerned with the invasiveness of typical biomedical care

KnowledgeCheck 40–2

- How does holism incorporate spirituality?
- What type of person is most likely to use CAM?

 Go to Chapter 40, **Knowledge Check Response Sheet and Answers,** on the Electronic Study Guide.

 ## CriticalThinking 40–3

The NCCAM (2004) findings identified people who have been hospitalized in the past year as more likely to use CAM. React to this finding. What do you think this finding suggests about traditional hospital care?

What Is Holistic Nursing?

Nursing, like medicine, has been fragmented by ever-increasing technological and bureaucratic demands. As we see in the case of Lisa Jackson and Mrs. Riddell ("Meet Your Patient"), nurses and patients feel the strain of hurried, disconnected, and unsatisfying contact. In fact, nurses often leave a workplace, and even the profession, when they feel that care is being dehumanized. Holistic nursing practice is a theory-based, relationship-centered, potent solution to such problems facing contemporary nursing and health care.

Holistic Theory

Holistic nursing is not new. Principles of holistic nursing are found in Florence Nightingale's vision of health and nursing. She described the work of nursing as putting patients in the best condition for nature to act upon them, emphasizing touch and kindness along with the healing influences of fresh air, sunlight, warmth, quiet, and cleanliness. Nightingale viewed people as multidimensional beings inseparable from their environment.

More recently, three prominent nursing theorists have contributed to the evolution of holistic nursing: Martha Rogers, Margaret Newman, and Jean Watson (Bright, 2002).

- *Rogers*. In Rogers' view, the environmental energy field is in constant and meaningful interaction with the human energy field. Nurses exert influence on these energy fields to effect change in health status.
- *Newman*. Newman, a student of Rogers, identifies disease as disequilibrium, which stimulates the person toward growth and regaining wholeness. From a holistic perspective, disease is an inevitable part of

the human condition and is necessary and beneficial for growth, adaptation, and maturation.
- *Watson*. Watson's theory of nursing identifies caring as the primary focus of nursing. She describes "authentic presencing," which facilitates the "caring moment" between the nurse and the client.

Holistic Concepts

Among the concepts found in holistic nursing are *meaning, therapeutic use of self, role modeling,* and *integrated lifestyle and practice.*

- *Meaning*. Barbara Dossey (Dossey, Keegan, & Guzetta, 2000), a leader in the field of holistic nursing, asserts that it is important to know the meaning inherent in a disease and its symptoms. **Meanings** are individual constructions that reflect a person's values, belief system, expectations, and the unique way in which the person experiences health and illness.
- *Therapeutic use of self*. Conventional nursing education emphasizes the therapeutic use of self. Holistic nursing expands the therapeutic use of self to include awareness of the effects of *presence* and *intention* on the healing process. The presence of the nurse is an integral part of the patient's environment. The mutual energetic process that is present in every caring act enhances health outcomes.
- *Role modeling*. A holistic nurse serves as a role model for her patients. Practically speaking, a holistic nurse understands that unless her own health is balanced, it is difficult to sustain the energy necessary to be a constructive presence and an effective practitioner.
- *Integrated lifestyle and practice*. Healthful nutrition, sleep, rest, and relaxation benefit your function as a healthcare provider. In addition, a support network of like-minded colleagues serves as a resource. A major source of support is the American Holistic Nurses Association (AHNA), founded in 1980. AHNA connects you with like-minded colleagues, provides opportunities for scholarly development, and offers an affiliation that facilitates renewal of core nursing values.

WHAT HEALING MODALITIES ARE COMMONLY USED?

A wide variety of alternative health traditions, practices, and therapies is available. Most require at least some advanced training, and often certification, prior to practice. NCCAM organizes CAM into five categories (Figure 40–1), which we discuss in the remainder of this chapter:

1. Alternative systems of medical practice
2. Mind-body interventions
3. Biologically based therapies
4. Manipulative and body-based methods
5. Energy therapies

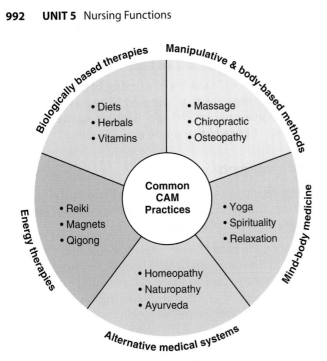

FIGURE 40–1 **NCCAM organizes CAM into five categories.**

Figure 40–2 illustrates the ten most commonly used CAM therapies. Prayer specifically for health reasons is the most commonly used CAM therapy. CAM is most often used to treat or prevent musculoskeletal conditions or other conditions involving chronic or recurring pain.

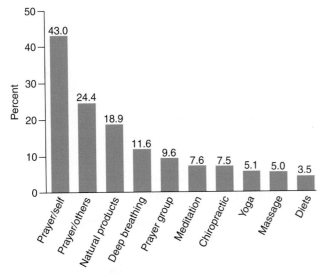

FIGURE 40–2 **The most widely used CAM therapies in the United States.**
Source: National Center for Complementary and Alternative Medicine. (2004). Understanding complementary and alternative medicine. Retrieved August 18, 2004, from http://nccam.nih.gov/news/images/campractice.htm

KnowledgeCheck 40–3

- Identify the five categories of CAM identified by NCCAM.
- What are the most commonly used CAM therapies?

Go to Chapter 40, **Knowledge Check Response Sheet and Answers,** on the Electronic Study Guide.

Alternative Medical Systems

Alternative medical systems predate the traditional Western health system. They have been used for centuries throughout the world, and their use in Westernized countries is currently increasing. Examples include ayurveda, Chinese medicine, acupuncture, homeopathy, and naturopathy.

Ayurveda

Ayurveda, a healing system derived from ancient India, covers all aspects of health and wellness. Ayurveda's core belief is that a sense of harmony with nature and our inner being produces health. Ayurveda attributes health to balance between three forces: creation (*kapha*), preservation (*pitta*), and destruction (*vata*). Imbalance between these forces leads to illness and disease.

Humans have a physical and psychological constitution made up of each of these three forces. This constitution is known as a *dosha*. The ideal dosha is vata-kapha-pitta in equal proportions. During an ayurvedic consultation, the practitioner assesses the patient's dosha and uses diet, exercise, breathing, meditation, visualization, therapeutic massage, and herbs to treat illness and maintain health. Color therapy, sound therapy, and aromatherapy are also used to create balance. If you are caring for a patient who follows ayurvedic treatments, offer these changes in conjunction with traditional health care.

Traditional Chinese Medicine

Chinese medicine is the oldest continuously practiced medicine in the world. **Traditional Chinese medicine (TCM)** is based on writings that originated between 200 B.C.E. and A.D.E. 200. TCM practitioners consider that each person has his own balance of yin and yang energies (complementary but opposing life forces) and the five elements of earth, water, wood, fire, and air/metal. If these balances are disturbed, ill health will result. Each element is associated with specific characteristics, such as color, smell, flavor, sound, and so on.

TCM practitioners base their therapies on information gathered from examination. They may look closely at your face, mouth, tongue, skin, nails, and hair. They may listen to sounds you make through your voice, breathing, or digestive system. The nature

| toward evidence-based practice |

Richardson, J. (2004). What patients expect from complementary therapy: A qualitative study. *American Journal of Public Health, 94*(6), 1049–1053.

Patients attending a British National Health Service outpatient department that provided acupuncture, osteopathy, and homoeopathy were asked to complete a qualitative survey about their expectations of complementary therapies. Patients expected symptom relief, information, a holistic approach, improved quality of life, self-help advice, and wide availability of such therapies.

Perry, R., & Dowrick, C. F. (2000). Complementary medicine and general practice: An urban perspective. *Complementary Therapies & Medicine, 8*(2), 71–75.

General practitioners in Liverpool were mailed a survey evaluating their attitudes about eight common complementary therapies and whether they treat with, refer to, or endorse each therapy. During the previous week, 56% of respondents had been involved in complementary medical activity with their patients: 13% had treated directly, 31% had referred patients to a practitioner, and 38% had endorsed one or more complementary therapies. Acupuncture was the most popular option, along with osteopathy, and chiropractic was the therapy most highly regarded by general practitioners in terms of effectiveness. Homeopathy and hypnotherapy received a mixed reaction, and herbalism, aromatherapy, and reflexology were viewed skeptically. Sixty-two percent of respondents reported successful outcomes of complementary treatments. Respondents were generally uncertain about the theoretical validity of these therapies: 50% thought acupuncture had a valid basis, compared with only 23% for homeopathy and 8% for reflexology.

Barrett, B., Marchand, L., Scheder, J., Appelbaum, D., Plane, M. B., Blustein, J., et al. (2004). What complementary and alternative medicine practitioners say about health and health care. *Annals of Family Medicine, 2*(3), 253–259.

A sample of 32 local CAM practitioners were selected for face-to-face in-depth interviews. Interviews were taped, transcribed, and reviewed by all coauthors. The CAM practitioners stressed the holistic, empowering, and person-centered nature of CAM. They described themselves as healers, employing attentiveness, touch, and love to increase self-awareness and strengthen the healing process. They felt goodwill and respect toward conventional medicine and desired greater integration of traditional and complementary health care. They expressed concern about the accessibility of CAM and stressed that attitudes and beliefs were often larger impediments to integration than were economic or scientific considerations.

---

1. What similarities exist among these study findings?

2. Identify the different points of view. How will these attitudes affect the integration of conventional and CAM therapies?

 Go to Chapter 40, **Toward Evidence-Based Practice Suggested Responses,** on the Electronic Study Guide.

---

of urine and stool are important. A major part of a diagnostic workup is the taking of pulses. TCM practitioners identify a large number of pulses and will almost certainly take three pulses (shallow, medium, and deep) at three points on each wrist. After observing, asking questions, listening, and feeling the pulses, they will put this information together and determine your balance of yin and yang, of the five elements, and of the *qi* (sometimes written *chi*), or energy, flowing in your body. Finally, they will decide on the appropriate form of treatment. This will almost certainly involve lifestyle modifications and herbal remedies but may also involve acupuncture. Your prescription, taken to a Chinese herbal pharmacy, will be prescribed as weights of a variety of dried herbs. These will be combined, and you will be asked to infuse and drink them as a tea.

Patients of diverse cultural backgrounds use TCM. Be sure to ask patients whether they are using any herbs or TCM products, because they may interact with other prescribed therapies.

Acupuncture

Acupuncture is the penetration of the skin with thin metallic needles (Figure 40–3) to stimulate anatomical structures of the body. Acupuncture was derived from TCM; however, some practitioners also use teachings from Japanese, Korean, and other medical systems. As a result, it deserves particular attention.

Energy, or *qi,* is believed to travel through the body along channels, known as *meridians.* A total of 72 meridians traverse the body (Figure 40–4). Points along these meridians, known as *acupoints,* are centers

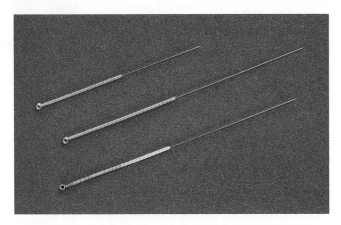

FIGURE 40–3 Acupuncture uses thin metallic needles to stimulate acupoints to restore the flow of *qi*.

of nerve and vascular tissue. The acupuncturist selects acupoints based on examination of the patient's pulses, appearance, tongue color, odors, and complaints. Stimulation of these points restores the flow of *qi* along the meridians.

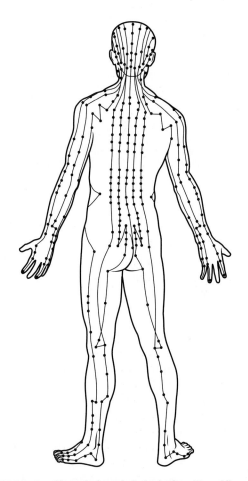

FIGURE 40–4 Qi travels through the body along 72 meridians. Acupuncture stimulates points along these meridians to restore health.

An NIH Consensus Report concluded that acupuncture triggers the release of opioids and other peptides in the central nervous system (CNS) and periphery, activates the hypothalamus and pituitary gland, produces changes in the secretion of neurotransmitters and neurohormones, alters immune function, and changes blood flow. The report concludes there is "sufficient evidence of acupuncture's value to expand its use into conventional medicine and to encourage further studies of its physiology and clinical value" (NIH, 1997, p. 6). Although some people choose acupuncture and TCM in lieu of traditional health care, there is a growing trend toward using them in conjunction.

Homeopathy

Homeopathy was developed in the 5th century B.C.E. by Hippocrates, the famous Greek physician. In the late 18th century Dr. Samuel Hahnemann rediscovered this effective, natural form of medicine. Homeopathy is based on an understanding of how the body heals itself and an acceptance that all symptoms represent the body's attempt to restore itself to health. The practice of homeopathy is based on the following three principles:

1. *The law of similars,* or "like cures like." The substance that would cause the patient's symptoms in a healthy person is the substance that is most likely to produce a curative response in the patient who already has the symptoms.
2. *The law of minimum dose.* Hahnemann developed his theory as a result of his own experience with the malaria treatment quinine, which in large doses causes symptoms of the disease in healthy individuals. He reasoned that if large doses can simulate disease, minute doses would stimulate the body's defenses against that disease, resulting in a cure. The smallest dose possible is used to limit side effects. Medicines are prepared by repeatedly diluting them in water or alcohol and mixing by succussion, a form of vigorous shaking. Hahnemann hypothesized that vigorous shaking potentiated the remedy's healing effect. Recent discoveries in quantum physics about the transfer of energy at the subatomic level appear to support the idea that succussion increases the energy of particles.
3. *The single remedy.* This principle guides the homeopathic practitioner to select one remedy that encompasses the totality of the person's symptoms and constitutional characteristics. Thus a homeopathic medication is person-specific rather than disease-specific.

Homeopathic treatments are readily available. One of the most frequently used treatments is Rescue

Remedy—a treatment derived from flower essences. It is believed to help alleviate stress.

Naturopathy

Naturopathic medicine is based on the healing power of nature. Health is the outcome of understanding nature and allowing the body to heal itself. Diseases and aging result from ignoring the laws of nature. The principle belief behind naturopathy is that nature and each living being have the innate ability to establish, maintain, and restore health. Naturopathic practitioners support the healing ability of nature through nutrition and lifestyle counseling, dietary supplements, medicinal plants, and exercise.

KnowledgeCheck 40–4

Which of the alternative systems of medical practice:

- Is based on the philosophy of restoring balance?
- Involves stimulation of points along meridians to restore *qi* flow?
- Involves medications given in minute doses?

 Go to Chapter 40, **Knowledge Check Response Sheet and Answers,** on the Electronic Study Guide.

Mind-Body Interventions

Think back to the last time you experienced heartbreak—perhaps it resulted from the end of a relationship, the death of a loved one, or the realization that you cannot achieve something you aspired to. What kind of physical sensation did you experience? Most people report feeling physically exhausted, with tremors or even a painful feeling in the chest. This is an example of an emotion generating a physical sensation. Mind-body therapies are based on awareness of the unity of the mind and body and on the ability of social, familial, and economic factors to affect all aspects of health and illness. Its interventions target the patient's mood and reaction to stress to enhance health. Several widely known practices are discussed below.

Prayer

Prayer, a dialogue with a spiritual being, is the most commonly used CAM modality. Prayer exists in all religions and forms of spirituality and may take the form of recited prose, meditation, or personal requests. Prayer may be a personal request or a request on behalf of another. In a recent study (McCaffrey, Eisenberg, Legedza, Davis, & Phillips, 2004), researchers found that 35% of respondents used prayer for health concerns. Approximately 75% prayed for wellness, but 22% prayed about specific medical conditions. Individuals over the age of 33 and those with chronic health concerns were more likely to pray. Although prayer resulted in a high degree of satisfaction, only 11% of the participants informed their primary care provider of their use of prayer. Chapter 14 further discusses prayer and provides examples of prayers across many faiths.

Meditation

Meditation encompasses practices that help to quiet and focus the mind. There are two major forms of meditation: concentration meditation and mindfulness meditation. The two types are distinguished by their relationship to the object of meditation. In *concentration meditation*, the focus is on the breath, a sound *(mantra),* or an object (e.g., a flower). *Mindfulness meditation* involves directing attention to thoughts, feelings, and sensations—opening up to all stimuli.

People who meditate report that they feel calmer, more focused, and more relaxed. Health benefits of meditation include lowered blood pressure and metabolic changes that correlate with reduction in the effects of stress. Research demonstrates positive effects on various disease states, for example, diabetes, asthma, fibromyalgia, premenstrual syndrome, Crohn's disease, psoriasis, cancer, and chronic pain (Bright, 2002). As little as 20 minutes per day of meditation can have positive effects on health. Meditation can be practiced alone or with a group. Teaching and guidance from an experienced meditation teacher helps establish effective practice.

Meditation is often incorporated into other healing systems, such as ayurveda and yoga. Hospitalized patients may find that meditation helps control stress and promote relaxation. To facilitate meditation, assist patients to a comfortable position, and create a quiet pleasant environment free of interruptions.

Imagery

Imagery, also known as *visualization,* uses the imagination to create an event or scenario that is desired. A successful visualization incorporates all the senses. Imagery has been successfully used to reduce pain, increase healing of joint injuries, enhance immune system function, reduce asthma symptoms, enhance breast milk production, decrease anxiety, and improve outlook among patients with chronic illness (Bright, 2002). The consistent use of imagery has also been shown to improve the performance of athletes.

As a nurse, you can use imagery to enhance your own energy state and performance. Visualizing yourself providing good care may increase your confidence and reduce stress. You may also use imagery with patients. For example, if you are caring for a patient experiencing pain and anxiety, ask the patient to imagine lying comfortably in the sun in a restful meadow. Successful visualization includes imagining sights,

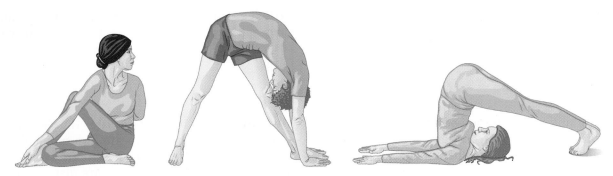

FIGURE 40–5   Yoga is designed to integrate body, mind, and spirit through the use of postures, or asanas, that increase flexibility, strength, body alignment, stamina, balance, and concentration.

sounds, tastes, and feelings of warmth and comfort. Often this imagery allows patients to relax and sleep. You may offer suggestions to patients or recommend guided visualization tapes.

Humor

Reading and telling jokes, viewing funny movies, and simply appreciating the humor of situations all help release tension and increase coping abilities (Phipps, 2002; Johnson, 2002). Laughter releases endorphins and relieves feelings of stress (Cousins, 1979). Laughter stimulates increases in pulse, respirations, muscle tension, and oxygenation; relaxation follows laughter.

Yoga

Yoga is a 5000-year-old traditional art, science, and philosophy that emphasizes a lifestyle of awareness, integrity, and compassion. Though many people practice yoga as exercise, yoga is designed to integrate body, mind, and spirit. Popular images of yoga focus on postures, or *asanas,* that increase flexibility, strength, body alignment, stamina, balance, and concentration (Figure 40–5). But the *asanas* are part of a practice intended to regulate the life force (called *prana* in the Hindu language) through breathing, meditation, reading sacred scriptures, and participating in a community of students who seek the teaching of yogi masters. As a result, many people classify yoga as an alternative medical system. The ultimate goal of yoga is to awaken the spiritual identity and experience happiness. A person of any age may practice yoga individually or as part of a group.

Hypnosis

Hypnosis is a trance-like state characterized by relaxed brain waves, hyper-suggestibility, and heightened imagination. A hypnotist may induce the state, or people can learn self-hypnosis. Hypnosis has been used to promote relaxation, weight loss, and smoking cessation and to suppress various symptoms (e.g., anx-

iety, pain). It has been used to modify pain in childbirth and as an adjunct to, or in place of, anesthesia for surgery. Hypnosis is widely used in traditional psychiatric care, but it is still not completely accepted.

Biofeedback

Biofeedback is a technique by which some people can learn voluntary control over typically involuntary activities, such as heart rate. Biofeedback techniques use electronic instruments to measure neuromuscular and autonomic nervous system activity. Visual or auditory cues provide information in the form of sound or light. For example, as the heart rate slows, the feedback sound might become quieter. Immediate feedback helps the person become aware of and learn how to voluntarily control certain physiological responses, such as those produced by stress. We do not understand how people use the feedback to learn control, but in general it teaches them to achieve a state of relaxation in which the parasympathetic nervous system dominates. Some traditional medical practitioners have been using biofeedback for many years. However, it is not completely accepted. Biofeedback practitioners require special training, and most are credentialed.

CriticalThinking 40–4
- Do you believe yoga is a mind-body intervention or an alternative system of health care?
- Which, if any of the alternative health systems or mind-body interventions would you be most comfortable facilitating for a patient?

Biologically Based Therapies

Biologically based therapies use substances found in nature, such as food, herbs, vitamins, and aromatherapy. These therapies are readily available and are often practiced as self-care measures and in conjunction with traditional health care and other CAM.

TABLE 40-1 The Pros and Cons of Herbs

Issue	Pro	Con
Safety	Many herbs are relatively safe.	Herbal products are not regulated (e.g., by the U. S. Food and Drug Administration), so their safety cannot be guaranteed.
Effectiveness	Numerous pharmaceuticals have been derived from herbs (e.g., aspirin, digoxin, morphine).	Unregulated products may claim benefits they do not offer.
Cost	Herbs are often readily available at health food stores.	Inappropriate use of herbs may actually increase healthcare costs if they prove to be ineffective or harmful.
Convenience	Readily available without a prescription.	May discourage clients from seeking care from a practitioner when they truly need it.
Privacy concerns	Allows clients to privately treat concerns.	May discourage clients from seeking care when they truly need it.

Dietary Therapies

Dietary therapies are used in traditional health care as well as with CAM. For example, a low-sodium diet is part of the treatment plan for patients with hypertension. Dietary modifications may also be part of treatment in alternative health systems. For example, in ayurvedic medicine, a patient with a *pitta dosha* is represented by the element of fire. Foods that are cool in nature are recommended to balance the fiery nature. Traditional Chinese medicine also uses diet to treat disease. In TCM, illness results when there is an excess of wind, cold, fire, summer heat, dampness, or dryness. Foods that have opposite qualities are used to counteract these excesses.

Naturopathy stresses the importance of pure food (unprocessed), recommending generous servings of raw food to prevent disease and aging. Mainstream research has repeatedly demonstrated that as foods have become more processed, the incidence of chronic disease has increased. This is an example of a CAM approach that has been incorporated into traditional health care.

Herbs

Herbal preparations have existed since the beginning of time. In fact, many prescription medications in use today are derived from herbs. Herbal products are often viewed as "natural" and, therefore, are sought out by people who wish to avoid exposure to chemicals. Table 40–1 presents some of the pros and cons associated with herb use. The National Center for Complementary and Alternative Medicine (NCCAM) offers extensive material on herbal products for healthcare consumers and professionals.

Herbal therapy is undergoing intense scrutiny in many countries. Because most herbs contain several components, it is difficult to study their pharmacology. In addition, herbs may change based on the soil and weather conditions in which they grow. In Germany, a health commission has reviewed the safety and efficacy of many herbs and created a monograph detailing their findings (German Federal Institute for Drugs and Medical Devices, 1998). The United States Food and Drug Administration (FDA) has also begun to investigate how to study and regulate herbal products.

Because herbal products are readily available and widely used, you need to question your patients about their use. Many herbs are known to interact with medications and to adversely affect some disease processes (e.g., to aggravate hypertension).

Vitamins

Vitamin therapy is widely used. In fact, many people consider it a nutritional "insurance policy." Vitamin therapy ranges from taking a daily multivitamin to a full megavitamin regimen. Vitamin therapy receives mixed reviews. For example, there is widespread use of antioxidants (beta-carotene, vitamin C, and vitamin E) to limit heart disease and cancer. However, *chelation therapy,* a megavitamin therapy that claims to reverse the effects of atherosclerosis and aging, has been classified as one of the top ten health frauds (American Heart Association, 2004; Ernst, 2000). This is an area of active research, so you can anticipate learning of new studies on a regular basis.

BOX 40-1 Common Aromatherapy Treatments

- *Basil:* Used to improve concentration, aid digestion, and relieve stress.
- *Eucalyptus:* Protects against respiratory problems, such as coughs, colds, and asthma; believed to boost the immune system and relieve muscle tension.
- *Ylang ylang:* Used to induce relaxation and reduce muscle tension.
- *Geranium:* Used to balance hormones in women and improve skin clarity. Can be both relaxing and uplifting.
- *Peppermint:* Extremely effective in treating digestive disorders, such as flatulence, nausea, and heartburn. A natural painkiller, peppermint can help treat headaches and general muscular aches. It also helps relieve morning sickness.
- *Lavender:* Used to induce relaxation and for superficial wounds, burns, and skin care.
- *Lemon:* An excellent essential oil for treating oily skin, acne, sluggish circulation, and digestive disorders. It is emotionally uplifting, with a zingy, fresh scent. It is used to treat insomnia and nightmares. It is a diuretic and can be used in a spray as a disinfectant.
- *Clary sage:* A balancing oil that can lift depression. It is calming, restores tranquility, and can lower blood pressure.
- *Tea tree:* Used to treat fungal infections and clear the skin.
- *Chamomile:* Used to induce relaxation, reduce muscle tension, and promote sleep.
- *Rosemary:* Used for mental stimulation and stimulation of the digestive and immune systems.

Aromatherapy

Aromatherapy is the use of essential oils, which are concentrated extracts of roots, leaves, or blossoms, to enhance physical and mental well-being. It is one of the fastest growing CAM therapies. Essential oils are most often used with touch therapy and massage. Researchers believe that the scent of essential oils activates the amygdala and hippocampus, the storage site for emotions and memories (Buckle, 2002). Fontaine (2000) states that aromatherapy may be used for stress reduction, mood regulation, sleep enhancement, immune support, first aid, enhanced energy, reduction of pain, and accelerated wound recovery. Research is currently underway at several major universities on the effects of essential oils on inflammation, infection, depression, and dementia, as well

as for alleviating side effects resulting from radiation treatment. Box 40–1 describes a number of commonly used aromatherapies.

KnowledgeCheck 40-5
- Compare and contrast mind-body and biologically based therapies.
- Identify at least four CAM interventions or therapies that could be easily practiced by a patient confined to bed.

 Go to Chapter 40, **Knowledge Check Response Sheet and Answers,** on the Electronic Study Guide.

Manipulative and Body-Based Methods

Manipulative and body-based therapies focus on manipulating and moving the body to improve health. Several types of therapies are widely practiced. We discuss the most common therapies below.

Chiropractic

Chiropractic focuses on the relationship between the structure and the function of the human body. The premise of chiropractic is that disease is caused by irritation of the nervous system. A total of 31 pairs of spinal nerves branch off the spinal cord to innervate all the organs in the body. *Subluxation* (loss of proper position or motion in a joint) of the vertebrae impinges on these nerves and leads to disease. Manipulation of body structures, especially the spinal column, realigns the vertebrae to allow nerve impulses to flow without interruption, thereby improving health. Realignment is referred to as an *adjustment.*

Chiropractors use health history, x-ray studies, and examination of the spine and posture to make a diagnosis. They treat primarily by performing adjustments; however, they may also use ice, heat, ultrasound, electrical stimulation, herbs, and nutritional supplements.

Massage

Massage involves the manipulation of muscles and other soft tissues. It is one of the oldest forms of healing. Massage works to relieve pain in a number of ways: by promoting muscle relaxation, by increasing lymphatic circulation and thereby reducing inflammation, by breaking up scar tissue and adhesions, by promoting blood flow through the muscles, and by promoting drainage of sinus fluids (Bright, 2002).

Swedish massage is used to induce relaxation and restore flexibility. It consists of five basic strokes: *effleurage* (touching lightly, with a gliding long stroke), *petrissage* (kneading for intensive work in small areas), *tapotement* (tapping with the fingertips), *vibration* (shaking), and *friction* (rubbing).

Sports massage is a specialized form of Swedish massage that facilitates maximum physical performance. Pressure, movement, and cross-fiber massage in a vigorous manner are used to warm up athletes before events, to relieve soreness after exertion, and to help repair athletic injuries.

Myofascial release restores balance, alignment, and mobility to the body by releasing tension in the soft connective fasciae through trigger point release, strumming, and muscle stretching. The therapist applies pressure and stretching to the edge of the client's tolerance level. Myofascial release may produce more long-lasting effects than other forms of massage because fasciae surround, support, and interweave every muscle, organ, and bone in the body.

Shiatsu massage is a finger-pressure method that balances the energy force in the body. The therapist applies pressure to specific points that lie along energy meridians, the same meridian points used in acupuncture. Meridian points are thought to be areas of energy concentration that influence organ and neuromuscular functioning.

Reflexology is a massage technique that promotes unblocking a terminal nerve to improve function along that nerve pathway. Nerve endings on the hands and feet have been identified that relate to every structure of the body. Research demonstrates that manipulating the reflex zones stimulates the same energy balancing that occurs when acupuncture points are used (Burton Goldberg Group, 1994).

Although massage is relaxing, it is not advisable for everyone. People with a history of phlebitis or vascular disorders should not receive deep muscle massage. As a nurse, you can provide simple massage (e.g., a back rub), but complex forms of massage require special training to perform. Massage therapists are licensed or credentialed in many states.

Osteopathy

Osteopathy is a manipulative modality that has been in existence for more than a century. Because osteopaths (DOs) are granted the same privileges as MDs, they may be considered part of the traditional healthcare system. In fact, many function as mainstream providers. However, their training includes osteopathic manipulation, a method of diagnosis and treatment focused on normalizing joint function, eliminating strains, and facilitating the function of the primary respiratory mechanisms.

Energy Therapies

Energy therapies involve the use of energy fields. Biofield therapies affect energy that surrounds and penetrates the body. Examples include therapeutic touch, Reiki, and Qigong. Bioelectromagnetic therapies involve the use of electromagnetic fields for healing purposes. They are among the most widely used forms of CAM.

Therapeutic Touch

Therapeutic touch (TT) uses the hands on or near the body to provide comfort, pain relief, and healing. The premise of TT is that human beings consist of energy fields that penetrate the body and extend 5 to 15 cm (2 to 6 inches) beyond the physical structure. In health, energy flows freely through the system in a balanced manner. But in illness or pain, the free flow of energy is disrupted. TT practitioners are able to repattern the energy field to produce a more healthful state. TT was co-developed by Delores Kreiger, RN, PhD, and Dora Kunz, a medical intuitive. It is now taught in 60 countries and practiced by over 70,000 nurses worldwide (Bright, 2002).

TT has been the subject of scientific inquiry for more than 25 years. Research has demonstrated a variety of beneficial effects, including decreased anxiety, reduced pain, accelerated healing, enhanced immune functioning, reduced agitation among dementia patients, and enhanced well-being. Many of these studies are available for review.

 Go to the **Nurse Healers–Professional Associates International (NH–PAI)** web site at www.therapeutic-touch.org

TT is noninvasive and can be used as primary or adjunctive treatment in many settings, with clients of any age, and for a variety of conditions. Box 40–2 briefly describes how therapeutic touch is practiced.

T'ai Chi and Qigong

T'ai chi and qigong are ancient Chinese practices that enhance health in many ways. T'ai chi (Figure 40–6) is a nonaggressive martial art, and qigong is a series of movements, breathing, and meditation. Both modalities develop body strength and flexibility, improve balance, increase physical stamina, and enhance mental alertness and muscular control.

There are many styles of t'ai chi and qigong. However, each strives to balance energy and cultivate the life force, known as *qi,* or *chi. Chi* cultivation involves relaxing the body, regulating or controlling breathing, and calming the mind. T'ai chi and qigong facilitate energy flow through the meridian system so that *qi* can be strong and balanced to support health. Consistent practice over time is said to have the most benefit. Because t'ai chi and qigong are gentle, they may be practiced throughout the life span.

Reiki

Reiki is an energy therapy that seeks to balance energy. Like TT, it involves the laying on of hands;

BOX 40-2   Therapeutic Touch

Centering

To practice TT, you must establish and maintain a state of conscious awareness that fosters sensitivity to energy field phenomena. This state of awareness is developed by a meditative practice that TT practitioners call "centering"—a quiet focused state. Being centered fosters sensitivity to your own energy as well as that of the patient's. Centering is simple and easy to learn and has an immediate calming affect. Do the following:

- Sit in a quiet, comfortable place. Close your eyes, and breathe deeply in and out.
- Allow your muscles to relax.
- Concentrate on your breathing. Visualize taking in energy with each inspiration and releasing tension with each exhalation.
- Focus on your breath, and allow outside stimuli and thoughts to pass.
- Now turn your attention to your professional role while concentrating on your breathing.
- Approach your client with renewed focus and calm.

Using Therapeutic Touch

Once you have centered, healing occurs by:

- Using your hands near the body surface to assess the patient's energy field. This is done by detecting the forces emanating from the patient.
- Unruffling (smoothing) the field by sweeping away stagnant energy in sweeping motions toward the periphery.
- Repatterning the field by transferring energy from the practitioner to the patient.

Source: Adapted from Bright, M. A. (2002). *Holistic health and healing.* Philadelphia: F. A. Davis Company.

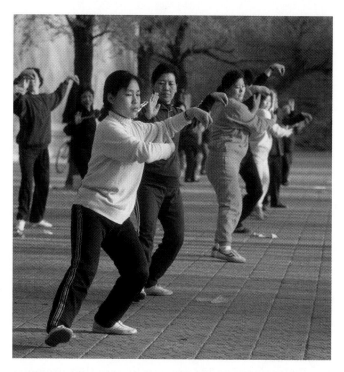

FIGURE 40–6 T'ai chi strives to balance energy and cultivate the life force.

Magnet Therapy

Magnet therapy uses the property of magnetism to treat a variety of human conditions. The most widely claimed effect is improvement in musculoskeletal pain for patients with injury or arthritis. Magnet therapy operates on the premise that the iron in hemoglobin is attracted to a magnet placed on the skin. Application of a magnet to an injured or fatigued area increases blood flow, which aids in healing. Studies on the efficacy of magnet therapy show mixed findings. Many magnet products (e.g., mattresses, arm wraps) are available without prescription and without the need to consult a healer.

KnowledgeCheck 40–6

Compare and contrast manipulative and body-based methods with energy therapies. How are they similar? How are they different?

 Go to Chapter 40, **Knowledge Check Response Sheet and Answers,** on the Electronic Study Guide.

CriticalThinking 40–5

Which, if any, of the therapies previously discussed would be appropriate for use with Mrs. Riddell ("Meet Your Patient")? Do you believe that TT would be helpful for this patient? Explain your answers.

however, in Reiki, the patient draws the needed energy from the hands of the practitioner rather than the practitioner imparting energy. Most Reiki treatments do not involve actually touching; instead, the hands are positioned a few inches away from the body. Reiki is administered by practitioners who have undergone an initiation process in which the Reiki master employs ancient sounds and symbols to attune the nervous system to a higher level of energy. Practitioners pass through three levels of attunement. With each level change, the ability to heal improves.

Practical Knowledge
knowing how

You may be wondering, "What do all these exotic therapies have to do with *me*? I certainly don't have time to get a massage therapy license or learn t'ai chi." Actually, there are three very practical applications to your practice.

1. You can, and should, facilitate communication about CAM between your patients and their healthcare providers.
2. You can use self-care practices to promote your own health and wholeness.
3. You can, with minimal training, use some of the less complex CAM therapies as independent nursing interventions.

We will address these applications briefly in this section.

| Assessment |

To make a holistic assessment, inquire about CAMs the patient may be using when conducting a nursing history.

- When taking a medication history, add questions such as, "What nonprescription medications do you take? What natural or herbal remedies do you use? What nutritional supplements, vitamins, and minerals do you use?" Explain to the patient that some remedies might interact with prescribed medications or treatments.
- Ask the patient, "How do you usually take care of yourself at home when you are ill?" This will help you to obtain information about self-prescribed modalities.
- Ask the patient, "Many people see more than one kind of doctor or healer. Other than Dr. Jones [the traditional medical doctor], who do you go to for advice and healing when you are ill?"

Above all, be neutral, accepting, and nonjudgmental in your interview. Patients may suspect that traditional caregivers will not approve of their alternative practices, so they must feel safe with you if they are to share information freely.

| Nursing Diagnosis |

The NANDA taxonomy includes physical, cognitive, emotional, spiritual, individual, family, and community diagnoses. So taken as a whole, the NANDA *set* of diagnoses is holistic. However, the only diagnosis that might be interpreted specifically as an alternative diagnosis is Disturbed Energy Field. Disturbed Energy Field is defined as "disruption of the flow of energy surrounding a person's being that results in disharmony of the body, mind, and/or spirit" (NANDA, 2005, p. 63).

You need not fear that labeling a problem makes you less holistic. All CAM practitioners identify the patient's condition or status so that they can determine what treatment is needed. For example:

- An ayurvedic practitioner might diagnose an imbalance in the *dosha*.
- A TCM practitioner might diagnose an imbalance of emotion, or too much wind.
- A nurse might diagnose Chronic Pain before prescribing imagery.

It is your attitude, approach, and interventions that make you a holistic nurse, not the words you use to describe your patient's problem.

| Planning Outcomes/Evaluation |

Patient outcomes are those which, when achieved, demonstrate resolution of the identified problem, regardless of whether you use traditional interventions or CAM. For example if you diagnose Acute Pain, the NOC outcome would be Pain Level, regardless of whether you treat the pain with narcotics or with imagery. One example of a holistic *individualized goal/outcome statement* is as follows:

Freely shares information about folk practices and over-the-counter medications with the primary care provider.

NOC standardized outcomes for Disturbed Energy Field might include Personal Health Status, Personal Well-Being, and Spiritual Health.

| Planning Interventions/Implementaton |

NIC standardized interventions and activities that you may implement in the clinical setting include the following:

- Autogenic Training
- Calming Technique
- Humor
- Meditation Facilitation
- Simple Guided Imagery
- Simple Massage
- Simple Relaxation Therapy
- Therapeutic Touch

For descriptions and use of each of these techniques,

VOL 2 Go to Chapter 40, **Techniques 40–1 to 40–8,** in Volume 2.

Additional *NIC standardized interventions and activities* include the following:

- *Aromatherapy* is the "administration of essential oils through massage, topical ointments or lotions, baths, inhalation, douches, or compresses (hot or cold) to calm and soothe, provide pain relief, enhance relaxation and comfort" (Dochterman & Bulechek, 2004, p. 171). You should have some education and training in the philosophy and use of essential oils. Assess for discomfort and nausea and obtain baseline vital signs before and after the treatment. Then monitor for contact dermatitis and exacerbation of asthma, as appropriate.

- *Biofeedback* requires special training. Once the patient has been taught about it, you can assist the patient to use instrumentation she has previously been instructed on.

- *Hypnosis* is defined by NIC (Dochterman & Bulechek, 2004, p. 426) as "assisting a patient to induce an altered state of consciousness to create an acute awareness and a directed focus experience." You will need advanced training to perform hypnosis. However, you can give your patient information about hypnosis.

As with all interventions, you must obtain consent from your patient to use CAM and evaluate and document the patient's physiological and psychological responses. There are other (non-NIC) interventions you can perform independently:

- *Self-care practices for nurse.* As you have learned, the vitality and health of the healer is a powerful force in the healing process. Holistic healing interventions are more effective when the healer is whole. Maintain your physical health by wise lifestyle choices, manage your stress, and develop a support network of colleagues, family, and friends. Take satisfaction in your work, but balance it with a healthy personal life.

- *Music therapy* can be used to induce relaxation. Music can have a healing effect on the body, mind, and spirit. You will need some advanced knowledge of music therapy to use it to its fullest, but even now, you can suggest that patients listen to music, and you can help them obtain the type of music they prefer.

- *Pet therapy* has been used extensively in long-term care and is just beginning to be used in other settings. Pets induce a feeling of relaxation.

- *Evaluating credibility of information sources and providers.* Be sure patients are aware that not all practitioners who provide CAM therapy are equally qualified to do so. They should examine credentials and ask for referrals. The same is true of books and information taken from web sites. For suggestions on how to evaluate CAM information,

 Go to the **National Center for Complementary and Alternative Medicine** web site at http://nccam.nih.gov/health/webresources/

 Go to Chapter 40, **Resources for Caregivers and Health Professionals,** on the Electronic Study Guide.

 Suggested Readings: Go to Chapter 40, **Reading More About Holistic Healing,** on the Electronic Study Guide.

 Bibliography: Go to Volume 2, Bibliography.

Promoting Health

Learning Outcomes

After completing this chapter, you should be able to:

* Define *health, health promotion,* and *health protection.*

* Identify health prevention activities and categorize them as primary, secondary, or tertiary levels of prevention.

* Discuss the Healthy People 2010 report in relation to leading causes of death and to health promotion strategies: nutrition, exercise, lifestyles, and environment.

* Apply Pender's Health Promotion Model to plan activities designed to change unhealthy behavior.

* Identify Prochaska and DiClemente's four stages of change.

* Identify specific health promotion strategies (including immunizations and screenings) across the life span.

* Discuss nurses' roles in health promotion, and list health promotion activities that a nurse may conduct in acute care facilities, in the workplace, in local communities, and schools.

* Identify the areas of assessment in relation to developing a health promotion plan.

* Assess a client's cardiorespiratory function, muscle strength and endurance, joint flexibility, and nutrition (body mass index or body fat percentage).

* Construct a health promotion plan of care using the nursing process, NANDA taxonomy, Nursing Outcomes Classifications, and Nursing Interventions Classifications.

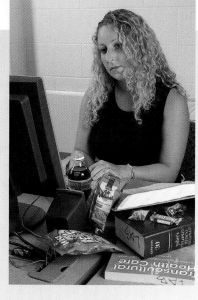

MEET Your Patient

You have completed all your prerequisites and are now enrolled in your first nursing course. Aside from classroom work, you have a skills course and clinical rotation. You spend a lot of time reading, studying, preparing for clinical work, writing care plans, and completing follow-up assignments from your clinical rotation. You have other non-nursing course work and family responsibilities, as well. Often, you stay up late and get up early. By the end of the week, you're exhausted. You eat fast food several times a week. You know it's not the healthiest choice, but you pass the place each day on your way to school. At least this way you can get something to eat. You have little time to exercise, and when you do have time, you feel too tired.

You spend most of your time learning about health and illness. Given your current lifestyle, do you consider yourself healthy? How did you make that decision? Your answer is based on your personal beliefs about health and what you have learned in your nursing course work. In this chapter we explore health promotion. As you learn more about this topic, you may develop a plan to promote your own health as well as the health of clients.

Theoretical Knowledge
knowing why

In Chapter 10 we explored the meaning of health, wellness, and illness. In this chapter, the emphasis is on exploring strategies to promote health and prevent disease. To begin, we explore what others have written about the concepts. Various descriptions and definitions use the terms *health* and *wellness* interchangeably, and we do the same in this chapter.

WHAT IS HEALTH PROMOTION?

To promote health, we must first identify what we mean by *health* and *wellness*. The World Health Organization (WHO) defines health as "a state of complete physical, mental and social well-being and not merely the absence of disease or infirmity" (WHO, 1948). Other professionals have also reflected on the meaning of health.

Nursing theorist Jean Watson (1979) proposes that health consists of three elements: (1) a high level of overall physical, mental, and social functioning; (2) a general adaptive-maintenance level of daily functioning; and (3) the absence of illness (or the presence of efforts that lead to its absence). She also refers to health as being a state of mind, the perception of the individual person. A person may have a terminal illness and yet consider himself healthy.

Another nursing theorist, Betty Neuman (1995), views health as an expression of living energy available to an individual. The energy is displayed as a continuum with high energy (wellness) at one end and low energy (illness) at the opposite end. The individual is said to have varying levels of energy at various stages of life. When more energy is generated than expended, there is wellness. When more energy is expended than is generated, there is illness, possibly death.

Myers, Sweeney, and Witmer (2000) define wellness as "a way of life oriented toward optimal health and well-being in which body, mind, and spirit are integrated by the individual to live more fully within the human and natural community" (p. 252). This definition includes lifestyles and habits as components of health and permits people who have been diagnosed with disease to be considered healthy.

Applying aspects of these reflections on health, **health promotion** means finding ways to help individuals develop a state of physical, spiritual, and mental well-being. Health promotion activities are useful to all individuals, whether well or sick, because they encourage optimal function.

Health Promotion versus Health Protection

On the surface, it appears that activities that promote health also protect health, and, for the most part, that

is true. Nevertheless, the ideas behind health promotion and health protection differ subtly but significantly. Pender, Murdaugh, and Parsons (2002) explain that the motivation behind the two activities distinguishes them. Health promotion is motivated by the desire to increase well-being, whereas health protection is motivated by a desire to avoid illness. Health promotion is related to individual lifestyle and involves making choices that affect one's health prospects. In contrast, health protection is directed at preventing illness. The 40-year-old who begins an exercise program to improve strength and endurance is motivated by the benefits of health promotion. But if he starts exercising because his father died of a heart attack at age 50, he may be motivated to protect his health.

Levels of Prevention

Leavell and Clark (1965) identified three levels of activities for health protection (illness prevention): primary, secondary, and tertiary. Interventions are classified according to the point in the disease process at which they occur. This timing directs the types of interventions needed.

- *Primary prevention* activities are designed to prevent or slow the onset of disease. Activities such as eating healthy foods, exercising, wearing sunscreen, obeying seat belt laws, and immunizations are examples of primary level interventions.
- *Secondary prevention* involves screening activities and education for detecting illnesses in the early stages. Health activities such as breast self-examination, testicular exams, regular physical examinations, blood pressure and diabetes screenings, and tuberculosis skin tests are examples of secondary interventions.
- *Tertiary prevention* focuses on stopping the disease from progressing and returning the individual to the pre-illness phase. Rehabilitation is the main intervention during this level.

Patients and health providers move among these levels of prevention. For example, a patient hospitalized for a total hip replacement would receive tertiary prevention—care focused on helping her recover from surgery, preventing complications of surgery, and, later on, helping her regain her strength and learn to walk again. Secondary prevention strategies may have been used previously, for example, to screen for osteoporosis (which leads to bone fragility and fractures). When she goes home, if she decides to limit her salt intake and eat a balanced diet, these activities would be primary prevention strategies.

Healthy People 2010

In 1994, McGinnis and Foege published a shocking report on the impact of an unhealthy lifestyle. They concluded that 54% of the years of life lost before age 65 was attributable to unhealthy lifestyles. An additional 22% was related to environmental factors, and a mere 16% was related to heredity.

Preliminary data for the leading causes of death for 2001 identify seven causes of death that can be linked to lifestyle issues of diet, exercise, smoking, immunizations, and substance abuse. For instance, costs of healthcare related to cigarette smoking increased by about $1.5 million annually in the United States during the years from 1995 through 1999 (Centers for Disease Control and Prevention [CDC], 2002). Imagine the total costs for all diseases affected by lifestyle. Imagine the savings if people altered their lifestyles to be more healthy.

Healthy People 2010 is a national initiative that addresses the effects of lifestyle by creating health improvement goals to reach by the year 2010. This is the third time that the U.S. Department of Health and Human Services (U.S. DHHS) has developed 10-year health objectives for the nation. The first document was released in 1979. Each plan incorporates new data and reflects progress achieved in the interim. Unfortunately, many lifestyle problems remain. The two overarching goals of the Healthy People 2010 initiative are to increase quality and years of healthy life and to eliminate health disparities. Interventions to achieve these goals are targeted at the 28 focus areas shown in Box 41–1. Public health agencies at the local, state, and federal levels use these focus areas as a blueprint to design programs aimed at improving the health status of the community.

KnowledgeCheck 41–1

- How does health promotion differ from health protection?
- Which level of prevention is represented by the following activities?

    mumps, measles, rubella (MMR) vaccination
    tuberculosis (TB) skin test
    physical therapy after repair of a hip fracture
- What is the purpose of the Healthy People 2010 initiative?

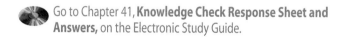 Go to Chapter 41, **Knowledge Check Response Sheet and Answers,** on the Electronic Study Guide.

Health Promotion Models

A model illustrates a system or framework to help explain what you see in the clinical arena. The most common frameworks used for designing health promotion programs are described next.

BOX 41-1 Focus Areas of Healthy People 2010

1. Access to quality health services
2. Arthritis, osteoporosis, and chronic back conditions
3. Cancer
4. Chronic kidney disease
5. Diabetes
6. Disability and secondary conditions
7. Educational and community-based programs
8. Environmental health
9. Family planning
10. Food safety
11. Health communication
12. Heart disease and stroke
13. HIV
14. Immunization and infectious diseases
15. Injury and violence prevention
16. Maternal, infant, and child health
17. Medical product safety
18. Mental health and mental disorders
19. Nutrition and overweight
20. Occupational safety and health
21. Oral health
22. Physical activity and fitness
23. Public health infrastructure
24. Respiratory diseases
25. Sexually transmitted diseases
26. Substance abuse
27. Tobacco use
28. Vision and hearing

Source: U.S. Department of Health and Human Services. (2000) *Healthy People 2010: Understanding and improving health* (2nd ed.). Washington, DC: U.S. Government Printing Office.

Pender's Health Promotion Model

Pender's Health Promotion Model (HPM) was introduced in the early 1980s and later revised (Figure 41–1). The model identifies three groups of variables that affect health promotion: (1) individual characteristics and experiences; (2) behavior-specific cognitions and affect; and (3) behavioral outcome. The HPM is based on seven assumptions that reflect both nursing and behavioral science perspectives (Pender, Murdaugh, & Parsons, 2002, p. 63):

1. Persons seek to create conditions of living through which they can express their unique human health potential.
2. Persons have the capacity for reflective self-awareness, including assessment of their own competencies.
3. Persons value growth in directions viewed as positive and attempt to achieve a personally acceptable balance between change and stability.
4. Individuals seek to actively regulate their own behavior.
5. Individuals in all their biopsychosocial complexity interact with the environment, progressively transforming the environment and being transformed over time.
6. Health professionals constitute a part of the interpersonal environment, which exerts influence on persons throughout their life span.
7. Self-initiated reconfiguration of person-environment interactive patterns is essential to behavior change.

Pender's model has been used extensively in research and professional practice focused on health promotion. As a nurse, you should find Pender's focus applicable to your work. Moreover, many professions have used her research and model.

 ### CriticalThinking 41–1

- How might peers influence health behaviors? At what age might peers have more influence?
- Apply Pender's model to a person trying to lose weight. What might be some perceived barriers (see Figure 41–1)?

Wheel of Wellness

Several authors have likened the different facets of health to the spokes of a wheel (Hettler, 1984; Witmer & Sweeney, 1982; Myers, Sweeney, & Witmer, 2000). If one of the spokes is weak, the whole wheel is weak. The "spokes" of the health wheel represent the dimensions of health: emotional, intellectual, physical, spiritual, social/family, and occupational (Figure 41–2). The level of wellness progresses from the center to the outer part of the wheel. The center represents the least amount of wellness, and the outer part represents optimal wellness. If one spoke on the wheel is not functioning at optimal level, the wheel will not roll properly. If one area of an individual's life is not functioning at optimal level, life will not be as fulfilling as it could be. As a nurse, you should assess each dimension for strengths and weaknesses.

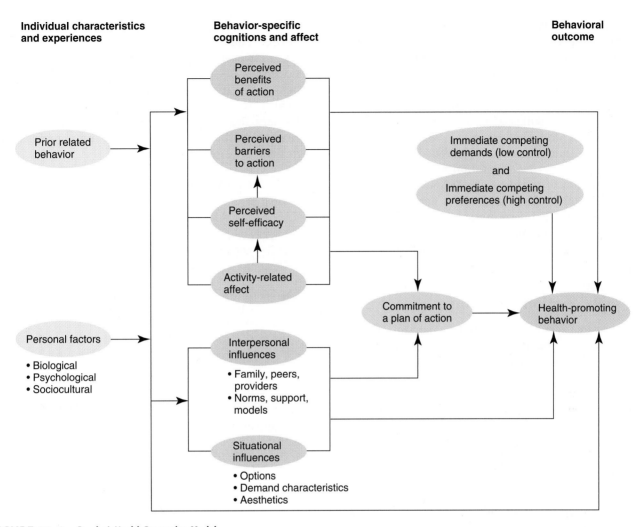

FIGURE 41–1 Pender's Health Promotion Model.

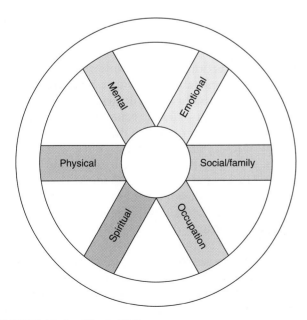

FIGURE 41–2 Wheel of Wellness.

Model of Change

The transtheoretical model of change (Prochaska & DiClemente, 1982) may serve as a means to alter unhealthy behaviors. Health promotion and protection involve either changing the individual's response to the illness-producing stimuli or changing the environment so that the person will be less likely to encounter illness-producing stimuli. Either idea involves change. In this model, change occurs in four stages:

1. *Contemplation* involves the decision-making process.
2. *Determination* is the stage in which the person makes a decision to change a behavior and prepares a plan.
3. *The action stage* is the implementation of the plan.
4. *The maintenance stage* allows the changed behavior to be reinforced.

Ideally the stages would progress in this order. Realistically, a person may progress and regress in any of the stages. The change process in persons with some unhealthy habits (e.g., cigarette smoking, substance

abuse, and unhealthy eating) may best be described as a revolving door. An individual may exit at any point from the revolving door. If the exit occurs during or at the end of the maintenance period, successful behavior change has occurred. If the exit occurs before the end of the maintenance period, relapse will occur, and the individual will return to the previous lifestyle.

Prochaska and DiClemente (1982) found additional stages that consistently preceded and followed the change. The *precontemplation stage* precedes the change and identifies those who are not aware of having a particular problem and so are not ready to contemplate change. The *termination stage* completes the maintenance. A person who enters the termination stage has changed the behavior and is not in danger of relapse.

Health Promotion Programs

Health promotion programs help a person advance toward optimal health. Below we discuss several types. For further discussion of individual activities that promote health,

 Go to Chapter 41, **Supplemental Materials: Individual Health Promotion Activities,** on the Electronic Study Guide.

• *Disseminating information.* To recognize a problem and understand their options for change, people need information. Information may be disseminated at the individual, group, or community level. For example, teaching a client about the Food Guide Pyramid is a form of disseminating information to an individual. Group-level programs include classes offered at the local hospital, prenatal education programs, and worksite programs. Community level health promotion programs are directed at the entire community. When you pass a billboard that presents the dangers of smoking, you are viewing a community-level health promotion program. Health columns in the newspaper and health fairs are other examples of ways to disseminate health information.

• *Programs for changing lifestyle and behavior.* These are group-level programs. They focus on such activities as weight loss, smoking cessation, exercise, nutrition, and stress management. These programs usually provide information and offer support. Many times they include a maintenance program to help solidify the change.

• *Environmental control programs. Environment* refers to air, water, and soil, as well as social and political surroundings. Environmental control programs promote health by working to create a healthy environment. Programs focus on air and water quality, toxic waste, healthy homes and communities, infrastructure and surveillance, global environmental health, and political advocacy.

• *Wellness assessment and health risk appraisal programs.* These programs focus on identifying behaviors that promote health and create risk for disease. A wellness assessment tends to focus on the healthy behaviors. It supports positive change to improve health. A health risk appraisal identifies risky behaviors that promote disease. These programs are readily available on the Internet, in magazines, and at fitness centers.

KnowledgeCheck 41–2

• What are the six dimensions of health represented by the spokes on the wellness wheel?
• Identify the stages of change identified by Prochaska and DiClemente.
• Describe the four main types of health promotion programs.

 Go to Chapter 41, **Knowledge Check Response Sheet and Answers,** on the Electronic Study Guide.

 ## CriticalThinking 41–2

J.T. has a mixed drink while eating lunch with his co-workers. He keeps a bottle of liquor in his office desk for sips during the day. Later, he stops at a local bar for a drink on the way home. At home, he has more drinks. What information do you need to determine which of Prochaska and DiClemente's stages of change he is experiencing? How would you get this information?

Settings for Health Promotion Programs

The most common sites for health promotion programs are health facilities, worksites, and schools. Healthcare settings, such as clinics, physician offices, or hospitals, are natural settings for health promotion because healthcare providers are in contact with clients. Each interaction is an opportunity for health promotion. Unfortunately, most interactions focus on the disease process and compliance with treatments (Engle & Kratt, 1999). You will need to make a conscious effort to help clients focus on behaviors that prevent illness and promote health.

Many nurses work in health clinics within large companies or may be contracted to provide specific programs. Programs may include smoking cessation, stress management, and fitness training (Brown, Weaver, Artz, & Hilyer, 1999). Employers have found that health programs decrease work-related injuries and sick leave. For instance, Appleton Papers, Incorporated, has an on-site wellness center aimed at reducing musculoskeletal injuries and illness. Staff at the center offer educational programs on topics such as ergonomics, low back injuries, breast cancer awareness, and child car seat safety. There is a fitness center for strength and endurance training. The goal is to decrease injuries, illness, and costs while increasing productivity (Halls & Rhodes, 2002).

One of the best settings for community health promotion is the local school district. Health teaching can begin at an early age, and nurses and teachers can regularly reinforce healthy behaviors and redirect unhealthy behaviors. Schools provide a setting that allows for continued exposure to information. Interventions may be directed at general health promotion issues, such as physical activity, or they may focus on specific health risks, such as tobacco use. Ideally, parents and families are included in the learning. School nurses work closely with teachers and parents to provide health promotion services in the schools.

Health Promotion Throughout the Life Span

Health promotion is a lifelong process that begins at conception. Table 41–1 describes the focus of health promotion programs at each developmental stage, as well the types of screenings recommended for each age group.

Practical Knowledge
knowing how

Pender, Murdaugh, and Parsons (2002) summarized the health promotion process as a series of nine steps that involve the client and the nurse. Notice that many steps of this process are similar to the nursing process:

1. Review and summarize data from assessment.
2. Reinforce the client's strengths and abilities.
3. Identify health goals and related behavioral change options.
4. Identify behavioral or health outcomes that will indicate that the plan has been successful from the client's perspective.
5. Develop a behavior change plan based on the client's preferences, on the stages of change, and on "state-of-the science" knowledge about effective interventions.
6. Reiterate benefits of change, and identify incentives for change from the client's perspective.
7. Address environmental and interpersonal facilitators and barriers to behavior change.
8. Determine a time frame for implementation.
9. Commit to behavior-change goals, and structure the support needed to accomplish them.

| Assessment |

A health promotion assessment involves obtaining a health history, physical examination, fitness assessment, lifestyle and risk appraisal, life stress review, analysis of healthcare beliefs, nutritional assessment, and screening activities.

History and Physical Examination

Assessment should begin with a thorough health history, review of body systems, and a physical examination. Gather the history directly from the client if possible; if not, gather information from the closest caregiver. As always, provide privacy and comfort while conducting the history and exam.

The level of detail of the physical examination depends on the health history. At a minimum, the exam should include vital signs, weight, BMI, auscultation and palpation of the chest and abdomen, inspection of the skin, and palpation of peripheral pulses. The exam may be accompanied by laboratory studies. Recommended lab work depends on the history and exam findings. For most adult clients, screening lab consists of a complete blood count, comprehensive metabolic panel (also known as a chem 20 panel), lipid panel, thyroid function panel, and urinalysis (American College of Sports Medicine [ACSM], 2000). In clients with known cardiac or pulmonary disease, additional disease-specific studies may be performed (e.g., electrocardiogram [ECG], carotid ultrasound, or pulmonary function tests).

Physical Fitness Assessment

Physical fitness is a major focus of health promotion. Although a sedentary lifestyle has been linked to increased risk for diabetes and heart disease, children and adults are nevertheless spending more time in front of television, video games, and computers than participating in physical activity. A physical fitness assessment includes the following:

- *Cardiorespiratory fitness.* Cardiorespiratory fitness is reflected in the ability to perform large-muscle, moderate- to high-intensity exercise for prolonged periods of time (ACSM, 2000). There are many different modes of testing, such as field tests (walking or running), motor-driven treadmills, stationary bicycles, and step testing. Results depend on age and gender. For more information,

 Go to Chapter 41, **Assessment Guidelines and Tools, Health Promotion: Physical Fitness Assessment,** in Volume 2.

- *Muscular fitness.* Muscular fitness refers to both muscle strength and endurance. Muscle strength is a measure of the amount of weight a muscle (or group of muscles) can move at one time. Muscle endurance refers to the ability of a muscle to perform repeated movements.

TABLE 41–1 Health Promotion Throughout the Life Span

Developmental Stage	Health Promotion Focus	Health Screenings
Conception to birth	Education about pregnancy Abstinence of alcohol, cigarettes, and illicit drugs Nutrition, including folic acid and iron requirements Exercise to maintain strength and muscle tone and to control weight gain Parenting education	Alpha-fetoprotein level Screening for gestational diabetes Prenatal care Abuse Additional screenings that may be offered: • Ultrasound • Amniocentesis • Chorionic villus sampling
Infancy	Nutrition (breast versus bottle) Introduction of solid foods Placing the infant on her back for sleep to reduce the risk of sudden infant death syndrome (SIDS) Sensory stimulation Safety Motor vehicle safety Oral health	Hearing evaluation Screening for birth defects Blood work to rule out certain metabolic conditions Monthly examinations until at least 6 months of age After age 6 months, visits every 2 or 3 months Growth and development Abuse
Toddler and preschool	Adequate supervision Safety, including storage of poisons Toilet training Motor vehicle safety Nutrition Immunizations Oral health Sleep and rest	Annual examinations Growth and development Cognitive skills Abuse Kindergarten readiness
School age	Nutrition Physical activity Safety Sexuality Stranger danger Oral health	Annual examinations Growth and development Cognitive skills Abuse
Adolescence	Peer pressure Motor vehicle safety Safety Self-esteem Physical activity Suicide and depression Firearm safety Violence Sexuality Alcohol and tobacco use Limiting sun exposure Update of immunizations Oral health	Growth and development Sexually transmitted infection (STI) screening Breast self-exam Testicular self-exam Mental health Stress Alcohol and drug use Abuse

TABLE 41-1 *(continued)*

Developmental Stage	Health Promotion Focus	Health Screenings
Young adult	Physical activity Motor vehicle safety Safety Violence Sexuality Alcohol and tobacco use Limiting sun exposure Update immunizations Oral health	Comprehensive exam at least every 3 years Lifestyle Pap smear STI screening Breast self-exam monthly Testicular self-exam monthly Mental health Stress Alcohol and drug use Abuse
Middle adult	Physical activity Safety Obesity Sexuality Lifestyle Update of immunizations Oral health	Comprehensive exam at least every 3 years to age 40, yearly after 40 BP screening Lipid panel Blood glucose Stress Mammograms yearly for women over 40 and clinical breast exam Digital rectal exam for prostate evaluation in men PSA for men yearly over age 50 Annual eye exam Sigmoidoscopy or colonoscopy Stool for occult blood with comprehensive exam Bone density Abuse
Older adult	Physical activity Nutrition Safety Obesity Sexuality Lifestyle Update of immunizations Oral health Changes associated with aging	Functional skills (ADLs and IADLs) Hearing Falls risk Stress Annual eye exam BP screening Lipid panel Blood glucose Mammograms and clinical breast exam Digital rectal exam for prostate evaluation in men PSA for men who have a life expectancy of at least 10 years Stool for occult blood Bone density Follow-up sigmoidoscopy or colonoscopy Mental health Abuse

- *Flexibility.* Flexibility is the ability to move a joint through its range of motion. The most common assessment is to evaluate low back and hip (trunk) flexion.

For information and guidelines for assessing physical fitness,

 Go to Chapter 41, **Assessment Guidelines and Tools, Health Promotion: Physical Fitness Assessment,** in Volume 2.

Lifestyle and Risk Appraisal

Lifestyle refers to the manner in which a person conducts his life: physically, emotionally, spiritually, and mentally. Personal habits, recreation, and occupation are part of one's lifestyle. In the context of health and wellness, lifestyle includes all of the activities that promote optimal living, such as taking responsibility for one's health, physical activity, nutrition, interpersonal relations, spiritual growth, and stress management. You can gather this information by interview or by using a variety of questionnaires. A health risk appraisal (HRA) is a questionnaire that evaluates risk for disease based on current demographic data, lifestyle, and health behaviors. There are many HRA tools available; many are online. For an example of an HRA,

 Go to Chapter 41, **Assessment Guidelines and Tools, Lifestyle and Risk Assessment,** in Volume 2.

 ## CriticalThinking 41–3

- Evaluate your own compliance with recommended health screenings for your age group. What activities should you incorporate into your own health promotion plan?
- Answer the questions in the "Lifestyle and Risk Assessment" in Volume 2. How did you score? What additional activities should be added to your health promotion plan?

Life Stress Review

In 1976, Hans Selye proposed that stress triggers physiological responses that may, over time, induce illness. Likewise, Richard Rahe (1974) identified some stress-inducing life change events and researched their possible effects on health. He attached numeric values for each change based on the degree of disruption or stress produced by the event. Rahe discovered that a high score on a life-change event scale is associated with a greater likelihood of a negative health change.

 Go to Chapter 25, **Assessment Guidelines and Tools, The Holmes-Rahe Social Readjustment Scale,** in Volume 2.

Other researchers have focused on daily stresses and their effects on actual health or on one's perception of health (Cassidy, 2000). Daily stresses involve travel to and from work, taking children to activities, daily chores, waiting in lines at shops, and traffic jams. Researchers have found that these stresses may gradually erode one's coping mechanisms, producing an inability to cope with daily events and an increased likelihood of illness.

Research has also demonstrated that in the face of life events, some people develop hardiness rather than vulnerability (Cassidy, 2000). Kobasa (1979) identified hardiness as a quality in which an individual experiences high levels of stress yet does not fall ill. There are three general characteristics of the hardy person: control (belief in the ability to control the experience), commitment (feeling deeply involved in the activity producing stress), and challenge (the ability to view the change as a challenge to grow). For additional information on hardiness, review Chapter 10.

 ## CriticalThinking 41–4

- Undoubtedly you are experiencing stress as a student in a nursing program. How would you rate your level of hardiness?
- What statements would demonstrate a hardy personality in each area (commitment, control, challenge)?

Health Beliefs

Health beliefs are embedded in one's culture and personal experiences. A health promotion assessment would not be complete without investigating an individual's culture and beliefs. Culture consists of characteristics, beliefs, and behaviors of an individual or group (Chapter 13)—all the experiences, biases, beliefs, and rituals. Culture includes beliefs and practices affecting wellness and disease prevention. For example, some people wear amulets or charms to ward off evil spirits. Others may use certain foods (e.g., garlic around the neck) or herbs to protect or restore health. It is important for you to respect cultural and religious views regarding health while working with clients to adopt personal health goals.

Early life experiences and culture help shape a person's sense of how health outcomes are achieved. Are health outcomes a result of actions the person takes, actions of powerful others, or chance? The Multidimensional Health Locus of Control scale (MHLC) developed by Wallston, Wallston, and DeVellis (1976), measures the person's perception of the extent of control from each source. The person rates her level of agreement with statements such as "I am in control of my health," "No matter what I do, if I am going to get sick, I will get sick" and "Regarding my health, I can only do what my doctor tells me to do." Identifying a

patient's locus of control is of practical importance for several reasons:

- People who feel powerless about preventing illness are least likely to engage in health promotion activities.
- People who respond to direction from respected authorities often prefer a health promotion program that is supervised by a health provider.
- Clients who feel in charge of their own health are the easiest to motivate toward positive change.

For a copy of the MHLC you can print out and use with your patients,

 Go to **the Vanderbilt University web site at http://www .vanderbilt.edu/nursing/kwallston/mhlcscales.htm**

Nutritional Assessment

A nutritional assessment is a key component of an overall wellness assessment. Poor eating habits occur across all ages, ethnicities, and socioeconomic classes. The assessment involves an evaluation of typical eating patterns correlated with physical examination findings and BMI. Body composition is important in identifying health risks. The usual methods for determining body fat composition clinically are by measuring height, weight, circumferences, and skinfolds (see Chapter 26).

The pattern of body fat distribution is an important predictor of health risks. People with fat stored around the trunk and abdominal area have a higher incidence of hypertension, hyperlipidemia, heart disease, type II diabetes, and premature death than those who have the fat stored in the extremities. Traditionally, the waist-to-hip ratio has been used as a method for determining fat patterns in the body. More recently, the focus has shifted to waist circumference alone. The more fat stored in the abdominal area, the greater the risk for disease.

Health Screening Activities

Health screening activities are secondary prevention activities designed to diagnose specific diseases at an early stage so that treatment can begin before there is an opportunity for the disease to spread or become debilitating. Many of these screening activities are part of your usual care. For example, each time you check a client's blood pressure, you are performing a screen for hypertension. Table 41–1 identifies the typical health screening activities with each developmental stage. Box 41–2 provides further information about selected health screening activities.

Currently, there is some controversy about whether we should encourage breast self-examination (BSE). Some studies indicate that it does not reduce death rates from breast cancer, but others found that more cancers are discovered and that the cancers are less advanced in groups who perform BSE (Green & Taplin, 2003; Hackshaw & Paul, 2004; Kösters & Gøtzsche, 2003; Thomas, et al., 2002; Weiss, N., 2003). So until evidence is conclusive, it seems reasonable to continue to encourage and teach BSE.

The issue of whether to perform mass prostate-specific antigen (PSA) screening for prostate cancer is also unsettled. The U.S. Preventive Services Task Force concludes that there is not sufficient evidence to recommend for or against routine PSA screening for prostate cancer. However, most experts and organizations agree that the most appropriate candidates for screening are men older than age 50 and younger men who have increased risk factors (Harris & Lohr, 2002).

For points to include when teaching breast and testicular self examination,

 Go to the expanded discussion of Chapter 9, **Figures, Boxes, Tables: ESG Boxes 9–6 and 9–7,** on the Electronic Study Guide.

KnowledgeCheck 41–3

- Identify at least three common sites for health promotion activities.
- What assessments are part of a health promotion assessment?
- What role does stress play in health promotion?

 Go to Chapter 41, **Knowledge Check Response Sheet and Answers,** on the Electronic Study Guide.

 ## CriticalThinking 41–5

Your 55-year-old aunt tells you she hasn't had a physical examination in 20 years. She is a registered nurse. "I don't need one because I feel fine and I can take care of myself." How would you respond?

| Nursing Diagnosis |

Wellness diagnoses are appropriate for health promotion activities. Such diagnoses describe healthy responses in areas where you can intervene to promote growth or maintenance of the healthy response. NANDA defines a wellness diagnosis as describing "human responses to levels of wellness in an individual, family, or community that have a readiness for enhancement" (2005, p. 245). The following are some NANDA labels you can use to describe wellness diagnoses:

- Anticipatory Grieving
- Effective Breastfeeding
- Effective Therapeutic Regimen Management
- Health-Seeking Behaviors (specify)
- Readiness for Enhanced Communication

BOX 41-2 Selected Health Screening Activities

- *Lipid screening.* The American Heart Association recommends that all adults age 20 years or older have a fasting lipid panel at least once every 5 years. If total cholesterol is 200 mg/dL or greater—or HDL is less than 40 mg/dL—more frequent monitoring is required.

- *Dental health.* Regular dental checkups can detect early signs of oral health problems, such as tooth decay, gingivitis (gum disease), and oral cancers. In addition to having regular dental examinations, drink fluoridated water and use a fluoride toothpaste to brush your teeth at least twice a day. Floss between teeth daily.

- *Colon screening.* Both men and women should have a fecal occult blood test every year beginning at age 50 and a screening colonoscopy based on risk factors. If there is a strong family history of colorectal cancer or polyps, screening should begin at an earlier age and be conducted more frequently. Anyone experiencing the following symptoms should check with their physician:
  - A change in bowel habits, such as diarrhea, constipation, or narrowing of the stool that lasts for more than a few days
  - A feeling that you need to have a bowel movement that is not relieved by doing so
  - Rectal bleeding or blood in the stool
  - Cramping or steady abdominal (stomach area) pain
  - Weakness and fatigue

- *Breast cancer screening.* Encourage women aged 20 or older to perform monthly breast self-examination (BSE). By doing the exam regularly, you will know the normal feel of breast tissue and more easily detect any change. Report any changes to a healthcare professional. Women between the ages of 20 and 39 should have a clinical breast examination by a health professional every 3 years. Women aged 40 and older should have a screening mammogram and a clinical breast examination by a healthcare professional every year. The clinical breast examination should be scheduled close to and preferably before the scheduled mammogram.

- *Cervical cancer screening.* A Papanicolaou (Pap) smear is used to detect cellular changes in the cervix. To limit the risk of cervical cancer, limit sexual partners, and avoid sex with people who have had many other sexual partners. The following guidelines are recommended for early detection:
  - All sexually active women should have an annual Pap smear.
  - Women 70 years of age or older who have had three or more normal Pap tests in a row and no abnormal Pap test results in the last 10 years may choose to stop having cervical cancer screening.
  - Women who have had a total hysterectomy (removal of the uterus and cervix) may also choose to stop having cervical cancer screening, unless the surgery was done as a treatment for cervical cancer or precancer. Women who have had a hysterectomy without removal of the cervix should continue to have Pap smears.
  - Women who have certain risk factors, such as diethylstilbestrol (DES) exposure before birth, HIV infection, or a weakened immune system due to organ transplant, chemotherapy, or chronic steroid use, should continue to be screened annually.

- *Testicular cancer screening.* The incidence of testicular cancer peaks at 30 to 34 years of age but is frequently diagnosed in males between the ages of 15 and 19 years or 50 and 54 years. Many men with testicular cancer have no symptoms that cause them to seek health care. In about 90% of cases (American Cancer Society, 2002) men have a painless or uncomfortable lump on a testicle, or they may have noticed swelling in the testicle. Monthly testicular self-examination leads to early detection.

- *Prostate screening.* Prostate cancer can be detected early with a blood test called the prostate-specific antigen (PSA) test or a digital rectal examination (DRE) by a trained healthcare professional. The American Cancer Society believes that healthcare professionals should offer the PSA and DRE yearly beginning at age 50 years. If there is a family history, testing should begin at the age of 45 years.

- Readiness for Enhanced Community Coping
- Readiness for Enhanced Coping
- Readiness for Enhanced Family Coping
- Readiness for Enhanced Family Processes
- Readiness for Enhanced Fluid Balance
- Readiness for Enhanced Knowledge (specify)
- Readiness for Enhanced Management of Therapeutic Regimen
- Readiness for Enhanced Nutrition

- Readiness for Enhanced Organized Infant Behavior
- Readiness for Enhanced Parenting
- Readiness for Enhanced Self-Concept
- Readiness for Enhanced Sleep
- Readiness for Enhanced Spiritual Well-Being
- Readiness for Enhanced Urinary Elimination

New NANDA wellness labels are preceded by the phrase *Readiness for Enhanced* and will be one-part statements (e.g., Readiness for Enhanced Parenting)

| toward evidence-based practice |

Hooper, L., Summerbell, C., Higgins, J., Thompson, R., Capps, N., Smith, G., et al. (2001). Dietary fat intake and prevention of cardiovascular disease: Systematic review. *British Medical Journal, 322*(31), 757–763.

This was a meta-analysis reviewing 27 randomized controlled studies that reduced or modified fat or cholesterol intake in healthy adult participants for at least 6 months. Alteration of dietary fat intake was found to have small effects on total mortality rate. Cardiovascular mortality was reduced by 9% and cardiovascular events by 16%. Trials with at least 2 years' follow-up provided stronger evidence of protection from cardiovascular events.

Soinio, M., Laakso, M., Lehto, S., Hakala, P., & Ronnemaa, T. (2003). Dietary fat predicts coronary heart disease events in subjects with Type 2 diabetes. *Diabetes Care, 26*(3), 619–624.

Dietary habits of 366 men and 295 women, aged 45 to 64 years, who were free from coronary heart disease (CHD) but were diagnosed with type II diabetes, were assessed with a 53-item food frequency questionnaire. Participants were followed for 7 years. A P/S ratio (ratio of polyunsaturated fat to saturated fat) was determined by comparing the dietary intake of polyunsaturated fats (vegetable fats) to saturated fats (animal fats). Men with a higher ratio of polyunsaturated to saturated fat (P/S ratio) had a significantly lower risk for coronary heart disease then men with lower ratios (higher saturated fat intake). The P/S ratio did not predict CHD events in women.

Kodali, V., Kodavanti, M., Tripuraribhatla, P., Ram, T., Eswaran, P., & Krishnaswamy, K. (1999). Dietary factors as determinants of hypertension: A case control study in an urban Indian population. *Asia Pacific Journal of Clinical Nutrition, 8*(3), 184–189.

This study involved 86 men and women diagnosed with hypertension and 79 who were not hypertensive. A detailed diet history was collected and validated. Among those classified as hypertensive, men reported higher intakes of dietary fat and salt, whereas women reported higher intakes of dietary protein and salt.

---

1. Based on these studies, would you alter your dietary habits? Explain your thinking.

2. What advice would you give your clients regarding decreasing the risk of cardiovascular disease and hypertension?

 Go to Chapter 41, **Toward Evidence-Based Practice Suggested Responses,** on the Electronic Study Guide.

---

with no etiology. Notice, however, that there are still some wellness labels that have different one-part formats (e.g., Effective Breastfeeding and Health-Seeking Behaviors).

| Planning Outcomes/Evaluation |

NOC standardized outcomes related to health promotion vary depending on the focus area. For example, if the nursing diagnosis is Readiness for Enhanced Nutrition, a NOC outcome might be Nutritional Status. For examples of other NOC wellness outcomes,

 Go to Chapter 41, **Standardized Language, Examples of NOC Standardized Health Promotion Outcomes,** in Volume 2.

The nurse's role in health promotion primarily is to motivate clients and facilitate change. Clients are independently responsible for most of their health promotion activities. You may need to help clients to identify their own goals, but it is essential that the goals be the clients', not yours. Examples of *individualized goals and outcomes* might include losing 20 pounds or exercising for 30 minutes five times per week.

You may need *aggregate wellness goals* for groups as well as individualized goals. Recall the two broad goals for the U.S. population set by the Healthy People 2010 initiative (U.S. Department of Health and Human Services [U.S. DHHS], 2000, Vol. 1, p. 2):

1. Increase quality and years of healthy life
2. Eliminate health disparities.

The focus areas for these goals are found in Box 41–1. Recall that there are 467 specific, measurable population objectives directed at achieving these two goals (U.S. DHHS, 2000). To view those objectives,

 Go to **the Healthy People 2010 web site at www.healthypeople.gov/Search/objectives.htm**

Whether standardized or individualized, expected outcomes for wellness diagnoses describe behaviors or

responses that demonstrate health maintenance or achievement of an even higher level of health. For example:

> Over the next year, Mr. Needham will continue to eat a balanced diet, with more emphasis on including whole grains and fiber.

By using the highest number (5) on the rating scale, you can use the NOC to write wellness outcomes. For example:

> Nursing diagnosis: Readiness for Enhanced Nutrition
>
> Expected outcome: Nutritional Status: (5) Not compromised

| Planning Interventions/Implementation |

Nurses have been recognized as leaders in health promotion for a long time. Community and public health nurses focus on the problems contributing to disease, such as poor housing conditions, poor sanitation, poor nutrition, poverty, and substance abuse. Nurses in acute care focus on educating patients about health and disease.

Once the client identifies his goals, help him to identify the steps that he must take to reach the goals. Recall that change occurs in stages. To create positive change, the client will need to understand the benefits of change, overcome the barriers to change, and make a commitment to follow through on the plan.

For *NIC standardized interventions* for health promotion,

 Go to Chapter 41, **Standardized Language, Selected NIC Wellness Interventions,** in Volume 2.

NIC does not have a special domain, or grouping, for wellness interventions. Instead, they are found throughout all areas of the taxonomy, particularly in the domains of Behavioral, Safety, Family, Health System, and Community.

Specific nursing activities for health promotion include those following. The remainder of the chapter provides some strategies to promote their use.

- *Nutrition.* To promote health and prevent disease, people need to make nutritional choices based on the United States Department of Agriculture (USDA) and the U.S. Department of Health and Human Services (U.S. DHHS) revised Dietary Guidelines for Americans and The Food Guide Pyramid (see Chapter 26). In short, this means eating a balanced diet and limiting the intake of fats, sweets, and salt.

- *Exercise.* Physically active people have fewer physician visits and hospital stays and use less medication than physically inactive people (U.S. DHHS,

2002). Programs such as the President's Challenge encourage the development of physical fitness lifestyle habits in people of all ages and abilities. A 30-minute walk five or more times a week, for example, may improve health (see Chapter 31). For more information,

 Go to the **President's Challenge web site at www.presidentschallenge.org**

- *Lifestyle changes.* Lifestyle changes focus on tobacco and alcohol use, substance abuse, and stress management.

- *Sleep.* In general, adults need 6 to 9 hours of sleep a night. Children need more sleep (see Chapter 33).

For an expanded discussion of these areas for health promotion,

 Go to Chapter 41, **Supplemental Materials: Individual Health Promotion Activities,** on the Electronic Study Guide.

Role Modeling

A role model teaches by example, demonstrating the behaviors and/or attitudes to be learned. Models provide inspiration and strategies for health promotion behavior. For example, a morbidly obese female joins a weight loss group led by a woman who has lost 100 pounds. She admires the leader and selects her as a role model.

Clients select their own role models, often without making a conscious decision to do so. But it may be helpful for you to facilitate the client's choice. When suggesting a model, consider the client's age, culture, values, and preferred activities. The model should be someone with whom the client identifies. Ideally, the role model should be someone accessible to the client during the early stages of change. This allows for interacting and for exchanging information. At times, however, a famous athlete or celebrity may be the model. This is more likely to be effective if the celebrity has written about her success or regularly speaks about her positive change.

Nurses also serve as role models. As a result, we should provide an example of healthy behaviors. It is difficult to advocate for healthy behavior if you do not follow the behavior you recommend to clients. Imagine the trust a client loses when he finds out that the nurse who tells him not to smoke cigarettes has a two-pack per day habit. How compelling is a discussion of the importance of weight loss given by an overweight nurse? To what extent do you role-model healthy behaviors?

Providing Counseling

Counseling is an interpersonal communication process that helps a client to identify problems and

make changes. In the context of health promotion, counseling promotes personal growth and helps clients change their lifestyle. Counseling may be formal one-to-one or small-group discussion, or it may be informal discussion with the client at a healthcare encounter. Each meeting with a client is a potential counseling session. In addition to face-to-face contact, counseling may be offered via telephone.

Individual Sessions

Face-to-face interaction may be helpful when clients are attempting major lifestyle change. In an individual session you can customize and map out the steps required to meet the client's goals. This may include writing a contract detailing the client's expected behaviors. Print out the contract, and have the client sign it to reinforce his commitment. Have the client post the plan in a location he sees often so that it serves as a frequent reminder.

During counseling sessions, remember to reinforce health promoting behaviors that have already been established. For example, the client who uses tobacco may eat a balanced diet; reinforce the healthy habit to boost self-esteem. Stress to the client that although the behavior to be changed may be unhealthy, you believe the client can succeed in making the change.

Telephone Counseling

Telephone counseling may be used as a primary counseling approach or as follow-up. Many clients with hectic schedules find it easier to arrange telephone counseling than to schedule a face-to-face interaction. The disadvantage is that telephone counseling does not allow you to see nonverbal communication.

When using telephone counseling, you will set goals and map out the strategy for change just as you would in individual counseling. Make sure to inform the client about how and when you can be reached if questions arise. If you are using the telephone for follow-up counseling, it is best to schedule a time to speak. Having an appointment helps to reinforce the expected behavior.

Providing Health Education

Health education may focus on self-care strategies, caregiver concerns, or how to be an effective health care consumer. Self-care programs typically focus on nutrition, exercise, stress management, or disease prevention. Programs may consist of lectures, printed material, billboards, or posters. For example, the accompanying Self-Care box might be reproduced and posted in the lounge, rest rooms, or locker areas of a worksite during cold and flu season to decrease absenteeism. Caregiver education programs may teach

Teaching Clients How to Prevent Upper Respiratory Infections

- Develop healthful lifestyle habits to help your body resist viral invasion. For example, get plenty of rest, exercise moderately, and eat a healthy diet.

- Wash your hands often; teach children to do so as well. This helps prevent spread of infection.

- Avoid touching your eyes, nose, and mouth, because doing so spreads any virus your hands have contacted (e.g., on doorknobs).

- Avoid crowds, especially when there is a cold or influenza epidemic.

- When using public restrooms, wash your hands. Then, turn off the faucet with a paper towel. Also use a paper towel to open the door as you leave the room.

- Throw away tissues as soon as you use them.

- When someone in the family has a cold, keep bathrooms and the kitchen very clean.

- When someone has a cold at home or at work, wipe telephone receivers with soap and water or an antiseptic solution.

- When choosing child care, look for a clean environment; ask what rules they have about keeping the children clean (e.g., washing hands before snacktime).

- Taking vitamin C has not been shown to prevent colds, but it may help symptoms to go away sooner.

- Recent studies suggest that there may be some benefit from taking echinacea, but no consensus on this has yet been reached. Consult your primary healthcare provider.

caregivers how to perform nursing tasks or prevent injuries, or they may provide a list of community resources for respite care. Classes focused on helping clients be effective consumers teach them how to interact with health providers and how to maneuver through the healthcare system. For a review of teaching and learning, see Chapter 24.

Providing and Facilitating Support for Lifestyle Change

Changing one's lifestyle is difficult. Clients need support to make the change. You will provide support during

your interactions and counseling sessions. Help the client identify available support in the community and in the client's immediate environment.

Group support exists for a variety of lifestyle changes. For example, Weight Watchers is a group support program for clients who want to lose weight; Alcoholics Anonymous is a group support program for clients who want to become and stay sober. Learn about programs available in your community. Provide clients with names and contact numbers during your interactions. Group support provides clients with a chance to meet people experiencing the same difficulties and perhaps to find a role model.

Studies have found that group support works. The Task Force on Community Preventive Services (2002) found group-level interventions to be effective in promoting physical activity. These interventions included making changes in school-based physical education programs, conducting community-wide campaigns, improving access to places for physical activity, and offering individually adapted behavior change programs in group settings.

Family, friends, and caregivers may help or hinder the change process. Help clients identify who can offer support and who may be threatened by the client's proposed change. For example, when a woman begins to lose weight, an insecure husband may secretly worry that she will become attractive to other men. Often you can provide information to family and friends that will help them support the changes the client is making.

KnowledgeCheck 41–4

Identify four strategies to help a client engage in positive lifestyle change.

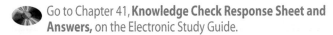 Go to Chapter 41, **Knowledge Check Response Sheet and Answers,** on the Electronic Study Guide.

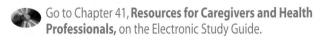 Go to Chapter 41, **Resources for Caregivers and Health Professionals,** on the Electronic Study Guide.

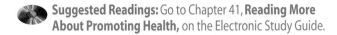 **Suggested Readings:** Go to Chapter 41, **Reading More About Promoting Health,** on the Electronic Study Guide.

 Bibliography: Go to Volume 2, Bibliography.

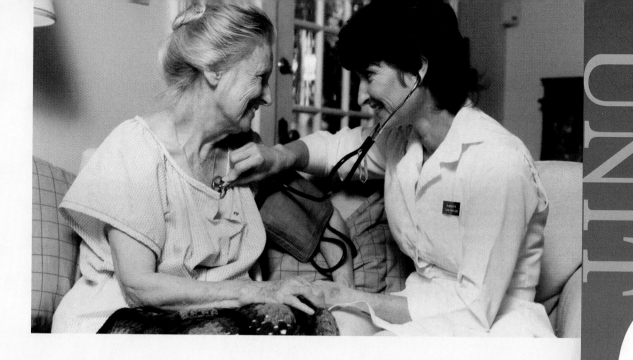

The Context
for Nurses' Work

42 CHAPTER

Community Nursing

Learning Outcomes

After completing this chapter, you should be able to:

❋ Define a community.

❋ Identify at least four factors that make populations healthy.

❋ Identify at least four factors that make populations vulnerable.

❋ Identify the major differences between community nursing and acute care nursing.

❋ Compare and contrast community-based nursing, community health nursing, public health nursing, and community-oriented nursing.

❋ Distinguish primary, secondary, and tertiary interventions in regard to a community health scenario.

❋ Discuss the dimensions of a community that are included in a nursing assessment.

❋ Describe the roles of nurses in the community setting.

❋ Identify at least five career opportunities for community nurses.

❋ Discuss at least three strategies that nurses use to gather community data.

❋ Explain how NANDA, NIC, and NOC taxonomies are used when the client is a community.

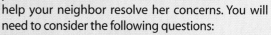

MEET Your Patient

You are nearing completion of your fundamentals course. One night while you are preparing for your next clinical, the telephone rings. It is your neighbor, Tanya. Her 5-year-old daughter, Tiffany, attends kindergarten at the local public school. Tiffany came home with a letter from the school nurse stating that another child in the class was ill with chickenpox and that all the students in the class had been exposed to the disease.

Tanya is concerned about the risks to Tiffany and the rest of the family. She does not recall whether Tiffany was vaccinated against chickenpox, and she is unsure whether she herself had the disease when she was a child. Tanya is 4 months pregnant, and the family has no health insurance. She states that because you are a nursing student, she thought you might know what she should do or where she might go for assistance.

Although you are flattered that your neighbor has consulted you, you need to consider whether you have the expertise to answer her questions. This complex situation requires knowledge from many aspects of nursing (e.g., immunizations, pregnancy,

microbiology, pathophysiology). Though you may not have all of the information you need to answer her questions, you should be able to help your neighbor resolve her concerns. You will need to consider the following questions:

- What is going on in the situation that may influence the outcome?
- Who should be involved to improve the outcome?
- What theoretical knowledge do I need to answer my neighbor's questions? Where would I find this information?
- What additional data do I need to collect from my neighbor?
- What suggestions and/or referrals should I offer to my neighbor?

In this chapter, we will discuss community nursing, a facet of nursing that frequently deals with problems such as this.

Theoretical Knowledge
knowing why

Nurses working in community and public health regularly deal with concerns about vaccinations and the risks of exposure to communicable disease. In this chapter, we discuss communities and community nursing care. We also explore the roles, interventions, and career opportunities for nurses who work within communities.

UNDERSTANDING COMMUNITIES

The word **community** comes from the Latin term *communis,* meaning the gift or fellowship of common relations and feelings (Hiemstra, 2000). In its medieval usage in Europe, it meant a body of like-minded people or the inhabitants of a town. Then and now, the term suggests a general sense of selflessness, sharing,

and doing good that comes from working together. Most members of a community share a common language, certain rituals, and special customs.

In contrast to community, a **population** is defined as all of the people inhabiting a specified area. For example, look at a map of Ohio and try to determine the approximate boundaries of the city of Dayton (Figure 42–1). To accurately determine the physical boundaries of the city, you would need local maps depicting exact roads, streets, rivers and other landmarks. As you can imagine, the characteristics and concerns of the 315,000 people living within Dayton vary greatly—there are many communities in Dayton.

The United States Bureau of the Census conducts a survey and count of the American people every 10 years. The last census was conducted in the year 2000. For results,

 Go to the **U.S. Census Bureau web site at www.census.gov**

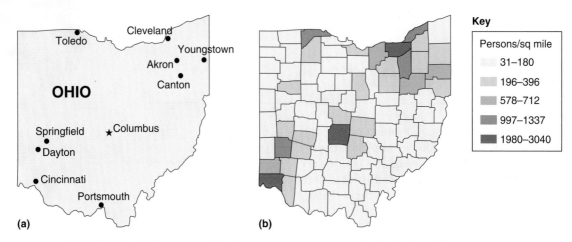

(a)

(b)

Key

Persons/sq mile

31–180

196–396

578–712

997–1337

1980–3040

FIGURE 42–1 *A,* Illustrates geopolitical boundaries. *B,* Census tract data provide more detail about communities.

Based on the data received from the completed census, the Bureau groups the information into sections of 1500 to 8000 people known as **census tracts.** The area of individual census tracts varies according to the density of the population. In urban centers, a census tract covers a small area. Rural census tracts are very large. Census tracts are useful to public officials, market analysts, and anyone—including community nurses—who studies the characteristics and concerns of smaller sections of people.

Maps and census tracts show the *geopolitical* boundaries of a community. But as we noted earlier, a community can also be a group of people with a common purpose. They may live in different geographical areas, but they have a "sense of belonging" to their group (community). An **aggregate** is a group of individuals with at least one shared characteristic, either personal or environmental. For example, a community health nurse may work with a class of high school girls to reduce the incidence of adolescent pregnancy. The shared characteristics of this aggregate are that they are female, of child-bearing age, and attend a particular school. As another example, the nursing students in your school are an aggregate. What characteristics and goals do you share?

CriticalThinking 42–1

• Why might the boundaries of a census tract change every 10 years?
• How could you figure out what census tract you live or go to school in?

KnowledgeCheck 42–1

• Give several examples of a community.
• How is a population different from a community?

 Go to Chapter 42, **Knowledge Check Response Sheet and Answers,** on the Electronic Study Guide

What Are the Components of a Community?

To understand a particular community and its needs, you will need information about its three components: structure, status, and processes.

1. **Structure** refers to the general characteristics of a community. These include demographic data, such as gender, age, ethnicity, and educational and income levels, as well as data about healthcare services, such as the number of primary care providers or emergency departments in the area.
2. **Status** describes the biological, emotional, and social outcome components of a community. *Biological* data includes morbidity (illness) and mortality (death) rates, life expectancy ratios, and risk factor profiles for the respective age groups within a community. *Emotional* data includes general indications of mental health and consumer satisfaction survey results about various aspects of the community as compared to other locales. *Social* data includes crime rates, citizenship involvement in community-wide activities, and general functioning levels of the community members.
3. **Process** describes the overall effectiveness level of the community. For example, do the members of the community perceive that they are part of a group with common interests? What is the extent of interaction among community members? Does the community have an established forum for conflict resolution?

What Makes a Community Healthy?

As with individuals, the meaning and perception of health varies among aggregates. For nurses, it is important to understand what a particular community defines (and values) as health rather than relying on

personal definitions. Health is whatever the client community defines it as.

When defining what makes a community healthy, the national consensus paper *Healthy People 2010* provides useful guidelines. The document (initially titled *Healthy People 2000* and now in a revised edition) was produced in response to a 1979 report from the surgeon general indicating that many of the health problems of Americans were preventable. *Healthy People 2010* identifies 28 focus areas and 10 leading indicators of health to guide planning and evaluation of programs. The broad goals of the plan are to (1) increase years of healthy life and (2) eliminate health disparities among different populations. The goals are to be achieved through promoting healthy behaviors, increasing access to quality health care, and strengthening community health resources. For more information,

 Go to the **Healthy People 2010 web site at www.healthypeople.gov**

KnowledgeCheck 42–2

- What makes up the "structure" of a community?
- What is community "status"?
- What is community "process"?
- Use the guidelines from *Healthy People 2010* to compile a list of several characteristics that make a community healthy.

 Go to Chapter 42, **Knowledge Check Response Sheet and Answers,** on the Electronic Study Guide.

What Makes a Population Vulnerable?

A **vulnerable population** is defined as an aggregate that is at increased risk of adverse health outcomes. Members of vulnerable populations have a higher probability of developing illness than do members of the general population. For example, pregnant adolescents are more likely to develop complications than pregnant women of all ages taken as a whole. Because of their increased risk of health problems, vulnerable populations are a major focus of community health efforts. Vulnerability involves multiple factors:

- *Limited economic resources.* Income is a major predictor of health risk. People with higher incomes typically have greater access to health services and wider choice of providers, treatment options, and location of health services. In contrast, the more limited a person's income, the more limited her healthcare options. Consequently, many persons of low income forego preventive or health maintenance care and seek healthcare services only when they are quite ill.
- *Limited social resources.* Friends and family are valuable resources to help a person deal with day-to-day stress as well as the stress associated with

illness. They provide feedback, listen to concerns, and offer emotional and physical assistance. Unfortunately, not everyone has social resources. Older adults who live alone and people with mental illness are examples of groups at increased risk because of social isolation.

- *Age.* The very young and the very old are less able to adapt to physiological stress and are at increased risk of disease. They are more prone to infections and may not be able to protect themselves from environmental hazards, such as cold or heat. These age groups are also more likely to be living in poverty.
- *Chronic disease.* People who have chronic diseases are at greater risk for many health problems. For example, people with HIV are at increased risk of opportunistic infections, as are people receiving chemotherapy for cancer.
- *History of abuse or trauma.* People who have experienced abuse or traumatic events often feel they have limited control over their health and circumstances. They may experience powerlessness and/or hopelessness and be unable to initiate activities that promote health or lead to early treatment of illness. These circumstances also place them at risk for mental health problems and tax their reserves.

Vulnerable populations include poor people, homeless people, migrant workers, people with disabilities, people with communicable disease, pregnant adolescents, people who abuse substances, members of particular ethnic/racial groups, victims of abuse or neglect, and the untreated mentally ill.

UNDERSTANDING COMMUNITY NURSING

A community can be either a *site* for healthcare delivery or a *recipient* of healthcare services. Throughout history, most care was provided in or for the community. In fact, the first hospitals in the United States were established only in the late 1860s to protect society from contagious disease. Several decades passed before hospitals and their satellite clinics became the predominant settings for providing health care. However, as the technological advances of the last 30 years have escalated the costs of delivering health services, health care—including complementary and alternative care—has again become more community focused, with an emphasis on lowering costs.

Community-Based Care

Community-based care refers to acute care or rehabilitative services performed in clinics, offices, and other facilities in the community—rather than in acute care settings such as hospitals (although acute

BOX 42–1   Ten Great Public Health Achievements—United States, 1900–1999

1. Vaccination
2. Motor vehicle safety
3. Safer workplaces
4. Control of infectious diseases
5. Decline in deaths from coronary heart disease and stroke
6. Safer and healthier foods
7. Healthier mothers and babies
8. Family planning
9. Fluoridation of drinking water
10. Recognition of tobacco use as a health hazard

Source: U.S. Department of Health and Human Services. (1999). Ten great public health achievements—United States, 1900–1999. *Morbidity and Mortality Weekly Report, 48*(50), 1141–1146.

care settings also exist within the community.) For example, more surgeries and diagnostic procedures are now performed in surgicenters, clinics, and physician's offices. Many people also receive mental, physical, cardiac, and pulmonary rehabilitation services in outpatient settings. Extended care facilities, or nursing homes, are also community-based facilities. They commonly provide rehabilitative care for patients after acute traumatic injuries, as well as continuous skilled care for older adults and people with chronic illness. The following section describes three approaches to community-based nursing care: community health nursing, public health nursing, and community-oriented nursing.

Community Health Nursing

Although many people use the terms *community health nursing* and *public health nursing* interchangeably, the two are not identical. **Community health nursing** focuses on the health of individuals, families, and groups and on how their individual health affects the community as a whole. Community health nurses strive to promote, protect, preserve, and maintain the health of the population through the delivery of personal health services to individuals, families, and groups. For example, a community health nurse may work in a prenatal clinic providing free services for low-income women. The nurse provides a direct service to each pregnant woman, yet she is doing that to improve the general health of the entire community. By

encouraging the mother to eat balanced meals, exercise, and avoid harmful substances, the nurse improves the health of both mother and baby—who are *members* of the community—and, therefore, improves the *overall* health of the community.

Public Health Nursing

Public health nursing focuses on the community at large and the eventual effect of the community's health status on the health of individuals, families, and groups. The goal of public health is to prevent individual disease and disability, in addition to promoting and protecting the health of the community as a whole. For example, a public health nurse may be employed by a county health department to provide tuberculosis (TB) surveillance services. The nurse helps to protect the entire community by screening for TB at the local school, by testing high-risk individuals for TB, and by identifying and tracking clients with active disease to insure that they complete the prescribed 6- to 9-month medication regimen.

Because public health focuses on large-scale programs that address the entire community, government-based agencies often provide these services. The United States Public Health Service (USPHS) is an example of a public health agency based within the federal government. Box 42–1 identifies ten major public health achievements of the 20th century. For additional information on the USPHS,

 Go to Chapter 42, **Supplemental Materials: United States Public Health Service,** on the Electronic Study Guide.

Community-Oriented Nursing

Community-oriented nursing combines components of community and public health. Nurses practicing community-oriented nursing are fluid in their approach. Their focus is a comprehensive look at the individual, family, group, and community at large. For example, a nurse with a community-oriented approach might work in a comprehensive adolescent prenatal program. The nurse provides individual care at the local clinic 2 days per week. While at the clinic, she gathers data from adolescent clients about the schools they attend, their knowledge of birth control, pregnancy, and childbirth, as well as the issues these girls face with pregnancy. On the remaining 3 days of the week, she engages in community-focused activities that are informed by her knowledge and experience with pregnant teens. For example, she meets with school officials to identify pregnant teens who need prenatal care, teaches a class about sexuality in the local high school, works with teachers to identify strategies to keep pregnant teens in school, provides parent education to adolescents who have children,

and advocates changing a bus route so that teens can easily get to the local clinic. Each aspect of care allows the nurse to gather more data about the needs of the individuals and the community as a whole. Figure 42–2 provides a schematic of the relationship of the various community-based nursing approaches identified in this section.

KnowledgeCheck 42–3

- What is the distinction between an aggregate population and a vulnerable population?
- Identify practice differences between a community-based nurse and an acute care nurse.
- How is public health nursing different from community health nursing? How is it the same?
- How is community-oriented nursing related to community health nursing and public health nursing?

 Go to Chapter 42, **Knowledge Check Response Sheet and Answers,** on the Electronic Study Guide.

CriticalThinking 42–2

Review the scenario of Tanya and Tiffany ("Meet Your Patient"). Which form of community-based nursing would be most appropriate to address their concerns?

Who Were Some Pioneers of Community Nursing?

The following are some of the most notable people who have contributed to the development of community-based nursing care.

- *Florence Nightingale*—Established the importance of promoting health by manipulating the environment (e.g., light, sanitation, cleanliness) and nursing the whole person.
- *Lillian Wald*—Known as the first community health nurse; founded the first visiting nurses association in New York.
- *Clara Barton*—Founder of the American Red Cross.
- *Margaret Sanger*—Founded the International Planned Parenthood Federation. Pioneered the use of family planning and birth control education.

For more information about the achievements of these community health pioneers,

 Go to Chapter 42, **Supplemental Materials: Pioneers of Community-Based Nursing,** on the Electronic Study Guide

WORKING WITHIN COMMUNITIES

In the community setting, nurses' roles vary depending on the community and its identified needs. The nursing care is by nature holistic, and it involves large

Relationship between community health and public health

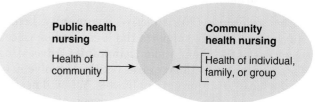

- Both nursing approaches aim to preserve, promote, and protect the community
- The public health approach focuses on protecting the community at large; protecting the health of individuals is a result of such efforts.
- The community health approach focuses on the health of each individual to promote the overall health of the community at large.

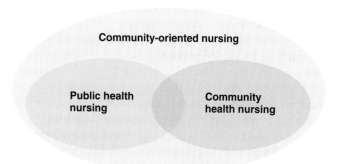

- Community-oriented nursing encompasses public health and community health approaches.
- It focuses on the illness-prevention needs of well clients and their perception of health.
- Practice is research-based and collaborative.

FIGURE 42–2   Schematic relationship of community nursing approaches.

numbers of clients. Therefore, one of the most effective nursing interventions is **empowerment.** This means assisting the client (individual or community) to recognize and use available resources to achieve or maintain the desired level of health, achieve autonomy, and maintain positive self-esteem.

What Are the Roles of Community Nurses?

Community health nurses function as client advocates, educators, collaborators, counselors, and case managers. All of these roles require excellent written and oral communication skills. Although personal computers have simplified the task of communicating with large numbers of people, not everyone in a community has computer skills and computer access. You will need to assess abilities and preferences in the

community and be creative in reaching out to clients through various means.

- *Client advocate.* The effective community health nurse consistently supports the identified or voiced concerns of the client and/or community. Advocating for a community often requires political involvement at the local, state, or national levels. You will need to be informed of the issues and their potential impact on a community and share this information with community members. But this is only the beginning. The challenge then is in knowing whom to approach for political support and how to gain their support. You can start becoming politically involved early in your career by becoming active in the local student nurses association, school boards, or citizen committees or attending council meetings.

- *Educator.* Because community nursing focuses on wellness and disease prevention, much of what the nurse does involves client education—of individuals, aggregates at risk of disease, politicians, or a community at large. Education is relatively inexpensive to provide. However, it is also difficult to evaluate the effect of the education because people may not act on the knowledge for months or years after the teaching moment. When planning teaching, you must be aware of the stage of development, educational level, and learning style of the community aggregate you intend to educate. The best learning programs are short; provide relevant, practical information; and can be easily incorporated into the learner's daily routine. For more information, see Chapter 24.

- *Collaborator.* A primary task of a community health nurse is to serve as a collaborator. Partnerships and coalitions can effectively address common concerns among different communities. Consider the following example: A community health nurse is concerned about the low level of immunization coverage among 2-year-olds in a particular community. He surveys some of the parents to determine their reasons for not obtaining vaccinations. The nurse discovers that the clinic's operating hours are inconvenient and that it takes several phone calls to get an appointment. The nurse also discovers that some offices are not reminding clients to return for missed appointments. The nurse schedules a meeting of the involved parents and area providers to resolve these issues. At the meeting, some larger issues are revealed, such as failure of state Medicaid agencies to reimburse the providers adequately and an insufficient number of providers in the community.

- *Counselor.* Once you have established rapport with a group, you may be consulted about a variety of health and non-health-related concerns. You must be cautious to offer counsel in areas within your scope of practice and make suggestions that are practical yet meet the needs of the community. Often, you may need only to serve as a witness to the group's concerns. Letting clients debate or work through issues empowers them.

- *Case manager.* Community nurses commonly make referrals to or collaborate with other health and social agencies. Be cautious in referring clients to these resources, because agency policies and financing change frequently. Also, because community agencies often operate on grants and time-restricted funding, a program that is available one month may be dissolved the following month. As a nurse, you will need to remain in contact with agencies to which clients are referred so that you remain aware of the current restrictions and availability of services. For example, a local group has established a free healthcare program for resident children who have no insurance. Volunteer pediatricians and nurses staff the free program. Pharmaceutical representatives provide the medical supplies and routine medications. Local specialists donate a limited number of hours to see children referred from the program. However, the available hours fill up very quickly, and often clients must wait more than a month for an appointment. Before enrolling families in the program, you would need to be aware of these limitations and share this information with clients.

KnowledgeCheck 42–4

Give an example of a nursing activity involved in each of the following community health roles: educator, advocate, case manager, counselor, and collaborator.

 Go to Chapter 42, **Knowledge Check Response Sheet and Answers,** on the Electronic Study Guide.

How Are Community Nursing Interventions Classified?

There are three basic levels of care in which nursing interventions can be classified: primary, secondary, and tertiary. Most community-oriented nursing practices are aimed at the primary (prevention) level.

Primary Interventions

The goal of primary (first-level) interventions is to promote health and prevent disease. Educating susceptible individuals with no known disease process is an example of a routine, primary intervention that community health nurses practice. For example, a nurse may educate junior high students about the risk of hepatitis B, the benefits of vaccination, and strategies to reduce the likelihood of exposure to contaminated body fluids. Other examples include collaborating with local agencies to provide clean and secure temporary housing for migrant farm workers,

and lobbying elected representatives for a ban on smoking in restaurants. Primary interventions are usually the least invasive and least expensive of the three levels of intervention.

Secondary Interventions

Secondary (second-level) interventions aim to reduce the impact of the disease process by early detection and treatment. For example, a community health nurse may screen a sexually active adolescent for hepatitis B and/or HIV. The adolescent has known risk factors but no apparent disease symptoms. The nurse will also educate the client on how to protect himself from sexually transmitted diseases, hepatitis B, and HIV in the future. Other examples of secondary interventions include providing outreach screening programs offering mammography, cholesterol testing, or PSA testing for prostate cancer.

Tertiary Interventions

The goal of tertiary (third-level) intervention is to halt disease progression and/or restore client functioning to the pre-disease state. The disease process is clinically apparent and client debilitation, including death, is likely without intervention. Tertiary level interventions are usually the most invasive and require the nurse to collaborate with other disciplines to provide treatment. For example, a student may report to a school nurse that he has been involved in unprotected sexual activities and is now complaining of generalized body aches and being tired all the time. The school nurse may refer the student to the public health clinic for sexually transmitted infection (STI), hepatitis B, and HIV screening. The student's blood work reveals that he has been exposed to the virus that causes hepatitis B. The nurse, in collaboration with the physician, provides medical treatment. There is no cure for hepatitis B, so the student also needs to learn how to prevent the spread of the disease to others.

 ## CriticalThinking 42–3

What level of intervention is required to address the concerns of Tanya and Tiffany ("Meet Your Patient")? Discuss your response.

KnowledgeCheck 42–5

For each of the nursing actions listed, identify the level of the nursing intervention as primary, secondary, or tertiary.

- Taking a client's blood pressure at a health fair.
- Administering insulin to an elderly person at an extended care facility.
- Teaching second-grade students to wash their hands correctly.

 Go to Chapter 42, **Knowledge Check Response Sheet and Answers,** on the Electronic Study Guide

What Career Opportunities Are Available for Community-Based Nurses?

The following are only a few of the many career opportunities for nurses who want to practice from a community-based perspective.

School Nursing

Nursing practice in the school setting began when educators realized that children with health problems had more difficulty learning. School nurses provide direct care for children with chronic health conditions such as asthma, hyperactivity disorder, and diabetes and for children who need routine procedures, such as catheterization, during the school day. School nurses perform mandated vision and hearing screenings and ensure that age-appropriate immunizations are documented. The nurse may also serve as a role model for students who lack parental support or who are struggling with peer pressure. For the most part, a school nurse is autonomous and must be capable of prioritizing and decision making.

Occupational Health

Occupational health nurses work primarily in industrial settings. Traditionally, occupational health nurses provided health teaching for employees and their families in an effort to reduce absentee hours and increase productivity. Few industries still use the occupational nurse in this manner. Instead, most retain nurses only to fulfill union contracts and to complete required medical paperwork. Thus, the responsibilities of the occupational health nurse may be limited to performing new-hire and annual screenings, tending to injured workers, completing random drug testing, and filing worker's compensation claims. To reduce costs, most large industries hire a staffing agency to provide trained occupational health nurses. Nursing autonomy and responsibility vary with the employer and the negotiated contract.

Parish Nursing

Parish nursing is a newly recognized community-oriented nursing specialty. However, for years nurse members of church congregations have been informally called on to provide consultation and participate in screening activities. The role of a parish nurse varies among congregations. For example, a large church of 1000 members may be able to appoint an official parish nurse from a group of willing, known nurse members. The nurse may donate her expertise and receive stipends to purchase needed supplies or educational materials. In another context, a nurse may facilitate a collaborative partnership

BOX 42–2 Parish Nursing on the Front Lines

Welcome Home Ministries

Reverend Carmen Warner-Robbins, MSN, RN, FAAN, MAT, established Welcome Home Ministries (WHM) in 1997 to help incarcerated women make the transition into a productive future. Warner-Robbins is a minister and holistic nurse practicing to meet the needs of the mind, body, and spirit, as well as the social and financial needs of incarcerated women.

Interventions

Many of the released women have a history of drug addiction and are estranged from their families, so making drug-free friends and having someone to be accountable to are vital steps in gaining control of their lives. Warner-Robbins counsels receptive women prior to release and again when they are actually leaving the prison. Most of the women are released at 5:30 A.M. with little money, nowhere to go, and no real friends to turn to. WHM provides a nurse or other member to meet with the woman and have breakfast to discuss "what to do now." The program has grown to offer weekly sessions for the participants.

Evaluation and Follow-Up

After the first 2 years of operation, the program conducted a follow-up of participants. Only one WHM participant had been reincarcerated. Members meet regularly to share their success stories of increased spiritual growth and strategies to maintain drug recovery, find a safe place to live, attend school, find a job, reestablish relationships with children and family, and actively help other previously incarcerated women succeed. The successful WHM participants are now generating new interventions to address common challenges they experience.

You can obtain the complete text of the June 2002 article "Holistic Nursing on the Front Lines" by Parsons and Warner-Robbins from the *American Journal of Nursing, 102*(6), 73–77.

Nursing in Correctional Facilities

Correctional facilities have a medical team that provides routine examinations and acute care to inmates on a scheduled, but intermittent, basis. Most facilities also have a nurse available 24 hours a day to administer medications and perform screenings for communicable diseases. The level of nursing autonomy is high in most prison facilities, and the nurse also tends to perform some occupational health duties for the assigned facility staff. For their own safety, nurses must meet certain physical requirements and complete special weapons training before working in most correctional facilities.

Public Health Clinics

Many community nurses practice within local and state departments of health, including public health clinics. The services offered by health departments can range from basic to comprehensive, based on financial constraints, such as the tax base of the community. Large cities tend to have many nurses. Each nurse may specialize in an area such as immunizations, prenatal health, or school health. Smaller communities may have only one full-time nurse providing all services. The autonomy and scope of practice of public health nurses are often limited by the philosophy of the political administration.

Disaster Services Nursing

A *disaster* is any event inflicting widespread loss of life and destruction of property. Disasters can be due to human activity, such as the terrorist attacks of 2001 or the West Virginia mining accidents of 2006, or can be natural, such as hurricanes, earthquakes, and floods. Community-oriented nursing emphasizes community assessment and education to prevent disasters when possible and to reduce the number of casualties when disasters occur.

In a disaster, the nurse's scope of practice depends upon her skills and competence level. If a disaster has been declared, the registered nurse may practice in any state under the direction of the American Red Cross. "Good Samaritan" laws protect nurses from liability provided that they are providing care on a volunteer basis and in a manner that another prudent nurse of the same educational level in the same circumstances would provide. In large-scale disasters, nurses are typically needed to staff first-aid stations, assess casualties, assign priorities for care, administer treatment to stabilize the wounded, facilitate transport to local hospitals, and provide health care in temporary shelters. For additional information on disaster preparedness and preparation for terrorist attacks,

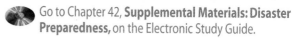

Go to Chapter 42, **Supplemental Materials: Disaster Preparedness,** on the Electronic Study Guide.

between a church and a community organization, such as a hospital. The partnership may allow for paying the nurse to provide a full-time ministry within the congregation and, at the same time, meet a hospital need for community service. The level of autonomy and responsibility of parish nurses varies with the expectations of the appointment or collaborative partnerships. One nurse's parish ministry is described in Box 42–2.

International Nursing

International nursing includes voluntary and paid positions for nurses in foreign countries. Voluntary positions are often time-limited missions to provide relief services after a disaster or to offer services that would otherwise be unavailable, such as providing specialty surgery. Doctors Without Borders and Heart to Heart are examples of voluntary opportunities. Paid positions include opportunities through the World Health Organization (WHO), the Peace Corps, and the Foreign Service Commission. These positions are challenging and require a high level of autonomy.

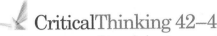 CriticalThinking 42–4

Increase your self-knowledge: Assume you are going to be a community-based nurse. Of the many career opportunities available, which work do you think you would rather do? Explain why.

Practical Knowledge
knowing how

Community nursing care should be delivered in a practical, culturally sensitive manner. The nursing process follows the same steps you have studied in the previous chapters but uses different forms and different language when your client is a community.

| Assessment |

Community assessment is usually ongoing and requires the nurse to collaborate with and compile information from a variety of sources. The assessment approach is based on the type of community, the purpose of the assessment, and personal preference. Most beginning students elect to assess a geopolitical community because the data are more readily available than data from aggregate groups. Therefore, we will focus on the geopolitical community assessment procedure.

- *Windshield survey.* Community assessment usually begins with a windshield survey. A **windshield survey** is performed by observing the community through your automobile window or otherwise being physically present in the area. It is similar to general observation of the individual client in that it provides an overview and allows you to see the community in its natural state. You may need to repeat the survey over a period of time at different times of the day to get an accurate picture of the community.
- *Databases.* You can also obtain data from publicly available resources, such as birth records, marriage licenses, newspapers, and community web sites. Internet search engines can help you obtain demographic information, morbidity and mortality data, vital statistics, educational levels, criminal activity, political leadership issues, and/or information about community resources.
- *Client perceptions.* You will also gather information about how individuals in the community perceive the community and its state of health. You cannot contact every person, but through community forums and informal conversations, you should be able to assess a cross-section of the population. This is not only an important part of your assessment, but also an excellent way to establish rapport, convey your concerns, and develop a working relationship with key community members. When you prepare to intervene in the community, you will find that this time was wisely spent, because community members are more likely to participate in the plan if they are involved from the beginning.

| Nursing Diagnosis |

After a thorough assessment, you will analyze the complete set of data and compile a list of community strengths and limitations. Prioritize the list, considering priorities that have been identified by the client, availability of funding, and the political feasibility of addressing the issue.

In community practice, you need nursing diagnoses that describe the health status of individuals, families, groups, and entire communities. Recall from Chapter 4 that the NANDA taxonomy of nursing diagnoses can be used in any nursing setting or specialty. You would simply add the term *community* to other NANDA labels when creating a community-based diagnosis: for example, Decisional Conflict (Community) related to safety needs of the homeless population. In addition, the NANDA taxonomy includes three diagnoses that specifically describe the health status of a community:

- Ineffective Community Coping
- Readiness for Enhanced Community Coping
- Ineffective Management of Therapeutic Regimen: Community

In contrast, the Omaha system was developed specifically for use in community settings (Martin & Norris, 1996). In addition to nursing diagnoses, it contains standardized terminology for outcomes and interventions. For a complete overview,

 Go to the **Omaha system web site** at www.omahasystem.org/

For an expanded discussion of the Omaha problem classification scheme,

 Go to Chapter 42, **Standardized Language, Omaha Problem Classification Scheme,** in Volume 2.

| toward evidence-based practice |

Kemper, A. R., Davis, M. M., & Freed, G. L. (2002). Expected adverse events in a mass smallpox vaccination campaign. *Effective Clinical Practice, 5*(2), 84–90.

Based on a review of historical data on adverse effects associated with smallpox vaccination, the researchers calculated anticipated risks associated with the current campaign to launch wide-scale smallpox vaccinations among the general public. Two vaccination strategies were compared: vaccinating individuals 1 to 29 years of age only; and vaccinating individuals 1 to 65 years of age only. To reduce the risk of vaccine-related complications, persons of high risk for complications were excluded. Researchers estimate that 25% of the general population meet those criteria and are therefore ineligible for vaccination. Known vaccine risks were applied to information about the general population. Fever (fewer than 1 case per 5 vaccine recipients) and rash (fewer than 1 case per 100 vaccine recipients) were among the most common complications. Serious adverse effects were encephalitis (fewer than 3 cases per million) and death (fewer than 2 cases per million).

Applying this data to known population figures, researchers concluded the following:

- Approximately 25% of the population would not be immunized because of high risk of complications.
- If a program were launched to immunize individuals aged 1 to 29, it is estimated that 1600 serious adverse events and 190 deaths would occur.
- Extending the immunizations to those aged 1 to 65 would result in 4600 serious adverse events and 285 deaths.

Bicknell, W., & James, K. (2003). The new cell culture smallpox vaccine should be offered to the general population. *Reviews of Medical Virology, 13* (1), 5–15.

Bicknell and James support the proposal to conduct mass immunizations against smallpox. They propose a decision-making model for countries to use to determine whether to undertake mass immunizations. The factors that the researchers maintain must be evaluated include the following:

- Perceived risk of attack with smallpox as a bioterrorist agent
- Risk of secondary spread from another country

- Known risks of vaccination
- Known effectiveness of vaccine in post-exposure vaccination
- The number of high risk individuals ineligible for vaccination in the general population
- The capabilities of the country's healthcare team
- The general economic status of the country

Based on this model, Bicknell and James support mass immunizations in the United States and propose a major role for the World Health Organization in developing immunization programs worldwide.

Mortimer, P. P. (2003). The new cell culture smallpox vaccine should not be offered to the general population. *Reviews of Medical Virology, 13*(1), 17–20.

Mortimer argues against wide-scale smallpox vaccinations. His argument is multifaceted:

- Any smallpox vaccination program should not be undertaken until there is credible evidence of a real risk from smallpox as an agent of terror.
- Vaccines grown from cell cultures have not been sufficiently tested to be shown to be safe and effective.
- The smallpox vaccine must have a better safety record before it is dispensed to the public.

Mortimer also discusses major concerns regarding the potential compromise of other vaccination programs in the United States. He favors an aggressive containment of epicenters of smallpox release. Data from previous smallpox outbreaks have shown that post-exposure vaccination within 4 days of contact and revaccination within 1 week for those vaccinated previously is highly effective against serious illness.

---

1. Based on the above research and accompanying interpretations of the data, are you for or against mass immunizations against smallpox?

2. Use the results of the study and the reviews to justify your opinion. What are the benefits of immunization of the general population? What are the risks?

 Go to Chapter 42, **Toward Evidence-Based Practice Suggested Responses,** on the Electronic Study Guide.

| Planning Outcomes/Evaluation |

In the community you will need to write goals and outcomes for aggregates. The Healthy People 2010 goals are aggregate goals. The NOC and Omaha taxonomies provide standardized terms for stating community goals.

For guidelines in using these two taxonomies,

 Go to Chapter 42, **Standardized Language, Using the NOC and Omaha Systems to Write Aggregate Goals,** in Volume 2.

| Planning Interventions/Implementation |

As a community health nurse, you will need interventions to promote and preserve the health of individuals, aggregates, and communities. Both NIC and the Omaha system provide standardized vocabularies for aggregate interventions.

The NIC taxonomy includes 16 interventions specifically designed for community health *The Omaha taxonomy* provides four *intervention categories* that can be used in community-oriented nursing practice. For guidelines,

 Go to Chapter 42, **Standardized Language, Using the NIC and Omaha Interventions Labels,** in Volume 2.

PUTTING IT ALL TOGETHER

The process for conducting a community assessment may appear overwhelming. This final section will attempt to apply the process to situations you are likely to encounter in the community.

As a community health nurse employed by the local health department within the immunization clinic, you have been hired into a new position created by federal and state grant monies to investigate why immunization levels are so low among 2-year-olds in Census Tract 15. How you would approach your new nursing career?

1. *Define the community.* Determine the physical boundaries of Census Tract 15, a geopolitical community.
2. *Learn the community.* Start interacting with the community to build rapport. Begin the ongoing assessment by conducting windshield surveys,

searching for information through reputable databases, and talking with community members.

3. *Focus the data collection.* Focus on the information that will help you determine possible causes of low immunization rates. In this case, the priority problem has already been defined by the financing agency.

 CriticalThinking 42–5

What data would you want to look at? What are possible reasons for low immunization rates?

4. *Analyze the data.* After working with the community for about 6 months, you have spoken at parenting classes about the need to vaccinate children. Several community members told you that they thought their child had already received all necessary vaccinations or that their doctor had said to wait until they have better insurance. You will need to arrange a meeting with the local doctors to discuss the low immunization status. The doctors explain that many vaccinations are very expensive and that they cannot afford to give them based on the reimbursement they receive from Medicaid.
5. *Plan care.* Using the Omaha system, you could generate a care plan to address some of the issues raised by the community members and the doctors.
6. *Assess results, and follow up.* The community assessment process is never actually complete because the community is fluid and constantly changing. However, you need to bring resolution to identified needs and desired outcomes. In this case, you would share your approach to addressing the suspected reasons for low immunization with the community members, area doctors, financing agency, and local health policy committee. You will also need to continue to monitor and evaluate the situation to provide communication updates to the appropriate groups.

 Go to Chapter 42, **Resources for Caregivers and Health Professionals,** on the Electronic Study Guide.

 Go to Chapter 42, **Reading More About Community Nursing,** on the Electronic Study Guide.

 Bibliography: Go to Volume 2, Bibliography.

43 CHAPTER Nursing in Home Care

Learning Outcomes

After completing this chapter, you should be able to:

✳ Identify the primary goal of home care.

✳ Explain some advantages and disadvantages of the home care environment.

✳ Categorize the various agencies that deliver home health care according to purpose, client served, and funding source.

✳ Identify four key roles of the nurse in home health care.

✳ Describe how home health care is reimbursed.

✳ Explain how clients are referred to home health care.

✳ Outline the steps required to prepare for a home visit.

✳ Explain the role of the nurse in treating caregiver strain.

✳ Describe the process for evaluating a home environment.

✳ Cite at least five examples of how care may be modified in the home setting.

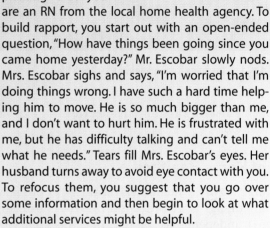

MEET Your Patient

Flora Escobar is a 78-year-old woman living at home with her 80-year-old husband, Roland. Until recently both have enjoyed good health. Roland suffered a cerebrovascular accident (CVA or stroke) 3 weeks ago. He was briefly hospitalized and then spent 2 weeks in a skilled nursing facility (SNF) for additional physical care and therapy. He returned home yesterday and will be followed by the local home health agency. You have been asked to make an initial visit today.

Flora Escobar greets you at the door. She is a petite woman who appears exhausted. She is wearing an apron over casual slacks and a sweater. She opens the door with her left hand but is carrying a glass of water with her right, and her apron pockets are stuffed with pill bottles. The hallway is narrow and partially blocked with a bedside commode, walker, and tray table. Mr. Escobar is in a hospital bed that has been placed in the living room. He is a tall, stocky man who is sitting up in bed but clearly listing to the left. He is dressed in pajamas and robe.

You begin your visit by introducing yourself and explaining that you are an RN from the local home health agency. To build rapport, you start out with an open-ended question, "How have things been going since you came home yesterday?" Mr. Escobar slowly nods. Mrs. Escobar sighs and says, "I'm worried that I'm doing things wrong. I have such a hard time helping him to move. He is so much bigger than me, and I don't want to hurt him. He is frustrated with me, but he has difficulty talking and can't tell me what he needs." Tears fill Mrs. Escobar's eyes. Her husband turns away to avoid eye contact with you. To refocus them, you suggest that you go over some information and then begin to look at what additional services might be helpful.

Imagine how stressed Mrs. Escobar must feel. How do you think you could best help this family? In this chapter we will answer these questions as we discuss home health nursing.

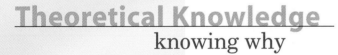

Theoretical Knowledge
knowing why

The first true home care agencies in the United States were established in the 1880s, and most nursing care was delivered in the home until the 1920s (National Association for Home Care [NAHC], 2001). But as the technical aspects of health care began to dominate, the hospital became the primary healthcare setting. By the early 1960s, there were just 1100 home care agencies in the United States. However, Medicare's enactment in 1965 prompted new growth in the home-care field by making skilled nursing care and therapy available to older adults and disabled people in their homes (NAHC, 2001). In the last two decades, home care has grown even more dramatically as the population has aged and the rising cost of care has led to shorter hospital stays and increased use of the home as a site for care delivery. The technology that has been used in the hospital—in modified form—has followed the patient home. The growing presence of healthcare technology in the home has led to increasingly complex care and growing concerns about quality of life. Home care, like hospital-based care, has become a mix of high-tech and high-touch.

WHAT IS HOME HEALTHCARE?

Home health care is the delivery of a variety of health-related services in the client's home. The National Association for Home Care (NAHC) reports that more than 20,000 providers deliver home care services to some 7.6 million clients each year in the United States, with annual costs estimated at about $40 billion in 2001 (NAHC, 2001).

Home healthcare is appropriate when a client needs ongoing care that exceeds the abilities of friends and family. Older adults may use home healthcare services when they need ongoing care but choose to avoid placement in a skilled nursing facility. People of any age may require home-care service when they are recuperating from illness or surgery or when they are terminally ill. Chronically ill adults and children may

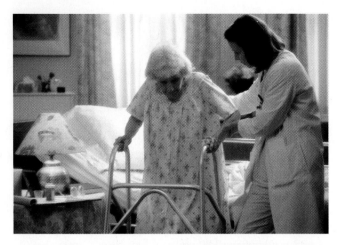

FIGURE 43–1   **The home is a window into the client's life.**

43–1 Skilled Nursing Services

- Patient assessment
- Ongoing monitoring of patient status
- Management and coordination of the patient's plan of care
- Evaluation of response to medications or treatment
- Medication instruction
- Teaching clients or caregivers to provide care or therapies
- Disease-related teaching (e.g., diabetes education)
- Complex tasks such as infusion therapy, wound care, or ventilator management

receive home health care for ongoing care or to avoid hospitalization.

Goals of Home Healthcare

The primary goal in home healthcare is to promote self-care. Nursing activities are directed at fostering the client's independence or teaching the family or other caregivers to assist the client with ongoing health needs. This approach may be very different from what you have experienced in other clinical settings. For example, in the hospital the nurses provided direct care for Mr. Escobar. This included bathing, toileting, giving medications, and ongoing assessment. In home health, the focus is to help the Escobars manage Mr. Escobar's care at home independently. Initially you may work with Mrs. Escobar, showing her how to administer medicines and explaining their function. However, your goal is to have her independently handle this task. Similarly, you may show the Escobars strategies for turning and moving that are comfortable for both of them, but you must be certain they understand how to use this information so they can handle these tasks when you leave.

Advantages and Disadvantages

The hospital environment is controlled. Surfaces are regularly disinfected, supplies are stocked, and foods, medications, and other therapies are readily available. Computers on the unit store information about the patient that is almost immediately accessible. In addition, the hospital-based nurse is a member of a large team of healthcare providers that includes other nurses, the primary care provider, various therapists, social workers, a pastoral care provider, and even a business office staff to ensure that reimbursement will be forthcoming.

In contrast, when you are in a client's home, surprisingly little is within your control. The home may be spotless or filthy, food plentiful or scarce, and supplies

readily available or unreliable. The television, radio, or stereo may be on at a loud volume, a dog may bark continually, or several young children may be playing nearby and repeatedly interrupt your conversations with the client or primary caregiver. Thus, to succeed in home health care, nurses must be able to improvise, to think and act quickly, to work independently, to adapt to the client's environment and needs, and to be flexible and resourceful.

One distinct advantage of home healthcare is that it allows you to see the client differently. The home is a window into the client's life through which you can see his personal environment—how he lives, eats, and negotiates his world (Figure 43–1). The photos, mementos, personal belongings, and other things the client values and cherishes provide clues to his strengths, resources, and motivation.

Nursing care in the home environment is also different in the following ways:

- The nurse is a guest in the patient's home. The patient and family determine whether they are willing to let the nurse enter the home to deliver care.

- The nurse is responsible for making the assessments and determining whether the primary care provider should be advised of patient changes.

- The nurse must bring all supplies or arrange to have them predelivered.

- The nurse must be able to distinguish between skilled services, which are eligible for reimbursement from Medicare, and homemaker services. **Skilled services** are services that must be performed or supervised by a licensed healthcare professional (Box 43–1). Homemaker services (e.g., cleaning, meal preparation) are available to clients only if the principal reason for home care is a skilled service. These services are provided by home health aides.

• The nurse is more self-sufficient. Often there are no other team members immediately available for support, assistance, or consultation. The nurse must enlist family to help in delivering care and to take over care when the nurse leaves the home.

Home health nursing also differs from community health care. Community health nurses provide care for individuals, families, and groups with an emphasis on population-based care. In contrast, home health nursing focuses on the individual in collaboration with the client's support system.

KnowledgeCheck 43–1

Identify at least four skilled services that may be provided in the home.

 Go to Chapter 43, **Knowledge Check Response Sheet and Answers,** on the Electronic Study Guide.

WHO PROVIDES HOME HEALTHCARE?

Home healthcare is provided by a wide variety of healthcare professionals employed by or working in cooperation with home healthcare agencies.

Home Health Agencies

The various types of agencies that deliver home healthcare may be categorized by purpose. *Direct care agencies* are the most common. They focus on direct client interaction by providing skilled care, associated therapies and health services, home health aides, chore workers, and delivery of **respite care** (relief for family caregivers). *Indirect service agencies* also play a vital role in home health care. Examples of indirect home services include pharmaceutical and infusion companies and suppliers of durable medical equipment.

Home health agencies may also be grouped according to the type of client served. The most obvious specialty home service agency is hospice care (discussed shortly). This may be a separate agency or a division of a home health agency. Still other agencies specialize in caring for patients with complex diseases, such as AIDS, or ventilator-dependent clients, or patients of a certain age group (services for older adults or chronically ill children).

These agencies may take on many forms based on funding source, profit or nonprofit status, and relationship with other healthcare organizations.

• *Public agencies* are official or governmental agencies. They may be organized at the city, county, state, or national level. Public agencies are usually funded by taxes along with reimbursement from insurance companies. The local health department is a good example of this type of agency. Health departments work chiefly at the community level, although these agencies often also conduct some home health services, especially when tracking clients in some of their disease management programs.

• *Voluntary agencies* are prominent in the delivery of home health care. These agencies are normally governed by a board of directors and funded by donations, endowments, and third-party (insurance) reimbursement. Many *hospice organizations* (groups that provide care for people who are frail, terminally ill, dying, or not expected to improve) are voluntary organizations.

• *Proprietary organizations* are corporate or privately owned businesses that aim to make a profit. These agencies receive payment from insurance companies but also accept private-pay clients. Proprietary organizations may provide traditional home health services as well as private-duty care and other services that assist individuals to remain independent.

• *Hospital-based agencies* serve as an extension of the services provided by the hospital. Clients who no longer meet the criteria for continued hospitalization may be transferred to home care for continued services. The benefit of this type of agency lies in the ease of transition between hospital and home.

The Home Health Team

In home healthcare, the registered nurse serves as the coordinator of health services, but other members of the healthcare team may also provide care. The team varies according to the needs of the client but is usually multidisciplinary. It may include physicians; nurse practitioners; registered nurses; licensed practical or vocational nurses; home health aides; physical, speech, or occupational therapists; respiratory therapists; nutritionists; social workers; pharmacists; podiatrists; dentists; chaplains; and family members.

The Home Health Nurse

Your principal roles as a home health nurse are discussed in this section. As you take on each of these roles, you will also need to function as a skillful communicator. Communication is crucial in home care because you must establish a good rapport with the client and family and communicate frequently with other members of the healthcare team.

• *Direct care provider.* As a direct care provider, you may administer medications, dress wounds, or perform other skilled, complex tasks.

• *Client/family educator.* Recall that the goal of home healthcare is to promote self-care. Instead of focusing on doing the care, you will be focusing on helping the client or family take over the care. You can easily see how you will need communication skills in

BOX 43-2

Home Healthcare and Home Hospice Care

Home Healthcare

- The purpose of home healthcare is to promote self-care.
- Nursing activities are directed at fostering the client's independence or teaching the family or other care-givers to assist the client with ongoing health needs.

Home Hospice Care

- The purpose of home hospice care is to promote comfort and quality of life.
- Nursing activities are directed at providing comfort and managing symptoms.

this role. You must be able to clearly explain the care required, the rationale for the care, and how to safely perform the care. This requires patience, skill, and repetition.

- *Client advocate.* As client advocate, you support the client's right to make healthcare decisions and protect the client from harm if he is unable to make decisions. In home care, the client and family are directly in charge of the plan of care. You must advocate for services the client needs. This may mean attempting to secure additional home health support to avoid hospitalization, or it may mean advocating for another level of service, such as referral to hospice or placement in the hospital based on your assessment of the client and discussion with the client and family.

- *Care coordinator.* As the *case manager,* you will need to gather data at an initial visit and develop a plan of care that addresses the client's needs. This plan may include additional visits by you, as well as delivery of therapies and services by other professionals in the home.

KnowledgeCheck 43–2

What roles does the nurse assume in home care? List and describe them.

 Go to Chapter 43, **Knowledge Check Response Sheet and Answers,** on the Electronic Study Guide.

Hospice Nurses

As you learned in Chapter 15, **hospice nursing** focuses on care of patients who are dying or whose condition is not expected to improve. Hospice services are provided in the home, in the hospital, in nursing homes, and in homes specifically designed as hospices. The goal of hospice care is to promote comfort and quality of life. For these reasons, the bulk of hospice services are provided in the client's home. Because the client is not expected to recover, home hospice care is quite different from traditional home care. Rather than focusing on promotion of self-care and independence, the focus of care shifts to providing comfort and managing symptoms (Box 43–2).

Generally, the hospice nurse assumes the same roles as the home health nurse, but the emphasis shifts. When functioning as a direct care provider, the hospice nurse assesses the client's condition, monitors the client's response to interventions to relieve distress, and teaches the client and family how to adjust medications and care to improve comfort. In the educator role, the hospice nurse teaches the client and family interventions to control pain and relieve symptoms. The roles of communicator and client advocate assume prime importance. As the patient's condition deteriorates, the nurse, in conjunction with the family, must continue to advocate for the client. Generally there is less coordination of multiple services in the home. Instead there may be greater emphasis on consultation for pain management. (For more information on hospice care, see Chapter 15.)

Home Health Reimbursement

Medicare, Medicaid, private insurance, and individual payments reimburse home care services. **Medicare** is a federally funded healthcare system designed to provide health coverage for persons who are over 65, disabled, or diagnosed with end-stage renal disease (chronic renal failure). Medicare is the largest payor for home health care. Reimbursement by Medicare for home care depends on the following criteria:

- *The client must need skilled care.* Other services may also be provided, but the primary purpose for establishing care must be based on a skilled need.

- *The client must be homebound.* Homebound is defined as having a condition that restricts the client's ability to leave the home. Leaving the home requires special assistance, transportation, supportive devices, and/or an escort.

- *The client must require care that is part-time and intermittent.*

- *The plan of care must be authorized by the physician and recertified every 62 days.* For the client to continue to receive care, there must be evidence of continued need that remains acute.

- *The care must be medically necessary and reasonable.* The plan of care must address the client's health concerns and have clearly delineated outcomes. The expectations of the patient must be reasonable.

Medicaid is a program jointly sponsored by the federal government and the state to provide services to people with limited financial resources. In many states the criteria for reimbursement are identical to those required by Medicare. However, each state determines what services will be part of its medical assistance plan. Private insurance companies may also offer home health services. The type and extent of covered services are specified in each separate insurance group and plan.

Many clients require assistance in the home but do not meet criteria for reimbursement from Medicare, Medicaid, or their private insurer. Others simply do not have health insurance. Services are available on a private pay basis, usually from a proprietary home health agency. Frequently, older clients require home health assistance but may not need skilled services. For example, they may need assistance with grocery shopping, meal planning, or transportation. The client or family may contact an agency to provide chore worker assistance for these services. Services are billed directly to the client. Unfortunately, these services are usually available only to affluent clients and families. Those with limited income may be forced to do without needed services. This disparity may lead to inadequate care and illness, hospitalizations, or death. This is one driving force behind the calls for healthcare reform.

 CriticalThinking 43–1

Review the scenario focused on Mr. Escobar. What members of the home health team may be required to provide care? Why?

WHAT IS THE FUTURE OF HOME HEALTHCARE?

Health care analysts have predicted several changes in home care over the next few decades:

- *Continued growth.* Over the next several decades, the use of home care is expected to rise sharply. The demonstrated cost effectiveness of home care, as well as the aging of the population, is sparking this rise.
- *Increased use of the home for hospice care.* The acceptance of the home as a place of comfort and care, as well as concerns about the cost of care, has increased the number of persons who choose this option for end-of-life care.
- *Increased technology.* Technological advances, such as online or telemedicine consultation, will make it safe and affordable to deliver complex care in the home and allow home health nurses to provide a growing array of services. Computerized monitoring and charting will allow home health agencies to bet-

ter coordinate care, receive needed supplies, and closely monitor costs.

- *Continued research.* Research on home care has been limited. Future research will focus on strategies to improve the effectiveness of care, identifying predictors of need for rehospitalization, and integrating home care into overall community-based services.

Practical Knowledge
knowing how

As a nurse working in home health care, your days will vary widely. Normally your caseload will be contained within a limited geographic boundary, so that you can concentrate on delivering care rather than driving. If you want to envision what it would be like to be a home health nurse, you need only to look at the list of services Medicare deems to be skilled, in Box 43–1.

HOW ARE CLIENTS REFERRED TO HOME HEALTHCARE?

Referrals to home health care come from a variety of sources. Hospital-based agencies have a built-in referral base. If the primary physician or nursing staff believe the client would benefit from home health services, they refer the patient to the agency for evaluation while he is still hospitalized. Often these agencies have intake coordinators who work in the hospital and review clients for suitability of services, gathering information from the chart, the client, the family, and the hospital team. Home services are arranged prior to discharge.

If the hospital does not have its own home agency, the client may still be referred to home health services during the hospital stay. Ideally, a discharge planner gathers information, secures the order from the physician, and makes arrangements. In some smaller hospitals, this task falls to the staff nurse on the unit.

Referrals may also come from doctors, nurses, primary care offices and clinics, mental health workers, and other health providers, as well as directly from families and clients. Most home health agencies evaluate clients to determine whether they are eligible for services that are reimbursable by insurance. They may also offer services that the client may pay for independently.

HOW DO I MAKE A HOME VISIT?

In home health care, services are brought to the client in the form of a home visit. The home visit has three phases: preparation before the visit, nursing care

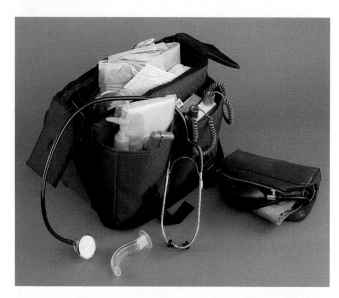

FIGURE 43–2   The home health nursing bag contains some standard items but is usually customized according to the requirements of the clients that the nurse will see.

during the visit, and evaluation after the visit. For the major activities in each phase,

 Go to Chapter 43, **Conducting a Home Visit,** in Volume 2.

Before the Visit

You should first review the client's chart and referral form to determine why you are making the visit. You may also need to review material on the client's disorder, medications, or treatment plan. Then you can begin to plan for the visit. What supplies will you need? What teaching materials will you need? What are the goals of the visit? Does the agency need additional client information, such as insurance data, to provide care?

You will need to find the address and get directions to the home. Telephone the client to notify him of the planned date and time of the visit and to determine whether his health status has changed since the referral was made. This will allow you to bring additional equipment along if you need it.

Supplies

Home health nurses usually carry a nursing bag (Figure 43–2). The nursing bag is often customized to the case load of the nurse and normally contains the following:

- Hand-washing supplies (e.g., soap, paper towels, or antibacterial solution)
- Stethoscope
- Sphygmomanometers in a variety of sizes
- Thermometers (oral and rectal)

- Small equipment (scissors, forceps, penlight, staple remover)
- Tape measure (with plastic coating that can be cleaned, or several disposable paper ones)
- Plastic apron
- Gloves, sterile and clean
- An assortment of gauze dressings
- Tape
- Cotton balls
- Occupational Safety and Health Administration (OSHA) supplies: mask, protective eyewear, disinfectant spray, disposable gowns to protect clothing
- A variety of syringes and needles (this varies widely among agencies because of safety concerns)
- Venipuncture supplies
- Airway and resuscitation mask
- Paper supplies (e.g., agency forms, business cards, local maps)

You may need other supplies, such as medications, scale, and transfer belt, depending on the requirements of the clients that you will see. (Note: In some states, nurses are not permitted to carry medicines because of safety concerns. You will need to check on the rules that apply to your state.) If the patient requires frequent dressing changes or treatments that require supplies (e.g., tube feedings) it is best to have the supplies delivered directly to the client's house to reduce the number of materials that you must carry.

Safety Considerations

As you drive to the home, begin to make your assessment. Locate the stores, hospital, and community resources. What is the overall character of the neighborhood? Does this appear to be a safe neighborhood? What are the conditions of the approach to the home?

Safety for yourself and the client is an essential consideration in home health care. Bring your impressions about neighborhood safety and home safety with you into the home. You must evaluate whether the environment contributes to the client's health problems. In addition, you must also provide for your own safety. For suggestions about the safe delivery of home health care,

 Go to Chapter 43, **Safety Considerations in Home Care,** in Volume 2.

KnowledgeCheck 43–3

What are the major tasks that must be completed before making a home visit?

 Go to Chapter 43, **Knowledge Check Response Sheet and Answers,** on the Electronic Study Guide.

At the Visit

When you arrive at the home, you must remember that this is the patient's domain. Knock, and wait to be invited in. Home health nurses are guests of their clients. Observe common courtesies. Introduce yourself to the client and family. Be respectful of their home, as well as their beliefs, values, practices, and cultural preferences.

The first few minutes of the initial visit set the tone for the relationship among client, family, nurse, and agency (Figure 43–3). This is your opportunity to develop rapport and trust. Introducing yourself, waiting for permission to enter, and treating the client and family members with respect help to establish rapport.

If this is an initial visit, you may need to verify or complete client data on the referral form. You should also offer your card, material on contacting the home health agency, and information on the client's rights, financial policies of the agency, and so on. As you do all this, you also gather data. Who answered your questions? What is the relationship between the caregiver and the client? How do they interact?

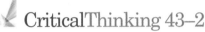 CriticalThinking 43–2
Review the case of Mr. Escobar. What information did you gain from the first few minutes of the visit?

| Assessment |

On the initial visit, you will need to perform an assessment, which establishes the baseline and determines the type of care required. This assessment might include health history, review of all medications—prescribed, over-the-counter, and alternative—pertinent family and social history, mental status, functional ability, availability of family and informal support and caregivers, nutritional status, and assessment of the home environment. Often a full assessment requires multiple visits.

In 1998, Medicare began requiring home health agencies to collect specific information for all Medicare clients they serve. This data set is called the Outcome and Assessment Information Set (OASIS). OASIS data must be collected at the start of care, with each recertification (every 60 days), and at the termination of care. For an example of the OASIS form,

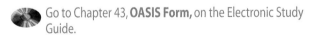 Go to Chapter 43, **OASIS Form,** on the Electronic Study Guide.

Medicare uses these data to determine the effectiveness of care and to monitor client outcomes. In addition to the required OASIS information, many agencies use additional assessment tools created specifically for their needs.

It is also important to assess the needs of the caregivers. These are the family members, friends,

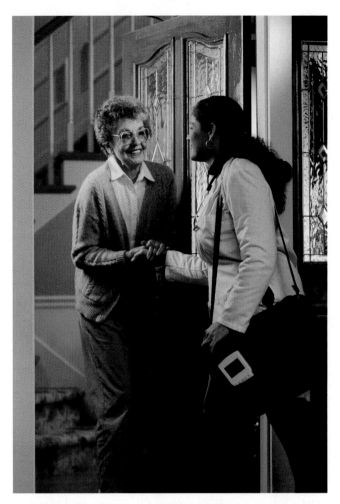

FIGURE 43–3 The first few minutes of the initial visit set the tone for the relationship among client, family, nurse, and agency.

and support system in the home. To be successful in home care, you must be willing to work *with* the caregivers. Take time at each visit to speak with them, making sure to include them in your assessment, plan of care, and teaching. Assessment of the caregivers often allows you to determine what services are needed in the home. Often, caregivers have health problems of their own that affect their ability to provide care for another. This is common among older couples.

| Nursing Diagnosis |

As in any setting, the nursing diagnoses are based on the client's responses to illness and care. As a nurse working in home healthcare, you will work with clients with numerous medical and nursing diagnoses. A frequent nursing diagnosis, Caregiver Role Strain, is discussed below. Other key concerns in the home are home safety, which we discuss at length in Chapter 21, and infection control, which we discuss in Chapter 20 and will address directly below.

Caregiver Role Strain

Providing care to a loved one at home is often a constant job, especially when finances don't allow a family to hire a home health aide. Round-the-clock caregiving duties can lead to physical exhaustion, social isolation, resentment, sadness, or depression. In addition, family members who become seriously ill are no longer able to function in their usual roles. These role changes may be difficult for both the ill person and the caregiver. For example, imagine that your mother suddenly became very ill and you became her primary caregiver. This would be a reversal of the roles you both are used to, and it may be emotionally taxing, especially if you are already exhausted and isolated from your friends.

Given these factors, it is not surprising that the two nursing diagnoses most commonly applicable to loved ones providing care at home are Caregiver Role Strain and Risk for Caregiver Role Strain. These diagnoses identify loved ones for whom the burden of delivering care has become—or is at risk of becoming—overwhelming. Common signs of caregiver role strain include difficulty adjusting to role changes, fatigue, isolation, and depression.

KnowledgeCheck 43–4

- Why are the first few minutes of the initial visit so important?
- Identify five things that should be assessed at an initial home visit.

 Go to Chapter 43, **Knowledge Check Response Sheet and Answers,** on the Electronic Study Guide.

 CriticalThinking 43–3

What, if any, evidence of caregiver strain does Mrs. Escobar exhibit?

Standardized Terminology for Nursing Diagnoses

Recall from the nursing process chapters of this text that various disciplines, including nursing, have developed classifications of standardized terminology (also called taxonomies, vocabularies, and languages) for describing their work and for planning and documenting care. You are familiar with the NANDA taxonomy of nursing diagnoses; however, home care nurses more commonly use the Clinical Care Classification (CCC) because it is linked to the OASIS reporting forms that are required for Medicare participation and payment. If you need to review the concept of standardized nursing language, see Chapters 4, 5, and 6. For complete information on the CCC and complete lists of diagnoses, outcomes, and interventions,

 Go to the **Clinical Care Classification** web site at **www.sabacare.com**

The CCC system consists of 21 care components and an accompanying coding structure that parallels the nursing process and links the CCC diagnosis and intervention systems. To see the CCC care components,

 Go to Chapter 43, **Standardized Language, CCC Care Components,** in Volume 2.

The CCC also contains 182 diagnostic categories—59 are derived from NANDA diagnostic categories, and the remaining 123 terms are subcategories that provide further definition of the problem. Approximately 50 of the 182 terms are criteria that are especially applicable to home care. Common CCC nursing diagnoses used in the home include Self-Care Deficit, Impaired Skin Integrity, Impaired Mobility, Altered Family Processes, Impaired Home Maintenance Management, Knowledge Deficit, and of course, Caregiver Strain. For other examples of CCC diagnoses,

 Go to Chapter 43, **Standardized Language, An Example of CCC Nursing Diagnoses and Interventions,** in Volume 2.

Planning Outcomes/Evaluation

CCC defines an outcome as "What really happened to the recipient of services in terms of the particular problem for which care was provided" (Head, Maas, & Johnson, 1997, p. 51). To formulate a goal/outcome in the CCC system, attach one of the three CCC "modifiers" (*improve, stabilize, deteriorate*) to the diagnosis. The outcome describes the *desired* client health status. To evaluate client progress, you again use one of the three modifiers to describe the client's *actual* health status. The following is an example:

CCC nursing diagnosis:	Knowledge Deficit
Goal/expected outcome:	Knowledge Deficit, Improve
Actual status on evaluation:	Knowledge Deficit, Stabilized

Medicare requires that the client's status be evaluated and coded as improved, stabilized, or deteriorated. In your nurse's notes, you would include additional narrative to support your evaluation.

The Nursing Outcomes Classification (NOC) can also be used in home health nursing (Moorhead, Johnson, & Maas, 2004). A few of the outcomes that pertain to home and families are Caregiver Home Care Readiness, Caregiver Performance: Direct Care, Caregiver Stressors, Family Coping, and Family Functioning. For more information about NOC,

 Go to the **Iowa Outcomes Project** web site at **www.nursing.uiowa.edu/centers/cncce/noc/index.htm**

Do you remember the overall goal of home care? That goal has implications for the kinds of activities you will perform after completing your assessment. To prepare the client and family for self-care, inform them of the needs you have identified, and involve them in setting goals and planning care. They may be able to identify strategies to solve problems or to help you identify needs that are not readily apparent.

| Planning Interventions/Implementation |

Once the plan of care has been agreed on, you will document it and forward it to the client's physician for certification. At the first visit, you will determine the specific skilled care required, make referrals to other required services such as physical, occupational, or speech therapy, social services, nutritional support, or home health aide services.

Often a client will have multiple services offered at the home. For example, Mr. Escobar is recovering from a CVA. He may require physical therapy, occupational therapy, and speech therapy as well as skilled nursing care and the assistance of a home health aide. As the Escobar's home health nurse, you would serve as the coordinator of this complex care.

The CCC contains 198 nursing interventions organized according to the care components. For an example,

 Go to Chapter 43, **Standardized Language, An Example of CCC Nursing Diagnoses and Interventions,** in Volume 2.

That list shows an example of an intervention for the Activity Component. An intervention consists of a label (e.g., Activity Care) and a definition (e.g., Actions performed to carry out physiological or psychological daily activities). In addition to the label, you must specify the type of intervention action from among four qualifiers:

Assess/Monitor
Care/Perform
Teach/Instruct
Manage/Refer

The CCC nursing interventions include only skilled services, because this type of service is the only type of care reimbursed by Medicare and most insurers in home health. In the case of the Escobars, Mrs. Escobar is clearly experiencing Caregiver Strain. This is a nursing diagnosis under the Care Component of Coping. Several interventions are possible:

Coping Support: Actions to sustain a person dealing with responsibilities, problems, or difficulties

Assess for Caregiver Strain

Provide (perform) emotional support

Refer to community services: caregiver support groups, Meals on Wheels, and respite care services.

The Nursing Interventions Classification (NIC) may also be used in home health nursing (Dochterman & Bulechek, 2004). A few of the interventions that pertain to home and families are Caregiver Support, Family Integrity Promotion, Home Maintenance Assistance, and Respite care. For more information about NIC,

 Go to the **Iowa Interventions Project** web site at www.nursing.uiowa.edu/centers/cncce/nic/index.htm

Infection Control in the Home

In the hospital there is ready access to supplies that facilitate infection control. The home presents unique challenges. You will need to follow Standard Precautions but recognize how to modify infection control techniques for the home environment.

Generally clients have developed some resistance to the microorganisms in their own homes and are less likely to acquire infections there than in the hospital environment. This makes the home an ideal site for care. However, homes vary widely. Do not assume that a client lives in a clean residence or that running water is readily available. Many people with limited financial resources, especially in urban environments, live in single-room occupancy hotels (SROs). Residents of SROs live in a small room with shared bath and shower areas. Conditions can vary from pristine to abysmal. To provide optimal care, you need to bring infection control supplies and personal protective equipment to the visit or order them to be delivered to the home.

The following suggestions can help you maintain infection control during a home visit.

- Keep antibacterial cleanser and OSHA-approved protective equipment in your nursing bag. Wash your hands using soap and warm water, if possible, at the beginning and end of each visit and before and after any treatment.

- Use a waterless antibacterial hand wash in place of soap and warm water if there is no sink or if the home conditions are filthy; wash your hands with soap and warm water as soon as possible after the visit.

- In homes that do not look clean, limit the supplies you bring into the home. For example, leave your nursing bag in the car, and bring only the supplies you need for the visit.

- Flush wound irrigation or potentially contaminated liquids down the toilet while wearing gloves and any other appropriate protective equipment.

| toward evidence-based practice |

Lee, T., & Mills, M. E. (2000). Analysis of patient profile in predicting home care resource utilization and outcomes. *Journal of Nursing Administration, 30*(2), 67–75.

Using a retrospective descriptive study design, researchers analyzed 244 patient records and data from a Washington, DC, home healthcare agency for resource use and care outcomes. It was found that the total number of nursing diagnoses and two specific nursing diagnoses (Alteration in Mobility and Knowledge Deficit: IV Therapy) were strong predictors of overall resource use. Prognosis (expected outcome), as recorded on the initial assessment form by the home health nurse, was the strongest predictor of discharge outcomes.

Goodman, C., Woolley, R., & Knight, D. (2003). District nurses' experiences of providing care in residential care home settings. *Journal of Clinical Nursing, 12*(1), 67–76.

Using small focus groups with district nurses in one county in England, researchers explored the contribution of primary care nurses in residential homes for older peo-

ple. The nurses interviewed regularly visited older adults residing in assisted living facilities. The original intent of this program was to improve the care delivered to this vulnerable population. In the focus groups, the nurses expressed concerns about the lack of consensus about their role and uncertainty about providing care in a setting that straddles health and social care. The authors conclude that until these issues are resolved, it is impossible to assess the impact these nurses could play in care of this population. They recommend including the views of the residents in future research.

---

1. How might a nurse working for a home health agency use the information from the first study?

2. How might an administrator at a home health agency incorporate information from the second study into her agency?

3. Would the second study be relevant in a Medicare-certified home health agency in the United States? Why or why not?

 Go to Chapter 43, **Toward Evidence-Based Practice Suggested Responses,** on the Electronic Study Guide.

- Double-bag dressings, equipment, or disposable supplies that have been contaminated with body secretions to prevent leakage. The bags should be labeled *Biohazard*.

- If necessary, use a 1:10 dilution of chlorine bleach in water to disinfect surfaces or equipment in the home. Some equipment may need to be disinfected by boiling in a covered pan of water for 15 to 20 minutes. Do not boil plastic or rubber items.

- You can disinfect hard plastic items by wrapping them with a wet paper towel and placing them in a zippered plastic bag. Microwave the entire bag on high for 10 minutes.

- Carry small biohazard sharps containers. Place syringes and sharps in the container without recapping. If clients or family must use syringes or sharps, you may wish to leave a sharps container in the home. An alternative solution is to have them use a metal coffee can with lid or a thick plastic milk jug with lid.

- If the client is immunocompromised, teach the signs and symptoms of infection and the process for immediate notification of the primary care provider.

- Provide instruction on home cleanliness, hygiene, hand washing, food preparation, and instructions to avoid contact with persons who are ill, as needed.

KnowledgeCheck 43–5

Identify three infection control supplies that you should bring in your nursing bag on a home health visit.

 Go to Chapter 43, **Knowledge Check Response Sheet and Answers,** on the Electronic Study Guide.

After the Visit

After you leave the home, there is still a lot of work for you to do. Often you will need to complete the documentation for the visit. In Chapter 16 you were introduced to documentation techniques, various forms of charting, and legal aspects of documentation. In home care all of these rules apply; however, some aspects of home care documentation are unique. For example, in the hospital, admissions personnel usually gather admitting data and obtain consent for treatment. In home care you will need to gather this information on the initial visit. Generally, agencies

have information packets that include the client's bill of rights, responsibilities, billing information, information on the frequency and duration of services, how to reach the agency, and the time of the next visit.

Home health agencies often use the OASIS data set to record initial assessment data. To continue to provide needed services to the client, you must include the following in your documentation:

• Evidence of homebound status.

• Continued need for skilled care.

Other post-visit activities include ordering supplies needed for the next visit, making referrals to additional services, coordinating care among the various services, and scheduling the next visit.

 Go to Chapter 43, **Resources for Caregivers and Health Professionals,** on the Electronic Study Guide.

 Suggested Readings: Go to Chapter 43, **Reading More About Nursing in Home Care,** on the Electronic Study Guide.

 Bibliography: Go to Volume 2, Bibliography.

44 Ethics

& Values

CHAPTER

Learning Outcomes

After completing this chapter, you should be able to:

* Define *morals, ethics, bioethics*, and *nursing ethics*.

* Discuss what is meant by ethical agency.

* Identify at least four factors that contribute to the frequency of nurses' moral problems.

* Differentiate personal values and morality from professional values.

* Explain how values, moral frameworks, professional guidelines, and moral principles affect moral decisions.

* Describe the major ethical principles that are used in reasoning about health care.

* Compare and contrast four moral frameworks: consequentialism, deontology, an ethics of care, and feminist ethics.

* Identify the moral issues and principles involved in a given ethical situation.

* Identify at least eight contemporary ethical issues in health care.

* Explain how nurses can use knowledge of values transmission and values clarification to facilitate the ethical decision making of clients.

* Describe a systematic approach for resolving ethical dilemmas.

* Discuss the concept of an integrity-producing compromise.

* Describe the nurse's obligations in ethical decisions.

* Discuss the roles of the nurse as client advocate in the delivery of ethical nursing care.

* Apply the steps identified in the MORAL model for ethical decision making to issues nurses encounter in patient care.

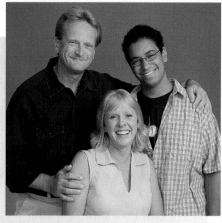

MEET Your Patients

Angie and Edward Frese are a couple with two teenaged children. They are a close and loving family with a large network of family and friends. Alan, 15 years old, has just been severely injured in a high school soccer game. Angie and Edward are summoned to the hospital, where they are told that Alan has multiple bone fractures and active internal bleeding.

The surgeon informs the distressed parents that Alan will need a blood transfusion to survive. Although genuinely devastated, the parents adamantly refuse to consent to a lifesaving blood transfusion, stating that they are Jehovah's Witnesses and that receiving blood is against their

religion. The surgeon asks you, Alan's nurse, to get the parents to change their minds right away. You talk with the couple, but they continue to refuse a blood transfusion. You immediately contact your charge nurse.

Try to answer the following questions about Alan and his parents. You may not have the experience or theoretical knowledge to answer them all—you will acquire that in this and the following chapter—but do your best based on the background you have.

CriticalThinking 44–1

- Do Alan's parents have the right to refuse a blood transfusion based on their religious beliefs?
- Do you think that the fact that Alan is a minor (under 18 years old) may make a difference in this situation?
- What actions do you think the charge nurse should take?
- Can an ethical conflict such as this be resolved to everyone's satisfaction?

Theoretical Knowledge
knowing why

The theoretical knowledge you will need to begin professional practice includes an understanding of the nature of morals and ethics (and especially nursing ethics) and basic information about factors that affect moral decisions (i.e., values, moral frameworks, professional guidelines, and ethical principles).

ETHICS AND MORALS

Although the terms *ethics* and *morals* are similar in meaning, in modern theory **morals** refers to private, personal, or group standards of right and wrong. **Moral behavior** is behavior that is in accordance with custom or tradition and usually reflects personal or religious beliefs. An example of morality might be a

person's opposition to or support of abortion. Another example is the "golden rule," that you should treat others as you wish to be treated.

Can you think of another example of moral behavior that you may have learned as a child?
Can you identify any morals that are evident in the scenario about Alan at the beginning of the chapter?
How are Mr. and Mrs. Frese's morals influencing Alan's care?

Ethics, in contrast, is a systematic study of right and wrong conduct in situations that involve issues of values and morals. Ethics is a formal process for making logical and consistent moral decisions. Morals consider in a broad, general manner what is good or bad, right or wrong (e.g., "In general, it is wrong to steal"). Ethics answers the question "What should I do in a given situation?" (e.g., "Is it wrong to steal if you have to do it to feed your children?"). Ethics uses specific rules, theories, principles, and perspectives to inquire into the justification of an individual's actions in a particular situation.

Ethics is rooted in the legal system and reflects the political values of a society. However, it is important to realize that ethics is not the same as law, religion, institutional practices, or customs. An action that is legal or customary may not be morally right or ethically justifiable. The same holds true of religion. You cannot assume that an accepted practice of a certain religion is an ethical practice in every situation.

TABLE 44-1   Kohlberg's Stages of Moral Development

I. Preconventional Level

The person conforms to cultural rules and labels of good and bad but interprets them in terms of punishment and reward or in terms of the physical power of those who enforce the rules. Children aged 4 to 10 years are usually at this level; some adults are, as well.

Stage 1—punishment-obedience orientation (right action is that which avoids punishment)

Stage 2—personal interest orientation (right action is that which satisfies personal needs)

II. Conventional Level

The person perceives that meeting the expectations of the family, group, or society is valuable in its own right, regardless of the consequences of the actions. More than just conforming, the person is loyal to the social order and identifies with those involved in it. The standards are set by others, but motivation to follow them is internal.

Stage 3—good boy–nice girl orientation (right actions are those that please others)

Stage 4—law-and-order orientation (right action is following the rules)

III. Postconventional, Autonomous, or Principled Level

The person makes an effort to define moral values and principles that have validity apart from society, groups, or persons in power. At this level, it becomes possible for conflict to occur between two socially accepted standards, and the person attempts to decide rationally between them. Both the standards and the decision are internal. Moral principles have validity apart from the authority of groups and persons.

Stage 5—legalistic, social contract orientation (right action is decided in terms of individual rights and standards agreed on by the whole society)

Stage 6—universal ethical principles orientation (right action is determined by conscience and abstract principles such as the golden rule)

Sources: Waugh, D. (1978). Moral development: Theory and process. In *Teaching and evaluating the affective domain in nursing programs* (pp. 17–30). New York: Charles B. Slack; Kohlberg, L. (1968). Moral development. In *International encyclopedia of social science*. New York: Macmillan; Kohlberg, L. (1981). *Essays on moral development*. Volumes 1–3. San Francisco: Harper & Row.

For example, there was a time in the United States when owning slaves was legal. That did not mean it was morally right. A more current example is that of abortion, which is legal under certain circumstances. However, many people argue that it is morally wrong in all circumstances.

In the case of Alan and his family ("Meet Your Patients"), the ethical decision making is quite different from the moral perspective of Alan's parents. The parents believe that a blood transfusion is morally wrong; this is congruent with their religious beliefs. The surgeon and the nurse, however, believe that withholding blood from Alan would be unethical.

Bioethics refers to the application of ethical principles to health care. Bioethics is concerned with every area of health care, including direct care of patients, allocation of resources, utilization of staff, and medical and nursing research.

How Are Morals Developed?

We learn and internalize our morals throughout the life span, beginning in childhood (Aiken, 2003). Building

on the classic developmental theory of Piaget (1932), Kohlberg (1968, 1981) theorized that moral development depends on one's ability to think and reason at progressively higher levels. Kohlberg's studies led to his view that children go through a sequence of moral reasoning ability, proceeding through several stages to a final level in adulthood, in which they base moral principles on universal and impartial principles of justice (Table 44–1). For an expanded version of Table 44–1 and examples of the stages,

 Go to Chapter 44, **Tables, Boxes, Figures: ESG Table 44–1,** on the Electronic Study Guide.

People progress through the stages as they grow older, mature, and interact with the environment. Progression is gradual, and the stages overlap. Kohlberg found that more than 50% of a person's thinking always reflects the stage he is in, with the remainder at the stage he is leaving or into which he is moving. Although some people never achieve Kohlberg's highest levels, progression through the stages is always forward—except in extreme trauma, it is never backward—and people do not skip stages.

Gilligan (1993) challenged Kohlberg's perspective of moral development, citing it as male-biased. Gilligan found through her research that girls develop morally by paying attention to community and to relationships, whereas boys tend to process dilemmas through more abstract ideals or principles (Beauchamp & Childress, 2001). For a review of Gilligan's three stages: caring for oneself, caring for others, and caring for self and others,

 Go to **Chapter 9** on the Electronic Study Guide.

What Is Nursing Ethics?

Nursing ethics, a subset of bioethics, refers to ethical questions that arise out of nursing practice. The first things to come to your mind may be the dramatic questions such as, "Should we shut off the ventilator and allow this patient to die? Should this baby have surgery even though his quality of life will probably never be good? Is abortion moral?" And so on. In reality, you will not make the final decision in such situations. You may have some input, but the patient, physician, and family will decide. As a nurse, you are responsible for deciding the nature and extent of your own participation in each situation, and you must support patients who are making ethical decisions or perhaps coping with the results of decisions made by others. Consider the following true story:

> *A woman took her 6-year-old son to the emergency department (ED) to have a scalp laceration sutured. On the way to the hospital, she tried to calm him by telling him that the doctors would "numb" him and no one would hurt him "on purpose." When they arrived in the ED, they were placed in a cubicle next to another little boy who was awaiting treatment for a similar laceration. His father was also trying to reassure his son, as the woman had done.*
>
> *A nurse entered the cubicle of the father and son. She roughly cleansed the cut with no explanation or words of comfort. The physician came and sewed the laceration without a word and without waiting for the local anesthetic to take effect. The boy screamed in pain and terror the whole time. The woman was horrified, and her son was scared. But when the very same nurse approached the woman and her son, she was kind and gentle. The same physician carefully injected a local anesthetic and waited for it to take effect before suturing (Curtin & Flaherty, 1982, pp. 3–4).*

Why do you think there was such difference in the treatment? Perhaps it was because the man and boy appeared to be of lower socioeconomic status; perhaps it was the presence of a father rather than a mother; and perhaps it was because the father and son were from a minority group and the lady and son were not. Regardless of why it happened, why is this case important?

Both boys received medical treatment; both incisions will heal; no one's life or health was threatened; no life-and-death decisions were made. But the first child's humanity and dignity were violated, and the actions were not fair. An important thing for you to recognize from this case is that *this is a perfect example of nursing ethics:* questions that have to do with *the nurse's* actions, not the actions of others. The nurse did not need a medical order nor permission from hospital administration to act ethically.

In the "Meet Your Patients" example, you, as the nurse, are not responsible for deciding the broad questions: "Is blood transfusion right or wrong?" or "Do the parents have a right to refuse blood transfusion?" Your decision is "What should *I* do? Should I try to persuade the parents to change their minds, as the surgeon directs, or not?" That is the *nursing ethics* question. And in that scenario, you will need to deal with the effects of the final decision on Alan. He may be frightened, he may be angry, he may die. The nurse is there for patients' most human and vulnerable moments.

Why Should Nurses Study Ethics?

Nurses should study ethics for a variety of reasons:

- *You will encounter ethical problems frequently in your work,* whether or not you are even aware of it. A consciously made, informed decision must surely be better than one made without awareness of the ethical issues involved. The most difficult question you will face will not be "How do I do this" but "Should I do this?"

- *Ethics is central to nursing.* Commitment to caring for other human beings supports the claim that nursing is a moral art (Curtin & Flaherty, 1982). Traditionally, people have expressed idealism by attending the sick; health and compassion are central values in nursing.

- *Multidisciplinary input is important.* No one profession is responsible for an ethical decision. As situations become more complex, multidisciplinary input becomes increasingly important. For example, physicians are responsible for knowing what surgery to perform and obtaining consent, but the nurse has a part in being sure the patient is adequately informed so that true consent is obtained.

- *Ethical knowledge is necessary for professional competence.* Being a professional includes being accountable to others in the profession for the ethical conduct of your work. Professions claim to use professional expertise for social good; therefore, to conduct our work well and have it stand the test of public scrutiny, we need to be clear about the ethics of our work.

- *Ethical reasoning is necessary for nursing to be taken seriously by other disciplines.* For your opinion

to be valued by others, you must be able to clearly express your moral position in a logical way. To be a truly accountable practitioner, you must be able to (1) understand your own values as they relate to basic morality and (2) use ethical reasoning to articulate your moral position.

- *Ethical proficiency is essential for providing holistic care.* Nurses deal with the whole person—that includes providing support for spiritual and moral concerns.

- *Nurses should be advocates for patients.* **Advocacy** is the communication and defense of the rights and interests of another. Since the 1960s, schools have socialized nurses to include patient advocacy in their role conceptions (Wilkinson, 1997). Currently, the American Nurses Association (ANA) Code of Ethics for Nurses (2001), provision 3, states:

  > *The nurse promotes, advocates for and strives to protect the health, safety and rights of the patient.*

  To advocate for patients in ethical situations, you must be able to identify the ethical issues and communicate the patient's wishes. Knowledge of ethical principles and decision making can give clarity to the aims of nursing practice and help us keep patients' interests foremost.

- *Studying ethics will help you to make better decisions.* Study of ethics prepares you to analyze moral problems from multiple perspectives rather than relying entirely on your personal values, intuition, and emotions. Practice in analyzing dilemmas will help you to become an informed decision maker, capable of understanding the perspectives of all the people in each situation—to understand, for example, why the Freses ("Meet Your Patients") are refusing a blood transfusion.

  Most nursing problems have more than one acceptable answer. This is especially true of ethical problems. Each situation is unique in its details. By thinking it through critically from several different angles, you will be assured that you have done all that you can to provide your client with the highest quality of ethical care.

KnowledgeCheck 44–1

- Define *morals*, and give an example that is not in the text.
- Define *ethics*, and give an example that is not in the text.
- How is bioethics different from ethics?
- Why do nurses need to study ethics?

 Go to Chapter 44, **Knowledge Check Response Sheet and Answers,** on the Electronic Study Guide.

What Is Ethical Agency?

Moral agency or **ethical agency** is the ability of nurses to base their practice on professional standards of ethical conduct and to participate in ethical decision making. Simply stated, it means that nurses have choices and are responsible for their actions. An ethical agent must be able to:

1. Perceive the difference between good and evil, right and wrong.
2. Understand abstract moral principles.
3. Reason and apply moral principles to make decisions, weigh alternatives, and plan ways to achieve goals.
4. Decide and choose freely.
5. Act according to choice (this assumes both the power and the capability to act).

For more an expanded discussion of ethical agency,

 Go to Chapter 44, **Supplemental Materials: Elements of Ethical Agency,** on the Electronic Study Guide.

 CriticalThinking 44–2

Consider the five components of ethical agency. To what extent do you believe nurses possess those abilities? Explain your thinking.

Moral Distress

In practice, nurses often make but are unable to carry out their moral decisions. A seminal study by Wilkinson (1987/88) identified this as **moral distress.** Ample literature documents that situational pressures (constraints) influence nurses' moral decisions as well as their ability to carry out their decisions (e.g., Corley & Minick, 2002; Erlen, 2001a; Georges & Grypdonck, 2002; Jameton, 1984). Whether these constraints are "real" or not, nurses in various studies have perceived the following as obstacles to carrying out their moral decisions: physicians, nurse administrators, other nurses, the law, threat of lawsuits, being socialized to follow orders, and doubting their own knowledge.

The fact is that even if you make a well thought-out moral decision, you may not be able to do what you believe to be right. This problem is not unique to nurses; no one is 100% "free" to choose and act. Actions always have consequences: for you and for others. Nevertheless, if you are confident you have made a good decision and can express it logically and clearly to others, you can at least enter into a dialogue with nurse administrators, physicians, and families about what ought to be done. Then you will be comfortable knowing that you have done all you could do, even if it is not all you wished to do.

For an expanded discussion of moral distress,

 Go to Chapter 44, **Supplemental Materials: Moral Distress,** on the Electronic Study Guide.

Whistleblowing

Nurses experience **moral outrage** when they perceive that others are behaving immorally (Wilkinson,

1987/1988). Moral outrage is similar to moral distress, except that in cases of moral outrage, nurses do not participate in the act. Therefore, they do not believe that they are responsible for doing wrong, but perceive that they are powerless to prevent it (Burkhardt & Nathaniel, 2002). A nurse may respond to moral outrage by "blowing the whistle."

A **whistleblower** is specifically defined as a person "who identifies an incompetent, unethical, or illegal situation, or actions of others, in the workplace and reports it to someone who may have the power to stop the wrong" (Ahern & McDonald, 2002, p. 314; Wilmot, 2000). The "others" in question may be an individual or an entire organization. When the wrongdoing involves an organization, the whistleblower must hold the situation up to public scrutiny, for example, by going to the news media or pursuing legal recourse.

At some point in your nursing career, you may become aware that a health team member is doing something illegal, unethical, or incompetent. It is difficult to know what to do. You will need to consider the consequence of the action, the competence of the person involved, and the completeness of your data about the incident. Before deciding to report the person, you will want to be sure that the information has been confirmed through another source and that reporting the problem will be likely to correct the wrongdoing or prevent future problems (Peternelj-Taylor, 2003).

Whistleblowing is difficult in the case of an impaired colleague. **Impaired nursing practice** occurs when the nurse's ability to perform the essential functions of nursing is diminished by chemical dependence on drugs or alcohol or by mental illness (Blair, 2001). Because this impairment affects patients, and because the impaired nurse may have difficulty being accountable to herself or in assessing her self-competence, you would need to report your co-worker's questionable behavior. The American Nurses Association proposes that as a colleague, you must ensure that an impaired nurse receives assistance in regaining optimal function by reporting the behaviors to the appropriate entity within the employment setting (ANA, 2001).

KnowledgeCheck 44–2
- Define *ethical agency*.
- What five abilities must be present for ethical agency to exist?
- List at least three constraints that can keep nurses from carrying out their moral decisions.

 Go to Chapter 44, **Knowledge Check Response Sheet and Answers,** on the Electronic Study Guide.

What Are Some Sources of Ethical Problems for Nurses?

Several factors contribute to the frequency of nurses' ethical problems, including societal factors, the nature of nursing work, and the nature of the nursing profession itself.

Societal Factors

Societal factors that give rise to ethical problems include increased consumer awareness, technological advances, transition from a homogeneous to a multicultural society, and efforts at cost containment in health care.

- *Increased consumer awareness.* As recently as 25 years ago, the healthcare system operated in a very paternalistic manner. Sick people sought the advice of a physician and then usually followed the physician's orders without question. Partly as a result of increased consumer awareness, professionals now are expected to share knowledge with patients and to obtain truly informed consent for treatments.

- *Technological advances.* With every new technology, new issues arise. For example, techniques of in vitro fertilization and embryo transfer have brought about questions of what should be done with embryos that are not implanted into a uterus. Can they be disposed of? What is their status as persons? Other ethical questions surround organ transplants, amniocentesis capable of revealing fetal defects, genetic engineering, cryogenics, and technical advances that allow loved ones to be maintained on life support beyond what anyone might have imagined 20 years ago (Rumbold, 1999).

- *Multicultural population.* In the not too distant past, it was safe to assume that your values and beliefs would be fairly consistent with those of your patients; we had a fairly homogenous society with a shared value system. We now live in a multicultural, multi-faith society, and that assumption is no longer valid. You will work with patients and colleagues from a variety of cultural backgrounds, who probably hold very different sets of values. You will need to respect a variety of belief systems, and you will need to serve as a patient advocate even when the patient's value system is very different from your own.

- *Cost containment.* The emphasis on cutting healthcare costs creates many morally questionable situations. For example, patients are being sent home from the hospital while they are still very ill. On being discharged, they discover that insurance payments are limited for services outside the hospital, including specialists, home care, and medical supplies (e.g., bandages, walkers).

Cost containment efforts and the nursing shortage have led healthcare agencies to increase the number of patients each nurse is expected to care for. As a nurse, you will undoubtedly find yourself in situations where fewer nurses are available than patient acuity requires. You will have to make personal decisions about how far you will stretch your own resources.

The Nature of Nursing Work

The nature of moral problems in nursing is that they are immediate, serious, and frequent. In the classroom, you have the luxury to leave questions unsettled. In the real world, you must always decide: Either you take action, or you do not. But for a nurse, deciding *not* to act is, in effect, an act. For example, suppose the family wishes a patient to have aggressive Code Blue (resuscitation) efforts; however, you know the patient does not wish to be "coded." When the patient dies, whether or not you know the "right" thing to do, you must decide immediately to carry out or not carry out the Code Blue. If you wait too long to ponder the ethical issues, it may be too late to carry it out. If you do not decide, the effect is the same as though you had decided *not* to code.

The nurse's unique position in healthcare organizations also creates problems. Nurses have multiple obligations and relationships, and sometimes conflicting loyalties. Nurses are employees (with a relationship with the agency) as well as professionals (with a special relationship with patients). In addition, they have peer relationships and a unique relationship with physicians. Although nurses are usually not employed by a physician, they are expected to follow physician orders regarding patient care. Additionally, in most organizations, physicians are higher on the power and status hierarchy than are nurses. Ethical questions arise when nurses experience conflicts among their loyalties to patients, families, physicians, employers, and other nurses. Consider the following example: A patient wants to know his test results; the physician is reluctant to tell him. What are the conflicting loyalties? Should the nurse give the patient the information or not?

1. *Tell*. The nurse could honor the principle of personal autonomy and her obligation to the patient by telling him his test results. But this might harm the patient's relationship with the physician, which is important to the patient's well-being. Furthermore, if the nurse tells the patient his test results, it may create problems between the physician and the employer (e.g., the hospital). Additionally, this action may in some instances violate hospital policies and therefore harm the nurse's relationship with the hospital. It will certainly affect her relationship with the physician.
2. *Don't tell*. The nurse could preserve the patient-physician relationship by withholding the test results from the patient. This choice does not honor her relationship with the patient. Also, if the nurse does not tell the patient his test results, the patient may find out anyway and be angry with the hospital, the physician, and the nurse.

According to professional ethics, your first allegiance is to the patient. However, the patient's needs often conflict with institutional policies, family desires, or even laws of the state. There may also be conflicts in your relationships with the patient and his family. You can see an example of this in the "Meet Your Patient" scenario, wherein the nurse finds it impossible to honor the parents' autonomy and at the same time advocate for Alan. You may also encounter this type of conflict when a patient does not want any heroic measures and wishes only to die peacefully, but the family has not yet been able to accept the imminent death and are insisting on full resuscitation.

The Nature of the Nursing Profession

Some ethical problems arise because of value conflicts and a lack of clarity within the nursing profession. We have unresolved questions about the nature, scope, and goals of our practice, as well as our professional values (values are discussed later in the chapter). Notice the conflicts of values in the following items:

- Nursing values caring, humanistic care, and nurse-patient relationships—however, nurses now spend less time at the bedside (with patients) than ever before. One reason is the nursing shortage and heavier patient loads, but there are other factors: the use of technology, the need for careful documentation, and the emphasis on leading, managing, and delegation instead of hands-on care.
- On one hand, we believe nurses should have autonomy and equal status with other healthcare professionals—on the other hand, many nurses want to escape hard choices by "letting the doctor decide."
- Most nurses believe we deserve higher pay—yet, we claim nurses are cost-effective because we work more cheaply than physicians.
- On one hand, we claim the nurse is a professional, citing critical thinking, knowledge, and management skills—on the other hand, we emphasize caring, with the nurse at the bedside offering comfort and doing hands-on tasks.

In most of those examples, we value both of the opposites. We would not wish to give up either one. But specific situations require us to choose between them, and that is one source of our discomfort.

WHAT FACTORS AFFECT MORAL DECISIONS?

By now you should have an idea of the nature of morals and ethics and of the need to study nursing ethics. We turn our focus now to some basic theoretical knowledge about factors that are involved in making moral decisions: values, ethical principles, moral frameworks, and professional guidelines.

Values, Attitudes, and Beliefs

Your values influence much of what you think and do. This is important to know because values are entangled in all ethical situations. If asked, could you say what your values are? Could you explain how they inform your decisions about right and wrong in a given situation? If so, that's a great beginning. If not, you will learn more as you move through this section.

A **value** is a belief you have about the worth of something; it serves as a principle or a standard that influences decision making. Values are ideals, beliefs, customs, modes of conduct, qualities, or goals that are highly prized or preferred by individuals, groups, or society (Burkhardt & Nathaniel, 2002). You can value an idea, a person, a way of doing things, or even an object (e.g., money). People express their values through behaviors, feelings, knowledge, and decisions. For example, the nurse who values compassion will interact with patients in a sensitive, caring manner. Some characteristics of values are that they:

- Are freely chosen
- Are often taken for granted
- Are learned in conscious and unconscious ways
- Are learned through observation and experience in social groups (e.g., the family, school, church)
- Become a part of a person's makeup
- Give direction to life
- Can be individual or shared
- Vary from person to person
- Can change over time.
- May be expressed overtly or manifested indirectly

Your **value set** is your "list" of values. It gives direction for your life and forms a basis for behavior. Your **value system** is your value set with the values ranked on a continuum from most important to least important. The total number of values a person has is rather small. The number of *significant* values is even smaller. It is easy enough to identify values—for example, love, freedom, courage, responsibility—but how many of your values have a consistent and predictable impact on your actions? Those are the significant values.

KnowledgeCheck 44–3
- What are values?
- What are three characteristics of values?

 Go to Chapter 44, **Knowledge Check Response Sheet and Answers,** on the Electronic Study Guide.

CriticalThinking 44–3
- Think about what you value personally in your own life. What are the five ideals, principles, or things that are most important to you?

- Now refer back to Chapter 13, where you were asked to list five ideals, principles, or things that were most important to you. What did you list then? Is your list any different now that you have gained some clinical experience and theoretical knowledge?

Attitudes are mental dispositions or feelings toward a person, object, or idea. Attitudes can include cognitive (thinking), affective (feeling), and some behavioral (doing) components. For example, you might have a positive attitude about cleanliness—that is, you may think it is a good thing (e.g., "The floor is clean. That's nice.") But if you *value* cleanliness, you would be willing to scrub the floor. You would also wash your hands at appropriate times, bathe regularly, and teach others about hygiene.

A **belief** is something that one accepts as true (e.g., "I believe that germs cause disease and that by washing my hands I remove germs"). Beliefs are sometimes based on faith and sometimes on facts. A belief may or may not be true. Beliefs may or may not involve values. Consider the following statements of belief. The first does not involve a value; the second one does.

"I believe the earth is round."

"Working hard to achieve goals is important to me; therefore, I believe that I must work during the summer to save money for college."

From those examples, can you see how values, beliefs, and behaviors are related?

CriticalThinking 44–4
- Think about Alan and his family ("Meet Your Patients"). What do you think were the values of Alan's parents that influenced their behavior at the hospital? First, identify their behaviors specifically. Then speculate about the values underlying each behavior.
- How do you think values can influence health?

KnowledgeCheck 44–4
- Define *belief;* give a new example.
- Define *attitude;* give a new example

 Go to Chapter 44, **Knowledge Check Response Sheet and Answers,** on the Electronic Study Guide.

Professional Versus Personal Values

Your **personal value system** is a set of values that you have reflected on and chosen that will help you to lead a good life (Purtilo, 1999). You have internalized some *societal values* and have come to perceive them as your own (e.g., good manners, such as saying "Please" and "Thank you"). In addition, you probably have some personal values (e.g., friendship, fairness, creativity) that are important to you but may or may not be important to society at large.

As you move forward in your profession, you will assimilate what you learn and experience and form **professional values** (Table 44–2), many of which will

TABLE 44-2   Professional Values and Behaviors

Values	Values Defined	Sample Professional Behaviors
Altruism	A concern for the welfare and well-being of others. Altruism is reflected by the nurse's concern for the welfare of patients, other nurses, and other healthcare providers.	• Demonstrates understanding of cultures, beliefs, and perspectives of others. • Advocates for patients, particularly the most vulnerable. • Takes risks on behalf of patients and colleagues. • Mentors other professionals.
Autonomy	The right to self-determination. Professional practice reflects autonomy when the nurse respects patients' rights to make decisions about their health care.	• Plans care in partnership with patients. • Honors the right of patients and families to make decisions about health care. • Provides information so that patients can make informed choices.
Human dignity	Respect for the inherent worth and uniqueness of individuals and populations. In professional practice, human dignity is reflected when the nurse values and respects all patients and colleagues.	• Provides culturally competent and sensitive care. • Protects the patient's privacy. • Preserves the confidentiality of patients and healthcare providers. • Designs care with sensitivity to individual patient needs.
Integrity	Acting in accordance with an appropriate code of ethics and accepted standards of practice. Integrity is reflected in professional practice when the nurse is honest and provides care based on an ethical framework that is accepted within the profession.	• Provides honest information to patients and the public. • Documents care accurately and honestly. • Seeks to remedy errors made by self or others. • Demonstrates accountability for own actions.
Social justice	Upholding moral, legal, and humanistic principles. This value is reflected in professional practice when the nurse works to ensure equal treatment under the law and equal access to quality health care.	• Supports fairness and nondiscrimination in the delivery of care. • Promotes universal access to health care. • Encourages legislation and policy consistent with the advancement of nursing care and health care.

Additional professional values frequently cited for nursing include the following:
Equality (having the same rights, privileges, or status)
Esthetics (qualities of objects or people that are pleasing)
Freedom (capacity to choose)
Truth (faithfulness to fact or reality)
Service (commitment to work useful to others)
Education (basic and lifelong continuing education for nurses)
Competence (skill, knowledge, performance of nursing work)
Loyalty (feeling of duty or attachment to other nurses)

Sources: American Association of Colleges of Nursing (AACN). (1998). *The essentials of baccalaureate education for professional nursing practice.* Washington, DC: Author, pp. 8–9; Jameton, A. (1984). *Nursing practice: The ethical issues.* Englewood Cliffs, NJ: Prentice-Hall; Watson, J. (1981). Socialization of the nursing student in a professional nursing education programme. *Nursing Papers, 13,* 19–24.

augment your own personal values. Personal and professional values are not always congruent, though. Consider the following situation:

Alexandra Jensen is a 17-year-old pregnant woman who comes in to your ambulatory surgical center for a voluntary termination of an early preg-nancy. You are assigned to admit her to your unit and get her ready for this procedure. Imagine that your personal value in this situation is that you do not believe in abortion but that your professional value is guided by the American Nurses Association (ANA) standards of professional practice, which state that the nurse "delivers care in a manner

TABLE 44-3 Modes of Value Transmission

Mode	Description
Modeling	Children learn values from a variety of role models (parents, peers, rock stars, significant others) by observation. This modeling may lead to socially acceptable or unacceptable behaviors.
Moralizing	"This way is the only way." Children are taught a complete set of values in an authoritarian approach. If the child does not conform, the parent may inflict guilt and fear on him. This approach by parents, teachers, church leaders, and other authorities may make it difficult for young people to make independent choices because they have no experience selecting values that are good for them.
Laissez-faire	"Doing your own thing." Children are allowed to explore differing sets of values on their own with little guidance or discipline. This may lead to conflict and confusion on the part of the child.
Reward and punishment	The child's behavior is controlled by offering rewards for certain valued behaviors and punishing the child who fails to comply. Rewards can strengthen behavior, whereas physical punishment may teach that violence is an acceptable behavior.
Responsible choice	A balance of freedom and restriction allows children to select the values, explore new behaviors, and experience the consequences. This can lead to personal satisfaction and parental support.

Sources: Gilligan, C. (1993). *In a different voice.* Cambridge, MA: Harvard University Press; Kohlberg, L. (1981). *Essays on moral development.* Volumes 1–3. San Francisco: Harper & Row; Piaget, J. (1932). *The moral development of a child.* New York: Free Press.

that preserves and protects patient autonomy, dignity and rights" (ANA, 2004). It is difficult to hold a personal value in high regard while under pressure to assume a conflicting professional value. How might you feel in the situation just described?

Do you think that your personal and professional values need to be compatible in order for you to be a competent nurse? Do you think that you should have the absolute right to refuse to participate in a situation (such as the one above) that may violate your personal values?

 CriticalThinking 44–5

- Name some other examples of societal values.
- What groups and social experiences have helped to form your values?
- Examine your personal values to see whether they match the professional values in Table 44–2.

   Which of those values, if any, do you *not* share? Explain your thinking.

   Name a few of your personal values that are not found on this list of professional values.

KnowledgeCheck 44–5

- What is the difference between personal and professional values?
- What is an example of professional values?
- What are some other types of values?

Go to Chapter 44, **Knowledge Check Response Sheet and Answers,** on the Electronic Study Guide.

How Are Values Transmitted?

As you have learned, we acquire values from social interaction. So how does that work? How are values transmitted? Table 44–3 outlines the methods of value transmission. A recent study adds to Table 44–3 the information that values transmission between parents and adolescents can be reciprocal and that the presence of a receptive and supportive parent makes value transmission more likely (Pinquart & Silbereisen, 2004).

What Is Value Neutrality?

You have probably been taught that nurses need to be nonjudgmental in providing health care to their clients. As a nurse, you have a duty to provide the best care to clients. You should not assume that your personal values are right, and you should not judge the client's values as right or wrong on the basis of whether they agree with your value system. Think back to the discussion regarding Alexandra, who was seeking an abortion. A nurse who does not believe in abortion could still provide competent nursing care to Alexandra even though his personal values regarding abortion are different from Alexandra's. **Value neutrality** means that we attempt to understand our own values regarding an issue and to know when to put them aside, if necessary, to become nonjudgmental when providing care to clients. However, some healthcare professionals (e.g., Beckwith & Peppin, 2000; Pellegrino, 2000) believe that value neutrality is neither possible nor desirable

| toward evidence-based practice |

Krishnasamy, M. (1999). Nursing, morality, and emotions: Phase I and phase II clinical trials and patients with cancer. *Cancer Nursing, 22*(4), 251–259.

In this qualitative study, the researcher conducted a semi-structured, tape-recorded group interview of three nurses' views of the moral dimensions of their work in caring for patients participating in cancer clinical trials. The nurses were not researchers. Three themes emerged:

- Being valued and moral distress
- Caring in a climate of scientific research
- Care, cure, and consequences for moral reasoning

One conclusion was that working in an environment suffused with moral conflicts can be painful and damaging for the professionals involved. Implications were (1) that to function effectively, nurses must be proactive in exploring the role emotions play in moral decision making, and (2) a commitment to valuing divergent ethical reasoning in and across professional cultures is necessary.

Severinsson, E. (2003). Moral stress and burnout: Qualitative content analysis. *Nursing and Health Sciences, 5*(1), 59–66.

In this qualitative study, the researcher performed an in-depth content analysis of an interview with one nurse regarding the nurse's experience of burnout. The main findings of the study concerned moral stress and burnout. All the themes identified were related to the nurse's identity, her personal experience of and reflections on ethical problems and suffering, and the responsibilities and difficulties nurses face. The researcher concluded that nurses need emotional support and the right to receive systematic clinical supervision to help them reflect on their work and interpret the needs of patients.

---

1. Based on these two studies, what can you do to help keep from experiencing moral distress and burnout? Do not go beyond what is suggested in these studies (although there are other actions that might be effective).

2. Imagine you are a nurse manager. You want to reduce burnout and turnover in your hospital. Which of the following actions are supported by these two studies?
   a. Make funds available for unit managers to attend ethics continuing education.
   b. Hire a nurse ethicist or a nurse counselor to work with individuals and groups of nurses who request this intervention.
   c. Work with other disciplines to include nurses on the agency's ethics committee.
   d. Conduct continuing education courses on ethical decision making.

 Go to Chapter 44, **Toward Evidence-Based Practice Suggested Responses,** on the Electronic Study Guide.

---

because it imposes an ethical obligation on healthcare providers to suppress or modify their own deepest moral and religious beliefs.

How Are Values, Morals, and Ethics Related?

As you may recall, values and morals are learned in conscious and unconscious ways and become a part of your makeup. When we evaluate right and wrong, or good and bad, we are using moral judgment. Therefore, our individual preferences (values) of right or wrong become our moral values. Whether or not you are aware of it, your morals and values shape the manner in which you make ethical decisions in your nursing practice (Burkhardt & Nathaniel, 2002).

So, although ethics are based on a structured set of principles and theories, and ethical decisions are publicly stated in terms of possible alternative behaviors, such decisions are always influenced unconsciously by our own personal values and morals. It is important to clarify the influence of your values and morals each time you enter into a situation where you

are called on to be objective in your ethical decision making. Later in this chapter, we will talk about practical strategies you can use to clarify your values and measure their influence on your ethical decisions.

KnowledgeCheck 44–6
- What are some ways that values can be transmitted?
- What is value neutrality?

 Go to Chapter 44, **Knowledge Check Response Sheet and Answers,** on the Electronic Study Guide.

Moral Principles

Moral principles are useful in ethical discussions because even if people disagree about which action is right in a situation, they may be able to agree about which principles apply. This agreement may provide common ground for a compromise or other resolution of the problem. Different moral frameworks (to be discussed later) use some of the same principles in ethical reasoning. We will discuss autonomy, nonmaleficence, beneficence, fidelity, veracity, and justice.

Autonomy

Autonomy refers to a person's right to choose and his ability to act on that choice. The principle of autonomy rests on the belief that every competent person has the right to determine his own course of action. Maintaining autonomy is one way to show respect for each person's humanity. You demonstrate respect for autonomy when you treat people with consideration, believe patients' stories about the course and symptoms of their illnesses, and protect patients who are unable to decide for themselves.

The principle of autonomy underlies informed consent—clients' right to decide for themselves whether or not they will agree to a proposed procedure or treatment. You also honor autonomy when you respect the patient's or surrogate's right to decide, even when you believe those choices are not in the patient's best interest. In the "Meet Your Patients" scenario, if you believed autonomy to be the most important principle in the situation, what would you think about Alan's parents' refusing to allow him to receive blood products? If you believed that respecting their autonomy gives them the right to choose on the basis of their religious beliefs, would you still try to persuade them to change their minds?

Nonmaleficence

The principle of **nonmaleficence** is the twofold duty to do no harm and to prevent harm. Nonmaleficence refers to both actual harm and risk of harm, as well as to intentional and unintentional harm. In nursing it is rare to find intentional harm, but unintentional harm due to lack of careful planning and consideration does occur (Husted & Husted, 2001).

When using the principle of nonmaleficence to guide treatment regimens, ask the question, "Does this treatment cause more harm or more good to the patient?" Nonmaleficence requires that you think critically about patient care and research situations, weighing the potential risks against the potential benefits. Risk of harm is not always clear. Suppose you are about to get a patient out of bed for the first time after surgery. The benefit clearly is that this will prevent postoperative complications such as pneumonia and thrombophlebitis, but the risks, in terms of excessive pain or unintentional damage to the operative site, may be less clear. Weighing risks and benefits is a value-laden exercise. Who is to say what amount of pain is excessive—you or the patient? To honor the principle of nonmaleficence in this situation, you would need to be sure to premedicate the patient and carefully assess his status as you are helping him to ambulate.

Nonmaleficence is a fundamental duty of healthcare professionals. Both the physicians' Hippocratic Oath and the nurses' Nightingale Pledge state that care providers are to cause no harm to patients. When you are careful to prevent medication errors, or provide a walker, or use an ambulation belt for ambulating patients, you are honoring the nonmaleficence principle.

 CriticalThinking 44–6

Think about the "Meet Your Patients" scenario in terms of nonmaleficence. The parents refuse to allow a blood transfusion. You, the nurse, have tried to persuade them to change their minds. You do not need to decide what you ought to do; just analyze the situation in terms of the risks.

- What is it that creates the risk for harm to Alan?
- What is the risk for harm to Alan's parents because of the nurse's actions?

Beneficence

Beneficence is the duty to do or promote good. You can think of this principle as being on a continuum with nonmaleficence. At one end of the continuum is the duty to do no harm; beneficence, at the other end, is the duty to bring about positive good (Milton, 2000). The following examples illustrate the duties in priority order:

- Do no harm. (Don't push the man into the river.)
- Prevent harm when you can. (If the man is getting dangerously close to the river's edge, warn him that he is about to fall into the river.)
- Remove harm when it is being inflicted. (If you see a struggle and someone is trying to push the man into the river, interfere and try to stop it.)
- Bring about positive good. (If the man has fallen in the river, jump in and try to save him.)

When weighing the risks and benefits of an action, you are actually balancing nonmaleficence with beneficence. It is well to remember that patients, family members, and other professionals may identify benefits and harms differently. A benefit to one may represent a burden to another. For example, in "Meet Your Patients," you may see a blood transfusion as a benefit to Alan, but to the parents it may represent harm.

In spite of the fact that "doing good" sounds like such a positive goal, beneficence can have negative consequences. One such outcome is **paternalism** (treating others like children). This would occur, for example, if you think you know what is best for a competent client and then coerce the client to act as you wish rather than to act as she wishes. Saying to a patient, for example, "Trust us; we know what is best for you to do in this situation," may seem to be beneficent because you are trying to support the patient. But it is actually paternalistic behavior that inhibits autonomy and lacks respect for the patient.

Fidelity

Fidelity (faithfulness) is the obligation to keep promises. In actual practice you will often find that competing tasks prevent you from being able to deliver

something exactly as you have promised. Fidelity requires you to make promises in a thoughtful, careful manner to maximize the likelihood that you can keep them. Instead of "I'll be right back with your medication," you might "waffle" a bit and say, "I'll get back with your medication as quickly as I can" or "I must go help another patient for a few minutes, but I'll get here with your medication as quickly as I can."

Being faithful to clients also means meeting their reasonable expectations. For example, clients should expect you to show them basic respect, to be competent, to follow the statements of your professional code of ethics, and to keep their information confidential. They will reasonably expect you to honor commitments you have made to them in terms of informed consent or verbal agreements.

Honoring fidelity is a basic part of every patient care situation. Sometimes the promises are of major significance, such as promising not to share certain information with other members of the healthcare team, and at other times it may be only a promise to come back to check the effectiveness of a pain medication or to bring a requested item back to the client's room. The commitment to fidelity is the same regardless of the level of significance of the promise.

Veracity

Veracity is the duty to tell the truth. This seems very straightforward, and you may wonder why it even needs discussion. However, there are times when veracity may present a challenge. For example, should you tell the truth when you know that it might cause harm to the client? Would it be appropriate to tell a lie in order to relieve extreme patient anxiety? Most nurses would agree that it isn't hard to tell the truth, but at times it may be very hard to determine how much of the truth to tell. For example, healthcare professionals feel uncomfortable giving families "bad news." So instead of saying, "Your father has a fatal illness and is unlikely to live for more than a month," they may say, "Your father is very ill, but we will do everything we possibly can for him." In this, as in most situations, the risk of losing patient trust outweighs any benefit of withholding the truth.

Although you always presume the value of telling the truth, there may be times when you are justified to withhold information. In some cultures, for example, families go to great lengths to protect a dying patient from the harsh truth of his prognosis, and the patient himself may not wish to know.

CriticalThinking 44–7

Review the "Meet Your Patients" scenario. Alan will not survive without a blood transfusion; the parents refuse. He asks the nurse, "Am I going to die?" You do not need to decide which response is best; just write an example that illustrates each of the following. What might the nurse say if she wishes to:

- Tell Alan the truth

- Withhold or partially disclose the truth
- Answer with an untruth

Justice

Justice is the obligation to be fair. It implies equal treatment of all clients. This principle is reflected in the first provision in the ANA Code of Ethics for Nurses (ANA, 2001) (Box 44–1). Questions of justice will become a part of your everyday experience in patient care, from deciding how to allocate your time among patients to larger decisions, such as how to allocate limited health care resources.

Distributive justice, which is one type of justice that is particularly relevant to health care, requires fair distribution of both benefits and burdens (Husted & Husted, 2001), as in the following issues.

- *Allocating resources.* Distributive justice questions come up when more than one person or group competes for the same resources. One example arises in determining how to spend federal and state tax dollars: Should money be spent to fund AIDS research or to find better treatments for Alzheimer's disease? Other examples surround organ transplantation. Human organs are scarce resources. How do we decide which patient should receive an available organ for transplantation? Is an 18-year-old more deserving of a kidney than a 75-year-old? Is a person with liver disease due to alcoholism less deserving of a liver than someone with liver disease not caused by alcoholism? The decision of who should live and who may die is never an easy decision. In the United States, we use a national committee to set criteria for how organs will be distributed so the standard of justice can be considered.

- *Fair access to care.* Access to care is a specific kind of healthcare resource. The principle of distributive justice holds that we should provide equal access to health care for all. As the baby boomer generation ages, the Medicare budget will be strained. At the same time, baby boomer nurses will be retiring in record numbers. There will be fewer nurses to care for more patients at a time when national healthcare dollars are stretched very thin. How will the nation decide where to spend the limited dollars? How will nurse managers decide how to provide adequate care when they do not have enough nurses on their staff? The ability to develop sound criteria on which to base the allocation of resources is the challenge of distributive justice.

Compensatory justice focuses on compensation for wrongs that have been done to individuals or groups. This is the type of justice considered when there are malpractice suits, for example, when a patient climbs out of bed and falls and breaks a hip. Groups of citizens may also be harmed, for instance, by a company's unintentional pollution of water in a community. If this

pollution were proven to cause cancer in members of the community, a monetary settlement might be made.

Procedural justice is relevant in processes that require ranking or ordering (Volbrecht, 2002). Often the unwritten rule of "first come, first served" is used as a basis for delivery of services. In many situations, this is considered fair. Institutional policies are written to ensure that the same procedures apply to all clients or employees in the same way (e.g., visiting hours, working on holidays, sick leave). Can you think of an example of procedural justice that you have experienced during your nursing education?

KnowledgeCheck 44–7

List each of the six ethical principles and its definition.

 Go to Chapter 44, **Knowledge Check Response Sheet and Answers,** on the Electronic Study Guide.

Moral Frameworks

Moral (or **philosophical**) **frameworks** are systems of thought (theories) that are the basis for the differing perspectives people have in ethical situations. Such frameworks have existed since ancient times, for example, in the works of the Greek philosophers Plato and Aristotle. No matter how well you know the theories and principles, though, they will not provide answers for specific patient situations. They simply offer a lens through which you can look to examine an ethical problem. See Chapter 8 if you need to review the purposes and uses of theories.

There is no single "best" theory that will give you all the answers or provide the one "true" answer to an ethical problem. Each provides a different perspective. By using more than one framework to analyze a situation, you will perform a more comprehensive analysis of the problem.

What Is Consequentialism?

In **consequentialist** theories, the rightness or wrongness of an action depends on the consequences of the act rather than on the act itself. Theories of this type are also called **teleology,** from the Greek word *telos,* meaning "end" or the study of ends (also called *final causes*) (Beauchamp & Childress, 2001). **Utilitarianism,** the most familiar consequentialist theory, takes the position that the value of an action is determined by its usefulness. The *principle of utility* states that an act must result in the greatest good for the greatest number of people. When we say "good" here, we mean positive benefit. Any act can then become the ethical choice if it delivers "good" results. In health care, the principle of "most of all, do no harm" is consequentialist in nature. Because of this principle, we are always concerned about weighing the risks and benefits of our

care (e.g., a medication may kill cancer cells, but side effects may harm the patient's quality of life).

Using utilitarianism to resolve an ethical problem, you would evaluate every alternative action for its potential outcomes, both positive and negative—similar to a technique you may already use when making a decision, that is, making a list of pros and cons. You would then select the action that results in the most benefits for the greatest number of people involved in the situation. The following is an example of utilitarian reasoning: The practice of triage is used in a disaster when emergency workers have to sort patients to determine who will be treated first or who will receive limited resources (e.g., oxygen or intravenous therapy). If a victim has little potential for survival, he may not be treated at all, or his treatment may be postponed to free the healthcare team to treat those victims (i.e., "the greatest number") with the greatest potential to survive.

CriticalThinking 44–8

- Describe a time in your life when you used consequentialism to resolve a difficult situation.
- What types of clinical dilemmas might be best resolved using this model?

What Is Deontology?

Deontology is almost the opposite of the utilitarian model in that it considers an action to be right or wrong independent of its consequences. This system of ethical decision making is also called **formalism;** decisions are based on moral rules and unchanging principles. A famous early philosopher, Immanuel Kant (1724–1804), established the principle of the **categorical imperative,** which states that one should only act if the action is based on a principle that is universal (or in other words, if you believe that everyone should act in the same way in a similar situation). Another deontology principle, also formulated by Kant, is to treat people as ends and never as means. Treating people as an *end* means that the person is more important than whatever else you may be trying to accomplish. Can you imagine the ethical concerns of research situations in which the research subjects were exposed to some amount of risk (e.g., a new surgical procedure) to find a drug or treatment that will benefit many other people?

When using a deontological model, you would critically examine a situation to determine which actions are right or wrong according to rules and principles such as justice, autonomy, doing good, and doing no harm. These principles are regarded as unchanging and absolute, and they come from the same universal values that underlie all major religions.

Deontological frameworks also emphasize rights (e.g., the right to freedom, the right of self-determination) and obligations (duties). For example, you must

help someone in need because you have a duty to help others, not because helping will produce good consequences. In fact, you have a duty to help even if your helping may produce some bad consequences.

One difficulty with deontology occurs when you must choose between conflicting universal principles. It is not always clear which principle to honor. Allowing Alan's parents ("Meet Your Patients") to refuse to provide him with blood honors the principle of autonomy, but their decision may interfere with a right, namely, Alan's right to life. Can you see that it might be difficult to decide which is the appropriate principle to honor?

In deontological models, it is also important to consider motives. It is one thing for Alan's parents to refuse blood transfusion because they are honoring a religious principle; it would be quite another thing if they refused the transfusion because they stood to inherit a large trust fund left to Alan by his grandfather. Motives may place more weight on one of the conflicting universal principles over the other and make a decision clearer. Unfortunately, it is sometimes hard to recognize your own motives, much less to be sure about the motives of others.

KnowledgeCheck 44–8
- Describe utilitarianism.
- Define *deontology*.

 Go to Chapter 44, **Knowledge Check Response Sheet and Answers,** on the Electronic Study Guide.

What Do We Mean by Feminist Ethics?

Feminist ethicists have created a model based on the belief that because traditional deontological models focus on abstract principles such as fairness, justice, and rights, they provide a mostly masculine perspective. In contrast, virtues such as love, relationships, caring, nurturing, and sympathy are more relevant to women but are rarely seen in traditional moral theories (Bandman & Bandman, 2002). They assert that focusing on deontological principles allows one to be distracted from dealing with larger social issues. Feminist ethics values relationships and stories about relationships over using universal principles. Feminists argue that it is impossible to avoid being influenced by one's relationships. They see that influence as positive and believe it should not be muted by an attempt to be objective—because objectivity is impossible anyway.

Feminist ethics does consider principles and the consequences, but it also asks you to look at social issues surrounding the ethical situation to ensure that social facts are not forgotten (Noddings, 2003). Feminist ethical reasoning addresses issues of gender inequality within each situation. Part of the reasoning would be to ask, "How is this decision affecting the woman?" An example of the feminist ethical approach arises in deciding whether to allocate federal healthcare resources to younger people or to older adults. Feminist reasoning might say that, all other considerations being equal:

- In the United States there are more older women than older men.
- Older women tend to be poorer and are more likely to be alone than are men.
- Therefore, if health care for older adults were to be rationed, it would negatively affect women more than men.
- Therefore, it would be unfair and unethical to allocate more healthcare resources to younger people than to older people.

What Do We Mean by the Ethics-of-Care?

The **ethics-of-care,** a nursing philosophy, directs attention to the specific situations of individual patients viewed within the context of their life narrative. Care theories are derived directly from the feminist ethics model and especially promote nurturing of patients and caregivers (Volbrecht, 2002). An ethics-of-care way of thinking emphasizes the role of feelings, but not at the expense of some of the principles that are part of conventional ethics, such as autonomy (self-determination) or beneficence (doing good).

In this model, nurses incorporate a responsibility to care as a part of their professional behavior. Leininger (1988) defines care as "the central unifying domain from the body of knowledge and practices in nursing" (p. 34). Some aspects of care include the ability and obligation to appreciate, understand, and even share the patient's pain or condition. Using a caring model, your ethical analysis would focus on relationships and client stories. The following are specific perspectives within the ethics-of-care model:

- Viewing caring as the central force in nursing
- Promoting dignity and respect for patients as people
- Attending to the particulars of each individual patient
- Cultivating responsiveness to others
- Redefining fundamental moral principles to include virtues such as kindness, attentiveness, empathy, compassion, and reliability

An advantage of including the caring perspective and client stories in ethical dialogue is that it tends to focus discussion at the level where the relationships are located, rather than in an intellectual plane. Critics of the ethics-of-care suggest that the term *caring* can be misconstrued to become too sentimental and, therefore, ineffective. If nursing is sentimentalized through overemphasis on caring, nursing will be seen as less strong than medicine.

An ethics-of-care model does provide an alternative to the heavily intellectual camps of utilitarianism and deontology. It can give a refreshingly new perspective into

moral situations. Some questions that might reflect this model of discourse include the following:

- Should we provide free medical care to the homeless? An ethics-of-care position would say yes, even though it might not, for example, provide the greatest good for the greatest number of people.

- Our healthcare system uses discharge criteria that allow patients to be sent home from hospitals while they are still too ill to care for themselves. What does that say about caring in the healthcare system?

KnowledgeCheck 44–9

- How does feminist ethics affect ethical decision making?
- What does the ethics-of-care model emphasize?

 Go to Chapter 44, **Knowledge Check Response Sheet and Answers,** on the Electronic Study Guide

Professional Guidelines

In addition to moral frameworks, consult professional guidelines when making ethical decisions. One of the characteristics of a profession is that it states publicly the ethical standards for its members. Professionals, especially those who provide health care, have an obligation to society to be competent in their field, to control entry into the profession to those who are qualified, to discipline members of the profession who do not practice at an acceptable level, to do no harm, and to use high moral and ethical standards to resolve dilemmas (Husted & Husted, 2001). You can find ethical standards for nurses in codes of ethics, standards of practice, statements of patients' rights, and in various laws.

Nursing Codes of Ethics

Professional codes of ethics are formal statements of a group's expectations and standards for professional behavior generally accepted by members of the profession. Codes of ethics set forth ideal behaviors and, of course, are only as effective as the behaviors of the members of the profession who live up to the codes. The purposes of a nursing code of ethics are to:

- Inform the public about the profession's minimum standards

- Demonstrate nursing's commitment to the public it serves

- Outline major ethical considerations of nursing

- Provide general guidelines for professional behavior

- Guide the profession's self-regulating functions

- Remind us of the special responsibility we assume in caring for the sick

Codes of ethics are open to public scrutiny. Therefore, others may observe and judge your professional behavior. The ethical aspects of your work, just as the technical aspects, are subject to review by professional groups and licensure boards, who may use sanctions to punish code violations. Nursing codes are not legally binding. However, codes often exceed legal obligations. In most states, the state board of nursing uses the nursing code of ethics as the standard against which to evaluate a nurse's ethical behavior. The board has the legal authority to censure or reprimand the nurse who does not practice within the boundaries of ethical practice.

Three nursing organizations have had longstanding codes to guide nurses' ethical decision making. The codes differ in specific details, but they are based on similar principles.

International Council of Nurses

The International Council of Nurses (ICN) first adopted its Code of Ethics for Nurses in 1953 as "a guide for action based on social values and needs" (ICN, 2000). It was revised in 2000. The Code has served as the standard for nurses worldwide since it was first adopted. The ICN Code stresses respect for human rights, including the right to life, right to dignity, and right to be treated with respect. The code is designed as a guide for nurses in everyday choices, and it supports their refusal to participate in activities that conflict with caring and healing. To see this code,

 Go to Chapter 44, **Tables, Boxes, Figures: ESG Box 44–1,** on the Electronic Study Guide.

American Nurses Association

The American Nurses Association (ANA) revised their Code of Ethics for Nurses in 2001 (Box 44–1). ANA used input from a wide range of nurses and groups to ensure that the revised code would be relevant in many practice settings and reflect current ethical situations. The code has nine provisions, followed by interpretive statements to explain what is meant by each provision. If you would like more information about the ANA Code for Nurses,

 Go to the **ANA web site at** www.nursingworld.org/ethics/ecode.htm

Canadian Nurses Association

The Canadian Nurses Association revised its Code of Ethics for Registered Nurses in 2002. Similar in purpose to the ANA code, it provides guidance for decision making, serves as a means for self-evaluation and reflection regarding ethical practice, and provides a basis for peer review. The Canadian code is organized around eight values central to ethical nursing practice. To review the values and their definitions, see Box 44–2. To review the full code with all of its interpretative statements,

 Go to the **Canadian Nurses Association web site at** www.cna-nurses.ca/pages/ethics/ethicsframe.htm

BOX 44-1 American Nurses Association Code of Ethics for Nurses

1. The nurse, in all professional relationships, practices with compassion and respect for the inherent dignity, worth, and uniqueness of every individual, unrestricted by considerations of social or economic status, personal attributes, or the nature of health problems.

2. The nurse's primary commitment is to the patient, whether an individual, family, group or community.

3. The nurse promotes, advocates for and strives to protect the health, safety and rights of the patient.

4. The nurse is responsible and accountable for individual nursing practice and determines the appropriate delegation of tasks consistent with the nurse's obligation to provide optimum patient care.

5. The nurse owes the same duties to self as to others, including the responsibility to preserve integrity and safety, to maintain competence and to continue personal and professional growth.

6. The nurse participates in establishing, maintaining and improving health care environments and conditions of employment conducive to the provision of quality health care and consistent with the values of the profession through individual and collective action.

7. The nurse participates in the advancement of the profession through contributions to practice, education, administration and knowledge development.

8. The nurse collaborates with other health professionals and the public in promoting community, national and international efforts to meet health needs.

9. The profession of nursing, as represented by associations and their members, is responsible for articulating nursing values for maintaining the integrity of the profession and its practice, and for shaping social policy.

Source: Reprinted with permission from American Nurses Association, *Code of ethics for nurses with interpretive statements,* ©2001, Nursebooks.org, American Nurses Association, Washington, DC.

BOX 44-2 Canadian Nurses Association Code of Ethics for Registered Nurses

Safe, competent and ethical care	Nurses value the ability to provide safe, competent and ethical care that allows them to fulfill their ethical and professional obligations to the people they serve.
Health and well-being	Nurses value health promotion and well-being and assisting persons to achieve their optimum level of health in situations of normal health, illness, injury, disability or at the end of life.
Choice	Nurses respect and promote the autonomy of persons and help them express their health needs and values and obtain desired information and services so they can make informed decisions.
Dignity	Nurses recognize and respect the inherent worth of each person and advocate for respectful treatment of all persons.
Confidentiality	Nurses safeguard information learned in the context of a professional relationship and ensure it is shared outside the health care team only with the person's informed consent, or as may be legally required, or where the failure to disclose would cause significant harm.
Justice	Nurses uphold principles of equity and fairness to assist persons in receiving a share of health services and resources proportionate to their needs.
Accountability	Nurses are answerable for their practice, and they act in a manner consistent with their professional responsibilities and standards of practice.
Quality practice environments	Nurses value and advocate for practice environments that have the organizational structures and resources necessary to ensure safety, support and respect for all persons in the work setting.

This code is organized around the above described eight values. In the code, each value is further described by explanatory responsibility statements based on each value.

Source: Canadian Nurses Association. (2002). *Code of ethics for registered nurses.* Ottawa: Author.

BOX 44-3 American Nurses Association Standards of Professional Performance: Ethics

Standard XII. Ethics

Definition: The registered nurse integrates ethical provisions in all areas of practice.

Measurement Criteria

The registered nurse:

- Uses the Code of Ethics for Nurses with Interpretive Statements (ANA, 2001) to guide practice.
- Delivers care in a manner that preserves and protects patient autonomy, dignity, and rights.
- Maintains patient confidentiality within legal and regulatory parameters.
- Serves as a patient advocate assisting patients in developing skills for self-advocacy.
- Maintains a therapeutic and professional patient-nurse relationship with appropriate professional role boundaries.
- Demonstrates a commitment to practicing self-care, managing stress and connecting with self and others.
- Contributes to resolving ethical issues of patients, colleagues, or systems as evidenced in such activities as participating on ethics committees.
- Reports illegal, incompetent, or impaired practices.

Source: Excerpted from American Nurses Association. (2004). *Nursing: Scope and standards of practice.* Washington, DC: American Nurses Publishing, American Nurses Foundation/ American Nurses Association. Reprinted with permission.

BOX 44-4 American Hospital Association: The Patient Care Partnership

Patients, when hospitalized, should expect the following:

- High-quality care, including the right to know the identity of caregivers.
- A clean, safe environment, including safety, freedom from abuse and neglect, and discussion of any changes in care.
- Respect for healthcare goals, values, and spiritual beliefs.
- To be involved in making decisions about their care and treatment. This includes receiving information about:

  Health condition and treatments

  The benefits and risks of treatments, and whether a treatment is experimental or part of a research study

  What the patient and family will need to do regarding treatment follow-up after leaving the hospital

- Information about the right to make decisions and to refuse care, including advance directives and counselors or chaplains available to help with decision making.
- Protection of their privacy and confidentiality.
- Help with the bill and filing insurance claims.
- Preparation and information when leaving the hospital, including:

  Identification of sources for follow-up care and whether the hospital has a financial interest in any of the referrals

  Coordination of hospital activities with caregivers outside the hospital

  Information and training about the self-care the person will need at home

Source: Excerpted and adapted from American Hospital Association. (2004). *The patient care partnership.* Chicago: Author.

ANA Standards of Care

In addition to its Code of Ethics, the American Nurses Association (ANA) sets standards for all aspects of clinical practice. In the newly revised *Nursing: Scope and Standards of Practice* (2004), standard 12 focuses on ethical practice. This standard (see Box 44–3) directs nurses to practice within the parameters described in the Code of Ethics for Nurses. Standard 12 speaks to the nurse's responsibilities to patients and directs nurses to manage ethical dilemmas and to report practices that are illegal, incompetent, or impaired.

The Patient Care Partnership

When clients are admitted to hospitals or to extended care facilities, they are entitled to specific rights in terms of their treatment: the right to make their own decisions, to be active partners in the treatment process, and to be treated with dignity and respect. Because rights are rooted in values, and because values are derived from culture, patient rights are different throughout the world. In the United States, the American Hospital Association (AHA) first published a model *Patient's Bill of Rights* in 1973 and then revised it in 1992. Recently, the AHA (2004) has replaced its *Bill of Rights* with a document called *Patient Care Partnership.* Instead of using "rights" language, this document is written in terms of patient expectations and responsibilities. For a summary, see Box 44–4. To view the entire document,

Go to the **American Hospital Association** web site at **www.aha.org/aha/ptcommunication/partnership/index.html**

The *Patient Care Partnership* encourages healthcare providers to be more aware of the need to treat patients in an ethical manner and to protect client rights.

KnowledgeCheck 44–10

- How would the nurse use a professional guideline or code of ethics to assist in the ethical decision-making process?
- What are some examples of such resources?

 Go to Chapter 44, **Knowledge Check Response Sheet and Answers,** on the Electronic Study Guide.

ETHICAL ISSUES IN HEALTHCARE

As a nurse, you are likely to encounter several ethical issues that occur in healthcare. For example, ethical questions arise in the following situations:

- Acquired immune deficiency syndrome (AIDS)
- Abortion
- Allocation of healthcare goods and services
- Confidentiality and privacy (e.g., reporting gunshot wounds and child abuse)
- Honoring advance directives
- Do Not Attempt Resuscitation (DNAR) orders
- Assisted suicide and euthanasia
- Using extraordinary (heroic) measures to prolong life
- Withdrawing or withholding life-sustaining treatments (e.g., ventilators, artificial nutrition and hydration)
- Informed consent
- Organ transplantation
- Reproductive technology (e.g., in vitro fertilization, surrogate mothering, sex preselection)

To learn more about these situations and the ethical conflicts surrounding them,

 Go to Chapter 44, **Supplemental Materials: Ethical Issues in Health Care,** on the Electronic Study Guide.

Practical Knowledge
knowing how

To fulfill your professional obligations for ethical practice, you will need practical knowledge of the processes of values clarification, moral decision making, patient advocacy, and integrity-producing compromise.

VALUES CLARIFICATION

Values clarification refers to the process of becoming conscious of and naming one's values (Burkhardt & Nathaniel, 2002). If you are clear about your values, you will make better decisions and be better able to

avoid imposing your values on others. Because each person has his own unique values set, it is important for you to appreciate others' values and how they influence their decisions. Clarifying values should be a positive process that leads to a human growth experience resulting in more awareness, empathy, and insight (Steele & Harmon, 1983). A values clarification process does not tell you what your values ought to be; it merely helps you discover what they are. Values change over time, so you may need to repeat the process more than once in your lifetime.

Raths, Harmin, and Simon (1978) identified seven criteria by which to identify a value as a "full" value (Table 44–4). A full value must be:

- Chosen freely from a list of alternatives after thoughtful consideration has been given to the consequences of each alternative
- Cherished and made known to other people
- Translated into behaviors that are consistent with the chosen value and integrated into the lifestyle

How Can I Clarify My Values?

As a nurse, you will need to examine your values regarding life, death, wellness, and illness. A good place to start is to ask yourself questions about situations that you think you may be uncomfortable with, such as caring for a substance abuser seeking drugs in the emergency department, an unwed adolescent mother pregnant for the second time in 11 months, or parents such as the Freses ("Meet Your Patients"), who refuse treatment for a child because of religious beliefs. Ask yourself questions such as:

- Could I take care of this person?
- Does this bother me?
- What would I do if confronted with such a situation?

For examples of exercises that can help you begin to clarify your values related to health care,

 Go to Chapter 44, **Supplemental Materials: Tables, Boxes, Figures: ESG Box 44–2: Rank-Ordering Values** and **Tables, Boxes, Figures: ESG Box 44–3: Values Preference Exercise,** on the Electronic Study Guide.

Remember that there are no right or wrong answers to these exercises. They are only to assist you as you identify your values and examine the relative importance of these values in your personal and professional life.

How Can I Help Clients to Clarify Their Values?

Some clients may exhibit behaviors that indicate that their values are not clear. Consider this example:

Jon White is the chief executive officer of a large healthcare facility. Jon has had two myocardial

TABLE 44-4 Values Clarification

Step	Description	Questions to Ask Your Patient
Choosing (cognitive)	Beliefs are chosen: • Freely (allows you to cherish your choice) • From alternatives • After considering all consequences (ensures that the alternative is right for you)	• Do (did) you have any choice about what you do? • Do you have any control over what happens? • What have you decided to do? • Can you list some alternative actions? • What are your options? • What could you do instead of . . . ? • What do you think will happen if you do that? • What will you gain by doing that? • What is the disadvantage of doing that?
Prizing (affective)	Beliefs and behaviors that are chosen are prized: • With pride (feeling good about your choice) • With public affirmation	• How do you feel about your decision? • People sometimes feel good after making such a decision. Others feel pressured. How is it for you? • How do you intend to tell your family (friends) about this decision? • What will you say to your wife (friends, family)? • When will you announce your decision to . . . ?
Acting (behavioral)	Beliefs are acted on: • By incorporating the choice into one's own behavior • With consistency and repetition	Try to determine whether the client will act on the decision: • How do you think your wife (significant other) will react when you do that? • When will you actually carry out this decision? Try to predict consistent behavior by asking: • How many times in the past have you . . . • What kind of schedule have you worked out? How often and when will you . . . ?

Source: Adapted from Raths, L. E., Harmin M., & Simon, S. B. (1978). *Values and teaching: Working with values in the classroom.* Columbus, OH: Merrill Publishing.

infarctions (heart attacks) in the last 5 years. He also has hypercholesterolemia (high cholesterol) and hypertension (high blood pressure). Jon's physician has prescribed a heart medicine, low-dose aspirin, and medications to control his hypertension and cholesterol. Jon has repeatedly been taught about his diet, medications, and activity. He insists he is compliant. Jon's wife tells you that he has stopped exercising and is eating whatever he wants, including saturated fats. Jon tells her it is OK to eat what he wants because he is taking a "cholesterol-buster" pill.

The following patient behaviors may indicate that a patient needs values clarification:

• Ignoring the advice of a health professional

• Communication that is inconsistent with behavior

• Numerous admissions to the agency for the same problem

• Uncertainty or confusion about which action to take

Which of those behaviors did Jon exhibit? To help Jon clarify his values, you might ask him to list the three things that are most important to him in life. Or you could help him work through the steps in Table 44–4 (choosing, prizing, and acting).

KnowledgeCheck 44–11

• What is values clarification?

• What are the steps in values clarification?

 Go to Chapter 44, **Knowledge Check Response Sheet and Answers,** on the Electronic Study Guide.

ETHICAL DECISION MAKING

Decision models used in bioethics do not offer pat, easily arrived at decisions, but they do provide a guiding structure to follow to arrive at the best answer in specific situations. Decision models can help you decide on a course of action even if they do not tell you absolutely that the action is right or wrong.

BOX 44–5   Nursing Process Compared to Purtilo Ethical Decision-Making Model

Nursing Process	Purtillo
Assessment	• Gather as much relevant information as possible to get your facts straight.
Nursing Diagnosis	• Determine the precise nature of the ethical problem (if data confirm that problem exists).
Planning	• Decide on the ethical approach that will best get to the heart of the problem. • Explore the practical alternatives: Decide what should be done and how it can best be done.
Implementation	• Complete the action.
Evaluation	• Reflect on and evaluate the process and outcome.

Source: Adapted from Purtilo, R. (1999). *Ethical dimensions in the health professions* (3rd ed.). Philadelphia: Saunders, pp. 81–89.

Problem or Dilemma?

In the best of all possible worlds, it would be easy to decide how to apply moral principles and decide what to do. However, it is common in moral situations for one ethical principle to be at odds with another equally important principle, or for a philosophical framework to produce more than one acceptable option. An **ethical dilemma** is a situation in which a choice must be made between two equally undesirable actions. There is no clearly right or wrong option. Such situations are emotionally painful for everyone in the situation, as you can see from the "Meet Your Patients" scenario presented at the beginning of this chapter. If you support Alan's parents' right to refuse blood transfusion, you honor the principle of autonomy, but at the expense of the principle of nonmaleficence, which says we should prevent harm to Alan.

However, not all moral problems are dilemmas. In fact, you will confront a true dilemma only occasionally (Cahn, 1987; Curtin & Flaherty, 1982; Levine, 1989; White, 1983). Not all moral problems are complex and difficult. Some questions are easily answered (e.g., "Should I take the patient's morphine to relieve my back pain?"). It is probably more accurate, then, to refer to "moral questions," "moral problems," or "moral situations" and not use the term *dilemma* loosely. Only those problems that pose a question between competing and equally valuable interests are true dilemmas.

What Are Some Decision-Making Models?

Once you have identified an ethical problem, a decision model will help you to think logically about the best action to take. Nonetheless, in the case of a true ethical dilemma, you will probably not be comfortable with any course of action, no matter how logically you think it through.

We have said it is important to be aware of the ethical issues in patient care situations, but how will you recognize them? The key is that there is usually a conflict. Conflict may occur:

• About the right action to take
• Between the duties and obligations of healthcare professionals (or they are unclear)
• Between the needs and interests of an individual and a group of clients
• Between what the family wants and what the client wants or needs
• Between the family and health professionals
• Between ethical principles or values (e.g., autonomy versus nonmaleficence, as in the "Meet Your Patients" scenario)

Ethical decision-making models will assist you to consider carefully multiple perspectives, guide your reasoning, and help you to explain the reasons for your final action (Cameron, Schaffer, & Park, 2001). As with the nursing process, you can adapt a basic problem-solving method when considering ethical problems (Box 44–5).

As already mentioned, different solutions will evolve with each approach. One of the easiest to remember and implement is the MORAL model. This model has been credited to two different authors: Thiroux (1977) and Crisham (in Scott, 1985). The letters MORAL will remind you of the steps in this model, which is described in the following section. Also,

VOL 2 Go to Chapter 44, **Technique 44–1: Using the MORAL Model for Ethical Decision Making,** in Volume 2.

How Do I Work Through an Ethical Problem?

Let's use the "Meet Your Patients" scenario to illustrate ethical decision making.

Use Problem Solving

As a first step in ethical decision making, use the problem-solving approach in Box 44–5 to describe the problem and alternative approaches:

Assessment—What are the relevant facts? Alan needs a blood transfusion to survive. Both the surgeon and the nurse (you) have tried to persuade the parents to consent, but they still refuse. The parents are Jehovah's Witnesses, a religion that prohibits blood transfusions. Alan is 15 years old (a minor), so you cannot administer a transfusion without his parents' consent.

Diagnosis—Identify the problem; state the conflict. There is a values conflict: The healthcare professionals value preserving physical life; the parents place more value on preserving the soul. There is a moral dilemma for the healthcare professional, as well. If no transfusion is given, then you have violated the principle of nonmaleficence (harm to Alan); if you somehow coerce or force the parents to consent, you have violated the principle of autonomy (respect for their values and their freedom to choose). So the decision to be made is whether to

1. follow the parents' wishes
2. find a legal way to transfuse without their consent, or
3. find some compromise that will work.

Use the MORAL Model

Now use the MORAL model to come up with alternative solutions for this family.

M—Massage the Dilemma

First identify and define the issues in the dilemma, and consider the values and options of all the major players: Mr. and Mrs. Frese, Alan, the surgeon, possibly a clergyman, and you, the nurse. You have already identified the values in the problem-solving approach: physical life versus spiritual life. You and the surgeon also value the principles of autonomy and nonmaleficence.

Then identify the information gaps. In massaging the situation, you should ask yourself:

• Do I fully understand the situation that is causing the need for blood?

• How much time is available to make this decision—do the parents have to decide within a few minutes, or do they have enough time to discuss this with their clergyman?

• Does the physician know that the family are Jehovah's Witnesses?

• Does the surgeon have any treatment that could be used to stabilize Alan while the parents discuss the situation?

• Do Alan's parents fully understand the nature of Alan's physical emergency?

• In the Freses' religious view, what is the consequence of receiving blood?

• Do they understand what might happen if blood is not administered (i.e., do they understand the consequence of their action or inaction)?

• Is this what Alan would want? Has Alan discussed in the past what he feels about blood transfusions? Have they ever had family discussions when other young Jehovah Witnesses have been faced with such a decision? Where did Alan stand in those discussions?

• How is this situation like other situations they have experienced in their lives?

• Have they thought about their opposing duties: the duty to uphold their religious values and the duty to protect their son from harm?

• Has everyone's voice been heard?

• Have the parents contacted their clergyman and discussed the situation?

• What emotions are coming into play in this situation?

• How is this decision affecting the parents as individuals? Are they in agreement on the issue, or is there dissension? If there is dissension, are both sides being supported?

• Is there some common ground between what the doctor wants and what the parents feel they need to do to uphold their religious convictions?

O—Outline the Options

At this step in the MORAL model, you (or the charge nurse or a member of the ethics committee) should outline all of the options to all parties, including those that are less realistic and conflicting. You might ask a member of the ethics committee or the hospital chaplain to help the family and the doctor understand the opposing viewpoints.

The surgeon will need to outline the state of emergency that exists for Alan and to clearly explain what the limited medical options are: to transfuse blood or, if no blood is given, what other treatments are available (e.g., volume enhancers). The surgeon will need to say how soon the decision must be made, based on Alan's condition. He should clearly describe the consequence of each action. Carefully, and with as little emotion as possible, explain the consequence of each action to the parents. The physician should state whether one administration of blood will likely fix the situation or whether continued administration may be required.

The family (or their clergyman) should explain for the doctor and nurse the basis for their refusal to consent and what they believe the consequence would be if blood were given.

R—Resolve the Dilemma

Now carefully review the issues and options. Apply basic moral principles. If you can, also look at the situation using alternate ethical frameworks.

Autonomy. By their refusing to give consent, the Freses are exercising their autonomy. How far will we go to honor their autonomy?

Beneficence and nonmaleficence. How are we defining "good" (beneficence) and "harm" (nonmaleficence) in this situation? The physician clearly defines "good" as Alan receiving the needed blood. He defines "harm" as the outcome for Alan without the blood, even if he uses a less effective alternative. Alan's parents would define "good" as following their religious mandates and making sure their son will remain pure in the eyes of God. They might explain that a Jehovah's Witness who willingly accepts a blood transfusion might forfeit his or her eternal life. The Freses might believe the taking of blood to be more harmful than death, because they believe that would affect Alan's eternal life, not just his physical life.

Fidelity. The surgeon is being loyal (exhibiting fidelity) to the principles of medicine and evidence-based practice, which mandate the administration of the blood. To the parents, their loyalty to their religious principles to ensure that Alan has eternal life may be more important than the loss of the physical life itself.

Veracity. The principle of veracity holds that the surgeon should not exaggerate the need for the blood, and he should be honest with the parents in terms of the consequences of the alternative actions. Another question of veracity involves the parents: Are they being honest with each other regarding their feelings?

Your role as a nurse is to be an advocate for the patient and the family.

- Talk with the family and their clergyman, if available, about what they are thinking about their opposing duties: the duty to uphold their religious values and the duty to protect their son from the physical harm of death.
- Ensure that everyone's voice has been heard.
- If you are in a position to do so, explain to the surgeon the reasoned position of Alan's parents.
- Always look for the opportunity for a good compromise (to be discussed later in this chapter).

A—Act by Applying the Chosen Option

This step is the first one that actually requires action. The hospital is bound to follow the parents' decision because Alan is a minor. However, if there is time, many agencies might refer this situation to the hospital ethics committee. Because Alan is a minor, the hospital might ask a legal court authority to resolve the situation. If an emergency requires an immediate decision, the only legal action is to follow the parents' decision, whether or not you consider it the best moral action.

Whatever happens, Alan's parents will need emotional support. If they decide to refuse the blood transfusion, you must remain nonjudgmental in supporting them, even if you do not agree with their decision. If they, or the court, decide that the blood will be given, they may need even more support. They may feel overwhelming guilt, and they may fear that Alan will be forever burdened with guilt at the realization that they broke church doctrine to save his life. If their extended family (recall that they have a large, supportive family) is not present, you could volunteer to call in extended family, friends, and clergy if they wish. They will need a quiet, private place to await the outcome of the treatment.

L—Look Back and Evaluate

This phase calls for evaluation of the entire process, not just the consequence of the decided action. How well did the process work? Were processes in place for the dilemma to be discussed respectfully without undue delay in treatment? Were all parties' expectations realistic? How are all of the affected parties feeling now (doctor, parents, family, Alan, you)? Regardless of the outcome of the decision, does everyone involved feel as though they had a voice and were respected? How well did you do in the situation? Did you act as an effective advocate for the rights of Alan and his parents? Were you unduly influenced by the power and authority of the physician or hospital in the situation? Were policies and procedures in place to guide you in the process of working out this situation? Has anything changed since the dilemma came to light? Has a greater good been achieved for future situations? Have future situations been made easier as a result of the things learned in this situation? Has any aspect of this ethical decision now become a universal policy at the institution? Are further actions required in terms of this or like situations?

For guidelines to help you avoid common errors when making moral decisions,

 Go to Chapter 44, **Supplemental Materials: Common Errors in Decision Making,** on the Electronic Study Guide.

Use the Notion of Compromise

As already mentioned, even if you believe you know the right thing to do, others may not agree with you, or there may be constraints that prevent you from

doing it. For example, in the case of Alan, even if you decided the right thing to do is give him a blood transfusion, (1) his parents do not agree with you, and (2) the law says you cannot do so without his parents' consent. This will happen often—much more often than a true dilemma, in which you cannot *decide* the right thing to do. No matter how well we work together, there will always be ethical problems and disagreements. Many cases are full of complexity and uncertainty, and sometimes the price of acting on your beliefs is extremely high. For example, what might have happened if the surgeon had infused blood without the Freses' consent? What might have happened if you had refused to talk to the parents as the surgeon asked you?

Many times it will be possible to reach a "good" compromise. A good compromise is one that preserves the integrity of all parties. This means that:

1. The discussions are carried out in a spirit of mutual respect—that all voices are heard.
2. The compromise solution itself should be ethically sound; that is, you should be able to provide principles-based rationale for the compromise, as well as for each of the opposing positions. In the case of Alan, there probably is no compromise position between "give blood" and "don't give blood." Perhaps the parents would agree to one, but no more than one, transfusion; but that is hard to justify ethically. If one transfusion is acceptable (to honor nonmaleficence), why not two or three? If two transfusions are against their religion, why would one be acceptable? Nevertheless, in many cases compromise is possible.

So how do you compromise without losing moral integrity? First, realize that there is more at stake than the issue itself ("Is a blood transfusion right or wrong?"). There are some things that are inherently good in making a compromise.

- First, it is never good to settle things by force (as you would if you got a court order to transfuse Alan without his parents' consent). You have probably heard the old saying, "Might doesn't make right." A compromise can preserve the rights of the less powerful party in a disagreement.
- Keeping peace on a nursing unit is good for both the nurses and patients. When there is upheaval and moral suffering, patient care can suffer. A compromise can bring peace.
- There is intrinsic good in taking part in a process in which we must try to see things from others' points of view. It may make us more open-minded, more creative, and less judgmental.
- Keep in mind that most issues do contain room for reasonable differences of opinion. In the "Meet Your Patients" scenario, can you see that both sides are

people of goodwill who have ethical justification for their opinion? Also, there is often room for doubt, on your own part, about the morally best action to take.
- A compromise may achieve mutual respect. It is a significant thing to reach a settlement in which each party feels assured of the other's respect for its seriousness and sincerity.

Given all those ideas, a person of goodwill might want to reexamine and back off a very strong opinion. Remember, sometimes your position isn't all that strong, and the other position isn't all that weak (as in the case of Alan). There is also always the chance that you may have made an error in your reasoning or have not completely understood some facts of the case. Ethical disputes can be settled only if you are willing to engage in discussion and admit that the other people might have a point! There may be cases where you cannot compromise (perhaps Alan's case is one), but don't listen to people who say "You can never reach agreement on ethical issues. They are too complex." It is possible to achieve integrity-producing compromises, and in nursing, it is often necessary.

What Are My Obligations in Ethical Decisions?

As you can see, in making ethical decisions, nurses rarely act alone. Usually you will be one of several healthcare professionals and family members who will jointly arrive at the best decision. What is your role when an ethical decision is needed?

- Be aware of and sensitive to issues, so you can identify them when they arise. Educate yourself—attend workshops, read, and talk to other nurses.
- Assume responsibility for your own moral actions. Even if you do not have the "last word" about what happens to a patient or about what others do, you are always responsible for your own actions in every situation.
- Function as a team member when ethical problems arise. Realize you should have input—no one profession has full moral expertise—and realize that your input can be valuable.
- Support the patient and family members while they are making the decision and afterward. Listen. Ask questions. Be helpful without being too directive or judgmental.
- Support patients who are not being allowed to decide. For example, in the "Meet Your Patients" scenario, you would want to be sure Alan's wishes were considered, if possible. However, if the parents insist on deciding for him, against his wishes, he may need a great deal of emotional support.
- Use and participate in institutional ethics committees if you are given the opportunity.

• Most important, advocate for your client. You may need to balance your client's autonomy with the wishes of family members or the responsibilities of other healthcare professionals to the patient. As an advocate, you may find yourself at odds with other team members or family members. Frequently you and the others involved will have different ethical perspectives.

Use and Participate in Institutional Ethics Committees

As you can see from the "Meet Your Patients" scenario, there is no easy way to decide which principle should outrank another principle, or which person's values are best in a given situation. For this reason, healthcare institutions have ethics committees. These typically interdisciplinary committees include nurses, doctors, clergy, ethicists, and lay representatives. Ethics committees write guidelines and policies, provide education and counseling, and, in the case of ethical dilemmas, review the case and provide a forum for the expression of the diverse perspectives of those involved (Salladay, 2002).

Ethics committees usually follow one of three distinct models when discussing a dilemma: the autonomy model, the patient benefit model, and the social justice model.

1. The **autonomy model** is useful when the patient is competent to decide. This model emphasizes patient autonomy and choice as the highest value. For example, if this committee knew Alan's ("Meet Your Patients") wishes, they might be inclined to try to persuade his parents to do as Alan wants.

2. The **patient benefit model** assists in decision making for the incompetent patient by using substituted judgment (i.e., what the patient would want for herself if she were capable of making these issues known). If Alan is unconscious and cannot say what he wants, this committee would probably ask Alan's parents, family, and friends, "What do you think Alan would want? Have you ever heard him talk about a situation such as this?"

3. The **social justice model** focuses more on broad social issues involving the entire institution, rather than on a single patient issue (Yoder-Wise, 2003). Such a committee might consider whether, in general, an institution ought ever to seek a legal order to act against the wishes of the parents. Or they might discuss whether supporting parents' religious beliefs in this instance might have implications for supporting other types of religious beliefs in future cases.

KnowledgeCheck 44–12

• Define *ethical dilemma*.
• How can you recognize an ethical problem?
• What is an integrity-producing compromise?
• What are the functions of an ethics committee?
• What does the mnemonic MORAL stand for?

 Go to Chapter 44, **Knowledge Check Response Sheet and Answers,** on the Electronic Study Guide.

Improve Your Ethical Decision Making

By now you should understand that you cannot avoid making moral decisions in nursing. The following suggestions will help you to be as well prepared as possible when ethical issues arise.

• *Use theoretical knowledge.* Review nursing and other literature for discussion of cases and experiences of other nurses. This will give you a broader view of the problems you may confront and the strategies for managing them. Become familiar with the various codes of ethics and the *Patient Care Partnership,* as well as the moral frameworks and principles.

• *Use self-knowledge.* Examine your personal value system. Explore the influences of your religion, cultural beliefs, and personal experiences. This will help you to recognize your comfort zone with specific ethical issues.

• *Use practical knowledge.* While still a student, you should ask to attend either ethical rounds or an ethics committee meeting. As a graduate nurse, you could benefit by volunteering to sit on your institution's ethics committee or plan to attend nursing ethics rounds to familiarize yourself with the types of ethical problems that occur at your institution.

• *Consult reliable sources.* Attend ethics education programs, and talk about issues with other healthcare providers. Attorneys, ethicists, and members of the clergy can provide helpful perspectives.

• *Share.* Regularly engage in discussions with the staff on your unit to determine differences in value systems and to collaborate proactively to work out methods that can be used to resolve ethical dilemmas effectively. When you are faced with a difficult moral decision, consult with peers, co-workers, and teachers. Seek guidance and support.

• *Evaluate.* After the situation is resolved, evaluate your decision and the effects of your actions. You should be able to learn from even the worst decision. And when everything goes well, you can file your strategies away to use in similar future situations.

Be a Patient Advocate

The role of advocates is to safeguard clients against abuse and violation of their rights. Why do you think

this is so important? Why can't patients do this for themselves? The following are some of the reasons.

1. *You have special knowledge that the patient does not have.* Diseases, treatments, and the health-care system are so complex that when clients become ill, they may not have the energy to deal with the complexity, even if they do have the necessary knowledge. You may need to help them to "jump through all the necessary hoops" to get what they need. When patients' rights are denied or when patients do not have the ability to exert their rights, nurses have a responsibility to step in (Rumbold, 1999). "Without the advocacy and protection of rights there really are no rights" (Bandman & Bandman, 2002, p. 23).

2. *One aspect of your professional role is to defend patients' autonomous decisions* (see Boxes 44–1, 44–2, and 44–3). Recall that the ANA Code of Ethics requires you to be a patient advocate. As a nurse, you will be called on to defend your patient's autonomous decisions even if you do not agree with them and even if they conflict with the opinions of others involved in the patient's care. You may find yourself the sole champion of a patient's right to choose for himself the direction of his care.

3. *Nurses have a special relationship with patients.* You may find that you are able to acquire information about a client that is not available to professionals of other disciplines. In general, nurses interact with patients over longer time intervals and are involved in very intimate activities, especially in inpatient settings. They often become the most trusted caregivers. Details about family life, coping styles, personal preferences, fears, and insecurities are all more likely to come out over the time involved in nursing interventions than in the brief minutes of interaction when the physician makes rounds. Additionally, patients may perceive less social distance between themselves and the nurse and, therefore, feel more free to confide in them. The nurses' point of view can be a valuable asset to resolving an ethical problem satisfactorily. Of course, many physicians

have long-standing relationships with their patients; however, this does not negate the importance of the nurse's input, which may provide a different perspective.

Your role as an advocate is to inform, support, and communicate. You should inform clients of their rights and provide the information they need to make informed decisions, if they are capable of doing so. Then you must remain objective and support them in the decisions they make, even when you believe it to be wrong. If others are not respecting client choices, you will need to intervene on the client's behalf. This may simply be a matter of conveying information and clarifying the client's wishes to family or healthcare professionals (e.g., "I know how hard it is for you to let him go, but Mr. Brown says he has made peace and is ready to die. His treatments make him feel even more ill, and he simply does not want to fight anymore.") Advocacy may require you to arrange for the client to consult with clergy or an attorney for advice and support or may require you to consult an institutional ethics committee.

For principles that will help you to function effectively as an advocate,

 Go to Chapter 44, **Technique 44–2: Using Guidelines for Advocacy,** in Volume 2.

KnowledgeCheck 44–13

- What are three reasons why patients may need a nurse advocate?
- Briefly describe the nurse's role as a patient advocate.

 Go to Chapter 44, **Knowledge Check Response Sheet and Answers,** on the Electronic Study Guide.

 Go to Chapter 44, **Resources for Caregivers and Health Professionals,** on the Electronic Study Guide.

 Suggested Readings: Go to Chapter 44, **Reading More About Ethics and Values,** on the Electronic Study Guide.

 Bibliography: Go to Volume 2, Bibliography.

Legal Issues

Learning Outcomes

After completing this chapter, you should be able to:

✳ Explain legal concepts basic to nursing practice.

✳ Identify federal and state laws regulating nursing practice.

✳ Discuss basic principles of criminal law controlling nursing practice.

✳ Discuss basic principles of civil law controlling nursing practice.

✳ Analyze major legal issues that arise within nursing practice.

✳ Identify measures to decrease the likelihood of committing nursing malpractice.

Disclaimer: The material contained in this chapter is intended to convey information on topics of interest to nursing students. Although prepared by a nurse attorney, this chapter should not be utilized as a substitute for legal counseling. No one should act upon the information contained in this chapter without professional guidance. These materials should not be considered legal advice or a legal opinion.

Your Nurse Role Model

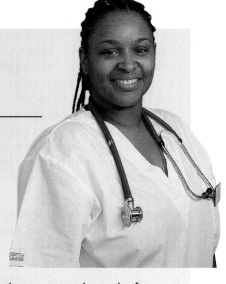

A nurse employed by a temporary agency is assigned to a nursing home for a 12-hour shift. On arrival, she discovers that the registered nurse assigned for the previous shift suddenly quit, leaving two unlicensed assistive personnel (UAPs) to provide patient care and complete the narcotics check. The UAPs inform her that she will be assigned to 20 patients requiring heavy care, with one UAP for the 12-hour shift. The nursing supervisor will not arrive for one hour, and the administrator for another hour and a half. The nurse decides not to accept the assignment, to report the decision and reasons to her agency supervisor, and to leave the nursing home facility immediately. Based solely on your past experiences and present knowledge, consider the following questions:

- Did the nurse do the right thing, from a legal perspective?

- What factors in this situation could create legal problems for the nurse?
- In addition to protecting her nursing license, what other factors should the nurse have considered in deciding whether to stay or leave the facility?
- The nurse's action (leaving the facility) might be viewed, under some laws, as abandonment of patients. What are some alternative actions the nurse might have taken to avoid that risk?

Theoretical Knowledge
knowing why

To answer the questions in the preceding scenario, you would certainly need to use the critical-thinking model in Chapter 2. In addition, you also need a working knowledge of laws designed to protect both patients and nurses.

Laws are sets of enforceable principles and rules established to protect society (O'Keefe, 2001). Legal principles form a framework within which you will practice the art of nursing. You need knowledge of laws, regulations, and standards of practice to understand legal issues you will encounter in practice and to avoid civil liability. Under the law, you are accountable not only to patients, employers, and professional colleagues, but also to the community at large.

WHAT ARE THE SOURCES OF LAW?

Laws are derived from four basic sources: (1) the constitutions of the state and federal governments, (2) state and federal legislatures, (3) administrative agencies, and (4) courts.

- *Constitutional law.* The U.S. Constitution is the document that sets forth the three branches of the government—the executive, legislative, and judicial. The Constitution grants the federal government only specific powers, leaving broad governing powers to the states. Under these powers, states also have the power to pass their own constitutions, as well as statutes. All laws and regulations must comply with the overriding dictates of the U.S. Constitution, however (Marchand, 2001). For a description of the seven Articles of the Constitution,

 Go to Chapter 45, **Tables, Boxes, Figures: ESG Box 45–1: Articles of the United States Constitution,** on the Electronic Study Guide.

- *Legislatures.* The laws enacted by federal and state legislatures are called *statutes*. States have **police powers:** the right to make laws necessary for the health, safety, welfare, and morals of the population (Marchand, 2001, p. 10). Nurse practice acts are examples of statutes. For examples,

 Go to the **Medi-Smart web site at http://medi-smart.com/ practice.htm**

- *Administrative agencies.* Rules, regulations, and orders developed by agencies (such as the board of nursing examiners, for example) to carry out administrative functions are defined as **administrative law.** After a statute is passed by the legislature, agencies develop specific regulations to enforce it. The legislature has delegated this authority to administrative bodies. For example, the board of nursing examiners may implement regulations and procedures to assess and penalize the conduct of a nurse suspected of violating the nurse practice act.

- *Courts.* Law developed through the court system via judicial decision is called **common law.** Common law is based upon the facts of each given case and on *precedent,* or prior decisions made by judges in the same or similar circumstances.

WHAT LAWS AND REGULATIONS GUIDE NURSING PRACTICE?

Various levels and types of laws, regulations, and standards guide nursing practice and protect both nurses and patients.

Federal Law

State nursing practice acts typically require you to have knowledge of federal laws affecting nursing practice. Some federal laws—both constitutional and statutory—affecting nursing practice are discussed below.

The Bill of Rights

The first 10 amendments to the U.S. Constitution are collectively known as the Bill of Rights. Some of these rights in particular play a critical role in health care and are the foundation of certain patient rights (Cammuso, Madden, & Wallen, 2001, p. 400):

1. The right to privacy
2. The right against self-incrimination
3. Protection from cruel and unusual punishment
4. Freedom of speech, religion, and the press
5. Protection of property rights
6. Equal protection under the law

To read the entire Bill of Rights,

 Go to Chapter 45, **Tables, Boxes, Figures: ESG Box 45–2: The Bill of Rights, Amendments 1–10 of the Constitution,** on the Electronic Study Guide.

Or,

  Go to the **infoUSA web site at http://usinfo.state.gov/usa/ infousa/facts/ funddocs/billeng.htm**

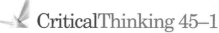 CriticalThinking 45–1

- Develop a scenario illustrating how a nurse might protect a patient's right to privacy.
- What is one thing a nurse can do to respect a patient's property rights?

Emergency Medical Treatment and Active Labor Act (EMTALA)

Enacted by Congress in 1986 and updated in 2003, the intent of the Emergency Medical Treatment and Active Labor Act (EMTALA) is to ensure public access to emergency services regardless of ability to pay. EMTALA prohibits "patient dumping"—transferring indigent or uninsured patients from a private hospital to a public hospital without appropriate screening and stabilization. When a client comes to the emergency department requesting examination or treatment for an emergency medical condition (including labor), the hospital must provide stabilizing treatment; the client cannot be transferred until he is stable. An exception is made if a hospital does not have the capability to stabilize a patient or if the patient requests a transfer. And in such circumstances, qualified personnel and equipment must be made available to transport the patient, and his medical records must be forwarded to the receiving hospital.

The Health Care Quality Improvement Act of 1986 (HCQIA)

The Health Care Quality Improvement Act of 1986 (HCQIA), implemented in 1990, created the National Practitioner Data Bank (NPDB). The NPDB collects and provides information related to (1) medical malpractice payments made on behalf of healthcare providers; (2) adverse actions taken against clinical privileges of physicians, osteopaths, and dentists; and (3) actions by professional societies adversely affecting membership. This law is designed to protect patients by providing knowledge of practioners who have been sanctioned for not meeting legal standards of care in the past. Reporting of this information to the NPDB is mandatory, and failure to do so will result in fines and penalties (Fedorka & Resnick, 2001, pp. 105–106).

The Americans with Disabilities Act (ADA)

The Americans with Disabilities Act (ADA) provides a national mandate for eliminating discrimination against people with disabilities (ADA, 1990, Section 2. Findings and Purposes). In general, the ADA provides that employees with disabilities must be provided reasonable accommodations within the work or healthcare setting to perform their jobs. For example, under this law, infection with the human immunodeficiency

virus (HIV) is considered a disability, and, as a rule, an infected worker has the right to decide whether or not to disclose his HIV status. It also means that care providers cannot discriminate against patients who are HIV positive. The ADA applies to patients as well, requiring that buildings be wheelchair accessible, for instance.

The Patient Self-Determination Act (PSDA)

The Patient Self-Determination Act (PSDA) requires healthcare agencies to give patients written information about their rights (which are specified under state law) to make healthcare decisions. For example, agencies must provide patients information about their rights to refuse treatments and to formulate advance directives. Specific laws regarding advance directives vary from state to state. It is important for you to understand the PSDA, the relevant laws of your own state, and the policies of your institution. Generally, there are two types of advance directives:

1. A *living will* is an advance directive that declares the patient's wishes regarding future health care, should the patient become unable to give instructions.
2. A *durable power of attorney* identifies a person who will make healthcare decisions in the event the patient is unable to do so.

The American Nurses Association position statement regarding the PSDA instructs nurses to provide the patient the following assistance: (1) information necessary for informed consent regarding treatment decisions; (2) opportunities to express decisions, verbally or in writing; and (3) opportunities to receive or refuse treatments (O'Keefe, 2001). As a nurse, you should document whether a patient has signed an advance directive.

A variety of legal issues arise in relation to advance directives. For example, a patient may specify actions in a living will that are not supported by family members, such as a desire for a "do not attempt to resuscitate" (DNAR) order or for organ donation. Still another problem is that even though a person has an advance directive, he may not bring it with him to the healthcare agency. Always ask the patient whether he has an advance directive. Under the PSDA, this question must be asked whenever a patient is admitted to any healthcare facility.

Some people fear that once an advance directive is signed, no further care will be provided. Explain to families and patients that this is not the case; instead, the purpose of the directive is to make sure that they will get however much or little care *they* wish. Such explanations are independent nursing activities, for which you are responsible. Also see Chapters 15 and 44 for further discussion of advance directives.

The U.S. Department of Health and Human Services (DHHS) "Privacy Rule," HIPAA

The so-called privacy rule consists of regulations that implement the Health Insurance Portability and Accountability Act (HIPAA) of 1996. The HIPAA initially intended to keep health plans from discriminating against people on the basis of their medical condition. An insurer may refuse to insure some preexisting conditions—for example, if a person with diabetes applies for insurance, they may insure him for all medical problems except diabetes. In most cases, HIPAA allows insurers to limit coverage for a preexisting condition for only 12 months.

The regulations provide comprehensive protection for the privacy of protected health information. Healthcare agencies must provide reasonable safeguards to protect the confidentiality of records. In addition, patients have the right to see and copy their medical records and to correct mistaken information. To read more about the HIPAA, see Chapter 39 and

 Go to the **Department of Health and Human Services web site at http://www.hhs.gov/ocr/hipaa/**

The Newborns' and Mothers' Health Protection Act of 1996 (NMHPA)

The Newborns' and Mothers' Health Protection Act (NMHPA) increases the length of stay for mother and newborn child following childbirth. In general, insurance plans may not restrict hospital stay in connection with childbirth to less than 48 hours following a vaginal delivery, or 96 hours following a delivery by cesarean section.

The National Labor Relations Act of 1935 (NLRA)

The National Labor Relations Act of 1935 (NLRA), an employment-related statute, gave legal recognition to collective bargaining. Collective bargaining is based on the principle that there is strength in numbers. Collective bargaining involves the right of nurses or other employees to bargain with the employer as a collective unit to achieve such objectives as securing better salaries or working conditions. Its goal is to equalize power between labor and management. In 1944, the American Nurses Association took the position that each state nursing association has a right to conduct collective bargaining for nurses. The ANA Code of Ethics for Nurses (2001) also says that nurses should use individual and collective action to promote a healthcare environment and conditions of employment conducive to providing quality health care that is consistent with the values of the profession. Under the NLRA, nurses have a right to (1) form and join unions, (2) designate representatives, and

(3) participate in negotiations and collective bargaining (O'Keefe, 2001).

KnowledgeCheck 45–1

- Which federal law requires healthcare agencies to provide patients with information about advance directives?
- Which federal law ensures that patients can receive emergency treatment regardless of their ability to pay?
- What protections are provided to patients by the Department of Health and Human Services "privacy rule" of the HIPAA?

Go to Chapter 45, **Knowledge Check Response Sheet and Answers,** on the Electronic Study Guide

State Laws

Some of the state laws affecting nursing practice include mandatory reporting laws, laws regarding patient abandonment, Good Samaritan laws, and nurse practice acts.

Mandatory Reporting Laws

Most states have mandatory reporting laws related to communicable diseases, immunizations, and abuse of children, the elderly, and the mentally disabled. To different degrees, nurses must report to designated authorities (e.g., Child Protective Services) suspected physical, sexual, emotional, or verbal abuse or neglect of patients by healthcare workers or family members.

Elder abuse laws provide protection to those persons over age 60 "from actions that cause serious physical or emotional injury, caretaker neglect, and financial exploitation" (Cammuso et al., 2001, p. 401). Similar protections are provided to children under the child abuse laws and to the mentally disabled.

You may be wondering how mandatory reporting is affected by privacy laws. To encourage reporting, states provide legal immunity if you have made the report in good faith. States vary in their requirements for mandatory reporting of abuse. However, in general, nurses who fail to report suspected abuse or neglect may be held liable under criminal or civil law (discussed later in this chapter). In some cases reporting is the responsibility of the employing agency rather than the nurse. Nevertheless, you should be familiar with agency policy and state laws for reporting.

Good Samaritan Laws

Good Samaritan laws provide protection for nurses who provide emergency care to people who have been injured (e.g., at the scene of an automobile accident). The specifics of these laws differ among states, so check your state's statutes. A few states may require

that citizens stop to render aid, but most do not. For these laws to apply:

1. The assistance provided must have been voluntary (and the person is not paid).
2. The person receiving the help must not object to being helped.
3. Your actions must be a good-faith effort to help.

In general, Good Samaritan laws protect you from civil liability for damages resulting from your attempt to help people in need. Keep in mind, however, that even in an emergency situation, negligence and gross misconduct are not defensible. These laws do not apply if the emergency occurs in a hospital. If you do provide emergency care, follow these guidelines to minimize your risk of liability:

- Call 911, or have someone else call, as soon as you can.
- Do not leave the person unless you transfer care to an equally competent professional. This may mean a trip to the Emergency Department in some cases.
- Place the person under the care of a physician or advanced practice nurse as soon as possible, and follow their instructions.
- Do not accept money or any form of compensation from anyone.

Nurse Practice Acts

Each state legislature has passed a law designed to enact the state nursing practice act. Nursing practice acts are designed to:

- Protect patients or society.
- Define the scope of nursing practice.
- Identify the minimum level of nursing care that must be provided to clients.

A nursing practice act provides for the regulation of nursing practice by an administrative board, such as the board of nurse examiners (or the "state board of nursing"). These boards generally have the authority to regulate nursing practice and education within the states (Fedorka & Resnick, 2001, pp. 100–101), including licensing, credentialing, and disciplinary procedures. For links to your state's nursing practice act,

Go to the **Nursing Power** web site at www.nursingpower .net/nursing/practice_acts.html or to the **National Council of the State Boards of Nursing** web site at www.ncsbn.org/

Licensing

Licensing is meant to ensure that practicing nurses have met the minimum competencies set by the state to protect the public. The licensing procedure varies

among states but usually involves some or all of the following steps. The applicant must:

1. Successfully complete an educational program in a state-accredited school of nursing.
2. Pass the NCLEX-RN, a computerized exam developed and administered under the direction of the National Council of the State Boards of Nursing.
3. Provide evidence of good mental and physical health.
4. Provide a statement of good moral character.
5. Pay a fee for entrance to the licensing examination.
6. Obtain a temporary license pending outcome of the first attempt at the licensure exam. (Note: not all states give a temporary license.)
7. Demonstrate competence in English (Fedorka & Resnick, 2001, p. 102).

All nurses must be licensed by the state in which they practice. Currently certain states, through a **multistate compact** (agreement), allow nurses to be licensed in one state and to practice in all states participating in the compact. Multistate practice often takes place through technology, such as video conferencing and telenursing, where the nurse is licensed in one state, yet gives advice to a patient in another state within the compact (Fedorka & Resnick, 2001, pp. 107–108).

Credentialing

Credentialing is a voluntary form of self-regulation used by many healthcare disciplines, including nursing. In the legal sense, credentialing includes accreditation and certification. Having credentials implies that the person or agency has met higher standards than the minimum (e.g., licensure).

- *Accreditation.* Most nursing boards establish educational requirements for nursing programs and continuing education courses within a given state. The board usually requires that for a nursing program to be **accredited,** it must meet the requirements for accreditation established by the National League for Nursing or the American Association of Colleges of Nursing and by the state nurse practice act. This helps ensure that students get a well-rounded education and that patients are cared for by safe practitioners.

  Accreditation also applies to noneducational facilities; for example, hospitals seek accreditation by the Joint Commission for the Accreditation of Healthcare Organizations (JCAHO). This is intended to ensure that a minimum standard quality of care is provided.

- *Certification.* **Certification** is another form of credentialing. Through certification and licensing, the board identifies nurses who are qualified for advanced practice (e.g., clinical nurse specialists, midwives, and nurse practitioners) or for certifica-

tion in a subspecialty, such as emergency nursing or pediatric nursing. In some states, the board establishes the criteria for certification, including (1) educational preparation, (2) clinical experience, and (3) certification by other professional organizations. In other states, the nurse may obtain an advanced practice license only if she is first certified by a national organization such as the ANA or a specialty organization (Fedorka & Resnick, 2001, pp. 102–103). Not all states require certification for advanced practice nurses.

Disciplinary Procedure

Along with specifying the requirements to be able to practice nursing, state boards commonly also enforce the requirements by establishing disciplinary procedures. The ANA generally recommends that the following unprofessional conduct result in disciplinary action: violation of the nursing practice act or rules, fraud, deceit, criminal activity, negligence, risk to clients, physical or mental incapacity, disciplinary action by another jurisdiction, incompetence, and unethical conduct.

The disciplinary procedure conducted by the state board may involve a series of all or some of the following steps (Fedorka & Resnick, 2001, p. 103):

1. Filing of the sworn complaint with the board by an individual, healthcare agency, or professional organization
2. Review of the complaint by the board of nursing
3. Hearing and decision by the board determining whether the nurse has acted unprofessionally and violated the state nursing practice act (Fedorka & Resnick, 2001, p. 103)
4. Disciplinary action issued if the board finds that the nurse acted unprofessionally
5. Request by the nurse that a state court review the decision of the nursing board.

Standards of Practice

Clinical guidelines, standards of professional performance, standards of practice, and *standards of care* are terms that are often used interchangeably. The legal definition of a **standard of care** looks to what a reasonable and prudent nurse would do in the same or similar situation. Standards of practice are developed by various legal and professional groups. Nurses are expected to follow the standards of care that apply to their area of practice, regardless of the source of the standards. In a court of law, various sources may be used to determine what constitutes reasonable care in a particular situation.

- *Nurse practice acts.* Standards of practice may have their basis in the state nurse practice act, which

BOX 45-1 ANA Standards of Professional Performance

Note: Standards 1 through 6, called Standards of Care, are found in Table 1–4.

Standard 7. Quality of Practice

The registered nurse systematically enhances the quality and effectiveness of nursing practice.

Standard 8. Education

The registered nurse attains knowledge and competency that reflects current nursing practice.

Standard 9. Professional Practice Evaluation

The registered nurse evaluates one's own nursing practice in relation to professional practice standards and guidelines, relevant statutes, rules, and regulations.

Standard 10. Collegiality

The registered nurse interacts with and contributes to the professional development of peers and colleagues.

Standard 11. Collaboration

The registered nurse collaborates with patient, family, and others in the conduct of nursing practice.

Standard 12. Ethics

The registered nurse integrates ethical provisions in all areas of practice.

Standard 13. Research

The registered nurse integrates research findings into practice.

Standard 14. Resource Utilization

The registered nurse considers factors related to safety, effectiveness, cost, and impact on practice in the planning and delivery of nursing services.

Standard 15. Leadership

The registered nurse provides leadership in the professional practice setting and the profession.

Source: American Nurses Association. (2004). *Standards of nursing practice.* Washington, DC: American Nurses Publishing. Used with permission.

minimal acceptable standards of care required in a typical state nursing practice act,

 Go to Chapter 45, **Tables, Boxes, Figures: ESG Box 45-3: Minimum Acceptable Standards of Care Required by a Typical State Nurse Practice Act,** on the Electronic Study Guide.

- *Professional organizations.* Standards of care are also identified by various professional organizations, such as the Joint Commission on Accreditation of Healthcare Organizations (JCAHO), the American Nurses Association (ANA), and nursing specialty organizations. The JCAHO standards are similar to clinical guidelines, or clinical steps for patient management. The first six ANA standards of care focus on interventions performed within the nursing process (see Table 1–4 in Chapter 1). ANA standards also focus on professional performance, or activities appropriately based on education and position. These are summarized in Box 45–1. Advanced practice nurses are held to the standards adopted by the specialty within which they practice and the standards of the certifying organization.

Other sources of standards of practice include medical and nursing literature, published practice guidelines, and expert practitioners.

Other Guidelines for Practice

Other practice guidelines may also factor into what constitutes reasonable and prudent nursing care.

Institutional Policies and Procedures

Institutional policies and procedures usually are more specific and detailed than standards set by professional organizations. They describe care that is reasonable, appropriate, and expected in the context of that facility, based, for instance, on the staffing and equipment available and the case mix of patients in the agency. Policies and procedures can be used as evidence of violation of the standard of care if a nurse fails to comply. So it is important that you know, follow, and question policies and procedures if they seem not to be working well.

Nursing Codes of Ethics

Although they are not laws, nursing codes of ethics (e.g., the American Nurses Association Code of Ethics, 2001; the Canadian Nurses Association Code of Ethics for Registered Nurses, 2002) specify ethical duties of the nurse to the patient, as related to corresponding patient rights. The ANA Code guarantees the patient the rights to dignity, privacy, and safety. The ANA Code also guarantees that the nurse will be accountable and competent, use informed judgment, maintain

identifies the minimum level of nursing care for a specific patient in specific circumstances. Standards set forth in nurse practice acts are mandatory; that is, they are set forth in statutes and enforced by authority granted by the state. For a summary of

employment conditions conducive to quality patient care, protect the client from misinformation and misrepresentation, and collaborate with other healthcare professions to meet the patient's healthcare needs. In a malpractice suit, these guarantees may sometimes be used as standards against which to compare the nurse's actions. For more information on nursing codes of ethics, see Chapter 44.

The Patient Care Partnership

The Patient Care Partnership was first adopted by the American Hospital Association in 1973. At that time, it was called the Patients' Bill of Rights. When clients are admitted to hospitals or to extended care facilities, they are entitled to certain rights in terms of their treatment: the right to make their own decisions, to be active partners in the treatment process, and to be treated with dignity and respect. For a summary of the Patient Care Partnership, see Box 44–4 in Chapter 44.

Although the rights are not necessarily legally binding, courts may look to this document as evidence by which to judge whether patient care has met the appropriate and reasonable standard of care. Various groups have created different versions of the old Patients' Bill of Rights to emphasize patient rights that are particularly applicable in their healthcare context. Examples include the Nursing Home Bill of Rights, the Veterans Administration Code of Patient Concern, and the Dying Person's Bill of Rights (Barbus, 1975). You should be familiar with the way in which different groups, and your agency, define patient rights.

The ANA Bill of Rights for Nurses

The American Nurses Association has developed a bill of rights for nurses to "protect the dignity and autonomy of nurses in the workplace" (ANA, 2002, p. 16). The ANA Bill of Rights for Registered Nurses, a policy statement, not a law, provides nurses the right to:

1. Practice in a manner fulfilling obligations to society and patients
2. Practice in accordance with professional standards and the nursing practice act
3. Practice within an ethical framework, as specified by the terms of the ANA Code of Ethics for Nurses
4. Advocate for patients or profession without retaliation
5. Fair compensation
6. A safe work environment
7. Negotiate conditions of employment

The intent of this document is to make clear the rights that are *not* negotiable in the workplace. The ANA supports nurses' rights through collective bargaining, political activism, and public education.

 ## CriticalThinking 45–2

Recall the opening scenario. You were asked: Did the nurse do the right thing when she decided not to accept the assignment and to leave the nursing home facility immediately?

- What standards, guidelines, and laws would apply to determine whether the nurse's behavior was in accordance with standards of practice?
- Which statements in the ANA Bill of Rights for Nurses might the nurse use to justify her actions?

KnowledgeCheck 45–2

How does each of the following protect patients?

- The Patient Care Partnership
- Nursing codes of ethics
- Mandatory reporting laws

Go to Chapter 45, **Knowledge Check Response Sheet and Answers,** on the Electronic Study Guide.

WHAT IS CRIMINAL LAW?

Two types of common law guiding nursing practice include criminal law and civil law. Although both types fall under both federal and state jurisdictions, there is a distinct difference in the purpose of civil and criminal laws. In a **criminal case,** the federal or state government seeks to penalize the accused for an offense against society. If found guilty under criminal law, a person may be fined, jailed, or even executed. Under civil law, in contrast, a defendant found liable pays money to the plaintiff.

A **crime** is whatever a legislative body has defined it to be. A **misdemeanor** is a minor crime, punishable by a fine and/or imprisonment for less than a year. For example, as a first offense, driving while under the influence of a substance would probably be a misdemeanor traffic violation. A **felony** is a crime punishable by death or more than one year's imprisonment. State laws may define felonies in other ways, as well. Homicide is a felony and generally leads to severe penalties under criminal law.

So-called mercy killing (active euthanasia) may result in charges of homicide in some states. The same is true of assisted suicide (O'Keefe, 2001). The American Nurses Association defines **assisted suicide** as providing a patient the means to end his life, with full knowledge of the patient's intentions to do so. Assisted suicide is therefore a form of active euthanasia. The ANA (1991) believes that nurses should not participate in active euthanasia (and assisted suicide) because such acts violate the Code of Ethics for Nurses and the ethical traditions of the profession. See Chapters 15 and 44 for more information about euthanasia and assisted suicide.

For an expanded discussion of criminal law,

 Go to Chapter 45, **Supplemental Materials,** on the Electronic Study Guide.

WHAT IS CIVIL LAW?

In a civil case, the courts seek to resolve a dispute between private parties, which may result in payment of money by the defendant to the plaintiff. The **plaintiff** is the person bringing the suit (or making the claim). In a civil case, the plaintiff must prove by a "preponderance of the evidence" that the defendant committed a wrong against him. This means that the person must prove to the jury that the *allegations* (charges or accusations) made against the **defendant** (the person being sued) are "more likely than not" true. Two types of civil law provide standards for nursing practice: contract law and tort law. We will focus more on tort law, which is seen more commonly in a nursing context.

Contract Law

Contract law controls legally enforceable agreements between individuals, such as employment contracts. A contract may be **explicit** (defined in writing) or **implicit** (defined by behavior and actions). Many nurses do not have explicit employment contracts.

Tort Law

Tort law deals with the duties and rights among individuals that are not covered by contractual agreements. A **tort** is a civil wrong, such as a claim for malpractice or negligence, usually with claims for damages (O'Keefe, 2001). **Damage claims** are money demands by the plaintiff for compensation for actual harm or injury inflicted by the defendant. Torts are generally identified under three categories, differing by intent of the defendant: (1) quasi-intentional torts, (2) intentional torts, and (3) negligence and malpractice (unintentional torts).

What Are Quasi-Intentional Torts?

Quasi-intentional torts all involve speech. There are three torts that fall into this category:

1. **Defamation,** which occurs when a false communication is made to a third person and the communication is harmful; holds the plaintiff up to hatred, contempt, or ridicule; or causes the plaintiff to be shunned or avoided
2. **Slander,** which is a defamatory statement made orally
3. **Libel,** which is a defamatory statement made in writing

What Are Intentional Torts?

"Intentional" conduct is designed to bring about a specific result in the mind of the defendant. Intentional torts include assault, battery, false imprisonment, fraud, and invasion of privacy. Intentional torts may also be prosecuted as misdemeanors or felonies under criminal law. For example, a nurse who has been sued for malpractice may also be charged with a homicide if a patient died as a result of the nurse's act or inaction. So, a patient may sue for damages for assault under civil law, and the government may charge the defendant with assault under criminal law—and the penalties differ.

Assault and Battery

Assault occurs when a nurse intentionally places a patient in a position of fear that he will suffer harmful or offensive contact (e.g., "Stop that, or I will restrain you"). Battery occurs when intentional, offensive physical contact actually takes place (Marchand, 2001, p. 31). In the healthcare context, claims for assault and battery most commonly occur when a nurse or doctor performs a procedure on a patient without informed consent. The physical contact need not result in a physical injury. For example, if you perform a procedure without informed consent, you may be sued for battery even though the patient suffers no physical harm (Columbia University, 2000, p. 4492). Keep in mind, however, that to prove a tort case, the plaintiff must make a showing of some kind of damages.

False Imprisonment

False imprisonment involves an intentional or willful detention of the patient without consent or authority to do so. Claims for false imprisonment most commonly occur in mental health or nursing home settings, when patients claim they were admitted and/or restrained against their will (Marchand, 2001, p. 31). Competent patients have a right to leave an institution, even if it is harmful to their health. If possible, you should have the person sign a form stating that they are leaving against medical advice (AMA). Restraining a patient without consent is another form of civil false imprisonment.

Fraud

Fraud is "willfully" or intentionally misleading another person, with the intent to cause legal injury or deprive the person of a right. The nurse may commit fraud when (1) telling a patient a lie; (2) failing to disclose material information, such as during informed consent; or (3) making a statement in reckless disregard of whether it is truthful or accurate. Because actual fraud requires intent, it can never be the

result of accident or negligence. In other words, ethics aside, lying to a patient rises to the level of fraud only if it is intended to cause him legal injury or deprive him of a right.

Invasion of Privacy

Invasion of privacy violates a person's right to be free from unwanted interference in her private affairs. The law holds that a person has a right to be left alone and not have her personal life held up for public scrutiny. The plaintiff must prove by a preponderance of the evidence that (1) her privacy was violated, (2) public disclosure of private matters occurred, and (3) a reasonable person would object to the intrusion. Examples are a breach of confidentiality, in which the nurse discusses the patient in the lunchroom; filming and making public disclosure of medical treatments without the patient's permission; searching a patient's belongings without permission (and disclosing search results); releasing medical information without the patient's consent; and releasing information to news media.

The right to privacy may conflict with the nurse's duty to report (e.g., reporting a sexually transmitted infection to public health authorities). Or the patient may be a public figure whose medical condition is of importance to the public (e.g., suppose the president has a heart attack). In such cases, you should consult with the agency's legal counsel, public relations department, and the nurse in charge of the unit to be sure that the patient's privacy is not violated.

Invasion of privacy is only one avenue protecting patient privacy. Patient privacy is also upheld by professional codes of ethics, nursing and institutional standards of care, and HIPAA. Note that writing in the patient's chart or discussing pertinent patient data with other involved professionals does not constitute public disclosure. Exceptions to privacy rules are made for mandatory reporting, for example, of suspected child abuse.

What Are Negligence and Malpractice?

Negligence and malpractice actions may be the torts most familiar to healthcare professionals. Clients and family members who believe that care was unprofessional and did not measure up to standard practice file claims for civil liability. Negligence and malpractice are unintentional torts—nurses can be negligent without intending to do harm. **Negligence** is simply the failure to use ordinary or reasonable care, as dictated by the standards of practice and/or by what a reasonable and prudent nurse would do in the same or similar circumstances. Intent is not an element of negligence. When a nurse or other licensed profes-

sional healthcare provider is negligent and fails to exercise ordinary care, it is called **malpractice.** In other words, malpractice is simply the professional form of negligence, so it is the form of negligence most relevant to nurses in a professional context.

Elements of Malpractice Liability

To recover damages in a malpractice claim, *all* of the following four elements must be proven by the plaintiff by a "preponderance of the evidence" (Marchand, 2001, pp. 26–27):

1. *Existence of a duty.* The nurse-patient relationship creates a duty by the nurse to the patient. This duty forms when the patient seeks care and treatment from the nurse (Marchand, 2001, pp. 27–28). Duty also arises when you see a patient in need or if you observe another provider committing malpractice.

2. *Breach of the duty.* The plaintiff may prove a breach of duty by demonstrating that the nursing actions failed to meet the standards of care. The standard of care will be established by a testifying expert, based on the state nursing practice act and a combination of any of the following sources of nursing care standards:
   a. the nurse's job description
   b. clinic or hospital policies, procedures, and protocols
   c. standards and guidelines adopted by professional organizations to which the nurse may belong, or
   d. a treatise or textbook that the expert witness views as authoritative (Marchand, 2001, pp. 28–30):
   As a nurse, you have a duty to assess, plan, implement, and evaluate care for your patients. You will find common breaches of duty in the "Practical Knowledge" section of this chapter.

3. *Causation.* Proximate cause must be demonstrated in two distinct steps. Plaintiff must prove that (1) the nurse's acts (or failure to act) actually *caused* the plaintiff's injury and (2) that the type of injury was foreseeable, or a logical consequence of the breach of the nursing standard (Marchand, 2001, p. 30; O'Keefe, 2001).

4. *Damages.* Plaintiff must also prove that there has been an actual injury or damage. For example, even though a nurse administers the wrong medication, if no injury occurred to the patient, then he will not be able to prove a negligence case and recover damages under civil law. The patient may, however, file a complaint before the board of nurse examiners to obtain sanctions against the nurse under administrative law.

KnowledgeCheck 45–3

- Distinguish negligence from malpractice.
- Distinguish civil from criminal law.
- Under which type of law (constitutional, statutory, administrative, or common law) does each of the following fall?

    A defendant claiming the right not to incriminate himself under the Fifth Amendment

    A nurse having her license revoked by the state board of nursing

    The wording of a state nurse practice act

- Define *plaintiff* and *defendant* in the context of civil law.

 Go to Chapter 45, **Knowledge Check Response Sheet and Answers,** on the Electronic Study Guide.

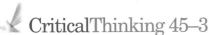 # CriticalThinking 45–3

- Give one nursing example of each: negligence, malpractice, damages.
- Can you think of one nonfraudulent example of a nurse's being untruthful with a patient? Do you think that the circumstances described in your example make the untruthfulness justifiable?
- Can you think of an example of a nurse's committing assault, other than the one given in the text?

The Nurse as a Witness

The nurse also may become a witness in a malpractice action. As a witness, the nurse may testify either for plaintiff or defendant, in the capacity of either a fact witness or an expert witness. For example, you may be called as a **fact witness** in a malpractice case if you were an **eyewitness** (present when the act or omission occurred). You could also be called to testify to information found in medical documentation. You can testify to the facts contained in the patient record, even if you do not remember what happened (e.g., "I see from the record that I took the patient's temperature at 8:00 P.M.")

The standard of care in malpractice cases is often brought into evidence by expert testimony (Aiken, 2004). In proving or disproving breach of duty, an **expert witness** has the role of testifying to (1) the actual standard of nursing care in the same or similar circumstances as the incident in question and (2) whether the defendant nurse adhered to the standard or acted as a reasonable and prudent nurse would have in the same or similar circumstances. An expert witness may be asked to summarize volumes of medical records or explain medical terminology to a jury (Mathews, 2001, p. 52). As a nurse, you may be called as an expert based on your specialized knowledge in an area. Experts are allowed to draw conclusions and form opinions regarding the facts in evidence (Mathews, 2001, p. 52).

Vicarious Liability

Each person is held responsible for his own acts of negligence. In certain circumstances, however, the law imposes vicarious liability. **Vicarious liability** is substitute liability, in which the employer is held responsible for injuries that occur as a result of an employee's negligent acts during the scope of employment. The most common legal theories of vicarious liability under which the nurse-employer relationship may fall include the following:

- *Captain of the ship.* Under this theory of legal liability, the doctor, not the actual employer, may be held liable for the acts of a nurse under the doctor's supervision (Hall, 2001, pp. 153–154). Even if the doctor is held liable, the nurse may still be liable for her own actions in the situation; this theory does not protect the nurse.
- *Borrowed servant.* In this instance, the first employer (e.g., an agency) directs the nurse to work for a second employer (e.g., a hospital), which has actual control over the nurse. The second employer then becomes answerable for negligent acts of the nurse (Hall, 2001, p. 154). This would apply, for example, to agency nurses.
- *Respondeat superior.* This is a Latin term meaning "let the master answer." Under this theory of liability, the healthcare employer (e.g., a hospital or clinic) becomes liable for the negligent acts of the nurse if the employer knew or should have known of the acts of the nurse (O'Keefe, 2001). Again, the nurse is still responsible for her own actions and may also be held liable.

KnowledgeCheck 45–4

- Define these terms: *assault, battery, fraud, slander, libel, negligence, malpractice.*
- State the four elements of malpractice.

 Go to Chapter 45, **Knowledge Check Response Sheet and Answers,** on the Electronic Study Guide.

LITIGATION IN CIVIL CLAIMS

Litigation is the formal process that adjudicates legal issues, rights, and duties between the parties. In brief, the litigation process begins when the **plaintiff** (party seeking damages or other relief) files a document called a **complaint,** claiming that a **defendant** (person, persons, or an entity) has violated his rights. If you are the defendant in a civil trial, you will need an attorney. If you have personal liability insurance or can afford to pay an attorney, you can have your own attorney. Alternatively, the employing agency can secure the attorney. You must also notify your employer and your liability insurance carrier if you are served with a complaint.

The litigation process follows several stages, including (1) pretrial, (2) discovery, (3) alternative dispute resolution, (4) trial, and (5) appeal.

1. *Pleading and pretrial motions.* After the plaintiff files the complaint outlining what the nurse did wrong and how the plaintiff was injured, the defendant files an "answer," admitting or denying each allegation (unproven accusation). If any of the four elements of malpractice are missing, the defendant may file a motion with the court to dismiss the lawsuit.

    Cooperate fully and be honest with your attorney. Do not discuss the case with anyone (not even co-workers) other than your attorney and the risk manager at your agency. Do not alter the patient records in any way, even if the documentation seems unfavorable to you in some way.

2. *Discovery phase.* The discovery process uncovers for both parties any facts and evidence of the case. Discovery is designed to make sure there are no "surprises" during the trial. Discovery may be obtained through written questions or interrogatories, requests for documents and other evidence, and by **deposition** (attorneys orally question parties to the suit under oath, as though the person were testifying in a courtroom).

    You may be deposed as a party to the lawsuit, as a fact witness, or as an expert witness. Prior to the deposition, you should review all pertinent medical records and other information. Keep in mind that opposing counsel can request a copy of anything you use in your preparation. If you are deposed, do not volunteer information; answer questions factually—if they can be answered yes or no, then do so. Take your time before answering a question; this allows your attorney to make any necessary objections. Tell the truth, but base your answers on facts, and do not speculate.

3. *Alternative dispute resolution.* Lawyers and involved parties typically seek to resolve disputes before going to trial. The three most common methods of alternative dispute resolution are negotiation, mediation, and arbitration. **Negotiation** takes place informally between the parties through their lawyers, in an attempt to settle the case prior to trial. **Mediation** is the attempt to resolve the dispute using a neutral third party; it is usually not binding. **Arbitration** is similar to mediation, but more formal and sometimes binding. A neutral third party with expertise in the area of contention hears the case and renders a decision.

4. *Trial process.* If the dispute cannot be resolved and is not dismissed by motions, the case proceeds to trial. Facts are presented and arguments made to a judge and sometimes a jury.

5. *Appeal.* After the judge or jury has rendered a decision, either party has the opportunity to (1) present post-trial motions, (2) move for a new trial, or (3) appeal the verdict and/or damages to an appellate court.

KnowledgeCheck 45–5

- Identify the phases of the trial process.
- How is arbitration different from mediation?

 Go to Chapter 45, **Knowledge Check Response Sheet and Answers,** on the Electronic Study Guide.

Practical Knowledge
knowing how

To decrease your chances of being involved in a malpractice suit, you should know the most common causes of malpractice claims and some practical preventive actions you can take. Keep in mind that causes are often difficult to categorize because they overlap; an error usually results from interlocking causes.

WHAT ARE THE MOST COMMON MALPRACTICE CLAIMS?

Malpractice claims generally result from negligence, a nurse's failure to maintain standards of practice. The most common causes of nursing malpractice claims (Box 45–2) can be categorized according to where they fall in the nursing process: failure to assess and diagnose, failure to plan, failure to implement, and failure to evaluate (O'Keefe, 2001).

Failure to Assess and Diagnose

The nursing duty to assess assumes four separate requirements. Failure to conduct any one of these four requirements will result in a breach of the duty to assess (Eskreis, 1998; Hall & Hall, 2001, pp. 136–146).

1. The nurse has the necessary knowledge and skills to observe the patient and interpret the symptoms in the form of a nursing diagnosis.
2. The nurse actually carries out the assessment.
3. When the assessment reveals adverse symptoms, the nurse reports the symptoms to the appropriate provider and carries out the standard nursing care and ordered medical interventions.
4. The nurse continues to assess and monitor until the patient is stable.

One of the most common breaches of the duty to assess is failure to identify and ensure client safety needs, especially involving falls. Others include failure

Common Causes of Nursing Lawsuits

Notice the overlapping in the following categories. For example, "failure to advocate" (by questioning medical orders) could easily lead to a "medication and treatment error." An error usually has many causes.

- Medication and treatment errors
- Failure to follow standards of care (e.g., institutional policies, medical orders)
- Failure to assess and monitor
- Failure to communicate (e.g., failing to report in a timely manner, failing to report significant changes in patient status; poor communication)
- Failure to use equipment in a responsible manner; use of defective technology or equipment
- Failure to act as a patient advocate (e.g., to question incomplete medical orders)
- Infections caused or made worse by poor nursing care
- Failure to document

Sources: Aiken, T. D. (2004). *Legal, ethical, and political issues in nursing* (2nd ed.). Philadelphia: F. A. Davis Company; Croke, E. M. (2003). Nurses, negligence, and malpractice. *American Journal of Nursing, 103*(9), 54–63. Faherty, B. (1998). Medical malpractice and adverse actions agains nurses: Five years of information from the national doctor or other prescriber data bank. *Journal of Nursing Law, 51,* 17–27; Northrop, C. E. (1987). Nursing actions in litigation. *QRB, 13*(10), 343; O'Keefe, M. E. (2001). *Nursing practice and the law: Avoiding malpractice and other legal risks.* Philadelphia: F. A. Davis Company; Physician Insurers Association of America (1993, June). *Medication error study.* The Association.

to perform an admission assessment, failure to complete a shift assessment, failure to make ongoing assessments of progress, and failure to listen to and act on a patient's complaints (Croke, 2003).

Failure to diagnose means not interpreting a patient's signs and symptoms or not recognizing when a patient's condition requires immediate notification of a physician.

Failure to Plan

The American Nurses Association standards specifically require nurses to formulate a plan of care. The plan of care may be written or unwritten, depending on state regulations. Agency policy and procedure may also require that the plan include or be based on protocols, critical pathways, or other tools, such as outcome objectives (Hall & Hall, 2001, p. 137). Negligence for failure to plan may arise, for example, if you fail to include a turning schedule in the care plan for an immobile, poorly nourished patient who subsequently develops a pressure ulcer.

Failure to Implement a Plan of Care

At the crux of nursing care are the interventions implemented on behalf of the patient. Failure to implement a plan of care may encompass the following:

1. *Failure to respond,* such as not intervening to care for the patient's specific symptoms or expressed request for care.
2. *Failure to educate,* such as not answering questions, not teaching self-care measures, or not explaining procedures or equipment adequately on the patient's discharge.
3. *Failure to follow standards of care and institutional policies and procedures.* This most commonly occurs in the form of medication errors and failure to follow a physician's orders. It also frequently occurs from failure to use equipment responsibly. Among other reasons, a nurse may fail to follow standards of care when the unit is understaffed or the nurse is inexperienced.
4. *Failure to communicate* often comes up when a nurse fails to seek medical authorization for a treatment or fails to notify a physician in a timely manner when a patient's condition warrants action.
5. *Failure to document* the following in the patient's record: assessment data (e.g., drug allergies), patient injuries, medication administration details, patient progress and response to treatment, physicians' orders, and telephone conversations with physicians.
6. *Failure to act as an advocate.* Nurses must frequently intervene to prevent harm to the patient by other healthcare providers and by relatives and significant others. The following are examples of advocacy errors:
   a. *Medical and discharge orders.* As an example of failure to advocate, suppose two physicians order the same drug for a patient, but under different brand names. The nurse does not recognize that two drugs are the same, so the patient receives twice the normal amount and has a toxic reaction. Other errors occur when the nurse does not question incomplete or illegible orders or does not question discharge orders when she believes the patient is not well enough to be discharged.
   b. *Impaired nurses.* You have a duty under most state nursing practice acts to report impaired nursing practice (e.g., as a result of alcoholism or mental illness) to the appropriate licensing agency. Failure to do so is a failure to advocate for patients.

c. *Family and significant others.* Advocacy includes reporting neglect and intentional injuries to children, the elderly, and the disabled. Failure to do so may constitute negligence and/or violation of state statutes.

Failure to Evaluate

The duty to evaluate requires an ongoing cycle of the following:

1. Observing for changes after interventions and treatments.
2. Recognizing significance of the change. For example, if Mr. Adkins's blood pressure (BP) is usually 140/88, a change to 150/90 after exercise would not be significant for him. But for Mrs. Jonas, whose BP is usually 100/64, a change to 150/90 would be cause for concern.
3. Documenting or reporting symptoms to the appropriate person. If a change is significant, you have a legal duty to report the change to the appropriate provider and to document this change in the appropriate medical record.
4. Follow-up. Following up on responses to nursing interventions requires you to know the expected outcomes and side effects of medications and treatments, so that you can accurately interpret and document anticipated and adverse responses.

Failure to perform any of these aspects of evaluation may rise to the level of negligence. See Chapter 7 for further discussion of implementation and evaluation in the nursing process.

KnowledgeCheck 45–6

- State the four requirements of the nurse's duty to assess.
- State four ways in which the nurse may fail to implement a plan of care.
- Give one example of the duty to advocate for a patient.
- List the four components of the nurse's legal duty to evaluate.

 Go to Chapter 45, **Knowledge Check Response Sheet and Answers,** on the Electronic Study Guide.

HOW CAN YOU MINIMIZE YOUR MALPRACTICE RISKS?

Your most important reference for avoiding malpractice and other legal risks is your state nurse practice act. The nurse practice act not only identifies mandatory standards of care, but also provides other legal safeguards for nurses. Be intimately familiar with the tenets of your state nurse practice act. For other tips,

VOL 2 | Go to Chapter 45, **Technique 45–2: Tips for Avoiding Malpractice,** in Volume 2.

Observe Mandatory Standards of Care

One way to avoid legal risks is to know and observe mandatory (compulsory) standards of care: those required by law. For the minimum acceptable level of patient care identified in most state nurse practice acts,

 Go to Chapter 45, **Tables, Boxes, Figures: ESG Box 45–3: Minimum Acceptable Standards of Care Required by a Typical State Nurse Practice Act,** on the Electronic Study Guide.

You must adhere to these standards to avoid sanctions by the board of nursing examiners and malpractice litigation.

You must be knowledgeable not only about standards of practice identified in your state's nursing practice act, but also about all federal, state, or local laws, rules, and regulations affecting your area of practice as an RN. Ignorance of the law is no excuse for failing to comply with the law, and it is no defense in a malpractice suit.

Use the Nursing Process and Follow Professional Standards of Care

You must use a systematic approach in providing patient care, generally referred to as the nursing process. Use of the nursing process is standard nursing practice and is the legally acceptable model of decision making to be used in nursing practice. It is also a part of the patient care standards of many professional organizations, such as the ANA (see Table 1–4 and Box 45–1). Your documentation should reveal that you have assessed, diagnosed, planned, implemented, and evaluated care. You should also keep current with healthcare literature, continuing education, agency policy, and so forth, so that you will know what current standards involve.

Avoid Medication and Treatment Errors

Medication errors are among the most common healthcare errors. You must accurately administer medications and treatments to avoid harm to your patients. Furthermore, as part of your direct duty to the patient, you must also know the rationale and side effects of the medications, and you should document desired, adverse, or side effects that occur. You can help prevent medication errors by:

- Following the "six rights" of medication administration (see Chapter 23)
- Investigating any patient concerns before giving the medication (e.g., the patient might say, "I didn't get one of those red pills yesterday.")
- Questioning physician orders that are incomplete or that seem inappropriate

| toward evidence-based practice |

Beckstead, J. W. (2002). Modeling attitudinal antecedents of nurses' decision to report impaired colleagues. *Western Journal of Nursing Research, 24*(5), 537–551.

This researcher studied the relationship between the attitudes of unimpaired nurses and the nurses' intentions to report impaired co-workers to nursing supervisors. Using a sample of 126 nurses, the study found that the following attitudes were significantly related to intentions to report impaired colleagues: a positive attitude toward the effectiveness of substance abuse treatment, and permissiveness. A moralistic attitude was not related to intention to report impaired nurses; however, it was strongly associated with a punitive attitude toward impaired nurses.

Haack, M. R., & Yocom, C. J. (2002). State policies and nurses with substance use disorders. *Journal of Nursing Scholarship, 34*(1), 89–94.

This study, using mailed surveys, compared two types of state policies regarding nurses with substance use disorders: (1) a traditional, disciplinary approach by the state regulatory board; and (2) an alternative approach, diverting the nurses to programs for treatment and for determining their suitability to return to practice. Following the nurses over 6 months, the study found:

- The nurses in the alternative approach group had more nurses with active licenses.

- The nurses in the alternative approach group had fewer criminal convictions.
- More of the nurses in the alternative approach group were employed in nursing.
- There was no difference in the rate of relapse between the two groups.
- Fewer than 15% of nurses in either group experienced one or more relapses in the 6 months.

---

1. The Beckstead study identified that some nurses had a "moralistic attitude." The summary does not define that term, but based on your own life experience, what do you think it means?

2. If your definition of "moralistic attitude" is correct, and if Nurse Adams measures high on the moralistic scale, which of the state policies in the second study would he probably favor?

3. Based only on the information in the studies, can you guess which state would probably have the highest reporting of impaired nurses by their colleagues: State A, with the traditional approach; or State B, with the alternative approach? Explain your thinking.

 Go to Chapter 45, **Toward Evidence-Based Practice Suggested Responses,** on the Electronic Study Guide.

Treatment errors also frequently occur from misuse of equipment. For tips to help you use equipment properly and safely,

 Go to Chapter 45, **Technique 45-1: Using Equipment Safely,** in Volume 2.

Report and Document

For every suggestion for minimizing malpractice risk given in this section, add the reminder: "Document what happened." Remember: "If it isn't documented, it wasn't done." If you are ever required to appear in court, the patient record may be the only proof you have of the care you gave. Do not make false entries or destroy entries in medical records, but do carefully record and detail all care you provide.

Charting

Be sure to make a record of all interaction with clients, as well as patients' refusal of or noncompliance with treatment. Document telephone conversations with physicians, including time, content of the conversation, and the action you took. Document the facts; do not editorialize (e.g., do not write, "I could not check on the patient as often as ordered because we were understaffed"). Refer to Chapter 16 for a review of your documentation responsibilities, and use the following mnemonic (FACT). Charting should always be:

Factual
Accurate
Complete
Timely

 Go to Chapter 45, **Technique 45-3, Guidelines for Documenting Patient Care,** in Volume 2.

Incident Reports

If a standard of care is breached or an unusual incident occurs (e.g., a visitor or patient falls or is somehow injured), you should complete an **incident report** (also called *variance report* or *occurrence report*).

These reports are used, in part, for quality improvement in the agency and should not be used to discipline staff members or be placed in employees' files. Do not write "Incident report completed" in the patient record. In some states, an incident report must be made available as a part of discovery in litigation. In other states, however, only the chart may be subpoenaed, but if the incident report is mentioned in the chart, the otherwise confidential report may be used as evidence.

When reporting an incident, be sure to identify the patient, date, time, and location clearly. Briefly describe the incident in factual terms. Quote the patient or persons involved if possible. Do not speculate, draw conclusions, or place blame. Identify any witnesses to the event or equipment involved.

Example

7:00 P.M. Demerol 50 mg given intramuscularly instead of Demerol 15 mg.

7:30 P.M. Patient's respirations: 8 per minute; BP 100/60; skin pale.

8:00 P.M. Called Dr. Smith. Orders for naloxone (Narcan) 1 mg IV STAT.

8:05 P.M. Narcan given as ordered. Resp 12/min, BP 118/70.

Chapter 16 presents additional information on occurrence reports.

Obtain Informed Consent

Informed consent is the necessary authorization by the patient for any and all types of care, given with full knowledge of the risks, benefits, costs, and alternatives. For hospital admission and for invasive or specialized treatments or diagnostic procedures, the consent must be written and signed by the patient or the person legally responsible for the patient. Written consent is not necessary in an emergency if experts would agree that there was an immediate threat to life or health.

Elements of Consent

To be legally valid, informed consent should include the following elements:

- *Completeness (disclosure).* Healthcare consumers need a great deal of information to make educated decisions, and they should be told everything they would consider important in making a treatment decision.
- *Comprehension.* The patient (or his surrogate decision maker) must understand the explanation. Ask the patient to describe in his own words the procedure to which he is consenting.

- *Voluntariness.* This means that the patient must be free to accept or reject the treatment. He must not be pressured or coerced to give consent. There must be no actual or implied threat (e.g., "Mom, if you don't let them do this, I am not coming back to see you ever again"). Otherwise, the consent is not valid.
- *Competence.* The person must have the capacity to understand the information and make a choice about *this* situation (e.g., the ability to decide what clothing to wear does not necessarily mean that the person is competent to decide whether to have a risky surgery). The law assumes that minors are not competent in this sense. If it is determined that the person is not a legally competent adult, parents, a legal guardian, next of kin, or a friend can make healthcare decisions, depending on the state's law.

Generally speaking, a competent adult has the legal right to consent to or refuse any treatment. However, this right does not always extend to situations where an adult is making the decision for a minor. A court sometimes will authorize treatment of a child against parents' wishes. In some states, a minor who is married, serving in the military, or living independently is considered *emancipated* and can consent to or refuse treatment.

Nurse's Role

As a nurse, your legal role regarding written consent is to collaborate with the primary provider, usually a physician. You may witness a patient's signature on a consent form, but you are not legally responsible for explaining the treatments and options, nor for evaluating whether the physician has adequately explained them. You must, however, determine that the elements of a valid informed consent are in place, communicate the patient's needs for more information to the care provider, and provide feedback if the patient wishes to change her consent.

In addition, you should be sure you have the patient's informal, verbal consent for interventions you perform (e.g., urinary catheterization). The patient's coming to the agency for health care implies that she consents to usual treatment, such as injections and catheters. Therefore, you do not need to say, "May I catheterize you?" or "May I take your temperature?" for example. But you should always tell the patient what you are preparing to do, the rationale for it, and what she will feel. If the patient objects, discuss it further with him. If the patient questions you or objects, do not proceed until you have the patient's permission.

In addition to state statutes, case law, and agency policy, the Joint Commission on Accreditation of Health Care Organizations (JCAHO) standards provide valuable guidance regarding informed participation in decision making. Also see Chapter 44 for

discussion of informed consent from an ethical perspective.

Attend to Patient Safety

Attend carefully to patient safety. Although institutional policies may address patient safety, following such policy is not an excuse for failing to meet this obligation to the patient. For example, even though you follow the agency's policy and keep the rails raised, you may still be found negligent if the patient falls because he called for help and no one came to assist him out of bed. Falls are a common cause of patient injury. You should assess all patients for falls risk on admission to the healthcare setting and institute falls precautions when needed. Several useful tools have been developed for assessing falls, including the Morse Fall Scale. See Chapter 21 for information about meeting patients' safety needs, including falls and use of restraints. Also,

 Go to Chapter 21, **Tables, Boxes, Figures: ESG Figure 21–1,** on the Electronic Study Guide.

Maintain Confidentiality and Privacy

Maintain patient confidentiality, unless directed by law to do otherwise (e.g., when a patient is threatening to harm someone). The patient's family and significant others do not have an automatic right to confidential information regarding the patient. For example, parents do not have an automatic right to see the medical records of their child if that child is married and/or declared legally competent to make independent decisions. Of course, you need to discuss clients' medical conditions with other health team members, but this does not include chatting about the client's personal life or talking about the patient in the lunchroom. Discuss only health status, and discuss it only with those involved in the patient's care.

Provide Education and Counseling

Educate and counsel your patients. This includes providing information about their illness and medications and other procedures so that the patient can give truly informed consent and perform adequate self-care. It is not adequate just to give information. You must be certain the patient has learned. Ask the patient to repeat instructions to you or to provide a return demonstration of a skill, such as self-injection of insulin.

Assign, Delegate, and Supervise According to Guidelines

As a nurse, you should undertake patient care and make assignments in accordance with your education,

knowledge, experience, and physical and emotional capability. You must also consider the skill level of the LVNs (or LPNs) and unlicensed assistive personnel to whom you delegate, as well as the condition of the patient. For example, it would be negligent to assign a practical nurse to care for a patient on a ventilator without checking to be certain that the nurse has had training or experience with such patients.

The duty to delegate has a corresponding duty to supervise the care. For example, if you assign an aide to take vital signs, you must check periodically to see that the vital signs are taken and reported accurately. For specific guidelines for delegating, see Chapter 7. For the ANA and other relevant web sites,

 Go to Chapter 45, **Resources for Caregivers and Health Professionals,** on the Electronic Study Guide.

As a rule, you will not be held responsible for harm that comes to a patient because of poor staffing, as long as the harm is not due to your own negligence.

Accept Assignments for Which You Are Qualified

As a nurse, when you accept an assignment consider whether the assignment is within your level of education, experience, and physical and emotional capability. According to the American Nurses Association (2000), refusal to *accept* an assignment does not constitute patient abandonment. Abandonment is a "unilateral severance of the established nurse-patient relationship without giving reasonable notice to the supervisor so that arrangements can be made for continuation of nursing care by others" (ANA, 2000).

You also have a duty to ensure adequate staffing and patient coverage to the extent that you are able to do so. This means that you must report to the nurse in charge when leaving the patient care unit. Failure to do this may result in charges of patient abandonment. Never leave a patient, for example, in the preoperative holding area without making certain there is a nurse there to attend to the patient. This does not mean that you must work overtime (e.g., a double shift), as long as you give notice and explain your reasoning (e.g., that you are too fatigued to provide safe care).

If you do work a double shift, or if a unit is understaffed, you are still liable for any malpractice that you commit. Unfortunately, being "busy" and overwhelmed is not a defense for error. In addition, you have the duty to tell supervisors that staffing is inadequate; be sure to do it in writing.

Participate in Continuing Education

As a nurse, you have a duty to participate in ongoing continuing educational training in your area of practice

and to keep up with new laws. Be sure to obtain documentation of your attendance. In some states, continuing education is mandatory for relicensure. In states where it is not mandatory, other standards of care still require that you obtain the education and training necessary to implement current nursing procedures and practices. Continuing education is available "for credit" through colleges and universities, hospitals and other healthcare agencies, in some nursing journals (e.g., *The American Journal of Nursing*), and online. For a web page providing links to free online continuing education for nurses,

Go to the **nurseCEU.com web site at www.nurseceu.com/**

Observe Professional Boundaries

Be careful to maintain professional boundaries, not only with the patient but also with other healthcare providers. Violations of professional boundaries may be physical, sexual, emotional, or financial in nature. Do not accept gifts from vulnerable patients or encourage attempts to have close personal relationships outside the healthcare setting.

Also be aware of and report the behaviors of staff members who commit sexual harassment. **Sexual harassment** involves the use of power over people lower in the power structure of the organization. It is defined as "unwelcome sexual advances, requests for sexual favors, and other verbal or physical conduct of a sexual nature" if submission to it (1) is a condition of employment, (2) interferes with job performance, (3) is the basis for employment decisions, or (4) creates a hostile and intimidating work environment (Equal Employment Opportunity Commission [EEOC], 2002).

If you witness or experience sexual harassment, your first step is to consult the agency's sexual harassment policy. Every agency receiving federal funding must have such a policy in place. It will tell you how to file a grievance, what forms you need to use, to whom the incident is reported, and what the procedure is for hearing and resolution.

Observe Mandatory Reporting Regulations

As noted earlier in the chapter, most states have laws requiring the nurse to report communicable diseases, known or suspected abuse of patients, and impaired or unsafe professional practice. When you observe violations of the state's licensing regulations, you have professional and legal responsibility to report them to the appropriate authority. The "authority" varies among states; it may be your immediate supervisor, the board of nurse examiners, or a peer assistance program, often sponsored by the state nurses association. See the section "Mandatory Reporting Laws," earlier in the chapter. Also see the following discussion regarding impaired nurses.

Impaired Nurses

One example of unsafe practice is practice by an impaired nurse. An **impaired nurse** is a nurse whose use of mood-altering substances renders him unable to carry out professional duties or responsibilities in a manner consistent with nursing standards. A recent national survey of 3600 nurses found that 17% reported heavy alcohol use, 6.9% reported inappropriate use of prescription drugs, and 3.8% reported illicit drug use (Trinkoff, Zhou, Storr, & Soeker, 2000). Most impaired nurses are identified by nonimpaired co-workers, yet in a recent study, only 37% of nurses who worked with impaired co-workers reported them to supervisors (Beckstead, 2002). See Box 45–3 for signs of chemical dependence in the workplace.

Unauthorized Practice

You must also report the **unauthorized practice** of nursing. This includes reporting persons practicing nursing without a proper license. Your state's nursing practice act will identify "minor" incidents that do not need to be reported. An example of a practice you should report is your observation of unlicensed personnel administering medications in an agency.

As a nurse, you have a duty to provide truthful information to the board of nurse examiners. This includes an obligation to correctly answer questions that affect the decision to license, employ, and certify the nurse.

Abuse

State laws also require you to report known or suspected abuse, rape, and communicable disease. Laws vary, so you will need to know what and to whom to report in your area. See Chapter 9 for a thorough description of how to assess for abuse. Also,

 Go to Chapter 9, **Procedure 9–1: Assessing for Abuse,** in Volume 2.

Legal Safeguards for Nurses

In addition to the Good Samaritan laws and the American Nurses Association Bill of Rights for Registered Nurses (both previously discussed), safe harbor laws and professional liability insurance offer some legal protection for nurses. The following are some legal safeguards provided to nurses.

BOX 45-3 Detecting Potential Chemical Dependence in the Workplace

The following may be signs of chemical dependence.

Absenteeism

- Frequent unscheduled absences
- Absences after payday or days off
- Higher than average absence for colds, flu, and minor illnesses

Absent "On the Job"

- Long coffee breaks
- "Locked door syndrome" (excessively long use of restroom)
- Frequent trips to Occupational Health Services for illness on the job

Difficulty Concentrating

- Medication errors
- Omitted, illogical, incomplete, or illegible charting
- Taking more time to carry out assignments than is expected given the nurse's skill and experience
- Deterioration of handwriting during the shift
- Overlooking the signs of patient's deteriorating condition

Inconsistent Work Patterns

- Alternating periods of high and low efficiency
- Minimal or substandard work compared to that of peers
- Frequent requests for help with patient assignments

Physical or Emotional Problems

- Nervousness, excessive sweating, tremors of the hands
- Physical or emotional condition changes during the shift
- Lack of attention to personal cleanliness or grooming

Decreasing Efficiency

- Omitting treatments; making bad decisions; showing poor judgment
- Requests to be changed to a less supervised shift

Poor Relationships on the Job

- Mood swings, from isolation to angry outbursts
- Uncooperativeness
- Avoidance of contact with supervisors
- Patient complaints of irritability, roughness, or verbal abuse

Medication-Centered Problems

- Excessive use of PRN psychoactive medications or narcotics recorded for patients
- Increased waste or breakage of controlled substances
- Missing drugs, unaccounted-for doses
- Omission of dates or times from narcotic sign-out sheets
- Patient complaints about lack of pain relief

Personal Life Interferes with Job

- Frequent or excessively long phone calls
- Visitors or unexplained errands during work shift

Source: Georgia Nurses Association. (2004). Checklist for detecting potential chemical dependence in an employee. Retrieved March 27, 2004, from *http://georgianurses.org/impaired_nurse .htm#tin* Used with permission.

Safe Harbor Laws

Safe harbor laws, found in the nurse practice act or other state laws, provide for exceptions to certain other laws. For example, they protect you from being suspended, terminated, disciplined, or discriminated against for refusing to do (or not do) something you believe would be harmful to a patient, for example, refusing to assist with a treatment when a patient has not given truly informed consent. Under these laws, the nurse also has a right to ask for a peer review of either the situation or directives that the nurse believes would violate the nursing practice act. When the situation occurs, you must tell your supervisor that you are invoking the safe harbor provision of the nurse practice act. As soon as possible, request and complete the appropriate safe harbor form (O'Keefe, 2001, pp. 82–83).

Professional Liability Insurance

Professional liability insurance provides some legal protection from nursing malpractice claims. If you are sued for malpractice, the insurance company pays for the attorney's fees and for any judgment or settlement, up to the limits of the policy. Most insurance policies have **exclusions** (items not covered by the policy). If the patient's claim arises out of excluded activities, the insurance company will not pay for the costs of litigation. The following are common exclusions (Aiken, 2004):

- Transmission of acquired immunodeficiency syndrome (AIDS) from the nurse to a patient
- Sexual abuse of a patient
- Injury caused while under the influence of drugs or alcohol

- Criminal activity
- Punitive damages (damages awarded to punish the defendant for egregious acts or omissions)

Types of Coverage

There are two types of malpractice coverage. **Occurrence-type** insurance is most often recommended for nurses, because the policy covers malpractice claims for any injury or damage occurring during the time the policy is in force, regardless of when the lawsuit occurs. **Claims made** insurance provides coverage only for malpractice claims made during the term of the policy *and* for injuries that occurred during that period. You should consult an attorney to decide which type of policy is best for you.

As a rule, if you work for a hospital or other institution, you will be covered by the institution's insurance. However, it covers you only while you are working within the scope of your employment. You would not, for example, be covered if you volunteer one day a week at a free health clinic. Some legal experts recommend that you purchase individual liability insurance in addition to the coverage provided by your employer. Again, consult a lawyer before making a decision.

Student Responsibilities

As a student, you are held to the same standards of care as are registered nurses. You must be familiar not only with your state's standards of practice, but also with the policies and procedures in which you have your clinical experiences. Your instructor is responsible for making assignments that are within your competence and for providing clinical supervision. However, this does not excuse you from your own legal responsibilities. To help protect yourself and your patients:

- Prepare carefully for each clinical experience.
- Never attempt a procedure or make a judgment about which you feel unsure. If you lack the theoretical or practical knowledge for an assignment, notify your clinical instructor immediately.
- Notify your instructor or a staff nurse if your patient's condition changes significantly.

Your nursing school may require you to carry personal professional liability insurance. The school's policy will cover you only for the nursing care you give in your educational experiences. If you work, for example, as an aide, the school's policy will not provide coverage for you at work. Furthermore, you are legally permitted to perform only the procedures contained in your job description. For example, even though you administer injections in your student role, you are not licensed to do so in your role as an aide.

WHAT ARE SOME MAJOR LEGAL ISSUES IN NURSING PRACTICE?

Ethical and legal issues are a major source of conflict for nursing practice. This chapter discusses only the legal aspects of the major issues. See Chapter 44 for ethical considerations. It is important to be clear in your mind that "legal" and "ethical" are not always the same thing. On the one hand, an act may be legal (e.g., abortion), even if you consider it unethical. On the other hand, you may believe that an action (e.g., assisted suicide) is ethically necessary, but the law may forbid it. You should be aware of the legal consequences that your ethical decisions may bring about. For a more detailed discussion of some major legal issues in nursing (organ donation, HIV/AIDS, abortion and other reproductive issues, life-sustaining medical treatment, DNAR orders, and advance directives,

 Go to Chapter 45, **Supplemental Materials: What Are the Major Legal Issues in Nursing Practice?,** on the Electronic Study Guide.

 Go to Chapter 45, **Resources for Caregivers and Health Professionals,** on the Electronic Study Guide.

 Suggested Readings: Go to Chapter 45, **Reading More About Legal Issues,** on the Electronic Study Guide.

 Bibliography: Go to Volume 2, Bibliography.

Text, Photo & Illustration Credits

Text Credits

Note: Unless cited below, text credits appear within the text.

CHAPTER 1

Table 1–1: March 2000. National Sample Survey of Registered Nurses, Division of Nursing, BHPR, Health Resources and Service Administration (HRSA).

CHAPTER 19

Table 19–1: Dillon, P. (2003). *Nursing Health Assessment: A Critical Thinking, Case Studies Approach.* Philadelphia: F.A. Davis Company, pp. 67–69.

Photo and Illustration Credits

Except as noted below, all illustrations are by Imagineering STA Media Services.

Author Photo, Karen Van Leuven: Richard Friedman

UNIT 1

Photodisc Green/Getty Images

CHAPTER 1

Meet Your Patients: (top) 1–1, 1–2, 1–3 etc. National Library of Medicine

Meet Your Patients: (bottom) Barros & Barros/The Image Bank/Getty Images

1–4 Hulton/Archive at Getty Images

1–5 Vietnam Women's Memorial Foundation, Inc., 1993. Glenna Goodacre, sculptor

1–6 Philadelphia Museum of Art. The William H. Helfand Collection, 1988

1–7 Keith Brofsky/Photodisc Green/Getty Images

CHAPTER 2

Meet Your Patients: © Royalty-Free/Corbis

CHAPTER 3

Meet Your Patients: Photodisc/Getty Images

3–3 Comstock/Getty Images

CHAPTER 4

Meet Your Patients: Jeff Cadge/Photographer's Choice/Getty Images

CHAPTER 5

Meet Your Patients: Xavier Bonghi/The Image Bank/Getty Images

CHAPTER 6

Meet Your Patients: Xavier Bonghi/The Image Bank/Getty Images

CHAPTER 7

Meet Your Patients: (top) Thinkstock/Getty Images

Meet Your Patients: (bottom) ThinkStock/SuperStock

CHAPTER 8

8–5 Anderson (2001). *Nursing Leadership, Management & Professional Practice for the LPN/LVN.* Philadelphia: F.A. Davis Company.

UNIT 2

© Royalty-Free/Corbis

CHAPTER 9

Meet Your Patients: Photodisc Blue/Getty Images

The following figures and photos appear only on the Electronic Study Guide:

9–1 adapted from Dillon, P. (2003). *Nursing Health Assessment,* p. 733, Philadelphia: F.A. Davis Company.

9–2 adapted from Dillon, P. (2003). *Nursing Health Assessment,* p. 755, Philadelphia: F.A. Davis Company.

9–3 adapted from Polan E. & Taylor D. (2003). *Journey Across the Life Span: Human Development and Health Promotion,* 2nd edition, p. 85, Philadelphia: F.A. Davis Company.

9–4 a-d adapted from Dillon, P. (2003). *Nursing Health Assessment,* pp. 767, 768, 770. Philadelphia: F.A. Davis Company.

9–5 Photodisc Green/Getty Images

9–7 © Royalty-Free/Corbis

9–9 Scott T Baxter/Photodisc Red/Getty Images

9–10 SW Productions/Photodisc Green/Getty Images

9–11 Photodisc Green/Getty Images

9–12 Anderson Ross/Photodisc Green/Getty Images

9–13 Photodisc/Getty Images

Tables 5–1–5–10: adapted from Polan, E. & Taylor, D. (2003). *Journey Across the Life Span: Human Development and Health Promotion,* 2nd edition. Philadelphia: F.A. Davis Company.

CHAPTER 10

Meet Your Patients: © Royalty-Free/Corbis

CHAPTER 11

11–4 Leanne Cowin

CHAPTER 12

Meet Your Patients: Keith Brofsky/Photodisc Green/Getty Images

12–1 Adam Crowley/Photodisc Green/Getty Images

12–2, 12–3, 12–4 Photodisc Green/Getty Images

12–5 SW Productions/Photodisc Green/Getty Images

CHAPTER 13

Meet Your Patients: Photodisc/Getty Images

13–1 adapted from Hanson, S., Gedaly-Duff, V., & Kaakinen, J. (2005). *Family Health Care Nursing: Theory, Practice, and Research,* 3rd edition, Fig. 17.01. Philadelphia: F.A. Davis Company.

13–2, 13–3, 13–4, 13–5, 13–6 Courtesy of Nancy Ahern, RN, MED, MSN.

13–7 adapted from Purnell, L. & Paulanka, B.J. (2003). *Transcultural Health Care: A Culturally Competent Approach,* 2nd edition. Philadelphia: F.A. Davis Company.

CHAPTER 14

Meet Your Patients: Photodisc/Getty Images

14–2 Tanji Hisamoto/©Royalty-Free/Corbis

CHAPTER 15

Meet Your Patients: Comstock/Getty Images

15–1 Skjold Photographs

15–2 ©Royalty-Free/Corbis

UNIT 3

David Buffington/Photodisc Green/Getty Images

CHAPTER 16

Meet Your Patients: PhotoLink/Photodisc Green/Getty Images

CHAPTER 17

Meet Your Patients: Amos Morgan/Photodisc Green/Getty Images

17–4 Dillon, P. (2003). *Nursing Health Assessment.* Philadelphia: F.A. Davis Company.

Tables 17–1 through 17–7 adapted from Dillon, P. (2003). *Nursing Health Assessment.* Philadelphia: F.A. Davis Company.

CHAPTER 18

Meet Your Patients: Amos Morgan/Photodisc Green/Getty Images

CHAPTER 19

Table 19–1, all except lithotomy position Dillon, P. (2003). *Nursing Health Assessment.* Philadelphia: F.A. Davis Company.

Table 19–1, lithotomy position.

19–2, 19–11, 19–12, 19–14, 19–15, 19–17a-d, 19–18, 19–19, 19–22, Dillon, P. (2003). *Nursing Health Assessment.* Philadelphia: F.A. Davis Company.

19–3, 19–4, 19–5, 19–6, 19–7, 19–8, 19–9, 19–13,19–16, 19–20, 19–21, 19–23, 19–24, 19–27 Imagineering STA Media Services.

19–10 Copyright ©ISM/Phototake

CHAPTER 20

Meet Your Patients: Digital Vision/Getty Images

20–2 adapted from Scanlon, V.C. & Sanders, T. (2003), *Essentials of Anatomy and Physiology* fig. 14–8, p. 316. Philadelphia: F.A. Davis Company.

20–3 adapted from Scanlon, V.C. & Sanders, T. (2003), *Essentials of Anatomy and Physiology,* fig. 14–7, p. 315. Philadelphia: F.A. Davis Company.

CHAPTER 21

Meet Your Patients: Jay Freis/Digital Vision/Getty Images

CHAPTER 22

Meet Your Patients: Amos Morgan/Photodisc Red/Getty Images

22–1a,b Courtesy of Caroll Health Care; London, Ontario, Canada

22–2 adapted from Dillon, P. (2003). *Nursing Health Assessment,* fig. 9–6, p. 199. Philadelphia: F.A. Davis Company.

22–3 adapted from Dillon, P. (2003). *Nursing Health Assessment,* fig. 9–7, p. 199. Philadelphia: F.A. Davis Company.

CHAPTER 23

23–17, 23–30 Courtesy of Medi-Dose ® Inc./EPS ® Ivyland, PA.

23–29 Courtesy of National Extravasation Information Service (*www.extravasation.org.uk*).

UNIT 4

Brand X Pictures/PictureQuest

CHAPTER 25

Meet Your Patients: Jay Freis/Digital Vision/Getty Images

25–5 adapted from Scanlon, V.C. & Sanders, T. (2003), *Essentials of Anatomy and Physiology* fig. 10–9, p. 227. Philadelphia: F.A. Davis Company.

25–6 Photodisc/Getty Images

CHAPTER 26

Meet Your Patients: Jay Freis/Digital Vision/Getty Images

26–1 adapted from Scanlon, V.C. & Sanders, T. (2003), *Essentials of Anatomy and Physiology*, p. 31. Philadelphia: F.A. Davis Company.

26–2 adapted from Scanlon, V.C. & Sanders, T. (2003), *Essentials of Anatomy and Physiology,* p. 35. Philadelphia: F.A. Davis Company.

26–3 adapted from Scanlon, V.C. & Sanders, T. (2003), *Essentials of Anatomy and Physiology,* p. 33. Philadelphia: F.A. Davis Company.

CHAPTER 27

Meet Your Patients: Jay Freis/Digital Vision/Getty Images

27–7a,b Courtesy of ATAGO U.S.A., Inc. Bellevue WA 98005

CHAPTER 28

Meet Your Patients: Amos Morgan/Photodisc Green/Getty Images

28–1 adapted from Scanlon, V.C. & Sanders, T. (2003), *Essentials of Anatomy and Physiology,* p. 351. Philadelphia: F.A. Davis Company.

28–2 adapted from Scanlon, V.C. & Sanders, T. (2003), *Essentials of Anatomy and Physiology,* p. 364. Philadelphia: F.A. Davis Company.

28–3 adapted from Scanlon, V.C. & Sanders, T. (2003), *Essentials of Anatomy and Physiology,* p. 366. Philadelphia: F.A. Davis Company.

28–4 adapted from Scanlon, V.C. & Sanders, T. (2003), *Essentials of Anatomy and Physiology,* p. 367. Philadelphia: F.A. Davis Company.

28–8 adapted from Williams, L. & Hopper, P. (2003). *Understanding Medical Surgical Nursing,* 2nd edition, fig. 31–10, p. 327. Philadelphia: F.A. Davis Company.

CHAPTER 29

Meet Your Patients: Amos Morgan/Photodisc Red/Getty Images

29–1 adapted from Scanlon, V.C. & Sanders, T. (2003), *Essentials of Anatomy and Physiology* fig. 29–1. Philadelphia: F.A. Davis Company.

CHAPTER 31

Meet Your Patients: Jay Freis/Digital Vision/Getty Images

31–1 adapted from Scanlon, V.C. & Sanders, T. (2003), *Essentials of Anatomy and Physiology* fig. 31–1. Philadelphia: F.A. Davis Company.

31–2 adapted from Scanlon, V.C. & Sanders, T. (2003), *Essentials of Anatomy and Physiology* fig. 31–2. Philadelphia: F.A. Davis Company.

31–3 adapted from Scanlon, V.C. & Sanders, T. (2003), *Essentials of Anatomy and Physiology* fig. 31–3. Philadelphia: F.A. Davis Company.

31–6 Williams, L. & Hopper, P. (2003). *Understanding Medical Surgical Nursing,* 2nd edition. Philadelphia: F.A. Davis Company.

CHAPTER 32

Meet Your Patients: Jay Freis/Digital Vision/Getty Images

32–1 adapted from Scanlon, V.C. & Sanders, T. (2003), *Essentials of Anatomy and Physiology* fig. 20–5, p. 441. Philadelphia: F.A. Davis Company.

32–2 adapted from Scanlon, V.C. & Sanders, T. (2003), *Essentials of Anatomy and Physiology* fig. 20–9, p. 447. Philadelphia: F.A. Davis Company.

32–3 adapted from Scanlon, V.C. & Sanders, T. (2003), *Essentials of Anatomy and Physiology* fig. 20–3, p. 438. Philadelphia: F.A. Davis Company.

32–4 adapted from Scanlon, V.C. & Sanders, T. (2003), *Essentials of Anatomy and Physiology* fig. 21–1, p. 455. Philadelphia: F.A. Davis Company.

32–5 Photodisc Blue/Getty Images

32–8 Bruce Burkhardt/Corbis

CHAPTER 33

Meet Your Patients:

33–1, 33–2 Courtesy of Debra Anne Schilleman, RN, BSN, LSAC

CHAPTER 34

Meet Your Patients: Amos Morgan/Photodisc Green/Getty Images

34–1 adapted from Scanlon, V.C. & Sanders, T. (2003), *Essentials of Anatomy and Physiology* fig. 5–1, p. 85. Philadelphia: F.A. Davis Company.

CHAPTER 35

Meet Your Patients: Digital Vision/Getty Images

35–1 adapted from Scanlon, V.C. & Sanders, T. (2003), *Essentials of Anatomy and Physiology* fig. 15–4, p. 330. Philadelphia: F.A. Davis Company.

35–2 adapted from Scanlon, V.C. & Sanders, T. (2003), *Essentials of Anatomy and Physiology* fig. 15–5, p. 332. Philadelphia: F.A. Davis Company.

35–3 adapted from Scanlon, V.C. & Sanders, T. (2003), *Essentials of Anatomy and Physiology* fig. 15–6, p. 332. Philadelphia: F.A. Davis Company.

35–5 adapted from Scanlon, V.C. & Sanders, T. (2003), *Essentials of Anatomy and Physiology* fig. 12–2b, p. 262. Philadelphia: F.A. Davis Company.

35–6 adapted from Scanlon, V.C. & Sanders, T. (2003), *Essentials of Anatomy and Physiology* fig. 12–6, p. 267. Philadelphia: F.A. Davis Company.

35–7 adapted from Scanlon, V.C. & Sanders, T. (2003), *Essentials of Anatomy and Physiology* fig. 12–4a, p. 263. Philadelphia: F.A. Davis Company.

35–9 adapted from Williams, L. & Hopper, P. (2003). *Understanding Medical Surgical Nursing,* 2nd edition, fig. 28–6, p. 453. Philadelphia: F.A. Davis Company.

35–19 adapted from Williams, L. & Hopper, P. (2003). *Understanding Medical Surgical Nursing,* 2nd edition, fig. 26–17, p. 423. Philadelphia: F.A. Davis Company.

35–21 Williams, L. & Hopper, P. (2003). *Understanding Medical Surgical Nursing,* 2nd edition, fig. 26–18, p. 424. Philadelphia: F.A. Davis Company.

CHAPTER 36

Meet Your Patients: Jay Freis/Digital Vision/Getty Images

36–1 adapted from Williams, L. & Hopper, P. (2003). *Understanding Medical Surgical Nursing,* 2nd edition, fig. 5–1, p. 46. Philadelphia: F.A. Davis Company.

CHAPTER 37

Meet Your Patients: Amos Morgan/Photodisc Green

37–4 Williams, L. & Hopper, P. (2003). *Understanding Medical Surgical Nursing,* 2nd edition, fig. 26–18, p. 424. Philadelphia: F.A. Davis Company.

37–6 Williams, L. & Hopper, P. (2003). *Understanding Medical Surgical Nursing,* 2nd edition, fig. 15–15, p. 247. Philadelphia: F.A. Davis Company.

UNIT 5

Stockbyte Platinum/Getty Images

CHAPTER 39

39–2 Photodisc Blue/Getty Images

39–3 ©Duncan Smith/Corbis

39–4 B Busco/The Image Bank/Getty Images

39–6 Picturequest/Bob Llewellyn

39–8a, b ©Image 100/Corbis

CHAPTER 40

40–6 Wolfgang Kaehler/Corbis

UNIT 6

Image Ideas/PictureQuest

CHAPTER 42

Meet Your Patients: Jay Freis/Digital Vision/Getty Images

CHAPTER 43

Meet Your Patients: ©Royalty-Free/Corbis

43–1 Jose Luis Pelaez, Inc./Corbis

43–3 The Image Bank/Getty Images

Index